Register Now for O
to Your Bo

SPRINGER PUBLISHING
CONNECT™

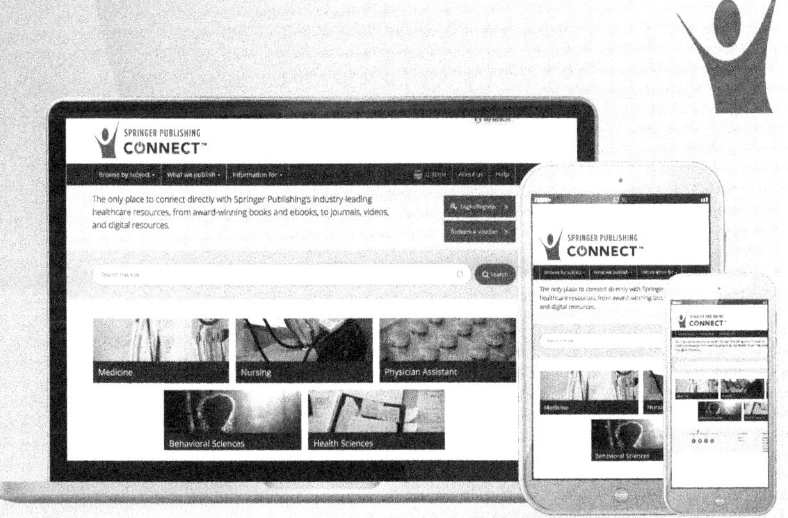

Your print purchase of *Emergency Nurse Practitioner Core Curriculum* **includes online access to the contents of your book**—increasing accessibility, portability, and searchability!

Access today at:
http://connect.springerpub.com/content/reference-book/978-0-8261-6091-5
or scan the QR code at the right with your smartphone. Log in or register, then click "Redeem a voucher" and use the code below.

KT5FUA4D

Scan here for quick access.

Having trouble redeeming a voucher code?
Go to https://connect.springerpub.com/redeeming-voucher-code

If you are experiencing problems accessing the digital component of this product, please contact our customer service department at cs@springerpub.com

The online access with your print purchase is available at the publisher's discretion and may be removed at any time without notice.

Publisher's Note: New and used products purchased from third-party sellers are not guaranteed for quality, authenticity, or access to any included digital components.

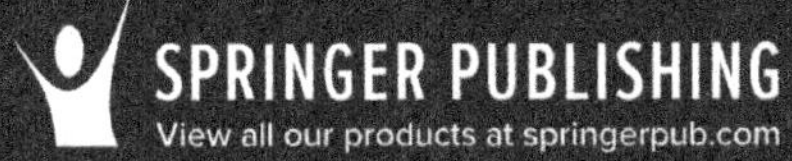

Emergency Nurse Practitioner Core Curriculum

Reneé Semonin Holleran, FNP-BC, RN-BC, PhD, CEN, CFRN, CTRN (Retired), CCRN (Alumna), FAEN, has practiced for over 30 years in emergency care. Dr. Holleran currently practices in Salt Lake City, Utah, where she serves as APRN Anesthesia Chronic Pain at George E. Whalen Veterans Health Administration and volunteers at the Hope Free Clinic, where she provides family practice and urgent care to the uninsured and immigrant populations.

Dr. Holleran is the former editor of the *Journal of Emergency Nursing* and *Air Medical Journal*, and currently serves on the editorial board for the *Advanced Emergency Nursing Journal*. Dr. Holleran was inducted as a Fellow of the Academy of Emergency Nursing in 2005 and earned a Lifetime Achievement Award from the Emergency Nurses Association. She is a past recipient of two *AJN* Book Awards in prehospital nursing and in air and surface transport nursing.

Theresa M. Campo, DNP, FNP-C, ENP-C, FAANP, FAAN, is Vice President of Education and Accreditation at the American Association of Nurse Practitioners and was previously Chair of the Department of Emergency Medical Services (EMS) and Director of the Emergency Nurse Practitioner Track as well as Associate Clinical Professor at Drexel University. Clinically, she is board certified as a Family Nurse Practitioner and Emergency Nurse Practitioner and works part time as a nurse practitioner in southern New Jersey.

Dr. Campo received her Doctor of Nursing Practice from Case Western Reserve University in Cleveland, Ohio. She earned her Master of Science in Nursing, Family Nurse Practitioner, from Widener University in Chester, Pennsylvania. Dr. Campo has over 30 years of experience in emergency medicine, including pre-hospital, emergency department/ quick care, and trauma. Dr. Campo is a founding Board Member of the American Academy of Emergency Nurse Practitioners, a national organization. She is a national and international lecturer on emergency and urgent care topics. Dr. Campo is the author of *Medical Imaging for the Health Care Provider: Practical Radiograph Interpretation;* editor of *Essential Procedures for Emergency, Urgent, and Primary Care Settings,* now in its third edition; and has authored several book chapters and peer-reviewed articles.

Dr. Campo was inducted as a Fellow of the American Association of Nurse Practitioners (AANP) in 2015 and as a Fellow of the American Academy of Nursing in 2017. She has received the alumni award for excellence from Case Western Reserve University and the state award of excellence from AANP.

Emergency Nurse Practitioner Core Curriculum

Reneé Semonin Holleran, FNP-BC, RN-BC, PhD, CEN, CFRN, CTRN (Retired), CCRN (Alumna), FAEN

Theresa M. Campo, DNP, FNP-C, ENP-C, FAANP, FAAN

Editors

Karen Sue Hoyt, PhD, RN, FNP-BC, ENP-C, FAEN, FAANP, FAAN

Elda Ramirez, PhD, RN, FNP-BC, ENP-C, FAEN, FAANP, FAAN

Consulting Editors

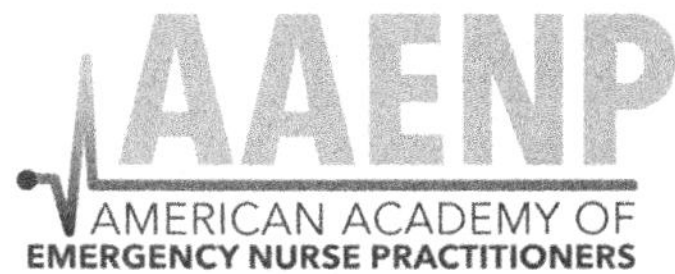

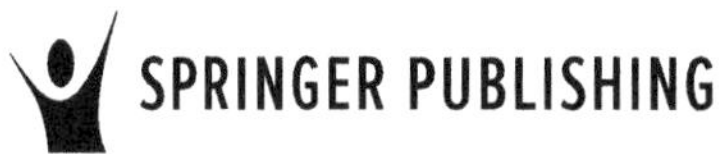

Springer Publishing Company, LLC
11 West 42nd Street, New York, NY 10036
www.springerpub.com
connect.springerpub.com/

Acquisitions Editor: Elizabeth Nieginski
Development Editor: Hannah Hicks
Compositor: diacriTech

ISBN: 978-0-8261-4125-5
ebook ISBN: 978-0-8261-4147-7
DOI: 10.1891/9780826141477

21 22 23 24 / 5 4 3 2 1

Medicine is an ever-changing science. Research and clinical experience are continually expanding our knowledge, in particular our understanding of proper treatment and drug therapy. The authors, editors, and publisher have made every effort to ensure that all information in this book is in accordance with the state of knowledge at the time of production of the book. Nevertheless, the authors, editors, and publisher are not responsible for any errors or omissions or for any consequence from application of the information in this book and make no warranty, expressed or implied, with respect to the content of this publication. Every reader should examine carefully the package inserts accompanying each drug and should carefully check whether the dosage schedules therein or the contraindications stated by the manufacturer differ from the statements made in this book. Such examination is particularly important with drugs that are either rarely used or have been newly released on the market.

LCCN: 2021908816

Contact sales@springerpub.com to receive discount rates on bulk purchases.

Publisher's Note: New and used products purchased from third-party sellers are not guaranteed for quality, authenticity, or access to any included digital components.

Printed in the United States of America by Gasch Printing.

Contents

25. Multisystem Trauma 363

Melinda K. Johnson

26. Head Trauma and Brain Injuries 373

Marisa Losavio

27. Spinal Injuries 377

Jane Holston

28. Neck Injuries 384

Allie T. Gilbert and Chris Gisness

29. Abdominal Trauma 394

Tiffany Andrews

30. Genitourinary Trauma 406

Tracy Brown and Tracie Gadler

31. Peripheral Vascular Injuries 409

Kelly Toffoli

32. Orthopedic Injuries 416

Mary Jo Cerepani and Michael Sweeney

33. Soft Tissue Injuries 445

Kristina Davis, Susanna Rudy, Audrey Snyder, and Reneé Semonin Holleran

IV. Environmental Emergencies

V. Toxicology, Overdose Management, Substance Use Disorder

VI. Emergency Medical Services, Patient Transport, and Disaster Preparedness

VII. Special Patient Populations

Contributors

Sarah Ackerman, DNP, FNP-C, CEN
Emergency Department
Thomas Jefferson University Hospital
Philadelphia, Pennsylvania

Colleen Andreoni, DNP, FNP-BC, ANP-BC, ENP-C
Assistant Professor
Loyola University Chicago, Niehoff School of Nursing
Med Express Urgent Care
Chicago, Illinois

Tiffany Andrews, MS BSN, BA, CCNS, CNE, ACNP-BC, ENP-C
U.S. Acute Care Solutions
Baltimore, Maryland

Vicki Bacidore, DNP, APRN, ACNP-BC, CEN, TNS
Assistant Professor of Nursing
Marcella Niehoff School of Nursing
Loyala University Chicago
Chicago, Illinois

Amy Bigham, D.N.P., RN, FNP-BC
Associate Professor
Family Nurse Practitioner Program
Moffett & Sanders School of Nursing
Samford University
Birmingham, Alabama

Tracy Brown, MSN, APRN, ACNP-BC, ENP-BC
University of Texas Southwestern Medical Center
Parkland Hospital
Dallas, Texas

Mary Jo Cerepani, DNP, FNP-BC, ENP-C, FAANP, FAEN
Nurse Practitioner
University of Pittsburgh Medical Center
Pittsburgh, Pennsylvania

Garrett K. Chan, PhD, ACNP-C, CNS-BC, FAEN, FPCN, FNAP, FCNS, FAAN
Nurse Practitioner
Stanford Health Care
Stanford, California
President & CEO
HealthImpact
Oakland, California

Kristina Davis, DNP, ENP-C, FNP-C, AGACNP-BC
Program Director, Emergency Nurse Practitioner Certificate Program
Rocky Mountain University of Health Professions
Provo, Utah

Wesley Davis, DNP, ENP-C, FNP-C, AGACNP-BC
Assistant Professor
Emergency Nurse Practitioner Specialty Coordinator
University of South Alabama
Mobile, Alabama

Nancy Denke, DNP
Instructor
Edson College of Nursing and Health Innovation
Arizona State University
Phoenix, Arizona

Dian Dowling Evans, PhD, FNP-BC, ENP-C, FAANP, FAAN
Clinical Professor and Emergency Nurse Practitioner Program Coordinator
Nell Hodgson Woodruff School of Nursing
Emory University
Atlanta, Georgia

Kathleen Flarity, DNP, PhD, CEN, CFRN, FAEN
Deputy Director CU Anschutz Center for COMBAT Research
Associate Professor
Department of Emergency Medicine
University of Colorado School of Medicine
Research Nurse Scientist, UCHealth
Brigadier General, US Air Force
Aurora, Colorado

Tracie Gadler, DNP, APRN, FNP-C, RNFA
Sharp Healthcare
Adjunct Assistant Professor
University of San Diego
San Diego, California

Allie T. Gilbert, MSN, RN, FNP-C, ENP-C
Nurse Practitioner
Department of Emergency Medicine
Grady Memorial Hospital
Emory University
Atlanta, Georgia

Chris Gisness, MSN, RN, FNP-BC, FNP-C, ENP-C CEN, FAEN
Nurse Practitioner
Department of Emergency Medicine
Grady Memorial Hospital
Emory University
Atlanta, Georgia

Hilary Ashton Glover, DNP, FNP-C, ENP-C
University of North Alabama
Florence, Alabama

Bradley Goettl, DNP, RN, AGACNP-BC, FNP-C, ENP-C, EMT-P
Department of Emergency Medicine
University of Texas Health Science Center at San Antonio
San Antonio, Texas

Michael D. Gooch, DNP, APRN, CCP, ACNP-BC, FNP-BC, ENP-BC, ENP-C, CEN, CFRN, CTRN, TCRN, NRP
Assistant Professor of Nursing
Vanderbilt University School of Nursing
Nurse Practitioner
Vanderbilt University Medical Center
Nashville, Tennessee

Chivas Guillote, MSN, APRN, AGACNP-BC, ENP-C, FNP-C, LP
Cizik School of Nursing
The University of Texas Health Science Center at Houston
Houston, Texas

Melanie Gibbons Hallman, DNP, CRNP, CEN, FNP, ACNP, ENP-C, TCRN, FAEN
Assistant Professor
Coordinator, Emergency Nurse Practitioner Program
University of Alabama at Birmingham School of Nursing
Birmingham, Alabama

Leigh Hart, PhD
Professor of Nursing
Keigwin School of Nursing
Jacksonville University
Jacksonville, Florida

Rodney W. Hicks, PhD, RN, FNP-BC, FAANP, FAAN
Associate Dean for Administration and Research, Professor
College of Graduate Nursing
Western University of Health Sciences
Ponoma, California

April T. Hill, DNP, FNP, ENP
College of Nursing and Health Innovation
Arizona State University
Phoenix, Arizona

Reneé Semonin Holleran, FNP-BC, RN-BC, PhD, CEN, CFRN, CTRN (Retired), CCRN (Alumna), FAEN
APRN Pain Medicine
Veterans' Health Administration
Salt Lake City, Utah
Nurse Practitioner
Hope Free Clinic
Midvale, Utah

Jane Holston, DNP, FNP-BC, ENP-C, COI
Associate Professor
Coordinator, Emergency Nurse Practitioner Track
Ida Moffett School of Nursing
Samford University
Birmingham, Alabama

David T. House, DNP, CRNP, APRN, FNP-BC, ENP-C, CNS
Assistant Professor
Emergency Nurse Practitioner Subspecialty Co-Coordinator
Department of Family, Community, and Health Systems
School of Nursing
The University of Alabama at Birmingham
Birmingham, Alabama

Karen Sue Hoyt, PhD, RN, FNP-BC, ENP-C, FAEN, FAANP, FAAN
Professor NP/DNP Programs
Hahn School of Nursing and Health Science
Beyster Institute of Nursing Research
University of San Diego
San Diego, California

Lori Hull-Grommesh, DNP, ACNP-BC, NEA-BC, FAANP
Assistant Professor
Cizik School of Nursing, UTHealth
Houston, Texas

John F. L. Jamison, MSN, FNP-BC, CFRN, CEN
Moses Lake Community Health Center
Moses Lake, Washington

Jasmine Johnson, MSN, APRN, FNP-C, ENP-C
Emergency Department
New York Presbyterian
Weill Cornell Medical Center
New York, New York

Melinda K. Johnson, DNP, AGACNP-BC, FNP-BC, ENP-BC, CEN, CCRN
Instructor of Nursing
Vanderbilt University School of Nursing
Nashville, Tennessee

Kathleen S. Jordan, DNP, RN, FNP-BC, ENP-C, SANE-P, FAEN, FAANP
Clinical Associate Professor
UNC Charlotte School of Nursing
Charlotte, North Carolina
Nurse Practitioner, APP Fellowship Director
Mid-Atlantic Emergency Medical Associates
Charlotte, North Carolina

Shannon M. Keating, DNP, APRN, ACNP-BC, FNP-BC, ENP-C
Emergency Department
St. Mary's Medical Center
West Palm Beach, Florida

Lisa Koser, DNP, ACNP-BC, CPNP-AC, RN, CCRN, CEN, CFRN, C-NPT, NREMT-P
Lead Advanced Practice Provider
Trauma and Acute Care Surgery
Department of Surgery
Division of Trauma, Critical Care and Burn
The Ohio State University Wexner Medical Center
Columbus, Ohio

Laura L. Kuensting, DNP, APRN, PCNS-BC, CPNP, CPEN
University of Missouri – St. Louis
Associate Teaching Professor
Director, MSN/DNP Programs
Mercy Children's Hospital – St. Louis
Advanced Practice Registered Nurse
Pediatric Emergency Medicine
Chesterfield, Missouri

Lisa Leonard, MSN, APRN, FNP-C, ENP-C
Prisma Health
Department of Emergency Medicine
Greenville, South Carolina

Marisa Losavio, MSN, AGACNP-BC
Department of Emergency Medicine
New York Presbyterian–Weill Cornell Medical Center
New York, New York

Virginia Mangolds, PhD, APRN, FNP-C, BSED, ENP-BC, CEN
Instructor, Emergency Medicine
Assistant Research Director
University of Massachusetts Medical Center
University of Massachusetts Medical School
Worcester, Massachusetts

Nicole Martinez, PhD, RN, FNP-BC, ENP-C, PHN
Hahn School of Nursing and Health Sciences
University of San Diego
San Diego, California

M. Allen McCullough, Ph.D., FNP-BC, ENP-BC
Instructor, Nursing
School of Nursing
Emory University
Atlanta, Georgia

Ronald D. Meador, DNP, ENP/FNP-BC, LP
Critical Care Transport Nurse Practitioner
Trans Aero Medevac 2
Artesia, New Mexico
Emergency Nurse Practitioner
UA Acute Care Solutions
Ascension Providence Emergency Department
Waco, Texas

Shana Metzger, AG-ACNP, FNP
Adjunct Instructor
Georgetown University
Washington, DC

Jill Ogg-Gress, DNP, ARNP, FNP-C
Assistant Professor
Family Nurse Practitioner Program
School of Nursing and Health Sciences
Georgetown University
Washington, DC

Edyta Pedlowska, DNP, FNP-C
Weill Cornell Medicine
New York, New York

Sharon R. Rainer, PhD, APRN, APN,BC, FNP-BC, ENP-C
Assistant Professor
Coordinator, Family-Individual Across the Lifespan Nurse Practitioner Program
Jefferson College of Nursing
Thomas Jefferson University
Philadelphia, Pennsylvania

Rick Ramirez, DNP, DPRN-Rx, AG/ACNP-BC, FNP-BC, ENP-C, CEN, CPEN
Assistant Professor
School of Nursing and Dental Hygeine
University of Hawai'i at Mānoa
Honolulu, Hawaii

Eric Roberts, DNP, FNP-BC, ENP-BC
Assistant Professor
Marcella Niehoff School of Nursing
Loyola University Chicago
Chicago, Illinois

Andrew Rotjan, MSN, APRN, FNP-BC, AGACNP-BC, ENP-C, EMT-P, CHSE
Director ACP Clinical Training and Education
Emergency Nurse Practitioner
Emergency Medicine Service Line
Northwell Health
Adjunct Faculty Instructor
Hofstra Northwell School of Nursing and Physician Assistant Studies
Lake Success, New York

Susanna Rudy, DNP, AG-ACNP, FNP, ENP, CCRN
Emergency Nurse Practitioner
Instructor, School of Nursing
Vanderbilt University
Nashville, Tennessee

Sheila Shea, RN, MSN, ANP
Long Beach Emergency Medical Group
Emergency Nurse Practitioner
Long Beach, California

Darlie Simerson, DNP, APRN, FNP-BC, CEN
Loyola University
Chicago, Illinois

Audrey Snyder, PhD, RN, ACNP-BC, FNP-BC, CEN, FAANP, FAEN, FAAN
Associate Dean for Experiential Learning
School of Nursing
University of North Carolina at Greensboro
Greensboro, North Carolina

Patricia M. Speck, DNSc, CRNP, FNP-BC, DF-IAFN, FAAFS, DF-AFN, FAAN
Professor
Coordinator of Advanced Forensic Nursing
Department of Family, Community, and Health Systems
University of Alabama at Birmingham School of Nursing
Birmingham, Alabama

Vincent Sperandeo, DNP
Orlin & Cohen Orthopedic Group
Suffolk County, New York
Adjunct Professor, Emergency Medicine and Family Medicine
Drexel University
Philadelphia, Pennsylvania

Michael Sweeney, MSN, FNP-BC, ENP-BC, NE-BC, CFRN, CEN, CCRN, CCNS, CTRN, PHRN
Emergency Department
Chestnut Hill Hospital
Tower Health System
Chalfont, Pennsylvania

Kelley Toffoli, DNP, APN-BC
Assistant Clinical Professor
Nurse Practitioner Program
College of Nursing and Health Professions
Drexel University
Philadelphia, Pennsylvania

Jennifer Wilbeck, DNP, RN, FNP-BC, ACNP-BC, ENP-C, FAANP, FAAN
Professor & Emergency Nurse Practitioner
Academic Director
Vanderbilt University School of Nursing
Nashville, Tennessee

Alexander F. Wrynn, DNP, FNP-C
U.S. Acute Care Solutions
Moon Township, Pennsylvania

Reviewers

Wesley Davis, DNP, ENP-C, FNP-C, AGACNP-BC
Assistant Professor
Emergency Nurse Practitioner Specialty Coordinator
University of South Alabama
Mobile, Alabama

Hannah R. Fudin, PharmD, BCACP
Clinical Pharmacist
George E. Wahlen VA Medical Center
Salt Lake City, Utah

Tracie Gadler, DNP, APRN, FNP-C, RNFA
Sharp Healthcare
Adjunct Assistant Professor
University of San Diego
San Diego, California

Juan M. Gonzalez, DNP, APRN, AGACNP-BC, ENP-C, FNP-BC, CEN
Associate Professor of Clinical
University of Miami School of Nursing and Health Studies
Coral Gables, Florida

Michael D. Gooch, DNP, APRN, CCP, ACNP-BC, FNP-BC, ENP-BC, ENP-C, CEN, CFRN, CTRN, TCRN, NRP
Assistant Professor of Nursing
Vanderbilt University School of Nursing
Nurse Practitioner
Vanderbilt University Medical Center
Nashville, Tennessee

Sondra Heaston, MS, NP-C, CEN, CNE, FAEN
Teaching Professor
College of Nursing
Brigham Young University
Salt Lake City, Utah

Kathleen S. Jordan, DNP, RN, FNP-BC, ENP-C, SANE-P, FAEN, FAANP
Clinical Associate Professor
UNC Charlotte School of Nursing
Charlotte, North Carolina
Nurse Practitioner, APP Fellowship Director
Mid-Atlantic Emergency Medical Associates
Charlotte, North Carolina

Virginia Mangolds, PhD, APRN, FNP-C, BSED, ENP-BC, CEN
Instructor, Emergency Medicine
Assistant Research Director
University of Massachusetts Medical Center
University of Massachusetts Medical School
Worcester, Massachusetts

Nicole Martinez, PhD, RN, FNP-BC, ENP-C, PHN
Hahn School of Nursing and Health Sciences
University of San Diego
San Diego, California

LaMon Norton, NP

Denise Ramponi, DNP, FNP-C, ENP-BC, FAANP, FAEN
Urgent Care Nurse Practitioner
Heritage Valley Health System & Professor
School of Nursing, Education & Human Studies
Robert Morris University
Pittsburgh, Pennyslvania

Sheila Sanning Shea, RN, MSN, ANP
Emergency NP
Long Beach Emergency Medical Group
Long Beach, California

Audrey Snyder, PhD, RN, ACNP-BC, FNP-BC, CEN, FAANP, FAEN, FAAN
Associate Dean for Experiential Learning
School of Nursing
University of North Carolina at Greensboro
Greensboro, North Carolina

Laura Truman, MSN, FNP-BC
Clinical Adjunct Professor
Hahn School of Nursing and Health Science
University of San Diego
San Diego, California

Preface

A Legacy Is a Gift

Dr. Frank Cole (deceased 2006), a visionary in the field of advanced practice emergency care, cofounded the first master's emergency nurse practitioner (ENP) program in the nation. Frank taught many highly impactful clinical nurse specialists (CNS) and ENPs in his phenomenal career. A product of his teachings included gifting us with the knowledge that everything has a *process*. This *process* included formation and implementation of the role of the ENP via scope, standards, curriculum, and extraction of competencies specific to the role by utilizing evidence-based research.

Dr. Cole left us with the legacy of continuing the process he initiated of establishing and realizing the ENP. In the years that followed his death, those of us who were his pupils had many obstacles to circumvent. The Consensus Model (CM; 2008) placed us in a precarious position strategically since the role, scope, and other defining characteristics of the ENP had not been taken into consideration. Key concepts of the CM—such as the effects of segregating the indivisible concepts of primary and acute care, which obstruct practice, and the lack of evolutional scope appropriations—have damaged the provision of emergency care by nurse practitioners across the country. Action had to be taken to set the ENPs apart to protect them and their patients and give them the recognition they worked for and deserved. A core curriculum was a must to solidify knowledge, skills, and abilities and to accompany our certification, scope, competencies, and practice standards.

The American Academy of Emergency Nurse Practitioners (AAENP) was established in 2013 to support ENPs in academic, clinical, and policy paradigms. The American Academy of Nurse Practitioner Certifying Board developed the ENP certification exam (2017) and now, in collaboration with Springer Publishing Company, the AAENP introduces *Emergency Nurse Practitioner Core Curriculum*.

This publication is a monumental step in the *process* Dr. Cole began, and is truly the pinnacle of success! The ENP is now acknowledged with a published core curriculum for the world to obtain. Dear Dr. Cole, your legacy has been realized.

AAENP Definition of Emergency Care

Emergency care encompasses the evaluation, management, and treatment of patients across the life span with unforeseen illness or injury of varying complexity. Emergency care is delivered by clinicians who are educated and trained to comprehensively address a wide variety of illnesses and injuries, ranging from resuscitation and stabilization of life-threatening health problems to management of minor injuries and illnesses. Emergency care is not defined by a practice setting, and takes place within urban, suburban, rural, and frontier/remote settings.

This publication specifically addresses and outlines ENP role and practice and is also the first core curriculum written specifically for ENPs.

Editors Reneé Semonin Holleran, FNP-BC, RN-BC, PhD, CEN, CFRN, CTRN (Retired), CCRN (Alumna), FAEN and Theresa M. Campo, DNP, FNP-C, ENP-BC, FAANP, FAAN have masterfully put forth the AAENP's most authoritative one-of-a-kind *Emergency Nurse Practitioner Core Curriculum*. This core is an evidence-based practice book for the ENP, which offers a holistic approach throughout. It also serves as a comprehensive review guide for the ENP studying for the ENP certification (ENP-C). The book can also be utilized for instruction by faculty in academia.

Two editors, two consulting editors, 57 authors, and 15 reviewers have worked to ensure content is up to date for AAENP's *Emergency Nurse Practitioner Core Curriculum*. Each chapter is organized in the following way:

- Content is written within the framework of the AAENP Certification Practice Analysis (Blueprint).
- This core curriculum provides succinct and pertinent details regarding management and care.
- This book also provides documentation information resources for the reader.

Section I, *Foundations of Practice*, includes the history of the development of the ENP, fundamental clinical skills (neonatal, pediatric, and adult), airway and ventilation management, anesthesia and acute pain management, ultrasound, cultural competency in the emergency care setting, patient and staff safety, postexposure prophylaxis, diagnostic and therapeutic procedures, evidence-based research and publication, clinical decision-making, emergency resuscitation and stabilization, pain management, leadership, team dynamics, and communication, ethics, bioethics, and legal aspects of emergency care, organ donation, and complementary and alternative modalities in the ED.

Section II, *Medical Emergencies*, comprises head, eyes, ears, nose, and throat; the neurologic patient; thoracic/respiratory, cardiovascular medical emergencies; vascular medical emergencies; esophagus, stomach, duodenum, renal, genitourinary, and reproductive conditions; metabolic and endocrinology; immunologic and inflammatory; hematology/oncology, infectious diseases, and psychiatric and mental health emergencies

Section III, *Shock and Trauma*, consists of shock: septic, cardiogenic, toxic, neurogenic, and hypovolemic; multiple trauma, head trauma, and brain injuries; spinal injuries; neck injuries; abdominal trauma; genitourinary trauma; peripheral vascular injuries; orthopedic injuries; and soft tissue injuries

Section IV, *Environmental Emergencies*, reviews frostbite and nonfreezing cold injuries, heat illness, lightning and electrical injuries, scuba diving and dysbarism, high-altitude medicine, drowning injuries, and radiation injuries.

Section V, *Toxicology, Overdose Management, Substance Use Disorder*, covers overdose management, substance use disorder, approach to the poisoned patient, toxicology, and other toxins.

Section VI, *Emergency Medical Services, Patient Transport, and Disaster Preparedness,* encompasses emergency medical services (EMS), patient transfer and transport, crisis and disaster management, chemical and biological weapons.

Section VII, *Special Patient Populations*, involves the pregnant patient, pediatric patient, geriatric patient, rural/austere patient population, gay/lesbian/bisexual/transgender patients in the ED, vulnerable populations in the emergency setting, and victims of violence.

The AAENP's *Emergency Nurse Practitioner Core Curriculum* provides a new approach to emergency medical care from the advanced nursing practice perspective, ensuring an all-inclusive approach to care in the emergency and urgent care setting. We hope you enjoy the read!

Consulting Editors

Karen Sue Hoyt, PhD, RN, FNP-BC, ENP-C, FAEN, FAANP, FAAN
Professor and Director, NP/ENP Programs
University of San Diego
Hahn School of Nursing and Health Science
Beyster Institute for Nursing Research
San Diego, California

Elda Ramirez, PhD, RN, FNP-BC, ENP-C, FAEN, FAANP, FAAN
Founder, American Academy of Emergency Nurse Practitioners
Director Emergency/Trauma Nurse Practitioner Program
The University of Texas Health Science Center
Houston, Texas

Introduction

Welcome to the ***first edition*** of the *Emergency Nurse Practitioner Core Curriculum* text! This book provides an outline of essential knowledge and information for the practicing nurse practitioner providing emergency care, emergency nurse practitioner (ENP) students, and ENP graduates of fellowship and academic educational programs. The *Core Curriculum* has been prepared to aid in gaining and renewing knowledge to care for patients across the life span, including addressing the complexity and acuity in the emergency care setting.

Development of the outline for the topics included in AAENP's *Emergency Nurse Practitioner Core Curriculum* was based on *Rosen's Emergency Medicine: Concepts and Clinical Practice, Ninth Edition* and *Tintinall's Emergency Medicine: A Comprehensive Study Guide, Ninth Edition.* Using the two "bibles" of emergency medicine as the foundation of the book, combined with current evidence-based research and guidelines, have made this text a comprehensive resource for clinical practice and education.

There are references to the Advanced Trauma Life Support (ATLS), Advanced Cardiac Life Support (ACLS), and Pediatric Advanced Life Support (PALS) resources; however, specific details have been omitted due to the regularity of changes and updates in guidelines. Citations to the most current editions are included.

The *Emergency Nurse Practitioner Core Curriculum* has incorporated diversity and inclusion throughout the book. Readers will notice that medication *classes* are noted unless only one particular medication is recommended within evidence-based guidelines. This decision was made due to the rapidly changing medical management recommendations, the new additions of medications, and to avoid inappropriate medication dosage recommendations.

You will find this core helpful, easy to understand, user friendly, and comprehensive. This project is the result of numerous emergency care professionals working together to provide you with the first-ever core for ENP practice.

Enjoy!

Reneé Semonin Holleran
Theresa M. Campo

I. Foundations of Practice

1. History of the Emergency Nurse Practitioner

DIAN DOWLING EVANS | KAREN SUE HOYT | JENNIFER WILBECK

Scope and Standards of Emergency Nurse Practitioner Practice

A. The first *Standards of Emergency Nursing Practice* were published in 1975 by the Emergency Department Nursing Association (EDNA). Established in 1970, EDNA was the first specialty organization for emergency nurses, and was renamed the Emergency Nurses Association (ENA) in 1985 in recognition that emergency nursing was role-specific rather than site-specific.[1–3] See Figure 1.1 for a historical timeline of key milestones in the development of the emergency nurse practitioner (ENP) specialty. The *Standards of Emergency Nursing Practice* spoke broadly regarding the emergency nursing profession but not specifically to the advanced practice emergency nursing role.

B. In 1998, ENA established an advanced practice registered nurse (APRN) committee to develop an APRN outline in the *ENA Core Curriculum, Fifth Edition* (K. S. Hoyt, personal communication, January 9, 2017). Shortly thereafter and by consensus of specialty nursing groups, the American Nurses Association (ANA) was designated as the official body to review scope-of-practice statements and standards of practice for nursing specialties.[4]

C. A resolution to the ENA General Assembly in 2004 requesting an APRN Validation Task Force led to the creation of an ENA Task Force in 2006 to review APRN practices in emergency care. A subgroup would later develop the competencies for nurse practitioners (NPs) in emergency care.[5]

D. In 2008, based upon a national Delphi study and a comprehensive practice analysis, ENA published the *Competencies for Nurse Practitioners in Emergency Care.*[5] These competencies were endorsed by the ANA in 2011[6] and the National Organization of Nurse Practitioner Faculties (NONPF) that same year.[4]

E. Also, in 2008, the *Consensus Model for APRN Licensure, Accreditation, Certification, and Education* (LACE) was published to provide guidance to state boards of nursing to improve regulation of APRN roles based on education and certification in a population foci while recognizing that NP practice "will evolve incrementally over time."[7(p6)] The Consensus Model is depicted in Figure 1.2.

F. In 2016, the American Academy of Emergency Nurse Practitioners (AAENP) published the *Scope and Standards for Emergency Nurse Practitioners*[8] based upon the 2016 role delineation study conducted by the American Academy of Nurse Practitioners Certification Board (AANPCB). These documents, a collaborative effort between the AAENP and ENA, defined ENP specialty scope and standards of practice subsequently informing the development of revised ENP practice standards/competencies and the ENP certification examination.

1. Recognition of specialty practice, including the ENP role, was further advanced in the Consensus Model's regulatory framework[7] and also within the National Council of State Boards of Nursing's position paper on NP specialty practice.[9] Consensus Model authors stated that NP practice will evolve to reflect changing healthcare workforce needs and trends, noting "specialties provide depth in one's practice within the established population foci."[7(p6)]
2. The Consensus Model further placed development and monitoring of specialty practice within the domain of specialty organizations that concluded that "competence at the specialty level will not be assessed or regulated by boards of nursing but rather professional organizations."[7(p6)]
3. Recognition of the ENP specialty by ANA, in conjunction with the national standards for APRN regulation in the Consensus Model and the endorsement of the ENP core competencies by NONPF in 2011,[4] solidified the need for development of ENP scope and standards of practice and specialty certification. Additionally, the ENP profession required a dedicated organization to promote ENP practice, which led to the formation of the AAENP in 2014.

Clinical Competencies and Practice Standards

A. In 2006, an ENA Task Force was developed to review APRN practice in emergency care. A subgroup from this Task Force conducted a national Delphi study and a comprehensive practice analysis. Data from this study

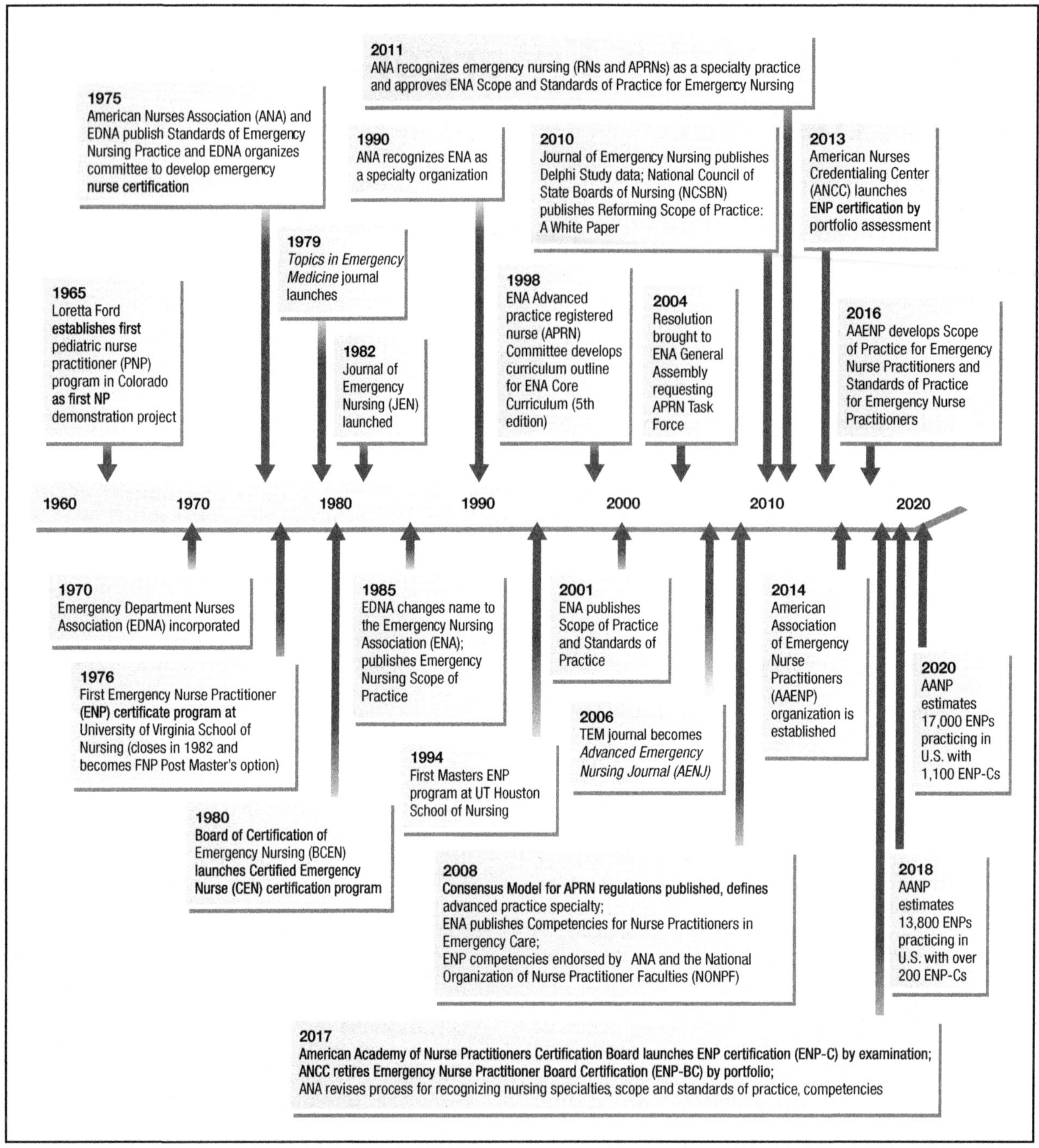

FIGURE 1.1 Emergency nurse practitioner historical milestones.

underwent a factor analysis which yielded ENP practice domains and competencies.[10]

B. In 2008, ENA published the results of the Task Force study as *Competencies for Nurse Practitioners in Emergency Care*.[5] These competencies were endorsed by ANA and NONPF that same year.[11]

C. In 2018, AAENP updated the decade-old 2008 ENA competencies using new practice analysis survey data obtained by AANPCB in preparation for development of the ENP board certification examination. The updated competencies were published as *Practice Standards for the Emergency Nurse Practitioner Specialty*.[12] These updated competencies for practice in emergency care were delineated using the structure outlined and knowledge identified from multiple sources, including the APRN Consensus Model,[7] the AANPCB ENP role delineation study,[13] and the ENP scope and standards of practice documents.[8] The current ENP competencies/

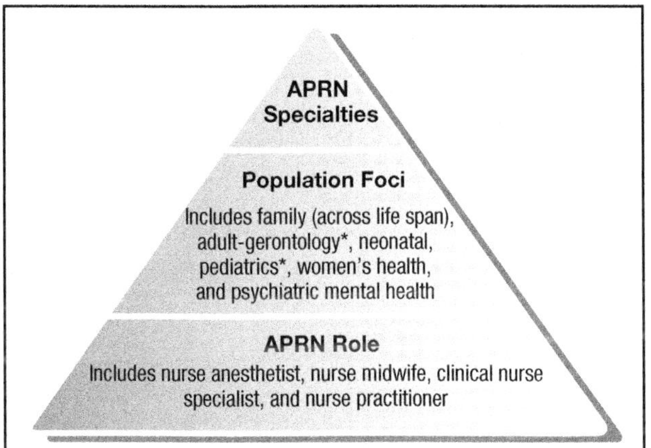

FIGURE 1.2 The Consensus Model for APRN Licensure, Accreditation, Certification, and Education.
*These populations are further divided into acute and primary care delineations.
Source: Adapted from APRN Consensus Work Group and NCSBN APRN Advisory Committee, 2008; https://ncsbn.org/Consensus_Model_for_APRN_Regulation_July_2008.pdf.7

practice standards reflect the specialty's unique care across the life span and levels of acuity and provide a measurable, objective means of assessing ENP competencies.

Educational Requirements and Preparation for Practice

A. Emergency department (ED) census trends and demographics informed the foundational competencies for an emergency nurse practitioner (ENP).[14] ED census data demonstrate that 83.2% to 92.1% of ED patients seen nationwide are discharged following evaluation and treatment.[15,16] Although ED admission rates vary based on region of the country and size of the facility, the ED admission national average in 2016 was 16.8%.[15] Additionally, only 1.6% of ED patients in 2014 required admission to the ICU.[15] These data support that ENPs must be grounded in the family nurse practitioner (FNP) role, able to care for patients of all ages and acuities, with additional knowledge in critical and resuscitative care.

B. Building upon FNP competencies, ENPs are prepared and licensed to assess, diagnose, and manage episodic illnesses, injuries, and acute exacerbations of chronic diseases in patients across the life span consistent with the core Nurse Practitioner Core Competencies.[17] Additional competencies in acute resuscitation and stabilization of emergent conditions for patients presenting to ambulatory, urgent, and emergent care settings are obtained through specialty education.[4]

C. Emergency care is not setting-specific, as defined by the Consensus Model: "The care provided by APRNs is not defined or limited by setting but rather by patient care needs" (p. 8).

D. ENP pathways to practice vary and include:

1. *Completion of a formal FNP/ENP academic program.* A current listing of graduate and postgraduate ENP programs is available on the AAENP website (aaenp.memberclicks.net/academic-programs). Academic programs incorporate core content to meet ENP practice standards and competencies.

2. *Completion of postgraduate emergency fellowship program.* These specialized fellowships range in length from 6 to 18 months and provide full-time clinical practice with intensive skills training and mentorship by emergency medicine physicians, expert ENPs, or physician assistants.

3. Some ENPs enter practice without emergency-specific training and obtain emergency competencies through continuing education and on-the-job training.

Educational Preparation for the ENP Role

A. The first academic ENP program was offered as a specialty certificate at the University of Virginia School of Nursing from 1976 to 1982.[18]

B. Board certification for nurse practitioners arose during the 1970s but did not extend to the ENP role.

C. From 1979 to 1981, the number of U.S. ENP programs accredited by the National League for Nursing grew from four to six.[19]

D. During the 1980s, specialty nurse practitioner educational programs shifted from postgraduate certificate to population-specific master's programs.[20] Consequently, the early ENP certificate programs were either discontinued or modified to meet changing population educational and board certification requirements.

E. In 1994, the first master's program for ENPs was started at the Cizik School of Nursing at the University of Texas Health Science Center in Houston, Texas.[21]

F. Following the establishment of the University of Texas–Houston program, other academic ENP programs were started within the United States. While the majority of programs were offered concurrently with FNP curricula or as postgraduate ENP specialty certificate programs for FNPs, a limited number of ENP programs were offered in combination with acute care nurse practitioner curricula.

G. Since 2016, following establishment of an ENP board certification examination by AANPCB, ENP academic preparation now requires completion of an FNP program of study with additional training as an ENP at the specialty level. ENP degrees are currently offered as master's degree, doctorate of nursing practice, or as postgraduate certificates for certified FNPs.

Certification

A. The first ENP certification was offered via a portfolio methodology by the American Nurses Credentialing Center (ANCC) in 2013.[22] The portfolio certification criteria were developed by a committee of diverse, expert ENPs representing a broad range of population foci and degree levels. Committee members used the 2008 ENP core competencies to identify the key domains of ENP practice and criteria for evaluating candidate qualifications. The portfolio approach offered a certification mechanism for any population-focused NP who met the criteria for expertise in emergency practice gained through clinical experience. ENPs awarded this certification were credentialed as Emergency Nurse Practitioner–Board Certified (ENP-BC). ANCC officially retired the ENP portfolio program on November 15, 2017, after granting 124 NPs the ENP-BC credential. Of the ENP-BC certificants, 68% were FNPs, 25% ACNPs, 2% PNPs, 2% adult NPs, 1% geriatric NPs, and 1% adult gerontology primary care nurse practitioners (Marianne Horahan, personal communication, September 13, 2017).

B. Due to concerns regarding the rigor of the portfolio certification program, in 2016 AAENP partnered with AANPCB to develop a valid and reliable board certification exam for ENPs consistent with the type of board certification recognized within the emergency medicine specialty. A large-scale practice analysis survey of NPs in emergency care obtained from ENA members and AANPCB certificants yielded a content outline for the ENP certification examination.[13] Using the national practice analysis of ENPs working in the role, the ENP certification examination was designed to align with the APRN Consensus Model for specialty nursing practice by measuring the unique body of knowledge specific to the ENP.

C. National ED census and workforce data further supported testing knowledge, competency, and scope of practice encompassing the life span.[16,23–27] Therefore, FNP certification was deemed essential as an eligibility requirement for the specialty examination.

D. The ENP certification exam was first offered in January 2017 through the AANPCB. ENPs awarded this certification are credentialed as Emergency Nurse Practitioner–Certified (ENP-C).[28]

E. The ENP-C is a postgraduate specialty examination. Eligibility requirements for the examination are outlined in the *ENP Specialty Candidate Handbook*[28] and include:

1. Certification as an FNP
2. Completion of an ENP academic or postgraduate fellowship program, or
3. Have at least 2,000 hours of clinical experience in emergency care in addition to documentation of advanced continuing education in emergency content and training in advanced procedural skills

F. In 2018, the Wyoming Board of Nursing officially acknowledged ENP specialty certification for FNPs as evidence of emergency specific education and competencies for practice within emergency settings.[29]

AAENP: The Organization

A. In 2014, a group of ENP clinicians and educators founded the AAENP to advance the ENP profession based on epidemiological evidence obtained from emergency census and demographic data and to validate ENP specialty competencies within existing regulatory frameworks.

B. Although the ENA represented the specialty of emergency nursing broadly, AAENP was established to represent the specific needs of the ENP specialty.

C. In 2015, the *Advanced Emergency Nursing Journal* (*AENJ*) became the official journal for AAENP. As a peer-reviewed journal, *AENJ* contains evidence-based, state-of-the-science content relevant to ENP practice.

Other Organizations

As the ENP specialty has received increasing recognition, following the establishment of AAENP, partnerships with interdisciplinary partners have been formalized and strengthened. In addition to more expansive efforts with diverse organizations, selected highlights of AAENP efforts with partner organizations include:

A. Nursing organization partnerships

1. *ENA:* Collaboration in 2016 yielded the *Scope and Standards for Emergency Nurse Practitioners*.[30] The number of sessions providing NP-level specialty content and procedural skills training at the ENA annual conferences has been increased with input from collaborative planning teams between AAENP and ENA. Ongoing collaboration with ENA on ENP initiatives seeks to strengthen the unified voice for ENPs nationwide and to offer mentorship for nurses interested in entering the ENP profession.
2. *AANP:* As an organizational partner of AANP, AAENP provides expert opinions for AANP on practice and policy issues facing ENPs nationwide. Additionally, AAENP was instrumental in establishing the AANP Emergency Special Practice Group to provide a forum for AANP members to network and receive updates on ENP practice issues.
3. *NONPF*: An Emergency Special Interest Group was established within NONPF to facilitate sharing of ENP teaching strategies, including curricular standards and best practices for simulation to assess ENP student competencies.

B. Physician organization partnerships

1. The American College of Emergency Physicians (ACEP) and the American College of Osteopathic Emergency Physicians (ACOEP) formally endorsed the establishment of AAENP at the 2014 ACEP Scientific Assembly, the inaugural AAENP Board of Directors annual meeting.
2. Since AAENP's inception, ACEP has provided mentorship, guidance, and financial support.
3. ACEP board liaisons have helped to guide AAENP initiatives and have facilitated appointment of AAENP members to key ACEP committees tasked with development of policy statements and advocacy initiatives.
4. The American College of Medical Toxicology invited partnership with AAENP during the COVID-19 pandemic to offer weekly webinars on emerging topics.

Development of the Profession

As emergency care continues to respond within healthcare systems to better meet population needs, the role of the ENP will similarly adapt. Changes within the role will be guided by innovation, science, cost-effectiveness, and best practice models. The ENP specialty can lead in improving emergency care delivery through continued interprofessional collaborations, which these efforts will likely result in changes within the role, scope, and standards of care as the profession evaluates health outcomes, quality, best practices, and access to emergency care.

References and Additional Reading

References and Additional Reading for this chapter are online only and can be found at https://connect.springerpub.com/content/reference-book/978-0-8261-6091-5/part/part01/toc-part/ch01.

2. Fundamental Clinical Skills (Neonatal, Pediatric, and Adult)

SARAH ACKERMAN | HILARY ASHTON GLOVER | CHIVAS GUILLOTE | RODNEY HICKS | APRIL T. HILL | SHARON RAINER | SUSANNA RUDY | RENEÈ SEMONIN HOLLERAN

2A: Airway and Ventilation Management

CHIVAS GUILLOTE

Learning Objectives

- Identify relevant airway structures with specific focus on difficult airway anatomy.
- Define airway adjuncts available for use in emergency airway management.
- Demonstrate the technique for endotracheal intubation.
- Explain the indications and process to establish a surgical airway.
- Describe common ventilator modes and settings used in the ED.
- Discuss indications for noninvasive ventilation and establishing initial settings.
- Identify necessary parameters to ensure safe ventilatory monitoring.

Predicting the Difficult Airway

A. Predicting the difficult airway[1]
  1. Mnemonic ROMAN—difficult bag-valve-mask (BVM)[2]
    a. *R:* Radiation/restriction
    b. *O:* Obesity/obstruction/obstructive sleep apnea (OSA)
    c. *M:* Mask seal/Mallampati/male sex
    d. *A:* Age
      i. Patients >55 years old are associated with a higher risk of difficult BVM.
    e. *N:* No teeth
  2. Mnemonic LEMON—difficult laryngoscopy
    a. *L:* Look externally.
    b. *E:* Evaluate 3-3-2.
      i. Interincisor distance
      ii. Thyromental distance
      iii. Hyoid to cricoid
    c. *M:* Mallampati score
    d. *O:* Obesity/obstruction
    e. *N:* Neck mobility
  3. Mnemonic RODS—difficult extraglottic airway
    a. *R:* Restriction
    b. *O:* Obstruction/obesity
    c. *D:* Disrupted or distorted airway
    d. *S:* Short thyromental distance
  4. Mnemonic SMART—difficult surgical airway
    a. *S:* Surgery
    b. *M:* Mass
    c. *A:* Access/anatomy
    d. *R:* Radiation
    e. *T:* Tumor

Airway Adjuncts Used in Emergency Airway Management

A. Basic airway adjuncts
  1. Oropharyngeal airway
  2. Nasopharyngeal airway
  3. BVM
  4. Nasal cannula (NC)
  5. Nonrebreather (NRB) mask
B. Supraglottic airway devices
  1. Indications/contraindications
    a. The RODS acronym (see A.3) is useful to determine difficult EGD (extraglottic device) placement.
  2. Laryngeal mask airway (LMA)
  3. King Airway
  4. I-Gel

Endotracheal Intubation

A. Advanced airway
  1. Preventing peri-intubation hypoxia
    a. Preoxygenation
      i. *Goal:* Maintain oxygenation saturation when able >93% SpO_2
        (1) Lower oxygen saturation associated with hypoxia
        (2) Increased risk for bradycardia and cardiac arrest 2/2 hypoxia
    b. Methods
      i. NC at flush flow + NRB mask at flush flow
      ii. BVM if unable to maintain oxygen saturation >93% SpO_2
      iii. Delayed sequence intubation (DSI) via ketamine induction
        (1) Utilized for the delirious/altered mental status (AMS) patient

(a) Gain immediate control of the airway.
(b) Goal is preoxygenation.
(c) Intubation continues after preoxygenation is achieved.
(d) Ketamine given at dissociative dose (1–2 mg/kg IV or 4–5 mg/kg intramuscular [IM])
(e) Continue intubation via muscle relaxants after peri-intubation oxygenation is achieved
- Associated with an improved first-pass success rate of the endotracheal tube (ETT).

iv. Apneic oxygenation (peri-intubation oxygenation)
(1) NC at flush flow while performing intubation
(a) Passive oxygenation may help prevent bradycardia, hypoxia, and cardiac arrest by providing alveolar oxygenation.
(b) Not effective in the presence of intrapulmonary shunt physiology

2. ETT
a. Sizes for adult versus pediatric
b. Different types of ETTs used in emergency medicine
i. Standard ETT with bevel
ii. Parker ETT with twin bevel
3. Bougie
a. Uses
i. Difficult airway placement in obstructed views
ii. ETT exchanger
iii. Surgical airway placement (scalpel/bougie/tube technique)
b. Indications
i. Difficult airway placement with obstructed views (Cormack–Lehane III and IV view)
4. Traditional laryngoscope
a. Miller blades
b. MacIntosh blades
c. Methods to improve laryngoscopic view
i. Positioning
ii. Head elevation
iii. Mouth opening
iv. Suctioning
5. Video laryngoscope
a. Standard geometry blades
b. Hyperangulated blades
6. Fiberoptic intubation
a. Indications
b. Contraindications

Surgical Airway Management

A. Needle cricothyrotomy versus surgical cricothyrotomy
1. Needle indicated
a. Pediatrics
b. Poor landmarks or contraindications for surgical crich
2. Surgical airway indications in adult patients based on
a. Cannot be intubated/cannot oxygenate (CICO) via ETT, EGD, BVM + adjuncts)
i. Vortex approach links
ii. Rapid progression toward surgical airway in presence of hypoxia
b. Distorted upper airway anatomy 2/2 anatomic variation or trauma
3. Surgical airway contraindications
a. SMART acronym (see above) revisited to identify difficult surgical airway

B. Front of neck access
1. Scalpel/bougie/tube technique

Mechanical Ventilation in the Emergency Department

A. Common modes
1. Invasive modes
a. Assist control (AC)
i. Rate
ii. Tidal volume (TV)
iii. Positive end-expiratory pressure (PEEP)
iv. Fraction of inspired oxygen (FIO_2)
b. Synchronized intermittent mandatory ventilation (SIMV)
i. Rate
ii. TV
iii. PEEP
iv. Pressure support
v. FIO_2
2. Noninvasive modes
a. Continuous positive airway pressure (CPAP)
b. Bilevel positive airway pressure (BiPAP)

B. Volume versus pressure cycled ventilation
1. Volume cycled
a. Volume is constant
b. Variable is pressure
2. Pressure cycled
a. Pressure is constant
b. Variable is volume

C. Lung protective strategy
1. ARDSnet Data
2. Reduced TV (6–8 mL/kg of ideal body weight)
3. Titration of PEEP based on FIO_2 requirement

Noninvasive Ventilation

A. CPAP
1. Uses—Hypoxia
a. *Example:* Classically used in dyspnea associated with congestive heart failure
2. PEEP
a. Set above physiologic PEEP (5 cmH_2O) and titrate upward
b. Range 5 to 20
i. Increased PEEP associated with improved oxygenation
ii. High PEEP can cause hypotension 2/2 increased intrathoracic pressure.
3. FIO_2

B. BiPAP
  1. Inspiratory pressure (pressure support)
  2. Expiratory pressure (PEEP)
  3. FIO_2

Patient Monitoring During Mechanical Ventilation

A. Monitoring parameters
  1. EKG
  2. SpO_2
  3. $ETCO_2$
  4. Respiration rate (RR)
  5. Temp
  6. Noninvasive blood pressure/invasive blood pressure (NIBP/IBP)
B. Ventilator parameters
  1. TV
  2. Peak inspiratory pressure (P_{IP})
  3. Plateau pressure (PPlat)
  4. Minute volume

2B: Anesthesia and Acute Pain Management

SARAH ACKERMAN

Learning Objectives

- Compare common anesthetic agents and their uses for topical/regional anesthesia as well as for procedural sedation in the ED setting.
- Evaluate common regional anesthesia procedures, including ultrasound-guided regional anesthesia, and their uses in the ED setting.
- Define safe preprocedure assessment, room preparation, and recommended monitoring guidelines for the administration of anesthesia in the ED.
- Demonstrate the nurse practitioner (NP) role in procedural sedation in the ED setting regarding safety, credentialing, and scope of practice.

Local Anesthesia

Local anesthesia is an important technique used frequently in the ED setting to reduce pain in the setting of acute injury or prior to performing painful procedures. This section will review: (a) commonly used topical anesthetic agents, (b) commonly used intradermal and subdermal anesthetic agents, and (c) techniques for administration of local anesthesia.

Common Topical Anesthetic Agents and Their Applications

A. Topical anesthesia can be used in three different clinical situations[3]:
  1. Intact skin (before dermal procedure)
    a. Eutectic Mixture of Local Anesthetics (EMLA), tetracaine gel, liposome-encapsulated lidocaine (LMX)
  2. Intact mucosa
    a. Benzocaine gel or spray, vapor coolants, viscous lidocaine
  3. Open skin (for pain control or prior to wound repair)
    a. Lidocaine, epinephrine, tetracaine (LET)
B. EMLA (lidocaine/prilocaine mixture)[3]
  1. First topical anesthetic that was formulated to penetrate intact skin
  2. Apply for at least 60 minutes under occlusive dressing.
  3. Ideal for peripheral IV insertion, lumbar puncture
  4. Approved for use on intact skin and mucous membranes
C. LET
  1. Usually compounded by institution's pharmacy
  2. Topical anesthetic used on open dermis
D. Ethyl chloride and fluoromethane sprays
  1. Vapor coolants that rapidly cool skin
  2. Rapid onset and short duration (less than one minute)[4]

Common Intradermal and Subdermal Anesthetic Agents

A. Lidocaine
  1. Addition of epinephrine allows for increasing duration of anesthesia, helps control bleeding, and slows systemic absorption of anesthetic agent.[3]
  2. Lidocaine with epinephrine has been found to be safe to use in end-arterial fields (fingers, toes) in healthy patients, but should be avoided in patients with potential vascular injury, or known vascular disease.[3]
  3. Sodium bicarbonate can be added to help reduce pain at the injection site. It also raises the pH of the tissue that acts to shorten the onset of action of the anesthetic agent.[3]
    a. Sodium bicarbonate can only be added to "amide" agents (e.g., lidocaine, bupivacaine, mepivacaine). Cannot be added to "ester" agents (e.g., procaine, chloroprocaine, tetracaine) as a precipitate will form with the esters.
B. *Bupivacaine and mepivacaine:* Longer-acting anesthetic agents
  1. Can also add epinephrine or sodium bicarbonate
    a. Be mindful that ratios for adding bicarbonate buffers ranges, depending on which anesthetic agent is selected—be sure to verify anesthetic agent and buffering agent dosages with institution pharmacy prior to administration.
      i. Bupivacaine can be buffered by adding 1 mL of sodium bicarbonate 8.4% (1 mEq/mL) to 29 mL of bupivacaine 0.25%.[3]
      ii. Lidocaine can be buffered by adding 1 mL of sodium bicarbonate 8.4% (1 mEq/mL) to 9 mL of lidocaine 1%.[3]
C. Diphenhydramine
  1. Can be used as an alternate anesthetic agent for patients that have true allergies to other local anesthetic agents.
  2. Short onset and duration of action
  3. Must be diluted to 1% solution—always verify dosage prior to administration.

Local Anesthesia Administration Techniques

A. Techniques that have been shown to decrease injection pain[4]
1. Slow injection of anesthetic agent
2. Keeping the solution warm
3. Addition of bicarbonate to amide agents in 1:10 ratio
4. Pinch skin at time of the injection.

B. Infiltrative anesthesia technique[4]
1. Rapid onset with low systemic toxicity
2. Inject at the wound margin—causes less pain than at epidermis.
3. Place needle just below epidermis at the level of superficial fascia—less painful and less tissue resistance.

C. Field-block anesthesia technique[4]
1. Local anesthetic agent is placed surrounding the wound, parallel to the wound edge.
2. Ideal for ear lacerations, where infiltrative anesthesia would be difficult to achieve

D. Calculating maximum dosage for anesthetic agents
1. Each anesthetic agent has a different maximum dosage.
2. Be mindful to carefully calculate the maximum dosage prior to administering local or regional anesthesia, especially for large wound repairs.
3. Dosage charts with onset, duration of action, max dose, concentration for both local and regional anesthesia are available from multiple online and text resources:
   a. *Tintinalli's Emergency Medicine: A Comprehensive Study*[3]
   b. *Essential Procedures for Emergency, Urgent, and Primary Care Settings: A Clinical Companion*[4]
4. Example calculation[4]:
   a. For a 70 kg patient, being given lidocaine with epinephrine (max dose 7 mg/kg).
      i. 100% solution is 1g/mL or 1,000 mg/mL so a 1% solution is 10 mg/mL
      ii. Maximum dose is 490 mg or 49 mL.

Procedural Sedation

"Procedural sedation" is a multifaceted term used to describe the act of giving analgesia and/or sedation in order to perform a specific procedure. Procedural sedation is used in various specialties for a wide range of clinical procedures, ranging from elective to emergent.

This text focuses on unscheduled procedures, which the American College of Emergency Physicians (ACEP) defines as "medical, surgical, or dental interventions that are emergent or urgent and, to optimize patient outcomes, must be performed within a short time frame unsuitable for that used to schedule elective procedures." The category of "unscheduled" procedures encompasses most of the procedures that are performed in the ED setting, and that are within the scope of the emergency nurse practitioner (ENP). There are several clinical practice guidelines regarding procedural sedation that have been published by various professional organizations such as the American Society of Anesthesiologists (ASA), the American Academy of Pediatrics (AAP), and the American Association of Oral Maxillofacial Surgeons (AAOMS). This text will focus on the most recent ACEP guideline, as this guideline gives the most comprehensive overview of the procedures and policies that are important for practicing ENP. This section will review: (a) the skill sets needed to perform sedation; (b) different levels of sedation; (c) presedation patient evaluation; (d) room set up and supplies; (e) common medications used in sedation; and finally, (f) monitoring guidelines. It is important to note that many states and most institutions regulate which clinicians can legally administer anesthetic agents. Although some states allow for NPs to administer anesthetic agents for procedural sedation, there are specific guidelines for each state regarding the necessity of physician presence during the administration, type of anesthetic agent used, and level of sedation. It is important for the practicing ENP to research both their own state and institutional regulations/credentialing process prior to administering any anesthetic agent for sedation purposes.

Skill Sets and Staff Requirements Necessary for Unscheduled Procedural Sedation

A. The sedation clinician should be able to manage a patient and address adverse events for any level of sedation, as the depth of sedation can change rapidly.

B. The Joint Commission states that "individuals administering moderate or deep sedation and anesthesia are qualified and have credentials to manage and rescue patients at whatever level of sedation or anesthesia is achieved, either intentionally or unintentionally."[5]

C. The guidelines by ACEP (Table 2.1) provides a set of clinical skills that clinicians who are administering sedation should be able to perform proficiently in order to provide safe and effective sedation care.

D. It is vitally important that the clinician administering sedation is proficient in airway rescue techniques and management of adverse events outlined below. A clinician who is not credentialed or proficient in rescue airway interventions should never provide sedation without the supervision or presence of a qualified clinician who can perform these rescue techniques.

E. It is reasonable to assume that there are circumstances where the ENP would be performing the procedure during procedural sedation, but not administering sedation. In this scenario, it appears it would be acceptable for the proceduralist to not be credentialed in rescue airway techniques as mentioned earlier, as long as the clinician administering sedation is available at the bedside to perform such procedures in case of an adverse event.

F. ACEP suggests that safe procedural sedation requires a two-person sedation team (see Table 2.1 for specific skills for each)
1. One sedation clinician (responsible for oversight of procedure)
2. One sedation monitor (responsible for patient monitoring and documentation)

TABLE 2.1 REQUISITE SKILL SETS FOR PROCEDURAL SEDATION

	PROCEDURAL SEDATION CLINICIAN	PROCEDURAL SEDATION MONITOR
Cognitive Skills	Must understand: ■ Airway, respiratory, and cardiovascular physiology and pathophysiology ■ The function and interpretation of continuous monitoring of cardiac rhythm, pulse oximetry, and capnography ■ Sedative and antagonist drug pharmacology (e.g., pharmacokinetics, pharmacodynamics, dosing, administration, contraindications, adverse event profiles) ■ Sedation adverse events and when intervention is appropriate ■ The principles of patient presedation evaluation and factors that increase sedation risk ■ The procedure to be performed and how it might impact the sedation course or sedation risk	Must be familiar with: ■ Airway, respiratory, and cardiovascular physiology and pathophysiology ■ The function and interpretation of continuous monitoring of cardiac rhythm, pulse oximetry, capnography, and blood pressure ■ The sedative drugs being used, including their dosing, administration, duration, and adverse event profiles ■ Sedation adverse events and when intervention is appropriate
Interactive Monitoring Skills	Must be able to: ■ Monitor airway patency, identify airway obstruction, and identify and distinguish obstructive and central apnea ■ Monitor ventilatory adequacy using continual observation of chest wall motion supplemented with pulse oximetry and capnography ■ Monitor cardiovascular stability using physical assessment supplemented with cardiac rhythm and blood pressure monitoring ■ Recognize when a patient is excessively or inadequately sedated	Must be able to: ■ Monitor airway patency and identify partial or complete airway obstruction ■ Monitor ventilatory adequacy using continual observation of the airway and chest wall motion supplemented with pulse oximetry and capnography ■ Monitor cardiovascular stability using physical assessment supplemented with cardiac rhythm and blood pressure monitoring ■ Recognize when a patient is excessively or inadequately sedated
Rescue Skills	Must be able to: ■ Relieve airway obstruction through appropriate application of head tilt, chin lift, or placement of nasal or oral airway ■ Perform bag-mask ventilation ■ Manage a patient who is excessively sedated, with or without active intervention as appropriate ■ Rapidly initiate resuscitative measures for hypoxia, apnea, laryngospasm, hypotension, bradycardia, anaphylaxis, seizure, or cardiac arrest ■ Rapidly summon additional resuscitation assistance, if required	Must be able to: ■ Assist the sedation clinician in resuscitation ■ Rapidly summon additional resuscitation assistance, if required

Source: From the American College of Emergency Physicians. Policy statement. Unscheduled procedural sedation: a multidisciplinary consensus practice guideline. Approved September 28th 2018. Available at: https://www.acep.org/globalassets/sites/acep/media/policy-statement/unscheduled-procedural-sedation-sept-28-2018-cp.pdf[3]

Levels of Sedation

A. The ENP performing procedural sedation should have a comprehensive understanding of the different levels of sedation and be able to rescue a patient from a deeper than intended level of sedation or move to a deeper level of sedation if desired level is not achieved initially.

B. Sedation can be considered a "continuum," as patients can quickly move between levels of sedation.

C. Levels of sedation[6]

1. Minimal sedation (anxiolysis)
   - **a.** Can respond normally to verbal commands
   - **b.** Cognitive function and coordination may be impaired
   - **c.** Airway reflexes, spontaneous ventilation, and cardiovascular function are unaffected.
2. Moderate sedation/analgesia (conscious sedation)
   - **a.** Depression of consciousness where patients maintain purposeful response to verbal or tactile stimulation (should be light tactile stimulation)
     - **i.** Reflex withdrawal from painful stimuli is NOT considered a purposeful response.
   - **b.** No intervention required to maintain airway
   - **c.** Spontaneous ventilation is usually adequate.
   - **d.** Cardiovascular function is usually maintained.
3. Deep sedation/analgesia
   - **a.** Depression of consciousness, patients are not easily arousable, but still respond purposefully with repeated or painful stimulus.
   - **b.** Patients not always able to maintain a patent airway or spontaneous ventilation.
     - **i.** May need ventilatory support
   - **c.** Cardiovascular function usually maintained
4. General anesthesia
   - **a.** Patients are not arousable even with painful stimulation.
   - **b.** Usually need intervention to maintain a patent airway
   - **c.** Often require positive pressure ventilation because of depressed spontaneous ventilation

d. Cardiovascular function may be impaired.

5. Dissociative sedation

a. Dissociative sedation is a different type of sedation not mentioned in the earlier guideline, typically only achieved with the use of the medication ketamine.

b. ACEP definition of dissociative sedation: "A trance-like cataleptic state induced by the dissociative drug ketamine characterized by profound analgesia and amnesia with retention of protective airway reflexes, spontaneous respirations, and cardiopulmonary stability."[7]

Presedation Evaluation and Preparation

A. Perform a focused history and physical.

1. Patients who are healthy or with mild systemic disease (ASA physical status I and II) generally make good sedation candidates.

2. Patients with severe systemic disease (ASA III and greater) are at greater risk for adverse events.

3. Use of Mallampati score has not been found to impact clinical outcomes.[8]

4. Anatomic/physiologic risks

a. The ACEP clinical practice guideline cites the importance of assessing for variants that might complicate ventilation such as:

i. Airway abnormalities

ii. Obstructive sleep apnea (OSA)

iii. Young age (infants under 3 months)

iv. Premature birth in an infant

5. Possibility of pregnancy for women of childbearing age

B. ASA recommendations for patient evaluation prior to sedation:

1. *Note:* Although these guidelines are quite thorough in their evaluation of the patient, it is important for the ENP to bear in mind that it may not be possible to gather this information prior to an urgent/emergent sedation.

2. Review previous medical records and interview the patient or family to identify:

a. Abnormalities of major organ systems (e.g., cardiac, renal, pulmonary, neurologic, sleep apnea, metabolic, endocrine)

b. Adverse experience with sedation/analgesia as well as regional and general anesthesia

c. History of a difficult airway

d. Current medications, potential drug interactions, drug allergies, nutraceuticals

e. History of tobacco, alcohol, or substance use/abuse

f. Frequent or repeated exposure to sedation/analgesic agents

3. Conduct a focused physical examination of the patient (e.g., vital signs, auscultation of heart and lungs, evaluation of the airway, and when appropriate to sedation, other organ systems where major abnormalities have been identified).

4. Review available laboratory results.

a. Order additional laboratory tests guided by a patient's medical condition, physical examination, and the likelihood that the results will affect the management of moderate sedation/analgesia.

b. Evaluate results of these tests before sedation is initiated.

5. If possible, perform the preprocedure evaluation well enough in advance (e.g., several days to weeks) to allow for optimal patient preparation.

6. Reevaluate the patient immediately before the procedure.

C. Time out

1. It is vital to perform a "time out" prior to initiating procedural sedation and is a requirement by The Joint Commission for universal protocol.[9]

2. Items to verify in "time-out" checklist

a. Verify patient identity.

b. Patient consent for procedure

c. Correct site of procedure

d. Verify roles of the sedation team.

D. Oral intake prior to procedural sedation

1. Aspiration is a rare complication of procedural sedation as it is uncommon for a patient to lose their airway-protective reflexes during procedural sedation.

2. Despite being a rare complication, last oral intake should be considered when choosing sedative agents, and desired depth of sedation.

3. It is important to consider the risks versus benefits of delaying a procedure secondary to recent oral intake.

a. Consider using a dissociative agent for sedation (such as ketamine) in order to avoid losing airway-protective reflexes[10]

4. Use caution in patients with increased risk of aspiration[3]:

a. History of serious underlying illness

b. OSA

c. Obesity

d. Age <12 months

e. Upper endoscopy as the procedure

f. Bowel obstruction

E. There is no evidence that "non-compliance with elective fasting guidelines increases the risk of aspiration or other adverse events."

Supplies and Room Setup

A. IV access (depending on medication selected and route of administration)

B. Supplemental oxygen

C. Suction

D. Cardiac/pulse oxygen monitoring equipment

E. Airway rescue equipment (e.g., oral airway kit [appropriate for age], nasal airway, bag valve mask)

F. Appropriate reversal agents (when using benzodiazepines)

G. Resuscitation medications (e.g., code cart/cardiac arrest medications in addition to anaphylaxis medications and antiemetics)

H. Capnography (if performing moderate/deep/dissociative sedation)

Common Medications Used During Procedural Sedation

A. There is an abundance of literature covering which medications (and combinations of medications) to choose when performing procedural sedation in the ED.

B. Helpful information to consider when selecting drug classes for sedation in the ED setting:

1. Opioids
   a. *Example of commonly used medication:* Fentanyl
   b. May cause respiratory depression
   c. No amnesic properties
   d. Varying levels of sedation based on individual
   e. Usually given in combination with sedatives that do not have analgesic properties[11]
2. Benzodiazepines
   a. *Example:* Midazolam
   b. Causes anxiolysis, sedation, amnesia, anticonvulsant activity, and to a lesser degree, muscle relaxation[12]
   c. No analgesic properties
   d. Preferable for longer procedures that require deep sedation[11]
   e. Increased cardiovascular and respiratory depression when combined with opioids[11]
3. Volatile agents
   a. *Example:* Nitrous oxide
   b. Very short acting
   c. Analgesic, anxiolytic, and sedative properties
   d. Noninvasive (not given intravenously)
   e. Relatively few contraindications
   f. Rapid onset
   g. Consider risk for staff exposure; use well ventilated room.
4. General anesthetic agents
   a. *Example:* Propofol
   b. Rapid onset, short acting
   c. Given intravenously
   d. Use for distressing or uncomfortable procedures—useful for orthopedic procedures
   e. No analgesic properties—should not be used alone for moderately painful procedures[12]
   f. Anticonvulsant properties
   g. May cause rapid sedation, apnea, respiratory depression, hypotension (increased risk for older patients)[11]
5. Phencyclidines
   a. *Example:* Ketamine
   b. Anxiolysis, amnesia, immobilization, profound analgesia[12]
   c. May have recovery agitation
      i. Avoid in patients with active/history of psychosis.
   d. Using a combination of ketamine and propofol (ketofol) may reduce adverse effects associated with using each agent individually
      i. Combination may be useful for prolonged procedures
   e. May be safer for patients with comorbid conditions as provides sedation/analgesia with cardiorespiratory stability[12]
   f. Useful for patients with risk for bronchospasm (ketamine is bronchodilator)[12]
   g. Respiratory depression possible if administered via rapid bolus push[11]
6. Etomidate
   a. Fast-acting anesthetic
   b. Minimal cardiovascular/respiratory depression
   c. Ideal for short procedures such as cardioversion
   d. No analgesic properties
   e. Adverse effect of etomidate—associated myoclonus (although not usually clinically relevant) and theoretical risk for adrenal suppression (no sound evidence to date)[7]

C. ACEP's policy subcommittee on procedural sedation and anesthesia evaluated the current literature regarding the safety of several common medications used for procedural sedation in the ED setting (ketamine, propofol, etomidate, dexmedetomidine, alfentanil, remifentanil):

1. Evidence was graded as Level A recommendations ("generally accepted principles for patient care that reflect a high degree of clinical certainty"), Level B recommendations ("recommendations for patient care that may identify a particular strategy . . . that reflect moderate clinical certainty"), and Level C ("Recommendations for patient care that are based on evidence from Class of Evidence III studies or, in the absence of any adequate published literature, based on expert consensus").[7]
   a. Level A recommendations:
      i. Ketamine can be safely administered to children for procedural sedation and analgesia.
      ii. Propofol can be safely administered to both children and adults.
   b. Level B recommendations:
      i. Etomidate can be safely administered to adults.
      ii. The combination of ketamine and propofol can be safely administered to both children and adults.
   c. Level C recommendations:
      i. Ketamine can be safely administered to adults.
      ii. Alfentanil can be safely administered to adults.
      iii. Etomidate can be safely administered to children.

Monitoring Guidelines

A. Telemetry, blood pressure monitoring, and pulse oximetry are commonly used.

B. Capnography is often used to provide "continuous, immediate, objective verification of the quality of ventilation, and is more reliable for this purpose than pulse oximetry or interactive monitoring alone."

C. Supplemental oxygen

1. "If apnea occurs, high-flow pre-oxygenation delays oxygen desaturation by up to 6 minutes in a healthy adult and 2 to 4 minutes in a healthy child with a patent airway."[10]

2. Preoxygenation may help patients tolerate periods of respiratory depression and avoid positive pressure ventilation.
3. When not using capnography or using solely pulse oximetry, avoid using supplemental oxygen so that respiratory compromise can be detected.
4. If using capnography, it is acceptable to deliver supplemental oxygen throughout the procedure.

D. Recovery
1. Patients may become unstable or encounter respiratory depression shortly after the procedure ends when the patient becomes more relaxed.
2. Monitor patient postsedation until:
a. The patient is no longer at risk for respiratory depression.
b. Vital signs return to presedation baseline.
c. Alert at age-appropriate baseline level of consciousness

E. Important documentation to include:
1. Original plan for procedural sedation
2. Patient evaluation
3. Procedural sedation course
4. Drugs/drug doses/ administration time
5. Adverse events and interventions
6. Sedation monitor (nurse or second clinician assisting with the procedure) should also keep separate monitoring documentation, in accordance with institutional guidelines.

Regional Anesthesia

Regional anesthesia has been widely used in the ED setting to aid in the treatment of complicated lacerations, fractures, joint dislocations, debridement, among others. Regional anesthesia can be achieved by clinicians using anatomic landmark identifiers, or by using ultrasound (US) technology to guide administration. US-guided regional anesthesia (UGRA) has been found to "shorten the block performance time, reduce the number of needle passes, minimize risk for vascular injury, and enable blocks to be performed using lower anesthetic doses."[11] Recent studies have found that "more than 30% of nerve blocks fail by anatomic landmarks alone, and US guidance has led to greater than 95% block success rates."[13] With the rise of opioid usage and issues surrounding narcotic prescriptions, UGRA offers a promising alternative for many clinicians in the ED setting. Some institutions do include UGRA in their credentialing pathway for physicians, however, this may be less common for nurse practitioner employees. This section outlines the core principles of regional anesthesia for common ED applications, including a review of the (a) preprocedure assessment, (b) common agents used for regional anesthesia, and (c) common nerve blocks performed in the ED setting; however, this text does not serve as a substitution for observed practice. It is important that the practicing ENPs advocate for both training and credentialing opportunities within their institution. The 2016 ACEP US guideline "practice-based pathway" could potentially be used to help guide further training for ENPs in UGRA. ENPs should not perform any type of regional or local anesthesia without significant preparation, training, and official institutional credentialing. In terms of what defines competency to perform UGRA, the definition ranges widely across organizations. Currently, there are no consensus guidelines with regard to UGRA training for emergency physicians nor for nurse practitioners. However, for reference, "anesthesia residents must perform a minimum of 20 nerve blocks to demonstrate competency."[13] Additionally, any clinician performing regional or local anesthesia should be comfortable with diagnosis and management of local anesthetic system toxicity (LAST), and should have access to intravenous lipid emulsion should this occur. The American Society for Regional Anesthesia (ASRA) provides a checklist for administration of lipid emulsion—this or other administration guidelines should be available to the clinician.[13,14]

Preprocedure Assessment

A. Clinician must document neurovascular status prior to administering regional anesthesia. Regional anesthesia may mask any underlying neurovascular injury.
1. Distal vascular function
a. Skin color
b. Temperature
c. Capillary refill
d. Distal pulses
2. Distal neurologic function
a. Sensation—for digital injuries, can use two-point discrimination to assess sensation[11]
b. Motor function (including range of motion and strength)

B. Contraindications for regional anesthesia[11]
1. Coagulopathy
2. Immune suppression (relative contraindication)
3. Multisystem trauma
4. Neuropathy
5. Neurologic deficit
6. Allergy to anesthetic agents

C. Special contraindications/considerations for UGRA[14]
1. Active infection at the injection site
2. Risk for compartment syndrome
3. Uncooperative patients
4. Preexisting neurologic deficit
5. Extreme obesity (might obscure either landmark or US visualization)
6. Anticoagulation or coagulopathy (relative contraindication)

D. Nerve block protocol/checklist
1. There are several protocols developed to help streamline the process of regional anesthesia administration in the ED.
2. See Figure 2.1 for example of protocol.

E. Safety checks
1. Mark appropriate extremity.
2. Two-person medication/dosage verification of anesthetic agent
3. Consent for procedure
4. Monitoring (per institutional protocol—usually telemetry, IV access, pulse ox, blood pressure)
5. Ensure availability of lipid emulsion in case of adverse event/LAST
6. Time out

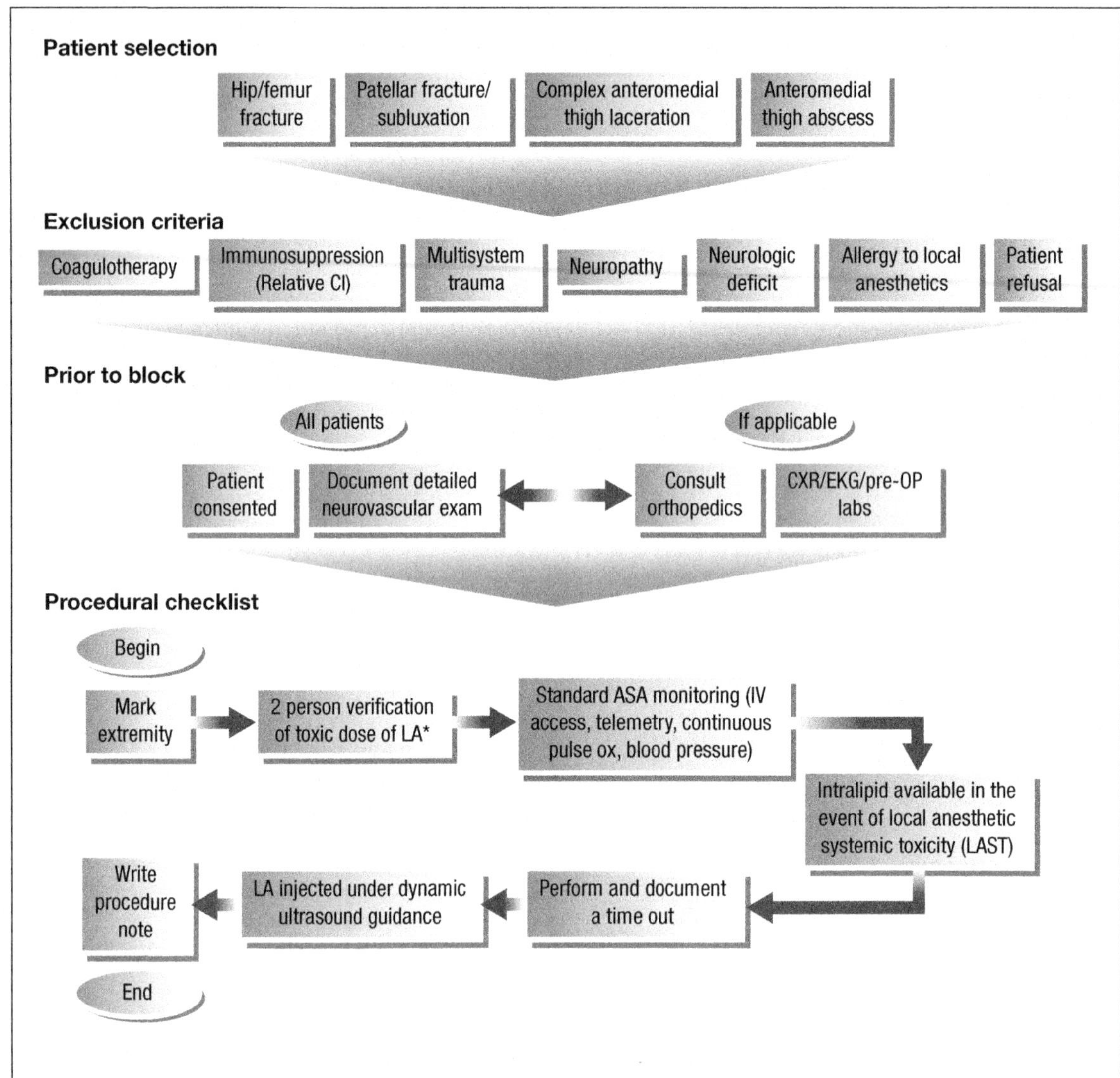

FIGURE 2.1 Regional anesthesia administration protocol for the emergency department setting.
Source: From Newton-Brown E, Fitzgerald L, Mitra B. Audit improves emergency department triage, assessment, multi-modal analgesia and nerve block use in the management of pain in older people with neck of femur fracture. *Australas Emerg Nurs J*. 2014;17:176-183.[15]

7. Patient-specific considerations
   a. If patient has fracture, consider orthopedics consult prior to block.

Common Anesthetic Agents Used for Regional Anesthesia

A. Lidocaine
   1. Popular agent for regional anesthesia
   2. Require approximately 10 to 20 minutes to achieve anesthesia[16]

B. Bupivacaine, levobupivacaine, ropivacaine
   1. Long-acting anesthetic agents
   2. Will require approximately 15 to 30 minutes to achieve anesthesia[16]

Common Nerve Blocks Performed in Emergency Department Setting

A. Many instructional videos and educational materials for performing regional nerve blocks are available online:
   1. *Tintinalli's Emergency Medicine: A Comprehensive Study Guide*[15] offers technical instructions as well as video access for performing most regional anesthesia procedures used in the ED setting.
   2. *Essential Procedures for Emergency, Urgent, and Primary Care Settings: A Clinical Companion*[13] provides step-by-step instructions for common regional and local anesthesia procedures used in the ED setting.
   3. *Essential Procedures for Emergency, Urgent, and Primary Care Settings*[4] provides step-by-step guidance

and illustrations to cover 60 commonly performed procedures in the ED and primary care settings.

4. iOS applications[13]:
   a. Block GuRU
   b. NYSORA
   c. SonoAccess
   d. Nerve Whiz
5. Websites[11]
   a. highlandultrasound.com
   b. 5minsono.com/vids/NYSORA.com
   c. Usra.ca (regional anesthesia section)

B. Digital nerve block

1. Provides anesthesia to an entire digit (fingers or toes)
2. Good for procedures such as finger lacerations, toenail removal/repair, paronychia drainage, finger, or toe reduction[16]
3. According to recent studies, there is less pain associated with injection of lidocaine 1% with epinephrine as compared to using bupivacaine for digital nerve blocks, however, the duration of action for lidocaine is about half as long as that of bupivacaine.[15,17]
4. Transthecal/flexor tendon sheath block can be used to anesthetize a digit as an alternative to a digital block; however, it may not anesthetize the entire distal fingertip.[15]

C. Hand and wrist blocks

1. Median nerve block
   a. Good for lacerations to lateral palm[11]
   b. Anesthetizes the "thumb, index, long, and half of the ring finger distal to the proximal interphalangeal joint, but not the dorsum of the thumb"[15]
2. Radial nerve block
   a. Good for distal radius fracture[11]
   b. Anesthetizes the "dorsal lateral half of the hand and dorsal aspect of the thumb"[15]
3. Ulnar nerve block
   a. Good for Boxer's fracture, injury to fifth digit, or injury to ulnar surface[11]
   b. Anesthetizes "entire fifth digit, half of the fourth digit, and medial aspect of hand and wrist"[15]

D. Foot and ankle blocks

1. There are five nerves that innervate the foot, four of which are branches of the sciatic nerve (superficial peroneal, deep peroneal, tibial, sural nerves) and the saphenous nerve, which is a cutaneous branch of the femoral nerve.[11]
2. Deep peroneal nerve and posterior tibial can be consistently found by anatomic landmarks, while the other three nerves (superficial peroneal, sural, and saphenous) are anatomically variable. Thus, for these three nerves, it is best to use a "field block" technique in the subcutaneous space in the general area where the nerve travels.[15]
3. US guidance suggested[15]
4. Sciatic branch blocks can be used alone or in combination for ankle dislocations, Achilles tendon rupture.
   a. Posterior tibial block
      i. Good for calcaneal fractures, laceration repair, or foreign body removal from the sole of foot[11]
      ii. Anesthetizes the plantar aspect of the foot
   b. *Superficial peroneal block:* Anesthetizes the dorsal lateral aspect of the foot
   c. *Sural nerve block:* Anesthetizes lateral aspect of the ankle—some extension of anesthesia to plantar aspect of the foot[15]
   d. *Deep peroneal block:* Anesthetizes web space between first and second toe as well as the small area just proximal to first/second toe on the plantar aspect of foot[15]
5. *Saphenous nerve:* Anesthetizes medial aspect of the ankle

E. Extremity blocks

1. Femoral nerve block
   a. Good for hip or femur fractures, patellar subluxation, tibial fracture, anterior/medial thigh lacerations[11]
   b. US guided strongly suggested[15]
   c. "Three-in-one" block technique
      i. Same injection location as femoral block, although uses special technique used to also block obturator and lateral femoral cutaneous nerves[15]
   d. Ropivacaine is commonly used for femoral blocks.[15]

F. Intercostal nerve block

1. Ideal for rib fractures, rib contusions, and post-chest tube thoracostomy, and thoracic herpes zoster
2. Anesthetizes the intercostal nerve above and below the affected rib in a "band-like fashion around the chest well"[15]

G. Head and neck blocks

1. *Supraorbital/supratrochlear nerve block:* Anesthetize the forehead, bridge of nose
2. *Infraorbital nerve block:* Anesthetizes lower eyelid, medial aspect of check, ipsilateral side of nose, and ipsilateral upper lip[15]
3. *Mental nerve block:* Anesthetizes the labial mucosa, gingiva, lower lip adjacent to incisors and canines[15]
4. Auricular nerve block
   a. Anesthetizes external ear using field block of the auriculotemporal, lesser occipital, and great auricular nerves[15]
   b. Does not anesthetize the concha and meatus—these are innervated by vagus nerve.

H. Dental nerve blocks

1. *Supraperiosteal (local) infiltration:* Ideal for toothache, not sufficient for avulsed tooth or dry socket usually[15]
2. *Palatal infiltration:* Infiltration of local anesthetic agent into the palate can help anesthetize individual maxillary teeth
3. Posterior superior alveolar (PSA) block
   a. Otherwise known as "zygomatic block"
   b. Anesthetizes the maxillary molar teeth up to the first molar[15](can possibly anesthetize the premolar region in some patients)
   c. This is a technique-sensitive block with many potential complications.
      i. Be sure to aspirate to avoid injecting into the maxillary artery or injecting into the

pterygoid plexus, which can cause hematoma formation.[18]

4. Infraorbital (anterior superior alveolar) nerve block
   a. Ideal for lacerations of upper lip and medial cheek
   b. Anesthetizes the maxillary central and lateral incisors, canine, surrounding buccal soft tissue, medial cheek, ipsilateral lower eyelid, lateral aspect of nose, and upper lip
   c. Helpful if multiple teeth are involved and if supraperiosteal infiltration does not achieve full anesthesia[18]
5. Inferior alveolar nerve (IAN) block
   a. Ideal for lacerations of the lower lip, providing pain relief for mandibular toothache, and some lateral tongue lacerations
   b. Anesthetizes the mandibular teeth on the ipsilateral side, lingual hard and soft tissue, and ipsilateral lower lip (often anesthetizes ipsilateral tongue as lingual, mental, and incisive nerves are proximal to the IAN)[4]
6. Buccal nerve block
   a. Ideal for buccal lacerations
   b. Anesthetizes buccal surface of ipsilateral mandibular molars and adjacent soft tissue
7. Mental nerve block
   a. Ideal for procedures involving buccal soft tissue that is anterior to mental foramen[18]
   b. Anesthetizes buccal soft tissue anterior to the mental foramen, ipsilateral lower lip, and chin[18]

2C: Diagnostic and Procedural Ultrasound

HILARY ASHTON GLOVER

Learning Objectives

- List the benefits of using ultrasound in the ED.
- Demonstrate emergency nurse practitioner (ENP) scope of practice as it relates to the use of emergency ultrasound (EUS).
- Explain basic ultrasound terminology, physics, and machine function.
- Describe basic ultrasound equipment including probes, main buttons, and modes of operation.
- List the potential indications of EUS by the ENP.
- Summarize the general approach, potential complications, and pitfalls of EUS.

Emergency ultrasound (EUS), also known as point-of-care ultrasound (POCUS), has been utilized since the 1980s.[1] Over the past two decades, EUS has become a fundamental skill in emergency care for both diagnosis and procedural guidance.[19,20] Since its inception, the use of EUS has increased and is now considered standard in the evaluation of the emergency patient. EUS is a diagnostic imaging modality that is not a component of the physical examination.[21] EUS differs from the traditional model of comprehensive ultrasound (US) in that it can be performed, interpreted, and integrated into the management of the patient at the bedside.[22] The text will review: (a) basic US terminology and physics, (b) scope of practice, c) basic principles of EUS that can be applied to any applications, d) indications, (e) general approach, (f) and potential complications and pitfalls. Specific US applications and procedures are outside the scope of this text.

Benefits

A. Due to its portability, an US machine can be brought to the bedside of an unstable patient.[22] This prevents the patient from being transported to radiology and potentially becoming more unstable there.[22]
B. EUS aids emergency nurse practitioners (ENPs) in obtaining a rapid diagnosis and developing a plan of care.[20]
C. EUS has transformed procedures performed in the ED.[20] Through the use of EUS, ENPs can now visualize the anatomy directly while performing a particular procedure. This added imaging increases procedural safety (e.g., central venous catheter placement) and decreases patient complications from these procedures.[22]
D. US devices use nonionizing radiation, unlike x-rays and CT scans.[22]
E. The use of POCUS has also contributed to quality improvement, timeliness of care, improved diagnostic accuracy, and decreased healthcare costs.

Scope of Practice

A. EUS is a fundamental skill for both diagnosis and procedural guidance.[20]

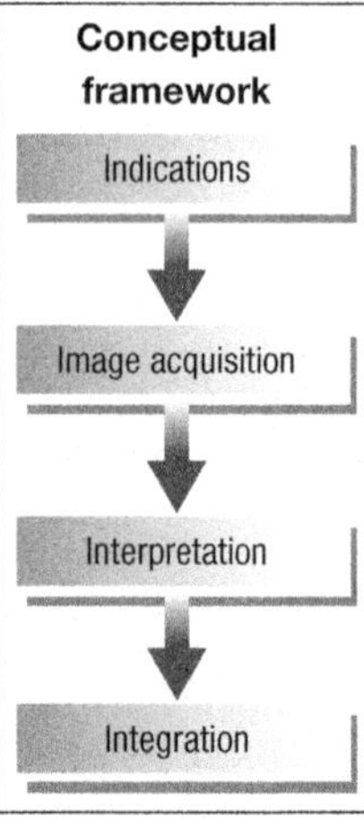

FIGURE 2.2 Conceptual framework of ultrasound skills. To master, emergency nurse practitioners (ENPs) must possess the knowledge and skills of emergency ultrasound: (a) indications, (b) image acquisition, (c) interpretation, and (d) integration of findings into practice.
Source: From Baston, C.M., Moore, C., Krebs, E.A., Dean, A.J., & Panebianco, N. (2019). *Pocket Guide to POCUS: Point-of-Care Tips for Point-of-Care Ultrasound.* McGraw-Hill Education, Inc.; 2019.[1]

B. These skills are both included within the practice standards of ENPs.[23]
C. To master EUS, ENPs must possess the knowledge and skills of EUS: an (a) indications, (b) image acquisition, (c) interpretation, and (d) integration of findings into practice.[19] (see Figure 2.2)
D. The American College of Emergency Physicians (ACEP) has outlined educational and competency standards for the use of EUS by advanced practice providers (APPs).[24]
E. According to the ACEP, APPs should successfully complete at least 100 to 300 total reviewed EUS examination in order to demonstrate proficiency. ACEP also suggests that trainees complete 25 to 50 reviewed examinations in a particular application prior to achieving competency.[24]
F. APPs should also adhere to the practice standards and scope of practice set forth by their individual institutions and state boards of nursing.[24]

Basic Terminology and Physics

A. In order to understand US, ENPs must have an understanding of basic physics, terminology, and how the machine operates.
B. Basic terminology[22] (see Table 2.2)
C. US is based on sound waves and the *pulse echo principle*.[20,22]

1. The US machine is plugged into an electrical outlet that creates electrical energy causing crystals in the tip of the probe to vibrate.[20,22] This is called the *piezoelectric effect*.[20]
2. The vibration results in mechanical energy or high-frequency sound waves, which are in turn emitted from the probe and transmitted into the patient's body. The sound waves are then reflected back to the probe.[20,22]
3. Depending on the type of structure or object encountered, a certain percentage of the sound waves will return back to the probe and convert back to electrical energy. The US machine is then able to translate this information and create the image on the screen.[20,22]

D. Wavelength and frequency

1. Wavelength and frequency are inversely related.[19,22]
2. Low-frequency waves are long, whereas high-frequency waves are short in wavelength.[19,22]

TABLE 2.2 BASIC ULTRASOUND TERMINOLOGY

TERM	DEFINITION
Ultrasound	Sound waves transmitted at a frequency greater than 20 kHz
Wavelength	The distance a wave travels in a single cycle, typically measured in meters (m)
Frequency	The number of times or cycles per second a wave is repeated. Measured in Hertz (Hz)
Pulse Echo Principle	Responsible for basic machine function
One Hertz (Hz)	One wave cycle per second

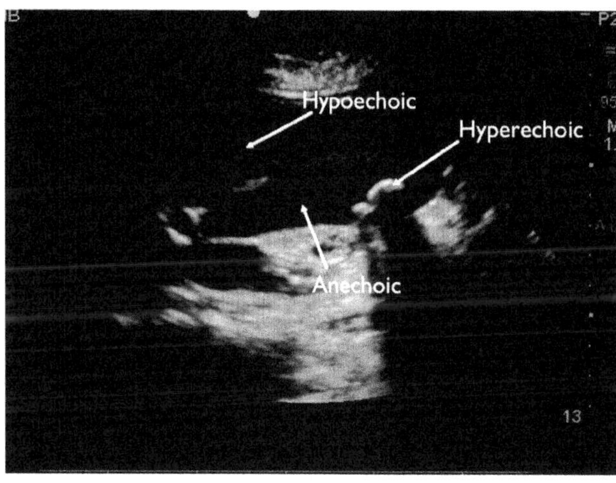

FIGURE 2.3 Echogenicity as Illustrated on an ultrasound image. *Anechoic* objects appear black on the ultrasound screen. *Hyperechoic* objects appear very bright on the ultrasound screen. *Hypoechoic* structures lie somewhere between these two extremes.
Source: From Blackstock, U., & Carmody, K. (2016). Transforming learning anatomy: Basics of ultrasound lecture and abdominal ultrasound anatomy hands-on session. *MedEdPORTAL, 12, 1–5*. https://doi.org/10.15766/mep_2374-8265.10446.[22]

3. The US probe transmits and receives waves.[25]

E. Basic concept of ultrasonography[25]

1. The image generated on the screen is based on (a) the probe used and (b) the type of tissue that the US wave is transmitted through.
2. Different probes generate US waves of different frequencies.
3. This impacts the resolution and depth of the image generated on the screen.

F. *Echogenicity* is defined as an object's ability to reflect sound waves or echoes (Figure 2.3).[22]

1. *Anechoic* objects appear black on the US screen.[20]
a. Sound waves travel well in fluid, resulting in most of the energy passing completely through them.
b. Therefore, fluid does not reflect echoes back to the US probe.
c. Examples of anechoic structures include blood vessels, a full bladder, and free fluid in the abdomen.[20,22]
2. *Hyperechoic* objects appear very bright on the US screen.
a. This is because dense objects reflect most of the sound waves back to the US probe.
b. Bone, gallstones, and nerves are all examples of hyperechoic structures.[20,22]
3. *Hypoechoic* structures lie somewhere between these two extremes.
a. These anatomic structures typically appear in varying shades of gray.
b. Hypoechoic structures reflect some echoes back to the US probe, depending on their water content.
c. Solid organs, like the liver and kidney, appear hypoechoic on US.[22]

G. Artifacts[19]

1. Acoustic shadow
   a. Occurs when sound waves cannot pass through a dense object causing all of the signal to be returned to the probe or absorbed.
2. Posterior acoustic enhancement
   a. Created when sound waves travel through fluid (e.g., urine, bile, effusions, purulent material) causing structures behind the material to appear brighter than the surrounding tissues of the same echogenicity and depth.
3. Reverberation
   a. Caused by sound bouncing back and forth in between two very reflective parallel surfaces that are perpendicular to the US (e.g., needle).
4. Mirror images
   a. Occurs when a high reflective surface results in an artifactual image, which is a reflection of an object.

Indications

A. EUS can be used for both diagnosis and procedural guidance.

B. While vascular access was one of the first indications for EUS, the list of emergent procedures that can be aided by ultrasound continues to grow[20] (see Box 2.1)

C. According to the ACEP (2016), EUS can be classified into the following categories:
   1. *Resuscitative:* Use directly related to an acute resuscitation
   2. *Diagnostic:* Emergent diagnostic imaging
   3. *Symptom- or sign-based:* Clinical pathway based on the patient's presentation (e.g., chest pain)
   4. *Procedural guidance:* Used as an aid to guide an emergent procedure
   5. *Therapeutic and monitoring:* Therapeutic or physiologic monitoring

D. Within these broad categories, the ACEP has identified 12 core EUS applications:
   1. Trauma
   2. Pregnancy
   3. Abdominal aortic aneurysm (AAA)
   4. Emergent echocardiography and hemodynamic assessment
   5. Hepatobiliary system
   6. Urinary tract
   7. Deep vein thrombosis (DVT)
   8. Soft tissue/musculoskeletal
   9. Thoracic-airway
   10. Ocular
   11. Bowel
   12. Procedural guidance

E. Focused Assessment with Sonography for Trauma (FAST) exam[20]
   1. One of the first applications of bedside US
   2. Introduced as an alternative to diagnostic peritoneal lavage (DPL) in patients with blunt trauma.
   3. Based on the principle that free fluid will collect in dependent areas of the peritoneum while the patient is in the supine position.
   4. The right and left upper quadrants, the pericardium, and the pelvis are evaluated in basic FAST exam.
   5. Extended FAST includes assessment of the lung and pleura.
   6. Nearly 100% sensitivity in the evaluation of free fluid in the hypotensive blunt trauma patient
   7. Very sensitive in identifying pneumothorax

BOX 2.1 EXAMPLES OF PROCEDURES PERFORMED USING EMERGENCY ULTRASOUND

Incision and drainage of soft tissue abscess
Arterial line placement
Arthrocentesis
Central venous catheter placement
Foreign body identification and removal
Nerve block
Paracentesis
Pericardiocentesis
Thoracentesis
Transvenous pacemaker insertion

Source: From Butts C. Ultrasound. In: JR Roberts (Ed.), *Roberts and Hedges' Clinical Procedures in Emergency Medicine and Acute Care*. 7th ed. Elsevier, 2018; 4695, Box 66.1.

Equipment[20,22]

A. US machine powered on

B. Conducting gel

C. Echogenic needle (if available and indicated)

D. Sterile transducer cover or sterile glove (if indicated)

E. Anesthesia
   1. Not required but can be considered to increase patient comfort and ease of scanning if the area of interest is painful.[26]

F. Transducer/probe[22]
   1. The type and quality of the image obtained depend on the type of transducer selected.
   2. High-frequency probes such as the *linear probe* are great for imaging superficial structures such as skin, soft tissue, and blood vessels.
   3. Low-frequency probes are better for imaging deeper structures.
   4. The *phased array* or cardiac probe leaves a small footprint and is excellent for intercostal scanning and cardiac exams.
   5. The *curvilinear*, curved array or abdominal probe has long wavelengths that penetrate deeply but have poor image resolution.

G. Important machine buttons[19,25]
   1. *Depth:* Used to adjust the depth of the displayed image (centers object of interest in the middle of the US screen)
   2. *Gain:* Used to amplify returning echoes (adjusts brightness of image)

H. Modes[1]
   1. *Two-dimensional (2D)/Brightness/B-mode/Grayscale:* Default on most machines, 2D image

2. *Motion or M-mode:* Used to measure movement over time. (e.g., fetal heart tones)
3. *Color flow Doppler:* Velocity and direction of blood flow using a color scale

General Approach[19,20,26]

A. Although each US application is unique, several general principles apply to all exams.
B. Lights dim and US powered on.
C. Enter the patient's information, so the scan can be saved on the machine.
D. The area of interest should be fully exposed and accessible to the sonographer.
E. Clothing should be removed for complete visualization, but optimal exposure must be balanced with appropriate draping of potentially sensitive areas.
F. Correct transducer and preset selection
G. Evaluate the area to be scanned.
H. Transducer hold/orientation
  1. All probes have an orientation marker or notch that cannot be moved. The US screen has a corresponding marker.
  2. Longitudinal scanning occurs when the probe marker faces the patient's head.
  3. Transverse scanning occurs when the probe marker faces the patient's right (similar to CT)
  4. Pencil hold
  5. Probe in the right hand, standing on the right side of the bed.
  6. Probe movements[19]
    a. Translation/sliding
    b. Angulation/sweeping
    c. Rocking/heel toe/tilt
    d. Rotating/twisting
    e. *Video example:* Coggins, A. (2013). *Ultrasound transducer movements* [video file]. Retrieved from http://youtube.com/watch?v=Q7yo1aDI4zw

Potential Complications or Pitfalls

A. EUS is a very safe imaging modality.[20]
B. The only absolute contraindication is lack of training or experience.[20] This may result in an incorrect diagnosis, patient harm, and potential complications.[20]
C. Although EUS has been described as a skill that is easy to learn, its utility is dependent upon sonographer competence.[27,28] Training is crucial for quality assurance and to ensure that EUS is being utilized correctly. Adequate training must be provided to ensure ENP competence and the delivery of high-quality, evidence-based care.

2D: Foreign Body Removal

SHARON RAINER

Learning Objectives

- Identify common patient presentations associated with foreign bodies.
- Identify common types and locations of foreign body material.
- Illustrate accurate assessment of a foreign body that needs removal.
- Utilize proper equipment and techniques for simple foreign body removal from skin, eyes, ears, and nose.
- Determine the appropriate plan and procedure for foreign body removal from the genitalia and rectum.
- Evaluate special foreign body removal considerations for children age ≤5 years.
- Assure informed consent and accurate documentation of foreign body removal procedures.
- Formulate patient education and instruction for continuing care and referrals as needed.

Foreign Body Removal

Foreign bodies (FBs) are a common problem for patients of all ages. Patients frequently present for emergency and urgent care with a known FB. However, FBs are often identified incidentally during the examination.[29,30] Moreover, one-third of soft tissue FBs are missed on initial examination.[29] As the name suggests, an FB is anything that does not belong to attached, inserted, ingested, or embedded in any part of the human body. Any object becomes an FB when it becomes lodged in soft tissue.[29] FBs vary from forgotten or lost contact lenses in the eyes to ticks embedded in the skin, insects in the ears, or material entering a body cavity during an accidental injury or intentional activity. Unwanted body piercings are considered for FB removal (FBR) when patients present requesting removal. Gunshots and traumatic injuries involving FBs are discussed elsewhere and not covered in this topic of simple FBRs (SFBRs). Other types of FBs such as body packing (packets with illicit drugs), implantable cardiac devices and wires, and intrauterine devices (IUDs) are considered FBs as well but are not considered SFBRs as they require specialist interventions for removal. Genital and rectal FBs will likely require specialty consultation for removal, but it is important to assess these FBs in order to develop the appropriate management plan and promptly consult a surgical specialist as indicated.[31]

SFBRs are those that can be performed readily in the ED or urgent care settings without surgical or other specialty interventions. SFBRs typically involve soft tissue, ears, nose, and vaginas.[29,30] The procedures are intended to remove the FB without causing damage to surrounding structures and preventing complications. Any FB with potential life-threatening complications such as those in the airway, esophagus, penis or rectum, must be referred immediately for expert consultation and treatment.[31] FBs are a common pediatric problem, especially in young children. Young children have unique considerations that must be considered when performing SFBRs.[32]

Overview of Foreign Body Removal[29,32]

A. Only a small percentage of wounds contain an FB.
B. Most FBs are discovered during wound examination.
C. Lacerating objects that splinter, shatter, or break increase the risk of a FB.
D. Infection is the most common complication of a retained FB.

E. The presence of FB should be confirmed by physical examination, radiography, or ultrasonography.
F. Most FBs do not present a medical emergency, however, FBRs are performed when the FB has the potential to cause further injury, infection, or when patients experience pain associated with the FB.
G. Vegetative materials and heavily contaminated objects should always be removed.
H. Most emergency clinicians will only be able to dedicate 15 to 30 minutes for SFBRs.
I. The severity of the problems caused by the presence of the FB depends on its size, composition, and duration of time in the body.
J. Before embarking on an FBR procedure, it is important to recall and review as needed the underlying anatomical structures. FBRs should only be attempted when the clinician can visualize, palpate, and confidently identify the location of the FB.
K. FBRs should only be attempted when the clinician ensures safety to avoid damage to underlying or surrounding structures such as tissue, nerves, and blood vessels.
L. Small button batteries that may be ingested or inserted into orifices have high morbidity as they rapidly induce ulceration and necrosis leading to perforation in, for example, the nasal septum or the esophagus and must be removed promptly.
M. Removal of a FB from a finger or toenail bed may require partial or full nail removal.
N. Consider referral to a surgical specialist when the cosmetic outcome is a priority.
O. Refer when a young child is uncooperative.

Assessment of Foreign Bodies

A. FBs are often found incidentally on examination for a variety of patient chief complaints.[29,30]
B. A thorough assessment, including imaging, is warranted so that an FB is not missed on the initial assessment and becomes a retained FB, which may lead to further tissue damage, pain, and potential infection.
C. Performing SFBRs in some anatomical locations in which the FB is found is not always possible due to safety concerns and will require surgical consultation and referral.
  1. It is imperative to fully assess the underlying structures and the extent to which FBs are embedded so that further damage is avoided when FBR is attempted.[29,30,31]
D. Patients do not always present for care, stating "I have a foreign body," so it is important to have a high level of suspicion of a possible FB for many head, eyes, ears, nose, and throat (HEENT) complaints, especially in young children as well as all ages presenting with cellulitis.[1]
  2. This is especially important when considering infection associated with IV drug abuse, wounds, sore throat, vaginal pain, and discharge as well as penile pain and discharge, rectal pain, and abdominal pain.[29,30]

Patient Presentations With Risk of Foreign Bodies[29,30,32]

A. Presentations that should be suspicious for FB include:
  1. Puncture wounds and lacerations with or without visible FB
  2. Puncture wounds and lacerations caused by glass
  3. Animal bites
  4. Clogged ears or feeling something inside of ear canal (possible insect)
  5. Discoloration or swelling of the skin at a new or old site of an injury
  6. Nonhealing wound
  7. Granuloma formation
  8. Cellulitis
  9. Abscess formation
  10. Vaginal discharge, vaginal pain
  11. Urethral or rectal pain, bleeding
B. The mechanism of injury and shape of the wound and FB increases the risk of a FB.
C. In adults, the perception of an FB more than doubles the likelihood of one being present.[29]
D. In the presence of a laceration or wound discoloration of the skin, palpable mass, sharp well-localized pain with palpation, and limitation of joint movement should heighten suspicion for an FB, although all puncture wounds and superficial wounds can hold FBs.
E. Deeper wounds (≥5 mm) and those whose depths cannot be investigated have a higher association with FBs.
F. Patients returning to the urgent care or ED with retained FBs may complain of sharp pain at the wound site with movement, a chronically irritated nonhealing wound, or a chronically infected wound.[29,31]
G. Indications for removal
  1. Not all FBs need to be removed.[29]
  2. Indications for FB removal include the potential for infection, toxicity, functional problems, or potential for persistent pain.
  3. Obtain the date of the patient's last tetanus booster. If the patient is unsure or if the date of tetanus booster is >10 years, the patient should be immunized for tetanus prophylaxis at the time of the visit for FBR.[33]
H. FB classification
  1. FBs are typically classified into two categories[29,30,31]:
    a. *Inert:* Nonreactive
    b. *Organic:* Reactive
      i. Soft tissue FBs are typically classified as organic (e.g., wood thorns, vegetative materials) and inorganic material (e.g., glass, metal, plastic, and rubber).
      ii. Metals that oxidize (rust) can cause tissue reaction.
      iii. Inert FBs that do not cause a localized tissue reaction often encapsulate within the soft tissue and can be left in place without causing further problems.
      iv. Glass FBs often cause significant pain and should be removed if possible.[33]
      v. Retained organic FBs such as wood, thorns, and spines may lead to a severe local inflammatory response.
      vi. Chronic local pain is associated with inert materials such as glass, metal, or plastic.

vii. A local toxic reaction may occur with such materials as sea urchin spines and catfish spines, so these should be removed promptly.[29,33]

Head, Eyes, Ears, Nose, and Throat Foreign Bodies

A. *Head:* Look for signs of injury or trauma, penetrating wounds, lacerations that may contain FBs.

B. *Eyes:* Perform a slit lamp examination and obtain visual acuity with and without correction. Observe for retained contact lenses, visible specks, or FBs; visualize inner eyelid by flipping eyelid. Consider Ophthalmology consultation when vision is affected or FB.

1. Ophthalmology should be consulted for FBs involving the following[34]:
   a. High-velocity FB
   b. Deeply embedded FB
   c. Any signs or symptoms of glove compromise such as loss of extraocular movement
   d. Changes in the contour of the globe, or positive Seidel sign (full-thickness corneal or scleral injury)
   e. Evidence of intraocular bleeding such as hyphemia
   f. Evidence of associated iritis
   g. Chemical alkaline burns

C. *Ears:* Observe the ear canal for vegetation such as beans, nuts, seeds, popcorn, paper balls, fabric, and modeling clay in children. Children may experience pain, drainage, decreased hearing when a FB is present. Patients may present with known insects (dead or alive) in the ear. Assess decreased hearing, especially unilateral hearing deficits for the presence of FBs. Live insects should be immobilized with 2% lidocaine solution instilled in the ear canal before attempting FBR.[30,31]

1. Small FBs such as beads in the ear can often be removed with irrigation. However, irrigation to remove organic materials may absorb water and swell. Otolaryngology consultation or referral is indicated for cases of FBs with tympanic membrane perforation or if the object cannot be safely removed.[29,31]

D. *Nose:* Observe for beans, beads, seeds, especially in young children. Nasal FBs should be suspected in patients with unilateral nasal obstruction, malodorous rhinorrhea, or persistent unilateral epistaxis.[29,31] Nasal FBRs should only be attempted when the FB can be directly visualized. Tools for removal include forceps, suction catheters, hooked probes, and balloon-tipped catheters. Assess for appropriate equipment for FBR.

1. Otolaryngology consultation is required for any unsuccessful removal.

E. *Throat:* Observe for swallowed objects. Fishbones may or may not be visible; consider imaging and prompt Otolaryngology referral as needed. Any difficulty breathing, speaking, or swallowing requires immediate emergency intervention before further assessment for FBs. Occasionally, the FB can be directly visualized in the oropharynx. Plain film lateral neck imaging may be useful. Further evaluation with CT scan may be needed.[29,31]

F. *Esophagus:* Young children age 1 to 4 years account for approximately 80% of cases of ingested FBs.[33] Adults with esophageal disease will often present with esophageal FBs. Adults with FBs generally complain of retrosternal pain, dysphagia, vomiting, choking, and inability to tolerate pooled secretions. An esophageal impaction can result in airway obstruction, stricture, or perforation, so prompt evaluation is recommended. Assessment must always start with the airway.[29,31]

Skin Foreign Bodies

A. Careful exploration of the depths of all wounds increases the likelihood of finding an FB.

B. Visualize and fully explore wounds through full depth and range of motion. Extending the edges of the wound is often necessary to thoroughly investigate for FBs. Blind probing with a hemostat is less effective but may be utilized if the wound is narrow and deep, and extending the wound is not desirable.[29,31]

C. Observe and feel for the presence of an animal tooth embedded in a puncture wound or laceration following an animal bite. Imaging is recommended to rule out the presence of FBs.

Genital Foreign Bodies

A. Presenting symptoms of a vaginal FB include itching, erythema, rash, and edema. There may be foul-smelling vaginal discharge.

B. Visualize the vaginal vault for retained FB such as a tampon, condom, or other objects during the vaginal speculum examination.

C. Vaginal FBs are a source of potential infection and may also result in ulceration, bleeding, and fistula formation.[31,35]

D. A child with repeated vaginal FBs raises suspicion of sexual abuse.[30] In cases of suspected child abuse, the emergency nurse practitioner (ENP) must notify child protective serves and seek appropriate referrals.

E. Objects in the vagina require removal to reduce the risk of complications.[31]

F. Urethral FBs are associated with bloody urine and slow, painful urination.

G. Radiographs of the bladder and urethral areas may disclose the FB.

H. Observe external genitalia for FB in the urethra and foreskin. Internal urethral FBs require prompt urology consultation.[36]

Abdominal Foreign Bodies

A. Consider packing or the ingestion of packs of contraband materials based on history and suspicion of ingesting objects.

B. Imaging is required and prompt surgical consultation recommended.[31]

Rectal Foreign Bodies

A. Patients may not be forthcoming with accurate history of rectal FB insertion.

B. Patients may complain of pain, cramping, bleeding, or discharge from the rectum.[33]

C. Perforation of the rectum may cause fever, leukocytosis, peritoneal signs, and bleeding.

D. Radiographs may be obtained to determine the position, shape, and number of FBs and the presence of perforation. Order a kidneys, ureters, and bladder (KUB) x-ray to localize and define FB and to assess for obstruction or perforation.[29,31]

E. Observe for external FBs and partial external objects.

F. Most FBs in the distal rectum can be removed in the ED with adequate sedation. Removal of rectal FBs should only be attempted if the FB is felt on digital rectal examination (DRE).[31]

G. Objects that are made of glass have sharp edges, or cannot be easily removed require prompt surgical consultation. If rectal perforation is suspected, broad-spectrum antibiotics should be administered promptly.[29,31]

Imaging of Foreign Bodies

A. Imaging studies should be obtained when a FB is suspected, keeping in mind that a single imaging modality is not ideal for all types of FBs.[29,31] Most FBs (80%–90%) can be seen on plain radiographs.[32]

B. Metal, bone, teeth, pencil graphite, glass, gravel, sand, aluminum, and a few types of plastic are visible on plain film.

C. Most plastics and organic materials such as wood, thorns, cactus spines, and some fish bones cannot be seen on plain film.

D. CT scan is more sensitive than plain film in detecting FBS.

E. Ultrasound is probably less accurate than CT but is reported to have high sensitivity (>90%) for detecting FBs >4 to 5 mm in size.

F. MRI can detect radiolucent FBs and is more accurate in identifying wood, plastic, spines, and thorns than the other modalities.

G. Fluoroscopy can be useful to detect metal, gravel, glass, and pencil graphite in real time.[29,30,31]

Diagnostic Reasoning

A. The decision to perform an SFBR procedure must first meet the criteria of doing no harm.[30] Emergency and urgent care clinicians must consider potential complications resulting from the procedure. SFBR in the ED or urgent care should take approximately 15 to 30 minutes.[29,31,37] Emergency and urgent care ENPs must consider consultation or referral for procedures that require longer time or require more complex procedures for removal of an FB.[29,31]

Simple Foreign Body Removal Procedures

A. Equipment and preparation for FBRs[29,30,31,36,38]

1. Verify safe removal possible without surgical intervention.

2. Ensure proper procedure environment (e.g., safety, lighting).

3. Ensure visualization or definite location of the FB.

4. Personal protective equipment (PPE; gloves, gown, mask with eye shield)

5. Analgesia (premedicate for pain control prior to starting the procedure)

a. *Local anesthesia:* 1% or 2% lidocaine without epinephrine for local infiltration in the skin or digital block for fingers and toes. Lidocaine with epinephrine may be used to help control bleeding in the area of the FB in the skin but never on fingers, nose, penis, or toes.

b. Antiseptic skin cleanser, such as betadine, chlorhexidine, and Hibiclens

6. Wounds thoroughly cleaned with saline or tap water

B. Eyes

1. *Equipment:* Slit lamp for examination, ophthalmoscope, 0.5% tetracaine or 0.5% proparacaine drops, cotton-tip applicator, fluorescein stain of the cornea (determine whether corneal abrasion or ulceration is present and helps to identify the presence of FB), eyewash station for irrigation. If an eyewash station is not available, use an alternative solution by attaching IV tubing to a bag of normal saline with a 22- or 20-gauge catheter at the tip. Once tetracaine has been

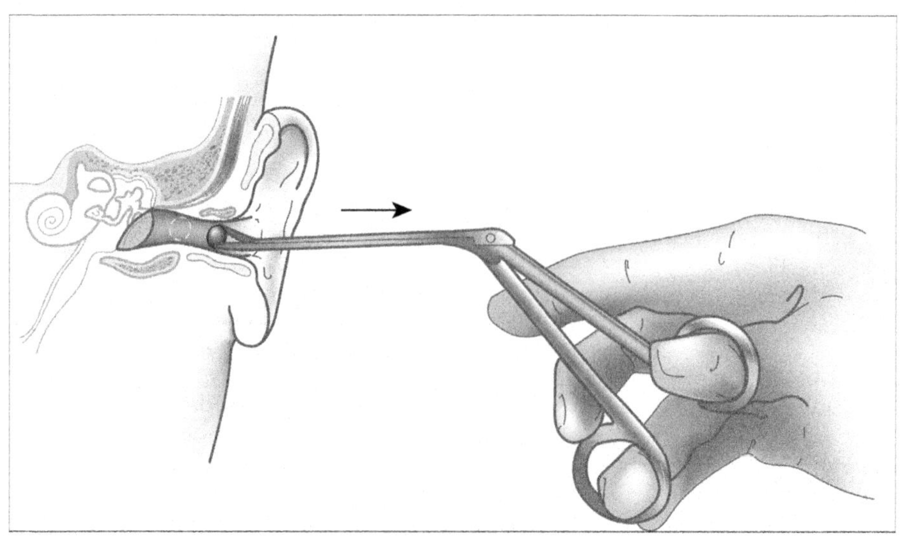

FIGURE 2.4 Ear foreign body removal (FBR). Grasp object with alligator forceps. Use caution and avoid puncturing the tympanic membrane during FBR. If direct removal is not successful, attempt to irrigate the ear canal to remove the FB.

administered to the eye, irrigate with normal saline. Copious irrigation will often dislodge the FB. If irrigation does not remove FB use the cotton-tip applicator handle to flip the eyelid and the cotton tip of an applicator to swab away the FB is readily visible and accessible.[31,34]

C. Ears

1. *Equipment:* Alligator forceps, otoscope, ear wax scoop or curette with flexible tip, and irrigation materials. A commercial ear irrigation kit (Rhino ear washer) or Waterpik-type device may be used. If this is not available, use a 20- to 60-mL syringe with a 14- to 20-gauge angio-cath or a butterfly needle tubing with the needle cut off attached to the syringe, room temperature tap water, or saline. Have the patient sitting upright to facilitate visualization. First attempt to grasp the FB with alligator forceps (Figure 2.4) or the scoop or curette depending on the type of object noted. A small suction tube attached to wall suction may also be used for objects such as beads. Use caution and avoid puncturing the tympanic membrane during FBR. If direct removal is not successful, attempt to irrigate the ear canal to remove the FB. Contraindication to irrigation includes patients with suspected or known tympanic membrane or tympanostomy tubes and organic FBs because they may cause the object to swell in the external auditory canal. To avoid vestibular stimulation, use water at body temperature.[29,31]

D. Nose

1. *Equipment:* Alligator forceps, otoscope, headlamp (to free up both hands), metallic ring curette (Figure 2.5).[36] Have patients sitting to facilitate visualization and removal. Parents of young children should be recruited to restrain the child. Remember that young children often place objects in their nose and often may be uncooperative during FBR, which can present a safety risk. A four-step approach has been shown to be successful in removing nasal FBs once directly visualized.[38]

a. *Step 1:* Use a headlamp for the procedure to free up both hands.

b. *Step 2:* Use a nasal speculum to examine the patient's nose and identify the FB. The speculum visualization is critical to avoid missing the nasal FB is not missed.

c. *Step 3:* Spray decongestant into the nose (Afrin nasal spray) as that will help to anesthetize and decongest the nasal cavity.

d. *Step 4:* Ensure the child is well-restrained. This is another crucial step, and the ENP should engage the caregiver for assistance. Only proceed with

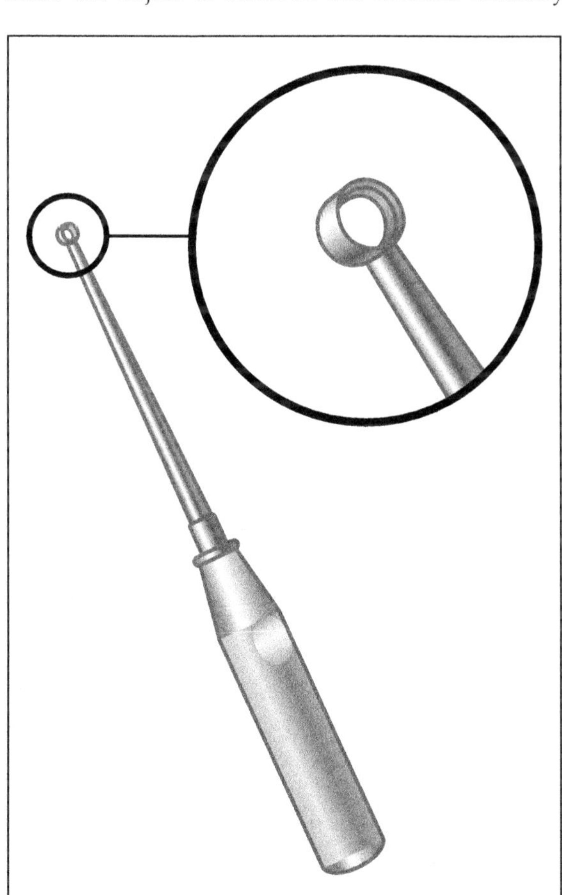

FIGURE 2.5 A metallic ring curette can be used in the removal of a nose foreign body.

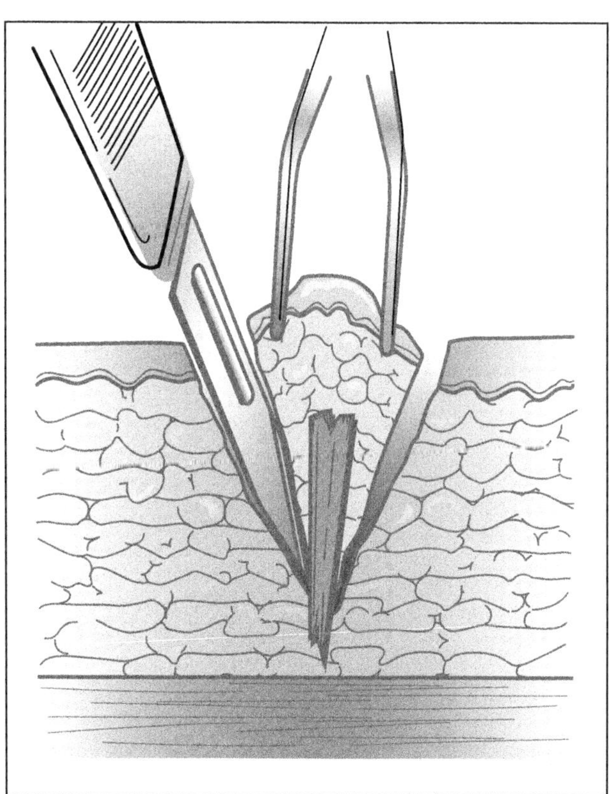

FIGURE 2.6 Removal of a deep foreign body (FB) requires an elliptical incision around the entry wound of the FB. Grasp the elliptical area of skin with forceps, then use an 11-inch scalpel blade to incise downward from the edges on both sides toward the center until the FB is felt with the tip of the blade. The entire elliptical area of skin and FB can then be grasped and removed by pulling upward.

FBR with the child quiet and well restrained due to the risk of injury to the child's nose with the instruments.

E. Soft tissue

1. Removal of a deep FB requires an elliptical incision around the entry wound of the FB. Grasp the elliptical area of skin with forceps then use an 11-inch scalpel blade to incise downward from the edges on both sides toward the center until the FB is felt with the tip of the blade. The entire elliptical area of skin and FB can then be grasped and removed by pulling upward (Figure 2.6).[29,30,31]

2. FBs lodged under the finger or toenails such as splinters require the nail to be either partially or fully removed. If there is a need for nailbed repair with suturing, then the wound must be fully visualized by removing the nail. In the case of FBR without the need for repair, partial removal of the nail should be enough to successfully remove the FB. A wedge-shaped incision into the nail as illustrated in Figure 2.7 will expose the FB so it can be pulled out with splinter tweezers or hemostat. In some cases, a scalpel blade or 18-gauge needle may be used to loosen and begin to pull a splinter out without breaking the FB with removal.[39]

F. Tick removal

1. Ticks burrow into the skin and may become buried, resulting in pain and infection. Removing ticks requires careful attention to avoid leaving parts of the tick's mouth behind. Do not attempt to apply any products, including petroleum jelly to smother, kill, or "stun" the tick. This may cause regurgitation that may spread infection.[33] With a fine tip forceps, grasp the tick as close to the skin as possible and pull it upward to remove it. If this technique does not work to fully remove the tick, including its mouth or other body parts, a punch biopsy technique can be attempted using local infiltration of anesthesia and a disposable biopsy punch or 11-inch scalpel. There are several tick removal devices on the market such as Tick Twister, which is an inexpensive set of instruments designed to remove ticks without compressing it and to remove the tick by twisting motion rather than pulling. However, in the emergency and urgent care setting, a set of fine-tipped tweezers work very well.[29,30,31]

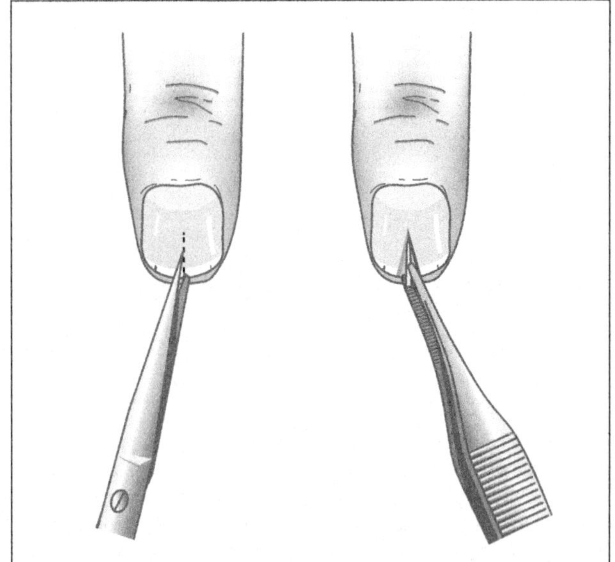

FIGURE 2.7 Splinter removal under the nail. A wedge-shaped incision into the nail will expose the FB so it can be pulled out with splinter tweezers or hemostat.

G. Needles

1. Needles may be difficult to locate and remove. The ENP must be careful to avoid a needle stick when attempting to locate and remove a retained needle. If the needle is superficial and can be palpated with a hemostat or forceps, an incision can be made over one end of the needle to remove it. If the needle is deeper, then an incision can be made at the midpoint of the needle and then grasp it.[29,31]

H. Piercings

1. Piercing removals are common in emergency and urgent care settings. Piercings often become embedded in the ear lobe and require removal by making a small vertical incision in the earlobe. The incision may need to be sutured to facilitate healing. Piercings in other parts of the body such as the umbilicus or nipples may be removed by making the smallest incision possible to remove. Often piercings have a horizontal backing that makes it necessary to extend the incision enough to facilitate complete removal. Imaging is recommended so that the location and placement of the piercing can be fully observed prior to attempting the FBR.

I. Fishhook removal

1. Approximately one million incidents of fishhooks becoming embedded in subcutaneous tissue occur every year.[31] The number seen in the ED and urgent care centers will depend largely upon geographic areas and season. Caution is advised when patients present with fishhooks in subcutaneous tissue as there is a risk of infection. Upon assessment, clinicians must identify whether the fishhook has been in saltwater or freshwater. The most common organisms found with secondary infections associated with fishhooks are[31]:

- **a.** *Gram-positive: Staphylococcus aureus*, streptococci
- **b.** *Gram-negative: Klebsiella, Proteus, Pseudomonas* (salt water)

2. Fishhooks lodged in or close to the eyes should be referred to a surgical specialist (Ophthalmology). If there is a ligament or arterial involvement the patient should be referred for surgical removal.

3. Three common methods are used to remove a fishhook from subcutaneous tissue[30]:

- **a.** Pull-through
- **b.** Barb sheath
- **c.** Angler's string-yank

4. Fishhook removal procedures

- **a.** Patients must be positioned with the fishhook easily accessible. Fishhook removal is done with an aseptic (not sterile) technique. Cleanse the skin around the fishhook with an antiseptic skin cleanser such as betadine. Inject 1% lidocaine using a 27- or 30-gauge needle at the point of the hook.
- **b.** Pull-through technique

i. Using pliers or hemostats, force the fishhook tip through the skin.
ii. Cut off the eye of the fishhook close to the skin with wire cutters.
iii. Attach pliers or hemostats to the sharp end of the hook and pull the hook out.

c. Barb sheath method
i. Insert an 18-gauge needle parallel to the embedded hook with the bevel of the needle toward the inside curve of the hook.
ii. Attempt to cover the barb with the bevel of the needle then back the hook and needle out as a unity.

d. Angler's string-yank method
i. Tie a silk or nylon suture or piece of string or fishing line around the hook where it enters the skin.
ii. With a gloved finger, push the hook further into the skin, then lift the shank of the hook parallel to the skin.
iii. The barb would disengage then using the suture quickly jerk the hook out.

J. Vagina
1. *Equipment:* Rng forceps, nasal speculum for the pediatric patient, culture swab, 60-mL syringe, warm sterile water, skin cleanser, weighted vaginal speculum.[29,35]
2. Small vaginal FBs may be removed in the ED or urgent care. Large objects in the vagina often need to be removed under anesthesia. Have the patient positioned in the dorsal lithotomy position and use a vaginal speculum to clearly visualize the vaginal vault to identify the FB. For infants and small children, position the patient in a frog-leg position and use a nasal speculum to visualize the vaginal vault. Small debris and small objects may be removed with vaginal lavage using a 60-mL syringe with warm sterile water and perform a gentle lavage. Small objects and retained tampons can be removed by busing ring forceps. Large objects may be removed with a weighted vaginal speculum.[29,31,35]

K. Urethra
1. Urethral FBs often require urologic consultation for endoscopy or open cystotomy. Removal of the FB may be achieved with a gentle milking action.

L. Rectum
1. Anorectal FBR should only be attempted in a stable, cooperative patient when the FB is palpable on DRE and the FB has no sharp edge. Surgical consultation is often required.[31]

Informed Consent

A. Informed consent must always be obtained verbally and/or in writing before beginning an FBR procedure. In addition, whoever is providing consent must be documented. This may be the patient, parent, spouse or guardian, or healthcare agent. Informed consent involves explaining and ensuring the patient understands the risk of the procedure he or she is about to undergo. Specific risks such as bleeding, damage to supporting structures, incomplete removal, infection, need for surgical removal even after SFBR is attempted, pain, and possible worsening of the condition. The full procedure must be explained in detail. Moreover, alternatives to the proposed FBR procedure must be presented to the patient. Alternatives include no treatment, delayed treatment, alternative treatments, observation, or referral.[30]

Post-Foreign Body Removal Procedure

A. Postprocedure considerations include copiously irritating the area where the FBR occurred. Sterile water or saline is usually preferred. The ENP must consider the need to prescribe antibiotics for suspected infections (if FB was retained) or prophylactically as indicated. Efficacy of prophylactic antibiotics has not been fully determined in current literature.[29,31] If multiple FBs are removed, a postprocedure x-ray should be obtained. If the FB is removed completely and the potential for infection is considered low, the wound may be closed primarily if needed. On the other hand, if there is a significant risk of infection, delayed primary closure is preferred. Patients should be instructed to return for any new or worsening symptoms or concerns related to the FBR specifically, bleeding, pain, redness, or other signs or symptoms of infection.

2E: Collection and Handling of Forensic Material

SUSANNA RUDY

Learning Objectives

- Define forensics and forensic evidence.
- Identify items that hold evidentiary value as forensic evidence to be collected.
- Discuss the role of the ED nurse practitioner in patient-centered forensic evidence collection.
- Outline the steps of documenting, collecting, and preserving types of forensic evidence.
- Describe basic evidence-collection guidelines, including evidence identification and documentation.
- Identify key rationale for forensic evidence collection by medical staff and clinicians.
- Explain the process for sexual assault examination using an evidence collection kit.

The World Health Organization (WHO) has recognized violence as a major public health problem as perilous as microbial diseases worldwide. "The devaluation of human life is inherent in the genesis of violence."[40]

The 2019 Federal Bureau of Investigation (FBI) crime statistics reported an estimated 1,203,808 violent crimes in the United States, a number that has collectively decreased over the past 3 years, and down 0.5% from 2018. There were 366.7 violent crime offenses per 100,000 inhabitants falling 1.0% from 2018, however, assault offenses, not resulting in death, rose 1.3% as identified by the FBI's Uniform Crime Reporting (UCR) Program.[41] The National

Center for Health Statistics updated in 2020 reports 139 million total visits to the EDs across the United States, 40 million were injury related.[42] Chances of a day in the life of an emergency clinician encountering a true forensic case is high. Patients who suffer violent crimes are most likely to seek evaluation and management in emergency care but may not disclose the true nature of their visit for fears of reprisal, embarrassment, or concern for getting themselves in trouble with law enforcement. This can consequentially lead to further miscarriage of justice with the loss of evidence that has not been properly identified, collected, and documented. The opportunity to preserve the patient's basic human right to justice can fall into the caring hands of a forensically trained nurse or provider, one who is visually astute, naturally suspicious, has awareness of the evidentiary value of forensic evidence, and is determined to ensure that the right to justice is not further violated by missing the point of the visit and loss of forensic evidence.

Over the past three decades, there have been significant scientific and technologic breakthroughs in how forensic evidence is handled. Forensic science as a discipline has made significant technologic strides in evaluating evidence through improved DNA typing, PCR, development of state and federal shared physical evidence databases, advanced instrumentation as well as forensic genetics to aid scientists in the investigation and adjudication of cases. Nurses and providers, frontline providers who care for patients in the ED, have the integral responsibility of playing many roles, one of which is the collecting and preserving of forensic evidence.

Approach to Forensically Significant Wounds

A. All forensically significant wounds require documentation and photographing at the time of presentation and preferably before any physical altering during medical management.
B. Body charts and American Board of Forensic Odontology (ABFO) No. 2 ruler should be used. See the section Forensic Documentation Guidelines.

Types of Injury

A. Shape, size, depth of injury can be related to the mechanism of injury.
B. Blunt and sharp trauma-related injuries
C. Ballistic injuries—firearms
D. Blast injuries—explosives
E. Electrical/energy injuries
F. Chemical injuries
G. Biological
H. Radiological
I. Thermal injuries—burns
J. Traumatic injuries—blunt and penetrating injury
- **1.** Blunt force trauma
- **2.** Blunt trauma
- **3.** Abrasions
- **4.** Avulsions—impact sliding injuries
- **5.** Bruises/contusions
- **6.** Suction wounds
- **7.** Burns
- **8.** Bites
- **9.** Dermal layers are torn away from the impact.
- **10.** Lacerations—caused by blunt force trauma
- **11.** Incised wounds—intentional, surgical

K. Defense wounds
- **1.** Blunt—abrasions or contusions on the back of the hands, wrists, forearms, and arms
- **2.** Sharp—less common, knife wounds
- **3.** May contain embedded fragments of instrument/weapon
- **4.** Fractures—less common as defense wounds, typically of the forearms

L. *Bruising:* One of the most common types of soft tissue injury noted on victims of violence or abuse. Can be caused by blunt, compressive, or squeezing trauma to tissues causing underlying damage to blood vessels.
- **1.** Injury to the tissue that results in rupture of small vessels from blunt impact causing subdermal bleeding.
- **2.** Typically observed on physical exam and visible by discoloration and associated inflammation.
- **3.** Deep bruising may not be immediately visible—important physical evidence in strangulation cases.
- **4.** Absence of a bruise does not mean there was no blunt force trauma. Get a good history.
- **5.** There is no standard terminology to describe a bruise and staging a bruise to determine the time of injury is forensically difficult.
- **6.** *Color of bruising varies:* Initially as red, dark blue, dark purple, violet, or black. As hemoglobin is broken down, the color can change to violet, green, dark yellow, and pale yellow before disappearing.
- **7.** Yellowing is visible sooner in superficial bruising than in deeper bruises.
- **8.** Bruising under loose thin skin appears almost immediately; deeper bruises take more time to be visible to the naked eye.
- **9.** Initial bruising may not be visible to the naked eye and requires an alternate light source (ALS) utilizing a yellow filter to visualize subtle or subclinical bruising in all skin colors. Recommended by The Department of Justice.[43]
- **10.** Impact areas should always be photographed regardless if there is obvious bruising or not
- **11.** Bruises evolve over time.
- **12.** Dating a bruise depends on histology and color changes.
- **13.** Bruising may be difficult to see in darker pigmentations.

M. Bite mark evidence
- **1.** Bite marks are as specific as a fingerprint and can be used to identify an assailant.
- **2.** Bite marks are a good source for forensic evidence.
- **3.** Forensic odontology is the forensic specialty that attempts to match bite marks to the dental impressions of suspects.
- **4.** Document bite marks in the physical assessment being as descriptive as possible in the medical record.
  - **a.** Size, shape, depth, and pattern of injury

5. Photograph the area of the bite mark utilizing the techniques of photographing wounds.
6. Utilize an angled ABFO No. 2 ruler for this type of injury.
7. Saliva and DNA analysis
   a. If saliva is wet, gently roll the cotton tip swab over the saliva area (two swabs).
   b. If the area is dry, moisten the cotton tip with sterile water and gently roll over the bite marks to capture any potential saliva.
   c. Air dry before packaging and sealing.
   d. Store swabs according to storage guidelines.
   e. Separate packaging for each swab

N. Ballistic injuries
1. Ballistic and missile injuries are those created by high-velocity projectiles, the speed at which a bullet, pellet, slug, ball/shot, or shell, that is, discharged from a firearm.
2. A general understanding of ballistics is necessary to evaluate and treat these traumatic injuries and preserve forensic evidence.

Ballistic Evidence Collection

A. In cases where patient presents with firearm in a trauma: any firearm should be the jurisdiction of local law enforcement and should be notified immediately.

B. Firearm should be secured by security or law enforcement immediately and assumed loaded.

C. All weapons go to law enforcement or hospital security and documented on chain of custody (COC) form.

D. If a weapon is legally registered to a patient and a crime is not involved, it goes to security until the patient is discharged.

E. Handle ballistic weapons with extreme caution and care.

F. Handle the firearm by avoiding common touchpoints where fingerprints can transfer.
1. If required to remove firearm from patient, handle the firearm from the areas least likely to retain latent fingerprints, the gnarled or checkered areas.
2. It should then be unloaded with care taken to preserve all types of possible evidence. Fingerprints, blood, hair or fibers, cylinder "halos," and debris in the barrel and/or cylinder.

G. Handle all ballistic evidence with gloves and appropriate personal protection equipment (PPE).

H. Bullet or cartridge evidence may be found around the patient with gunshot wounds or lodged in the clothing.
1. Valuable as it can link the crime to a firearm
2. Handle all bullets, cartridges, casings, shot wads, shot pellets, fragments, or shrapnel with the intent to preserve fingerprints.

I. Recovering bullets
1. Recovery of the bullet is important for comparison purposes can compare duplicate make, model, and age of ammunition.
2. Never retrieve bullet fragments or ammunition with metal objects as this can scratch the surface and negate its possibility as evidence.
3. Handle bullets with a soft cloth or gauze.

J. It is not generally recommended to wash off bullets.

K. Bloody bullets retrieved from the body can be rinsed under water.
1. If bullets are embedded with tissue, they should be washed off with running water.
   a. Do not use any detergents, scrubbing agents, pads or scrubbers, or anything abrasive.
2. All ballistic material washed should be allowed to dry entirely before packaging.
3. Dry the bullets by blotting (not rolling) with a soft dry facial cloth or toilet tissue prior to packaging.
   a. Sealing bloody or wet bullets in airtight packages promotes corrosion on the bullet.
4. Wrap recovered bullets in soft tissue and then paper and seal in a separate labeled box or envelop.
   a. Each bullet is wrapped separately.
5. Do not mark the bullet or allow it to be marked.
6. Mark sealed container with the description of the bullet.
7. Package according to evidence collection guidelines.
8. Handle with a cloth or rubber-tipped forceps to prevent any scratching or marking.
9. Do not mark or label any bullet or fragment directly.
10. Each piece of ballistic evidence should be packaged separately.
11. Do not place bullets, casings, pellets, fragments, or shrapnel in a metal container.
12. Seal in a labeled paper envelope, pillbox, or plastic urine container.
13. Do not place in a metal container.
14. Document on the COC form.
   a. Secure law enforcement to pick up in evidence locker.
   b. Appropriately package clothing in paper bags following COC and packaging guidelines.
15. Document all wounds and photograph.
16. Follow packaging and labeling protocols.

Gunshot Residue Evidence Collection

A. Gunshot residue (GSR)
1. Important evidentiary value providing indirect evidence of the distance from the firearm
2. Includes various primer residues and partially burned and unburned gun powder particles
3. Cannot always be seen but is assumed in crimes involving a firearm
   a. Bag both hands in brown paper bags that are prelabeled left/right. Secure at the wrist with tape.
      i. Ensure circulation is intact.
4. Document presence or absence of GSR that is visible
   a. Residue can last up to 6 hours on the skin but is like talcum powder and can easily be washed off, dusted off.
   b. Document dark powder, soot, particles on skin.

c. Document punctate hemorrhages.
5. Do not document the term "powder burns."
6. Preserve GSR evidence on the hands.
a. If associated with a wound and has a dressing overlay, save the dressing as evidence.
b. To obtain sample on hands use sterile water moistened swab to roll over the gunshot injury site and around the insertion site.
c. Do not use normal saline; it has salt in it and can destroy potential DNA evidence.
7. GSR should be collected within 3 hours of discharge of the firearm.
a. Considered fragile evidence; consistency of flour
i. Only stays on hands for approximately 4 to 6 hours
ii. Wiping hands on anything will transfer the GSR.
b. An item of clothing can contain GSR up to 5 years, if undisturbed.
i. The same quality the day it was deposited
c. If more than 6 hours since the weapon discharged and patient washed their hands, unlikely residue can be retrieved.
8. Protect the hands with paper bags until they can be photographed.
a. Hand preservation bags are available from law enforcement.
b. Place brown paper bags over both hands and tape them at the wrists within 3 hours.
c. Avoid plastic bags, hands will sweat and deteriorate biologic evidence.
9. Obtain photographic images prior to cleaning wounds if not life-threatening.
10. Law enforcement should be responsible for securing GSR.
a. An adhesive disc is used to press onto the back of the hands in a systematic pattern.
b. Do not slide or rotate the disc on the skin.

Toxicology as Evidence

A. Toxicology is relevant in cases involving suspected toxic ingestions or as requested in forensic cases.[44,45]
1. Urine or blood analysis
2. Obtain written and informed consent from the patient.
3. *Blood:* Draw blood first before administering medications through the line.
4. Do not draw a blood alcohol level (BAL) from a preestablished IV line.
5. Blood toxicology is collected in a gray-topped tube (contains sodium fluoride).
a. Document in the medical record any specimens obtained.
b. Carefully label specimen containers.
c. Document in the COC form and in the medical record.
d. Document exact time, date, and who secured the sample.
e. Urine toxicology requires a minimum of 30 mL of urine.

B. Drawing a BAL in the ED
1. Impaired driver brought in following a motor vehicle crash (MVC), law enforcement may legally request a BAL.
a. May be used as evidence for an investigation in suspected driving under the influence (DUI) cases.
2. Consents to diagnostic tests that could include serum ethanol level are given when patient signs consent.
a. Consent for drawing blood for evidence in a criminal case is not included in the standard consent for treatment.
b. Obtain a written request from law enforcement.
c. Obtain informed consent of the patient.
d. The nurse drawing blood for evidence cannot take part in the patient's active restraint when the draw is against their will.
e. Draw sample in front of law enforcement who requested procedure.
i. Do not use alcohol to clean the skin for a BAL; use an alternate cleanser (e.g., iodine).
f. Label each tube with the date-time, subject's name, location, the collector's name, and a case or evidence number (if available).
g. Hand the blood sample directly to the requesting officer.
h. Complete the COC form.
i. Document in the medical record the blood drawn and time.
3. A nurse can draw blood from a patient who is being restrained by law enforcement personnel and remain protected from civil and criminal liability.
a. The Supreme Court ruled that no warrant is required to draw blood from an unconscious patient suspected of driving intoxicated.
4. Requests for blood draws from a conscious patient
a. Law enforcement requests the results from a patient already being managed and blood alcohol was ordered in the process of treatment.
i. Those results cannot be released to the police or prosecuting attorney.
ii. Requires consent from the patient.
iii. Obtain consent or court order when possible.
iv. Consult with hospital attorneys or risk managers.
v. Document specifics on the urgency of the request.
vi. Review Health Insurance Portability and Accountability Act (HIPAA) regulations.
b. Storage of blood specimens
i. Refrigerate liquid blood specimens and toxicology specimens between 36°F and 46°F with less than 25% humidity.

Collection and Preservation of Forensic Evidence

Injury to a victim will almost always result in the presence of some type of trace evidence. The evaluation should begin with outward observation of the patient as they presented, taking note of overall presentation, demeanor, any obvious injuries, or evidence. The collection of forensic evidence begins with the initial interview which includes a detailed history and physical exam, this may be secondary to your immediate patient workup when managing life-threatening injuries. Interviewing the patient to obtain vital information related to circumstance and mechanism of injury, photographing the patient and injuries, properly collecting and preserving physical evidence, documenting and transferring physical evidence are all essential policies and procedures to maintaining chain of custody (COC).

Forensic evidence is of two types: material or physical. Material evidence is also called trace evidence. There are hundreds of types of trace evidence. It is inorganic, and anything that can be manufactured such as hairs, paint, glass, fiber, glitter, adhesives, chemicals, mineral, soil, plant spores, cosmetics, fire debris, or gunshot residue are the most common examples. Trace evidence can be visible, seen by the naked eye or invisible, requiring sensitive microscopes or forensic technology to extract and analyze. Physical evidence can be seen, smelled, or touched, is biologic or organic, and can be of varying types: blood, skin, hair, saliva, and semen. Fingerprints can be visible to the naked eye, be imprinted on the clothing or physical being of the patient. If they are not visible, they are called latent prints. GSR can be found on clothing, hands, and other items that present with the patient. The most common type of physical evidence is DNA, biologic markers known to all living species. This can be obtained from all sources of biologic evidence and often under fingernails in scrapings.

Locard's Exchange Principle is the foundation of trace evidence and asserts that "every contact leaves a trace."[46] It is important to note that not all contact will leave trace evidence and that absence does not conclude that no contact occurred. It is the transfer of forensic evidence during the commission of a crime that can be collected to identify a victim or suspect. The "Crime Scene Investigation effect" is a documented phenomenon attributed to the belief of the general population that expects the existence of evidence in order to convict. A 2006 study published by the National Institute of Justice concluded that 46% of jurors expect to see scientific evidence in every criminal case, and up to 36% expected fingerprints and ballistic evidence in every criminal case. DNA evidence is expected in 46% of all murder cases and 73% in rape cases. As a clinician, there are certain protocols for the collection of specific types of evidence that can be followed for any suspected forensic case. Lack of familiarity with forensic evidence collection protocols by untrained medical personnel can result in the unintentional loss or destruction of evidence, impeding the process of justice.[47]

Evidence Collection in the Healthcare Setting

Collecting evidence is a patient-centered nursing function. Caring for these patients requires medical management and preservation of evidence that must be properly collected, procedures witnessed, documented correctly and maintained by chain of custody to be successfully entered into civil or criminal legal proceedings. A lack of specialized education and training in the management of forensic cases may translate to errors in properly documenting injuries, preserving evidence with validated protocols and principles of forensic evidence collection that further victimizes the case. Understanding of the role and objective responsibilities when faced with a forensic case, provider actions can assist with the investigation of abuse, violence, or criminal activity that can link or eliminate a suspect or victim to a crime, exoneration of an accused suspect, or the corroboration of a crime.

A 2017 policy statement by the Emergency Nurses Association (ENA) recognizes the importance and value of professional nursing practice in the proper collection, preservation, and handling of evidence as integral to practice and recommends nursing professionals to be familiar with "the concepts and skills of evidence collection, written and photographic documentation, as well as testifying in legal proceedings."[48] In 1992, The International Academy of Forensic Nurses (IAFN) was established by a group of sexual assault nurse examiners (SANEs); today, it has grown into a worldwide network providing leadership in forensic nursing practice through the dissemination of information and support to forensic science and the medical profession. It is intermediary between medicine, law enforcement, and the justice system.[49]

A number of ED presentations could require evidence collection. It is imperative that emergency providers understand that proper methods of evidence collection and documentation in medico-legal cases are crucial, and may be the only source of information for the criminal justice system to work with[48] (Box 2.2).

The Forensic Presentation

The term "forensics" is defined by Merriam-Webster's Dictionary as: belonging to, used in, or suitable to the courts or to public discussion and debate and relating to or dealing with the application of scientific knowledge to legal problem. Evidence is defined by Webster's as something legally submitted to a competent tribunal as a means of ascertaining the truth of any alleged matter of fact under investigation before it. The forensic patient is defined as an individual who seeks treatment for a medical complaint that coincides with the laws or has the potential to interface with law enforcement and social services (Box 2.3[50]). All patient presentations to the ED have a potential to be a forensic case, and all cases should be treated as having evidentiary value until proven otherwise.

BOX 2.2 POTENTIAL AREAS OF INTERFACE FOR THE FORENSIC PATIENT

- Healthcare, psychiatric support
- Law enforcement
- Legal
- Social services
- Cultural practice
- Government agencies
- Community
- Legislation
- Forensic science
- Medical examiner
- Emergency medical services

Legal Implications

Occasionally, emergency nurse practitioners (ENPs) are called upon to provide testimony in a court case involving evidence they have collected. This is an established part of emergency nursing practice.[48] Often this testimony authenticates the evidence that was collected in the healthcare setting. Testimony can also confirm that the chain of custody was maintained during evidence collection procedures. Providing testimony in a legal case can be very stressful. If called upon to testify or provide a deposition for a legal case, be sure to make adequate preparation, including a review of the evidence and a discussion with the plaintiff or defense attorney who is calling for the testimony.

Preparing for Testimony

A. Juries consider both objective information and subjective presentation of the information.

B. Expert demeanor, then, is an important component of testimony.

1. Remain professional, thorough, and objective.
2. Never contrive information related to the case.
3. If you do not know the answer, state "I do not know" or "I do not recall."
4. It is important to provide information in a sincere and honest manner using direct eye contact and a calm voice.
5. Carefully listen to the questions that are asked and consider a response before answering.
6. Pausing to think about the question before answering demonstrates a thoughtful observer and reporter.
7. Answer questions with focused response, do not provide extraneous information unless encouraged to do so.

C. Jurors have certain expectations about the dynamics of sexual assault, including stereotypes about a victim's behavior.

1. Jurors expect the victim to be emotional and report the incident immediately to law enforcement. In cases where there is a delay in presentation to emergency care, the credibility of the victim may be called into question.
2. It is helpful for jurors to have a sexual assault expert explain the realistic dynamics of a crime and victim reaction.

D. Expert testimony is typically used in criminal cases to support the prosecution of a sexual assault; to demonstrate that the victim's behavior and injuries are consistent with a person who has been sexually assaulted.

E. Federal Rules of Evidence state that "if scientific, technical, or other specialized knowledge will assist the trier of fact to understand the evidence or to determine a fact in issue, a witness qualified as an expert by knowledge, skill, experience, training, or education may testify thereto in the form of an opinion or otherwise."

BOX 2.3 FORENSIC CASE PRESENTATIONS

Abuse of a child	Drownings	Mass casualty
Abuse of the elderly	Domestic violence	Occupation injury
Abuse of the disabled	Death-coroner cases	Organ donation
Abuse of the mentally impaired	Electrocution	Overdose
Assault and battery	End of life decisions	Personal injury
Asphyxiations Attempted/suicide	Ethanol poisoning	Police custody
Ballistic injuries	Falls	Product liability
Bites: Human and animal	Firearm injuries	Psychiatric clients
Blunt force trauma	Food and drug poisonings	Sharp force trauma
Bioterrorism	Gang violence	Substance abuse
Burns	Hangings	
Communicable disease control		

Source: Adapted from Darnell C, Michel C. *Forensic Notes.* 1st ed. F.A. Davis Company; 2012.[50]

F. Most experts called to testify in sexual assault cases include physicians, physician assistants, nurse practitioners, or sexual assault nurse examiners.

G. Critically important that the medical professional have specialized training and experience in sexual assault exams and experience in conducting "normal" gynecologic exams.

1. Asked to describe the process of examining the victims
2. The physical findings observed and interpretation of those results
3. Documented findings
4. Physical injury
5. Subjective tenderness described by victim
6. Stains or substances found on the victim's body
7. Physical evidence collected from sexual assault exam or on clothing
   a. Are the physical findings "consistent" or "congruent" with the victim's account of events?

H. Clinicians cannot "diagnose" a sexual assault.

I. Clinicians cannot make any definitive conclusions regarding the degree of force used by the assailant or if there was "consent."

J. Clinicians can make definitive conclusions as to whether there is evidence of sexual contact or recent trauma.

K. Clinicians can make statements regarding the conclusion of consistency between physical findings and the victim's account of events.

Principles of Evidence Collection

Forensic Process of Evidence Collection

A. Key processes and rules that dictate the forensic process of evidence collection

1. Do not contaminate the evidence.
2. Preserve the integrity of the sample.

B. General collection recommendations

1. Collect a sufficient sample.
   a. Hair
   b. Body fluids
   c. Vegetation
   d. Glass fragments
   e. Debris
2. Preserve each sample separately to avoid contamination.
   f. Avoid simultaneously collecting evidence from more than one patient.
   g. Evidence from one case should not be packaged with another case for transport.
3. Label and seal each sample.
   h. Evidence containing blood or body fluids should be labeled as biohazard.
   i. Glass or sharp objects should be labeled as such outside of the container.
   j. Access to storage should be sealed and signed and dated across tape line.

Forensic Evidence Collection Kit

A. Multiple ready forensic evidence collection kits are recommended to be on hand for potential forensic cases. General content recommendations include:

1. *Personal protective equipment (PPE):* owns, gloves, masks, eye protection, face shield
2. Chain of custody (COC) forms (triplicate)
3. Camera (digital) with memory card or film
4. Measuring ruler/American Board of Forensic Odontology (ABFO) No. 2 scale
5. Indelible pen/marker
6. Blank labels
7. Cotton swabs
8. Gauze pads
9. Sterile forceps/pickups
10. Paper envelopes of varying sizes (manila or plain white)
11. Paper bags of varying sizes (large and small)
12. Lab tubes (red, purple, and gray collection tubes)
13. Specimen cups
14. *Boxes:* Cardboard and metal
15. Styrofoam cups or pads (for drying specimens)
16. Sterile water (for moistening swabs)
17. Transparent tape
18. Tamper-proof tape or adhesive to secure evidence bags
19. *Camera:* Point and shoot, digital, light source (built-in flash)

Initial Encounter

Trauma presentations are innately complex and can present challenges to hospital staff. All patients are to be considered as forensic patients until proven otherwise. Emergency medical treatment and lifesaving care will always supersede forensic evaluation and evidence collection. Lynch asserted that clinicians have a responsibility to meet both the patient's medical and forensic needs and that management of violence is a mutual responsibility shared between healthcare and the law.[40] Management of these patients requires an organized and systematic approach involving multiple resources and interdisciplinary collaboration with multiple agencies, community resources, and social support.

The spectrum of abuse, violence, and trauma asserts psychological as well as physical harm. Socioeconomic, cultural, and social disparities require a sensitivity to a patient's psychological well-being requiring patient advocacy when interacting with other members of the healthcare team and law enforcement professionals.

A. Patient-centered principles for compassionate care[44]

1. Demonstrate respect and patience.
   a. Supports psychologic trauma
   b. Transition into the traumatic event through dialogue, allowing the patient to discuss at their own pace.
2. Maintain patient confidentiality.
   a. Health Insurance Portability and Accountability Act (HIPAA)

3. Establish a rapport.
   a. Empathetic and understanding, compassionate, and caring
   b. Listen to the patient.
   c. Pay attention to "verbal forensics," taking note of what the patient states, or dialog with patient and family members.
      i. State only the facts using "direct quotes."
   d. Speak slowly; explain things in simple terms.
   e. Assess understanding of circumstance and answer any questions related to the process of evidence collection, exam, and overall management plan.
   f. Keep eye contact (unless culturally unacceptable).
4. Obtain patient consent.
   a. Patients must agree to evidence collection.
   b. If a patient refuses an exam against medical or legal advice, evidence cannot be collected.
   c. In sexual assault cases, most states require a minor under the age of 16 to have parental consent for an exam. Age $\geq$16, the patient can decline an examination.
   d. Many facilities incorporate this consent into their general treatment consent form.
      i. Some may use a separate, specific form for a forensic consent.
   e. Specifically include consent for photographs.
5. Respect cultural and religious norms and considerations.
6. Respect privacy.
   a. Offer comfort measures and privacy barriers.
   b. Offer visual and sound privacy during the interview process.
7. Explain the forensic procedures.
8. Offer the option of a male or female examiner.
9. Allow family member or support person to be with the patient as they request.
10. Watch for evidence of distress during interview, in particular with cases of sexual assault.
11. Trained rape advocate should complete exam alone with a victim of sexual assault if possible.

B. Documentation
1. The exam begins with a detailed history and physical examination by the clinician.
   a. All documentation needs to be legible, in ink or electronic medical record.
   b. All sketches or notes will become part of the medical record.
   c. History of presenting illness or problem
   d. Statements should be exact words, unedited, unsanitized, and put into direct quotations.
   e. Statements should be documented as "patient states," "patient reports," "patient declines."
   f. Avoid statements such as "patient refuses" or patient is "unwilling."
   g. Document patient account in terms of facts without elaboration.
   h. Note the patient's overall behavior, attitude, emotional status, ability to communicate, preoccupation with other persons or items.
   i. Pay attention to patient statements to provider and family members. "Excited utterances," "present sense impressions," "then-existing mental, emotional or physical condition" are all accepted under the Federal Rules of Evidence and defined as a statement (s) that concern a startling event, made by the declarant when the declarant is still under the stress or excitement from a traumatic event. It is admissible under an exception to the hearsay rule (Federal Rules of Evidence, Rule 803; retrieved from law.cornell.edu/rules/fre/rule_803).
   j. Use the name of the person described by the patient as the alleged perpetrator.
   k. Document the names of anyone else in the room during this interview or history.
2. Documenting the review of systems
   a. Documenting a full review of systems can differentiate the previous statements of problems or injury in specific systems. Be as detailed as possible as it relates to the presenting problem, complaint, and injury.
3. Documenting the head-to-toe physical exam
   a. If managing a medical emergency, conducting the primary and secondary survey takes precedence over any forensic evaluation.
   b. Maintain privacy and cultural sensitivity with the physical exam.
   c. Involve the patient in the process by explaining all procedures related to the physical exam.
   d. Wear PPE to maintain universal precautions.
   e. Conduct an overall observation of the patient in the current state of presentation and document observations.
   f. Note any unusual or overwhelming odors that could indicate contamination with volatile or chemical agents that could be harmful to patient or hospital staff.
   g. Patient should be fully undressed for a full physical exam with considerations of protecting the privacy and patient comfort dictating the exam.
   h. Conduct a detailed head-to-toe assessment.
   i. Document any obvious injuries utilizing documentation charts/body diagrams.
4. Body diagram (Figure 2.8)
   i. Effective tool to document anatomical location of observed injuries or biologic evidence in the medical record narrative and on body diagram
   ii. Helpful for documenting multiple injuries
   iii. Size, pattern, shape of multiple wounds
   iv. Documented wounds should be in proportion to anatomical chart size.
      (1) Do not overexaggerate size of wounds.
      (2) Maintain shape of wound or mark.
      (3) Round, elongated, elliptical, jagged, pear-shaped
   v. Do not label wounds with your interpretation.

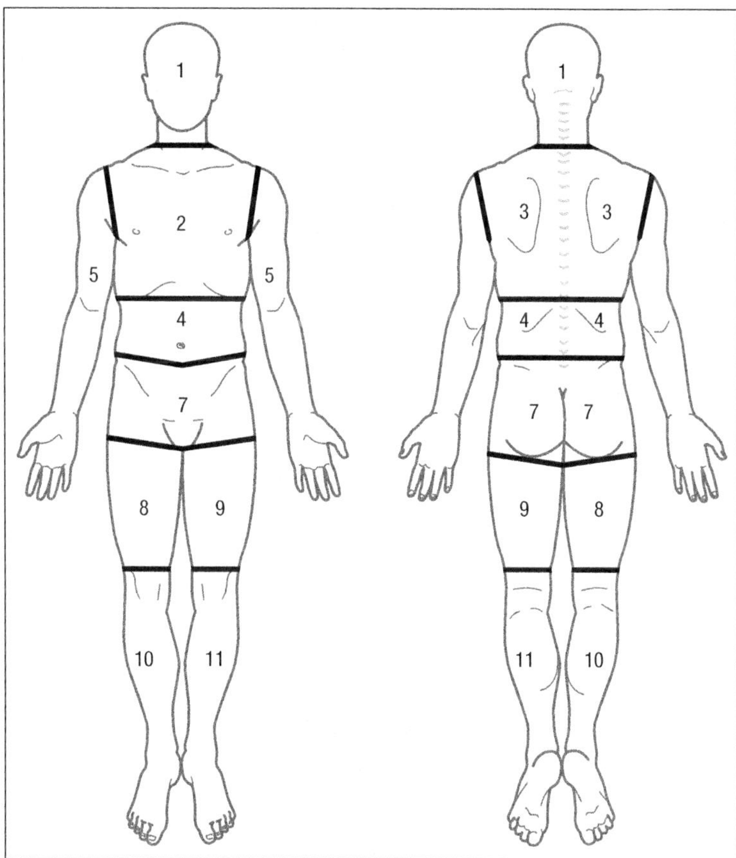

FIGURE 2.8 Body diagram.

vi. Do not identify entrance and exit wounds.
(1) Clinicians incorrectly document entrance/exit wounds >50% of the time.
(2) Include burns, bruising, abrasions, soot, imprint marks.
(3) Measure and photograph.
(4) Powder residue samples can be taken at both sites to determine.

vii. Document wounds in terms of shape, pattern, and in proximity to anatomical locations, do not use other wound locations to describe orientation or proximity to other wounds.

viii. Document the size, location, and appearance of defects before alteration by time or medical intervention.

ix. If any medical intervention altered the appearance of a wound, it should be documented.

x. Document the placement of surgical drains, IVs, chest tubes, intubation, endotracheal tube (ETT) placement, nasogastric (NG) tube, urinary catheter, central line access, or any invasive procedure.

xi. Circle all IV and blood draw puncture sites.

xii. EDs may have standard documenting diagrams.

xiii. Age- and sex-specific diagrams are available.

Taking a History and Conducting a Physical Assessment

A. Initial interviewing principles
1. Apply patient-centered principles for compassionate care.
2. A detailed interview and history will dictate the physical exam.
3. Information obtained should be forensically relevant.
   a. Pay attention to the words the patient uses, descriptors, locations, and mechanism of injury.
   b. Implications of responses guide assessment, prioritize the areas of the body that may have physical evidence for collection and corroboration of the history and complaints.
   c. Helps determine the differential causes for injury
4. Findings can be consistent or inconsistent with a patient's statement of events.
5. The medical record will be considered a legal document.
   a. Document the facts as they are stated or observed.
   b. Document in complete, nonjudgmental, and objective statements.
   c. Use medical terminology.
   d. Avoid abbreviations unless they are nationally approved.

B. Conducting a physical assessment

1. Complete after the interview and history.

2. Use a systematic approach to the physical assessment.

- **a.** Requires written and a graphic documentation
- **b.** Utilize medical record.
- **c.** Utilize sex- and age-related body charts to document physical injuries or statements of injury.

3. *General overview:* How does the patient look?

- **a.** Is the patient sick, not sick, emotional, smiling, tearful, withdrawn?

4. Document appearance, behavior, and psychologic and emotional state on initial assessment.

5. Document wounds—describe by appearance, color, and location.

- **a.** Document presence of obvious debris or foreign bodies within wounds.
- **b.** Document presence of tattoos or piercings and any interruptions of those.

6. Document the smell of any odors.

- **a.** Can indicate intoxication
- **b.** Can indicate underlying disease processes: festering wounds, diabetic ulcers, necrosis

7. Exposure to chemical substance

8. Exposure to fire

9. Exposure to gasoline

10. Document overall hygiene-homelessness.

11. Document exactly as seen; do not attempt to age determine the age of wounds.

C. Photographing evidence

1. A well-composed photograph can be worth a thousand words. Forensic photography implies that when legally and properly obtained, it can be used in legal proceedings.

2. Forensic photography supplements the medical history and physical findings. Captures the initial injuries observed and managed by the provider on initial assessment.

3. Importance of photographic evidence in medical forensic cases

- **a.** Record and document injuries.
- **b.** Record and document evidence that may be destroyed through the normal process of medical management.
- **c.** Permit the courts or jurors to see the presentation in captured "real-time" and to corroborate that against the presented testimony.
- **d.** Document injuries or conditions before and after medical treatment.
- **e.** To show the condition of evidence or injuries at the time of discovery or examination
- **f.** To demonstrate the absence of injury or alleged findings
- **g.** Illustrate and supplement the written and medical record.
- **h.** To demonstrate malice or criminal intent
- **i.** To dispute or exonerate testimony based on discrepancy

4. Obtain consent for photographing patient, injuries, and evidence.

- **a.** Some operative or consent form language may be included on operative consent or admission forms.
- **b.** Patients must give consent for photography unless they are unconscious, under arrest, and/or there is a court order for photos to be taken, or they are in a public place.
- **c.** Clinicians are obligated by law to obtain consent (implied or informed).
- **d.** Forms should be dated/timed and include the clinician or nurse and patient signatures.
- **e.** If patient is unable to sign due to injury but able to give consent, form can be signed by next of kin or patient representative (relationship).
- **f.** *Informed consent*: Explaining the purpose of taking forensic photographs and patient has the right of refusal.
- **g.** *Implied consent*: Legal construct to adopt what a reasonable person would adopt under normal circumstances. Implied consent secures "consent" from unconscious or patients unable to give comprehensible consent due to their medical condition or injury
  - **i.** When applied, clinicians must obtain consent from patient or their next of kin at a later time.
- **h.** Consent form becomes part of the permanent medical record.
- **i.** Consent should address release of image information to law enforcement or district attorney's office.
- **j.** Medical record should reflect how many images were taken, how and where they were stored (server/image storage system/memory card).

5. Admissibility and substantive evidence

- **a.** *Accurate depiction of the subject:* Photograph (digital or film) must be accurate and an objective depiction of subject.
- **b.** *Authentic*: Photographer and the photograph must be able to withstand the legal standard of integrity, credibility, and authenticity or it will be inadmissible.
- **c.** Photographer must be available to speak to the image. A photograph cannot stand alone as evidence in court; it must be explained and verified by the photographer.
- **d.** A photograph may be accepted into evidence if it fairly and accurately depicts what the healthcare professional witnessed.
- **e.** Not unduly gruesome or inflammatory
- **f.** In focus
- **g.** Depicts a ruler to show size
- **h.** Feature of the wound is clearly visible
- **i.** Properly exposed with color range
- **j.** Does not have extraneous surgical or medical instruments
- **k.** Corresponds to the verbal and written documentation of the provider.

6. Admissibility challenges that clinicians will be required to speak to:
   a. Where, when, and why was the photograph taken?
   b. Was consent (informed or implied) obtained?
   c. What type of camera and film, lenses, or filter was used?
   d. What does the photograph represent?
   e. What is the orientation, landmarks, and exact anatomical location?
   f. Where the film was developed or system images were stored, and if that correlates with hospital protocol.
7. Photograph patient when patient is medically stable and treatment allows.
8. Maintain consideration and comfort of patient when photographing.
9. Photographs, evidence collection, and documentation are always secondary to primary medical management and should not compromise patient care.
10. Photographs are part of the medical record and should not be turned over to law enforcement.
11. Take as many images as needed to document the most information about the injury/wound.
12. Never delete a photo once a forensic series has started (no matter how poor the quality).
13. Basic working knowledge of forensic photography is necessary.
   a. Initial photo will be identifying the case images in a series.
   b. Photograph the patient's armband/hospital ID and the photographer ID.
   c. Patient name/case number, date, time
   d. Photograph the patient with a head shot/full body shot
      i. Removes doubt as to the person being photographed
   e. Photograph any evidence that has a potential to be lost or altered.
   f. Photographs are best taken at a 90-degree angle to the injury.
   g. Photograph wounds or injuries before and after alteration/intervention if possible.
   h. Forensic "series" of images should be taken.
   i. Every injury is photographed at least four times.
   j. *Overview:* Photograph each wound with an orientation to body part and anatomic structures (two anatomical locations)
   k. Midrange (to include at least one anatomical landmark)
      i. Within three feet
   l. Closeup (macro setting)
      i. Within one foot of wound/injury
   m. For smaller wounds <3 cm, take two additional photos. Zoom in.
      i. Only include a single injury.
         (1) Remove anything else in image view if possible.
      ii. *Two or more images:* One with and one without the reference scale.
         (1). An ABFO No. 2 scale or measuring tape/ruler or a known size standard (coin).
      iii. *Use a color guide:* Can attach to the ruler or also have in same frame.
         (1). Place on the same plane as the injury 1 to 2 inches from the skin by an assistant helps to assess size.
         (2). Do not place directly on the skin and bending shape of ruler to align with curvature will distort image.
   n. *Intermediate shot:* Closer to the patient capturing identifying landmarks in proximity to the injury or wound for orientation purposes
   o. Close shot
      i. Digital camera
      ii. Lighting source
      iii. Photograph with identifying information and ruler in image
      iv. *Capture long-range images:* Everything in view
         (1). Good for orientation
      v. Capture closeup images, focus close up.
         (1). Good for detail
         (2). Upload images in medical records.

D. Photographing the forensic patient (Di Maio, 2011).[51]
1. Subjective and objective evidence will be documented.
   a. Description of injuries should be documented in the patients' medical chart.
   b. Anything photographed should be consistently described in the chart.
   c. Same injuries should be described under the physical exam or in the history of presenting illness as are being photographed.
2. Reference to the person who is taking the photos should be noted in the chart.
3. Obtain witnessed, written consent for photographing patient or evidence.
   a. Consent for release to law enforcement
   b. Considered HIPAA-protected and cannot be shown to anyone not on the treatment team
4. If possible, and not in process of immediately life saving measures, photograph the initial condition of the patient immediately on arrival.
5. Attempt to photograph all wounds prior to cleaning or repair of the wounds to preserve the injury.
6. All photographic images will contain patient's demographic information.
   a. Name, age, date of birth, time, the area being imaged
7. All images must be cataloged and labeled for introduction into evidence.
8. All institutions should have a policy that protects image storage in a printed, electronic, or cloud-based form.
9. Type of camera used, magnification, lighting limitations should be documented.
10. First image in the series
   a. Taking a picture of the patient demographic name label will start the series of images.
11. Second image in the series establishes identity
   a. Take a photo of the patient's face.

12. Can separate out sections of locations by photographing another label with a different location and changing the labels in the sequence to correspond with body location.
13. This sets the image sequence for recall when cataloging the images.
14. Color images can be called into question.
15. Consider a color card standard.
16. Be as detailed as possible when documenting any photographic evidence for recall if the case goes to trial.

E. Photographed wound:
  1. Measured
  2. *Recommended to use an ABFO #2 scale ruler:* Size (in centimeters) and shape
     a. "L"-shaped scale with two arms perpendicular to each other (see Figure 2.9)
  3. *Alternate scale:* Setting something of known size against the wound (e.g., setting a dime next to a wound can provide approximated size
  4. Take four photographs of every wound.
     a. General orientation shot
        i. Captured from 3 to 5 feet away and include enough information to see exactly where the injury on the body is.
        ii. Anatomic location in relation to surrounding areas
     b. *Intermediary photo:* Closer images from different angles to capture the size and shape and surrounding areas.
     c. Close-up of the injury
        i. One image with the ruler and one without

Chain of Custody[52]

A. The process used in forensic science to maintain an accurate record of information about the collection and preservation of forensic evidence to protect it from tampering or contamination. COC is a record in triplicate that documents every person that has had custody of the item of evidence from the time it was collected until the time it was introduced into court. It is closely scrutinized, and improperly handled or undocumented evidence can be legally challenged or inadmissible.

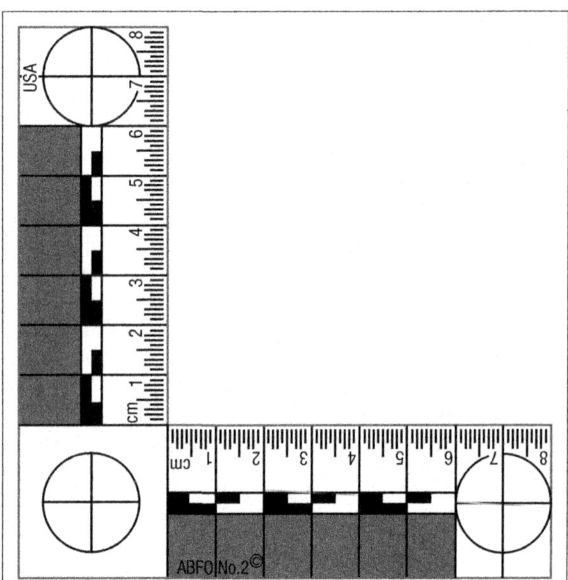

FIGURE 2.9 American Board of Forensic Odontology (ABFO)-2 photomicrographic scale (© American Board of Forensic Odontology).

B. Maintain COC for all physical evidence
  1. The COC evidence form must be filled out in its entirety and follow the evidence from start of collection to transfer of evidence to law enforcement
  2. Triplicate form (white, yellow, pink)
     a. *White form*: Goes to law enforcement when they come pick up evidence
     b. *Yellow form*: Stays with the patient
     c. *Pink form*: Goes to hospital security. If law enforcement has not yet arrived, both white and pink forms will go to security.
  3. Anyone handling evidence will be listed in the COC.
  4. *Keep it as short as possible:* Limit persons who handle the evidence.
     a. Person collecting evidence
     b. Person accepting evidence into locker for storage while awaiting law enforcement or law enforcement accepting hospital evidence.
     c. Person transporting evidence
     d. Person who receives evidence in the lab
     e. Person who examines evidence
     f. Person retrieving it from the lab

C. COC is documented in chronological order
  1. COC forms
  2. Keep a copy of the COC in the medical record.
     a. Copy goes with the evidence.
     b. Located in forensic evidence kits
        i. Located in the ED or brought by law enforcement
           (1) Use paper forms.
           (2) Electronically stored
           (3) Always used when obtaining and securing physical and trace evidence
  3. Case identification
     a. Includes the patient's information
        i. Name or trauma name, number, or unique case number assigned by trauma/law enforcement
        ii. Unique case number assigned
           (1) Applied to all evidence samples
     b. Where the evidence was collected?
     c. Who collected the evidence?
        i. *First and last name:* Printed and signed
     d. Transferring of evidence
        i. Name of persons in possession of the evidence (collecting, receiving, securing, releasing) and reason for access to it?
        ii. Evidence never released without documenting on the form.
        iii. Law enforcement receiving evidence: name, badge number, date, time, sign COC form.
        iv. What was done to the evidence?
           (1) Forensic analysis
           (2) Comparison

(3) Packaging
v. Date and time of information
4. Ensures integrity of evidence is secure
a. Through labeling, packaging, and processing
b. Protects integrity of evidence for use in court
i. Provides defense for legal challenges to the authenticity of the evidence.

D. Maintaining security of evidence[53]
1. Evidence collected should be kept by the person who collected it, never to be left unattended.
2. Avoid multiple staff members handling evidence.
3. Evidence collection limited to one clinician/nurse
4. Keep evidence in plain view of the collector.
a. Keep in a preestablished and dedicated place in the ED.
b. Never place evidence in your pocket or on your person.
c. Never leave evidence unattended. This increases the risk of tampering, which may result in lost evidence.
d. If evidence cannot be in constant view, it must be secured in a locked area until it is turned over to law enforcement. This provides the best security of the evidence.
e. Avoid long custodial holds of evidence in the ED.
i. Keeps COC short
f. Eliminate unnecessary transfers of evidence.
i. Reduces dispute over integrity of the evidence

Packaging: Labeling Guidelines

A. Packaging forensic evidence should be done to protect the items from damage, contamination, tampering, or alteration.
1. Each piece of evidence should be packaged separately.
2. *Plastic containers:* Label separately.
3. *Plastic bags:* Only to be used to carry evidence already packed in paper envelopes or other storage containers.
a. Wet clothes that are not completely dry are to be packaged in paper bags (sealed) and then placed in plastic biohazard bags and left open.
b. Plastic traps moisture and accelerates decomposition, destroys DNA evidence, and can alter evidence.
c. Plastic can cause static electricity and trace evidence to stick to the bag.
4. Paper is poros and allows breathability of airflow to prevent moisture buildup.
a. Hair, fibers, paint chips, and vegetation
b. Plants and mushrooms
c. Powdery evidence
d. Must be folded securely multiple times to prevent the escape of trace evidence.
5. Brown paper bags
a. Most evidence will go in brown paper bags to prevent the breakdown of evidence.
b. Choose the bag appropriate to the size.
6. Envelopes of different shapes and sizes
a. Manila coin envelopes for small-item evidence
b. Large manila envelopes for larger evidence
c. Avoid power in envelopes unless all sides are sealed.
7. Cardboard boxes or containers for bulky or heavy items
a. Do not use for "trace evidence" or small evidence.
b. Allow air circulation and moisture to pass through.
8. All DNA evidence should be packaged in paper or cardboard, even articles that appear dry.
9. Glass vials and jars
a. Liquid evidence can go in glass sealed containers.
b. Blood, alcohol, flammable liquids, and water.
10. *Metal cans:* Flammable liquids, fire debris, accelerants (gasoline, charcoal lighter fluid-soaked clothing), vapor hazards, paints, must go in a vapor-tight container (usually metal).
11. Volatile materials should only ever be stored in metal, never plastic.
12. Plastics are durable and transparent.
a. Water vapor does not freely pass through plastic so evidence that has moisture will be adversely affected.
b. Gaseous materials are permeable.
c. Used for needles, knives, samples that are prepackaged

B. Sealing and closure procedures
1. Any evidence turned over to law enforcement and received by the crime lab must be sealed properly indicating that it has not been accessed, altered, or contaminated during storage or transport. If sealed properly, it would be easy to detect tampering
2. To close and secure the brown paper bags
a. Heat sealing in plastic
b. Tamper-evident tape—destroys the tape when attempted to be removed.
i. Some tapes change color or change words when disturbed.
c. Tamper-proof adhesive strips
d. Cellophane, cloth tape, or tape with agency name or indication (e.g., "evidence tape" or "do not tamper").
e. *Do not stable the evidence closed:* Not acceptable method of securing evidence
f. Do not lick envelopes shut. Moisten with a gloved finger.
g. Use an indelible pen to write your name/initials across the junction (oblique) of the tape and the packaging.
h. Close the opening of the bag by folding tightly over, the opening more than once.
i. Seal with tamper-proof/evidence tape over all edges.
j. Write across the tape with time, date, and initial of person collected it.
k. On outside of bag, label with patient's name.
i. What clothing is in the bag
ii. Identifying item information (what is in bag)
iii. Person collecting evidence

iv. Date and time it was collected and sealed

Methods of Evidence Collection

A. Clothing
  1. Can be vital to a criminal investigation
  2. To fully evaluate and manage any patient involved in forensically significant case, all clothing must be removed.
  3. In trauma cases, clothing work by individuals can contain physical and biologic evidence that must be preserved, requiring the patients' clothes to be cut off the patient.
  4. At the crime lab, the preserved clothing is photographed and can be placed on a mannequin to identify wound patterns and help corroborate testimony.
  5. All clothing must be preserved.
    a. If still wearing clothing, they will need to be cut off and secured.
    b. Remove obvious gross physical evidence.
      i. Secure any physical evidence removed off clothing.
      ii. Carefully label the container used for trace evidence.
    c. Avoid cutting through bullet holes, knife wounds, tears, blood, or other stains.
    d. Cut around areas that are near the point of entry/exit bullet or stab wounds.
    e. Cut down seams, around holes, tears, and buttons.
    f. Cut the posterior part of the clothing if injuries are on front.
    g. Make as few cuts as required to remove the clothing.
    h. One person should be responsible for cutting off clothing and package it according to the guidelines of packaging.
  6. If patient is able to stand and take off clothing
    a. Cover the floor with two large layers of exam paper or white sheets.
    b. Bottom layer is against the ED floor and will be discarded.
    c. Top layer will collect any evidence that falls from patient while they undress.
      i. Can be folded up to protect dropped evidence
      ii. Do not drop clothing on top of the evidence on the floor.
      iii. Each article of clothing will be placed in a separate bag.
      iv. Each bag is labeled with the full name of the person collecting, date, and time.
      v. Full name of patient and case number assigned
      vi. Fold over each bag and secure with tamper-proof tape.
      vii. Sign across the tape to overlap tape and bag to ensure integrity that the seal will not be broken without explanation.
    d. Have patient take off shoes and step onto the paper in socks or bare feet.
      i. Bag shoes in a single paper bag.
    e. Have patient take off their clothes from top down, allowing the clothes and any evidence to fall on the paper.
      i. Remove top and then put on patient gown.
      ii. Remove bottom layer of clothes.
      iii. Do not shake out the clothing.
      iv. Do not let clothing fall on the floor.
      v. Leads to cross contamination
      vi. Decreases evidentiary value
  7. Wear gloves when touching the clothing.
    a. Separate pair of gloves for each article of clothing
  8. Inspect the clothing for damage, tears, stains, evidence.
  9. Dry any moist or wet material before packaging if possible.
  10. Package articles of clothing separately in paper bags.
  11. If clothes cannot be dried fully prior to turning over to law enforcement, place in brown paper bag and then in a plastic "biohazard" bag.
  12. Do not close the plastic bag; allow it to remain open to circulate air.
    b. Trapped moisture facilitates fungal growth and degradation of DNA evidence.
    c. Notify law enforcement that the clothing remains "wet."
  13. Once all clothes are removed, the patient can step off paper.
  14. Fold the top paper inward so that any debris or evidence is secured within.
  15. Hospital linen and emergency medical services (EMS) linen should also be secured in the same manner as outlined for clothing.
  16. Place each piece of clothing/linen in separate paper bag and close.
    a. Secure in same manner as outlined for documentation and securing of evidence.
    b. Document on the COC form.
  17. Do not put articles of clothing in plastic bags.
    a. Plastic degrades evidence and process starts immediately.
  18. Carefully label the container used to package clothing.
  19. Document the evidence on the COC form.

B. Biological evidence
  1. The most important biological evidence will yield DNA, a human biomarker that verifies the identify of an individual with incredible odds. The chances of two individuals having identical DNA is approximately one in one billion. Advanced in forensic technology are capable of identifying minute traces of DNA that are often central to criminal investigations.
  2. There are multiple types of biological evidence.
    a. Body fluids
      i. Semen, saliva, urine, tears, bile, perspiration
      ii. For specimen samples, use cotton tip applicators.
      iii. Buccal swabs, oral swabs, perineal, perianal, vaginal, cervical Os, penile, scrotum, rectum, bitemarks
      iv. Emesis, fecal matter

b. *Soft tissue:* Hair, skin, fingernails, organs
c. *Structural tissue*: Bone, joints, teeth
d. *Other nonhuman sources:* Microbial, animal, vegetative
e. *Objects that can retain DNA:* Makeup, lipstick, toothbrush, razor, articles of clothing, cigars, cigarettes, bottles, cans

3. Collecting trace evidence
   a. Hairs, fibers, paint, gravel, dirt, soil, grass, leaves, twigs, adhesive tape, glass
   b. Document and photograph all evidence.
   c. Follow documentation and photographing guidelines.
   d. Collect evidence properly using tweezers or tape transfer.
   e. Secure the evidence per guidelines.
   f. Place in a paper bag or envelope.
   g. Close and seal the evidence envelop or bag with tape.
   h. Write date, time, initial, and examiners name across the sealed tape area
   i. Label the bag with the contents on the outside.
   j. Document in the COC form
   k. Secure in the storage locker and call law enforcement for pickup.
4. Collecting biologic evidence
   a. Maintain universal precautions when handling biologic or blood evidence.
   b. All biologic fluid is considered biohazard.
   c. Risk of exposure to pathogens, bloodborne illnesses (e.g., HIV, hepatitis B, or hepatitis C)
   d. *Wear appropriate personal protection equipment (PPE):* Gloves and gown, face mask and eye protection, head covering or clean lab coat if concern for contamination
   e. Collect specimens and swabs in appropriate containers that are labeled with the patient's case number and identifying information.
   f. Packaged separately in a plastic evidence collection bag and then sealed, sealed on the outside with tape.
   g. Name and date of the person collecting and sealing evidence across the tape
   h. Document the type of sample on the evidence form.
   i. Sign name of person collecting specimen on the COC form.
   j. Package that in a clean brown paper bag.
      i. Folded, sealed with tape with sign name and date on the bag across the tape.

Methods of Storing Biological Evidence

A. Dedicated evidence storage locker
   1. All EDs should have a dedicated evidence storage locker.
   2. *Biologic evidence:* Blood, urine, semen, vaginal swabs, oral secretions, buccal, nasal, anal swabs
   3. Sexual assault kits should be kept in the storage lockers.
   4. Lockers should be kept closed, locked.
      a. Only charge nurses should have access to the key and knowledge of access should be limited to designated persons and law enforcement.
   5. All collected evidence will go into the storage locker immediately after collection to await law enforcement pickup and transfer to the crime lab.
      a. Evidence goes to law enforcement within the jurisdiction the crime was committed. Get a good history of the location where injuries or incidents occurred.
   6. Document date/time/person reaching out to law enforcement on COC form.
   7. Document time law enforcement arrived to pick up the evidence.
   8. Document this on the COC form.

B. Ideal locker conditions:
   1. Temperature-controlled room
   2. Ambient temperature or 60°F to 75°F
   3. Humidity <60%
   4. Higher humidity or warmer temperatures promote the growth of mold and bacteria and can degrade biologic evidence.

C. Blood or other biological liquid specimens should be kept refrigerated in a secure area free from tampering.

D. Wet clothes, swabs, or blood evidence
   1. Allow clothes to dry as much as possible before placing in a dry paper bag.
   2. Dry swabs thoroughly with cool air only—no heat.
      a. Package swabs in a vented swab container or boxes.
      b. Do not package swabs in paper or plastic.

E. Seal items in the dry paper bag.
   1. Mark the bag as "WET EVIDENCE."
   2. Notify law enforcement that evidence is "wet" for safety precautions.

F. Package wet clothes in paper, never plastic.
   1. Plastic accelerates the degradation process of blood and DNA.
      a. Promotes the growth of mold or mildew

Sexual Assault Presentations in the Emergency Department

Sexual assault is an act of violence that includes victims of rape, incest, intimate partner violence, and human sex trafficking. The allegation of sexual assault is medically and psychologically complex. The demographics and statistics of sexual assault and rape is a nondiscriminatory sex-based crime reported annually by the Centers for Disease Control and Prevention (CDC) under Sexual Violence statistics. In 2019, there was a reported annual estimate of 1.5 million women and 834,700 men who had been sexually assaulted with a lifetime average rate of sexual assault being between 17% and 18% for U.S. women and 3% of men having reported rape or attempted rape. According to 2019 data collected by the U.S. Department of Justice, sexual assault occurs every 73 seconds in the United States and every 9 minutes for pediatric patients. Many assault victims will suffer posttraumatic stress in the form of disorders of anxiety, suicidal ideations, eating disorders, and substance abuse. Cochran (2019) determined the risk of suicide increased 10-fold for victims of sexual assault, 45% had suicidal ideation and 23% completing attempt. Close interdisciplinary collaboration between medicine and law is essential to achieving the best outcomes for all victims of sexual assault.

Management of sexual assault cases is complex and time intensive to do correctly. The assault has medical, psychologic, and legal implications. An evidence collection exam is one of the most challenging processes encountered by an emergency nurse. A level of sensitivity and attention to detail is crucial to conducting a forensic exam that maintains chain of custody (COC). Capturing the patient's history and story that collaborates with a physical exam is crucial for crime reconstruction. Documentation is completed on evidence collection forms and approximately 90% of forensic examinations for evidence collection in assault cases happens in an ED, the remaining 10% in OB/GYN, urgent care or primary care offices combined. There is pressure on ED staff to have awareness and training or a dedicated staff trained in sexual assault evidence collection. All assault victims should be evaluated by a trained medico-legal examiner or forensic sexual assault nurse who is experienced in exams to limit repeat or suboptimal exams that do not meet the quality standard of legal scrutiny.[54] In 2013, Senate Bill 1191 was passed, allowing forensic evidence to be collected in the hospital EDs by nurses who have received training in sexual assault exams in order to improve access to care for patient in critical access areas. In that same year, Congress passed the Sexual Assault Forensic Evidence Reporting (SAFER) Act, considered a reauthorization of the Violence Against Women Act. The Debbie Smith DNA Backlog Grant Program was created to develop practices appropriate for the accurate, timely, and effective collection and processing of DNA evidence and the steps required to investigate cases involving DNA evidence prioritizing sexual assault kits (SAKs) to be forensically analyzed, and expedient collaboration between healthcare, law enforcement, crime lab and the criminal justice system.

Sexual Assault Evidence Collection Methods

A. Every emergency care center should have on hand or access to sexual assault evidence collection kits (SAECK).
  1. Collection procedures are complex, having a plan and following an established standard for head-to-toe and external-to-internal approach documentation and evidence collection will help the examiner stay organized.

B. All aspects of the evidence collection should be documented in both medical and forensic records.
  1. Each item will be listed on a form and signed by both the nurse who collected the evidence and the law enforcement officer who receives the evidence.

C. National standard guidelines for evidence collection in adults and pediatrics sexual assault can be consulted.

D. *A National Protocol for Sexual Abuse Medical Forensic Examinations: Pediatric* can be found at www.justice.gov/ovw/file/846856/download.

E. *Sexual Assault Evidence Collection Procedure* (similar to general evidence collection rules)
  1. A collaborative multidisciplinary approach should be implemented for sexual assault cases.
  2. Utilize victim-centered and trauma-informed approach when managing victims of sexual assault.
  3. Involve victim advocates early in the process for ongoing management and follow-up.
  4. Evidence collection should be performed by an experienced sexual assault nurse examiner (SANE) nurse or trained medical professional.
  5. Guided by the victim, sexual assault samples should be collected up to ≥5 days postassault.
  6. Reimbursements should be provided for the forensic medical exam independent of timeframe.

F. Toxicology testing should be done within 72 hours (urine and blood) to prevent the loss of potential
  1. Drugs responsible for drug-facilitated sexual assault (DFSA)
  2. Alcohol (38%), marijuana (18%), cocaine (10%), benzodiazepines (10%), amphetamines (5%), gamma-hydroxybutyrate (GHB; 4%), Rohypnol (0.5%) and ketamine
  3. Timely collection of specimens warranted
  4. Victim should not urinate until it can be collected.
  5. Collect 100 mL of urine and 30 mL of blood—best opportunity for detection in the first 24 hours of alleged assault.
  6. Rohypnol (Flunitrazepam), a benzodiazepine
    a. When mixed with alcohol it will incapacitate. Also known as the "date rape drug" or "roofie"; not approved for medical use
    b. Effect within 15 to 20 minutes, lasting 12 hours
    c. Similar to Xanax and valium but 7 to 10 times more potent
    d. *Incapacitating:* Disinhibition, passivity, muscle relaxation, anterograde anesthesia
    e. Levels can remain in the system for 3 to 5 days.
      i. Short half-life of 10 to 15 hours
        1 *Outside lab:* Gas chromatograph (GC) mass spectrometer can detect minute levels
      ii. Level >50 ng/mL is considered positive.
    f. Urine levels detected up to 5 days
    g. GC mass spectrometry lab can detect levels.
      i. Blood, up to 24 hours
      ii. Hair, up to 30 days
  7. GHB
    a. A central nervous system depressant similar to benzodiazepines
    b. It is a hallucinogen ("liquid ecstasy").
    c. Occurs naturally in the gut. Cutoff level of 5 mg/L distinguishes it from exogenous GHB ingestion. Normal levels in the body are <5 mg/L.
    d. Blood levels >50 mg/L lead to euphoria, uninhibited behavior, lightheadedness, and arousal.
    e. Levels >250 mg/L can cause seizures, coma, and death.
    f. Elimination half-life is only 0.3 to 1.0 hours.
    g. Peak levels are reached in only 20 to 60 minutes.
    h. Detectable in plasma for 6 to 8 hours
    i. Should be measured in blood serum rather than urine

G. Patient must provide written and verbal consent for a forensic evidence collection exam.

1. Patient can elect to decline any part of the exam process.

2. Encourage patient to ask questions throughout the exam.

H. Utilize the SAECK.

1. Only someone trained in sexual assault evidence collection should perform the exam.

2. Discuss each aspect of the exam with the patient prior to starting the exam and before each step.

3. Important medical questions for interview/evaluation

4. History of presenting assault (e.g., time, date)

5. Loss of consciousness, memory of event, memory lapse, amnesia

6. Symptoms since assault

7. Any recent genital procedures

8. Details of assault

9. Specific threats

10. How many assailants

11. Types of penetration

12. Nongenital acts

13. Activities postassault (e.g., shower, cleansing)

I. Collection procedures

1. Masks and gloves should be worn by the examiner to prevent contamination of DNA when collecting and packaging evidence samples.

2. Fully examine the body for injuries, lesions, secretions.

3. Conduct general physical and anogenital exam and document the physical findings on body diagram forms.

4. Conduct general physical exam. Obtain vitals, physical appearance, general demeanor, behavior, orientation, and condition of clothing on arrival.

5. Record all physical findings.

a. *Observable or palpable tissue injuries:* Physiologic changes, foreign material (e.g., grass, sand, gravel, stains, moist secretions, dried secretions)

b. Utilize black light or Wood's lamp fluorescence to assist with visualizing secretions.

c. Note redness, abrasions, bruises, swelling, lacerations, fractures, bites, burns, and other physical trauma

d. Special attention should be given to assessing injury on dark-skinned individuals and be directed by the patient to identify areas of injury.

6. *Clothing collection:* Follow outlined forensic evidence collection methods

7. *Photographing:* Follow outlined forensic photography protocols

8. *Position patient for exam:* Females require a lithotomy position. Take external genital swabs, vaginal swabs, and perianal swabs

9. Male patients should have penile and anal injuries examined prior to obtaining penile, urethral, or anorectal swabs. Swab each area twice.

10. Photography in this area is extremely sensitive and personal and requires additional consent and discussing the process with the victim.

11. Two control swabs

12. *Sample swabs:* No more than two swabs per collection area as not to dilute the biologic sample.

13. *Bite marks:* Swab the area twice.

14. Blood or saliva swabs for DNA analysis

a. Oral swabs/smears if <24 hours of presentation since oral penetration

b. *Buccal swabs*: Air dry swab before packaging.

c. *Dry blood:* If no blood samples are drawn, a pinprick sample can be drawn.

d. Cleanse with betadine and then prick finger and drop onto blood collection card. Allow to dry before packaging.

e. *Blood draw:* Lavender-top, yellow top, red top, gray top

f. Keep medical samples separate from evidentiary samples.

g. Package and document by forensic collection guidelines.

15. Head-hair combings

16. Pubic-hair combings

17. Fingernail scrapings if the patient was able to scratch perpetrator

J. Complete forms and seal envelopes inside the SAECK with specimens.

1. Once evidence collection completed and medically stable proper hospital monitoring and follow-up should be considered.

K. Pain control

L. Psychiatric consult to address immediate emotional and psychologic well-being

M. Rape trauma syndrome in the immediate postassault can present in 16% of patients.

N. *Acute phase (disorganized phase):* Sleep disturbances, generalized physical pain, mood and eating disturbances, sense of disorganization, fear, and self-blame.

O. Delayed phase-phobias, nightmares, flashbacks (posttraumatic stress disorder [PTSD]), sexual dysfunction

P. *Long term:* Depression, chronic pelvic pain, diminished quality of life

Q. Antibiotic prophylaxis for sexually transmitted diseases (STDs)

R. Nutritional services

S. Sleep improvement strategies addressed

T. Discharge considerations

1. Follow-up for infections, pregnancies, or administration of vaccinations

2. Schedule a follow-up appointment within 2 weeks to check for sexually transmitted infections (STIs).

3. Schedule a 6-week appointment for repeat pregnancy testing, HIV screening, and hepatitis C.

4. Schedule follow-up appointments at 12 and 24 weeks to follow-up on HIV and hepatitis C screening.

5. OB/GYN follow-up

6. Psychiatric care follow-up

7. Primary care (PCP) follow-up

8. Offering legal counseling

9. *National Sexual Assault Telephone:* Call 800.656.HOPE (4673).

2F: Cultural Competency in Emergency Care

RENEÉ SEMONIN HOLLERAN

Learning Objectives

- Define the concept of cultural competence including sensitivity to gender and race.
- Describe the impact of cultural diversity on the care of patients and families seen in the emergency care setting.
- Use education and interventions that allow the emergency nurse practitioner to understand the effects of a patient's culture on their beliefs related to medical care.

The practice of emergency care involves assessing and managing a culturally diverse patient population. The mobility of the world's population has brought people from many countries and cultures to the United States. Many of these patients do not have access to healthcare and use the ED as a portal into the health care system. One of the most important ideas related to cultural competence in the ED is for the emergency nurse practitioner (ENP) to be aware that there are disparities in health care access within the United States. Lack of universal healthcare, financial support, and overall access has increased the role of the ED in the primary care of many diverse populations. Unfortunately, unless there are major changes in the healthcare system, this is not going to change. The ENP must be prepared and willing to provide safe and competent care to the diverse patient population they will be exposed to.

The Emergency Medical Treatment and Labor Act (EMTALA; www.cms.gov/Regulations-and-Guidance/Legislation/EMTALA) requires that EDs that accept Medicare funding provide appropriate services, including the transfer to a higher level care center if needed, to patients who seek care regardless of their ability to pay. The ED is accountable for patient-centered care that includes the need for clinicians to be culturally competent to provide fitting and safe care.

There are multiple definitions that define and describe cultural competence. Primarily, cultural competence includes the ability of the ENP to provide care to diverse patients of different cultures and consider how the patient's culture impacts the care that the patient may need.[55,56] The need to be sensitive to the patient's culture allows for the development of a therapeutic relationship and, hopefully, an improvement in the patient's health based on their care in the ED.[57]

In summary, the American Academy of Emergency Nurse Practitioners (AAENP) Standards of Practice for the ENP specialty note the following[58]:

- Integrate cultural competence into patient care.
- Identify needs of vulnerable populations and intervene appropriately.

Components of Cultural Competence[55,56,57]

A proposed conceptual model of cultural competence includes the following:

A. *Cultural awareness:* Understanding of the effects of one's own beliefs and prejudices about the patients the ENP is caring for in the ED.

B. *Cultural knowledge:* Acquisition of knowledge related to different cultures.

C. *Cultural sensitivity:* The need to value, respect, and admire cultural diversity. This will help the ENP to understand how the patient views their illness or injury and how it may be treated.

D. *Cultural skill:* Ability to establish effective communication with patients from different cultures.

E. *Cultural proficiency:* Describes the ability to acquire new information about specific cultures and adapt to practice.

F. *Dynamicity:* Allows the ENP to become culturally competent through caring for multiple patients from different cultures.

Culturally Sensitive Communication[57,59]

A. Encourages the patient and their family to participate in their care. This includes using the patient's belief systems and language so that there is open and trusted communication between the patient and the ENP.

B. Include cultural considerations by asking sensitive questions related to the patient's values, believes and practices, and patient's perception related to their illness or injury. The ENP should include an assessment of the patient's psychological, physiological, and sociocultural needs, nonverbal communication cues, understanding of other languages, religion, and food preferences.

C. ENP must be aware of their response to the patient so that a trusting relationship can be developed. In the stresses of the ED this can be challenging, but it must be considered or the patient or the family will feel safe with the clinician.

D. The ENP should communicate with the patient and family with dignity and respect.

E. Laws that require healthcare clinicians and institutions to have interpreters available for patients include:

1. *The Civil Rights Act of 1964:* The civil rights act is widely known for title VI—outlawing discrimination based on race, color, religion, sex, or national origin. Access to language services is covered by antidiscrimination laws regarding national origin.

2. *Executive Order 13166:* In 2000, antidiscrimination efforts for individuals with limited English proficiency (LEP) were further solidified when then President Bill Clinton signed Executive Order 13166. This order mandated laws requiring interpreters in healthcare when institutions were provided with federal funding. It also applies broadly to all agencies receiving federal money. (*Source:* interpretertrain.com/laws-requiring-interpreters-in-healthcare/)

F. The Joint Commission developed a document entitled *Advancing effective communication, cultural competence, and family-centered care: a roadmap for hospitals*, published in 2010. (www.jointcommission.org/resources/

patient-safety-topics/health-equity/#t=_Tab_StandardsFAQs&sort=relevancy)

G. A professional interpreter should be used. The use of someone in person is the best practice. Body and facial expressions are an important component of communication in many cultures.

H. Avoid using "medical jargon," especially since it may not be able to be interpreted to the patient's primary language.

I. Do not discuss inappropriate issues in front of the patient that may put the interpreter in a difficult situation.

J. Allow the patient and family to participate in the conversation as much as possible.

K. Always identify who is talking with the patient and family, including what their responsibilities are with the patient's care.

L. Allow collaboration with the patient and family when possible. This can be particularly challenging in the ED when decisions need to be quickly made. If a trusting relationship has been development, this may be easier for the clinicians, patient, and family.

Cultural Competence Education[60]

A. Cultural Awareness in Emergency Care (https://www.acep.org/patient-care/policy-statements/cultural-awareness-and-emergency-care/)

B. Cultural competence: Are you prepared. On-Line Education (ed-areyouprepared.com/patients-care/cultural-competence/).

C. Marion, L., Douglas, M., Lavin, M., Barr, M., Gazaway, S., Thomas, E., Bickford, C. (2017). Implementing the new ANA Standards 8: Culturally congruent practice. OIJN. Accessed July 12, 2020, from http://ojin.nursingworld.org/MainMenuCategories/ANAMarketplace/ANAPeriodicals/OJIN/TableofContents/Vol-22-2017/No1-Jan-2017/Articles-Previous-Topics/Implementing-the-New-ANA-Standard-8.html

2G: Patient and Clinician Safety in the Emergency Department

RODNEY HICKS

Learning Objectives

- Identify significant patient and clinician safety concerns unique to the ED.
- Identify at least two systems approaches for reducing error opportunities.
- Identify at least two high-risk populations for adverse events.

A. All healthcare, regardless of where such care is delivered, shares six domains of quality.[61] The domains of healthcare quality include:

1. Timely care
2. Effective care
3. Efficient care
4. Safe care
5. Patient-centered care
6. Equitable care

B. Failing to satisfy any of the domains gives rise to the broader concept of patient safety, given that all patient care should be quality care.

C. Patient safety emerged as a professional and organizational responsibility following the release of the November 1999 Institute of Medicine (IOM) report, *To Err Is Human: Building a Safer Health System.*[62]

1. This report provided evidence that as many as 98,000 individuals lost their lives directly due to interactions with the healthcare system. Merely seeking healthcare harmed thousands more.
   a. The authors called for a national agenda of making healthcare and the healthcare system safer.
   b. A notable finding was that the clinicians themselves were not the source of medical error problems, but rather, the system itself was inefficient, ineffective, and bore most of the responsibilities for patient harm.
   c. Another notable finding was pervasive culture of secrecy and silence surrounding error-causing events.
   d. The report springboarded larger discussions on quality, safety, and patient outcomes across the various locations where patients and clinicians interact.
2. The ED setting remains one setting where patient harm can occur. In fact, medical errors in the ED are thought to occur more frequently and result in more serious outcomes in ED patients as compared to errors in non-ED settings.[63,64] While awareness of the need for a patient safety culture emerged following the IOM report, the unpredictable nature of the ED, coupled with the high pace of work, does at times negatively impact operations.[65,66]

D. Amplifying the opportunities for medical error in the ED stems from overcrowding.[67,68,69] Understanding the causes of medical error allows clinicians to adopt proven methods to reduce patient harm. According to the Agency for Healthcare and Quality (AHRQ), eight categories of factors contribute to errors[69]:

1. Communication problems
2. Inadequate information flow
3. Human problems
4. Patient-related issues
5. Organizational transfer of knowledge
6. Staffing patterns and workflow
7. Technical failures
8. Inadequate policies and procedures

Emergency Department Clinicians and Concerns

A. ED clinicians have identified the importance of patient safety factors. While the rankings of the safety factors vary between urban, suburban, and rural settings, the list of topics is noteworthy.[70] ED clinicians can utilize such a list with hospital leaders to share concerns and plan for solutions.

1. Crowding from inpatient boarding
2. Availability of specialty consultation
3. Nurse shortages
4. Lack of follow-up for ED care
5. Laboratory/radiology time
6. Information systems and ability to share information between institutions
7. Aspirin and beta-blockers for myocardial infarction
8. Handoffs
9. Availability of language interpreters
10. Handwashing
11. Nonurgent use of the ED
12. Atibiotics within 4 hours for pneumonia
13. Medication errors
14. Ambulance diversion
15. Clinician order entry systems
16. Time-outs to verify correct side and site of procedures

Other Leading Areas of Concern for Patient Safety

A. Diagnostic errors

1. The ED setting is a generalist setting, due in part to serving as the safety net of the healthcare system. The flow of patients might be erratic; patients with life-threatening conditions are interspersed with patients having common medical complaints. Regardless of patient acuity, timely and accurate diagnosing is the standard of performance. Threats to accurate diagnosing arise from not having prior medical records. As a result, the opportunity for diagnostic errors may be higher in the ED than in other structured settings.[16,71] Leading diagnoses associated with diagnostic errors include[63]:

   a. Fracture
   b. Myocardial infarction (MI)
   c. Intracranial bleed
   d. Stroke/cerebrovascular accident (CVA)
   e. Acute abdomen
   f. Pulmonary embolism (PE)
   g. Ectopic pregnancy
   h. Appendicitis
   i. Ischemic limb
   j. Deep vein thrombosis (DVT)
   k. Meningitis
   l. Pneumonia

Pediatric Patients

1. Pediatric patients are another population susceptible to adverse events, especially in settings that care for both adults and children.

2. Pediatric care is considered high risk due to special considerations such as the lack of standardized dosing of many medications, weight-based dosing, incomplete medical history, having electronic medical records without pediatric specialization, a generalized formulary, the absence of a clinical pharmacist, and multiple transitions in care.[72,73] Common adverse events in the pediatric population include:

   a. Medication errors[72,73]
   b. Adverse events associated with sedation[74]
   c. Suicide attempt[75]
   d. Patient misidentification[76]

Mental Health Patients

1. Mental health illnesses are common across the lifespan. Many individuals with mental illness present to the ED, either voluntarily or involuntarily.

2. Treatment of psychiatric patients does not follow treatment norms of other ED patients; medical care is directed by the presenting complaint and the psychiatric history.[77] Common presenting complaints include mood disorders, personality disorders, substance abuse disorders, anxiety disorders, and altered mental status. The presence of a mental health disorder positions both the patient and the staff at higher risk of adverse events. Adverse psychiatric events include:

   a. Suicide or other self-directed harm
   b. Elopement
   c. Violence toward staff

3. The potential for patient safety adverse events extends beyond psychiatric events. ED clinicians should recognize the potential for adverse drug reactions that may arise with patients taking psychiatric medications and other medications.

Systems Approaches to Reduce Medical Errors

A. Opportunities to improve patient care and reduce errors are now part of every ED clinician's responsibilities. The patient safety movement has adopted preventative strategies from industries outside healthcare to reduce variation and improve outcomes. Many of these strategies have time-tested tools that facilitate problem identification, determine practical solutions, and evaluate the level of change across the system. Common to most of the tools is the systems-level approach that addresses organizational flaws as opposed to human-based or people-based approaches. Systems-level changes are more likely to yield sustained change as compared to people-level approaches. Systems-level approaches and tools include:

1. Root cause analysis
2. Plan-Do-Study-Act (PDSA) cycle[78]
3. TeamSTEPPS®[79]
4. Lean Six Sigma for Health Care[80]
5. Failure Mode and Effects Analysis (FMEA)[81]
6. Process mapping[81]
7. Pareto charts[81]
8. Incident reports[64]

Patient-Centered Strategies to Improve Patient Safety

A. Patient encounters are interactions between a patient, a clinician, and the healthcare system. With the goal of improving the quality of care and reducing opportunities for errors, patients become part of the process and solution. ED clinicians should consider and adopt policies and processes that support patient-centered safety initiatives. Such initiatives could include:

1. Sharing of clinician notes, electronic medical record (EMR) notes
2. Encourage family and caregiver engagement in understanding the treatment plan.

Organizational Patient Safety Initiatives Applicable to Emergency Department

A. The ED is a microsystem within the larger hospital or health system. Many patient safety priorities and initiatives are organization-wide activities. The ED clinician should contribute to policies and procedures that facilitate implementation of the activities, considering the unique needs of the department. Examples of where the ED clinician influences and supports policies include:

B. Improving transitions of care
1. Transitions from Emergency Medical Services (EMS) to ED[82]
2. Transitions from referring hospitals
3. Transitions from nursing homes or assisted living centers[83]
4. Handoffs from ED to other hospital units or other departments[84,85]

C. Reducing adverse medication events
1. Utilize a computerized provider order entry (CPOE) system with clinical decision support[73]
2. Ensuring pharmacist availability
3. Performing medication reconciliation[86,87]
4. Developing standardized order sets based on evidence-based guidelines
5. Eliminate the use of abbreviations

D. Minimizing risk of healthcare-acquired infections (HAIs)[87]
1. Adherence to hand hygiene protocols
2. Catheter-associated urinary tract infection (CAUTI) protocols
3. Central line-associated bloodstream infections (CLABSI) protocols
4. Appropriate antibiotic use

E. Adhering to principles of the Universal Protocol[87]
1. Preprocedural checklist for intubation[88]

F. Improving the accuracy of patient identification[87]
1. Patient identification through barcode procedures[76,87]
2. Utilizing barcode labels for specimens[76,87]

G. Minimizing interruptions[89,90]

H. Developing a fall prevention program[91]

I. Incorporating suicide prevention program[87,92]

J. Implementing safe patient handling program[93]

K. Participating in safety culture surveys[94]

L. Developing a culture of reporting errors and near misses[95]

M. Participating in walk-rounds[95]

Workplace Violence

A. An organization's culture of safety must include protection of the healthcare workforce in the ED setting. The organization bears the legal and ethical responsibility for ensuring a safe workplace.[96] Workplace violence (WPV), an occupational hazard,[97] does occur in the ED and workers in this setting are at higher risk than other healthcare workers.[98] WPV ranges from verbal assault to physical assault to homicide, and the rate of violence against nurses (8.1 per 1,000) and physicians (10.1 per 1,000) is higher than that of the general population (5.1 per 1,000).[96] WPV can come from the patient or the family member. Commonly reported examples of WPV include[10,98]:
1. Verbal abuse
2. Name calling
3. General threats
4. Threat of a lawsuit
5. Spitting
6. Grabbing
7. Physical violence
8. Sexual groping or sexual innuendo
9. Injuries
   a. Bruising
   b. Bites
   c. Abrasions
   d. Scratches

B. Some patient and family factors associated with WPV among ED employees include[98]:
1. Alcohol or other substance use
2. Psychiatric illness
3. Dementia
4. Gang involvement
5. Situational and environmental factors that contribute to physical assault include[98,99]:
6. Inadequate staffing
7. Hours of 7p to 7a
8. Being alone with the patient
9. Long wait times to be seen
10. The ease of having weapons in the ED/lack of metal detectors
11. Lack of security personnel
12. Lack of policies, procedures, and training on WPV
13. Easy access to nonsecured medical equipment as weapons
14. Lack of privacy
15. Facility design

Conclusion

A. The ED setting is a setting that serves many people with diverse medical needs and varying levels of patient acuity.
1. Reducing medical errors enhances patient safety.
2. Applying systems-levels tools and having established protocols, policies, and procedures help to mitigate risk that is inherent in an uncontrollable, unpredictable workload environment.

2H: Postexposure Prophylaxis

APRIL T. HILL

Learning Objectives

- Define different types of exposures.
- Differentiate types of postexposure risks.
- Describe the advantages of available postexposure prophylaxis options.
- Determine appropriate testing in response to exposure.
- Perform appropriate follow up in response to exposure events.

Exposure prevention remains the primary strategy for reducing occupational bloodborne pathogen infections; however, occupational exposures will continue to occur. Healthcare organizations should make available to their personnel a system that includes written protocols for prompt reporting, evaluation, counseling, treatment, and follow-up of occupational exposures that might place healthcare personnel (HCP) at risk for acquiring a blood-borne infection. HCP should be educated concerning the risks and prevention strategies against blood-borne infections, including the importance of vaccination against hepatitis B and postexposure prophylaxis (PEP).

Definition

For transmission of bloodborne pathogens HIV, hepatitis B virus (HBV), or hepatitis C virus (HCV) to occur, an exposure must include both of the following:

A. Infectious body fluid
   1. HIV, HBV, and HCV can be transmitted via blood, semen, vaginal fluid, amniotic fluid, breast milk, cerebrospinal fluid, pericardial fluid, peritoneal fluid, pleural fluid, and synovial fluid.
   2. Note that saliva, vomitus, urine, feces, sweat, tears, and respiratory secretions do not transmit HIV, unless visibly bloody.
   3. The risk of HBV and HCV transmission from non-bloody saliva is negligible.

B. A portal of entry
   4. Percutaneous, mucous membrane, cutaneous with nonintact skin

   If both of these factors are not present, there is no risk of transmission and further evaluation is not required.

Exposure Transmission Risk

A. Probability of HIV transmission from a percutaneous needle stick is approximately 0.3% (1 in 300) and 0.09% from mucous membrane exposure.

B. Probability of HCV seroconversion after percutaneous needle stick is 1.8%. Transmission rarely occurs from mucous membrane exposures to blood, and no transmission to HCP has been documented from intact or nonintact skin exposures to blood.

C. HBV infection is a well-recognized occupational risk for HCP. The risk of HBV infection is primarily related to the degree of contact with blood in the workplace and also to the hepatitis B e-antigen (HBeAg) status of the source person. In studies of HCP who sustained injuries from needles contaminated with blood containing HBV, the risk of developing clinical hepatitis if the blood tested positive for both HBeAg and hepatitis B surface antigen (HBsAg) was 22% to 31%; the risk of developing serologic evidence of HBV infection was 37% to 62%. By comparison, the risk of developing clinical hepatitis from a needle contaminated with HBsAg-positive, HBeAg-negative blood was 1% to 6%, and the risk of developing serologic evidence of HBV infection, 23% to 37%.

D. PEP provides a transmission reduction of approximately 79%.

E. Common side effects are constitutional and gastrointestinal (GI).

High-Risk Exposures

A. Source
   1. Symptomatic HIV/AIDS
   2. Acute seroconverison
   3. High viral load

B. Exposure
   1. Deep injuries
   2. Visible blood on device
   3. Injuries sustained while placing a catheter in a vein/artery

Low-Risk Exposures

A. Dried blood on an old needle

B. Human bites

C. Table 2.3 summarizes the estimated risks of HIV transmission following exposure to blood. Risk for transmission from infectious fluids other than HIV-infected blood is considerably lower than for blood exposures.

Postexposure Prophylaxis Recommendation

A. PEP is recommended when occupational exposures to HIV occur.

B. The HIV status of the exposure source patient (SP) should be determined, if possible, to guide the need for HIV PEP.

C. Optimal time to start PEP is within hours of exposure, rather than days. Do not wait for SP test results, unless results will be available within an hour or two. Goal is <2 hours after exposure.

D. PEP medication regimes should be continued for a 4-week duration.

E. PEP medication regimes should contain three or more antiretroviral (ARV) drugs for all occupational exposures to HIV.

F. Expert consultation is recommended for any occupational exposures to HIV at a minimum for special situations, such as pregnancy or breastfeeding.

TABLE 2.3 ESTIMATED RISKS OF HIV TRANSMISSION FOLLOWING EXPOSURE TO BLOOD

ROUTE OF EXPOSURE	RISK OF EXPOSURE WHEN SOURCE PERSON IS HIV POSITIVE	FACTORS INCREASING RISK
Percutaneous	Approx. 1/435 episodes (0.23%)	Hollow bore needles, visibly bloody devices, deep injury, and device used in an artery/vein
Mucous membrane	Approx. 1/1,000 episodes (0.09%)	Large volume
Cutaneous	<1/1,000 episodes (0.09%)	Must involve nonintact skin integrity

G. >36 hours is normally deferred, unless particularly high risk

H. 72 hours postexposure is the outer limit of opportunity to initiate PEP; however, a delay of that scale is believed to compromise PEP efficacy.

I. If initiation is delayed, the likelihood increases that benefits may not outweigh the risks inherent in taking ARV medications.

J. Close follow-up for exposed HCP should be provided, including counseling, baseline, and follow-up HIV testing, and monitoring for drug toxicity.

K. If newer fourth-generation combination HIV p24 antigen-HIV antibody test is utilized for follow-up HIV testing of exposed HCP, HIV testing may be concluded 4 months after exposure. If a newer platform is not available, follow-up HIV testing is typically concluded 6 months after an HIV exposure.

Diagnostic Testing

A. Source-patient laboratory studies

1. Rapid HIV (or HIV Ag/Ab). Rapid HIV testing preferred if accessible.

2. *Consider hepatitis panel:* HBsAg (active infection), HBV core antibody immunoglobulin M (HBcAb IgM, window period).

3. Consider rapid plasma reagin (RPR).

4. HCV antibody (HepCAb), or HCV RNA (HCV viral load). Centers for Disease Control and Prevention (CDC) recommends HCV RNA.

B. Exposed-patient laboratory studies

1. In some systems, no immediate lab testing is performed. If no exposure occurred or SP is confirmed negative on baseline testing, no baseline testing is clinically indicated for the exposed person (EP).

2. Testing may be considered for other purposes including medico-legal concerns or as per institutional protocols.

3. In many systems, a standardized baseline laboratory panel is sent in the ED and then followed up at employee health the next day.

4. If giving HIV PEP:

a. Rapid HIV, to confirm EP does not already have HIV

b. Complete blood count (CBC), basic metabolic panel, liver function tests, pregnancy test

5. Most HCP and public safety personnel have been vaccinated against hepatitis B.

a. If EP was previously vaccinated and responded to the vaccination series (a positive titer is ≥10 mIU/mL), individual is considered to have lifelong immunity and requires no further testing or treatment.

Medical Decision-Making/Differential Diagnoses

A. PEP is generally recommended when an exposure to an HIV-positive person has occurred.

B. Additional source person information (e.g., the SP's current or most recent viral load, HIV treatment, history of resistance to HIV medications) can be helpful in PEP decision-making including regimen selection. Initiation of PEP should not be delayed if this information or consultation is not available. Additionally, for an HIV-positive SP who has been durably suppressed on HIV medications, transmission risk to the EP is significantly lowered.

C. PEP is generally not warranted in cases of an SP with unknown HIV status. However, consider PEP for exposures from a source with HIV risk factors. If questions exist, seek expert consultation.

D. In cases of uncertainty of the SP (e.g., sharps box), PEP is generally not warranted. However, consider PEP in settings where exposure to HIV-infected persons is likely.

E. If uncertain whether the exposure constitutes significant risk and expert consultation is not available within a few hours, PEP can be started and then consultation may be obtained at a later time. Note, however, timely and comprehensive assessment is key.

F. *Window period:* If the SP's HIV test is negative at the time of exposure, they are generally considered uninfected and HIV PEP is not recommended. The "window period" for HIV Ab seroconversion can cause patient and clinician anxiety. To date, no transmission to HCP from an SP during the window period has been detected in the United States.

G. If acute HIV is highly suspected, PEP should be started while an HIV RNA polymerase chain reaction (PCR; viral load) is sent for the SP.

H. *Found needle:* Exposure to a sharp device from an unknown source outside the healthcare setting. This common occurrence falls into the classification of exposure to blood/body fluid from an unknown SP. No documented cases of HIV transmission from a "found needle" outside of a healthcare setting in the United States have occurred. Therefore, PEP is generally discouraged.

I. Human bites can result in exposures for both the biter and the bitten person. The bitten sustains a cutaneous exposure to HIV if blood was present in the mouth of the biter before the bite. The biter sustains a mucous membrane exposure to HIV if blood from the bitten person enters the oral cavity of the biter.

1. If the saliva is nonbloody, there is no HIV transmission risk to the bitten. The risk of HBV and HCV transmission from nonbloody saliva is negligible.

Patient Management

A. HIV exposure management

1. Follow evidence-based guidelines when prescribing.

2. Three-drug PEP regimens are recommended for all exposures.

3. No longer required to assess the degree of risk for the purpose of choosing between basic/two-drug regimens versus an expanded/three-drug regime.

4. There are some special circumstances in which a two-drug regimen can be considered. Especially when recommended ARV medications are unavailable, or there is concern about potential toxicity or adherence difficulties.

5. Preferred HIV three-drug occupational PEP regimen. Duration: 28 days.

a. Truvada
b. Coformulated Tenofovir DF (Viread; TDF) + emtricitabine (Emtriva; FTC)
PLUS
c. Raltegravir (Isentress; RAL)
or
d. Dolutegravir (Tivicay)

6. Alternate regimens (Table 2.4).
a. May combine one drug or drug pair from the left column with one pair of nucleoside/nucleotide reverse transcriptase inhibitors from the right column.

7. ARV drug dosing and toxicity monitoring (Table 2.5)

8. PEP is taken for 28 days. If SP testing is negative for HIV, PEP can be stopped before 28 days.

9. Monitoring and side effects of PEP
a. Side effects can be a limiting factor in PEP adherence. Side effects are generally self-limited but sometimes last the duration of the 28-day PEP course.
b. GI side effects are most common. Headache, fatigue, and insomnia are other side effects. Antiemetic and antidiarrheal medications can be prescribed to help with adherence.
c. If side effects are severe, consider changing to a different regimen. Toxicities are rare with the preferred regimen and are generally not life-threatening and are reversible once PEP medications are stopped.
d. The most important side effect of the preferred regimen, tenofovir DF + emtricitabine (Truvada) plus raltegravir, is renal toxicity from tenofovir. This regimen should be used with caution in those with impaired renal function or at high risk for impaired renal function.
e. Laboratory monitoring for drug toxicity: CBC, renal and hepatic function at baseline and 2 weeks after starting PEP.
f. Exposures in pregnant women
i. Starting PEP in pregnant EPs should be based on consideration similar to those of non-pregnant exposed persons.
ii. When deciding to start PEP, a pregnant EP should discuss with the treating clinician the potential risks of exposing her fetus to ARV medications.
iii. All pregnant women initiating ARVs should be entered in the ARV pregnancy registry, a database designed to collect information

TABLE 2.4 ALTERNATE REGIMENS FOR HIV EXPOSURE MANAGEMENT

DRUG OR DRUG PAIR	+	NUCLEOSIDE/NUCLEOTIDE REVERSE TRANSCRIPTASE INHIBITORS
Raltegravir (Isentress: RAL)	+	Tenofovir DF (Viread; TDF) + emtricitabine (Emtriva; FTC); available coformulated as Truvada
Dolutegravir (Tivicay; DTG)		Tenofovir DF (Viread; TDF) + lamivudine (Epivir; 3TC)
Darunavir (Prezista; DRV) + ritonavir (Norvir; RTV)		Zidovudine (Retrovir; ZDV; AZT) + lamivudine (Epivir; 3TC); available coformulated as Combivir
Atazanavir (Reyataz; ATV) + ritonavir (Norvir; RTV)		Zidovudine (Tetrovir; ZDV; AZT) + emtricitabine (Emtriva; FTC)
Lopinavir/ritonavir (Kaletra; LPV/RTV)		
Etravirine (Intelence; ETR)		
Rilpivirine (Edurant; RPV)		

May combine one drug or drug pair from the left column with one pair of nucleoside/nucleotide reverse transcriptase inhibitors from the right column.

TABLE 2.5 ANTIRETROVIRAL DRUG DOSING AND TOXICITY MONITORING

HIV MEDICATION	ADULT DOSING	COMBINATION FORM	TOXICITY MONITORING
Tenofovir disoproxil fumarate (DF)	300 mg PO once daily	Truvada	BUN, creatinine, LFTs
Emtricitabine	200 mg PO once daily		Rash
Raltegravir	400 mg PO once daily		Headache, nausea
Dolutegravir	50 mg PO once daily		Headache, insomnia
Zidovudine	300 mg PO twice daily	Combivir	CBC, LFTs
Lamivudine	150 mg PO twice daily		Rash
Lopinavir/ritonavir	Two tabs PO twice daily	Kaletra	GI toxicity, especially diarrhea. Many drug–drug interactions with common medications; use with caution.

Note: Always consult most recent evidence-based recommendations.
BUN, blood urea nitrogen; CBC, complete blood count; GI, gastrointestinal; LFT, liver function test; PO, orally.

on the outcomes of ARV-exposed pregnancies regardless of HIV status: www.apregistry.com

iv. The pregnant EP and her fetus are at risk for HIV acquisition.

v. Acute HIV in pregnancy incurs a high risk of vertical transmission.

vi. The use of most PEP medications can be justified when the benefits outweigh the risk of infant and maternal exposures to ARVs.

vii. Based on limited data, use of ARVs in pregnancy, including in the first trimester, does not appear to increase the risk of birth defects compared to the general population.

viii. Toxicities of currently recommended PEP medications are not believed to increase in pregnancy.

ix. PEP options in pregnancy (Table 2.6)

g. HIV exposures in lactating persons

i. Breastfeeding is not a contraindication for PEP.

ii. When deciding to start PEP, lactating EPs should discuss with the treating clinician the potential risks and benefits of infant exposure to ARV medications through breastmilk. The decision to take PEP and/or continue breastfeeding is complex and individualized, and expert consultation is recommended.

10. Consultation/collaboration

a. Consultation with the PEPline or a PEP-experienced clinical pharmacist/clinician is advised.

b. National Clinicians' PEP Hotline 1-888-448-4911

B. HBV exposure management

1. SP testing for HBsAg

a. If SP is known to be hepatitis B uninfected, no hepatitis B testing or PEP treatment of the EP is needed

b. If EP is known to be immune (notified of a positive response to a complete HBV vaccine series, postvaccination HBsAb titer ≥10 mIU/mL), they are considered to have lifelong immunity and require no hepatitis B testing or PEP treatment.

2. PEP after HBV exposure (Table 2.7)

3. *Hepatitis B immune globulin (HBIG):* 0.06 mL/kg ASAP. Max dose: 5 mL.

4. HBIG is considered effective up to 1 week after occupational exposures.

C. HCV Exposure Management

1. The risk of HCV transmission after percutaneous exposure is about 1 in 56 (1.8%) when the source person is HCV-infected.

2. There is no PEP currently available/approved for HCV prevention.

3. Table 2.8 summarizes HCV exposure management.

Patient Disposition

A. HIV

1. If SP is HIV negative, no follow-up testing is clinically indicated for the EP.

2. If SP is HIV positive, retest EP for HIV at 6 weeks and at 3 to 4 months.

a. Follow-up testing can be with either a third- or fourth-generation HIV test. Both reliably identify whether HIV infection has occurred, although the fourth-generation HIV Ag/Ab test is preferred for diagnosing acute HIV.

b. A fourth-generation test would not necessarily provide important advantages in postexposure follow-up beyond the first month after an exposure.

c. Follow-up HIV testing is not needed out to 6 months, as final testing at 3 to 4 months is sufficient to identify whether transmission has occurred.

3. Extended HIV testing to 12 months is indicated only for HCP who acquire HCV infection after exposure to HCV–HIV coinfected SP.

4. Symptoms of acute HIV should prompt immediate evaluation.

TABLE 2.6 POSTEXPOSURE PROPHYLAXIS OPTIONS FOR PREGNANT PATIENTS

TENOFOVIR DF/EMTRICITABINE (TRUVADA, TDF/FTC) 1 PO DAILY + RALTEGRAVIR (ISENTRESS, RAL) 400MG PO TWICE DAILY	
Pros **(1)** Well-tolerated **(2)** TDF/FTC and RAL are both preferred agents in treating HIV + pregnant women per DHHS Perinatal Guidelines **(3)** Very low potential for drug–drug interactions	Cons **(1)** Need for twice daily dosing with RAL
or	
Zidovudine/lamivudine (Combivir, also available as generic, AZT/3TC), 1 tab PO twice daily + Darunavir (Prezista, DRV), 800 mg once daily + ritonavir (Norvir, RTV), 100 mg PO daily OR Atazanavir (Reyataz, ATV), 300 PO daily + ritonavir (Norvir, RTV), 100 mg PO daily	
Pros **(1)** Extensive experience with use of AZT/3TC in pregnancy **(2)** Darunavir/ritonavir as well as atazanavir/ritonavir are preferred agents in treating HIV + pregnant women per DHHS Perinatal Guidelines	Cons **(1)** More side effects: nausea, vomiting, diarrhea, headache, fatigue **(2)** AZT associated with hematologic toxicity **(3)** High drug–drug interaction potential with darunavir/ritonavir, atazanavir/ritonavir

Note: Always consult most recent evidence-based recommendations.

3TC, lamivudine; AZT, azidothymidine; DHHS, United States Department of Health and Human Services; FTC, emtricitabine; PO, orally; TDF, tenofovir disoproxil fumarate

TABLE 2.7 POSTEXPOSURE PROPHYLAXIS FOLLOWING HEPATITIS B VIRUS EXPOSURE

EXPOSED PERSON VACCINATION STATUS	TEST RECOMMENDED FOR EXPOSED PERSON	TREATMENT
	Previously Vaccinated	
Responder after complete series (HBsAb ≥10 mLU/mL)	None	No action needed
Response unknown after three doses	HBsAb	If ≥10 mLU/mL: No action needed. If <10 mLU/mL: Check HBcAb (total) as well, administer HBIG × one and revaccinate
Nonresponder (HBsAb < 10 mLU/mL after two series of three doses)	HBcAb (total)	HBIG two one month apart
	Unvaccinated or Incompletely Vaccinated	
Unvaccinated or incompletely vaccinated	HBcAb (total) Follow-up at 6 months: HBcAb (total) and HBsAg	HBIG × one vaccine/revaccinate

Note: HBcAb, hepatitis B core antibody; HBIG, hepatitis B immune globulin; HBsAb, hepatitis B surface antigen.

TABLE 2.8 HEPATITIS C VIRUS EXPOSURE MANAGEMENT

RECOMMENDATION	BASELINE TESTING	INITIAL FOLLOW-UP	FINAL FOLLOW-UP
HCV + SP or SP has potential HCV risk factors	HCV Ab	6 weeks HCV RNA (HCV viral load)	≥6 months HCV Ab

Note: Always consult most recent evidence-based recommendations.
HCV, hepatitis C virus; SP, source person.

B. HBV

1. If SP is HBV negative, no follow-up testing is clinically indicated for the EP

2. Follow-up testing is only necessary for EPs who do not have hepatitis B immunity.

3. Symptoms of acute hepatitis should prompt immediate evaluation.

C. HCV

1. If SP is HCV negative, no follow-up testing is clinically indicated for the EP.

2. Symptoms of acute hepatitis should prompt immediate evaluation.

Counseling

1. HCP who experience occupational exposure to HIV should receive follow-up counseling, postexposure testing, and medical evaluation regardless of whether they take PEP.

2. It is important for HCP to follow-up on HIV PEP within 72 hours of exposure to improve care provided to exposed HCP.

a. Follow-up provides another opportunity for the EP to ask questions and for the counselor to make certain that the EP has a clear understanding of the risks for infection and the risks and benefits of PEP.

b. Ensures continued treatment with PEP is indicated

3. Increases adherence to HIV PEP regimes and manages associated symptoms and side effects more effectively

4. Improves the likelihood of follow-up serologic testing for larger proportion of exposed personnel to detect infection

5. Closer follow-up should in turn reassure EPs who become anxious after these events. The psychological impact of needlesticks or exposure to blood or body fluid should not be underestimated for HCP.

6. EP should be advised to use precautions (e.g., use of barrier contraception and avoidance of blood or tissue donations, pregnancy, and if possible breastfeeding) to prevent secondary transmission, especially during the first 6 to 12 weeks after exposure.

7. Providing HCP with psychological counseling should be an essential component of the management and care of EP.

8. Follow-up appointments should begin within 72 hours of an HIV exposure.

References and Additional Reading

References and Additional Reading for this chapter are online only and can be found at https://connect.springerpub.com/content/reference-book/978-0-8261-6091-5/part/part01/toc-part/ch02.

3. Diagnostic and Therapeutic Procedures

LISA LEONARD

Learning Objectives

- Identify the role of the emergency nurse practitioner (ENP) related to performing procedures in selected patient populations within their scope of practice.
- Identify the components of informed consent.
- Explain how to discuss the need for procedures with patients.
- Describe shared decision-making.
- Identify low-, moderate-, and high-risk procedures.
- Describe what makes procedures more high or low risk.
- Identify the steps needed to minimize procedure risks.
- Describe the Universal Protocol.

According to The Joint Commission, in a survey performed by the National Hospital Medical Ambulatory Care Survey, there were 139 million ED visits in 2017 in the United States. Procedures account for almost half of these visits. The most common procedures performed during these visits included administering IV fluid, splinting fractures, laceration repairs, wound care, incision and drainage of an abscess, foreign body removal, endotracheal intubation, lumbar puncture, central lines, joint reduction, and tube thoracotomy.[1]

An emergency nurse practitioner (ENP) has had additional training in order to perform multiple procedures including complicated ones such as invasive procedures (e.g., central lines, intubation, chest tubes, lumbar puncture, paracentesis), ultrasound, and more straightforward procedures (e.g., suturing, reductions, splinting). This chapter explores what each of these procedures entails as well as the ENP role in performing these procedures, the indications and contraindications for these procedures, and how to consent a patient including emergency consent.[2]

An ENP is a vital clinician in the ED. They can be a part of a physician-led team working in conjunction with the physician team, or they can be a solo clinician in an ED and be the head of the team taking point on all aspects of care of the patient. When working in conjunction with the physician-led team, the ENP can be a useful resource doing time-consuming procedures while allowing the physician to focus on resuscitation and stabilization of more critically ill patients.[2] When an ENP is a solo clinician, they must be proficient in performing these sometimes lifesaving procedures because there is no back up. It is very important that ENPs in this role have sufficient training and be highly skilled clinicians with experience. ENPs have a scope of practice that is based on nationally recognized licensure, education, and certification, with inclusion of specialty educational content. The scope of practice though may be limited by state policies, and organizational, credentialing, and privileging entities.

Informed Consent[4]

A. This is a critical step in the process unless it is an imminent life or death situation

1. Patients should be able to ask questions about any procedure that is about to be performed. It is important that patients be able to make a well-informed decision about the care they are receiving.
2. When informed consent is obtained, there has been effective communication between the clinician and the patient about the procedure to be performed; they understand the risks and benefits of the procedure.
3. If the patient is not capable of providing informed consent, then they may have an assigned proxy or surrogate who is able to make their medical decisions.[4] Per the American Medical Association (AMA), "As a provider we must assess the patient's ability to understand the relevant medical information and the implications of treatment alternatives and to be sure that the patient can make an independent and voluntary decision."

B. The clinician must also present relevant information accurately and sensitively, in keeping with the patient's preferences for receiving medical information. Information that must be provided is the diagnosis if it is known, and the nature and purpose of recommended interventions, and the burdens, risks, and expected benefits of all options including forgoing treatment.[4]

C. Documentation

1. The clinician must document the consent conversation as well as how the consent was obtained. It should be documented if the patient was unable to make their own decisions, including why the patient did not have the capacity to consent, and if a medical surrogate consented for the patient.
2. How the consent was obtained (verbal or written) needs to be in the medical record. If there is an emergent situation that arises where a patient is

incapacitated and unable to make their own decisions, and their surrogate medical decision-maker is not available for consultation, then it is within the clinician's right to initiate emergent lifesaving treatment. As soon as the patient or medical decision-maker is available, the treatment should be discussed with the designated person and consent obtained.[4]

D. Discussion with the patient[5]

1. Clinicians may perform multiple procedures throughout their work shifts. Some procedures have a low risk where other procedures require a higher level of skill and training. These types of procedures will require more explanation prior to proceeding with the procedure.

2. Every time a procedure is performed, it needs to be thoroughly explained to the patient. The explanation should include:

a. Why the procedure is being performed

b. Alternative options to the procedure

c. Risks and benefits

3. The more invasive and risky the procedure is, the more discussion is necessary with the patient or their healthcare proxy. As always in emergent situations, the clinician must act in the best interest of the patient.

4. Ensuring patient understanding[1]

a. Procedures that seem mundane to clinicians may be frightening to the patient and family. Clinicians need to be sure that procedures are explained in a manner that the patient can understand.

b. Many patients who have been interviewed have felt that they were not given a full explanation of what the procedure was, what it entailed, or availability of other options.

c. The clinician performing the procedure needs to be sure that the person discussing and explaining the procedure to the patient is educated about the procedure, its risks, and its possible complications.

5. Health literacy[1]

a. Providing written material when possible can be of help. Discussion with the patient should include an assessment of the inherent risks of the procedure along with the benefits of the procedure. If options are available for a less invasive procedure, these should also be discussed, including the benefit and risk of this route. All discussions with the patient need to be based on their health literacy.

b. If there is a language barrier, a trained interpreter must be used. The patient who is being discharged should have a clear idea related to their follow-up and what signs and symptoms, as well as complications, would indicate a need to be seen back in the ED. All discussions of this nature should be documented in the medical record.

Procedural Risks[1,3,4]

A. There is a difference in risks among procedures. The more invasive and technically complex the procedure, the more risk that is involved.

1. The clinician needs to be aware of the specific risks involved in each procedure and be able to describe these risks to the patient or their healthcare proxy.

2. Table 3.1 summarizes procedures commonly performed in the ED and their associated risk. Some of these procedures carry less risk than the others for both the clinician and the patient.

B. Verbal versus written consent

1. The less risky procedures can normally proceed with verbal consent compared to written consent.

a. Ask the patient or the one providing consent to state they understand and are willing to move forward with the procedure.

2. When obtaining a verbal consent, discuss with the patient or their healthcare proxy the procedure, and the risks and benefits.

a. A written consent form should have a description of the procedure as well as its potential benefits and risks detailed in writing. The patient or their healthcare proxy should sign the consent form as well as a hospital representative such as the nurse or clinician. When the consent is clearly written, this creates a standardized process for moderate- to high-risk procedures as well as a clearly defined document that can be referenced later if needed. Patients need to be informed of the most common risks of the procedure as well as the specific risks they may face.

Determining the Level of Acuity

A. Bucher et al. (2018) determined the most and least commonly performed procedures in the ED by following residency procedures throughout a year in practice.[6]

1. Most commonly performed procedures included ultrasound, adult medical resuscitation, intubation, adult trauma resuscitation, and laceration repair.

2. Least commonly performed procedures included intraosseous access paracentesis, lateral canthotomy, pericardiocentesis, and thoracotomy.

3. For procedures that are not performed often, it is still extremely important to maintain skill sets. This can be achieved in a variety of ways, such as skills labs, procedure conferences, self-study with videos as well as frequent visualization of the procedure.

B. Four questions can help to determine the acuity level of a procedure.

1. What is the risk of procedural complications?

2. What is the risk of poor outcomes from com plications?

3. What are the patient factors augmenting risk?

4. What are the care factors that may augment the risk?

C. The conceptual model of ED procedural safety also addresses what should be done in the case of an emergency exception.[4]

1. *Emergency exception:* Preprocedure checklists and time-outs will be aimed at addressing specific hazards such as verbal confirmation of the side into which the chest tube is being placed.

2. *No emergency exception:* Life and limb are not on the line, and the procedure-specific interventions, checklists, and time-outs should be directed at mitigating all potential hazards.

D. Expert consult

TABLE 3.1 PROCEDURAL RISK LEVEL AND SAFETY CONSIDERATIONS

ED PROCEDURE	GENERAL RISK LEVEL OF PROCEDURE	SPECIFIC SAFETY HAZARD[a]				RECOMMENDATIONS				
		Wrong Patient	Wrong Site	Medication Allergies/ Interactions	Equipment Issues (Inadequate/ Malfunctioning)	Emergency Procedure	Time-Out[b]	Preprocedure Check	Equipment Check by Type of Procedure	Postprocedure Check
Procedural Sedation	High	X		X	X		X	X	X	X
Rapid Sequence and Tracheal Intubation	High			X	X	X	(X)[c]	X	X	X
Cricothyrotomy	High				X	X		X	X	X
Tube Thoracotomy	High	X	X		X		(X)	X	X	X
Thoracentesis	High	X	X		X		(X)	X	X	X
Thoracotomy	High				X	X		X	X	X
Cardioversion	High			X	X	X	(X)	X	X	X
Pericardiocentisis	High				X	X		X	X	X
Pacing										
Transvenous	High				X	X	(X)	X	X	X
Transthoracic	High				X	X	(X)	X	X	X
Vaginal Delivery	High				X	X			X	X
Central IV Access	Medium	X			X		X	X	X	X
Arterial Line	Medium	X			X		X	X	X	X
Aspiration of a Peri-tonsillar Abscess	Medium		X		X		X		X	
G-Tube Replacement	Medium				X					X
IV Placement										
Peripheral	Low	X								
External Jugular	Low	X								
Access Indwelling Port	Low									
Access AV Fistula	Low									
Anesthesia Blocks										
Local	Low	X		X						

(continued)

TABLE 3.1 PROCEDURAL RISK LEVEL AND SAFETY CONSIDERATIONS (*CONTINUED*)

ED PROCEDURE	GENERAL RISK LEVEL OF PROCEDURE	SPECIFIC SAFETY HAZARD[a]				RECOMMENDATIONS				
		Wrong Patient	Wrong Site	Medication Allergies/ Interactions	Equipment Issues (Inadequate/ Malfunctioning)	Emergency Procedure	Time-Out[b]	Preprocedure Check	Equipment Check by Type of Procedure	Postprocedure Check
Regional	Low	X	X	X			X			
Suture Laceration	Low				X				X	
I&D Abscess	Low				X			X	X	
Fracture Reduction	Low									X
Joint Reduction	Low									X
Arthrocentesis	Low		X				X			
Splint Placement	Low		X						X	X
Removal of Foreign Body	Low									
Skin/Subcutaneous	Low									X
Ear/Nose/Mouth	Low				X				X	X
Eye	Low				X				X	X
Lumbar Puncture	Low	X			X		X		X	X
Urinary Catheter	Low	X								X
Nasogastric Tube	Low	X								X
Nasopharyngoscopy	Low				X				X	
Epistaxis Control	Low				X	X			X	
Hernia Reduction	Low									

AV, arteriovenous; I&D, incision and drainage; IV, intravenous.

a. Safety hazard implies specific safety hazards and risks, not general medical and surgical complications from the procedure.

b. **Time-out involves preprocedure verification of patient, procedure, and site.

c. Parentheses indicate a semi-elective procedure.

Source: Reproduced with permission from Pines JM, Kelly JJ, Meisl H, et al. Procedural safety in emergency care: A conceptual model and recommendations. *Jt Comm J Qual Patient Saf.* 2012;38(11):AP1. https://www.jointcommissionjournal.com/article/S1553-7250(12)38069-0/fulltexthttps://www.elsevier.com/__data/promis_misc/JCJQPSPines.pdf

1. The scope of emergency medicine is extremely broad, and clinicians in the ED can be faced with any kind of medical emergency at any time.
2. For a procedure not routinely performed (e.g., having OBGYN along with a NICU team present for an emergency postmortem C-section), expert consult should always be utilized when immediately available.

Universal Protocol[4]

A. The Universal Protocol went into effect on July 1, 2004, for all hospitals including the ED, ambulatory care, and office-based surgical facilities that are accredited by The Joint Commission.[4]

B. There are three main principles to the Universal Protocol, including:

1. A preprocedure verification process
2. Marking the procedure site
3. Performing a time-out before the procedure
   a. The results of these processes have been shown to reduce equipment problems and lower the rates of wrong site surgical procedures.
   b. It has also improved the confirmation of patient allergies as well as the availability of blood products.
   c. In 2009, the Universal Protocol was broadened and revised to include all invasive procedures that put patients at a more-than-minimal risk—regardless of the location within an organization—to include all surgical and nonsurgical invasive procedures.
   d. In 2010, The Joint Commission surveyed hospitals showed the updated protocols to be beneficial by 94% of operating room (OR) respondents, 93% of ambulatory surgery respondents, and 90% in hospital units where invasive procedures were performed.[4]

C. *Emergency exception:* An emergency exception can be made to the Universal Protocol when a patient presents with a severe and imminent life-threatening illness or injury. If there is an immediate need, and that need is not met as quickly as possible, then the patient may have adverse outcome or even death.

1. Situations that may arise in the ED may include the patient in severe respiratory distress, needle decompression of a tension pneumothorax, limb-threatening trauma with ischemia requiring immediate reduction and splinting, or defibrillation for cardiac arrest.
   a. Although these are life-threatening emergencies, and all protocols may not be followed during this time, the risk for error (e.g., placing a chest tube on the wrong side) is increased. It is always helpful to try and take a pause prior to performing any procedure to verify the right site as a team; however, emergency exceptions are in place so as to not delay the delivery of care by going through a checklist of steps prior to performing a procedure.

D. Preparation

1. Due to the nature of patients coming into the ED with life-threatening illnesses, there are steps that can be taken to ensure equipment and clinicians are ready at a moment's notice.
   a. Rounding and making sure code carts, airway boxes, and trauma rooms are stocked appropriately, and that all staff is trained regarding the location of items, will reduce equipment issues.

BOX 3.1 STRATEGIES FOR RISK REDUCTION IN THE ED SETTING

- Training
  - Ensures the healthcare team is skilled; maintains proficiency in current practices and standards of care
- Equipment
  - Ultrasound-guided IV or central line placement can have decreased risk and lower rates of complication
- Simulation
  - Ensures equipment, staff, and protocols are in place when higher risk situations arise
  - Increases procedural skills

E. All team members should be trained and maintain competence in procedures, techniques, and protocols. Verification methods following performance of a procedure may include a chest x-ray (CXR) after an intubation, central line, or chest tube placement.

F. Risk reduction

1. Risk reduction can be achieved via various additional training strategies, as summarized in Box 3.1.

Shared Decision-Making

A. Shared decision-making is described as "an approach where clinicians and patients share the best available evidence when faced with the task of making decisions, and where patients are supported to consider options, to achieve informed preferences."[7] Shared decision-making allows the patient to help guide their care, and sometimes results in patients not making the decision recommended by the healthcare agent.

1. This leads to doubt among clinicians who believe that patients may make poor decisions, or that patients do not truly wish to have a decision-making role in their care.
2. Other clinicians believe they already perform shared decision-making; however, patient surveys indicate that patients do not necessarily feel they are being included in the decision-making process.
3. When performing shared decision-making, the clinician needs to summarize the problem and propose choices and steps that can be taken. It is the clinician's responsibility to fully explain—at a level the patient can understand—the treatment options; the risks and benefits of procedures, assessment, and diagnostic tests; the clinician recommendation as the best course of treatment; and why it is recommended.
4. After the discussion, the patient should be able to agree with the plan as recommended or may choose not to. The clinician will need to provide alternate

options and also fully explain the risks involved in not following the recommended treatment course.

Procedural Risk Level and Safety Considerations

A. Table 3.1 summarizes procedural risk level and specific safety hazards associated with key ED procedures.

B. Low-risk procedures

1. In stable awake patients, risk is low as there is lower chance of procedural mistakes (e.g., wrong site, medication allergies, wrong procedure).

2. Appropriate to have a verbal conversation with the patient or their healthcare proxy and obtain verbal consent to the procedure.

3. As the clinician, you should explain the benefits of the procedure, risks, and potential side effects. You also need to discuss what follow-up may be needed after the procedure.

4. Examples of low-risk procedures include a simple laceration repair or an incision and drainage. These are obvious pathologies; patients are generally awake and able to speak with you about history and allergies. It also makes it difficult to have the wrong site because the injury, and thus where to perform the procedure, can be visualized. Preprocedure checklists can be helpful even with simple procedures to be sure all the equipment is available and brought to the room.

C. Medium-risk procedures

1. Medium-risk procedures are procedures that have more inherent risk of harm but are commonly performed. When able, the clinician needs to have a verbal conversation with the patient, explaining the risks, the benefits, alternatives to the procedures, and risk of infection. A written informed consent should be obtained from the patient or their healthcare proxy.

2. An example of a medium-risk procedure is a central line. When performing the central line, a patient may or may not be conscious, which increases the risk of wrong patient. Utilization of tools such as ultrasound help to improve the safety of the procedure. Proper training of the personnel performing the procedure is critical, and staying up to date on these procedures is also important. There are also increased risks of this procedure, such as hitting an artery or causing a tension pneumothorax. If a procedure is not performed frequently, staff may not know where equipment is located, or it may be missing from the department. This may lead to a delay in the patient care or cause the procedure to not be able to be performed. Having checklists in place and ensuring all tools and supplies are readily available are important in helping the workflow of the ED, and increasing the safety for both the clinician and the department.

High-Risk Procedures

A. High-risk procedures are complicated procedures that require a great deal of training, and sometimes are specialized. Some high-risk procedures are very infrequently performed, and therefore it can be difficult to maintain appropriate proficiency. If appropriate consults are available to help perform specialized procedures, these resources should be utilized.

B. An example of a high-risk procedure frequently performed in the ED is placing a tube thoracotomy. This can be very high risk if a patient is unconscious, as they are not able to verify their information and increases the risk of wrong patient. There may not be an obvious pathology to indicate site of procedure. The equipment required to successfully perform the procedure may be missing or unavailable (e.g., correct tubes, scalpel, hemostat). This is a procedure that frequently falls into the category of an emergency exception, and Universal Protocol may be deferred. Even in a life-threatening emergency such as a tension pneumothorax, a brief time-out should be performed to verify the correct side with everyone in the room. After the procedure is performed, a brief time-out should also be performed to check equipment is working properly and to obtain a chest x-ray (CXR) to verify proper placement.

C. High-risk procedures may require equipment that is infrequently utilized, so it is important that checklists be in place that are rounded on daily to be sure equipment is properly stocked and available at all times. Staff should also know to replace used equipment as soon as possible to ensure it is available for the next emergency. For procedures that may be infrequently performed, staff should maintain training through simulation, self-guided learning with videos, or procedure conferences in order to maintain proficiency.

References

References for this chapter are online only and can be found at https://connect.springerpub.com/content/reference-book/978-0-8261-6091-5/part/part01/toc-part/ch03.

4. Evidence-Based Research and Publication

DIAN DOWLING EVANS | KAREN SUE HOYT | JENNIFER WILBECK

Learning Objectives

- Define the research process as it relates to advancing the emergency nurse practitioner (ENP) role and profession.
- Describe how research is applied to determine the best evidence to guide clinical practice and tailor patient treatment to achieve optimal outcomes.
- Identify appropriate research methods and processes, including the ethical conduct of research to answer clinical questions.
- Discuss how to select a quality journal for publication.
- Understand the key components for a successful publication.

Inherent in the emergency nurse practitioner (ENP) role is engagement in continuous evolution of the specialty to reflect changing population health needs and healthcare delivery trends. This evolution ensures that emergency care and clinician roles are data-driven and consistent with scientifically derived best practices. Specialty practice, as described within the Consensus Model for APRN Practice, is unique and adds depth of knowledge and competency within a population foci to align with changing workforce needs and trends.[1] Therefore, it is imperative that ENPs understand the research principles of evidence-based research to incorporate new knowledge into practice.

A. *The research process:* Research is a process of systematic inquiry: a question exists, investigation occurs, and conclusions are reached. Nursing research and evidence-based practice (EBP) are an integral aspect of emergency nursing practice. Research is essential to ensure that the care provided to patients will result in safe and optimal clinical outcomes. Using EBP, the ENP considers what is known about a specific clinical condition or circumstance, evaluates the evidence, and derives best practices from the interpretations. Research outcomes are also used to develop and evaluate educational programs, to develop health policy, and to adapt nursing roles.

B. *Embedding research within nurse practitioner (NP) education:* Schools of nursing, consistent with the American Association of Colleges of Nursing's (AACN) master's and doctorate of nursing practice *Essentials,* delineate the core educational outcomes for the NP role across educational levels from baccalaureate to doctorate with research competencies designed to align with increasing levels of education and practice expertise.[2,3] Research activities are integrated into ENP master's nursing programs to familiarize students with the research process to prepare them to lead changes to improve quality outcomes, design innovative nursing practices, and translate evidence into practice.[3(p3–4)] Master's-educated ENPs are prepared to participate as active research team members; assume the role of clinical expert collaborating with experienced investigators in proposal development, data collection, data analysis, and interpretation; appraise the clinical relevance of research findings; create a climate in the practice setting that supports scholarly inquiry, scientific integrity, and scientific investigation of clinical nursing problems; and provide leadership for integrating findings in clinical nursing practice.[3]

Research competencies are differentiated for ENPs preparing at the doctoral level. Research-focused programs granting the PhD prepare ENPs as nurse scientists. This preparation emphasizes development of theory to guide investigation, gaining proficiency in research methodology and statistics to generate new knowledge, and competency in obtaining funding to support research activity and dissemination of findings.[2] In contrast, ENPs preparing at the doctorate of nursing practice (DNP) level focus on application of evidence-based findings to improve health system processes and outcomes and in translation of research to practice to improve patient clinical outcomes using program evaluation and quality improvement (QI) methodologies.[4,5]

For example, a PhD ENP may conduct field research using statistical analysis and hypothesis testing to examine the effects of heat stress on biomarkers to better understand the physiology of heat illness to improve treatment. A DNP/ENP might take the findings from the heat stress study to evaluate and compare clinical outcomes among patients receiving different approaches for reversing adverse effects of heat stress to determine best EBPs. A master's-prepared ENP may lead the implementation of novel evidence-based treatment approaches for heat stress, while the ENP educator will design curricula using research-derived evidence to ensure ENP students are able to recognize signs of heat stress, prioritize care, and order appropriate evidence-based treatments to improve patient outcomes.

C. *Basic research curricula for ENPs:* Regardless of level of education, all ENPs require a fundamental understanding of the research process and methods, study design, and how research is interpreted and applied to practice.[5] ENPs also need basic skills in conducting a literature search to locate reliable sources of evidence as well as skill in evaluating and critiquing research findings and appraising levels of evidence.

D. *Overview of EBP*

1. *Definition of EBP:* "The integration of best research evidence with clinical expertise and patient values and circumstances."[6(p1)]

2. *The research process:*

a. The basic steps in conducting any type of research proceeds with a question or understanding of a concept of interest.[7,8]

i. Conduct a concept analysis to identify a phenomenon of interest.

ii. Conduct a literature review, searching valid scientific databases (e.g., PubMed, CINAHL, Web of Science) to understand the state of the science and to identify knowledge gaps related to the concept.

iii. Develop a research question or problem statement based on a systematic review of the literature (e.g., PICO pneumonic: **P,** population; **I,** intervention; **C,** comparison; **O,** outcomes).

iv. Collect the most relevant and best evidence.

v. Evaluate research findings for bias, quality, and levels of evidence.

vi. Develop hypotheses or study aims.

vii. Select the appropriate research design and sample population.

viii. Determine the most appropriate methods of data collection and analysis.

ix. Conduct the study, analyze, and interpret results or evaluate the practice decision or change.

x. Disseminate study conclusions.

xi. Integrate evidence into practice.

3. *The DNP project process:*

a. The DNP EBP project incorporates many of the steps involved in basic clinical research with key differences related to incorporating stakeholder involvement related to feasibility and sustainability.[9] The EBP project framework includes the following:

i. Background and evidence for the problem based on external evidence and gap analysis

ii. Description of evidence-based intervention including benchmark and rationale and critique, rating, and grading of intervention evidence

iii. PICO question or EBP question

iv. Project plan process, including tasks and activities, timeline, key stakeholders, target population, communication plan, evaluation methods, project costs and savings, and sustainability

v. Evaluation results addressing all aspects of the project plan

vi. Conclusions including cost/benefit analysis and sustainability

vii. Implications for clinical practice and future study

E. *Research methodologies*

The selection of a specific research approach depends on the study questions and purpose. Approaches are categorized as follows:

1. *Quantitative nonexperimental design*

a. Variables are examined and compared, but the investigator does not introduce an intervention or manipulate variables of interest.[7,8] Nonexperimental designs include the following:

i. Descriptive studies

ii. Correlational

iii. Predictive versus explanatory

iv. Cross-sectional

v. Case-control

vi. Cohort

vii. Repeated measures

viii. Secondary data analysis

ix. Big data analysis

x. Meta-analysis

2. *Quantitative experimental/quasi-experimental designs*

a. Studies in which the researcher introduces and examines the effects of an intervention on variables of interest and uses statistical analysis and deductive reasoning to interpret results.[7,8] These designs are classified as experimental or quasi-experimental.

b. Experimental designs include randomization in sampling and assignment to comparison groups to test cause and effect relationships between study variables.

i. Randomized controlled trials

ii. Clinical trials

iii. Comparative effectiveness trials

c. Quasi-experimental designs involve manipulation of variables but without randomization or comparison/control groups.

i. Observational pre–post design

3. *Qualitative research*

a. Purpose is to understand how individuals or groups experience or assign meaning to a phenomenon or variable of interest. Qualitative research methods are tied to philosophical interpretive frameworks that are used to explain research findings.[10,11] Qualitative methodologies include:

i. Narrative

ii. Case study

iii. Grounded theory

iv. Phenomenology

v. Ethnography

vi. Interpretive frameworks include postpositivism, social constructivism, feminist theories, critical theory and critical race theory, queer theory, disability theory, transformative frameworks, pragmatism, and postmodern perspectives.[10]

4. *Mixed methods*
   a. A study design that integrates both qualitative and quantitative data in the interpretation of results providing contextual meaning to statistical results.
5. *Systematic reviews*
   a. This type of study involves using a reproducible database's search and selection criteria to examine existing research evidence, to appraise the evidence's quality and risk of bias, and synthesize the findings to answer a specific research question.[12]
   b. Because a systematic review uses a systematic and reproducible approach to examine high-quality studies the findings from these reviews are considered to provide reliable evidence related to the topic of interest. The Cochrane Reviews are an example of a systematic review synthesis.
6. *Meta-analysis*
   a. A meta-analysis is a type of systematic review that uses statistical methods to pool and integrate the statistical results from a group of individual randomized controlled trials. Meta-analysis investigations are considered to have the highest level of clinical evidence.[13]
7. *QI and patient safety methods*
   a. These studies employ data-based process improvement approaches to improve clinical or systems outcomes.[9] Examples of QI and patient safety methods include the following:
      i. Plan-Do-Check-Act cycle, Lean, or Six Sigma
      ii. Choosing Wisely
      iii. Quality Measures-Agency for Healthcare Research and Quality
      iv. National Quality Forum[14]
8. *Program evaluation*
   a. This approach examines the results of evidence-based interventions on variables of interest and may incorporate QI or quasi-experimental research methods.

F. *Appraising research:*

To evaluate the quality of evidence-based research, an ENP needs to understand how to evaluate a research study for quality and level of evidence so that the findings can be used to inform practice change. Polit and Beck[8] suggest the following components for critiquing research:

1. *Title*
   a. Related to the content of the study
2. *Abstract*
   a. Briefly summarizes the background, purpose, methods, data analysis, findings, and conclusions
3. *Problem statement/purpose*
   a. Specific, clear, and concise
4. *Review of the literature*
   a. Reviews information relevant to the problem and purpose of the study, is logically organized and analyzed, and concludes with a summary and implications for the purpose of the study.
5. *Theoretical/conceptual framework*
   a. May or may not be included. If so, it should be relevant to the research topic, providing a context or framework for interpretation of results.
6. *Study aims/hypotheses/questions*
   a. Each question or hypothesis describes relationships between the study variables that will be examined or tested.
7. *Methods*
   a. Includes a description of the type of study design; how subjects will be sampled, including inclusion/exclusion; describes study procedures/interventions, includes descriptions of data collection procedures, the instruments or tools used to measure variables of interest, and methods for data analysis.
8. *Results*
   a. Results are clearly presented and described; tables and figures are concise.
9. *Discussion*
   a. Results are discussed in the context of existing literature, methodologic problems and limitations, interpretation and conclusions drawn from data analysis, and implications for clinical practice and/or further study as appropriate and feasible.

G. *Components of evaluating research:*

1. *Evaluating the ethics of research*
   a. Evaluating whether the research study was legal, feasible, and conducted ethically with appropriate protection of human subjects. Indicators may include:
      i. Collaborative Institutional Training Initiative (CITI) human subject training
      ii. Institutional review board approval
      iii. Informed consent
      iv. Subject rights to be maintained while participating in a research study
      v. Treatment of vulnerable populations
      vi. Types of and methods for reducing bias in research
2. *Evaluating levels of evidence*
   a. Figure 4.1 depicts the levels of evidence, with the strongest level of evidence being meta-analysis and systematic reviews of randomized controlled trials. The lowest level of evidence is expert opinion/consensus statements.
3. *Evaluating clinical recommendations*
   a. Examines how evidence is graded and used to develop evidence-based clinical guidelines for application to practice settings for process and QI and patient safety. If an outcome of a research investigation, do the findings present new evidence for practice change?
      i. Clinical practice guidelines: AHRQ and professional organizations
      ii. *GRADE* (Grading of Recommendations, Assessment, Development, and Evaluations) framework provides a systematic approach for evaluating clinical practice recommendations.[15]

H. *Role of the ENP in evidence-based research*

1. *Exemplars of how research has been used to inform the ENP role, education, regulation, certification, and policy*
   a. The ENP role[16,17]
   b. ENP scope and standards of practice[18]
   c. ENP competency development[19,20]

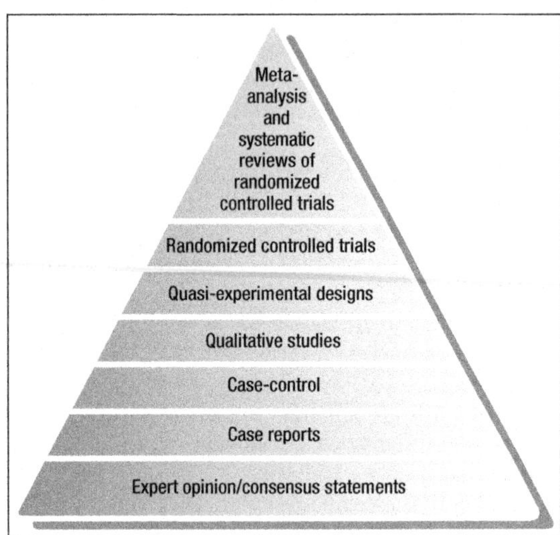

FIGURE 4.1 Levels of evidence. Meta-analysis and systemic reviews of randomized controlled trials represent the highest level of evidence, followed by randomized controlled trials, quasi-experimental designs, qualitative studies, case-control, case reports, with expert opinion/consensus statements representing the lowest level of evidence.

   d. ENP certification examination development[21]
   e. ENP curricular standards[22]
   f. ENP care outcomes research[23]
2. *Future research initiatives for the ENP may include:*
   a. Re-evaluating ENP scope and standards of practice
   b. Analyzing workforce trends for relevancy of practice and role adaptation
   c. Assessing ENP clinical care outcomes
   d. Evaluating validity of ENP competency assessment measures
   e. Evaluating ENP program outcomes consistent with workforce and practice trends
   f. Generating new knowledge related to emergency care

I. *Publication*
1. *Choosing the right journal*
   a. Aims and scope
   b. Prestige and visibility
   c. Review and publication process
2. *Choosing the right publication*
   a. Audience
   b. Impact factor
   c. Journal circulation
   d. National/international
   e. PubMed indexing
   f. Ovid/CINAHL usage
   g. Article views
   h. Sessions
3. *Journals frequently used for ENP-focused manuscripts*
   a. Send a query letter to determine if the journal editor is interested in your manuscript; review the past five years of previous articles on your topic in that journal.
   b. See Table 4.1 for a summary of ENP-focused journals.
   c. See the Comprehensive List of Nursing Journals at nursingschool.org/ultimate-list-of-nursing-journals/
4. *Understanding publication terminology*
   a. *Manuscript:* Term used until your article is published.
   b. *Page proofs:* Also *galley proofs*, the process of locating any mistakes in spelling or in text composition prior to publication.
   c. *Editorial management systems:* Manuscript submissions are done through a submission service on a website (e.g., Editorial Manager).
   d. Open access
      i. *Gold open access:* Available to anyone on the internet without any subscription fees or sign-in (e.g., author pays a fee, usually holds copyright).
      ii. *Green open access:* Self–archiving (e.g., free copy of an electronic document post by an author); near-final version is called a post-print.
      iii. *Hybrid open access:* Mixture of open and closed access.
   e. Predatory journal typical practices
      i. Rapid, minimal review process (e.g., 1–2 days)
      ii. Acceptance for publication includes a fee
      iii. Loosely assembled editorial board
      iv. Near-copycat of legitimate journal titles
5. *Top 10 avoidable mistakes as an author*
   a. https://nursingeditors.com/2017/03/29/top-10-avoidable-mistakes-as-an-author/[24]

TABLE 4.1 SUMMARY OF EMERGENCY NURSE PRACTITIONER-FOCUSED JOURNALS

NAME OF JOURNAL	JOURNAL CHARACTERISTICS
Advanced Emergency Nursing Journal (AENJ)	Published 4 times per year (quarterly) Peer-reviewed Practical information for APRNs/ENPs to integrate into clinical care and implement system changes
Journal of American Association of Nurse Practitioners (JAANP)	Published monthly Peer-reviewed Addresses NP clinical practice, clinical management, health policy, research, education, and other issues affecting NPs
Journal for Nurse Practitioners (JNP)	Published 10 times per year Peer-reviewed Provides a resource to NPs regarding clinical and policy concerns affecting NP practice

i. Ignoring the journal's instructions for authors
ii. Presenting inconsistent data
iii. Ignoring a journal's reference citation policy
iv. Revealing participant identity
v. Presenting exaggerated conclusions
vi. Making punctuation and style errors
vii. Leaving footnotes unexplained
viii. Submitting incomplete or incorrectly filled out forms
ix. Engaging in duplicate submission
x. Not understanding the copyeditor's changes

b. Note each journal has specific instructions and guidelines for submitting manuscripts.

6. *Reasons why journals reject manuscripts*
   a. Mismatch with journal's scope
   b. Lack of originality/significance
   c. Flaws in study design/poorly formulated research question
   d. Poor writing and organization
   e. Language and spelling issues
   f. Poorly presented visual elements
   g. Unintentional ethical issues
   h. Lack of adherence to journal submission guidelines
7. *Ethical and legal considerations*
   a. A submitted manuscript:
      i. Is an original contribution not previously published (except as an abstract or a preliminary report)
      ii. Must not be under consideration for publication elsewhere
      iii. If accepted, must not be published elsewhere in similar form/any language, without journal consent
      iv. Does not pose conflict of interest
      v. Honors patient anonymity and informed consent
      vi. Adheres to copyright/copyright transfer agreement
      vii. Complies with research funding agencies (e.g., National Institutes of Health)
8. *Scholarly collaboration networks*
   a. Sites provide tools for scientific social networking and researcher workflow; generally are free services related to common tasks
      i. Group sharing of research materials (e.g., CVs, bibliographies, article links, drafts)
      ii. Interaction with potential collaborators
      iii. Dashboards (e.g., Mendeley, Academia.edu, ResearchGate, SSRN)
9. *Editorial services*
   a. Discovery services
   b. Citation sharing services
   c. Peer-review sharing
   d. Data mining and collation
   e. Artificial intelligence
10. *Manuscript preparation and submission*
   a. Manuscripts are submitted online through a website.
   b. QI/Process Improvement Projects: See squire-statement.org/guidelines for specific information.
   c. Use plagiarism software prior to submission (e.g., iThenticate).
11. *Typical manuscript contents*
   a. Title
   b. Author name(s)
   c. Author biography
   d. Acknowledgments, credits, or disclaimers
   e. Abstract
   f. *Keywords:* include the most relevant keywords to find your paper
   g. Disclosure of funding received for this work
   h. Copyright transfer agreement
   i. Written permission for any borrowed text, tables, or figures
12. *Manuscript text*
   a. No identifying author information
   b. Use generic medication names followed by trade names in parentheses
   c. Cite values (e.g., weight and temperature in both metric and nonmetric terms)
   d. Avoid error-prone abbreviations by consulting the Institute for Safe Medicine Practices website www.ismp.org/Tools/errorproneabbreviations.pdf
   e. *Abbreviations:* Write out the full term for each abbreviation at its first use unless it is a standard unit of measure. See www.ismp.org/Tools/errorproneabbreviations.pdf
   f. References (use style dictated by journal [e.g., seventh edition of the *Publication Manual of the American Psychological Association*])
   g. Illustrations
   h. Digital artwork
   i. Figures
   j. Captions
   k. Tables
13. *Manuscript review process*
   a. Articles should not previously have been published.
   b. Manuscripts are reviewed (e.g., blind reviewed, peer reviewed) for concise, logical flow of ideas, content accuracy, and consistency with journal purpose.
   c. Evaluation and comments are sent to the editor for final decision.
   d. If chosen, reviewer comments and editor's summary, indicating the editor's evaluation of the article, are returned to the author.
14. *After acceptance*
   a. Page proofs and corrections made.
   b. *Reprints:* Authors will usually be provided a reprint order form from the publisher.
   c. Manuscript becomes an article and is published according to each journal's timeline.

References

References for this chapter are online only and can be found at https://connect.springerpub.com/content/reference-book/978-0-8261-6091-5/part/part01/toc-part/ch04.

5. Clinical Decision-Making

BRADLEY GOETTL

Learning Objectives

- Apply the diagnostic process when evaluating and treating a patient seeking emergency care.
- Effectively gather and organize clinical information that allows the clinician to recognize patterns and diagnostic cues.
- Develop and prioritize a differential diagnosis that is patient-specific and prevents diagnostic error.
- Use an evidence-based approach when ordering diagnostic tests and prescribing treatment.
- Incorporate evidence-based references and decision-making tools into the diagnostic process.
- Integrate shared decision-making to make the diagnostic process patient centric.
- Effectively document medical decision-making that describes the diagnostic process and complexity of care provided.
- Standardized the handoff and disposition process to provide safe transitions of care.
- Recognize cognitive biases and implement strategies to prevent diagnostic error.

The Committee on Diagnostic Error in Health Care[1] describes the diagnostic process as a collaborative and patient-centric activity that includes gathering information, analyzing data, and making medical decisions (Figure 5.1). This cyclical process is used by emergency nurse practitioners (ENPs), during every patient encounter, to diagnose correctly, prescribe treatment, and make appropriate patient dispositions. The ENP should use this standardized approach to prevent cognitive bias and diagnostic error.

Gathering and Organizing Clinical Information

While obtaining the history and performing the physical examination, the ENP will recognize patterns and pick up on diagnostic cues. Obtaining a clinical history is the first step in determining the etiology of a patient's complaint. A thorough clinical history will guide and improve the value of the physical examination. Signs, symptoms, and presentations will help determine acuity (Table 5.1). The information

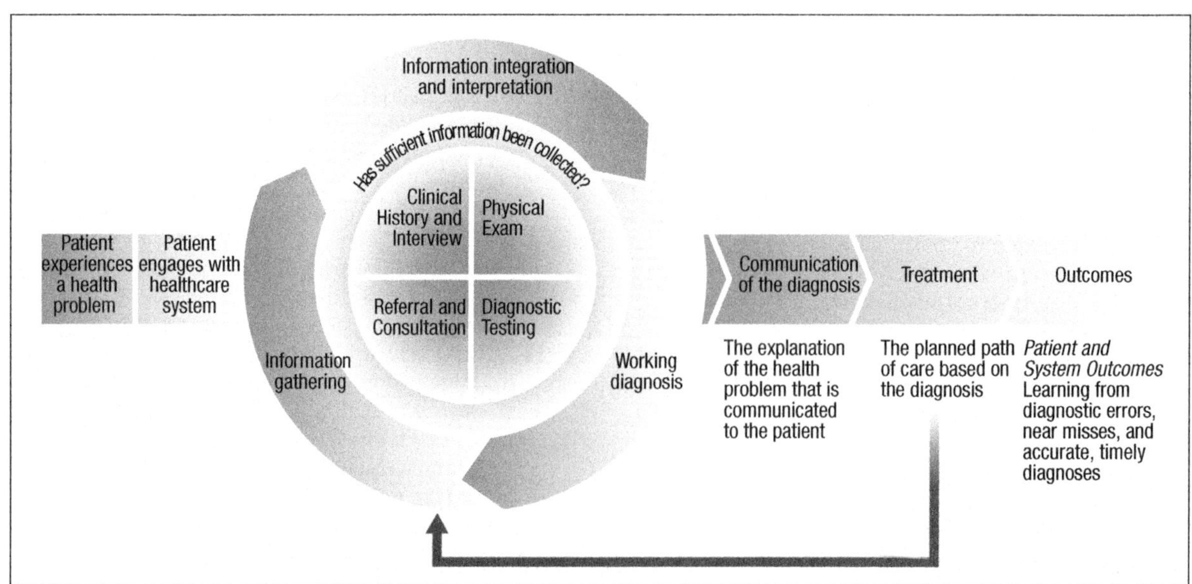

FIGURE 5.1 The diagnostic process.
Source: From National Academies of Sciences, Engineering, and Medicine. Improving diagnosis in health care. The National Academies Press; 2015. Reprinted with permission.[2]

TABLE 5.1 SIGNS, SYMPTOMS, AND PRESENTATIONS

SIGNS, SYMPTOMS, PRESENTATIONS	CRITICAL	EMERGENT	LOWER ACUITY
Abnormal Vital Signs			
Hypothermia	X	X	X
Fever	X	X	X
Bradycardia	X	X	X
Tachycardia	X	X	
Bradypnea/Apnea	X	X	
Tachypnea	X	X	
Hypoxia	X	X	
Hypotension	X	X	
Hypertension	X	X	X
Pain			
Unspecified	X	X	X
Headache	X	X	X
Eye pain		X	X
Chest pain	X	X	X
Abdominal pain	X	X	X
Pelvic pain	X	X	X
Back pain	X	X	X
Chronic pain			X
Extremity pain	X	X	X
Other Symptoms			
Altered mental status	X	X	X
Anuria		X	
Anxiety		X	X
Ascites		X	X
Ataxia		X	X
Auditory disturbances			X
Bleeding	X	X	X
Congestion/rhinorrhea			X
Constipation			X
Cough		X	X
Crying/fussiness		X	X
Cyanosis	X		
Dehydration	X	X	
Diarrhea		X	X
Dysmenorrhea			X
Dysphagia		X	X
Dysuria			X
Edema		X	X
Failure to thrive		X	X
Fatigue/malaise		X	X
Feeding problems			X
Hematemesis	X	X	
Hematuria		X	X
Hemoptysis	X	X	
Hiccup			X
Jaundice		X	
Joint swelling		X	X
Lethargy	X	X	X
Lightheadedness/dizziness		X	X
Limp		X	X
Lymphadenopathy			X
Mechanical and indwelling devices, complications (e.g., left ventricular assist device [LVAD])	X	X	X
Nausea/vomiting		X	X
Occupational exposure		X	X
Palpitations	X	X	X
Paralysis	X	X	
Paresthesia/dysesthesia		X	X
Poisoning	X	X	X
Pruritus		X	X
Rash	X	X	X
Rectal bleeding	X	X	X
Shock	X		
Shortness of breath	X	X	
Sore throat		X	X
Stridor	X	X	
Syncope	X	X	X
Tinnitus			X
Tremor		X	X
Urinary incontinence			X
Urinary retention		X	
Vaginal bleeding	X	X	X
Vaginal discharge			X
Vertigo		X	X
Visual disturbances	X	X	X
Weakness		X	X
Wheezing	X	X	
Toxidromes	X	X	X
Sudden unexpected infant death	X		

Source: From Counselman FL, Babu K, Edens MA, et al. The 2016 model of the clinical practice of emergency medicine. *J Emerg Med.* 2017;52(6):846–849. https://doi.org/10.1016/j.jemermed.2017.01.040. Reprinted with permission.[3]

gathered will provide a foundation for the diagnostic process and help guide diagnostic testing and decision-making.

Clinical History

A. Chief complaint (CC)

  1. The CC is a brief statement that indicates why the patient is seeking medical attention.

B. History of present illness (HPI)

  1. The HPI is a detailed description and timeline of the patient's symptoms.

   a. Location
   b. Radiation/migration
   c. Quality
   d. Severity
   e. Duration
   f. Timing
   g. Context
   h. Modifying/aggravating factors
   i. Associated signs and symptoms

C. Review of systems (ROS)

  1. The ROS is an inventory of body systems. The purpose of the ROS is to identify any signs and/or symptoms that the patient may be experiencing. The ROS should include both pertinent positive and negative findings. A negative finding can be as important as a positive finding. Negative findings will help rule out some suspected problems.

D. Past, family, and/or social history (PFSH)

Physical Examination

A. In emergency medicine, a physical examination can range from focused to comprehensive.

B. *Focused physical assessment:* Specific assessment focused on the patient's system or systems involved in the patient's problem.

C. Comprehensive physical assessment includes evaluating not only the specific problem but what other systems are or will affect the patient's physical problem or problems.

D. The extent of the physical examination is often dictated by the patient's complaint and clinical history.

E. The assessment begins by observing the general appearance of the patient, obtaining vital signs, and identifying any immediate life threats.

F. The remainder of the physical examination should be done systematically and must include observing, palpating, percussing, and auscultation.

Differential Diagnoses

A. Usually, there are multiple diagnoses that could match a patient's CC. Developing and documenting a differential diagnosis, or list of potential diagnoses, is essential and proves that the clinician has considered potential and life-threatening causes for the patient's condition. Anatomical and physiologic causes should be considered.

B. Mnemonics and differential diagnosis generators can help ensure that possible physiologic processes are considered (Table 5.2).

C. The differential is an evolving list of diagnostic considerations. The initial differential is often broad and made with limited information. After obtaining a clinical history and performing a physical exam, the differential can be narrowed to become more patient specific. As more information is obtained, the ENP can prioritize the list of potential diagnoses (Table 5.3).

TABLE 5.2 EXAMPLES OF MNEMONICS THAT CAN BE USED TO HELP DEVELOP A DIFFERENTIAL DIAGNOSIS

GENERAL SYSTEMS	
VINDICATE	
V	Vascular
I	Infection and Inflammation
N	Neoplasm
D	Degenerative
I	Iatrogenic and Intoxication
C	Congenital/Developmental
A	Autoimmune and Allergic
T	Trauma
E	Endocrine/Metabolic and Exposures (environmental, occupational)
SPECIFIC SITUATION—ALTERED MENTAL STATUS	
AEIOU TIPS	
A	Alcohol
E	Endocrine/Electrolytes
I	Ischemia/Infarction
O	Oxygen (Hypoxia; Hypercapnia)
U	Uremia
T	Trauma/Tumor/Temperature/Toxin
I	Infection
P	Psychiatric
S	Seizure/Syncope

TABLE 5.3 PRIORITIZING A DIFFERENTIAL DIAGNOSIS

SPIT Mnemonic		
S	Serious Diagnosis	Exclude or rule-out any life-threatening diagnoses
P	Probable Diagnosis	Evaluate and treat likely diagnoses
I	Interesting Diagnosis	Consider uncommon and complex diagnoses
T	Treatable Diagnosis	Consider diagnoses with specific and effective treatment regimens

Source: Adapted from Chinai SA, Guth T, Lovell E, Epter M. Taking advantage of the teachable moment: A review of learner-centered clinical teaching models. *Western J Emerg Med.* 2018;19(1):28–34. https://doi.org/10.5811/westjem.2017.8.35277[4]

Diagnostic Testing

A. The clinical history, physical examination, and differential diagnosis will guide diagnostic testing.

Diagnostic testing should be methodical and purposeful. The goal is to provide safe, yet cost-effective, patient care. In some circumstances, clinical decision rules (CDRs) can be used to help determine the need for diagnostic testing. The clinician should be familiar with the risks associated with performing certain testing. Prior to ordering a diagnostic test, the clinician should ask a few questions:

- Does the patient need a test to help me confirm or exclude a diagnosis?
- What diagnostic test(s) should be performed?
- Is this the best available test for the patient's condition?
- What is the risk to the patient?
- What is the cost of the test and does it provide diagnostic value?
- How will the test results affect the patient's management and final disposition?

Clinical Reasoning

A. Clinical reasoning is the cognitive method that the ENP uses to analyze and interpret a clinical situation. Reasoning will differ based on the experience and knowledge of the clinician. ENPs should use a combination of analytical and nonanalytical reasoning in their practice.[5]

1. *Nonanalytical reasoning:* Nonanalytical reasoning is automatic, based on intuition and pattern recognition. This type of reasoning is fast, sometimes done unconsciously, allowing the clinician to take mental shortcuts.[6] These cognitive shortcuts are known as gestalt or heuristics. Heuristics are applied by experienced clinicians, after repeated exposure to certain types of patients.[7]

2. *Analytical reasoning:* Analytical reasoning is a slow and more deliberate thought process. This type of reasoning is applied when there is diagnostic uncertainty and will help prevent diagnostic errors. Analytical reasoning is a cyclical process of considering a diagnosis, gathering data, then testing that diagnosis.[6] This process continues until the ENP is confident in a diagnosis.

Medical Decision-Making Resources

A. Decision-making tools are evidence-based resources that can help direct the plan of care.

B. Decision-making tools are meant to help reduce the clinician's cognitive load and prevent the clinician from relying on memory. Clinical practice guidelines, CDRs, and clinical scores are examples of diagnostic tools. These tools are available through various online resources, phone applications, and may be imbedded in electronic medical records.

C. Clinical practice guidelines

1. Clinical practice guidelines are often established by professional organizations and associations. When practice guidelines are developed, the authors perform an extensive review of the available literature. After complying and reviewing the evidence, recommendations can be made for best practice. Clinical practice guidelines help direct clinicians when managing specific medical conditions. Guidelines are meant to standardize and optimize patient care.[8]

D. Clinical decision rules

1. CDRs are validated tools that are used to help make diagnostic and treatment decisions. These tools help improve efficiency and standardize emergency care. CDRs are developed to answer simple questions about common complaints. Ideally, a CDR will have a limited number of clinical variables and can be applied quickly. CDRs are only valid if they are applied exactly how they were designed. It is important to be familiar with all inclusion and exclusion criteria, when considering a CDR.[9]

E. Some CDRs are designed to rule out a disease process (one-way), while others help determine the need for a diagnostic test (two-way). Pulmonary Embolism Rule-out Criteria (PERC) is an example of a one-way CDR. A patient who is PERC negative has a low likelihood of pulmonary embolism (PE) and does not require further workup. However, a patient who is PERC positive does not necessarily have a PE or require further workup. This rule was only designed to rule out a PE.[10] The NEXUS Cervical Spine Rule is an example of a two-way CDR. The NEXUS Cervical Spine Rule has two endpoints, to determine whether or not a patient requires diagnostic imaging of their cervical spine.[11]

F. Clinical scores and risk stratification

1. Many clinical situations are too complex to be solved using a single CDR. Clinical scores or risk stratification scales/tools are used to help predict the likelihood of a bad outcome. These scoring tools are often used to help determine whether a patient can be safely discharged with close follow-up or if the patient needs additional services.

a. One example, the HEART score is used to help predict the risk of a major adverse cardiac event in undifferentiated chest pain (Table 5.4).[13] The HEART score calculates points from five variables, including clinical gestalt, to determine whether the patient is low-, medium-, or high risk. Patients with a low HEART score may be candidates for early discharge. However, higher HEART scores may require additional observation, diagnostics, or cardiology evaluation.[12] As with any decision-making tool, clinical scores should not replace good clinical judgment.

G. Shared decision-making

1. The diagnostic process is a patient-centered activity. Therapeutic communication is used to build a trusting relationship with the patient and learn about their healthcare priorities. When patients are engaged in the decision-making process, they will better understand their health conditions and the diagnostic and treatment options.[14] Often, there is no single or "right" answer when treating a patient. Shared decision-making allows the ENP and the patient to work together to determine the plan of care (Figures 5.2 and 5.3). Shared decision-making improves patient and clinician satisfaction.

TABLE 5.4 HEART SCORE FOR MAJOR CARDIAC EVENTS

HEART SCORE				
H	History	Slightly suspicious	0	
		Moderately suspicious	1	
		Highly suspicious	2	
E	EKG	Normal	0	
		Nonspecific repolarization disturbance	1	
		Significant ST deviation	2	
A	Age	<45 years old	0	
		45–64 years old	1	
		>65 years old	2	
R	Risk factors	No known risk factors	0	
		1–2 risk factors	1	
		3 or more risk factors or history of ACS	2	
T	Initial troponin	Normal	0	
		1–3x normal limit	1	
		>3x normal limits	2	
			TOTAL	

0–3 points: Risk of cardiac event 0.9%–1.7%.
4–6 points: Risk of cardiac event 12%–16.6%.
> or = 7 points: Risk of cardiac event 50%–65%.
ACS, acute coronary syndrome.

Source: Adapted from Six AJ, Backus BE, Kelder JC. Chest pain in the emergency room: Value of the HEART score. *Neth Heart J.* 2008;16(6):191–196. https://doi.org/10.1007/BF03086144.[13]

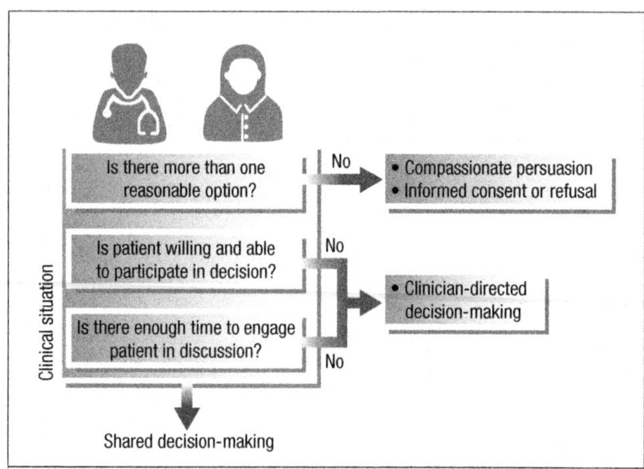

FIGURE 5.2 Shared decision-making.
Source: From Probst MA, Kanzaria HK, Schoenfeld EM, et al. Shared decision-making in the emergency department: A guiding framework for clinicians. *Ann Emerg Med.* 2017;70(5):688–695. https://doi.org/10.1016/j.annemergmed.2017.03.063. Reprinted with permission.[14]

Consultation

A. Consultation is one of the components of patient management in the practice standards for the ENP specialty. The ENP needs to "collaborate and consult with other healthcare clinicians to optimize patient management." The five Cs of consultation are summarized in Box 5.1:

1. Contact
2. Communication
3. Core Questions
4. Collaborate
5. Closing the Loop

Disposition Decision

A. ENPs should start thinking about the patient's disposition from the beginning of the patient encounter.

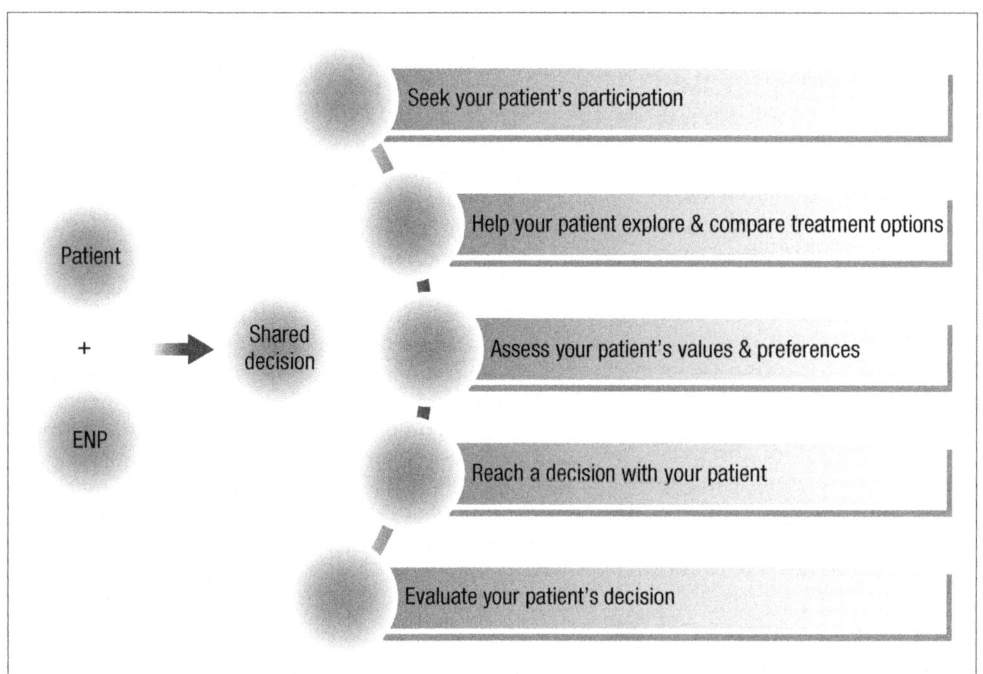

FIGURE 5.3 The SHARE approach to shared decision-making.
Source: Adapted from The SHARE Approach. Agency for Healthcare Research and Quality; August 2018. http://www.ahrq.gov/professionals/education/curriculum-tools/shareddecisionmaking/index.html.[15]

BOX 5.1 5 Cs OF CONSULTATION

Contact
Introduction of consulting and consultant physicians and building of relationship. Identify with full name, rank, service, and name of supervisor.
Communicate
Give a concise story and ask focused questions. Communicate concerns, urgency of matter, timeline.
Core Questions
Have a specific question or request of the consultant. Decide on reasonable time frame for consultation.
Collaborate
A result of the discussion between the emergency physician and the consultant, including any alteration of management of patient or testing.
Closing the Loop
Ensure that both parties are on the same page regarding the plan and maintain proper communication about any changes in patient's status.

Source: Adapted from Kessler CS, Tadisina KK, Saks M, et al. The 5Cs of consultation: Training medical students to communicate effectively in the emergency department [published correction appears in *J Emerg Med.* 2016 Aug;51(2):222. Deiorio, N [corrected to Deiorio, Nicole]]. *J Emerg Med.* 2015;49(5):713–721. https://doi.org/10.1016/j.jemermed.2015.05.012[16]

B. When considering the disposition of the patient, the following can influence the decisions related to patient disposition in the ED.[17,18]

C. Contributors to disposition errors

1. Incorrect triage
2. ED overcrowding (pressure to quickly decide a disposition due to increased patients)
3. Inadequate testing because the wrong exam or testing is missed
4. Diagnostic error
5. Lack of recognition of patient resources—i.e., no transportation for discharge
6. Patient's ability to communicate his or her problem, language barriers
7. Patient triaged to the wrong section of the ED, for example, a trauma patient in the cardiac area

D. Possible decisions

1. Treat and release:
   a. Discharge against medical advice (AMA)
2. Admission
   a. Requiring inpatient observation
   b. Observational medicine is a growing emergency medicine subspecialty and many EDs have a designated observation unit. Observation is a patient status that is used to provide extended monitoring, serial physical examinations, additional diagnostic testing, and/or treatment to determine the final disposition. This option is good for patients who are not safe for an immediate discharge, however, also do not meet admission criteria. Successful observation units use diagnosis-based protocols that have clearly defined inclusion/exclusion criteria and admission/discharge criteria (Box 5.2). Patients are typically observed up to 24 hours. Following the observation period, patients are either discharged or admitted to the hospital.
   c. Benefits of having a designated ED observation unit:
      i. Reduction in inappropriate discharges
      ii. Prevents unnecessary hospital admissions
      iii. Decreased cost
      iv. Improve hospital throughput metrics
      v. Patient satisfaction
3. Transfer
   a. Patient transfers occur when a facility lacks the capacity or resources to manage a patient's emergency medical condition. Patients are typically transported to a facility with specialized capabilities. All patient transfers must be done in accordance with the Emergency Medical Treatment and Labor Act (EMTALA).

BOX 5.2 EXAMPLE OF AN EMERGENCY DEPARTMENT OBSERVATION PROTOCOL

Inclusion Criteria
- Allergic reaction with need for continuing therapy
- Observation after epinephrine therapy
- Local skin eruptions or skin breaks
- Swelling of face or neck
- Mild respiratory problems

Exclusion Criteria Potential Interventions:
Disposition Criteria
- Hypotension, significant tachypnea, or other unstable vital signs
- Pulmonary complications or SpO_2 <90%
- EKG changes
- Stridor, respiratory distress
- Significant ongoing upper airway involvement
- IV fluids
- Antihistamines (H1 blockers)
- H2 receptor antagonists
- IV or PO corticosteroids
- Cardiac monitoring
- Respiratory treatments
- Pulse oximetry monitoring
- Repeat doses of SQ epinephrine (1:1,000–0.3 mL)

Discharge: Home Admission
- Improvement in clinical condition
- Stable vital signs
- Resolution or improvement in local skin irritations and/or respiratory function
- Delayed reaction or recurrence of symptoms
- Significant respiratory problems, persistent wheezing, or stridor
- Inability to take oral medications

b. Stabilize the patient, within the capabilities of the facility.
c. The sending clinician should initiate the transfer process and communicate with the accepting facility/clinician.
d. Unless they lack capacity, hospitals with specialized capabilities are obligated to accept transfers from hospitals that are unable to treat unstable emergency medical conditions.
e. Whenever possible, obtain a signed patient consent for the transfer.
f. Complete a Memorandum of Transfer (MOT).
g. Certify that the medical benefits outweigh the risks of transfer.
h. The sending facility should provide copies of medical records and imaging.
i. The mode of medical transportation and level of care is determined by the sending facility and should be based on patient acuity.
j. EMTALA violations should be reported to the Centers for Medicare & Medicaid Services (CMS) and appropriate state agencies.

E. *Discharge:* Components
1. Focus on a team approach
2. *Patient education:* Including significant others if indicated
3. Confirm patient or family member of understanding the plan of discharge care
4. Teach back method
5. Health literacy
6. Notify primary care
7. Referral to appropriate follow-up clinician
8. Characteristics of high-quality ED discharges include[19]:
a. Informs and educates patients on their diagnosis, prognosis, treatment plan, and expected course of illness. This includes informing patients of the details of their visit (e.g., treatments, tests, procedures).
b. Supports patients in receiving post-ED discharge care. This might include medications, home care of injuries, use of medical devices/equipment, further diagnostic testing, and referral for further clinician evaluation.
c. Coordinates ED care within the context of the healthcare system (e.g., other healthcare clinicians, social services).
9. Interventions that can improve the ED discharge process[19]
a. Discharge instructions and education
b. Telephone follow-up
c. Scheduled follow-up appointments
d. Prescription assistance
e. Transportation assistance
f. Care coordination

F. Against medical advice
1. Occasionally, a patient will refuse a specific treatment, diagnostic test, observation, or hospital admission. When a patient refuses a recommended plan of care, it is referred to as "against medical advice" or "AMA."

Documentation—Medical Decision-Making

A. The medical record serves as a method of communication between healthcare clinicians. In addition, the medical record provides the necessary data for reimbursement, research, quality improvement, and risk management. Documentation of the clinical history, physical exam, and medical decision-making (MDM) are required for each patient encounter.[20]
B. The MDM is meant to reflect the thought process of the clinician. From a medicolegal perspective, the clinician wants to support their decision-making process while proving they did not miss anything important. From the reimbursement and productivity side, the clinician wants to validate the need for medical services and describe the complexity of their decision-making.[20]
C. Starting the MDM note with a summary statement helps support diagnostic and management options for the patient. The summary statement includes pertinent patient information and a differential diagnosis. For example: A 20-year-old-male with an acute right ankle injury that has severe pain, swelling, and is unable to bear weight—concerned for fracture versus sprain. This statement indicates the medical necessity for an emergency evaluation, pain control, splinting, and radiographs.
D. The following information is commonly documented, as a part of MDM:
1. Data reviewed
a. Laboratory studies
b. Radiology
c. Consultation
d. EKG interpretation
e. Independent review of an image, tracing, or specimen
f. Review of past medical records, including nurse and EMS notes
2. Decision-making tools (CDRs, scores, pathways)
3. Crucial conversations with the patient and/or family (Code status, Against Medical Advice)
4. Shared decision-making
5. Consents to treatment and/or procedures
6. Treatment and response to treatment
7. Discharge teaching, prescriptions, and follow-up instruction

E. The amount of information a clinician must obtain, analyze, and/or review should be reflected in the medical record. This information helps describe the complexity of the case.[20] Diagnostic data can help the clinician work through the list of differential diagnoses. Documentation should support a diagnosis and rule out other causes for the patient's complaint.

Transitions of Care

A. Transitions of care, also known as patient handoffs, is an interactive process of passing essential patient information from one caregiver to another. Transitions of care happen when patients move between healthcare locations, clinicians, or different levels of care. Transitions of care can be one of the most dangerous parts of patient care. Communication failures can lead to medical errors. For this reason, improving the handoff process has become a national safety priority.

B. Setting up for successful transitions of care:

1. Develop a culture that emphasizes effective and safe transitions of care.
2. Hardwire a standardized process within your system.
3. Standardize content and delivery.
   - **a.** Identification of patient
   - **b.** Identification of admitting/primary/supervising physician
   - **c.** Diagnosis and current condition of the patient
   - **d.** Recent events, including changes in condition or treatments current medication status, recent lab tests, allergies, anticipated procedures, and actions to be taken
   - **e.** Outstanding tasks
   - **f.** Outstanding laboratories/studies
   - **g.** Changes in patient condition that may occur requiring interventions
4. Allow opportunity for questions.
5. Minimize interruptions.
6. Ensure patient confidentiality and privacy.
7. When appropriate, incorporate teaching, training, and coaching.

C. High-risk transitions of care

1. Clinical circumstances
   - **a.** Diagnosis that requires immediate treatment
   - **b.** Diagnosis or that requires specific follow-up
   - **c.** Initiation of high-risk medications
   - **d.** Comorbidities
   - **e.** Young and geriatric
   - **f.** Mental illness
2. Psycho-social-environmental circumstances
   - **a.** Lack of financial recourses or poverty
   - **b.** Lack of access to healthcare resources
   - **c.** Homelessness or unsafe living conditions
   - **d.** Cultural consideration
   - **e.** Substance abuse
   - **f.** Opioid use disorder

Preventing Diagnostic Error

A. Working in the ED has unique challenges. Patients are commonly moved from one treatment area to another leading to transitions of care. Clinicians are confronted with distractions, frequent interruptions, and competing priorities. There is diagnostic uncertainty, and medical decisions often must be made rapidly or with limited information. The busy and somewhat chaotic environment can predispose patients to medical and diagnostic errors.

B. Heuristics are mental shortcuts that allow clinicians to make quick decisions. When applied appropriately, the clinician can be more efficient. When applied inappropriately, heuristics can lead to cognitive bias (Table 5.5). Cognitive bias is a leading cause of diagnostic error. All clinicians are vulnerable to bias. Having self-awareness, taking a step back, and reproaching a situation can help prevent diagnostic errors.[7,21]

C. Strategies to prevent diagnostic error include:

1. Using cognitive aids and diagnostic tools, rather than relying on memory
2. Making time for quality decision-making
3. Engaging in safe transitions of care
4. Implementing a diagnostic checklist for high-risk situations (Box 5.3)
5. Participating in performance improvement and feedback opportunities

TABLE 5.5 COGNITIVE BIAS

Anchoring	Jumping to conclusions. Fixating on a single diagnosis. Not considering an alternative diagnosis, despite new information.
Ascertainment bias	Stereotyping. Seeing what you want to see. This is common with "frequent flyers."
Availability bias	Making a diagnosis on a current patient, based on a recent or memorable patient presentation.
Confirmation bias	Only seeking or acknowledging information that supports your preconceptions.
Diagnosis momentum	Once a diagnosis is applied to the patient, it is difficult to see past it.
Framing effect	How information is "framed" or presented can impact decision-making.
Overconfidence bias	Believing that you know more than you do. The tendency to act on intuition instead of data.
Search satisfying	ENP, emergency nurse practitioner. Once you find something, you stop searching. Example: Missing a second fracture.
Example: A patient with a history of diabetes and hypertension arrived at the ED via ambulance. Although the patient's chief complaint was chest pain, it was reported to the triage clinician as shoulder and back pain, a secondary complaint (*framing effect*). The patient was a "frequent flyer," having been to the ED several times for pain-related complaints. The patient was seen the day before and received a pain shot (*ascertainment bias*). The initial clinician focused on back pain, rather than chest pain (*anchoring, confirmation bias, diagnosis momentum*). The ENP used information from the triage clinician's note, indicating "back pain" (*framing effect, diagnosis momentum*), and did not evaluate the patient independently. Shortly after arrival, the patient had a cardiac arrest, in the minor care area.	

ENP, emergency nurse practitioner.

BOX 5.3 CHECKLIST: HIGH-RISK SITUATIONS FOR DIAGNOSTIC ERROR

HIGH-RISK SITUATIONS FOR DIAGNOSTIC ERROR

Have I ruled out must-not-miss diagnoses?
Did I just accept the first diagnosis that came to mind?
Was the diagnosis suggested to me by the patient, nurse, or another clinician?
Did I consider other organ systems besides the obvious one?
Is there data about this patient I haven't obtained and reviewed?
Old records? Family? Primary care clinician?
Are there any pieces that don't fit?
Did I read the x-ray myself?
Was this patient handed off to me from a previous shift?
Was this patient seen in the ER or clinic recently for the same problem?
Was I interrupted/distracted excessively while evaluating this patient?
Am I feeling fatigued right now, or cognitively overloaded?
Is this a patient I don't like for some reason? Or like too much (friend, relative)?

What to Do in High-Risk Situations:

1. Pause to reflect—take a diagnostic "timeout"
2. Consider the universal antidote: What else could this be?
3. Make sure the patient knows when and how to get back to you if necessary (e.g., if their symptoms change or worsen)

Source: From Graber ML, Sorensen AV, Biswas J, et al. Developing checklists to prevent diagnostic error in emergency room settings. *Diagnosis (Berlin, Germany).* 2014;1(3):223–231. http://doi.org/10.1515/dx-2014-0019. Reprinted with permission.[22]

References and Additional Reading

References and Additional Reading for this chapter are online only and can be found at https://connect.springerpub.com/content/reference-book/978-0-8261-6091-5/part/part01/toc-part/ch05.

6. Emergency Resuscitation and Stabilization

VINCENT SPERANDEO

Learning Objectives

- Describe the concept of resuscitation.
- Define basic life support.
- Define advanced life support.
- Describe the assessment and management of airway, breathing, and circulation related to patient resuscitation
- Describe basic and advanced airway management.
- Describe basic and advanced ventilation management.
- Describe basic and advanced management of circulation.

Emergency resuscitation has been practiced for many centuries. The first reported use was in the mid-18th century when mouth-to-mouth resuscitation was recommended for drowning victims by the French Academy of Sciences; in 1767, the Society for Recovered Drowned Persons became the first organized effort to deal with sudden death. It was another 120 years before Dr. Friedrich Maass performed the first documented use of chest compressions in 1891. In 1903, Dr. Crile was the first person to successfully use chest compressions in resuscitating a human being. In the mid-1950s, Safar and Elam formally invented mouth-to-mouth resuscitation, which was adopted by the U.S. military to revive unresponsive victims. This invention led to the formation in 1960 of what is known today as cardiopulmonary resuscitation (CPR). The American Heart Association started a CPR committee in 1963 led by cardiologist Dr. Leonard Scherlis to assist in standardizing a training regimen for CPR. It was not until 1972 that CPR was taught to the general population, and within the first two years over 100,000 people were trained. As time passes and research continues, modifications have occurred in both the basic and advanced measures used in resuscitation.

Assessment—Airway, Breathing, and Circulation

Airway

A. The first step in the approach to the unresponsive/arrested patient is to follow the ABCs.

B. For resuscitative measures to be effective, there must be a patent airway.

1. Airway management can vary from simple to complex, depending on the situation presented.
2. On the basic level, make sure there is no obvious obstruction, and if one is present, remove it immediately.
3. Consider other possible causes of airway obstruction:
   a. Trauma
   b. Allergic reactions, such as a reaction to a bee sting
   c. Side effects of medications
   d. Congenital abnormalities
   e. Burns

Basic Life Support

A. Multiple airway adjuncts are available for basic and advanced air management.

1. *Oral airway (OA):* The first and easiest to use.
   a. Inserted into the mouth of an unresponsive individual with nontraumatic injuries
   b. Lifts the tongue off the posterior pharynx of the patient to ensure there is no obstruction caused by the tongue resting on the posterior pharynx
2. *Nasopharyngeal airway (NPA):* A flexible tube usually made of latex/rubber
   a. Inserted through one of the patient's nostrils
   b. Similar to the OA, it is used to maintain an airway though the nasal turbinate so air can pass with less restriction.

Advanced Life Support

A. *Laryngeal mask airway (LMA):* An advanced device that requires training in its use

1. Supraglottic device—once it is inserted, it is seated just above the epiglottis.
2. The purpose of this device is to maintain an individual's airway, but is more secure than an oral or nasal airway as the cuff is inflated to maintain proper position once inserted.[1]

B. *Combitube or esophageal tracheal double-lumen tube:* Device placed blindly through the mouth and has multiple cuffs that are inflated above and below the glottis

1. Since it is easy to intubate the esophagus, the principle behind this tube is that when it is inserted into

the unresponsive patient, the tube will slide easily into the esophagus.

2. The two cuffs hold the tube in place and obstruct the esophagus, allowing ventilation through a proximal lumen, which terminates at side ports overlying the laryngeal inlet.

C. Other devices, such as the esophageal obturator airway (EOA) and the esophageal gastric tube airway (EGTA), were used but replaced by the above-described devices, as these devices had very high complication rates associated with their insertion and use.

D. *Endotracheal (ET) intubation:* Requires specific training and proficiency.

1. Training and continued practice by clinician are necessary to maintain proficiency.

2. It is commonly believed that ET intubation is a recent advancement because of the advanced equipment used to perform this technique, however:

a. The first documented use of ET intubation was found on an Egyptian tablet dating back to approximately 3600 BC.[2]

b. Late in the 20th century, ET intubation became safer due to advances that allow for direct visualization of anatomical landmarks instead of blindly intubating the patient, and now with the use of fiber optics, the procedure is safer and easier than ever before.

3. Directly inserting a tube into the trachea to allows control of the airway helps prevent possible aspiration.

4. Aside from different-size tubes used for this procedure, the main difference in intubation devices is whether the tube has a cuff or not.

a. In general, an uncuffed tube is used in the pediatric population, but this decision comes down to the size of the patient's airway.

b. In the patient over the age of 18, tube size usually is considered based on gender and height.

i. For male patients, the ET tube size usually ranges between 7.5 mm and 8.5 mm.

ii. For female patients, the ET tube size usually ranges between 6.5 mm and 7.5 mm.

c. *Pediatric population:* Box 6.1 can be used as a guide for ET tube size, but variations may occur. A Broselow tape or similar reference should be used to determine the appropriate ET tube size.

BOX 6.1 TRACHEAL TUBE SIZE GUIDE FOR PEDIATRIC PATIENTS

- *Newborn:* 2.5–4.0 mm
- *Infant <6 months:* 3.5–4.0 mm
- *Infant between 6 months and 1 year:* 4.0–4.5 mm
- *Child 1 and 2 years:* 4.5–5.0 mm
- *Child >2 years:* Divide the child's age by 4 and add 4 mm.

Source: Duff JP, Topjian A, Berg MD, et al. American Heart Association focused update on pediatric advanced life support: An update to the American Heart Association Guidelines for Cardiopulmonary Resuscitation and Emergency Cardiovascular Care. Circulation. 2018;138:e731-e739.

E. *Emergency cricothyroidotomy (surgical airway):* This procedure requires specific training and practice. Indications for an emergency cricothyrotomy include inability to intubate, inability to ventilate, inability to maintain a SpO_2 >90%, and severe trauma to the upper airway or face.

1. An incision is made approximately two finger widths above the sternal notch.

2. The landmarks used to guide the clinician through this process are the area between the cricoid cartilage and the thyroid cartilage.

a. Note a vertical incision is preferred for this procedure due to the vascularity of the neck; horizontal incisions may be used, but extra caution is warranted (Figure 6.1).

3. Emergency airways are only temporary until the patient is stabilized enough that a sterile surgical procedure can be performed to secure a permanent airway.

F. *Breathing*: Once a patent airway is established, ventilation will be needed in order to maintain patient oxygenation.

G. Basic life support (BLS)

1. Patient breathing requiring limited assistance

a. Supplemental oxygen is an excellent adjunct.

b. A nasal cannula, Venturi mask, or nonrebreather mask may be indicated.

c. Slightly more invasive options, such as bilevel positive airway pressure (BiPAP) or continuous positive airway pressure (CPAP), may be highly successful and spare patients from being placed on mechanical ventilation.

2. The use of these techniques requires the patient to be awake and somewhat alert, breathing on their own.

3. Patients requiring significant intervention to breathe

a. Clinicians must consider where they are practicing and what equipment may be available.

i. The simplest form of ventilation is standard "mouth-to-mouth" for patients in both respiratory and cardiac arrest. Clinicians should always consider the safety of this practice if protective devices are not available.

ii. *Bag valve mask (BVM):* Should be used as soon as available for appropriate ventilation

(1) The BVM is a better option than mouth-to-mouth resuscitation due to better ventilation control, as well as allowing the use of adjunctive oxygen to increase oxygen saturation.

(2) Use BVMs with patients in respiratory and/or cardiac arrest, patients with respiratory distress, or patients requiring elective intubation to provide supplemental oxygen.

H. Advanced life support

1. *Mechanical ventilation:* Assisted artificial ventilation, intermittent or mandatory

a. The practice took form in the early 18th century.

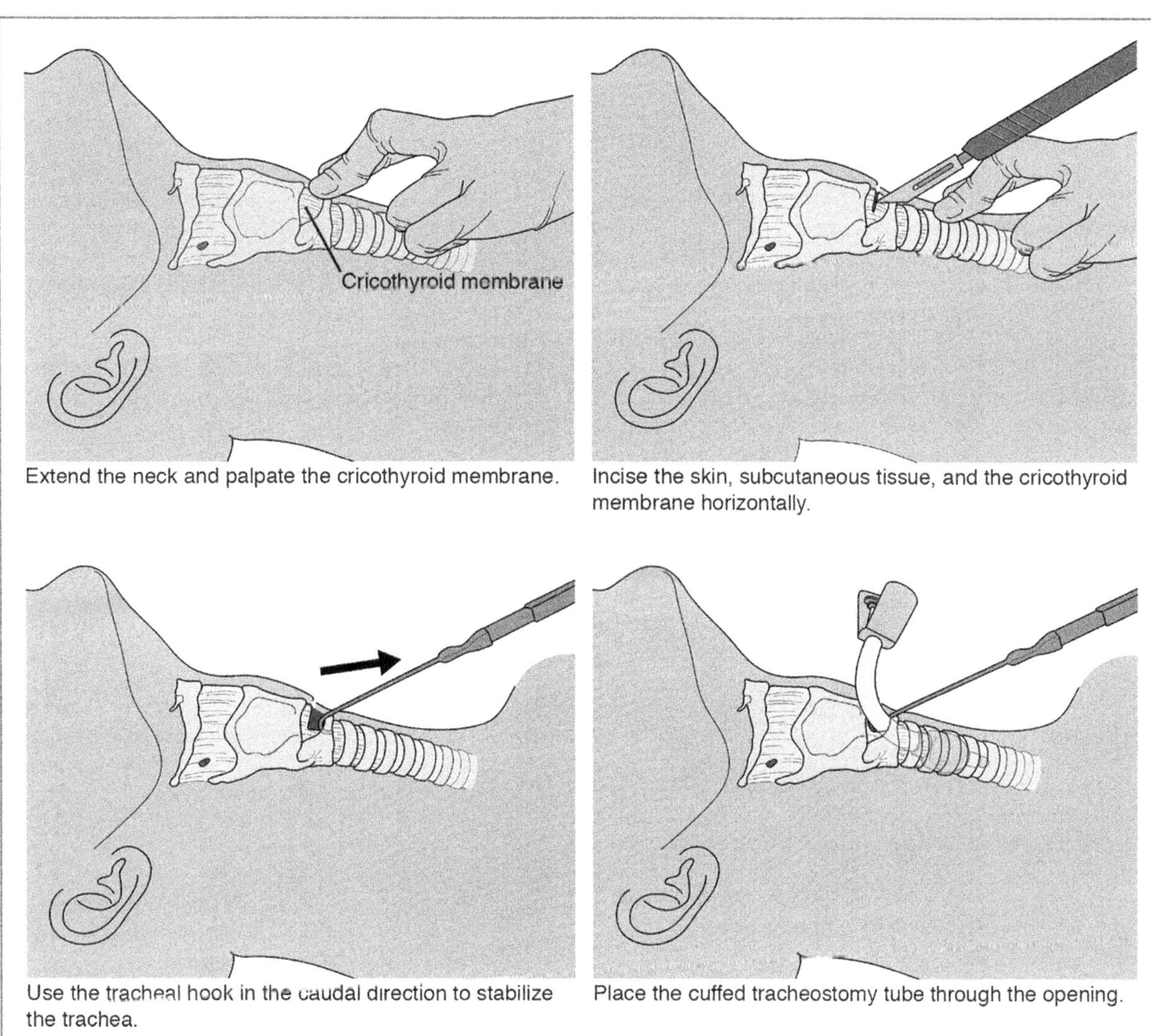

FIGURE 6.1 Open surgical cricothyrotomy.
Source: Betz D, Wald DA. Cricothyrotomy. In: Campo T, Lafferty K, eds. *Essential Procedures for Emergency, Urgent, and Primary Care Settings*. 3rd ed. Springer Publishing Company; 2021. Fig. 8.4.[3]

b. Initially, the thought behind artificial ventilation was to decrease the pressure around the lungs, accomplished by placing a patient into a large airtight chamber, which became known as the "iron lung." This chamber created a negative pressure that allowed the lungs to inflate.

c. Late in the 1800s, thought shifted from the "negative" pressure approach to the "positive" pressure approach. The Humane Society of England began to use bellows similar to that of a blacksmith to provide positive pressure respirations but found it difficult to control pressure.[4]

d. The 1950s saw the first use of a positive pressure device. Surprisingly, this device was not used for medicine but for pilots flying old World War II–era planes that required supplemental oxygen. The past 20 to 30 years have brought significant changes in the use of mechanical ventilation, with research even today continuing to make changes.

e. Three common ventilator settings:

i. *Assist-control (AC) ventilation:* Helps the patient to breathe by initiating a cycle when a drop in pressure from the patient attempting inspiration occurs. The ventilator also delivers a breath in the event the patient does not initiate one spontaneously. Settings can be adjusted for both sensitivity of patient inspiration as well as controlled rate in the event spontaneous inspiration does not occur.

ii. *Controlled mechanical ventilation (CMV):* Used for apneic patients.

iii. *Intermittent mandatory ventilation (IMV):* Similar to AC, but with this setting a predetermined number of ventilations are applied in an unsynchronized or synchronized (synchronized intermittent mandatory ventilation [SIMV]) manner.

f. Positive end expiratory pressure (PEEP) or constant positive airway pressure (CPAP):

i. These settings are used to increase lung volumes or if there is persistent low oxygenation levels despite the use of 100% FiO_2.

ii. If PEEP or CPAP is not used, ventilator sighs should be considered.

iii. In a normal healthy patient, sighs occur on average 12 times per hour.

iv. Sighs are a normal mechanism needed for healthy lung function. Their main purpose is to inflate alveoli in the lower lung fields where normal respirations may not effect. This inflation becomes crucial in the critically ill patient since lung compliance is already compromised and lung expansion is significantly impeded due to immobility.

Circulation

A. The latest recommendation in one-person CPR is to ONLY perform chest compressions for the first 2 minutes (cpr.heart.org/en/resuscitation-science/cpr-and-ecc guidelines).

B. Associated research alongside these changes have caused a push to reorganize ABC (airway, breathing, and circulation) into "CAB."

C. The proper depth of a compression is important in order to be successful.

1. Recommended depth for an adult is 2.5 inches; in children 1.5 to 2 inches, or 1/3 the depth of the anterior/posterior distance chest to back.
2. The main concern in this phase of resuscitation is to ensure cerebral perfusion.

D. Cerebral anoxia occurs quickly during cardiac arrest, giving someone approximately 10 to 12 seconds to perform CPR prior to the patient's oxygen levels hitting zero.

E. Glucose and glycogen stores are triggered as well as a cascade of other factors ultimately allowing between 5 and 10 minutes of compensatory time prior to complete cell death.

F. By providing external measures to assist in circulation, or the return of spontaneous circulation even temporarily, interrupts this cascade failure and preserves potential brain function.

G. Cerebral perfusion is a direct result of blood pressure and intracranial pressure; the average perfusion pressure lies between 50 and 100 mmHg. Proper compressions are needed in order for perfusion to occur and be effective.

H. In the event of partial or complete loss of circulation due to cardiac arrest, external influence must be provided in order for circulation to occur:

1. Physical chest compression by an individual
2. A compression device such as the Lund University Cardiopulmonary Assist System (LUCAS)

a. Extracorporeal membrane oxygenation (ECMO) may be used to assist patients with circulatory failure. The principle behind this machine is to not only use an external pump to bypass the heart but also provide reoxygenation of blood in patients. Although rarely used, ECMO may be a consideration if available at the institution where the clinician practices.

3. Defibrillation and pacing

a. Primarily considered to restore or maintain cardiac output in order for proper perfusion to take place

b. Techniques are used to not only help restore a regular rhythm in a patient experiencing rhythm abnormalities but also to assist in maintaining a regular rhythm.

c. Defibrillation and pacing are both in the BLS and ALS algorithms, with ALS having additional indications and procedures for patients with dysrhythmias.

d. Defibrillation

i. The automatic external defibrillator (AED) in recent years has become the cornerstone of resuscitation. The National Institutes of Health (NIH) approximates that nearly 18,000 people who suffer from sudden cardiac arrest have shockable rhythms.[5] The NIH study and others, additional studies sparked a move to improve access to devices that bystanders with even minimal knowledge can place on a patient and follow automated instructions based on computer analysis to potentially save lives. The use of the AED is taught both in BLS and ALS protocols.

I. Advanced life support

1. Defibrillation technology continues to advance away from the manual approach. Devices are available to deliver hands-off defibrillation.
2. Advances in electrophysiology have led to better understanding of the effects of monophasic (shocking the patient in a single direction) versus biphasic (rectilinear approach to delivering a current to the patient) shock.

a. Monophasic devices use either paddles or pads and deliver a current through the patient.[6] The amount of energy used in the monophasic devices varies from 200 to 360 joules, whereas in the biphasic devices the energy use is between 120 and 200 joules. The biphasic device's less energy was found to be safer to the patient by decreasing skin burning, myocardial damage, and dysfunction, and was also noted to allow for a more rapid return of ejection fraction and mean arterial pressure to baseline.[7]

b. *Open chest cardiac defibrillation:* A third approach is used only in rare situations.

i. Mostly seen in cardiac surgery, but may be seen in the trauma setting as well

ii. Defibrillation is applied directly to the myocardium, resulting in the need for much less energy. The recommended energy setting is between 10 and 20 joules. Studies show less than this setting seems to be ineffective and more tends to increase the likelihood of myocardial damage.[8]

3. Shockable rhythms

a. *Three rhythms to consider when attempting defibrillation:* Ventricular tachycardia, ventricular fibrillation, and supraventricular tachycardia.

b. Multiple underlying etiologies may cause each of these arrhythmias; correction of those causes will help in successful defibrillation.

c. Arrhythmias that are not considered shockable are asystole and pulseless electrical activity (PEA). In these cases clinicians must continue with good CPR, attempt to identify the underlying cause or causes of the arrhythmia, and administer epinephrine.

d. *Atrial fibrillation:* In most cases, this condition is treated with medication and may even be self-limiting, but in rare situations it may require cardioversion where a patient is sedated, medicated, and electrical shock is used in an attempt to correct the dysrhythmia.

4. Pacing

a. There are multiple indications for a patient to require pacing. The goal is to maintain or restore normal depolarization to regulate heart rate. Situations that may be considered for pacing include tachy-/bradyarrhythmias or asystole.

b. *There are two types of emergency pacing*— transcutaneous and transvenous:

i. Transcutaneous pacing is the most frequently used technique due to its ease in application.

(1) It delivers predetermined intervals of energy through the intact chest wall.

(2) The amount of energy used varies and the recommended setting is between 50 and 100 mA.

(3) Sedation may be necessary during pacing. The external shock required for adequate pacing can be traumatic and not tolerable for some patients.

(4) In order to maintain adequate pacing, energy output is recommended at 1.25 times the threshold of initial electrical capture.[1]

ii. Transvenous pacing is a highly specialized procedure and should not be attempted without the proper training and equipment.

(1) Consists of inserting a catheter into a central vein and introducing a pacing wire into the apex of the right ventricle

(2) Transvenous pacing requires far less energy than transcutaneous pacing. The maximum amount of energy required is 20 mA, and with proper catheter placement capture should occur at approximately 2 mA.[1]

(3) Limitations due to the difficulty in pacing performing are dependent on successful placement and having appropriate equipment at hand.

(4) Procedure is significantly more time-consuming than transcutaneous pacing and, if performed blindly, has a very low rate of success and a high rate of complication.

(5) Advancements in transcutaneous pacing have been so successful that transvenous pacing in the emergency setting is rarely if ever used.

5. Pharmacotherapy during resuscitation

a. The clinician should follow the most recent ACLS Guidelines from the American Heart Association.

b. Additional medications may be indicated but should be used based on the institution guidelines where the clinician practices.

6. Postresuscitation measures

a. Once spontaneous circulation has returned, the focus needs to change from saving to maintaining the patient's life.

b. Box 6.2 outlines an excerpt from Pediatric Advanced Life Support (PALS), which holds true not only in pediatrics but also in adult medicine.

c. Considerations surrounding care postemergency resuscitation are numerous, complex, and must take into account myriad factors and monitor multiple aspects of the patient.

i. Controlled postarrest hypothermia

(1) This technique was initially used in the late 1950s but due to lack of evidence supporting its use it was abandoned until recently when further research was performed supporting its use.[9]

(2) The reasons why hypothermia can be effective are still not clear. One explanation is that hypothermia results in the slowing of chemical reactions, another that the lowering of the body temperature may assist in reducing swelling in the brain, helping to reduce damage and maintain brain function.[10]

(3) Protocols should be in place for hypothermia for the postarrest patient. The core aspects of each institution's protocols should be consistent with the possibility of slight variations due to availability of equipment. In order for a patient to be considered for hypothermia treatment after return of spontaneous circulation, the patient must be intubated, be comatose or have significant neurologic deficits, be hemodynamically stable either with or without the use of medications, and be within an 8-hour window

BOX 6.2 POST-RESUSCITATION MEASURES

Respiratory System

- Chest x-ray to verify ET tube placement
- Arterial blood gas (ABG) and correct acid/base disturbance
- Pulse oximetry (continuously monitor)
- Heart rate and rhythm (continuously monitor)
- End-tidal CO_2 (if the patient is intubated)
- Maintain adequate oxygenation (saturation between 94% and 99%)
- Maintain adequate ventilation to achieve PCO_2 between 35 and 45 mmHg, unless otherwise indicated
- *Intubate if:*
    - Oxygen and other interventions do not achieve adequate oxygenation
    - Needed to maintain a patent airway in the child with a decreased level of consciousness
    - Ventilation is not possible through noninvasive means, e.g., CPAP
- Control pain with analgesics and anxiety with sedatives (e.g., benzodiazepines)

Cardiovascular System

- ABG and correct acid/base disturbances
- Hemoglobin and hematocrit (transfuse or support as needed)
- Heart rate and rhythm (continuously monitor)
- Blood pressure (continuously monitor with arterial line)
- Central venous pressure (CVP)
- Urine output
- Chest x-ray
- 12-lead EKG
- Consider echocardiography
- Maintain appropriate intravascular volume
- Treat hypotension (use vasopressors if needed and titrate blood pressure)
- Pulse oximetry (continuously monitor)
- Maintain adequate oxygenation (saturation between 94% and 99%)
- Correct metabolic abnormalities (chemistry panel)

Neurological System

- Elevate head of bed if blood pressure can sustain cerebral perfusion
- Temperature
    - Avoid hyperthermia and treat fever aggressively
    - Do not rewarm hypothermic cardiac arrest patient unless hypothermia is interfering with cardiovascular function
    - Treat hypothermia complications as they arise
- Blood glucose
    - Treat hypo/hyperglycemia (hypoglycemia defined as less than or equal to 60 mg/dL)
- Monitor and treat seizures
    - Seizure medications
    - Remove metabolic/toxic causes
- Blood pressure (continuously monitor with arterial line)
- Maintain cardiac output and cerebral perfusion
- Normoventilation unless temporizing due to intracranial swelling
- Frequent neurological exams
- Consider CT and/or EEG
- Dilated unresponsive pupils, hypertension, bradycardia, respiratory irregularities, or apnea may indicate cerebral herniation

Renal System

- Monitor urine output
    - Infants and small children: >1 mL/kg an hour
    - Larger children: >30 mL an hour
    - Exceedingly high urine output could indicate neurological or renal problem (diabetes insipidus)
- Routine blood chemistries
- ABG and correct acid/base disturbances
- Urinalysis (when indicated)
- Maintain cardiac output and renal perfusion
- Consider the effect of medications on renal tissue (nephrotoxicity)
- Consider urine output in the context of fluid resuscitation
- Toxins can sometimes be removed with urgent/emergent hemodialysis when antidotes fail or are not available

Gastrointestinal System

- Monitor nasogastric (NG)/orogastric (OG)tube for patency and residuals
- Perform a thorough abdominal exam
    - Tense abdomen may indicate bowel perforation or hemorrhage
- Consider abdominal ultrasound and/or abdominal CT
- Routine blood chemistries including liver panel
- ABG and correct acid/base disturbances
- Be vigilant for bleeding into the bowel, especially after hemorrhagic shock

Hematological System

- Monitor complete blood count and coagulation panel
- Transfuse (as needed)
    - Correct thrombocytopenia
    - Use fresh frozen plasma to replenish clotting factors
    - Consider calcium chloride or gluconate if massive transfusion required
- Correct metabolic abnormalities (chemistry panel), especially after transfusion

Source: From Duff JP, Topjian A, Berg MD, et al. American Heart Association focused update on pediatric advanced life support: An update to the American Heart Association Guidelines for Cardiopulmonary Resuscitation and Emergency Cardiovascular Care. Circulation. 2018;138:e731-e739.

ABG, arterial blood gas; CPAP, continuous positive airway pressure; CVP, central venous pressure; ET, endotracheal; NG, nasogastric; OG, orogastric.

from return of circulation. Exclusion criteria include severe cardiogenic shock, terminal illness, severe uncontrollable bleeding, underlying coagulopathy, or infection/sepsis.

(4) The goal of hypothermia treatment is to rapidly cool the patient within 1 to 3 hours to a temperature of 32 to 34° C, which should be maintained for 24 hours. Medications for sedation, neuromuscular blocking, and DVT prophylaxis should be considered and started. After 24 hours, rewarm should occur slowly over the course of 17 to 20 hours (0.2–0.33°C per hour). Goal temperature is 36.5°C to 37.5°C.[11]

(5) Special attention to the patient is needed to avoid rebound hyperthermia while maintaining the goal temperature. The clinician needs to closely monitor the patient's electrolytes as hypothermia could cause significant shifts in values. Conservative management needs to occur since rewarming can cause a rebound and result in elevated levels.

Overview of Resuscitation

A. Resuscitation is a procedure to support and maintain breathing and circulation in a person in respiratory arrest and/or cardiac arrest.

B. Regardless of the underlying cause of respiratory or cardiac arrest, the basics of CPR must be performed.

C. BLS

1. Training available to licensed and unlicensed learners alike

2. Enables the individual to perform basic techniques that are usually used outside the hospital setting

3. Topics taught in BLS encompass all ages from the infant through the adult years.

4. Focuses on cardio or pulmonary arrest but also includes the choking victim

D. Advanced cardiac life support (ACLS)

1. Incorporates the fundamentals learned in BLS; designed for the trained medical professional

2. Skills are used both in the hospital and the prehospital care environment by emergency medical services (EMS).

3. Proper application and utilization of ACLS skills significantly increase chances for survival; effective training is important to success.

Role of the Emergency Nurse Practitioner

A. Emergency resuscitation touches on every aspect of medicine and the ultimate goal is the return of spontaneous circulating and respiration.

B. Emergency nurse practitioners (ENPs) can assist in the short term with these functions, and the ENP needs to make every attempt to return the patient to a normal state as quickly as possible in order to ensure the best possible patient outcome.

C. ENPs must remember to correct the underlying medical issue, otherwise the resuscitation is temporary at best.

D. Advances in resuscitative measures will continue to advance and evolve. Clinicians have a responsibility to stay up to date in order to provide the highest level of care and give patients the best possible chance at survival.

References

References for this chapter are online only and can be found at https://connect.springerpub.com/content/reference-book/978-0-8261-6091-5/part/part01/toc-part/ch06.

7. Pain Management

SHANA METZGER

Learning Objectives

- Describe the pathophysiology of pain and explain the use of analgesics to manage pain.
- Develop strategies for managing acute pain that utilizes both nonopioid and opioid medications.
- Evaluate a patient with an acute pain complaint and develop a comprehensive, patient-centered treatment plan.
- Identify patients who are at high risk of opioid overdose and identify risk-mitigation strategies in prescribing.
- Determine when it is appropriate to use procedural sedation and discuss how it is safely performed.
- Identify the indications and contraindications of commonly used analgesic medications.

Age and Developmental Considerations

A. *Pediatric*

1. Humans are able to perceive pain from birth.

2. Infants and children have decreased pulmonary reserve due to higher rate of oxygen consumption, smaller caliber airway, reduced capacity for accessory muscle use, and increased rate of fatigue.

3. Pain control techniques should be family-centered, and the family should be involved in patient care when possible.

4. Nonpharmacologic techniques to distract the patient and induce relaxation are preferred.

5. Dosing of pharmacologic agents must be precise and is based on patient weight.

6. Pediatric patients may benefit from procedural sedation for common bedside procedures such as laceration repair, incision and drainage of cutaneous abscess, lumbar puncture, and arthrocentesis.

B. *Pregnancy*

1. Selection of strategies and medication for pain management in the pregnant patient depends on the risks versus benefits to both the mother and the fetus. In general, the well-being of the mother must be preserved in order to preserve the well-being of the fetus. Consider potential teratogenic effects and pregnancy class of medications prior to administration.

2. Local or regional anesthesia is preferred over systemic agents when possible.

3. Discuss with the parents all risks and benefits to both mother and fetus with the patient in order to ensure informed consent.

4. Physiologic changes of pregnancy that may affect analgesia and sedation

i. Supine position may exacerbate hypotensive side effects due to aortocaval compression of the uterus and compress the major vessels in late pregnancy.

ii. Respiratory rate and minute ventilation increases while vital capacity decreases, increasing risk of hypoxia during sedation.

iii. GI motility decreases, increasing the likelihood of presence of gastric contents and thereby increasing aspiration risk.

C. *Geriatric patients*

1. Older adults tend to underreport pain and may have diminished sensation and interpretation of pain.

2. Older adults are often prescribed a number of medications that may interact with analgesics to potentiate harmful side effects.

3. Older adults are more prone to falls related to a natural decline in muscle mass and strength and slowing of reflexes. Furthermore, antihypertensives and normal cardiovascular changes of aging may increase the risk of orthostatic hypotension and subsequent falls due to dizziness and syncope.

4. A natural decline in kidney and liver function prolongs the half-life of many analgesics, resulting in increased rate of adverse effects such as sedation, respiratory depression, and nausea and vomiting.

5. Older adults with underlying dementia may experience an acute delirium from centrally acting analgesics and muscle relaxers. Older adults in general are more susceptible to the CNS side effects of medications.

6. The natural decline in pulmonary function and cardiopulmonary reserve increases risk of hypoxia during sedation.

7. Individual older adults may have underlying conditions or suffer drug–drug interactions that preclude the use of common analgesics, such as NSAIDs, IV lidocaine, muscle relaxers, or opioids.

Management of Acute Pain

Medical Screening

A. *Chief complaints*

1. Pain may present anywhere in the body and stem from a variety of etiologies.

2. The patient often presents with a chief complaint that localizes the pain, such as headache, neck pain, back pain, chest pain, abdominal pain, and so on.
3. The patient will express what they are feeling, and the clinician must diagnose the cause in order to treat the pain.
4. Management of acute pain is focused around the treatment of the underlying cause. This requires the collection of a detailed history of present illness, including accurate characterization of the pain itself and possible proximal causes.
5. Some patients may have difficulty describing or localizing pain based on the etiology, or may use alternative terms such as "soreness, discomfort, ache, bother, or misery."

B. *Signs and symptoms*
1. Signs and symptoms of acute pain vary widely and depend on the etiology of pain.
2. Furthermore, the expression of pain varies greatly from one person to another depending on age, gender, culture, and prior experience with pain.
3. Gathering a focused pain history includes asking the patient to describe the onset, location, duration, characteristics, severity, and timing of the pain, as well as aggravating and alleviating factors and whether the pain radiates.
4. A number of standardized pain scales exist to quantify the severity of pain, including for pediatric patients (e.g., Wong-Baker FACES™ Scale).
5. In focusing on acute pain, some possible signs and symptoms include the following:
a. Objective signs
i. Tachycardia
ii. Elevated blood pressure
iii. Tachypnea and hyperventilation
iv. Diaphoresis
v. Grimacing
vi. Guarding
vii. Pacing or shifting
viii. Changes in mood or affect (e.g., anger, agitation, flat affect, excessive talking, or lack of verbal response)
ix. Crying, moaning, or yelling
x. Signs of pain in pediatric patients can vary from restlessness to diminished movement
b. Associated symptoms
i. Nausea and vomiting
ii. Mood changes
iii. Sleep disturbance
iv. Fatigue
v. Limited mobility
6. Important to remember that some patients may present with the above signs and symptoms, while others may present with no discernable signs of pain. It is therefore critical to obtain a detailed subjective and objective assessment of the reported pain complaint.

C. *Medication history*
1. Current pain medications
a. Topical preparations (e.g., capsaicin cream, diclofenac gel, lidocaine patches)
b. Over-the-counter oral medications (e.g., acetaminophen, ibuprofen, aspirin)
c. Antiepileptics (e.g., gabapentin, pregabalin, lamotrigine, carbamazepine)
d. Selective serotonin reuptake inhibitors (SSRIs), serotonin-norepinephrine reuptake inhibitors (SNRIs), and other antidepressants (e.g., fluoxetine, bupropion, paroxetine, duloxetine)
e. Nonsteroidal anti-inflammatory drugs (NSAIDs; e.g., diclofenac, celecoxib, naproxen)
f. Opioids (e.g., oxycodone, morphine, Dilaudid, fentanyl patches)
g. Opioid receptor partial agonists and antagonists (e.g., methadone, buprenorphine, naltrexone)
2. Chronicity and frequency of medication use
3. Effectiveness of each medication
4. Past history of pain medication use, including chronicity and efficacy

D. *Past medical history*
1. The clinician should get a complete medical history with emphasis on the particular pain complaint. With regard to acute pain management specifically, the clinician should focus on the following:
a. Current and historical patterns of alcohol and illicit drug use. Tolerance, dependence, addiction/abuse, and dependence on particular substances may affect analgesic dosing and choice of pain control. Patients taking high-dose opioids, methadone, buprenorphine, and naltrexone present a particular challenge in managing acute pain, as mu receptors are occupied and nonopioid strategies must be considered. In addition, recent consumption of centrally acting sedatives of any kind may preclude the use of procedural sedation or any other central nervous system (CNS) depressant.
b. History of chronic painful conditions, such as fibromyalgia, complex regional pain syndrome, chronic orthopedic pain, sickle cell, neuropathy, and so on. Patients who experience chronic pain may have higher or lower tolerances to pain and analgesics or express preferences for analgesic therapies.
c. History of allergic reactions to pain medications or adverse reactions to anesthesia
d. History of respiratory disorders such as obstructive sleep apnea, obesity hypoventilation syndrome, chronic obstructive pulmonary disease, and congestive heart failure. The risk of oversedation and respiratory depression from CNS depressants may preclude their use. If procedural sedation must be used, be prepared to manage the airway emergently.
e. History of kidney or liver impairment. This may affect the pharmacodynamics of medications and influence the choice of analgesic and dosing.

Physical Examination

A. *Focused assessment*
1. The physical assessment should focus on the chief complaint in order to determine the underlying cause of the pain.

2. The suspected etiology of pain should guide the choice of pain control. For example, pain management for a patient with leg pain from a sprained ankle should include joint immobilization, ice, and NSAIDs.

3. A patient with leg pain from an ischemic limb will require IV opioids and emergent revascularization. Leg pain from a laceration requires regional or local anesthesia. Each of these patients requires an assessment that focuses on the chief complaint of limb pain in order to determine the underlying cause of pain.

4. The key to obtaining effective analgesia is to tailor therapy to the underlying cause and the patient's medical history.

5. Objective findings associated with acute pain vary widely from one person to another.

  a. Findings depend on the patient's own expression of pain, underlying medical problems, and current medications.

  b. A patient with a pacemaker or who is taking a beta-blocker may not present with tachycardia.

  c. A person who is intoxicated may not be able to psychologically process the pain stimulus.

  d. Because pain itself is a subjective complaint, it is difficult to rely on a physical exam to determine the presence or severity of pain. Physical assessment should instead focus on determining the cause of a patient's pain.

6. For a patient who requires procedural sedation for a painful condition (e.g., a joint reduction), thorough ENT and cardiopulmonary examinations are required.

  a. Evaluate the structures of the airway to determine whether or not the clinician is likely to have difficulty securing the airway in the event of an emergency.

  b. A detailed cardiopulmonary examination is required to evaluate the risk of respiratory failure during the sedation.

  c. If a patient is at high risk of respiratory failure and is likely to be difficult to intubate, the clinician may conclude that the patient would be managed more safely by an anesthesiologist.

7. Prior to administering sedating analgesics, the clinician must perform a complete baseline neurologic examination. Patients who present with altered mental status from CNS pathology (e.g., head injury, stroke) that requires serial neurologic exams may not be candidates for sedating analgesics, such as IV opioids.

8. Patients who present with neuromuscular disorders such as Guillain-Barré syndrome, myasthenia gravis, or amyotrophic lateral sclerosis may have a compromised respiratory capacity and are at high risk of respiratory failure with CNS depressants. Furthermore, sedating analgesics should be avoided in patients with respiratory compromise of any etiology unless the airway is secured and managed mechanically.

Diagnostic Testing

A. There are no diagnostics to detect or quantify the perception of pain.

B. Diagnostics should focus on determining the underlying cause of the pain in order to appropriately manage the patient's presenting condition.

  1. For example, order x-rays for traumatic extremity pain, abdominal imaging for suspected appendicitis, and so on.

Medical Decision-Making and Differential Diagnoses

A. Severe, intractable pain that is difficult to manage even with IV opioids may indicate a serious, potentially life-threatening underlying problem.

  1. For example, clinicians are traditionally taught that "pain out of proportion to exam" may be an indicator of an ischemic bowel, aortic dissection, or ischemic limb.

  2. Each patient presenting with a pain complaint, particularly severe pain, warrants a detailed history and physical exam in order to elicit potentially life-threatening causes of pain.

  3. Once life-threatening conditions have been ruled out, the clinician should then focus on adequate pain management strategies.

B. Every clinician will encounter patients who are suspected of drug-seeking behavior.

  1. Now that greater awareness has been brought to the opioid epidemic and the dangers of prescribing opioids in excess, many clinicians and institutions are on the lookout for drug-seeking behavior and refuse to prescribe them controlled substances.

  2. To date, the literature has not demonstrated a validated tool or list of behaviors that can correctly identify patients who are presenting to the ED for the sole purpose of obtaining prescriptions for controlled substances.

  3. Even one of the more common tools used to predict risk of opioid misuse and abuse, the Opioid Risk Tool, has not consistently been shown to have high sensitivity or specificity for predicting aberrant drug behaviors.

C. Rather than seeking to identify patients who present with painful complaints for the purpose of obtaining controlled substances, it is better to approach all patients with a painful complaint in the same manner.

  1. Evaluate the chief complaint medically with a complete history and physical examination.

  2. If a diagnosis for the patient's pain can be determined in the ED, then treat the underlying cause using evidence-based therapies, preferably with non-opioid therapies as first-line agents.

  3. If a diagnosis for the patient's pain cannot be determined in the ED, initiate non-opioid pain strategies and refer the patient to the appropriate specialist who can further diagnose and manage the patient's pain.

  4. Studies have demonstrated that discussing reasonable, patient-centered goals for pain management and educating patients about the realistic dangers of

opioid analgesics improves patient outcomes and satisfaction scores.

5. The Centers for Disease Control and Prevention (CDC) has identified the following as risk factors for opioid overdose:
   a. Patients with a history of overdose or a history of substance use disorder (SUD)
   b. Patients taking high-dose opioids
   c. Concurrent benzodiazepine use

6. The CDC also recommends searching state prescription drug monitoring programs to identify patients who are at high risk of opioid overdose (patients prescribed high-dose or long-acting opioids, or patients who receive prescriptions from multiple prescribers).

7. It is reasonable to discuss the high likelihood of harm with patients who are identified as high-risk when determining the best analgesics to administer or prescribe.

8. Focusing on keeping patients safe while also using nonopioid analgesics to address the patient's complaint is much more effective than attempting to determine who is presenting to the ED for secondary gain.

Management

A. *Nonpharmacologic therapies*
   1. Whenever possible, nonpharmacologic therapies are preferred over pharmacologic therapies and should be considered first.
      a. Include cryotherapy, elevation and immobilization of an injured extremity, repositioning, massage, and distraction, mindfulness exercises, battlefield acupuncture, manual medicine, and therapeutic touch.
      b. Adverse effects associated with these interventions, if any, are generally mild, and they can be implemented by nursing staff or the layperson with minimal training and direction and are a good method to encourage family involvement in care.
      c. These interventions work particularly well for patients with musculoskeletal pain.

B. *Pharmacologic therapies*
   1. *Topical*
      a. *Overview*
         i. *Benefits:* Limited systemic effects and low risk of adverse drug reactions. Reactions are typically limited to local skin irritation or allergy.
         ii. *Limitations:* Some formulations may be expensive or not covered by insurance. Use is limited to local or regional pain control, such as neuropathy, soft tissue injury, joint pain, and back pain.
      b. *Capsaicin cream*
         i. Commonly used for arthralgia due to arthritis and postherpetic neuralgia
         ii. Evidence demonstrates limited efficacy but low rate of adverse events.
      c. *Topical NSAIDs*
         i. Used for arthralgia due to arthritis, strains, and sprains
         ii. Evidence indicates topical diclofenac gel 1% and ketoprofen are effective for managing pain due to sprains and strains.
      d. *Lidocaine transdermal*
         i. Extended-release (12-hour) transdermal system
         ii. Used for arthralgia and localized pain
         iii. Evidence demonstrating efficacy is limited.
   2. *Local/regional*
      a. *Medications*
         i. *Topical (dermal, mucosal):* Lidocaine, bupivacaine, tetracaine, benzocaine, proparacaine
         ii. *Intradermal, subdermal, intra-articular:* Bupivacaine, lidocaine, mepivacaine, prilocaine, procaine, tetracaine
         iii. Epinephrine may be mixed 1:100,000 with anesthetic. Induces vasoconstriction to reduce bleeding and rate of absorption, thereby prolonging time of anesthesia.
            (1) Contraindicated in areas with poor vascularization, but can be used safely in hands and fingers
         iv. *Mechanism of action:* Inhibits depolarization of nerve cell membrane by blocking the sodium channels.
      b. *Indications*
         i. Corneal eye pain, oral mucosal pain
            (1) Nebulized lidocaine (3 mL of 4% lidocaine) works well to anesthetize the nasopharynx prior to nasogastric tube insertion or drainage of a peritonsillar abscess.
         ii. Dermal application prior to painful procedures, such as venipuncture or injection of local anesthetic
         iii. Intradermal injection for local anesthesia for incision and drainage of cutaneous abscesses, laceration repair
         iv. Hematoma block for orthopedic reduction of fractures, dislocations
         v. Nerve block for regional anesthesia prior to painful bedside procedures. See Table 7.1 for types of regional blocks.
         vi. Intra-oral nerve blocks for dental and oral pain
      c. *Benefits*
         i. Rapid onset of near-complete anesthesia with duration of 2 to 6 hours
         ii. May preclude the use of procedural sedation
         iii. Generally considered safe with few systemic adverse effects when administered in recommended doses
         iv. Bypasses the opioid receptor in patients with opioid tolerance or who are taking mu receptor blockers
      d. *Limitations*
         i. Will need alternate form of pain control after anesthetic effects subside
         ii. Limited to areas of peripheral nerve innervation

TABLE 7.1 COMMON TECHNIQUES FOR REGIONAL ANESTHESIA AND USES

BLOCK TECHNIQUE	INNERVATION	BODY REGION	USES
Ear field block	Trigeminal and cervical plexus branches	Ear	Ear lacerations, abscesses
Infraorbital	Maxillary branch of trigeminal nerve	Upper lip, nares, upper incisors/lateral incisors/premolars	Lacerations, abscess of upper lip and lateral nose, dental pain
Mental nerve block	Mental nerve	Lower lip	Lip lacerations
Alveolar nerve block	Dental nerves	Maxillary molars	Dental pain
Mandibular nerve block	Mandibular branch of trigeminal nerve	Anterior ⅔ of tongue, maxillary teeth	Dental pain, tongue lacerations
Ulnar nerve block	Ulnar nerve	Ulnar aspect of hand, 5th and ulnar side of 4th fingers	Reduction of fractures/dislocations of 5th digit and metacarpal, lacerations, abscesses
Median nerve block	Median nerve	Palmar side of hand from 4th finger to the thumb, dorsum of 2nd, 3rd, and 4th fingers	Lacerations, abscesses
Radial nerve block	Radial nerve	Dorsum of hand from thumb to 4th finger	Lacerations, abscesses
Digital nerve block	Digital nerve	Any finger or toe	Lacerations, amputations, dislocations, fractures, nail bed injuries
Penile block	Pudendal nerve	Penis	Lacerations, paraphimosis reduction, penile fracture
Anterior ankle block	Superficial and deep peroneal nerves, saphenous nerve	Dorsum of foot and toes	Lacerations, metatarsal and toe fractures/reductions (when combined with posterior ankle block)
Posterior ankle block	Posterior tibial, sural nerves	Plantar aspect of foot	Lacerations, metatarsal and toe fractures/reductions (when combined with posterior ankle block)

3. *NSAIDs*
   a. *Medications*
      i. *Topical:* As given in Management/B.2.a.i
      ii. *IV:* Ketorolac
      iii. *Oral:* Aspirin, ibuprofen, naproxen, celecoxib, diclofenac, ketorolac, etodolac, indomethacin
      iv. *Mechanism of action:* Inhibits cyclooxygenase 1 and/or 2, thereby inhibiting prostaglandin synthesis
   b. *Indications*
      i. NSAIDs have a wide variety of uses and are particularly effective in the management of primary headache, musculoskeletal pain, postoperative pain, renal colic, biliary colic
   c. *Benefits*
      i. NSAIDs have been shown to provide noninferior and sometimes superior pain control in the ED when compared with opioids for acute extremity pain, renal colic, primary headache, biliary colic, and back pain.
      ii. They are nonsedating and have no abuse potential.
      iii. They come in a variety of preparations and formulations.
      iv. NSAIDs are generally inexpensive and covered by most insurance plans.
   d. *Limitations*
      i. NSAIDs are platelet inhibitors and may increase bleeding risk in patients who are anticoagulated, have an underlying bleeding disorder, or have had a recent surgery.
      ii. May cause peptic ulcers and increase the risk of gastrointestinal (GI) bleeding
      iii. Use with caution in patients with underlying cardiovascular disease. Prolonged use may increase the risk of heart attack or stroke.
      iv. Use with caution in patients with history of or current renal disease. May cause or worsen acute kidney injury
      v. Contraindicated in the third trimester of pregnancy
4. *Opioids*
   a. *Medications*
      i. *Examples:* Codeine, tramadol, morphine, hydromorphone, fentanyl, meperidine, oxycodone, hydrocodone, methadone
      ii. *Routes of administration:* IV, oral, transdermal, epidural/intrathecal
      iii. Onset and duration of action depends on the route of administration, oral formulation, and pharmacologic properties of each medication.
      iv. *Mechanism of action:* Mu-receptor agonist mitigates the transmission of pain signals in the CNS.
   b. *Indications*
      i. Acute, severe pain
         (1) Opioids should not be used in patients with mild pain or pain that can be safely managed with alternative modalities.

(2) Parenteral opioids are indicated when the risk of harm does not outweigh the potential benefit.

(3) Opioid doses should be titrated to efficacy at intervals of 20 to 30 minutes.

ii. Management of chronic pain is generally considered outside the general practice of the emergency clinician. However, patients will present to the ED with chronic pain complaints. The American Academy of Emergency Medicine (AAEM) does not recommend the routine use or prescription of opioids in managing acute exacerbations of chronic pain.

iii. The use of opioids in the treatment of acute pain should be limited to short-acting formulations and administered in the lowest effective dose for the shortest period of time possible to limit the risk of harm.

c. *Benefits*

i. Rapid analgesia when administered appropriately

ii. Low risk of harm if parenteral opioids are used cautiously

iii. Oral opioids may be an effective alternative analgesic in patients who cannot tolerate other oral analgesics, such as NSAIDs.

d. *Limitations*

i. The risk of overdose, addiction, abuse, and misuse has been clearly demonstrated in the literature. This risk increases with prolonged use and high doses of opioids.

ii. The efficacy of opioids in managing acute back pain, migraine headache, neuropathic pain, and a multitude of chronic pain complaints has not been established in the literature.

5. *Gabapentinoids*

a. *Medications*

i. Gabapentin, pregabalin

ii. *Mechanism of action:* Poorly understood, but gabapentinoids work similarly to GABA to decrease neurotransmission. It is theorized that they act on transmembrane channels to cause hyperpolarization and prevent nerve transmission.

b. *Indications*

i. Neuropathic pain, such as neuropathy and chronic back pain

ii. Adjunctive therapy for acute postoperative pain to reduce opioid consumption

c. *Benefits*

i. May reduce the consumption of opioids postoperatively

ii. Provides an alternative to opioids in the management of neuropathic pain

d. *Limitations*

i. Most of the studies evaluating the use of gabapentinoids in pain management originate from the peri-operative and chronic pain literature. There are no randomized controlled trials evaluating the efficacy of gabapentin in the ED setting.

ii. Studies show that gabapentin and pregabalin may be diverted and abused, especially among opioid abusers. They may become controlled substances in the future.

6. *Ketamine*

a. *Mechanism of action:* N-methyl-D-aspartate (NMDA) receptor antagonist blocks glutamate neurotransmission.

b. *Indications*

i. Acute, severe pain in the ED

ii. Ketamine for the treatment of acute pain should be administered in low, subdissociative doses; consult current evidence-based guidelines.

c. *Benefits*

i. Shown to be non-inferior to parenteral opioids in clinical trials

ii. May be used as an adjunct to morphine to reduce overall consumption and opioid-related side effects

iii. Safe for use in patients who are hypotensive and tachycardic. Does not cause respiratory depression

d. *Limitations*

i. Higher rate of mild adverse effects, including hallucinations, emergence phenomenon, and dysphoria. These adverse effects are transient and may be controlled with benzodiazepines if necessary.

ii. May transiently increase blood pressure and intracranial pressure

7. *IV lidocaine*

a. *Indications*

i. Renal colic

ii. Acute extremity pain due to trauma

b. *Benefits*

i. Comparable to morphine for acute pain control with mild side effects

ii. Effective analgesic alternative for patients with opioid tolerance or who are currently taking mu receptor blockers

c. *Limitations*

i. Not for use in patient with structural heart disease or dysrhythmia. Use with caution in pregnant women

ii. Low risk of side effects when given in the recommended doses. Consult current guidelines for recommended doses.

8. *Procedural sedation*

a. *Background:* Procedural sedation is a pain management technique used to temporarily decrease consciousness in order to allow a patient to tolerate a painful procedure. Examples of indications include dislocation of a fractured bone or dislocated joint or cardioversion. It is done at the bedside under close monitoring.

b. *Sedation type:* Procedural sedation is commonly characterized by the level of consciousness induced by the drug of choice. Different institutions use different terminology, and often the lines are blurred as the clinical effect on the patient varies by the patient's drug tolerance, the drug of choice, and dose given. Occasionally, a clinician may intend to induce moderate sedation, but the patient will slip into deep sedation. This possibility underscores the importance of close cardiopulmonary monitoring during the procedure and readiness to provide ventilatory support. A variety of scales are available to quantify the level of sedation. One commonly used scale in the United States is the Richmond

TABLE 7.2 RICHMOND AGITATION–SEDATION SCALE

SCORE	TERM	DESCRIPTION
+4	Combative	Overtly combative or violent; immediate danger to staff
+3	Very agitated	Pulls on or removes tube(s) or catheter(s) or has aggressive behavior toward staff
+2	Agitated	Frequent nonpurposeful movement or patient–ventilator dyssynchrony
+1	Restless	Anxious or apprehensive but movements not aggressive or vigorous
0	Alert and calm	
−1	Drowsy	Not fully alert, but has sustained (more than 10 seconds) awakening with eye contac, to voice
−2	Light sedation	Briefly (less than 10 seconds) awakens with eye contact to voice
−3	Moderate sedation	Any movement (but no eye contact) to voice
−4	Deep sedation	No response to voice, but any movement to physical stimulation
−5	Unarousable	No response to voice or physical stimulation

Procedure: Patient has eye opening and eye contact, which is sustained for more than 10 seconds (score −1).

1. Observe patient. Is patient alert and calm (score 0)?
   Does patient have behavior that is consistent with restlessness or agitation (score +1 to +4 using the criteria listed above, under DESCRIPTION)?
2. If patient is not alert, in a loud speaking voice state patient's name and direct patient to open eyes and look at speaker. Repeat once if necessary. Can prompt patient to continue looking at speaker.
   Patient has eye opening and eye contact, but this is not sustained for 10 seconds (score −2).
   Patient has any movement in response to voice, excluding eye contact (score −3).
   Patient has any movement to physical stimulation (score −4).
3. If patient does not respond to voice, physically stimulate patient by shaking shoulder and then rubbing sternum if there is no response to shaking shoulder.
   Patient has no response to voice or physical stimulation (score −5).

Source: With permission from Sessler, CN, Gosnell, MS, Grap, MJ, et al. The Richmond Agitation–Sedation Scale. *Am J Respir Crit Care Med.* 2002;166(10):1338–1344. https://doi.org/10.1164/rccm.2107138.

Agitation–Sedation Scale (RASS; Table 7.2). The following is one system of nomenclature for describing the levels of sedation:

i. *Minimal sedation:* Promotes anxiolysis. Patients can respond normally to verbal commands. No effect on cardiopulmonary function

ii. *Moderate sedation:* Somewhat depressed level of consciousness. Patients can respond to verbal commands with light stimulation. Minimal effect on cardiopulmonary function

iii. *Deep sedation:* Decreased level of consciousness. Patient cannot be aroused but can respond to painful stimuli. Ventilatory function may be impaired, and some drugs may induce bradycardia or hypotension.

iv. *General anesthesia:* Complete loss of consciousness. Patients are not arousable and do not respond to painful stimuli. This state is not a goal for bedside procedural sedation and should be performed under the supervision of an anesthesiologist or certified nurse anesthetist.

c. *Patient evaluation before, during, and after sedation*

i. *Preprocedural patient evaluation:* Prior to sedation, it is critical to obtain a medical history, which will guide the clinician in selection of agent as well as level of sedation (light, moderate, or deep sedation).

(1) Subjective patient assessment
(a) Informed consent
(b) Medical history, especially pertaining to diseases of the heart, lungs, liver, kidneys, and neurologic system
(c) Medications and when they were last taken
(d) Alcohol and illicit substance use
(e) History of prior adverse reactions to anesthesia
(f) Last oral intake to determine aspiration risk

(2) Physical assessment
(a) Preprocedure diagnosis
(b) Baseline vital signs, including baseline cognition
(c) American Society of Anesthesiologists Physical Status (ASA PS) Classification (Table 7.3)
(d) Airway Mallampati Score (Table 7.4)

(3) Preparing the environment
(a) Ensure that an adequate number of staff are able to respond quickly should the patient require resuscitation
(b) Functional cardiopulmonary monitoring equipment to include 3-lead EKG, pulse oximetry, automatic blood pressure cuff, and ideally end-tidal CO_2
(c) Supplemental oxygen
(d) Bag-valve mask for ventilatory support
(e) Emergency airway management equipment

TABLE 7.3 AMERICAN SOCIETY OF ANESTHESIOLOGISTS PHYSICAL STATUS CLASSIFICATION SYSTEM

ASA PS CLASSIFICATION	DEFINITION	ADULT EXAMPLES, INCLUDING, BUT NOT LIMITED TO:
ASA I	A normal healthy patient	Healthy, nonsmoker, no or minimal alcohol use
ASA II	A patient with mild systemic disease	Mild diseases only without substantive functional limitations. Examples include (but not limited to): current smoker, social alcohol drinker, pregnancy, obesity (30 < BMI < 40), well-controlled (diabtes mellitus) DM/HTN (hypertension), mild lung disease
ASA III	A patient with severe systemic disease	Substantive functional limitations; one or more moderate to severe diseases. Examples include (but not limited to): poorly controlled DM or HTN, COPD, morbid obesity (BMI ≥40), active hepatitis, alcohol dependence or abuse, implanted pacemaker, moderate reduction of ejection fraction, ESRD undergoing regularly scheduled dialysis, premature infant PCA <60 weeks, history (>3 months) of MI, CVA, (transient ischemic attack) TIA, or CAD/stents
ASA IV	A patient with severe systemic disease that is a constant threat to life	Examples include (but not limited to): recent (<3 months) MI, CVA, TIA, or CAD/stents, ongoing cardiac ischemia or severe valve dysfunction, severe reduction of ejection fraction, sepsis (disseminated intravascular coagulation) DIC, ARD, or (end stage renal disease) ESRD not undergoing regularly scheduled dialysis
ASA V	A moribund patient who is not expected to survive without the operation	Examples include (but not limited to): ruptured abdominal/thoracic aneurysm, massive trauma, intracranial bleed with mass effect, ischemic bowel in the face of significant cardiac pathology or multiple organ/system dysfunction
ASA VI	A declared brain-dead patient whose organs are being removed for donor purposes	

ASA PS, American Society of Anesthesiologists Physical Status; BMI, body mass index; CAD, coronary artery disease; CVA, cerebrovascular accident; COPD, chronic obstructive pulmonary disease; DM, diabetes mellitus; ESRD, end-stage renal disease; HTN, hypertension; MI, myocardial infarction; PCA, postconceptional age.
Source: With permission from ASA House of Delegates/Executive Committee. ASA physical status classification system. https://www.asahq.org/standards-and-guidelines/asa-physical-status-classification-system. October 14, 2014.

TABLE 7.4 MODIFIED MALLAMPATI SCORING

Class I	Soft palate, uvula, fauces, pillars visible
Class II	Soft palate, major part of uvula, fauces visible
Class III	Soft palate, base of uvula visible
Class IV	Only hard palate visible

Source: With permission from Samsoon GL, Young JR. Difficult tracheal intubation: A retrospective study. *Anaesthesia.* May 1987;42(5):487–490. https://doi.org/10.1111/j.1365-2044.1987.tb04039.x.

(f) Patent peripheral IV access

(g) Infusion of IV fluids at bedside

ii. *Intraprocedure monitoring:* During sedation, the patient should have continuous cardiopulmonary monitoring, and one person (either a registered nurse or advanced practice clinician) should be dedicated solely to patient monitoring. Monitoring parameters include:

(1) Level of sedation using a validated tool (e.g., RASS)

(2) Blood pressure every 3 to 5 minutes

(3) Continuous monitoring of 3-lead EKG and respiratory rate

(4) Continuous pulse oximetry

(a) Keep in mind that pulse oximetry may be limited by poor quality readings, and that an adequate pulse oximetry reading does not correlate with adequate ventilation

(5) Continuous end-tidal CO_2

(a) Capnometry provides a more sensitive indicator of respiratory depression than pulse oximetry. The $ETCO_2$ correlates closely with $PaCO_2$.

iii. Postprocedural recovery

(1) Monitoring parameters and criteria for establishing full recovery vary among institutions. In general, the goal is to ensure that the patient has returned to their baseline mental status and vital signs without risk of regressing back into a state of sedation. Doses of all agents vary depending on desired clinical effect, patient characteristics, and route of administration. Confirm the appropriate dose for each individual patient.

(2) A number of validated tools exist to aid in the evaluation of full patient recovery postprocedure. In general, the patient should meet the following criteria prior to discharge from the ED:

(a) Return to baseline vital signs and mental status.

(b) Return to baseline ambulatory status.

(c) Patient must be able to tolerate oral fluids.

(d) Patient or supervising adult must be able to return if complications arise.

(e) Patient must be discharged to the care of a responsible, sober adult who can provide a ride and monitor the patient at home.

(3) The length of the recovery period depends on the choice of drug(s) used during procedural sedation. Propofol, ketamine, and etomidate have short durations of action and therefore a relatively short recovery period (as little as 15 minutes).

d. *Medications*

i. *General information:* The medication of choice for procedural sedation depends on patient characteristics, desired level of sedation, and available route of administration. Typically, medications are administered intravenously and titrated to effect. If IV access is unavailable, agents such as ketamine and benzodiazepines can be given intramuscularly or even orally.

ii. Propofol

(1) *Pharmacology:* Prolongs binding of gamma-aminobutyric acid (GABA) and its receptor. Acts as short-acting sedative hypnotic. No analgesic effect

(2) *Benefits:* Rapid onset of action, within 1 minute of administration. Duration is approximately 5 to 15 minutes.

(3) *Limitations:* Cardiopulmonary depression can result in bradycardia, hypotension, hypoxia, and apnea. These effects typically resolve after propofol is metabolized, but the patient may require ventilatory support or fluid resuscitation.

iii. Etomidate

(1) *Pharmacology:* Short-acting sedative hypnotic with amnestic properties. No analgesic effects

(2) *Benefits:* Limited cardiopulmonary depression. Does not cause hypotension or respiratory depression. Decreases intracranial pressure. Onset <1 minute, duration 3 to 10 minutes

(3) *Limitations:* May cause myoclonus, nausea and vomiting, pain with injection that can be minimized by first injecting 1% lidocaine through the IV site

iv. Ketamine

(1) *Pharmacology:* Dissociative anesthetic. Results in sedation, analgesia, amnesia

(2) *Benefits:* No cardiopulmonary depression, provides analgesia; sympathomimetic effects can counteract hypotension and bradycardia. Onset in 1 minute, duration 15 minutes

(3) *Limitations:* Emergence phenomenon may occur, but severe symptoms can be managed with benzodiazepine. Nausea and vomiting, avoid use with head injury or increased ICP

v. Benzodiazepine plus opioid

(1) *Pharmacology:* Benzodiazepines bind to GABA receptors to decrease neurotransmission. Onset and duration of action vary depending on the choice of agent. Midazolam has a faster onset and shorter duration than diazepam or lorazepam, which makes it ideal for use during procedural sedation. Benzos have anxiolytic, amnestic, sedative, and muscle relaxant properties but do not provide analgesia. If analgesia is needed, a fast-acting opioid such as fentanyl can be administered concurrently.

(2) *Benefits:* Minimal effects on the cardiovascular system. Dose may be titrated to effect.

(3) *Limitations:* May cause respiratory depression and apnea. May cause adverse effects such as paradoxical agitation and vomiting. Onset and duration of action varies greatly depending on the agent(s) of choice.

C. *Consultation/collaboration*

1. Consultation with specialty services will depend on the etiology of acute pain and severity of the patient's condition.

2. Anesthesiology

a. Patients who require epidural or intrathecal administration of analgesics

b. Patients who may benefit from regional anesthesia of an entire limb

c. Patients who require procedural sedation but are at high risk of respiratory failure or may have a difficult airway to manage

3. Pain management team

a. May provide expert advice in managing acute pain in patients who are opioid tolerant or are taking mu receptor antagonists

b. May be an excellent resource in managing patients in palliative care or who frequently present to the ED with severe pain of any etiology

The Management of Pain in the Emergency Department

Pain is one of the leading complaints that brings patients to the ED to seek medical care. Furthermore, studies have shown that a large proportion of patients presenting to the ED with a pain complaint expect their symptoms to be mostly or completely relieved. As a result, the emergency nurse practitioner (ENP) must be comfortable using a wide variety of methods and medications to manage pain in patients presenting to the ED. The etiology of a patient's pain may stem from any variety of acute or chronic conditions, or from multiple overlapping conditions resulting in an exacerbation. The perception of pain is a complex physiologic process that involves the peripheral and central nervous systems (CNS), the expression of which varies widely from one individual to another.

It is important to differentiate acute and chronic pain, as the management of each is quite different. The emergency clinician is primarily focused on the management of acute pain conditions; however, patients will commonly present with chronic pain complaints, or acute pain that is complicated by chronic underlying painful conditions. Acute pain is rapid onset, short-term pain in response to a mechanical, chemical, or thermal insult. It is a normal physiologic response. Chronic pain is considered a pathology in and of itself, characterized by pain lasting longer than three months or the expected healing time of the initial painful insult. It is a general dysfunction of the pain processing of the nervous system.

The safe and effective management of pain has been a long-time challenge for emergency clinicians, and practice standards continue to evolve as the safety and efficacy of available pain medications are being closely examined. The content of this chapter serves as a general guideline for managing acute pain complaints, as well as a resource for the emergency clinician who requires a diverse toolbox of pain management strategies.

Pathophysiology of Pain

In order to understand how to adequately manage pain, it is critical to understand how pain is perceived, processed, and expressed in the human nervous system. In the setting of acute pain, damage to body tissue from a mechanical, chemical, or thermal insult stimulates the peripheral nociceptors (pain receptors), which transmit the pain signal through peripheral nerve pathways to the dorsal horn of the spinal cord. Nociceptors are expressed throughout the human body, including the skin and mucosa, muscles, joints, and major visceral organs. Signal transmission of the pain signal occurs through the A fibers and the C fibers. The A fibers transmit acute, sharp pain rapidly along myelinated nerve fibers via the primary neurotransmitter glutamate. The C fibers transmit dull, throbbing pain more slowly along unmyelinated nerve fibers via the primary neurotransmitter substance P. These signals enter the spinal cord through the dorsal horn and cross over to the spinothalamic tract, where the signal is transmitted up the spinal cord to the brain.

In the brain, the pain signal is processed in multiple locations. The signal stimulates the reticular formation, which results in a heightened level of awareness. In the thalamus, the pain signal is sorted and transmitted to the somatosensory cortex, where the brain localizes the source of the pain, and to the limbic system, where an emotional response is generated. The brain responds by increasing alertness, responding emotionally (e.g., anger, anxiety, crying), and signaling a motor response to mitigate the cause. Additionally, the pain signal stimulates the periaqueductal gray, which triggers the release of the endogenous opioids (e.g., enkephalins, dynorphin, endorphins) that travel down the spinal cord and activate the mu receptors in order to block further transmission of pain. This is the physiologic process that exogenous opioids simulate in order to achieve anesthesia. See Figure 7.1 for an illustration of this process.

Exogenous and endogenous opioid ligands stimulate a group of opioid receptors located throughout the CNS and gastrointestinal tract, as well as on mast cells, microglia, and astrocytes. These opioid receptors include the mu, kappa, delta, and opioid-like receptor 1 (OLR-1) receptors. Stimulation of these receptors in the CNS and gastrointestinal tract results in the decreased release of glutamate, substance P, acetylcholine, norepinephrine, and serotonin. The effects of stimulation of these receptors are listed in Table 7.5. Paradoxically, the stimulation

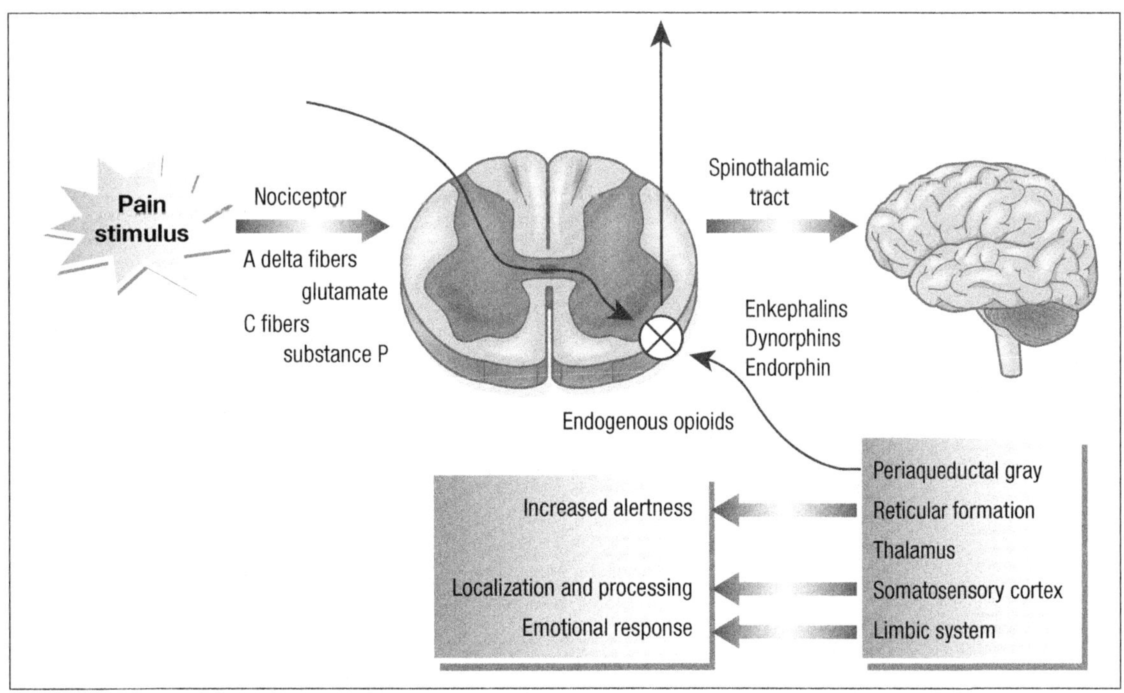

FIGURE 7.1 The perception of pain.

TABLE 7.5 PHYSIOLOGIC EFFECTS OF OPIOID RECEPTOR STIMULATION	
LOCATION OF OPIOID RECEPTOR	PHYSIOLOGIC EFFECT
Central nervous system	Analgesia Respiratory depression Euphoria Sedation Miosis Memory impairment Nausea Cough suppression
Peripheral systems	Decreased gastrointestinal motility Reduced intestinal absorption Decreased blood pressure and heart rate Urinary retention Diuresis Itching/flushing Suppression of immune function
Mast cells, microglia, astrocytes	Allodynia, hyperalgesia

of opioid receptors expressed on mast cells, microglia, and astrocytes results in an increased release of proinflammatory cytokines, resulting in the phenomenon of hyperalgesia in the setting of chronic opioid use.

Chronic Pain

Chronic pain is defined as persistent pain lasting longer than 3 months or longer than the expected time of "healing" from an illness or injury. Patients with chronic pain frequently present to the ED for multiple reasons. It is important for the ENP to be familiar with and sensitive to the patient with chronic pain. EDs need to have policies and procedures to consistently provide competent and safe care for these patients.

Additional Reading

Additional Reading for this chapter are online only and can be found at https://connect.springerpub.com/content/reference-book/978-0-8261-6091-5/part/part01/toc-part/ch07.

8. Leadership, Team Dynamics, and Communication

KATHLEEN FLARITY

Learning Objectives

- Compare and contrast leadership styles in healthcare.
- Describe team dynamics and its role on high-functioning healthcare teams.
- Apply principles of crew resource management in healthcare.
- Demonstrate practices that support effective conflict resolution.
- Discuss the impact of personal values on healthcare leadership.

Effective leadership, teamwork, and communication are vital to optimal patient outcomes and patient safety. In 2000, the Institute of Medicine (IOM) published *To Err Is Human*, and subsequently, organizations have been examining practice methods, team dynamics, and attributes needed to improve quality outcomes.[1,2] Healthcare has also studied and adopted many safety practices from the aviation industry,[3] specifically crew resource management (CRM), which focuses on effective communication, situational awareness, and team dynamics.[2,4]

Effective teamwork and communication in healthcare, like aviation, are essential to achieve best safety practices and optimal clinical outcomes. APRNs, as key members of interprofessional teams, impact clinical practices and patient outcomes when they communicate effectively, operate reliably as a team, and model these behaviors.[5–7]

Introduction to Team Dynamics

Team dynamics describe how unconscious, psychological influences affect the behavior and impact the performance of groups of people working together.[2] The need for high-functioning and high-performing teams is widely recognized as essential for creating a more patient-centered, coordinated, and effective healthcare delivery system. The ED is a dynamic, challenging, complex, and high-risk environment. Beyond patient safety issues, positive team dynamics have been shown to have a significant impact on job satisfaction and staff turnover. It has also been correlated with reduced sick leave taken by healthcare professionals.[2]

To promote effective team functioning, several models have been developed and implemented to coordinate the activities of healthcare teams. One model used in healthcare is termed "team-based care." Team-based healthcare is the delivery of health services to individuals, families, and/or their communities by at least two health clinicians who work collaboratively with patients to accomplish shared goals within and across settings to achieve coordinated, high-quality care.[8]

Crew Resource Management

The healthcare industry has adopted many safety practices from the aviation industry, which has an exemplary safety record after identifying the role of human error in airplane crashes during the 1970s and 1980s.[3] In particular, crew resource management (CRM) is used in environments where human error can have devastating effects. CRM is used for improving safety and focuses on effective interpersonal communication, leadership, situational awareness, team dynamics, and decision-making.[4] Human errors, communication failures, leadership problems, and cockpit decision-making were found to be major contributors to errors in aviation. In many cases, other crew members in the aircraft knew a mistake was being made and did not speak up. CRM values input from all sources—including personnel and equipment—to ensure efficient and safe flights. CRM has been shown to improve safety in multiple industries, including longstanding use in military and civilian medical flight programs. It has shown efficacy when applied to medicine to promote teamwork and patient safety in Veteran's Administrations, and in operating rooms.[2,4,9] Studies have shown that in teams using CRM, communication barriers are reduced and problems are solved more efficiently, leading to increased safety.[2,3] Effective teamwork and communication in healthcare, like aviation, are essential to achieve best safety practices and optimal clinical outcomes. APRNs, as key members of interprofessional teams, influence safety practices when they communicate effectively, operate reliably as a team, and model these behaviors for others on the team.[5–7] Specifically, CRM aims to foster a culture where authority may be respectfully questioned, particularly valuable in EDs. It recognizes that a discrepancy between what *is* happening and what *should be* happening is often the first indicator that an error is occurring. This is a delicate subject for many organizations, especially ones with traditional hierarchies such as healthcare.

A CRM expert, Todd Bishop, developed a five-step assertive statement process that encompasses inquiry and advocacy steps.[10]

1. ***Opening or attention getter:*** "Captain Miller or Dr. Little" or whatever name or title will get the person's attention.

2. ***State your concern:*** Express your analysis of the situation in a direct manner while owning your emotions about it.

3. ***State the problem as you see it:*** "We're showing only 30 minutes of fuel left" or "we are unable to obtain venous access on this trauma patient."

4. ***State a solution:*** "Let's divert to another airport and refuel," or "I think we should put in an **intraosseous** or central line."

5. ***Obtain agreement (or buy-in):*** "Does that sound good to you, Captain?" or "Dr. Little, how would you like to proceed for venous access?"

These are often difficult skills to master, as they may require significant changes in personal habits, self-awareness, interpersonal dynamics, and organizational culture.[10]

Situational Awareness

Situational awareness (SA) is advocated in both civilian and military medical flight programs. SA was first developed from investigations of airline accidents and has expanded to other healthcare arenas such as EDs.[10,11] SA—a component of CRM—is the ability to identify, process, and comprehend the critical elements of information about what is happening to the team with regard to the environment of care.[10,12] Most airline crashes were found to be preventable and due to inappropriate responses to changing situations exacerbated by poor communication between crew members.[2] Human factors are responsible for most airplane crashes rather than instrument or mechanical failures. These errors can be broken down into decisional, procedural, or operational, and perceptual/motor or technical. Having good SA requires constant monitoring of all facets of a dynamic environment such as EDs. Ideally, all team members possess high levels of SA and CRM and work synergistically to identify and treat the complexity of patient care.[11]

Interprofessional Teams

Effective interprofessional teams have been well articulated in the literature and the present-day model is founded on the following elements[2,4,8,13,14]:

- Involvement of multiple healthcare professions, each with relevant areas of expertise
- Division of duties and responsibilities
- Shared goals
- Shared decision-making among team members
- Effective respectful communication among team members
- Patient-centered care
- Shared accountability
- High-performing healthcare team synergy
- Enhanced quality of care and patient outcomes
- Team learning and continuous improvement

Clinical Expertise

Each team member must be able to effectively contribute their specific areas of expertise to the team and understand how each member's expertise is best operationalized in patient care. Each team member relies upon information and action from other team members. The roles of the physician, advanced practice clinician, RN, pharmacist, respiratory therapist, ED technician, and other team members need to be distinct, clear, and synergistic to the clinical situation. In high-performing teams, leadership is dynamic and decision-making is shared.[8,13]

Interdisciplinary Teamwork

Interdisciplinary team work has been described as a dynamic process involving two or more health professionals with complementary backgrounds and skills, sharing common goals and interdependent collaboration in assessing, planning, or evaluating patient care.[15] This open communication and shared decision-making generates positive patient, organizational, and staff outcomes.[15]

Team Values

In the process of considering and refining the principles of team-based care, it is important to note that while teams are groups, they are also made up of individuals. In addition to behaviors that facilitate the team functioning, certain personal values are necessary for individuals to function well within the team. This complements the core competency domain of "values/ethics" put forward in Interprofessional Education Collaborative (IPEC) Team-Based Competencies.[8]

Table 8.1 outlines six personal values that characterize the most effective members of high-functioning teams in healthcare.[8,13]

Principles of Interdisciplinary Teamwork

In a 2013 systematic review of the literature on interdisciplinary team work, Nancarrow, Booth, Ariss, Smith, Enderby, and Roots, identified 10 principles of high-functioning interdisciplinary teams that were later reformulated as competency statements.[16] Applying these principles will serve ED leaders and teams well.

1. Identifies a leader who establishes a clear direction and vision for the team while listening and providing support and supervision to the team members.

2. Incorporates values that clearly provide direction for the team; these values should be visible and consistently portrayed.

3. Demonstrates a team culture and interdisciplinary atmosphere of trust where contributions are valued and consensus is fostered.

4. Ensures appropriate processes and infrastructures are in place to uphold the vision.

5. Provides quality patient-focused services with documented outcomes; utilizes feedback to improve the quality of care.

6. Utilizes communication strategies that promote intrateam communication, collaborative decision-making, and effective team processes.

TABLE 8.1 VALUES OF EFFECTIVE MEMBERS IN HIGH-FUNCTIONING HEALTHCARE TEAMS

VALUE	DESCRIPTION
Honesty	■ Transparency about goals, decisions, uncertainty, and errors. ■ Contributes to continued improvement and maintenance of mutual trust.
Discipline	■ Roles and responsibilities are performed with discipline despite challenges. ■ Members seek and share new information to improve individual and team function. ■ Members are disciplined in developing, following, and improving standards and protocols.[10,14]
Creativity	■ Mistakes and undesired outcomes are regarded as opportunities to learn and improve.[10,14] ■ Members are motivated by solving new or emerging problems creatively.
Humility	■ Differences in training and education are recognized, but no one individual's perspective is seen to be superior to that of another. ■ Members recognize that they are human and will make mistakes. ■ Members rely upon one another to identify and avoid mistakes, regardless of one's position in a hierarchy.
Integrity	■ Members possess strong moral principles and values. ■ Members provide collaborative decision-making and insulation against challenges.
Inquisitiveness	■ Members are dedicated to reflecting upon lessons learned in the course of their workday. ■ Members apply insights gained for continuous development of the individual and improvement of the team.

Source: From Mitchell P, Wynia M, Golden R, et al. Core principles and values of effective team-based health care. Discussion Paper, Institute of Medicine; 2012. www.iom.edu/tbc. https://www.nationalahec.org/pdfs/VSRT-Team-Based-Care-Principles-Values.pdf; Mabiker A, Husseini ME, Nemri AA, et al. Health care professional development: Working as a team to improve patient care. *Sudan J Paediatr*. 2014;14(2):9–16. https://www.ncbi.nlm.nih.gov/pmc/articles/PMC4949805/pdf/sjp-14-9.pdf

7. Provides sufficient team staffing to integrate an appropriate mix of skills, competencies, and personalities to meet the needs of patients and enhance smooth functioning.
8. Facilitates recruitment of staff who demonstrate interdisciplinary competencies including team functioning, collaborative leadership, communication, and sufficient professional knowledge and experience.
9. Promotes role interdependence while respecting individual roles and autonomy.
10. Facilitates team personal development through appropriate training, recognition, rewards, and opportunities for career development and advancement.[16]

Principles of Team-Based Healthcare

- *Shared goals:* The team includes the patient and, where appropriate, family members or other support persons work to establish shared goals that can be clearly articulated, understood, and supported by all team members.[8,11]
- *Clear roles and responsibilities:* Establish clear expectations for each team member's functions, responsibilities, and accountabilities, which optimize the team's efficiency.[8,11]
- *Mutual trust and respect:* Team members earn each other's trust, creating models of reciprocity and greater opportunities for shared success. They respect and appreciate each other's roles, talents, and beliefs.[8,11]
- *Effective communication:* The team prioritizes and continuously improves its communication skills. The team has consistent channels for candid and complete communication, which are used by all team members, using closed-loop communication.[8,11]
- *Measurable processes and outcomes:* The team agrees on and implements reliable and timely feedback on successes and areas of growth in both the functioning of the team and achievement of the team's goals. These are used to track and improve performance immediately and over time.[8,11]

Effective Communication and Teamwork

The literature has shown a direct correlation between effective communication, teamwork, and patient safety.[6,17–19] Nurses who are more likely to demonstrate effective communication behaviors, such as listening to understand and listening with intent—repeating and validating the information received—and seeking to understand, are more likely to foster teamwork.[6]

Teamwork is a critical concept for units to possess in order to have a highly reliable and safe environment of care.[20] In the literature, researchers found that multiple elements contributed to and/or inhibited the effective communication patterns of a team. The elements were often related to the dynamics of the team and the leadership behaviors, which serve as modeling influences.[21] Leaders who had a high degree of confidence and integrated effective team behaviors saw improved results in higher quality outcomes.[22] Leaders, who modeled and upheld the safety behaviors, while reinforcing them without punitive consequences, were also noted to have fewer and less adverse safety events.[19]

Additionally, regulatory requirements have been based on improving patient outcomes as evidenced by the Centers for Medicare & Medicaid Services (CMS) and The Joint Commission. These programs have proven that the culture of safety and patient outcomes were related to effective communication and team dynamics.[23–27]

Leadership influences the tone and establishes the expectation of performance. An effective leader who values the contributions of all staff regardless of years of experience or tenure is able to hear all staff voices equally. Leaders, both formal and informal, influence the peer and social norms of the team that promotes safety and quality as high-value targets.[5] When leaders have a positive correlation with safety practices, the effectiveness of the team has been demonstrated by improved patient outcomes, a reduction of serious safety events, and improved staff engagement.[5,20,21]

Interprofessional Conflict

It is important for healthcare leaders to be able to prevent, negotiate, and resolve interprofessional conflict.[8] The following practices are shown to support conflict resolution[8]:

1. Demonstrate a respectful attitude toward other colleagues and members of the team.
2. Work with other professionals to prevent conflicts.
3. Employ collaborative negotiation to resolve conflicts.
4. Respect differences, misunderstandings and limitations in other professionals.
5. Recognize one's own differences, misunderstandings, and limitations that may contribute to interprofessional tension.
6. Reflect on interprofessional team function.[8]

High Reliability and the Culture of Safety

The literature on high reliability and best safety practices emerged from the science of high reliability and the nuclear power and aviation industries. High reliability is a mindfulness where all workers look for and report small problems or unsafe conditions before they pose a substantial risk to the patient.[28] High-reliability theory has established the actions, behaviors, and improvements in the safety culture that will only occur when there are tangible improvements in team performance occurring at both micro and macro levels of an organization.[24] Behaviors specific to high-reliability organizations are SA, use of SBAR (situation, background, assessment, and recommendation), closed-loop communication, and a shared team vision.[15,24,26,28]

Additional context from the high-reliability literature emerged as the power distance or gradient and SA. Power distance or gradient refers to the way in which power is distributed and the extent to which the less powerful accept that power is distributed unequally.[29] The features of SA include the perception, comprehension, and projection of the appropriate actions based on the clinical findings, which are how the behavioral factors influence communication, teamwork, and the culture of safety.[29,30] The connection between high reliability and effective teamwork to improve safety outcomes is well described in the literature.

A "Just Culture" is a culture in which staff are encouraged to speak up regardless of rank or position if they have a concern. A Just Culture takes into account organizational system and process failures that contribute to errors. Team members are not punished for actions, omissions, or decisions taken by them which are commensurate with their experience and training.[29]

High-reliability organizations (HROs) commonly use daily safety huddles. Safety huddles are an evidence-based practice standard that allow teams to exchange safety information, build empowerment, and create a sense of community, which together form a culture of collaboration that increases the collective awareness for eliminating patient harm.[4,29,31]

Leadership Influences

Leadership sets the tone and establishes the expectations for team performance. An effective leader who values the contributions of all staff regardless of years of experience or education is able to hear all staff voices equally. Leaders, both formal and informal, also influence peer and social norms of the team that promotes safety and quality as a high-value targets.[5] When leaders had an affirmative correlation with safety practices, the effectiveness of the team was demonstrated by a reduction of serious safety events, improved patient outcomes, and improved staff engagement.[5,20,21,32,]

TeamSTEPPS®

A division of the U.S. Department of Health and Human Services, the Agency for Healthcare Research and Quality (AHRQ), also provides training based on CRM principles to healthcare teams at no cost. This training is called Team Strategies and Tools to Enhance Performance and Patient Safety (TeamSTEPPS).[1,2] The TeamSTEPPS program has demonstrated an improvement in team dynamics, communication, and decreased serious safety events in organizations who have utilized this content.[24] The program has been implemented in hospitals, long-term care facilities, and primary care clinics around the world. Specifically, TeamSTEPPS was designed to improve patient safety by teaching healthcare clinicians how better collaborate with each other by using various tools such as huddles, debriefs, handoffs, and check-backs.[1,2,24] Implementing TeamSTEPPS has been shown to improve patient safety.[5,6,24,33–35]

Moral Courage and Empowerment

Moral courage is the expression of a belief or opinion without the fear of reprisal and part of personal integrity.[36] The significance of moral courage as an element to improving communication or speaking up for safety is that moral courage informs how fear, previous experience, peer support, and the institutional culture that results in the practice of courage or what is also described as empowerment. Additionally, moral courage is seen as a related influence in the literature when communication barriers and teamwork are being studied.[22]

Nurse empowerment was the key characteristic described in speaking up on behalf of patient safety or advocacy.[34] The two critical elements supported in the literature to improve on this practice problem were empowerment and skill acquisition. Laschinger, a nurse scientist, has conducted extensive research on nurse empowerment and the link to improved patient outcomes. Laschinger described powerless nurses are ineffective nurses, and the consequences of nurses' lack of power as less satisfied with their jobs and more susceptible to burnout and depersonalization. The lack of nursing power may also contribute to poorer patient outcomes.[33] When nurses are empowered to speak up for patient safety, patients have better outcomes and the quality of care is improved.[7,34,35]

Resilience for Emergency Department Leaders

Evidence validates that ED leaders are at high risk for suffering from compassion fatigue (CF) as a result of the many challenges of the profession mentioned in previous chapters, such as caring for the critically ill/injured, witnessing the pain and suffering of others, high patient acuity, overcrowding, unrealistic patient expectations, violence, trauma, death, and the need to respond to rapidly changing time-sensitive situations.[35,37,38] The effects of cumulative exposure to other's distress and suffering (secondary trauma) may lead to an altered worldview, emotional withdrawal, depersonalization, and empathy blunting in ED leaders.[35,37,38] CF affects not only the ED leaders in terms of job satisfaction and emotional and physical health but also the organization by decreasing productivity, increasing errors, and increasing turnover.[37] It is vital that individuals and organizations take measures to mitigate the risk and negative resulting effects of CF, and increase resiliency. ED leaders should role model personal self-care, empathy, and consider organizational interventions aimed at well-being and resiliency.[38]

Leadership in Healthcare

Over the past decade, a growing body of evidence has developed surrounding the importance of human factors in healthcare and particularly within complex/high demand environments such as the ED.[2] Effective leadership is vital to team performance and optimal patient care. Effective interprofessional health care teams require members to be prepared for a team approach, including clear roles, closed-loop communication, and an understanding of team dynamics. The leader role in a high-performing team must include an understanding of shared decision-making and respect for diversity, while applying individual clinical expertise. All team members must possess both appropriate clinical expertise and teamwork abilities, including team dynamics, conflict prevention, negotiation, communication, and conflict resolution.[13] There should be a commitment to mutual respect, excellence, continuous improvement, and the strength of diversity by all team members.[13,14]

The IOM has stressed the importance interprofessional team-based healthcare.[8]

> Given this complexity of information and interpersonal connections, it is not only difficult for one clinician to provide care in isolation but also potentially harmful. As multiple clinicians provide care to the same patient or family, clinicians become a team—a group working with at least one common aim: the best possible care—whether or not they acknowledge this fact. Each clinician relies upon information and action from other members of the team. Yet, without explicit acknowledgment and purposeful cultivation of the team, systematic inefficiencies and errors cannot be addressed and prevented. Now, more than ever, there is an obligation to strive for perfection in the science and practice of interprofessional team-based healthcare.[8]

Leadership Styles in Healthcare

Leadership of healthcare professionals is critical for providing quality care and has correlations on patient outcomes. Although there are many styles of leadership, a 2017 systematic review identified six common types of leadership in healthcare settings. These include: transformational, transactional, autocratic, laissez-faire, task-oriented, and relationship-oriented leadership. Transformational leadership is characterized by the ability to motivate, develop, and maintain relationships among staff members. Transformational leaders are well-respected, inspire confidence, and communicate loyalty through a shared vision, resulting in increased productivity, strong staff morale, and job satisfaction.[39] In transactional leadership, the leader drives change by influencing staff, which results in improvement in productivity. An autocratic leader makes all decisions without taking into account the thoughts or opinion of staff or team members. With the autocratic leader, mistakes are often not tolerated. The laissez-faire leader does not make decisions and instead, staff members act without direction or supervision. The laissez-faire leader practices a hands-off approach that rarely results in positive change. Task-oriented leaders are involved in planning of work activities, clarification of roles within a team, setting objectives, and continuously monitoring performance and processes. Lastly, relationship-oriented leaders prioritize support for and development, and recognition of the team and team members.[39] Often, healthcare leaders function within various leadership styles depending on the situation.

Summary

Leading in a dynamic, fast-paced environment such as EDs is not easy. It is important to put the team at ease, encourage communication, and empower team members to think critically and function effectively in their role. This requires self-awareness, self-confidence combined with humility The following concepts support the healthcare leader in performing optimally.[36]

Know yourself: It is important to have a strong sense of personal ethics or a moral compass to build upon in your profession. Knowing who you are and what you stand for personally and professionally allows you to speak up when needed.[36]

Live your values: Knowing your values and ethics isn't enough, you must practice this through your actions. This is not always easy in the challenging work environment of the ED. This takes wisdom, courage, integrity, and resilience.[40] Obligation to care for ourselves before caring for others. Include your personal well-being in your definition of success.

Listen to your intuition: If you are consistent about living your values and ethics, you will be able to rely on that internal voice.[40]

Check in with others: Translating ethical decision-making into daily professional practice is challenging. Building and maintaining a network of colleagues who can help navigate through situations is vital.[40]

Practice with respect: Create a climate of respect and dignity.[40]

References

References for this chapter are online only and can be found at https://connect.springerpub.com/content/reference-book/978-0-8261-6091-5/part/part01/toc-part/ch08.

9. Ethics, Bioethics, and Legal Aspects of Emergency Care

SHANNON M. KEATING | JOHN JAMISON

Learning Objectives

- Differentiate between concepts of ethics and bioethics, and how to apply these concepts to emergency care.
- Compare and contrast the difference in fundamental bioethical principles and apply in an appropriate clinical scenario.
- Demonstrate knowledge of the three most common medical negligence lawsuits (i.e., failure to diagnose, delay in critical diagnosis, and wrong diagnosis) and put into practice methods to avoid these unfortunate events.
- Describe ways to reduce the risk of litigation: Listen to patient concerns, specialty consultation when needed, review prior documentation, and rule out worst-case scenario.
- Recognize the important components of decision-making capacity (i.e., knowledge of available options, awareness of consequences of choosing the option or not choosing it, cost vs. benefit of the options) and apply to practice.

Ethics and Bioethics in Emergency Care

Both ethics and bioethics play an important role in emergency care. The principles that make up these concepts are the cornerstone of decision-making at the bedside and guide legal discussions regarding the delivery of care. This section will focus on the basics of ethics and bioethics in emergency care, including a discussion of basic medicolegal terminology and issues.

Ethics Versus Bioethics

Ethics are an individual's moral principles, guiding them in how they conduct themselves and behave. Hence, medical ethics encompasses justice, charity, generosity, and the concept of duty to act in one's own best interest, as well as the best interest of society, or singularly, a patient. Bioethics is simply the ethics of medicine and research. It is the application of values and morals to find reasonable solutions for dilemmas faced by clinicians. The very basis of emergency care naturally focuses on the medicine, often brushing the ethical piece to the side. However, when it comes to the law, ethics and bioethics are most certainly considered as the law is not always black and white. Laws are simply rules of conduct that may vary by geographic location. Ethics incorporate the broad values and beliefs of conduct that are believed to be correct within a culture. The societal values that make up ethics and bioethics must be incorporated into the law. Therefore, a good understanding of this relationship and how the concepts intermingle will help clinicians make the best decisions—both medical and ethical—for their patients.

Most individuals have a personal system of values learned at a very young age through indoctrination into the culture of their birth, behaviors observed, and secular and religious education and experience. Clinicians care for and treat patients with various value systems requiring them to be sensitive to beliefs that are different from their own. A vital element to ethical, bedside decision-making is an understanding of the patient's values. This may be challenging as some people struggle to honestly articulate their personal values when it comes to health and healthcare. However, a working solution is to ascertain the patient's goal of medical treatment and why they seek certain interventions. In some instances, such as with patients who are incompetent or too young or to express their values, clinicians may need to make general assumptions about what a normal person would want in a particular situation. Certain values that are generally accepted by the medical community, legal system, and society include the following fundamental bioethical principles.

Nonmaleficence. Do no harm, prevent harm, remove harmful conditions.

Beneficence. Be beneficial to the patient, do good, take steps to prevent harm.

Autonomy. A patient's right to self-determination, including the right to accept, or reject, medical care even if it is in direct conflict with the clinician's recommendations, including the refusal of care.

Justice. Although not necessarily a confusing definition, justice is a controversial societal issue. Simply put, justice is fairness; however, determining who decides what is fair can be controversial. Justice implies distributing goods in society and enabling entitlement. Generally, persons who are equal should qualify for equal treatment and fairness in the allocation of resources and obligations. It is a value applied in the formation of healthcare policy. One example is how Medicare was formed for all persons over 65 years of age, but only taking into account that one common factor, age, and not the other variety of factors used for distributive justice; to each an equal share according to need, effort, contribution, merit, and free market exchanges. Many believe society must help even the playing field by providing resources to those not to blame by the natural, cultural, or societal factors one has been born into. An example of this is Medicaid, healthcare designed to help those at poverty level. Justice will continue to create confusion and debate in our healthcare communities and among those forming the policies. It must be understood and discussed openly to make the best possible decisions for patients and society as a whole.

Truth-telling. A concept basic to ethical thought and reasoning is truth-telling. Therefore, it is a wonder that this might be considered controversial in certain medical circles. Whereas some clinicians may see the truth as absolute and a patient's right to know, others may believe withholding certain information is of more benefit to the patient's health than the absolute truth. An example where withholding the truth may benefit the patient is that of the news of critical illness. The clinician may believe that if the patient loses hope, or does not find it due to their grave illness, they may not have the chance to find the strength within themselves to survive. The clinician may feel that withholding information may benefit the patient in the long term, and therefore, feel as if they are upholding the Hippocratic Oath by protecting them from emotional harm. On the other hand, withholding information may be in direct contrast with other pertinent values, namely informed consent and autonomy, for without the truth, a patient cannot make an informed decision autonomously.

Confidentiality and privacy. Patient confidentiality is imperative to the clinician–patient relationship as it presumes whatever the patient tells the clinician will not be revealed to any other person or entity without permission. This value is an obligation and duty on the part of the clinician and a critical component to earning and maintaining patient trust and confidence, which ultimately upholds other values, particularly that of beneficence and nonmaleficence. Privacy is the right of the patient to have physical and auditory isolation during an examination or interview with medical personnel. The Health Insurance Portability and Accountability Act (HIPAA), discussed in the next section, works to protect both of these patient values. Barriers in the ED to these values are also discussed in the next section.

The Basics From a Legal Perspective

Consent

Implied Consent and Presumed Consent

Different sources cite varying, but closely linked, definitions of these two terms, and some use them interchangeably. Implied consent means the patient actively cooperates with a procedure. Presumed consent is when the patient is informed of what will occur, and they do not refuse treatment; therefore, the clinician can presume consent has been given. Some examples are closely linked and include a patient that actively places her legs in stirrups for a gynecological examination or one that holds still for suturing of a wound. It could also be implied that a person who is unconscious would want medical care if they were able to communicate for themselves. Neither presumed nor implied consent indicate the patient is unconcerned about the treatment or condition, but they may not verbalize this under several scenarios, such as inability due to incapacitation, the belief they know enough about the treatment or procedure and do not need to ask questions, or they are too embarrassed to ask questions. Regardless, a clinician must act in the patient's best interest under the circumstances given.

Informed Consent

This concept requires clinician to give patients adequate information about proposed treatments and requires two conditions: adequate decision-making capacity and ability to make voluntary choices free of undue influence.

Capacity and Competency

A patient's capacity is the ability to make an informed medical decision based on personal values and comprehension regarding the consequences of their decision. Competence is a legal term referring to an individual's ability to manage his or her own affairs as ruled by a court of law. The clinician must informally assess the patient's ability by taking their health history without any barriers to communication, such as language or intoxication, and ask why they have made a specific choice, particularly if it does not seem like a reasonable choice to the clinician. A patient can be deemed competent but not have the capacity to make a decision. An example of this is an intoxicated patient who may have the competence to refuse a small laceration be sutured, but not the capacity to refuse a life-saving procedure or operation. Components of decision-making capacity include:

- Knowledge of the available options
- Awareness of the consequences of choosing or not choosing an option
- Cost versus benefit of the options and their consequences

Advance Directives

If a patient is no longer able to communicate their wishes, thus they no longer have the bioethical principle of autonomy, an advance directive may be put into place prior to incapacitation, which can outline their wishes in writing. This is usually done in anticipation to avoid the inevitable, whether painful or nonpainful, dying process. Examples of such documents include a living will, durable power of attorney for healthcare, prehospital and mental health advance directives.

Living Will

A living will outlines treatment preferences or rejections if a person is incapacitated. Examples include medical procedures or treatments that serve only to prolong, not prevent, death, such as a feeding tube, endotracheal intubation, or use of a ventilator.

Durable Power of Attorney for Healthcare

Multiple terms may be synonymous with this definition including power of attorney for healthcare, surrogate decision-maker, and healthcare proxy or agent, all of which are appointed by the patient prior to incapacitation to assist in healthcare decisions.

Prehospital and Mental Health Advance Directives

These documents take into account the established fact that certain interventions may not be appropriate in all instances and the activation of emergency medical services (EMS) may not be necessary. An example would be a patient who is in hospice care with impending death. It may be more appropriate to contact the patient's personal clinician as opposed to call for EMS.

Against Medical Advice

Despite a clinician's best efforts, some patients may choose to leave the ED against medical advance (AMA). Multiple reasons have been cited for this decision, including fear of the proposed testing or treatment, concerns regarding cost of the visit, or outside obligations. Regardless of the reason to leave AMA, the clinician should make every attempt to inform the patient, in good faith, about their diagnosis or potential diagnoses and the concerns or possible outcomes. If a patient has the mental capacity to make an informed decision, the clinician can proceed with an AMA discharge. Documentation of the aspects of the discharge should include decisional capacity with specific examples, discussion of risks associated with diagnoses that are being considered, documentation that the patient wanted to leave AMA and what treatments, procedures, or recommendations they were refusing, any offers made of alternative options (e.g., agreeing to delay a CT scan while labs and repeat examinations are pending), and efforts to involve relatives of the patient. Furthermore, if there are concerning labs or other diagnostic values in the chart that may lend doubt on the decision-making capacity of the patient (such as an elevated blood alcohol level or positive toxicology screen), documenting that the patient is clinically sober with a specific follow-up physical examination is important. Other elements of documentation should include an offer to treat, with a prescription for antibiotics, for example, and the fact the patient is welcome to return to the ED at any time. Lastly, the patient should sign the AMA form as this can help relieve the clinician of the duty to treat, create assumption of risk on the part of the patient, and record the evidence of the patient's refusal. If they refuse to sign the AMA form, this should be documented as well.

Issues Regarding Minors

Clinicians are given great leeway to determine what constitutes an emergency medical condition under EMTALA (Emergency Medical Treatment and Active Labor Act). Once an emergency condition is stabilized, attempts to obtain informed parental consent need to be made and documented. An adult relative, such as a grandparent or adult sibling, can grant permission to render care, but attempts should still be made to reach the parents. State laws vary regarding treatment of minors, but in general, most states have some common exceptions allowing clinicians to treat minor patients in the ED, including emancipated minors (living independently, married, or with children of their own), mature minor law (older than 14 years and able to understand the nature of the illness and treatments), sexually transmitted diseases, prenatal and pregnancy care, and sexual or physical abuse.

Maintaining Privacy and Confidentiality

Upholding patient privacy and confidentiality in the ED is of utmost importance as it affirms a patient's dignity and value. Originally adopted by physicians at the advent of the profession, the Hippocratic Oath is a moral code of conduct and ethical practices that encompass the duty to preserve a patient's privacy. It is widely followed by all clinicians. However, despite the best of intentions, several barriers exist that make this rather challenging for clinicians. Examples of such barriers include ED layout (e.g., using curtains instead of doors), ED overcrowding leading to patient placement in areas not meant for treatment (e.g., hallways), and presence of visitors, students, or technology (e.g., cell phones for video recording). If a patient requests a private area to speak to the clinician, this should be granted, and the clinician should refrain from discussing anything that may be overheard by others. Additionally, clinicians need to be cautious in how they discuss personal information. For example, if a patient's family member is in the room, the clinician should ask permission to discuss diagnoses, treatments, or any other information. At times this can be challenging, and the clinician may need to be creative with their approach. For example, an 18-year-old girl in the ED for abdominal pain and vomiting may not want her mother to know that she could be pregnant nor feel comfortable saying in front of her mother that she wants privacy to discuss personal information. The clinician should take any opportunity to discuss this information when the patient is alone, and the mother has left to use the restroom, for instance.

Another challenging situation that frequently arises in the ED is a patient who is in police custody, particularly if they are deemed dangerous, and the officer is unable to leave the examination room while the clinician speaks with or examines the patient. Safety of everyone must be balanced with the individual's right to privacy and confidentiality. The clinician should provide unbiased care and privacy to the fullest extent possible to all patients regardless of the circumstances. Communication to law enforcement regarding treatment of the medical condition would be warranted and appropriate.

Advancing technology has provided many more opportunities for the recording of real-time situations in the ED. The question of technology's use in healthcare, particularly regarding patient information inclusive of written documents as well as pictures, of wounds for example, requires permission by the patient. Specific laws and hospital policies can vary by geographic region. A prudent clinician should be aware of the specific laws of their state in addition to the organizational policy regarding use of electronic devices including phones and tablets in the ED.

Health Insurance Portability and Accountability Act

Originally signed into law in 1996, HIPAA includes administration simplification processes that require the U.S. Department of Health and Human Services (HHS) to adopt national standards for electronic medical records, identifiers, and security of individual's personal health information. It protects an individual's healthcare privacy and confidentiality, including any information that may be shared, whether in writing, electronically, or verbally regarding an individual's past, present, or potential future mental or physical health. This protected health information (PHI) is shared only to the extent that is necessary to accomplish the purpose of the disclosure and allows for open discussions between clinician—such as emergency clinician or primary care clinicians—and consultants. It also allows health information to be shared for the purpose of reimbursement or for the release of medical records to a patient or authorized representative. In an emergency situation, PHI can be discussed with family or friends if the patient is unable to consent and the information may be helpful to the patient. Conversely, discussing PHI in public areas or in front of others without permission is prohibited. Leaving a logged-in computer unattended with PHI or accessing records by a nontreating clinician is also prohibited, unless needed for law enforcement or another legitimate reason and should be documented in the chart.

There are certain instances that PHI will be shared if the needs of the public supersede the privacy and confidentiality of the individual. These laws may vary by state but typically include abuse, particularly child or elder abuse, injury by a deadly weapon such as gunshot wounds, driver impairment such as with epilepsy, and infectious diseases. Civil penalties in the form of monetary fines, ranging from $100 to $1.5 million per violation, may be instituted depending on whether the breach was intentional or neglectful. Furthermore, Federal law allows criminal penalties of up to 10 years in jail and $250,000 in fines. If a breach is suspected, the clinician should discuss it with legal counsel immediately to minimize the risk of penalties.

Emergency Medical Treatment and Active Labor Act

A legal area unique to emergency care is the Emergency Medical Treatment and Active Labor Act (EMTALA), passed in 1985 as part of the Consolidated Omnibus Budget Reconciliation Act (COBRA). Also known as the "anti-dumping act," EMTALA was enacted to address the unsafe transfer and discharge of uninsured and underinsured patients and to ensure all patients receive appropriate care regardless of ability to pay. EMTALA has four core components; three directed at originating facilities, and one directed at receiving facilities:

- *Medical Screening Exam (MSE):* All patients presenting to a facility with an ED requesting evaluation must receive an MSE to determine whether an emergent medical condition or active labor are present.
- *Stabilizing Treatment:* Patients must be provided all necessary stabilizing medical treatment within the facility's capability for their identified emergency medical conditions.
- *Appropriate Transfer*: Patients must be appropriately transferred. Facilities are required to care for patients within their capability and capacity until they are stable for discharge. Patients can only be transferred if the facility lacks capacity or capability to care for the patient. The patient must be transferred to the closest most appropriate facility and have an accepting clinician at that facility. Unstable patients can only be transferred if the benefit outweighs the risk.
- *Transfer Acceptance:* Receiving facilities with appropriate capability and capacity to care for referred patients are required to accept appropriate transfers from referring facilities.

On its face, the purpose, intent, and requirements of EMTALA are straightforward; however, compliance has several complexities and risks for both the clinician and the facility. Certain types of patients and situation increase the risk of EMTALA violations.

EMTALA does not specify what exactly constitutes an MSE, only those patients with similar complaints and conditions cannot receive disparate examinations. The MSE needs to be sufficient to determine whether an emergency medical condition exists, and if the patient is stable but does not require a correct final diagnosis. Situations that can result in an MSE violation include delayed triage or clinician assessment of a patient, explicit or implicit referral of low acuity patients to alternative treatment destinations, minimal assessment of frequently seen or drug-seeking patients, ambulance diversions, direct referral of a pregnant patient to OB triage or a facility with OB services, and inadequate assessment of a psychiatric patient to determine whether an underlying medical condition exists.

Under EMTALA, stabilizing treatment is defined as the treatment—within the capability of the facility—necessary to prevent, with reasonable medical certainty, the patient's condition from deteriorating on discharge or during transfer. This includes necessary procedures and interventions, assessment by on-call specialists as indicated, and admission to an appropriate medical unit. For pregnant women in active labor, stabilization includes delivery of the baby and placenta. Stabilization violations primarily occur due to premature discharge of a patient or failure of on-call specialist to respond. The one exception to the stabilization mandate is if the facility does not have the capability to provide definitive stabilizing treatment. In this case, a patient can be transferred in a less than stable condition if the patient or representative consents to the transfer and the clinician certifies that the benefits of the transfer outweigh the risk.

EMTALA has several requirements to ensure transfers are appropriate. Facilities can only transfer patients if they lack the capability or capacity to care for the patient. Patients must be sent to the closest appropriate facility. Patients must be stable for transfer. A clinician at the receiving facility must accept the patient. The patient must be sent by appropriate mode of transport. Appropriate transfer violations can occur by failing to admit an appropriate patient due to on-call specialist not responding, transferring a patient to a farther or insurance-preferred destination without proper justification, transferring a woman in active labor without clear justification of the risk versus benefit (e.g., breech baby with no surgery available for a C-section), transferring a patient to an accepting facility prior to getting acceptance from a receiving clinician, or sending a patient by private vehicle or medical crew whose skill level is below that indicated by the patient's condition (e.g., BLS [basic life support] vs. ALS [advanced life support] vs. critical care).

Transfer acceptance under EMTALA, sometimes called the "reverse dumping provision" requires that a receiving facility with the specialized capability required by the patient accepts the transfer if it has the capacity. Transfer acceptance is not a direct violation issue for referring facilities or clinicians; however, it can potentially result in patient harm through delayed transfer or the need to transfer the patient further. Clinicians should be aware of the capabilities not only of the closest referral facilities but also alternative referral facilities so as to help facilitate timely and appropriate transfers.

EMTALA compliance is regulated and investigated by the individual State Survey Agency (SA) using the published interpretive guidelines and sent forward to the Regional Office (RO) of CMS (Centers for Medicare & Medicaid Services) for review. EMTALA requires that violations be reported within 72 hours and provides monetary fines and possible loss of CMS certification for both the facility and the responsible clinician. The original maximum fine per EMTALA violation (not just per patient) was $50,000 for facilities with less than 100 beds and $100,000 for facilities with greater than 100 beds. In 2015, new legislation added an annual cost of living adjustment to the fines. The current 2020 maximum fines for EMTALA violations are $55,800 and $111,597, respectively. EMTALA violations are only a regulatory violation and do not directly constitute malpractice but can increase the risk of malpractice and negligence claims. Improper management of certain patient types such as indigent patients, frequent ED utilizers, obstetric patients, and psychiatric patients are more likely to result in EMTALA violations. EMTALA is also not always uniformly interpreted and enforced. Various application by the 10 CMS Regions and court interpretations by the 13 federal circuit courts has resulted in some regional variations. Over the years, CMS had added revisions and interpretive guidance regarding EMTALA compliance. This has included definitions expanding EMTALA coverage to Hospital Urgent Care Centers and certain inpatient situations as well as the "250-yard rule," requiring anyone presenting on the campus of a facility requesting emergency examination to be seen and evaluated, even if they do not initially present directly to the ED. The most recent guidance is the March 2020 memorandum on the application of EMTALA to COVID-19 drive-up testing, COVID-19 isolation, and telemedicine. CMS provides general interpretive guidance in Appendix V of the *State Operations Manual* (CMS publication 100-07). The best defense against EMTALA violations is good staff training on EMTALA and what constitutes violation, reading and following facility policies on MSE, and transfer procedures and thorough documentation. When in doubt, the best policy is to do what is in the best interest of the patient. Many EMTALA violations are related to poor policies or institutional violations of policy. Courts and CMS inspections will generally take motive into consideration when contemplating fines or judgments against individual clinicians.

Civil Law

Unlike criminal cases, civil cases typically involve a dispute between two or more parties where compensation to the suing party (plaintiff) is the ultimate goal for an alleged injury, or wrongdoing, by the sued party (defendant). The burden of proof is on the plaintiff for medical malpractice cases, or those claiming professional negligence.

Negligence

Negligence is the failure to do or not do something that a reasonable person in a similar situation or setting would or would not do. The plaintiff must prove four elements against the defendant to be successful in a medical malpractice case:

1. *Duty of care:* Clinicians are obligated to provide the standard of care (knowledge, skill, and care ordinarily provided by a reasonably well-qualified clinician in similar circumstances).
2. *Breach of that duty:* The clinician did not provide the standard of care.
3. *Proximate cause:* The negligence of the clinician more than likely caused the injury sustained by the patient. Furthermore, this connection must be reasonably foreseen and probable in a similar course of events.
4. *Damages:* Compensation awarded for loss or injury suffered due to the negligence of the clinician. This will include damages for disability or disfigurement, pain and suffering, past and future medical expenses, lost wages, funeral expenses, and any other damages deemed appropriate by the court.

Risk Management

There are numerous factors in the ED setting that could create the potential for error despite best efforts put in place for checks and balances. Areas of risk that have been identified in malpractice lawsuits time and again in the ED show several potential errors regarding particular chief complaints and medical diagnoses, such as but not limited to the following:

- Chest pain and the potential missed acute myocardial infarction (MI)
- Abdominal pain and potential missed appendicitis or abdominal aortic aneurysm
- Open wound with foreign body or tendon injury
- Cerebrovascular accident (CVA)
- Ectopic pregnancy
- Embolism
- Spinal cord injuries
- Traumatic injuries
- Meningitis
- Pediatric fever
- Missed fractures

In addition to issues related to missed, failed, or delayed diagnosis, the potential for error could manifest as delay in treatment, improper treatment, and failure to consult or refer. It is important to note that almost two-thirds of errors occur when there is more than one clinician involved in the patient's care, such as the case with end of shift sign out. In one study of malpractice claims by four insurers, cognitive errors such as judgment, memory, and knowledge contributed to 96% of claims with medical errors. The supervision of students and residents is also important, as the performance of procedures, where they may not be as skilled, was the second highest category of error.

Clinicians can take certain steps to reduce the risk of medical errors. Introducing oneself to the patient and family and sitting down to talk and listen to their concerns is very well received by the patients. Professional attire and speaking in clear, simple language is inviting and comforting to patients and family members. Showing empathy and giving emotional support when appropriate is also helpful. Lastly, discussing the patient's expectations and personally providing discharge instructions while giving the patient the opportunity to ask questions helps reduce anxiety and makes them feel important to the clinician. If a clinician takes sign out from another clinician, it is good practice to meet the patient and evaluate for themselves.

Unique Ethical Issues in Emergency Care

Due to the environmental and patient distinctiveness of the ED, there are multiple unique situations that may arise and can pose challenging ethical questions for clinicians. Oftentimes, these situations require as much uniqueness in their approach as is required for treatment attempts and solutions. Some examples include ethics in resuscitation and the question of futility. Resuscitation is the most time-dependent activity in the ED, and any patient who requires this care has implicitly been guaranteed that all available knowledge and resources will be utilized for life-saving purposes. However, resuscitation is also one of the best scenarios for a healthcare student to learn so that they may one day be able to perform life-saving treatments. This bears the question of futility. If a resuscitation is deemed futile, it may be considered an appropriate opportunity for students to practice skills on a patient who is not salvageable, as they cannot cause any further harm. Futile circumstances in an ED can only be used in certain situations, those that have a recognizable less than 1% chance of survival based on the literature (e.g., thoracotomy for blunt chest trauma), known physiological futility (e.g., decapitation), and when the treatment or intervention will not achieve the patient's goal of therapy. This last example would require the clinician have prior knowledge of the presenting patient to the ED, which would be uncommon. An example would be the patient who is well known to the ED for multiple prior visits and a chronic, fatal health problem.

In a disaster, the normal process of the ED is interrupted and often overwhelming. History has proven that healthcare needs will far outweigh available resources. Thus, ethical procedures must be in place well before a disaster occurs in order to efficiently activate a response, which includes mobilizing personnel, equipment, setting up rapid triage, assessment, and stabilization of patients. Safety of staff is a top priority and can start with restricting patient entry to only one location, the triage area for rapid assessment, identification, registration, priority management, and distribution to the appropriate treatment areas. Clinical care will be altered based on available supplies and personnel, but staff should perform the roles that are familiar to them.

Multiple research studies have been conducted on ethical considerations in a disaster situation. The principles of utilitarianism (maximize the greatest number of lives), beneficence (do no harm), and justice (provide care to all) are the common results. Simply put, patient prioritization should be based on patient needs, the sickest patient receives the highest priority to avoid worse outcomes unless that care is deemed futile, in which case, redirecting resources from those without high chances of survival to others with greater chance of survival is essential. Palliative care may be implemented for someone not likely to survive. This approach aims to achieve individual as well as public health ethics by achieving the most good for the most people. Therefore, clinician engagement through continuing education and disaster preparation training is critically important in order to be familiar with triage protocols regarding scarce allocation. Having strict guidelines in place can help navigate through ethical decision-making and prioritization during a disaster response.

Legal Issues in Emergency Care

Medicolegal issues are a great concern to clinicians and healthcare institutions. Most clinicians expect to become involved in litigation to some degree at some point during their career. Medical negligence lawsuits create great emotional stress for the named defendant. Because there are so many different insurers in the United States, data on the exact amount of malpractice cases are uncertain. However, it is estimated that there are 125,000 active cases at any given time in the United States. Nearly 57% are related to diagnosis issues: failure to establish a diagnosis, delay of critical diagnosis, or forming the wrong diagnosis. Coupled with a high-stress environment in today's ED with episodic care and little time for leisurely contemplation, unfortunately, the overall effect of malpractice cases has caused clinician to practice defensive medicine by obtaining more supportive diagnostics than what might otherwise be obtained with clinical presentation. This includes ordering a test when the likelihood of an emergency diagnosis is low (e.g., CT chest for pulmonary embolism in a patient in no distress with normal vital signs or CT head in minor head injury vs. education and reevaluation).

Nurse Practitioners and Malpractice

As of August 2018, there were 248,000 nurse practitioners (NPs) licensed in the United States. Malpractice rates as a primary defendant for these clinicians remain at a low 1.9%. However, studies for NP medical malpractice claims are statistically limited due to the low number of claims made. This number is expected to rise as the number of physicians retiring from primary care rise and more

NPs fill the role. Being named in a medical malpractice case can cause a great deal of stress for the named clinician, including time away from work and family, lost wages, depression, anxiety, and feelings of worthlessness or incompetence.

To avoid mistakes in clinical care, it is important for NPs to be present in the moment, which can be challenging with multiple different stimuli in the ED at any given second. Focusing on the patient, giving them the time and attention they deserve by really listening to their concerns, seeking consultation when needed, reviewing other clinician's documentation or previous findings, and ruling out the most dangerous or worst scenario first are all ways to diminish the risk of litigation. Documentation provides a picture of what the clinician was thinking. The medical decision-making (MDM) portion of the chart is the window into the brain of the NP who is treating the patient. It is a synopsis of the care received and the patient's response to treatment. The opportunity should be taken for the NP to explain why certain treatment modalities were sought and others avoided. It should paint a picture of the patient's ED visit and the NP's line of thinking and include the history, physical examination findings, and explanation of what took place in the ED. It should include what differentials were considered and ruled out. Documentation of discussions with patients and family members should include medical advice and decisions regarding disposition. A reassessment prior to discharge should always be documented. Abnormal findings should be noted as attorneys look for abnormalities that were not addressed accordingly. It is not uncommon to have multiple abnormal findings with an ED patient even if they are being discharged. If a patient is being sent home with diagnostic abnormalities, explain this in the documentation. For example, an adult patient sent home with an abnormal heart rate of 110 beats per minute could be documented as "heart rate noted to be tachycardic at 110 beats per minute commensurate with mild dehydration, which has been treated in the ED and the patient is now tolerating oral fluids and has improved." Additionally, documentation should include a conversation with the patient regarding their diagnosis and the importance of hydration, in this case, including symptoms they may suffer from dehydration and directions to return to the ED for worsening symptoms. Some things that may not be so obvious, but can result in malpractice issues as well as criminal offenses, include presigning prescriptions, prescribing scheduled drugs without proper documentation (examination and diagnosis that necessitate the medication, and in some states checking the state's prescription drug monitoring site), taking kickbacks (receiving anything of value from a vendor in return for making a referral or prescribing certain medications), and billing inappropriately. Fortunately, the last example is not frequently encountered in the ED setting as the clinician does not independently do the billing.

Conclusion

This chapter sought to give a brief and succinct overview of ethics and bioethics in emergency medicine and how they tie into legal aspects pertaining to emergency care. Specific examples aim to help the reader to understand how to apply certain aspects into their personal practice style while upholding principles important for personal integrity and safety as it pertains to both the clinician and the patient. Overall, as with any healthcare, emergency care is a helping profession, and in order for one to achieve the goal of helping people, they must understand the ethical principles and how it relates to maintaining and upholding the law.

Additional Reading

Additional Reading for this chapter are online only and can be found at https://connect.springerpub.com/content/reference-book/978-0-8261-6091-5/part/part01/toc-part/ch09.

10. Organ Donation

RENEÉ SEMONIN HOLLERAN

Learning Objectives

- Discuss the determination of brain death.
- Identify the barriers to organ donation in the emergency department (ED).
- Identify patients in the ED who may be suitable for organ donation.
- Discuss ways to approach a family to consent for organ donation.

It is estimated that over 112,000 people in the United States are on the waiting list for an organ to save their lives. One organ donor could save up to eight lives (www.organdonor.gov/statistics-stories/statistics.html).

Most brain death determination occurs in the ICU. The ED is a challenging setting for approaching families for organ donation consent, but it has been found that not doing so could be a missed opportunity for patients who have agreed to organ donation and the families who would like their family member's life to be of value to someone else.[1–3]

A study of organ donation after cardiac arrest found that patients resuscitated from cardiac arrest with irrecoverable neurological injury nonetheless have the potential to be organ donors.[2,4]

Unfortunately, asking a family who has lost a loved one to consider organ donation in the ED can be very difficult for many reasons. The emergency nurse practitioner (ENP) does have a role in assisting the family in making this difficult decision.

Determining Brain Death[5,6]

A. Clinical history, etiology of illness or injury, and neuroimaging demonstrate an irreversible, devastating brain injury that leads to the loss of all brain functions.
B. No confounding variables such as hypothermia, pharmacological paralysis, central nervous system (CNS) depressing medications or toxins, or severe metabolic, acid–base, and endocrine derangements (e.g., hypoglycemia or hyperglycemia)
C. Apnea testing

Barriers to Organ Donation in the Emergency Department[3]

A. Limited resources in the ED and facilities to keep the patient alive until a decision can be made by the family or person responsible for making decisions on behalf of the patient
B. Lack of standardization of the local and state guidelines for determining brain death
C. Determining the transition from life to death
D. Religious beliefs of the patient and family
E. Fear of negative reactions from the patient's family
F. Cause of death
G. Negative effects of the mass media
H. Fear of legal problems
I. Sudden unexpected death
J. Death of a child

Recognition of Patients in the Emergency Department Who May Be Suitable for Organ Donation

A. Patients who are at the end of life.
B. Patients who are taken off mechanical ventilation in the ED.
C. Patients who have given consent for organ donation. In many states consent can be found on the patient's driver's license.
D. Family who request that the patient become an organ donor.
E. Patients post cardiac arrest with lower rates of shockable rhythms, fewer witnessed cardiac arrests, and more epinephrine.
F. Failed use of automation resuscitation equipment or placing the patient on extracorporeal membrane oxygenation (ECMO).
G. Out-of-hospital cardiac arrest.

Approaching the Family of the Patient for Organ Donation

A. Check to see if the patient has any identification that may indicate they have elected organ donation (e.g., state driver's license).
B. Bring the family to the bedside when possible and speak with them about what is happening. Answer all questions as best as possible.
C. Involve other support persons, such as clergy, mental health, and social work professionals.
D. Involve organ procurement professionals to answer any questions about organ donation.
E. It is important that the family does not feel any undue pressures, and the advanced practice registered nurse (APRN) needs to be seen as the clinician participating in the resuscitation of the patient.

References

References for this chapter are online only and can be found at https://connect.springerpub.com/content/reference-book/978-0-8261-6091-5/part/part01/toc-part/ch10

11. Complementary and Alternative Modalities in the Emergency Department

RENEÉ SEMONIN HOLLERAN

Learning Objectives

- Define integrative therapies.
- Identify integrative therapies that can be used in the emergency department (ED).
- Describe the use of these therapies in the management of patients in the ED.

Integrative therapies, also described as complementary and alternative medicine, have gained increasing popularity in clinical care.[1] One of the primary reasons has to do with the failure of current medical modalities to meet the needs of ill patients, especially those with a chronic illness. Integrative medicine is healing—and holistic—oriented. It focuses on relationship-centered care and integrates complementary and conventional medical treatments. It incorporates Western and Eastern care philosophies. It uses both naturalistic and invasive interventions if needed. It engages all components of an individual, including the physical and emotional environment in which the patient lives. The focus is on healing, even if it is toward a "good" death.[2,3]

These approaches, however, are not new to the practice of nursing. Nursing has always been based on caring for the "total" person: mind, body, and spirit.[4,5]

In 2007, the National Center for Complementary and Integrative Health (NCCIH) estimated about one-third of all Americans had used some type of complementary health modalities (nccih.nih.gov/research/statistics/2007/camsurvey_fs1.htm).

The recognition of the effectiveness of integrative therapies can be of significant use in the care of patients in the ED with such complaints as pain, anxiety, and chronic illnesses such as asthma and chronic obstructive pulmonary disease (COPD).

There are multiple integrative therapies in use all over the world. Box 11.1 contains a list of these integrative therapies. It is important to remember when obtaining a history from a patient who presents to the ED to question the patient's use of integrative therapies. The following discussion presents some of the integrative therapies that may be used in the ED.

BOX 11.1 EXAMPLES OF INTEGRATIVE THERAPIES

- Acupuncture
- Alpha
- Ayurveda
- Biofeedback
- Chelation therapy
- Chiropractic or osteopathic manipulation
- Deep breathing exercises
- Energy healing therapy/Reiki
- Essential oils
- Guided imagery
- Homeopathic treatment
- Hypnosis
- Massage
- Meditation
- Mindfulness
- Movement therapies
- Naturopathy
- Progressive muscle relaxation
- Qi gong
- Tai chi
- Traditional healers
- Yoga

Acupuncture

Acupuncture has been used for over 3,000 years in traditional Chinese medicine. Over the past 40 years, it has gained popularity in the United States. There are a variety of people who practice it. Acupuncture involves inserting needles into specific areas of a patient's body, known as meridians, to manage a person's life-force energy or qi. Disease states interfere with the qi, blocking the energy flow. By studying the physiological effects of acupuncture, Western medicine has found that the technique likely activates the sensory system with regulation of neurotransmitters, neurohormones, and other neuromodulators.[6]

Acupuncture should be performed by clinical providers who have been appropriately trained. This will vary from state to state. Emergency nurse practitioners (ENPs) need to be familiar with the requirements in the state where they practice. Acupuncture will generally require credentialing as well as any other procedure the provider is permitted to perform.

One form of acupuncture, known as auricular or "battlefield" acupuncture, has been used by some clinicians in the ED for acute pain management. Battlefield acupuncture involves the use of five auricular acupuncture points per ear in a specific sequence. There are small needles available for this procedure, or traditional acupuncture needles may be used.[7–9]

Indications

A. Neck pain
B. Low back pain
C. Osteoarthritis
D. Headaches
E. Postoperative pain
F. Abdominal pain
G. Cancer pain
H. Neuropathic pain

Adverse Effects

A. Bleeding/hematoma
B. Dizziness
C. Syncope
D. Nausea
E. Somnolence
F. Euphoria
G. Hysteria
H. Central nervous system (CNS) injury
I. Infection
J. Broken needles

Management

A. Determine whether the patient is appropriate for the intervention based on indications.
B. Explain the intervention to the patient.
C. Obtain written or verbal consent for procedure based on hospital or location policy.
D. Perform the time-out procedure.
E. Cleanse the area where the needles are to be placed.
F. Monitor the patient closely for adverse effects and intervene as needed.

Patient Disposition

A. Advise the patient to drink plenty of fluids.
B. Return to the ED for evaluation of any adverse effects.
C. Record the location of the needles and patient response.

Energy Therapies

Energy therapies are based on the manipulation of energy fields within the body. Some of the therapies that may be used in the ED include Reiki therapy, therapeutic touch on the affected areas, and intentions that allow the patient to relax.[10] One study found that patients receiving emergency care who experienced healing touch perceived a feeling of energy that supported their body; a nourishing feeling of being aware of the body without pain; and a sense of unconditional compassion.[10]

Indications

A. Pain management
B. Anxiety
C. End-of-life care

Adverse Effects

A. Increased anxiety
B. Ambivalence
C. Embarrassment

Management

A. Determine whether the patient is appropriate for the intervention based on indications.
B. Explain the intervention to the patient and family.
C. Monitor the patient closely for adverse effects and intervene as needed.

Patient Disposition

A. Advise the patient to drink plenty of fluids.
B. Return to the ED for evaluation of any adverse effects.
C. Record the location of the therapy and patient's response.

Essential Oils

Essential oils are created from plants. These oils can be ingested or used topically. In the ED, topical application is the foundation of aromatherapy and offers another example of a holistic nursing intervention. Inhalation or absorption of the oils triggers changes in the limbic system. This results in stimulation of the nervous, endocrine, and immune systems. Aromatherapy can positively affect the patient's heart rate, blood pressure, and breathing. The essential oils can be delivered by massage, inhalation, compresses, or in water.[11,12]

Examples of essential oils that are useful in the ED are lavender, which has sedation, calming, antidepressant, antiseptic, analgesic, and antispasmodic properties, and rose, which assists with circulation and can encourage deep and calm breathing. Rose oil also has antidepressant properties.[11,12]

Indications

A. Pain management
B. Relaxation
C. Depression
D. Decreasing anxiety
E. Decreasing heart rates, blood pressure, and respiratory rates
F. Wound healing
G. Antiseptic/antifungal
H. Xerosis
I. Pruritus
J. Cough

Adverse Effects

A. Headache
B. Constipation
C. Changes in appetite
D. May cause miscarriage
E. May increase headaches

Management

A. Determine whether the patient is appropriate for the intervention based on indications.
B. Explain the intervention to the patient and family.
C. Monitor the patient closely for adverse effects and intervene as needed.

Patient Disposition

A. Advise the patient to use the essential oils as prescribed.
B. Return to the ED for evaluation of any adverse effects.
C. Record the location of the therapy and patient's response.

Guided Imagery

Guided imagery encompasses various techniques that are used to promote relaxation, relieve pain relief and anxiety, stimulate healing, and help patients tolerate treatments and procedures.[13] It can be a useful technique in the ED. Guided imagery allows the patient to "draw on their own inner resources to support healing and understand what their symptoms may be signaling." Guided imagery is a form of directed daydreaming that involves all of one's senses.[14] One technique that may be of use in the ED involves mental and physical relaxation. Patients are guided to "imagine" a place of safety, beauty, or peacefulness, which can allow them to "heal." Being led to this place can help them relax. Guided imagery should be used with caution in patients who have active psychosis, diffused dissociative disorder, history of a suicide attempt, history of physical or sexual abuse, and unstable medical problems. This intervention can be used after the patient is discharged from the ED, or if admitted, throughout their hospitalization. The use of this technique requires that the clinicial provider receive education and training in order to effectively use it.

Indications

A. Pain management
B. Relaxation
C. Decreasing anxiety
D. Preparing a patient for a procedure such as suturing a wound or draining an abscess
E. Reducing or relieving symptoms after a diagnosis has been made

Contraindications

A. Inability to hold a train of thought
B. Impaired cognition, delirium, or dementia
C. Strong religious beliefs

Management

A. Determine whether the patient is appropriate for the intervention based on indications.
B. Explain the intervention to the patient and family.
C. Monitor the patient closely for adverse effects and intervene as needed.

Patient Disposition

A. Advise the patient of possible adverse events (e.g., increased anxiety, disorientation).
B. Return to the ED for evaluation of any adverse effects.
C. Record the patient's response to the intervention.

Massage

Various types of massage might be used in the ED. Massaging muscles and soft tissues can increase blood flow and relieve stress in muscles and overall. Touching also plays a part in the relaxation response that may result from massage. There are several types of massage, including Swedish massage, which involves kneading and compression of tissues as well as deep circular movements, vibration, and tapping.[15] Shiatsu massage is a form of acupressure to certain points of the body.[15]

Indications

A. Neck pain
B. Low back pain
C. Headaches

Adverse Effects

A. Dizziness
B. Syncope
C. Somnolence

Management

A. Determine whether the patient is appropriate for the intervention based on indications.
B. Explain the intervention to the patient and family.
C. Monitor the patient closely for adverse effects and intervene as needed.

Patient Disposition

A. Advise the patient to drink plenty of fluids.
B. Return to the ED for evaluation of any adverse effects.
C. Record the location of the massage therapy and patient's response.

References

References for this chapter are online only and can be found at https://connect.springerpub.com/content/reference-book/978-0-8261-6091-5/part/part01/toc-part/ch11.

II. Medical Emergencies

12. Head, Eyes, Ears, Nose, and Throat

RODNEY W. HICKS | LISA KOSER | JILL OGG-GRESS | SHEILA SHEA | RENEÉ SEMONIN HOLLERAN

Learning Objectives

Dental Emergencies

- Identify leading causes of dental abscess, fracture, and avulsions.
- Formulate a focused assessment plan for clients with dental injuries.
- Recognize unsafe practices for storage of displaced teeth.

Ocular Emergencies

- Identify common ocular medical and traumatic conditions seen in the urgent or emergency setting.
- Differentiate between emergent and nonurgent ocular conditions in order to preserve vision.
- Conduct an appropriate ophthalmologic history.
- Utilize a systematic approach to the examination of the eye.
- Describe the pathophysiology, clinical presentation, natural history, and therapy for the selected ophthalmologic conditions.
- Identify when urgent or emergent ophthalmology consultation is indicated.
- Formulate differential diagnoses for the red eye and visual loss.
- Outline selected procedures needed as part of the ocular examination such as fluorescein stain and slit lamp examination.
- Discuss initial management common ocular emergencies.

Ear Conditions

- Identify the common ear conditions seen in the ED.
- Identify when urgent or emergent ear, nose, and throat (ENT) consultation is indicated.
- Discuss the management of acute otitis externa, acute otitis media, labyrinthitis, and foreign body in the ear.

Nasal Conditions

- Identify the common nasal conditions seen in the ED.
- Identify when urgent or emergent ENT consultation is indicated.
- Discuss the management of epistaxis, nasal foreign bodies, nasal fractures, and sinusitis.

Throat Conditions

- Identify the common throat conditions seen in the ED.
- Identify when urgent or emergent ENT consultation is indicated.
- Discuss the management of pharyngitis, laryngitis, epiglottitis, and laryngeal foreign body.

DENTAL EMERGENCIES

RODNEY W. HICKS | JILL OGG-GRESS

Dental Abscess/Cellulitis

According to the National Health and Nutrition Examination Survey (NHANES), from 2011 to 2012, 91% of Americans aged 20 to 64 had dental caries with approximately 27% of adults aged 20 to 64 with untreated tooth decay. Dental infections are a direct result of dental caries that destroy the dental enamel and dentine line. These lesions often penetrate the dental pulp, causing inflammation and necrosis. With untreated dental necrosis patients are at higher risk for developing abscesses or worsening infections such as cellulitis.[1]

Medical Screening

A. *Chief complaint:* Patients typically present with a complaint of "dental pain," "tooth pain," or "pain in the gums."

B. Signs and symptoms

  1. Apical abscess is typically localized to the area of pain.

  2. Fever may accompany if cellulitis is suspected.

  3. Foul taste in the mouth if abscess is draining

C. Focused assessment

  1. While utilizing universal precautions, clinician should examine the area of concern in which the patient is complaining of pain.

    a. Specifically note any buccal or palatal swelling, drainage, and regional adenopathy.

Medical Decision-Making and Differential Diagnoses

A. Not all patients with dental pain require empiric antibiotic therapy.

B. If cellulitis was not appreciated, antibiotics are typically not necessary.

C. If cellulitis is suspected, prophylactic antibiotic therapy as indicated

D. Referral to general dentistry is warranted for consideration of incision and drainage, root canal treatment, or extraction.

1. **Differential diagnoses**
   a. Fistula
   b. Maxillary/mandibular infection

Diagnostic Testing

A. Consider complete blood count (CBC) with differential and/or sedimentation rate, and c-reactive protein (CRP).
B. Medical imaging should be considered when there is considerable swelling and risk for potential deep-seated infection or airway compromise.

Management

A. Procedures
1. Incision and drainage by trained clinician in the setting of abscess if indicated.

B. Pharmacological therapies:
1. Not typically indicated for abscess; however, local anesthesia may be indicated.
2. In the setting of cellulitis
   a. Penicillin
   b. Penicillin-allergic adult patients should receive clindamycin.
3. Pain control options include acetaminophen, tramadol, or codeine.

C. Consultation and collaboration:
1. Referral to general dentistry to be seen in 24 to 48 hours.

Patient Disposition

A. Patient may be discharged to home.
B. Transition of care information
C. Referral to dentistry as appropriate:
1. Discharge instructions
2. Take antibiotics as prescribed.

D. Prevention and education
1. Patient and family education and counseling
   a. Signs and symptoms of dental infections
   b. Consideration of who and where the patient should seek treatment
2. Daily dental care including twice daily brushing and flossing, as well as routine dental care; seek dental care for acute dental problems.

Dental Avulsions

Dental avulsions, or "teeth knocked out," are common dental conditions that warrant urgent/emergent evaluation and treatment.[2] Oral injuries account for up to 5% of ED visits. A dental avulsion results from the traumatic displacement of a tooth from the alveolar socket; such injury involves the periodontal ligament, pulpal tissue, blood supply to the dental pulp, the alveolar bone, and the gingiva. In avulsion injuries, the number of teeth affected can range from 1 to 3, with a mean number of 1.4.[3,4] Dental avulsions are a worldwide phenomenon.[5] Common etiology of traumatic injuries includes[6–8] falls (36.4%); traffic accidents (22.7%); bicycle accidents (18.2%); collisions (9.1%); and other nonspecified causes, including skateboard injuries, sports-related injuries, altercations, and physical abuse.

Incidence and Etiology

A. The pediatric age group represents the largest patient population affected.
B. The incidence within this population, attributed to the etiologies above, has steadily increased over the past decade.
C. In adults, the trauma profile is similar to that of children, with sports-related injuries being the most common.
D. The absence of a mouth guard contributes to these injuries.
E. Adults are also more likely to be victims of assault.
F. A less common etiology pertains to endotracheal (ET) intubation where the laryngoscope blade is not appropriately used.[9,10]

Medical Screening

A. Dental injuries are traumatic injuries. The etiology of the trauma may affect more than one body system.
B. Emergency clinicians should be skilled in rapid triage, gathering health history, and performing physical assessments given the time-sensitive nature of preventing tooth loss.
C. Subjective assessment
1. *Chief complaint:* Localized pain in the oral region, with onset often just prior to the ED visit
2. Patient history
   a. *History of present illness:* Probing questions that follow include onset, location, duration, quality, and precipitating factors.[11]
   b. Additional tasks would include reviewing the medication and allergy list, immunization history, and past medical history.
   c. Identify if the patient has a primary dental clinician.

Physical Examination

A. The emergency clinician, while wearing gloves, visually inspects the oral cavity for a missing or loosely displaced tooth (Figure 12.1).
B. Avulsed tooth is identified by tooth number (Figure 12.2).
1. Notation should be present if the tooth is a primary (baby) or secondary (permanent) tooth.

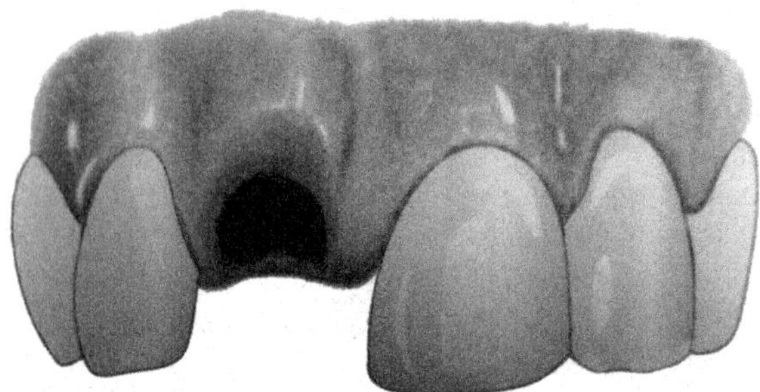

FIGURE 12.1 Dental avulsion.

C. Concurrent examination of the oral cavity to note the presence or absence of bruising, lacerations, and facial fractures
D. Evaluate the patient for bite, occlusion, mobility, and other abnormalities.
E. The tooth itself is examined with care not to touch the roots.[12]
F. Assess for other injuries as directed by history, chief complaint, and examination findings.

Medical Decision-Making and Differential Diagnoses

A. In the absence of overt other trauma injuries that result in loss of limb or life, the emergency clinician's decision-making primarily targets tooth preservation.
B. The clinical setting should have ready access to appropriate media.
C. All ED team members should recognize the advantages/disadvantages of each type of medium (Table 12.1).

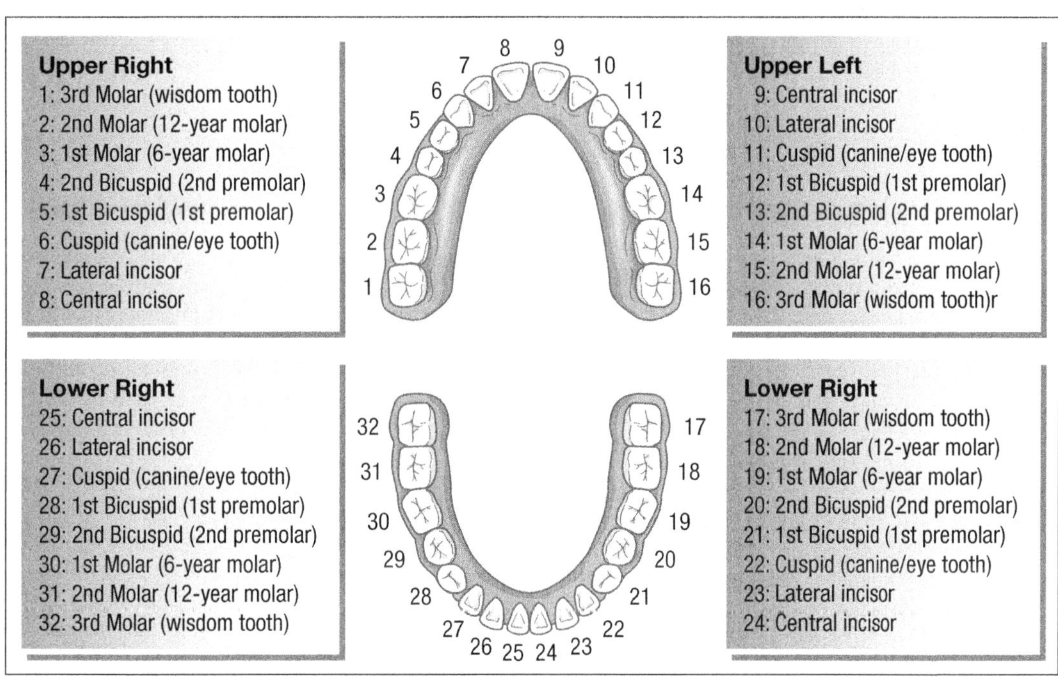

FIGURE 12.2 International tooth chart.

TABLE 12.1 RECOMMENDED MEDIA FOR DENTAL AVULSIONS

MEDIA	DESCRIPTION	MAXIMUM STORAGE TIME	COMMENTS
RECOMMENDED MEDIA			
Hank's Balanced Salt Solution (HBSS)	A pH-balanced salt solution with essential metabolites and glucose	24 hours	• Available to consumers in first aid kits • Common in clinical settings • No prescription required • No refrigeration required
Isotonic (Normal) Saline	An isotonic neutral sodium chloride solution, but lacks nutrients and does not maintain cell metabolism	1 hour	• No refrigeration required • Widely available in clinical settings
Milk	A solution of amino acids and vitamins capable of inactivation of enzymes harmful to APDL cells; does not replace cell metabolites	2–3 hours	• Readily available • Should be fresh and refrigerated
Saliva	Natural; able to store tooth in buccal sulcus	30 minutes	For immediate, interim (short term) storage
DISCOURAGED MEDIA			
Water (tap, distilled, sterile)	Hypotonic solution	NOT recommended	Incompatible with PDL cells, resulting in cellular lysis

Source: Hicks RW. Dental avulsion. In: Hollier A, ed. *Clinical Guidelines in Primary Care.* 2nd ed. Advanced Practice Educational Associates Inc; 2016:174–175.[6]

Diagnostic Testing

A. Diagnostics are of limited value. Consider chest and abdomen radiographs when the index of suspicion suggests aspiration or swallowing of the displaced tooth/teeth.
B. The extent of trauma on other body systems may affect the decision to utilize other diagnostics.

Management—The First Hour

A. The emergency clinician should proceed in a timely fashion.
   1. The first priority is to replant the tooth in the socket (if possible) within 40 minutes of injury.
   2. Tooth viability diminishes as the time outside the socket increases.
   3. When replantation of the tooth in the socket is not immediately possible, secure the tooth in a clean container with appropriate media solution.

B. Clinicians concurrently consider pharmacologic decision-making activities.
   1. Initiating antimicrobial prophylaxis, when indicated, can decrease the risk for endocarditis.
      a. First, consider the class of penicillin-based products.
      b. Alternatively, consider doxycycline or metronidazole. Clinicians update tetanus prophylaxis as indicated.
   2. May also consider nonaspirin analgesic products

C. Collaboration and consultation
   1. Patients with dental avulsions will need emergent dental consultation and/or referral.
   2. The ED should maintain a list of on-call dental clinicians skilled at treating and following patients with such injuries.
   3. In the ideal setting, the dental clinician should be able to evaluate and initiate treatment while the patient is in the ED setting.
      a. When this evaluation is possible, the setting should have an examination chair, a room with appropriate lighting, and access to the proper equipment.

Patient Disposition

A. Transition of care information
   1. The final ED treatment plan should anticipate releasing the patient from the ED.
   2. Patients should receive written discharge instructions that direct the follow-up with the dental clinician.

B. Prevention and education
   1. Emergency clinicians have an opportunity to improve the oral health of the community through education about prevention of infections and good dental health.
   2. Emergency clinicians should serve as advocates and promote access to Save-A-Tooth for schools, recreation centers, ambulances, and other places where people congregate. Early reimplantation of the avulsed tooth has the greatest viability.[6]

Dental Fracture/Luxation

Dental fractures are common injuries in which patients present to the ED for evaluation and treatment. In children, fractures are typically sports-related and typically more prevalent among males than females. Adult dental fractures are more likely to occur due to poor oral hygiene resulting in periodontal disease and bone loss or trauma. Any traumatic avulsion, lateral or extrusive luxation, or alveolar or displaced root fracture is considered a serious dental injury because they compromise the nerve tissue within the tooth and periodontium that anchors the tooth to the bony socket. Traumatic fractures and avulsions require immediate dental referral.

Medical Screening

A. *Chief complaint:* Tooth pain
B. Signs and symptoms
   1. Inability to eat secondary to pain, temperature intolerance (especially cold)

C. Focused assessment
   1. While utilizing universal precautions, the clinician should inspect and transilluminate the reported area of discomfort, palpate the area with a tongue blade to assess for worsening discomfort, and document physical examination findings in addition to appearance of tooth including tooth number in the electronic medical record.

Medical Decision-Making and Differential Diagnoses

A. Considerations
   1. Patients will likely require pain medication as an outpatient until dental care can be received.
   2. Antibiotics are not indicated in this situation.
   3. Consider dental block if travel time to dentist is significant.

B. Differential diagnoses
   1. Cracked tooth syndrome

Diagnostic Testing

A. No diagnostics beyond focused assessment are necessary.

Management

A. Procedures:
   1. Referral to dentistry
   2. Consider dental block.
   3. If tooth "fell out," replace or place tooth into milk to maintain viability (see "Dental Avulsions").

B. Pharmacological therapies
   1. Opioids
      a. Scheduled narcotics will likely be warranted for pain control with careful consideration of limited supply until dental appointment can be made.
   2. *Dental block:* Consider if distance to dentist is significant, severe pain, history of narcotic abuse.

C. Consultation and collaboration
   1. Referral to dentistry
   2. Immediate referral if traumatic fracture or luxation
   3. 24- to 48-hour referral if "cracked tooth"

Patient Disposition

A. *Discharge instructions:* Take pain medication as prescribed, room temperature fluids and soft foods, and referral to dentistry
B. *Immediate referral:* Traumatic fracture, avulsion, lateral or extrusive luxation, alveolar or displaced root fracture
C. Prevention and education
  1. Patient and family education and counseling
  2. Encourage the use of mouth guards for athletes.
  3. Encourage proper dental care daily, in addition to dental visits every 6 months.
D. *Documentation:* Document initial presentation, mechanism of injury (if applicable), treatment, consultation, and referral (if applicable).

Age and Developmental Considerations

A. Children typically start to lose deciduous teeth at approximately 6 years of age.
B. Dental implants can fracture and cause damage to surrounding teeth and bone structure.

OCULAR EMERGENCIES

SHEILA SHEA

Acute Anterior Iritis

A. The uveal tract comprises the tissue between the cornea and sclera, and the inner retinal layer of the eye.
B. The anterior part of the uveal tract contains the iris and ciliary body.
C. When the iris is inflamed, this painful condition is called iritis or iridocyclitis.
D. Uveitis is the term for inflammation of both the iris and contiguous ciliary body. Inflammation of these structures is often idiopathic but can become inflamed due to trauma, infection, postoperative, or a large number underlying systemic diseases.
E. Some medications such as sulfonamides are also associated with iritis. A search for other causes of a painful red eye is important in the evaluation of anterior iritis.
F. Evaluate carefully for corneal abrasion or ulcer, foreign body, or epithelial defects due to herpes simplex virus (HSV) or herpes zoster virus (HZV) infection.
  1. While some cases of iritis are of unknown etiology, a search for systemic infection such as tuberculosis, sarcoidosis, and syphilis should be considered.
  2. For patients with dramatic iritis, dramatic rental detachment or hyphema is possible.
  3. Iritis involves a deeper structure of the eye and a hallmark finding is lack of relief with topical anesthesia drops unless there is an associated corneal epithelial defect.

Medical Screening

A. *Chief complaint:* Acute onset of a red, painful eye; mild to severe. Possible history of blunt eye trauma or autoimmune diseases.
B. Physical examination
  1. Upper lid edema, tearing
  2. Direct and consensual photophobia (often severe)
  3. Visual acuity usually mildly decreased or blurred. Partial or circumferential ciliary flush. Extraocular movements (EOMs) intact without pain or limitation.
  4. Pupil may be smaller than midrange and irregular with sluggish reaction; trauma can cause tears in iris sphincter and cause pupil to dilate.
  5. No relief with topical anesthetic drops is an important finding and indicates there is deeper structure involvement such as iritis.

Diagnostic Testing and Management

A. Procedures
  1. *Slit lamp examination:* Cells (white blood cells [WBCs]) and flare (protein) in anterior chamber; keratitic precipitates made of WBC on endothelium that appear round and white; hazy and swollen cornea due to inflammation; hypopyon; possible corneal abrasion, ulcer, or foreign body.
  2. Intraocular pressure measurement is initially normal or slightly lower than normal
B. *Laboratory:* not indicated unless concern for granulomatous etiologies such as syphilis, tuberculosis, sarcoidosis, or herpetic infection. If no clear history, trauma or systemic disease to explain onset consider: complete blood count (CBC), erythrocyte sedimentation rate (ESR) and C-reactive protein (CRP), antinuclear antibody (ANA), rapid plasma reagin (RPR), VDRL, HIV, purified protein derivative (PPD), and urinalysis; Lyme titer for endemic areas; HLA-B27 for ankylosing spondylitis.
C. *Imaging:* Chest x-ray (CXR) can indicate tuberculosis or sarcoidosis.
D. Treatment
  1. *Advise eye rest:* Dark room, sunglasses, and topical cycloplegia for pain control
  2. Consult ophthalmology for initiation of steroids to decrease inflammation.

Conjunctivitis

A. Conjunctivitis, or "pink eye," is a frequent and usually benign and self-limiting inflammation of the transparent bulbar and tarsal conjunctiva that covers the white part of eye and lines the eyelids.
B. The eye is generally well protected from infection and the natural tear flow helps disperse and wash away debris and organisms.
  1. Organisms that may cause bacterial infection include streptococci, *Haemophilus influenzae,* staphylococci, pneumococci, and gonococci or chlamydia.
  2. It can be a viral (adenovirus), allergic, or bacterial condition.
  3. Inflammation can also be caused by chemical contact or burn, actinic injury, or systemic illness.
C. Conjunctivitis in contact lens users can lead to a vision-threatening corneal ulcer.
D. Eye problems may be a sign of a systemic disease or may be the portal for serious conditions such as meningitis or sepsis.

Medical Screening

A. *Chief complaint:* Red eye(s) often starts in one eye and involves other eye in a few days, except if it is caused by allergies.

1. Itchy, gritty, and foreign body sensation with minimal pain

2. Matted discharge, often worse in morning

B. Possible low-grade fever, rhinorrhea, pharyngitis, and cough

C. Sudden and severe onset symptoms and copious purulent drainage of less than 1 day suggests serious gonococcal conjunctivitis.

D. Symptoms of conjunctivitis that persist for over 3 weeks and are associated with follicular "cobblestones" on inner eyelids may indicate chlamydial conjunctivitis.

E. Physical examination

1. Visual acuity is usually normal or slightly decreased.

2. Mild eyelid swelling with minimal erythema

3. Watery to whitish or yellow-green mucoid drainage to purulent if bacterial

4. Conjunctival follicles or papillae

5. Chemosis (scleral edema) may be marked if allergic etiology

a. Corneas are grossly clear and pupils normal; a minimally reactive or fixed pupil may indicate glaucoma.

b. Palpable preauricular lymphadenopathy common if viral etiology. Look for associated lesions of scalp, face, periorbital, or nose that may indicate herpetic etiology.

c. Photophobia increases concern for keratitis or iritis.

d. Eye pain associated with headache and nausea or vomiting may indicate acute angle closure glaucoma.

Diagnostic Testing and Management

A. Procedures

1. Fluorescein stain for epithelial defect such as corneal dendrite with herpes simplex virus (HSV) or corneal abrasion from scratching at eye

2. Slit lamp examination

3. Possible one-time eye lavage with normal saline for gonococcal conjunctivitis

B. *Laboratory:* Possible culture of discharge if etiology not clear

C. Routine screening for associated sexually transmitted infections (STI) if concern for gonococcal etiology with possible chlamydial immunofluorescence test

D. Point-of-care testing (POCT) for adenovirus may be helpful in distinguishing viral from bacterial conjunctivitis and avoiding unnecessary antibiotic therapy.

E. Treatment

1. Gentle cleansing of eyes medially to laterally to remove debris, cool compresses to decrease swelling if allergy; warm compresses for bacterial infection

2. Advise patient to wash hand frequently, avoid touching eyes, and discard eye makeup and avoid cosmetics use until symptoms resolve.

3. Discontinue contact lens use for at least 2 weeks and discard disposable contact lenses.

F. Supportive measures

1. Artificial tears for comfort and lubrication if viral conjunctivitis

2. Topical vasoconstrictor/antihistamine for severe itching

3. Oral antihistamines or topical mast-cell stabilizers or steroids may be useful for allergic conjunctivitis. If steroid is prescribed, patient should be referred to an ophthalmologist for follow-up.

4. Topical steroids may exacerbate local infectious processes and are not indicated in acute conjunctivitis but may be ordered after consultation with ophthalmology for presence of pseudomembrane or subepithelial infiltrates.

G. Bacterial conjunctivitis (if gonorrhea and chlamydia not suspected) usually treat 7 days:

1. Polymyxin B/trimethoprim solution or erythromycin 0.5% ointment ½ inch or sulfacetamide 10% solution drops

2. More serious or refractory cases may require fluoroquinolones such as levofloxacin 0.5% solution.

H. Gonococcal conjunctivitis requires aggressive antibiotic coverage with ceftriaxone or ciprofloxacin if penicillin allergic and the patient is not pregnant; also use topical erythromycin ointment.

I. Chlamydial conjunctivitis should be treated as a possible coinfection with gonorrhea with azithromycin.

J. Herpetic eye infection antiviral medications such as acyclovir, both drops and oral medications, may be prescribed; patient should be referred to an ophthalmologist for follow-up.

K. Neonatal conjunctivitis is presumed to be due to chlamydia and treated with ceftriaxone *and* erythromycin.

Corneal Ulcer

A. A corneal ulcer (ulcerative keratitis) is a serious and painful condition that causes open sore on the cornea usually due to inflammation or viral or bacterial infection.

B. The cornea has no blood supply and gets oxygen from the air, so contact lens use is a risk factor.

C. Corneal ulcers related to contact lens use are often caused by *Pseudomonas aeruginosa* and require appropriate antibiotic coverage.

D. The loss of corneal tissue in an ulcer allows bacteria to enter the deeper corneal layers.

1. In the ED setting, corneal ulcers are presumed to be infectious until evaluated by an ophthalmologist.

E. Corneal ulcers are an ophthalmologic emergency because of the risk of corneal perforation and loss of vision.

Medical Screening

A. *Chief complaint:* Usually unilateral red eye with moderate to severe pain

B. Corneal ulcer is a significant complication of soft or extended contact lens.

C. Corneal ulcers may also follow chemical burn or corneal foreign body or following ocular surgery and with systemic diseases such as HIV, rheumatoid arthritis, or systemic lupus erythematosus or dry eye syndrome.

D. Physical examination

1. Eyelid erythema and swelling, mucopurulent drainage

2. Decreased visual acuity. EOMs and pupils usually normal

3. Conjunctival and scleral injection with possible ciliary flush

4. Painful pupillary constriction due to ciliary muscle spasm

5. Possible visible whitish opacity on cornea. Evert eyelid for possible foreign body.

6. Foreign body (FB) sensation usually indicates an epithelial defect.

Diagnostic Testing and Management

A. Procedures

1. Fluorescein stain may show single or multiple punctate infiltrates in epithelium, but if overlying corneal epithelium is intact there will be no dye uptake. Possible dendrites, pseudodendrites, foreign body.

2. *Slit lamp examination:* Opaque round or oval grayish ulcer, usually >1 mm; slit lamp light beam will not pass through the ulcer; epithelial defects such as punctate lesions. Inflammatory reaction in surrounding stromal layers and cell and flare in anterior chamber if iritis is present. *Hypopyon:* Whitish exudate or pus in the anterior chamber. Intraocular pressure measurement.

B. Treatment

1. Corneal ulcers related to contact lens use are often caused by *Pseudomonas aeruginosa* and require appropriate antibiotic coverage.

2. Very small infiltrates (<1 mm) that are not over the visual axis and without epithelial disruption: Fluoroquinolone (moxifloxacin or gatifloxacin) drops.

a. For contact lens users, add tobramycin or ciprofloxacin ointment at bedtime.

3. Ulcers with epithelial defects, mucopurulent discharge, or cells and flare in the anterior chamber and "dirty" ulcers (fingernail injury, soil, or plant matter):

a. Fluoroquinolone (moxifloxacin or gatifloxacin) drops

4. Larger ulcers (1.5 mm), ulcers over the visual axis, or with purulent drainage and significant anterior chamber reaction require double antibiotic coverage with aminoglycoside (tobramycin or gentamycin) drops or vancomycin drops; or fluoroquinolone (moxifloxacin or gatifloxacin) drops.

a. For contact lens users, add tobramycin or ciprofloxacin ointment at bedtime.

5. Cycloplegic drops are helpful for pain management of ciliary spasm.

Dacryocystitis

A. Acute dacryocystitis is an acute inflammation or infection of the lacrimal sac located in the nasal aspect of the lower lid.

B. Inflammation is caused by nasolacrimal duct obstruction that is prone to infection given the close proximity of bacteria from the conjunctival and nasal mucosa.

C. Acute dacryocystitis is rare in newborns but an acquired form of the condition may be seen in middle age and older adults. Dacryocystitis may also be congenital or acquired.

D. Other conditions to consider include preseptal cellulitis, facial cellulitis, acute sinusitis, or orbital cellulitis.

E. Cavernous sinus thrombosis is a rare and potentially fatal complication.

Medical Screening

A. *Chief complaint:* Focal, tender, raised, erythematous lesion of medial aspect of lower eyelid that may extend to the side of the nose

B. Possible fever, increased tearing, or mucopurulent drainage that may be expressed using a cotton tip applicator and gentle pressure over lower punctum

C. Possible blurred or decreased vision due to increased tear film—unilateral epiphora (excessive tearing) with visible tears draining onto the cheek and matter on lashes

D. Conjunctival injection or conjunctivitis

E. The lacrimal sac may rupture, leading to a fistula of the skin. Confirm extraocular movements (EOMs) are intact without limitation or pain and no signs of preseptal cellulitis.

F. Perform nasal examination to rule out tumor or distal lacrimal duct obstruction.

1. Avoid assessment by manual exploration or irrigation.

Diagnostic Testing and Management

A. Laboratory:

1. Cultures of discharge, nose, and possibly blood

2. Complete blood count (CBC) if seriously ill-appearing

B. *Imaging:* Consider CT scan of orbits and sinuses for severe or refractory cases.

C. *Procedures:* Fluorescein stain may show an increase in dye level in affected eye due to obstructed outflow

D. Treatment

1. Conservative measures and patient teaching include saline nasal sprays, warm compresses several times a day, and close follow-up with ophthalmology.

2. The most common organisms are staphylococci and streptococci, and while antibiotics are first-line treatment, surgical management may be required.

3. Amoxicillin/clavulanate (pediatric outpatient)

4. Cephalexin or amoxicillin/clavulanate (adult outpatient)

5. Topical ophthalmic antibiotics such as trimethoprim/polymyxin B solution or gentamicin ointment

6. Possible topical ophthalmic steroids to decrease inflammation after consultation

Patient Disposition

A. Admit for IV antibiotics for severe infection such as orbital cellulitis.

Endophthalmitis

A. Endophthalmitis is a rare and potentially vision-threatening condition that causes inflammation in the cavities of the eye.

B. Disruption of the normal protective barrier between the blood and eye allows invasion of pathogens into the eye.

C. It is usually due to infection, especially in immunocompromised hosts and is associated with IV drug use.

- **1.** Other risks are ocular surgery or malignancy.
- **2.** Endophthalmitis can also be spread by the blood from distant infections such as endocarditis.

D. Penetrating injury of the eye and retained foreign body are also associated with traumatic endophthalmitis.

- **1.** Any invasive procedure may become a source for bacteremia such as dental procedures, indwelling catheters, or hemodialysis.
- **2.** Staphylococcus and streptococcus are common organisms but penetrating ocular injuries may be caused by Gram-negative organisms such as Pseudomonas or *Escherichia coli.*

E. Viral endophthalmitis is rare, but fungal infections are likely in patients with diabetes, malignancy, renal or heart failure, or AIDS.

Medical Screening

A. *Chief complaint:* Red, painful eye, drainage, eyelid swelling, headache, light sensitivity

B. *History:* Ocular or invasive procedures, immunosuppression, or IV drug abuse (IVDA)

C. Physical examination

- **1.** Photophobia, visual acuity markedly decreased; only hand movement, light perception, or complete loss of vision
- **2.** Purulent discharge, scleral and conjunctival injection with possible chemosis
- **3.** Decrease or loss of red reflex; inflammatory cells prevent visualization of retina
- **4.** *Funduscopic examination:* Possible flame-shaped retinal hemorrhages or cotton-wool spots
- **5.** If infection has spread to all layers of the eye, panophthalmitis may develop and cause proptosis and restriction of extraocular movements (EOMs).

Diagnostic Testing and Management

A. Procedures

- **1.** Fluorescein stain usually normal
- **2.** *Slit lamp examination:* Cells and flare in anterior chamber and possible hypopyon
- **3.** Intraocular pressure measurement

B. *Laboratory:* Complete blood count (CBC), basic metabolic panel (BMP) with blood urea nitrogen (BUN) and creatinine, erythrocyte sedimentation rate (ESR)

- **1.** *If unknown source:* Blood, urine, stool, throat cultures

C. Ophthalmology consult for vitreous humor culture

D. *Imaging:* Consider orbital CT scan or ocular ultrasound if retained foreign body possible or cannot rule out endophthalmitis; CXR to determine source of infection.

E. Treatment:

- **1.** Once endophthalmitis is the most likely diagnosis, emergent ophthalmology consultation is required for aspiration and intraocular medication administration to preserve vision.
- **2.** Broad-spectrum antibiotics selection is based on suspected organism:
  - **a.** Vancomycin or gentamicin or ceftriaxone
  - **b.** *IVDA:* Use an aminoglycoside PLUS clindamycin.
  - **c.** *Suspected fungal etiology:* Amphotericin B
- **3.** Topical cycloplegic agent can help with pain control.
- **4.** Confirm tetanus immunization status.
- **5.** Ophthalmology consultation for management of traumatic endophthalmitis and repair of globe rupture if indicated

Episcleritis and Scleritis

A. Both of these conditions cause redness of the sclera and conjunctiva.

B. Episcleritis

- **1.** Self-limiting condition due to a localized inflammation involving the vascular deep subconjunctival layer of tissue under the conjunctiva and superficial to the sclera (episcleral)
- **2.** May be seen in isolation or be associated with a viral or autoimmune disorder or dry eye syndrome and is more frequently occurs in adults between the ages of 40 and 50 years of age.
- **3.** Must be distinguished from scleritis, which is a much more serious inflammation of the sclera itself

C. Scleritis

- **1.** Usually associated severe systemic vasculitic conditions such as rheumatoid arthritis or irritable bowel disease.
- **2.** Can cause thinning and perforation of the cornea leading to blindness
- **3.** More serious red-eye problems include uveitis or iritis.
- **4.** Disorders of the bulbar conjunctiva that cause redness are conjunctivitis, pinguecula, pterygium, and infectious keratitis.

Medical Screening

A. Chief complaint is eye pain; deeper and more severe with scleritis. Visual acuity may be normal or decreased.

B. Episcleritis

- **1.** Associated with abrupt onset of focal bright erythematous injection of the bulbar conjunctival and episcleral vessels associated with clear tearing, irritation, and photophobia
- **2.** Superficial vessels of episcleritis may be moved slightly with gentle pressure using a moistened cotton tip applicator; deeper scleral vessels will not move.
- **3.** Phenylephrine or neosynephrine eye drops will cause constriction and blanching of blood vessels in episcleritis but do not affect scleritis.

C. Scleritis
1. Often accompanied by severe eye pain that radiates to same side of face and head. The thin sclera may take on a bluish hue due to visible uvea.
2. Symptoms associated with episcleritis may wax and wane while scleritis has a gradual onset that leads to decrease in vision.

Diagnostic Testing and Management

A. Procedures:
1. *Slit lamp examination:* Microscopy reveals edema and injection of episcleral vessels; cell and flare in the anterior chamber may be seen if iritis is present.
B. *Laboratory:* Complete blood count (CBC), chemistry, urinalysis (UA), erythrocyte sedimentation rate (ESR), and serum C-reactive protein
C. *Imaging:* Chest x-ray (CXR) if underlying systemic condition suspected
D. Treatment
1. Artificial tears for lubrication

Patient Disposition

A. May need ophthalmologist consultation to confirm presence/absence of scleritis or decision to initiate corticosteroid or anti-inflammatory medications.
B. Primary care clinician to discuss rheumatology consultation if underlying systemic illness suspected.

General Approach

Concerns and fear about possible loss of vision make visits to the ED very stressful for patients and their families. The complex anatomical structures of the eye and familiarity with specialized equipment such as the slit lamp or tonometer can make ocular complaints also stressful for many clinicians. Eye pain and changes in vision are frequent patient presentations in the ED and a strong understanding of anatomy and meticulous assessment skills are essential for the recognition of ocular emergencies. While many eye problems are actually not vision-threatening in nature, such as conjunctivitis or minor corneal abrasions, timely and accurate evaluation is needed to identify more serious eye emergencies such as retinal detachment, acute angle-closure glaucoma, or chemical burns. A consistent approach to the history and systematic assessment of patients with eye complaints will provide a strong basis for early identification of ocular emergencies and improve vision and patient outcome.

Anatomy

A. External eye (Figure 12.3)
1. Eyebrows and lashes; upper eyelid skin crease (superior palpebral sulcus)
2. Medial and lateral canthus (commissure), upper and lower puncta, lacrimal caruncle, and papilla
3. Extraocular movements (EOMs)
a. *CN III—Oculomotor:* Look up, look midline, look down and out
b. *CN IV—Trochlear:* Superior oblique (SO), top of eye toward nose

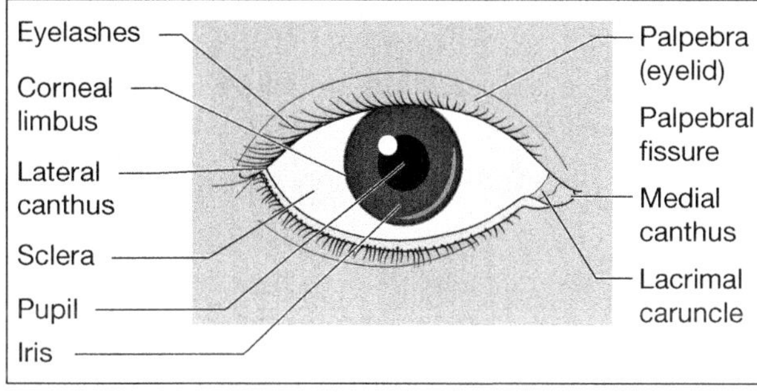

FIGURE 12.3 External anatomy and accessory structures of the eye.
Source: Guida KM. Advanced health assessment of the eyes and ears. In: Myrick KM, Karosas LM, eds. *Advanced Health Assessment and Differential Diagnosis.* 1st ed. Springer Publishing Company; 2020. Fig. 4.1.[13]

c. *CN VI—Abducens:* Lateral rectus (LR), look away from nose
d. CN III innervates all extraocular movements with the exception of SO (CN IV) and LR (CN VI).
4. *Eyelids:* Tarsal plates form and support eyelids.
a. *CN 3:* Innervates levator palpebrae to open eyelid
b. *CN 7:* Facial nerve closes eyelid.
B. Eyeball (focused anatomy)
1. *Cornea:* Most anterior structure and highly innervated; refracts light and transmits to the lens and retina; five layers, 0.5–0.8 mm thick that protects against infection or injury of deeper structures
2. *Sclera:* Connective tissue layer that provides shape and protection
3. *Limbic margin:* Connects cornea and sclera
4. *Conjunctiva:* Transparent covering of visible part of sclera; bulbar conjunctiva covers cornea and palpebral conjunctiva lines upper lid.
5. *Iris:* Controls the size of the pupil and light to the retina
6. *Ciliary body:* Connects iris to choroid body; ciliary muscle controls the shape of the lens and produces aqueous humor
7. *Choroid:* Vascular layer between the retina and sclera; provides nutrients and oxygen to retina
8. *Retina:* Complex layer that receives and processes light
9. Chambers of the eye
a. *Anterior:* Between cornea and iris
b. *Posterior:* Between iris and lens
c. *Vitreous:* Between lens and retina

Pathophysiology

A. See selected etiologies.

Predisposing Factors

A. Older age, smoking, alcohol use, history of hypertension (HTN), rheumatologic or vascular problems, diabetes, and family history may predispose individuals for eye problems.
B. Use of contact lenses is an important predisposing factor for eye infection.
C. Chronic skin conditions such as seborrhea or rosacea may cause recurrent chalazion due to obstruction as the Meibomian glands.

D. Local trauma can cause subconjunctival hemorrhage or corneal abrasion; blunt eye or facial trauma result in detached retina, traumatic iritis, retrobulbar hemorrhage, or damage to the globe.

Assessment

A. Primary and secondary assessment/resuscitation (see Chapter 6).

B. *Focused history:* History of the present illness and chief complaint:

1. History of the present illness or injury/chief complaint

a. *Pain PQRST:* Provoking or palliative factors, quality, radiation/region, severity, timing

b. Details regarding onset of complaint or symptoms

c. Swelling, redness, itching, tearing, or drainage

d. *Changes in vision:* Blurred or cloudy, double vision (diplopia), photophobia, grittiness or foreign body sensation, scotoma, flashes or floaters, transient blindness

e. Painful or restricted eye movement

f. Recent cold or sinus infection, cough, fever, vomiting, lesions of eyes or face, mouth, genitals

g. Mechanism of injury, chemical exposure, blunt or penetrating trauma

h. Baseline visual acuity; use of contact lenses; use of protective or corrective glasses; past eye problems, injuries, surgeries

i. *Past medical history:* Diabetes, hypertension (HTN), cardiovascular disease, migraines, hematologic, immunologic, or connective tissue disease

C. *General:* Level of consciousness, vital signs, skin signs, level of distress

D. Ocular assessment:

1. *Visual acuity:* Must be included on every eye complaint patient but initially deferred if irrigation is indicated

a. Best corrected vision of each eye; use pinhole chart if needed.

b. Snellen chart, count fingers (CF), hand motion (HM), light or shadow perception, no light perception (NLP)

c. Topical anesthetic may facilitate examination.

d. Normal visual acuity does not exclude potentially serious condition.

2. Visual field loss

a. *Bitemporal hemianopsia* (visual loss of each temporal field): Possible aneurysm

b. *Homonymous hemianopsia* (visual loss of nasal field on side of lesion and temporal field of other eye): Consider stroke.

3. Visual changes

a. *Diplopia:* Perception of two images of an object that can be horizontal, vertical, or diagonally displaced

b. *Floaters:* Common problem as shadows are cast on retina; usually due to age-related changes as vitreous becomes more liquid

c. *Flashes ("photopsia"):* Perceived flashes of light due to separation of the posterior vitreous from retina or migraine

d. *Amaurosis fugax:* Painless, transient loss of vision in one or both eyes that may be seen with vascular, ocular, or neurologic problems

e. *Scotoma:* Blind spot that is surrounded by normal vision

f. *Scintillating scotoma:* Band of loss of vision with shimmering, zigzag border often associated with migraine

4. *Face and periorbital area:* Erythema, swelling, lesions, bony tenderness, crepitus

5. *Eyelids:* Erythema, swelling, lesions, tearing, crusting, drainage, ptosis, foreign body, or lesions upon eyelid eversion

6. Eyeballs: Position, enophthalmos or exophthalmos, tenderness to palpation

7. *Pupils:* Equal, round, reactive to light and accommodation

a. *Afferent pupillary defect (APD):* also referred to as "swinging light test" or "Marcus Gunn Pupil"; is most common pupillary defect

b. Eye needs intact pathway from globe to retina and optic nerve for light to be "sensed."

c. Shine light into one eye and then the other—both pupils should constrict. If the pupil dilates, the affected eye cannot "sense" light so there is no constriction. When the light swings back to normal eye, the pupil will constrict as light is sensed.

8. *Corneas:* Clear or hazy, obvious foreign body, hyphema, or hypopyon

9. *Sclera:* Clear, scleral injection, ciliary/limbic flush

10. *Conjunctiva:* Palpebral and bulbar conjunctiva, subconjunctival hemorrhage, chemosis

11. *Extraocular movements (EOMs):* cardinal fields of gaze

12. *Lacrimal system:* Canthus, papilla, puncta

13. Funduscopic examination

E. Other pertinent assessment

1. *Head:* Surface trauma, tenderness, lesions

2. *Ears:* Surrounding lesions, canals, tympanic membranes (TMs)

3. *Nose/face:* Symmetry, sinus tenderness, bony abnormality, erythema, warmth or swelling, tenderness or decreased pulsation over temporal area

4. *Mouth/throat:* Mucous membranes, posterior pharynx

5. *Neck:* Supple, lymphadenopathy, meningismus

Herpes Simplex Virus Keratitis

A. The herpes simplex virus (HSV) type-1 virus can affect either the epithelial layer and is called "epithelial keratitis" with the hallmark dendritic lesions or geographic ulcers.

1. "Stromal or interstitial keratitis" occurs when deeper layers of the cornea are affected and may involve ulceration or necrosis.

2. The distinction is important for accurate medication management with the use of steroids.

3. Primary HSV usually occurs in childhood and is dormant in the trigeminal nerve and reactivated to cause facial lesions and cold sores.
4. HSV keratitis is often overlooked in patients with unilateral follicular conjunctivitis. There are many precipitating causes of viral reactivation such as by exposure, stress, fever.
5. When the virus affects the cornea it is called herpetic keratitis and is often seen in conjunction with infection of the eyelids and conjunctiva.
6. The condition most often affects middle-aged and older adults but can affect children. HSV keratitis is a frequent cause of blindness due to corneal infection if the virus affects the nerves of the cornea.
7. The painful red eye of HSV keratitis must be distinguished from conjunctivitis or keratoconjunctivitis, corneal abrasion, herpes zoster keratitis, corneal ulcer, contact lens use, and systemic diseases that may cause similar symptoms.

Medical Screening

A. *Chief complaint:* Painful, red eye (usually unilateral) with tearing and possible rash
B. May have had a possible history of similar red eye problems or herpetic disease
C. Physical examination:
  1. Decreased visual acuity, blurred vision, photophobia, and tearing
  2. Conjunctival injection with possible ciliary flush
  3. Possible decreased corneal sensation to cotton swab. Palpable preauricular lymphadenopathy
  4. Herpetic vesicular lesions in periorbital, facial, oral, or genital area

D. Test corneal sensation (cotton tip applicator or dental floss) in all four quadrants of eye and over lesion prior to topical anesthesia; as the virus replicates, it damages the cell in which it replicated and causes hyposensitivity.

Diagnostic Testing and Management

A. Procedures
  1. Fluorescein stain
    a. Irregular appearance of corneal surface and small punctate erosions
    b. Classic dendritic ulcer (linear branching lesion with terminal bulbs at ends that stain brightly under fluorescein); possible central ulceration and possible central ulceration
    c. Small, raised, clear corneal vesicles (usually resolved by the time of patient presentation)
    d. Geographic ulcers appear as dendrite grows and looks more swollen with irregular, blurred, and scalloped borders.
    e. Marginal ulcers are located near the limbic border and appear smooth and oval; often seen in the mid-lower cornea.
  2. Slit lamp exam for cell or flare in anterior chamber. Intraocular pressure measurement

B. Treatment
  1. Prompt and aggressive treatment is needed to prevent extension of infection into deeper corneal layers.
  2. HSV epithelial keratitis (dendritic or geographic ulcers present) is treated with topical antivirals but not steroids because treatment is focused on live virus eradication rather than inflammation.
    a. Topical antiviral drops such as trifluridine ophthalmic or ganciclovir ophthalmic gel 0.15%
    b. Oral acyclovir or valacyclovir
    c. Deeper stromal infections have little live virus and require steroids to reduce inflammation and prophylactic oral antivirals to prevent recurrence after ophthalmology consultation.
    d. Prednisolone 1%
      i. *Pediatrics:* Use acyclovir in divided doses.
  3. Treat skin lesions with topical acyclovir to decrease viral shedding into the eyes.
  4. Cycloplegic drops are effective and reduce pain caused by ciliary spasm.

Herpes Zoster Virus Ophthalmicus

A. Herpes zoster virus (HZV) ophthalmicus is a form of keratitis that is caused by reactivation of the varicella zoster virus (VZV) that lies dormant in the first division of the trigeminal nerve.
B. Spread by direct contact or droplets
C. Vesicular eruptions occur as the virus travels to the sensory neurons of the skin or eye.
D. The condition more commonly affects adults over 60 years of age but can be seen at any age.
  1. Immunocompromised patients such as those with HIV are at much higher risk for HZV ophthalmicus.
  2. Increased compliance with shingles vaccination for patients over 60 years has played a role in prevention of the disease.

E. HZV ophthalmicus must be distinguished from HSV ocular infection, which more commonly affects younger patients, does not follow a specific dermatome, and lesions may cross the midline.
F. Other differential diagnoses include conjunctivitis, corneal abrasion or ulcer, episcleritis or scleritis, optic neuritis and retinitis.
  1. Ramsay Hunt syndrome involves herpes zoster lesions of the auricular area or inside of the mouth
  2. Patients should be evaluated for immunosuppression such as HIV especially if under 40 years of age.
  3. Occasionally a contact dermatitis of the face may mimic HZV keratitis.

Medical Screening

A. *Chief complaint:* Viral prodrome such as headache, low-grade fever, malaise. Painful red eye (unilateral) and photophobia with blurred vision. Painful, tingling, burning rash
B. Physical examination
  1. Visual acuity usually decreased. Vesicles, pustules, crusts around eyes, forehead, face, or scalp (consider Ramsay Hunt syndrome if periauricular lesions).
  2. Lesions follow dermatome of fifth cranial nerve and do not cross the midline.

3. Hutchinson's sign—(lesion on tip of nose indicating involvement of the nasociliary branch of the trigeminal nerve) suggests ocular involvement.
4. Conjunctival injection or possible ciliary flush
5. Evaluate EOMs (cranial nerves III, IV, and VI) for cranial nerve palsy.

Diagnostic Testing and Management

A. Procedures
 1. *Fluorescein stain and slit lamp examination:* Multiple small punctate epithelial erosions (superficial punctate keratitis) without epithelial erosion. *Pseudodendrites:* Elevated or "stuck-on" appearing lesions with no end bulbs and minimal fluorescein uptake; usually on corneal periphery without central ulceration. Possible cell and flare in anterior chamber. *Intraocular pressure measurement:* May be elevated.
B. *Laboratory:* Screen for HIV.
C. Treatment
 1. *Oral antiviral medication to limit duration:* Acyclovir or valacyclovir; or famciclovir
 2. Treat epithelial involvement such as corneal dendrites or geographic ulcers with topical antiviral drops such as Viroptic (trifluridine ophthalmic) or ganciclovir ophthalmic gel 0.15%.
D. Consult ophthalmology if stromal disease present to initiate prednisolone 1%; requires slow taper (months to years). Pain related to HZV may require opioid analgesia; neuropathic pain may respond to amitriptyline.

Hordeolum ("Stye")

A. A hordeolum is a painful cause of a red eye that causes external inflammation or abscess of the eyelash follicle of lid margin and involves the gland of Zeis. This is a sebaceous gland located on the margin of the eyelid (Figure 12.4).

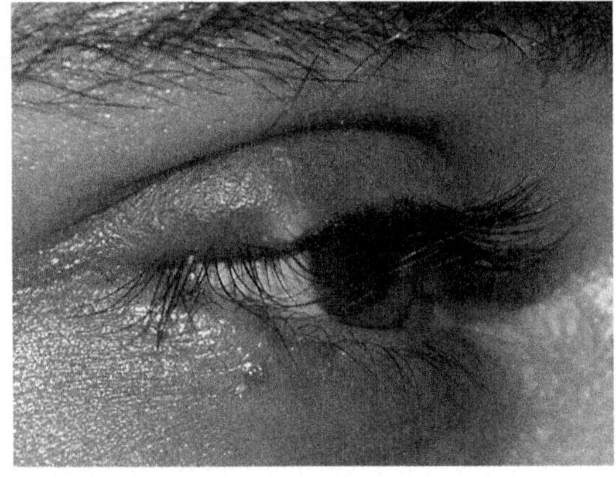

FIGURE 12.4 Hordeolum.
Source: Guida KM. Advanced health assessment of the eyes and ears. In: Myrick KM, Karosas LM, eds. *Advanced Health Assessment and Differential Diagnosis.* 1st ed. Springer Publishing Company; 2020. Fig. 4.30.[13]

B. An internal hordeolum is called a chalazion and is an inflammation of the deeper meibomian glands in the eyelid. *Staphylococcus aureus* is the most common organism but patients with chronic skin conditions such as seborrhea or rosacea may experience recurrent chalazion due to obstruction as the meibomian glands.
C. Consider preseptal cellulitis in patients with periorbital soft tissue swelling, erythema, warmth, and possible fever or sebaceous gland malignancy in older patients with recurrent chalazion.

Medical Screening

A. *Chief complaint:* Unilateral, red, painful eyelid with mild tearing
B. Palpable or visible focal swelling or pustule at the lid margin. May be mildly diffuse conjunctival injection without ciliary flush
C. Patients are usually well-appearing and afebrile with normal visual acuity.
D. A chalazion will be seen on lid eversion as a minimally tender, firm erythematous nodular lesion that points toward the underlying conjunctiva and is often caused by *Staphylococcus aureus*.
E. Patients with chronic skin conditions such as seborrhea or rosacea may experience recurrent chalazion due to obstruction as the Meibomian glands.
F. Fever, periorbital soft tissue swelling, erythema, and warmth may indicate preseptal cellulitis while painful or restricted EOMs may suggest orbital cellulitis.
 1. Consider sebaceous gland malignancy in older patients with recurrent chalazion.
 2. A moderately erythematous raised lesion within the conjunctiva may indicate a benign pyogenic granuloma that often occurs following mild trauma and often requires surgical excision.

Management

A. Procedures
 1. *Fluorescein stain:* No epithelial defect
 2. *Slit lamp examination:* Anterior chamber clear
B. Treatment
 1. Acetaminophen or NSAIDs for pain
 2. Consider topical antibiotic.
 3. Artificial tears for lubrication
 4. Conservative measures and patient teaching include warm compresses 3 to 4 times a day, do not attempt to squeeze pustule and primary care follow-up for acute hordeolum if symptoms do not improve in 1 week.
 5. If no improvement, patient should be referred to an ophthalmologist for follow-up.

Patient Disposition

A. Aftercare instructions include good handwashing, warm compresses, and careful contact lens care. Avoid use of makeup or anything that may contribute to causing additional irritation.

Keratitis

A. Keratitis is a serious condition that causes inflammation of the transparent cornea that covers the iris and pupil.
B. Caused most often by infection that causes disruption of the corneal epithelium and allows organisms to invade the deeper corneal stromal layers
  1. Also caused by UV light exposure, dry eye syndrome, contact lens use, mild trauma, and adverse topical medications or chemicals
  2. Can also be a sequelae of conjunctivitis
C. The cornea is about 0.5 to 0.8 mm thick, and keratitis may be superficial or deep; spreading infection can lead to iritis.
D. Superficial keratitis causes epithelial defects seen with fluorescein stain but some noninfectious forms of keratitis originate in the deeper corneal layers and do not cause epithelial damage.
E. Keratitis must be identified and treated aggressively to prevent possible loss of vision due to scarring, perforation, or progression of infection to endophthalmitis which can occur in 1 to 2 days.
F. History of contact lens use

Medical Screening

A. Chief complaint is usually a unilateral red eye with moderate to severe pain (foreign body [FB] sensation or grittiness), photophobia, and slight blurred vision.
B. *May also have history of exposure to ultraviolet light:* Sunlight, sunbed use, welder's arc, seafoam, snow blindness, or high-altitude environment.
C. Physical examination:
  1. Visual acuity normal or may be decreased.
  2. Blepharospasm, watery or mucoid discharge, crusting, or swelling of lid margins
  3. Conjunctival injection and possible ciliary flush
  4. FB under upper eyelid on lid eversion

Diagnostic Testing and Management

A. Procedures:
  1. If only superficial cornea affected, topical anesthesia should provide significant pain relief and is reassuring that deeper structures are not affected.
  2. *Fluorescein stain:* Superficial punctate lesions or "stippling" is seen as multiple tiny dot-like epithelial defects with uptake of fluorescein; may be diffuse and confluent or band-like if partially open eye exposed to ultraviolet light (actinic keratitis).
    a. Corneal ulcer may be present.
  3. *Slit lamp examination:* Clear anterior chamber or may see "cell and flare" or hypopyon caused by a proliferation of inflammatory cells in anterior chamber.
    a. Cornea may appear opacified if deeper stromal infiltrates present. *Seidel sign:* Leakage of aqueous humor if corneal perforation.
B. Treatment
C. Keratitis must be identified and treated aggressively to prevent possible loss of vision due to scarring, perforation or progression of infection to endophthalmitis which can occur in 1 to 2 days.
D. Artificial tears for comfort and lubrication
E. Topical fourth-generation fluoroquinolones such as moxifloxacin provide better Gram-positive bacteria coverage than ciprofloxacin or ofloxacin for mild to moderate keratitis.
F. Can alternate with erythromycin ointment to provide streptococci coverage
G. Tobramycin alternated with fortified cefazolin or vancomycin if severe keratitis
H. Cycloplegic drops to paralyze ciliary muscle may help with pain.
I. Systemic medications if *N. gonorrheae* suspected
J. Topical corticosteroids to reduce corneal inflammation remain controversial and consultation with ophthalmologist is recommended prior to prescribing.

Preseptal/Orbital Cellulitis

A. Patients with periorbital erythema (usually unilateral) must be evaluated for preseptal (periorbital) or orbital cellulitis to determine if the infection has extended to the deeper structures and globe.
B. Since the orbital septum acts as a physical barrier, bacterial transfer is most likely due to local skin infections, trauma, dental infection, sinusitis, or systemic infection.
  1. Though *Staphylococcus aureus* and streptococci are typical, *H. influenzae* is commonly seen in children under 5 years of age.
  2. Both preseptal and orbital cellulitis are rare in adults and more likely in immunosuppressed hosts, especially diabetics.
  3. Periorbital and orbital cellulitis can be a continuum of the same disease process, and patients must be monitored closely for extension of infection to the deep structures posterior to the orbital septum.
  4. Orbital cellulitis can lead to loss of vision and so a high index of suspicion must be maintained in the assessment of all periorbital erythema and soft tissue swelling associated with eye pain.

Medical Screening

A. Preseptal cellulitis
  1. History of recent viral illness, otitis media, sinus infection or break in skin integrity due to insect bite, skin infection, lacrimal system infection
  2. Periorbital soft tissue swelling and redness with mild, diffuse conjunctival injection without ciliary flush
  3. Possible chemosis
  4. Extraocular movements (EOMs) intact without limitation or complaint of pain, no proptosis or diplopia
  5. May have difficulty opening eyes due to local swelling; edema may be significant in younger children with *H. influenzae* infection
  6. Local erythema and warmth, may have break in skin integrity, insect bite, herpes simplex, or herpes zoster lesions in periocular area

7. Possible low-grade fever but generally looks well. Visual acuity and pupils are normal.

B. Orbital cellulitis

1. Pain with movement of eyes and associated with periorbital soft tissue swelling and redness; patient appears ill and is often febrile.
2. Headache with eye pain, blurred vision, and possible diplopia.
3. Visual acuity is decreased.
4. Possible afferent pupillary defect (APD) if optic nerve affected. Restricted and painful EOMs
5. Chemosis of conjunctiva with diffuse injection; possible purulent discharge
6. Periorbital soft tissues often more deeply erythematous or violaceous in color and proptosis may be present.

Diagnostic Testing and Management

A. *Laboratory:* Complete blood count (CBC), comprehensive metabolic panel (CMP), blood cultures, CRP (elevated in patients with concern for necrotizing fasciitis), conjunctival discharge culture

B. *Imaging:* Orbital CT scan (thin axial sections orbits and sinuses) is indicated for periorbital swelling and erythema if associated eye pain, restricted or painful EOMs or proptosis but is not indicated for clear cases of preseptal cellulitis.

1. CT scan of the orbits and head is indicated for patients with orbital infection and new neurological findings.
2. MRI if cavernous sinus thrombosis or orbital abscess suspected.

C. Procedures:

1. Incision and drainage of cutaneous abscesses that may be the origin of infection. Consider lumbar puncture if abnormal neurological findings present after CT has been performed.

D. Treatment

1. Well-appearing patients with preseptal cellulitis may be treated as an outpatient with clindamycin plus amoxicillin/clavulanic acid.
   a. *Pediatrics:* Clindamycin; or trimethoprim-sulfamethoxazole (TMP/SMZ) plus amoxicillin/clavulanic acid
   b. Orbital cellulitis requires admission for broad-spectrum IV antibiotics or antifungals based on suspected organism.
   c. Vancomycin plus clindamycin or ceftriaxone
   d. Amphotericin for fungal infection initiated after test dose
2. Emergency canthotomy indicated for signs of orbital compartment syndrome

Subconjunctival Hemorrhage

A. A subconjunctival hemorrhage is a collection of blood between the thin sclera and the conjunctiva.

1. May occur spontaneously or following mild trauma
2. Mechanisms include Valsalva such as vomiting, coughing, or sneezing.
3. Patients may have a history of hypertension, blood dyscrasias, or HIV.
4. Subconjunctival hemorrhages may also be seen in neonates following a vaginal delivery.
5. Also consider if redness may be due to foreign body, hyphema, conjunctival laceration, globe disruption, or retrobulbar hemorrhage.
   a. A red sclera may also be caused by episcleritis or scleritis, hordeolum, conjunctivitis, endophthalmitis, Kaposi's sarcoma, or conjunctival neoplasm.

Medical Screening

A. *Chief complaint:* Redness of the white part of the eye that is asymptomatic or mild irritation or foreign body sensation.

B. Vital signs (VS) are usually normal, but hypertension (HTN) may be seen in elderly or anticoagulated patients.

C. Hemorrhage appears as localized, flat scleral erythema often localized to one aspect of the eye. Pupils equal, round, and reactive to light and accommodation (PERRLA) and visual acuity normal.

D. Circumferential, raised, or dense-appearing erythema or bloody chemosis is suspicious for scleral tear or globe disruption and a lateral subconjunctival hemorrhage with a history of local trauma may indicate an associated zygomatic arch fracture.

E. Chemosis, proptosis, limited EOMs suggest retrobulbar hemorrhage.

1. A red sclera may also be caused by foreign body, episcleritis or scleritis. Other etiologies to consider include hordeolum, conjunctivitis, endophthalmitis, Kaposi's sarcoma, or conjunctival neoplasm.

Diagnostic Testing and Management

A. Procedures

1. Intraocular pressure measurement to rule out ruptured globe
2. *Fluorescein stain:* No epithelial defect
3. *Slit lamp exam:* Anterior chamber clear to rule out hyphema

B. Laboratory

1. Consider complete blood count (CBC) and prothrombin time/partial thromboplastin time (PT/PTT), international normalized ratio (INR) to rule out blood dyscrasias.

C. *Imaging:* Consider orbital CT based on history.

D. Treatment:

1. Artificial tears for mild irritation

E. Patient education:

1. Patient teaching to avoid aspirin and NSAIDs to prevent bleeding and the importance of hypertension and anticoagulant management

Patient Disposition

A. Urgent referral for traumatic subconjunctival hemorrhage if there is significant bulging of conjunctiva to rule out open globe injury

TRAUMATIC OCULAR EMERGENCIES

SHEILA SHEA

Blowout Fracture With Entrapment

A. Blowout orbital fractures are caused by a sudden increase in intraorbital pressure or compression of the inferior orbital rim and causes the weaker orbital floor or medial wall to break.
B. Extraocular muscles and periorbital fat may prolapse through the fracture into the open air-filled maxillary sinus and become "entrapped."
C. The inferior infraorbital nerve and artery run through orbital floor which account for some or the patient symptoms with blowout fractures.
D. Maxillary fractures can include orbital floor fracture and also cause entrapment of the inferior rectus muscle.
E. As with other traumatic injuries, younger males are more likely to experience eye injuries, but older adults have an increased risk of falls resulting in eye trauma.
F. The potential for assault and domestic violence must also be considered.

Medical Screening

A. *Chief complaint:* Blurred or decreased vision, light sensitivity, flashing lights (associated with possible detached retina, tinnitus, history of blunt or penetrating periocular or eye trauma
B. Physical examination
- **1.** *Visual acuity:* Blurred, decreased, or complete visual loss
- **2.** *Pupils:* Round, reactivity both direct and consensual; may be teardrop shaped if laceration; possible afferent pupillary defect (APD)
- **3.** Photophobia is more common with traumatic iritis.
- **4.** *Extraocular movements (EOMs):* Limited or painful upward gaze most common, may be present with downward gaze, and may be due to muscle entrapment, nerve damage, or soft tissue injury
- **5.** Diplopia especially on lateral or upward gaze
- **6.** Funduscopic examination
- **7.** Associated eyelid laceration, periorbital soft tissue swelling, ecchymosis, bony stepoff, or tenderness. Mechanical ptosis. Enophthalmos due to prolapse of orbital soft tissues into maxillary sinus; may be difficult to appreciate if significant periorbital swelling present. Subconjunctival hemorrhage and scleral injection; possible ciliary flush if traumatic iritis.
- **8.** Possible obvious hyphema
- **9.** Decreased sensation or anesthesia of the infraorbital area, periorbital subcutaneous emphysema due escape of air from sinus fracture; more commonly seen with medial wall fracture. Epistaxis or cerebrospinal fluid (CSF) rhinorrhea, nasal tenderness. Malocclusion or intraoral trauma or facial bony injuries such as tripod fracture of the zygomaticomaxillary complex.

Diagnostic Testing and Management

A. Imaging
- **1.** Orbital CT scan to evaluate fracture location and size, possible intraocular foreign body, EOMs, optic nerve.
- **2.** Head CT as indicated based on history of mechanism of injury and physical examination.

B. Fluorescein stain; corneal epithelial damage or positive Seidel sign
C. *Slit lamp examination:* Epithelial injury, foreign body, corneal laceration
D. Treatment
- **1.** Avoid blowing nose, elevate head of bed, local ice packs
  - **a.** Saline rinses and nasal decongestants are helpful in addition to oral analgesia.
  - **b.** Empiric antibiotic coverage is usually recommended.
  - **c.** Referral to ophthalmology or plastics, for follow-up

Chemical Burns

A. Ocular chemical burns are an ophthalmic emergency and require immediate and aggressive treatment.
B. Copious irrigation should be initiated regardless of the type of chemical substance involved.
C. Ocular burn severity depends on the chemical involved and the duration of exposure.
D. In general, acid burns, other than hydrofluoric acid, which is used to clean swimming pools, denature the tissue proteins, and creates a barrier against further extension of damage and so are less destructive.
E. Alkalines such as drain cleaners, lye, plasters, or cement cause immediate and more serious damage to ocular structures due to liquefactive necrosis and cellular death.
F. Alkali exposures often require prolonged irrigation and can continue to penetrate the eye long after the initial exposure.
G. Complications of ocular burns include glaucoma or blindness.

Medical Screening

A. *Chief complaint:* Severe eye pain; unilateral or bilateral, foreign body sensation, blurred vision, tearing, blepharospasm, light sensitivity
B. *History:* Chemical exposure by liquid, gas, or particles. Duration of exposure, acid, or alkali
C. Physical examination
- **1.** Detailed examination is deferred until irrigation completed.
- **2.** Visual acuity usually decreased. Diffuse scleral and conjunctival injection with possible ciliary flush.
- **3.** Chemosis, eyelid edema, photophobia
- **4.** Cornea may be grossly clear but a hazy or opaque appearance; increased risk for impaired vision or blindness.

5. Presence of perilimbic ischemia or blanching indicates a more serious burn.
6. Periorbital soft tissue burns

Diagnostic Testing and Management

A. *Fluorescein stain:* Superficial punctate keratitis

B. *Slit lamp exam:* Possible focal epithelial tissue loss or sloughing, corneal haziness, anterior chamber reaction. Intraocular pressure measurement

C. Procedures:

1. Immediate eye irrigation with copious normal saline or any available noncaustic liquid using Morgan Lens if available
    a. Amount and duration of irrigation is based on ocular pH (7.0–7.3).
    b. Measure pH with litmus paper after irrigation has been discontinued for 5 to 10 minutes and recheck every 30 minutes until it is within normal limits.
    c. Sweep or irrigate conjunctival fornices for retained chemical liquids or particulate matter.
    d. Re-instill topical anesthesia as needed.

D. Treatment:

1. Topical anesthesia and cycloplegic drops for pain control.
2. Topical antibiotics such as erythromycin ointment ½" ribbon q2h while awake or moxifloxacin or polymyxin B trimethoprim.
3. Topical steroid such as prednisolone drops qid after consultation with ophthalmology
4. Artificial tears for lubrication; chemical damage can interfere with normal tearing and delay healing.
5. NSAIDs, acetaminophen, or narcotic oral analgesia as needed. Confirm tetanus immunization status.

E. The use of an eye patch is controversial but is sometimes used as a therapeutic bandage while the epithelium heals.

Corneal Abrasion

A. Corneal abrasions can be painful and are a very common emergency complaint typically caused by a scratch of the cornea or other mild trauma.

1. Contact lens use is an important historical element and raises concern for complication of corneal ulcer.
2. A search for occult foreign body can help identify the cause of the abrasion.
3. A history of ultraviolet light exposure or contact lens use increase the risk for corneal epithelial defect.
4. Children with what appears to be conjunctivitis may actually have a corneal abrasion, and identification can help explain the child's discomfort.
5. The prognosis for most superficial corneal abrasions is very good.

Medical Screening

A. *Chief complaint:* Sharp pain, tearing, blinking, grittiness or foreign body sensation, sensitivity to light; possible minor eye trauma history

B. Physical examination:

1. Visual acuity usually normal unless large abrasion over pupil.
2. Mild to moderate diffuse conjunctival injection; no ciliary flush
3. Mild lid edema and blepharospasm
4. Pupils normal
5. Possible foreign body on upper lid eversion

Diagnostic Testing

A. Procedures:

1. *Fluorescein stain with uptake of dye:* Describe size and location and presence/absence of Seidel sign.
2. *Slit lamp examination:* Minimal to no anterior chamber reaction

Management

A. *Treatment:* Eye rest, sunglasses, darkened room, and lubrication with artificial tears

B. *Topical antibiotics for affected eye:* Erythromycin ointment ½ inch ribbon every 6 hours; or polymyxin B/trimethoprim drops

C. *Contact lens users:* Cover for possible pseudomonas with tobramycin, ofloxacin, or ciprofloxacin drops or ointment.

D. Tetanus immunization if needed

E. Oral analgesia with NSAIDs, acetaminophen, or short-term opioid for severe pain

F. Topical steroids are not indicated and can impair healing of epithelium.

G. Patching generally not needed and is to be avoided in corneal abrasions caused by contact lens use, plant matter, "dirty" fingernails.

H. Depending on the size of the abrasion, patient may require a referral for follow-up with an ophthalmologist.

Corneal Foreign Body

A. Superficial corneal foreign bodies (FBs) adhere to the surface of the cornea or embedded in the outermost corneal layers.

B. FBs are often specks of dirt or makeup but can be glass, plastic, or other materials.

1. Metallic objects can cause a rust ring to form on the cornea that must be removed to preserve vision and to avoid permanent staining.

C. Infection or necrosis can result from retained FBs. Details regarding the injury such as grinding or other high-velocity mechanisms can help identify potential globe perforation.

Medical Screening

A. *Chief complaint:* Eye pain, tearing, blinking, grittiness or foreign body sensation, sensitivity to light

B. History of ocular trauma; document use of protective lenses.

C. Physical examination:

1. Visual acuity usually normal unless FB is over pupil
2. Mild to moderate diffuse conjunctival injection; possible ciliary flush
3. Mild lid edema with blepharospasm
4. Pupils normal

5. Evert upper lid for possible FB. It is often possible to visualize foreign body or retained rust ring with bright light.

D. There is usually good pain relief with topical anesthetic.

Diagnostic Testing and Management

A. Procedures:

1. *Fluorescein stain:* Uptake of dye at site of foreign body
2. Slit lamp examination to determine location and depth of foreign body, depth of anterior chamber, Seidel sign if perforation, cell and flare if anterior chamber reaction or hyphema, residual rust ring from metallic foreign body. Consult ophthalmologist as needed.
3. *Intraocular pressure measurement:* May be decreased

B. *Imaging:* Ultrasound or orbital CT scan with thin cuts if there is any question of intraocular foreign body.

C. Treatment:

1. FB removal with moistened cotton swab or needle tip
2. Apply eye shield (not patch) if unable to remove multiple, deep, or large retained FBs and obtain urgent ophthalmology consultation.
3. Treat as for corneal abrasion with lubrication and topical antibiotics after corneal FB removal.
4. Confirm tetanus immunization status.

Eyelid Laceration

A. Eyelid lacerations may result from blunt or penetrating forces and can be superficial or affect deeper structures and seemingly innocent lacerations can mask more serious injuries.

B. Injuries to surrounding tissue can affect the eyelid margins, extraocular movements (EOMs), lacrimal drainage system, or globe and can lead to both cosmetic and functional problems.

C. The upper lid is most commonly affected, and eyelid lacerations may be seen at any age.

D. A detailed history of the mechanism of injury can help determine the possibility of retained foreign body (FB).

E. Emergency management is directed at identifying injury to the globe or cornea, excluding foreign body, preventing infection, and achieving optimal cosmesis.

Medical Screening

A. *Chief complaint:* Pain, bleeding, possible blurred or decreased vision

B. History of local trauma

1. Animal and human bite wounds present increased risk for contamination and infection and usually require antibiotic coverage.

C. Physical examination:

1. Visual acuity normal or decreased
2. *Eyelid laceration:* Lid margin, inner canthus, tarsal plate, tissue loss, protrusion of orbital fat
   a. Note location and extent—lacerations involving the medial one-third of the eye are often associated with damage to the puncta and canalicular system and usually require emergent repair by an ophthalmologist.
3. Ptosis due to damage to elevator or superior rectus muscles
4. Subconjunctival hemorrhage or scleral injection
5. Possible FB or hyphema or extrusion of vitreous humor
6. Funduscopic exam, EOM function. Periorbital soft tissue swelling, stepoff, or deformity. Assess facial motor function and sensation.

Diagnostic Testing and Management

A. *Imaging:* Orbital CT scan with thin cuts for concerning eyelid lacerations to identify intraocular FB, globe disruption, retrobulbar hemorrhage or orbital fracture. Possible head CT based on mechanism of injury

B. *Procedures:* Protect globe with metal shield and avoid any pressure on orbit.

C. Fluorescein stain for epithelial defect or FB

D. Slit lamp examination may show cell and flare if anterior chamber reaction, hyphema, or Seidel sign ("waterfall" of aqueous humor) if full thickness corneal injury.

1. Magnification may reveal a corneal or scleral laceration and orbital fat may be seen if injury extends through orbital septum.

E. *Treatment:* Topical anesthetic drops, systemic analgesia; confirm tetanus immunization status.

Ruptured Globe and Penetrating Injury

A. Penetrating injuries to the globe are an immediate threat to loss of vision or loss of the eye itself and are a major ophthalmologic emergency.

B. Full-thickness damage to the sclera and cornea may represent an open globe injury. The globe is susceptible at where the sclera is thinnest at the limbic margin.

C. Damage to the globe can result from blunt forces that cause a sudden compression of the eye and increase intraocular pressure.

D. Penetrating injury mechanisms include high velocity objects, grinding, fists, baseballs, or sharp objects such as sticks or knives.

E. Younger males are much more likely than females to sustain trauma that causes disruption of the globe.

Medical Screening

A. *Chief complaint:* Pain (minimal to severe), foreign body (FB) sensation, red eye, blurred vision, possible diplopia. History of blunt or penetrating trauma

B. Physical examination

1. Extensive periorbital soft tissue swelling may make the eye examination difficult, but immediate confirmation of visual acuity and pupillary reaction is essential.
2. Red reflex may be absent due to vitreous hemorrhage.
3. Visual acuity decreased, limited to light perception or absent
4. Possible diplopia; may be due to lens dislocation, cranial nerve palsy or entrapment of extraocular movements (EOMs) associated with orbital floor fracture.

5. Eyelid swelling, ecchymosis, laceration. Subconjunctival hemorrhage; complete hemorrhage is highly suspicious for globe disruption.
6. Pupil shape, size, reactivity, light reflex
   a. Possible afferent pupillary defect (APD)
   b. Pupil may be teardrop shaped and pointing toward rupture. EOMs function.
7. Obvious hyphema may be visible. Iris deformity (iridodialysis) as iris separates from ciliary body
8. Extrusion and visible intraocular contents; aqueous or vitreous humor.
9. Asymmetry of globes due to enophthalmos or exophthalmos.
10. Periorbital soft tissue swelling, ecchymosis, crepitus, or stepoff deformity and associated facial injury or intracranial injury.

Diagnostic Testing and Management

A. Imaging
   1. Orbital CT scan with thin cuts to detect globe rupture, foreign body or optic nerve damage.
   2. Orbital ultrasound is contraindicated due to pressure on globe.
   3. CT of head or cervical spine as indicated based on mechanism of injury

B. Procedures
   1. Protective eye shield to avoid any pressure on globe, elevate head of bed, and stabilize embedded FBs.
   2. Avoid instillation of anesthetic eye drops if concern for open globe.

C. Fluorescein stain is deferred in cases of obvious ruptured globe but may demonstrate full-thickness corneal wound with positive Seidel sign ("waterfall" of aqueous humor).

D. Slit lamp examination may show a shallow or flat anterior chamber; may be only sign of globe rupture and is associated with poorer prognosis.
   1. Cell and flare in anterior chamber if microscopic or gross hyphema. Iris or lens deformities; prolapse, dislocation, subluxation

E. Intraocular pressure measurement is contraindicated if globe rupture suspected.

F. Treatment
   1. Analgesia and antiemetics if needed
   2. Confirm tetanus immunization status.
   3. Topical anesthesia and topical medications are contraindicated in cases of open globe.
   4. Prophylactic systemic antibiotics to prevent complication of endophthalmitis using ceftazidime, ciprofloxacin, gentamicin, or vancomycin.

Patient Disposition

A. Immediate ophthalmology consultation for definitive management and transfer to tertiary center if ophthalmology services are not available.

Traumatic Hyphema

A. A hyphema is the accumulation of blood in the aqueous humor of the anterior chamber.

B. It is usually caused by either blunt or penetrating trauma that damages the vessels of the iris and ciliary body.

C. Adults and children are at risk for injuries that cause a hyphema, and there are a wide variety of mechanisms of injury, including sports, toys, pellets, and airbags.

D. Assaults and closed-fist injuries are also common causes and more often involve males.

E. Postoperative hyphema formation is a surgical complication, and patients can experience a spontaneous hyphema in rare cases.
   1. The risk of rebleeding in the first 3 to 5 days occurs in more than 25% of patients.

Medical Screening

A. *Chief complaint:* Unilateral eye pain and blurred vision

B. *History:* History of head, facial, or orbital trauma

C. Physical examination:
   1. Visual acuity decreased, pupils normal; possible afferent pupillary defect
   2. Blood in anterior chamber that may be visible as it layers into lower portion of iris.
   3. Conjunctival and scleral injection; ciliary flush if associated with traumatic iritis. Extraocular movements (EOMs) intact unless there is an associated orbital blowout fracture.
   4. Also consider skull fracture, intracranial injury, and cervical injury based on the history of mechanism of injury.

Diagnostic Testing and Management

A. Slit lamp examination may show only haziness indicative of microhyphema.
   1. Hyphema grades
      a. Blood fills less than 1/3 of anterior chamber.
      b. Blood fills between 1/3 and 1/2 of anterior chamber.
      c. Blood fills between 1/2 and less than complete.
      d. Blood fills the anterior chamber completely and gives the appearance of an "8-ball" or "blackball."

B. *Intraocular pressure measurement:* May be decreased or elevated

C. *Imaging:* CT scan of orbits, face, head as indicated

D. Treatment
   1. Apply protective eye shield and elevate head of bed to decrease intraocular pressure and facilitate settling of blood inferiorly and improve vision.
   2. Avoid aspirin and NSAIDs to reduce bleeding risk; use acetaminophen or narcotic analgesia if needed. Cycloplegic drops for pain control related to iritis
   3. Topical steroids such as prednisolone drops to control inflammation after ophthalmology consultation. Antifibrinolytic agents such as aminocaproic acid may be ordered by ophthalmology to prevent risk of recurrent hyphema.

Patient Disposition

A. Anticipate admission for noncompliant patients with hyphema or those with associated ocular or other trauma.

LOSS-OF-VISION OCULAR EMERGENCIES

SHEILA SHEA

Acute Angle-Closure Glaucoma

A. Acute angle-closure glaucoma is an ophthalmologic emergency that can rapidly lead to irreversible optic nerve death within hours.
B. This type of acute glaucoma occurs when the angle between the cornea and iris suddenly narrows and prevents the normal outflow of aqueous fluid into the trabecular meshwork causing a rapid rise in ocular pressure.
C. Retinal damage follows impaired blood supply. There are many reasons for acute angle-closure glaucoma including accommodation of reading, sudden pupillary dilation that occurs in dim lighting or the with use of mydriatics.
D. Some people are predisposed to pupillary blockage because of anatomically shallow anterior chambers including Asians or Inuit or farsighted people with small eyes.
E. Acute angle-closure glaucoma can also be precipitated by emotionally stressful situations.
F. Medications that cause the eye to dilate such as over-the-counter cold medications, sympathomimetics, antidepressants, and cocaine, may be implicated in acute angle-closure glaucoma.
G. Women generally have a shallower anterior chamber than men and after 60 years of age are at significant risk for acute angle-closure glaucoma.

Medical Screening

A. *Chief complaint:* Sudden, severe deep eye pain
B. Nausea and vomiting are also very common symptoms upon onset of eye pain.
C. Some patients may complain more of unilateral frontal headache and blurred vision rather than eye pain.
D. Colored halos around lights due to corneal edema as aqueous humor moves under pressure into stromal layers may be present.
E. Physical examination
  1. Visual acuity decreased; may be limited to hand motion
  2. Pupils are midrange, sluggish, or minimally reactive, and may be irregularly shaped.
  3. Diffuse scleral injection and possible ciliary flush is common, and the cornea may appear hazy or steamy.
  4. Eye pain may increase with ocular movement.
  5. Visual field assessment and funduscopic examination are needed.
    a. Gentle palpation of the eyeball may feel firm or tense.

Diagnostic Testing and Management

A. Slit lamp examination may demonstrate corneal edema, irregular-shaped pupil.
B. *Estimate depth of anterior chamber:* Shine a strong light from temporal side of eye; a normally deep anterior chamber will allow light to shine over flat iris while a shallow anterior chamber pushes the iris forward to cast a shadow on nasal aspect of iris.
C. Intraocular pressure measurement will be elevated, often greater than 60 mmHg.
D. Fluorescein stain can confirm that eye redness is not due to corneal abrasion or foreign body.
E. Treatment
  1. Management is geared toward reduction of intraocular pressure and reduction of ocular inflammation.
  2. Antiemetics to control nausea and vomiting; also helps to decrease intraocular pressure associated with retching
  3. Oral analgesia as needed
  4. Acetazolamide to decrease aqueous humor production; systemic hyperosmotic agents such as mannitol may be used to produce osmotic diuresis may also be used.
  5. Topical beta-blocker such as timolol to decrease aqueous humor production
  6. Topical steroids such as prednisolone to decrease inflammation after ophthalmology consultation
  7. Topical miotic such as pilocarpine to constrict ciliary muscle; initiate 1 hour after other medications.

Central Retinal Artery Occlusion

A. Central retinal artery occlusion (CRAO) is an embolic event that causes unilateral sudden, painless loss of vision due to loss of blood supply to the retina.
  1. This ophthalmologic emergency requires prompt recognition and immediate action to preserve vision as a favorable outcome depends on the duration of arterial occlusion.
  2. The condition is much more common in elderly populations, and there is an increased risk of cerebrovascular accident or myocardial infarction following CRAO.
  3. Some patients with migraine headaches can experience transient visual changes. Central retinal venous occlusion (CRVO) can also present with unilateral painless loss of vision but is more gradual in onset over hours to days.
  4. This relatively common eye condition is seen more often in patients over 50 years of age and is associated with diffuse retinal hemorrhages that appear as "cotton-wool spots" or "blood and thunder."

Medical Assessment

A. *Chief complaint:* History of sudden (within seconds to minutes), painless loss of vision; often limited to light perception or complete loss
  1. Patients may report recent transient visual loss (amaurosis fugax) due to emboli from carotid or heart.
  2. Medical conditions such as systemic diseases such as atrial fibrillation (AF), hypertension (HTN), diabetes, atherosclerotic disease, valvular disease, systemic lupus erythematosus (SLE), polyarteritis nodosa, or conditions with predisposition for embolus formation or hypercoagulability

B. In younger patients, risk factors include history of sickle cell disease or oral contraceptive use.
C. Infective endocarditis can lead to embolic visual loss; patients usually also report fever, chills, malaise, anorexia, night sweats, and weight loss.
D. A history of prosthetic valve and IV drug abuse (IVDA) is also important.
E. Physical examination:
  1. Visual acuity is markedly decreased; hand motion or light perception or complete loss of vision.
  2. Pupils usually equal, round, and reactive; marked afferent pupillary defect (AFD)
  3. Funduscopic exam will reveal a pale retina with cherry-red spot at center of macula; changes may not be visible for hours after onset of symptoms.
  4. Vessels that look like "boxcars" due to impaired blood flow in veins and arteries if severe obstruction.

Diagnostic Testing and Management

A. Intraocular pressure measurement
B. Laboratory
  1. Complete blood count (CBC) and basic metabolic panel (BMP)
  2. Erythrocyte sedimentation rate may be elevated in giant cell arteritis; coagulation studies; blood cultures are indicated if there is concern for emboli due to bacterial endocarditis.
C. *Imaging:* Carotid artery Duplex Doppler ultrasound to establish patency of blow flow.
D. 12-lead EKG and possible echocardiogram
E. Treatment:
  1. Ocular massage to attempt to dislodge the embolus:
    a. Direct pressure to globe for 5 to 15 seconds, then release pressure and repeat several times.
  2. Acetazolamide to decrease aqueous humor production
  3. Topical beta-blocker such as timolol to decrease aqueous humor production
  4. Carbogen gas (95% oxygen plus 5% carbon dioxide)
  5. Anterior chamber paracentesis by ophthalmologist; intra-arterial thrombolysis is controversial; hyperbaric treatment may be helpful if initiated within 2 hours of onset of symptoms.

Optic Neuritis

A. Optic neuritis is caused by inflammation or damage to the myelin sheath of the optic nerve that impairs the transmission of visual information to the brain.
B. It is usually unilateral but may affect both eyes and lead to partial or complete loss of vision.
C. Visual changes are associated with painful movement of the eye due to irritation of the optic nerve.
D. The most common cause is multiple sclerosis and visual changes may be the first sign of the disease.
E. Optic neuritis can also be caused by local trauma or ischemia, infection, and can be associated with diabetes, metabolic derangement or autoimmune disorders.
F. Most cases of optic neuritis have an onset from ages 20 to 45 years and more likely involve women.
G. Uncomplicated optic neuritis has a good prognosis with visual recovery within 2 to 6 months.

Medical Screening

A. *Chief complaint:* History of time-specific onset of visual changes such as blurred, foggy, or dark vision with sudden partial or complete loss of vision
  1. May complain of periocular pain that precedes onset of visual changes by days
  2. Loss of vision, peripheral or central, that worsens over days; may report previous transient episodes lasting minutes
  3. Decreased color vision or clarity ("washed out"), especially red colors, decreased contrast/brightness of vision
  4. Pain with movement of the eyes; mild to severe and may be exacerbated by elevated body temperature
  5. Possible photopsia (flashes of lights), foreign body sensation or light sensitivity, reduced night vision, or eye redness.
  6. If multiple sclerosis is underlying etiology, patient may also report ataxia or lack of coordination and slurred speech.
B. Physical examination
  1. *Visual acuity:* Decreased and may be no light perception
  2. *Pupils:* Direct and consensual pupillary reflex is weaker in the affected eye with a relative afferent pupillary defect (APD).
  3. Painful extraocular movements (EOMs)
  4. Visual field defect; central scotoma is common.
  5. Color vision testing
  6. Funduscopic exam may show possible mild optic nerve swelling or disc edema; a normal optic disc on funduscopic examination and clinical signs of optic neuritis is called retrobulbar optic neuritis.

Diagnostic Testing and Management

A. Optic neuritis is generally a clinical diagnosis and fluorescein stain and slit lamp examination will be normal.
B. Imaging
  1. MRI is superior to orbital CT and will show enhancement of the optic nerve and should follow initial episode verify clinical suspicion of multiple sclerosis.
  2. Lumbar puncture may be helpful in identifying uncommon infectious or inflammatory causes of optic neuritis.
C. Treatment
  1. Ophthalmology evaluation and initiation of outpatient parenteral steroids, which have been shown to speed recovery but does not improve the final visual acuity.

Retinal Detachment

A. Retinal detachment is a time-critical emergency due to ischemia that results when the inner layers of the retina separates from the vascular choroid plexus causing impaired blood supply.

B. The retina can detach following eye surgery such as cataract removal.
C. In younger people, the causes are often due to sports-related trauma, assaults, or maltreatment.
D. Tears in the retina allow fluid to flow from the vitreous chamber and collect behind the retinal causing the detachment to spread.
E. Retinal tears may progress to complete retinal detachment.
F. Patients over 65 years of age may experience a posterior vitreous separation due to vitreous changes as the eye ages.
G. The gel-like vitreous liquefies and becomes contracted with a "stringy" consistency.
H. These strings are what the patient perceives as floaters, a hallmark of retinal detachment.
I. Some other conditions like diabetic retinopathy can cause traction on the retina and cause detachment.
J. It is important to refer for ophthalmology consultation for new onset of floaters with flashes of light or peripheral vision loss.

Medical Screening

A. *Chief complaint:* Patients report visual change most often in periphery of vision where most retinal tears occur.
  1. Flashes of light (photopsia) likely due to traction on the retina
  2. Floaters in vision due to hemorrhage or debris in vitreous; one large floater may indicate a posterior vitreous detachment, while a shower of floaters or black specks may indicate a vitreous hemorrhage.
  3. This may be followed by irregular blood clots that appear as "spiderwebs" in vision or a feeling of a dark shadow, curtain, veil, or spiderweb at periphery of vision.
  4. Possible visual field defect. There may be a history of recent trauma or family history of retinal detachment.
B. Physical examination
  1. Visual acuity usually decreased; if detachment affects the macula, vision will be markedly reduced.
  2. *Pupils:* Possible APD due to disruption of visual pathway.
  3. Visual field defects can help identify location of detachment.
  4. A normal funduscopic examination does not rule out detachment; many retinal tears are not visible without pupil dilation and indirect ophthalmoscopy.
  5. A large tear may be visible only as it "flaps" with eye movement.

Diagnostic Testing and Management

A. Fluorescein stain will be normal.
B. Slit lamp examination will show a "tobacco dust" due to a collection of pigmented cells in the anterior vitreous and often seen with posterior vitreous detachment. Intraocular pressure measurement
C. Imaging:
  1. Ocular ultrasound may assist with identification of detachment.
  2. Orbital CT scan is not helpful in the diagnosis of retinal detachment but may be indicated in cases of suspected fracture or intraocular foreign body.
D. Treatment:
  1. Definitive management of most retinal tears is surgical repair; keep patient NPO (nothing by mouth) if urgent surgery is planned.

EAR CONDITIONS

Acute Otitis Externa

A. Usually is caused by a bacterial infection of the external auditory canal. It is also known as "swimmer's ear."
B. An emergent problem is malignant otitis externa. It is an aggressive infection of the external auditory canal which involves the mastoid and base of the skull. Patients with diabetes or who are immunosuppressed are at greatest risk.

Medical Screening

A. *Chief complaint:* Localized ear pain to the external canal and the outer ear, discharge, swelling
B. Signs and symptoms:
  1. Pain with movement of the ear which may radiate to the neck, jaw, and head
  2. Swelling of the external canal and outer ear
  3. Discharge or debris in the external canal
  4. Itching which progressively gets worse
  5. Swelling of preauricular and postauricular lymph nodes
  6. Low-grade fever
C. *Medication history:* Immunosuppressive agents, on diabetic medications including insulin
D. *Past medical history:* Diabetes, cancer being treated with chemotherapy, patient on immunosuppressive medications
E. Physical examination
  1. Inspection:
    a. Swelling of the external canal and outer ear
    b. Purulent discharge or debris in the external canal
    c. Edema, erythema in the external canal
    d. Cellulitis
  2. Palpation
    a. Pain with movement of the year
    b. Palpable periauricular and postauricular lymph nodes

Differential Diagnoses

A. Otitis media
B. Cellulitis
C. Presence of a foreign body

Diagnostic Testing

A. Based on patient and history and exam as noted
B. Gram stain and culture of discharge

Management

A. Gather appropriate equipment and supplies, including personal protective equipment (PPE).

B. Otoscope with adequate lighting.
C. Ear suction under microscope may be needed.
D. Collaborate with ENT (ear, nose, and throat) as needed, especially if patient is acutely ill.
E. *Pharmacologic therapies:* Follow evidence-based guidance when prescribing.
F. Analgesia
G. Topical antibiotics (otic drops)
1. Ear canal needs to be cleaned before using ear drops.
2. If the patient has problems instilling the ear drops due to swelling and pain, a wick may be inserted so that the medication can get into the canal.
3. Ear drops that contain aminoglycosides and alcohol should be avoided in patients with possible tympanic perforations.
a. Ciprofloxacin/dexamethasone solution (may be used with a perforated membrane)
b. Ofloxacin (may be used with a perforated membrane)
c. Finafloxacin
H. Consultation and collaboration when indicated, especially when mastitis may be suspected

Patient Disposition

A. Provide patient with a referral for follow-up as needed.
B. Educate patient and family about signs and symptoms of mastitis.
C. Age and developmental considerations such as avoiding swimming pools, hot tubs, or ponds, avoid use of swabs or putting anything into the ear canal.
D. Prevention and education
E. Patient and family education and counseling

Acute Otitis Media

A. Acute otitis media occurs with inflammation or infection in the middle ear cleft and the mastoid cavity.
B. Otitis media can be either acute and chronic.
C. It is more commonly seen in children than adults.
D. Infections may be caused by *Streptococcus pneumoniae, Haemophilus influenzae,* and *Moraxella catarrhalis.*

Medical Screening

A. *Chief complaint:* Ear pain, recent upper respiratory infection (URI)
B. *Signs and symptoms:* Ear pain, pulling at the ear (as seen in children), sensation of fullness in the ear, fever, chills, diarrhea, vertigo, and dizziness
C. *Medication history:* None
D. *Past medical history:* Previous otitis media, immune deficiency, exposure to smoking, gastroesophageal reflux disease, craniofacial abnormalities, prolonged bottle feeding
E. Physical examination
1. *Inspect:* Diminished hearing, obvious discomfort, purulent ear or nose drainage, bulging or retracted eardrum, erythema of the tympanic membrane (TM), drainage from a ruptured TM
2. *Palpate:* Pain with movement of the affected ear

Differential Diagnoses

A. Mastoiditis
B. Otitis externa
C. Facial palsy
D. Meningitis
E. Brain abscess
F. Lateral sinus thrombosis

Diagnostic Testing

A. Otoscope evaluation
B. Culture and sensitivity of drainage, if appropriate

Management

A. Gather appropriate equipment and supplies, including personal protective equipment (PPE).
B. Otoscope with adequate lighting
C. Collaborate with ear, nose, and throat (ENT) if patient is acutely ill and may need admission.
D. Collaborate with Medicine or Neurology if acute infection is suspected (e.g., meningitis, brain abscess or lateral sinus thrombosis).
E. Analgesia
F. Fever management
G. Antibiotic treatment when indicated based on patient's age:
1. Amoxicillin
2. Amoxicillin/clavulanate
3. Cefdinir
4. Cefuroxime axetil
5. Azithromycin
6. Ceftriaxone

Patient Disposition

A. Provide patient with a referral for follow-up as needed.
B. Educate patient and family about signs and symptoms of possible complications including:
1. Acute mastoiditis
2. Facial palsy
3. Meningitis
C. Age and developmental considerations
D. Prevention and education
E. Patient and family education and counseling

Ear Foreign Body

A. A foreign body in the ear is more often seen in children but can occur in adults as well. Common objects include toys, candy, and popcorn. In adults, insects are more common.

Medical Screening

A. *Chief complaint:* Ear pain
B. *Signs and symptoms:* Purulent drainage, visible foreign body in the ear, "buzzing or a feeling of something moving in the ear
C. *Medication history:* None
D. *Past medical history:* Previous ear infections
E. Physical examination:
1. Inspection
a. Visible object
b. Red swollen ear canal
c. Bleeding or purulent drainage in the ear canal

Differential Diagnoses

A. Acute otitis media
B. Psychological problem (e.g., self-harm)
C. Cerumen impaction

Diagnostic Testing

A. Otoscope examination

Management

A. Gather appropriate equipment and supplies, including personal protective equipment (PPE).
B. Collaborate with ear, nose, and throat (ENT) if unable to safely remove the foreign body.
C. Topical anesthetic (nonviscous, usually lidocaine 1%); should be warmed before instillation.
D. Strong light (e.g., head lamp)
E. *Recommended equipment:* Suction; alligator forceps; cerumen loop
F. Consider analgesia and antibiotics as needed based on the foreign object and its effects on the ear canal.

Patient Disposition

A. Provide patient with a referral for follow-up as needed.
B. Keep ear canal clean and dry.
C. Educate patient and family about signs and symptoms of infection.
D. Age and developmental considerations/concern about abuse
E. Prevention and education
F. Patient and family education and counseling

Labyrinthitis

A. Labyrinthitis is an inflammatory response that effects the labyrinth in the cochlear and vestibular system of the inner ear.
B. Most common cause is a viral infection, but can also occur as a result of a bacterial infection related to otitis media.

Medical Screening

A. *Chief complaint:* Vertigo, loss of balance, and hearing loss
B. *Signs and symptoms:* Vertigo with head movement, hearing loss, nausea and vomiting, and headache
C. *Medication history:* Medications with side effects of dizziness
D. *Past medical history:* Viral upper respiratory infection (URI), previous ear infections, neurological disorders, hypertension (HTN), migraine headaches, Meniere's syndrome, smoking, alcohol, or substance abuse
E. Physical examination
F. Inspection
   1. Altered gait
   2. Spontaneous horizontal nystagmus with peripheral features, away from the side of disease, suppression of nystagmus with fixation
   3. Normal neurological examination

Differential Diagnoses

A. Cerebrovascular accident (CVA)
B. Infectious process such as meningitis
C. Intracerebral bleed

Diagnostic Testing

A. Complete blood count (CBC), basic metabolic pane (BMP), blood cultures may be considered, toxicology screen
B. *Dix-Hallpike test:* Positive test can indicate the diagnosis of Benign Paroxysmal Positional Vertigo (BPPV)
C. MRI of the brain

Management

A. IV fluids for nausea and vomiting
B. Pharmacological therapies:
   1. Antiemetic
   2. Sedatives/anxiolytics
   3. Antibiotics if indicated
C. Consider ENT or Neurology if unsure of the source of the vertigo.

Patient Disposition

A. Provide patient with a referral for follow-up as needed.
B. Educate patient to lie still with eyes closed during an acute exacerbation; encourage practice safety, for example, not driving until vertigo is gone).
C. Follow-up care should be arranged for the patient.

NASAL CONDITIONS

LISA KOSER

Epistaxis

A. Nasal circulation supply from branches of internal and external carotid arteries (Figure 12.5).
B. Arteries lie just under mucosa and require heat and humidification; vessels at risk for damage.
C. *Anterior vasculature:* Little's area or Kiesselbach's plexus are supplied by ethmoidal, greater palatine, superior labial, and sphenopalatine arteries.
D. *Posterior vasculature:* Occurs in noncompressible area. Woodruff's plexus supplied by sphenopalatine, posterior ethmoidal, and nasopalatine arteries.
E. Prevalence
   1. Incidence <10 years of age and between 50 and 80 years of age
      a. 6% to 10% seek medical attention.
   2. Can result from digital trauma, low humidity during winter
   3. Usually spontaneous, unilateral from a discrete lesion
   4. 90% are anterior, 10% are posterior (see Figure 12.5).
   5. Children
      a. Spontaneous or from rhinitis, cold, or trauma
      b. Usually from Little's area, anterior septum
   6. Adults

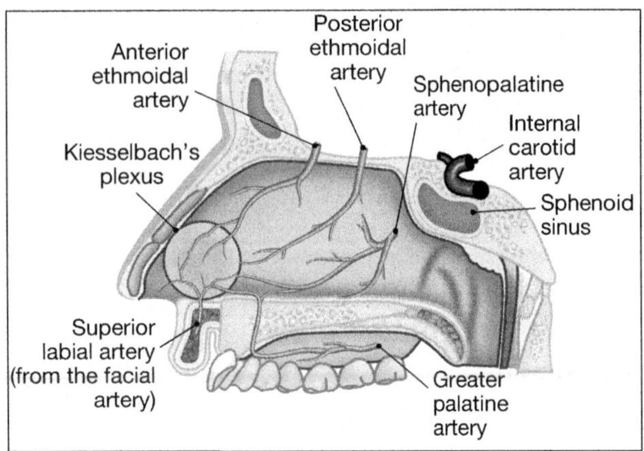

FIGURE 12.5 Vasculature of the nasal cavity.
Source: Colandrea M, Raynpor EM. Evidence-based assessment of the ears, nose, and throat. In: Gawlik KS, Melnyk BM, Teall AM, eds. *Evidence-Based Physical Examination.* 1st ed. Springer Publishing Company; 2021:341. Fig. 13.1.[14]

a. Usually posterior to Little's area, Kiesselbach's plexus
i. *Bleeding diathesis:* Anticoagulation, antiplatelet drugs

7. Elderly
a. Usually occurs in higher posterior part of nose from atherosclerotic vessels

Medical Screening

A. *Chief complaint:* Nose bleeding
B. Signs and symptoms
1. Nosebleed
2. Nausea
3. Hematemesis
4. Anemia
5. Hemoptysis
6. Melena
7. Lightheadedness
8. Fatigue
9. *Hypovolemic shock:* Tachycardia, hypotension, altered mental status (AMS; usually associated with severe trauma)

C. Medication history
1. Anticoagulants
2. Antiplatelet medications
3. NSAIDs
4. Steroid nasal spray
5. Illicit drug use (e.g., snorting cocaine)
6. Herbal supplements (e.g., garlic, ginkgo, ginseng, vitamin E)
7. Nasal trauma from excessive picking

D. Past medical history:
1. Previous episodes
2. Bleeding disorders and blood dyscrasias
3. HIV
4. Liver disease, heavy alcohol abuse
5. Kidney disease
6. Cancer, tumors
7. Splenomegaly
8. Recent nasal surgery or nasal procedure (NG, nasopharyngeal suctioning, nasal intubation)
9. Recent trauma (direct blow, picking, foreign body)
10. Recent or current upper respiratory infection (URI), sinusitis, allergic rhinitis
11. Exposure to environmental irritants, dry winter weather

E. Physical examination:
1. *General:* Fatigue
2. *Neurologic:* Altered mental status, dizzy
3. *Skin:* Pale, cool diaphoresis
4. *Cardiac:* Tachycardia, weak pulses, hypotension or hypertension (HTN)
5. *Head, eyes, ears, nose, and throat (HEENT):* nasal hemorrhage, postnasal drip
6. *Gastrointestinal (GI):* Hematemesis
7. *Respiratory:* Hemoptysis

Differential Diagnoses

A. Anterior epistaxis
B. Posterior epistaxis
C. Nasal tumor, known or new diagnosis
D. Nasal trauma
E. Coagulopathy
F. Cancer or pancytopenia, known or new diagnosis
G. Blood dyscrasia, known or new diagnosis

Diagnostic Testing

A. *Profuse bleeding:* CBC (complete blood count), international normalized ratio (INR), liver function test (LFT), type and cross
B. *Imaging:* CT face if facial trauma

Management

A. Supplies:
1. Gown, glove, eye protection
2. *Equipment:* Bright light, suction, nasal speculum, forceps, cotton swabs, cotton ball, medicine cup, silver nitrate sticks, Surgicel/Gelfoam, nasal tampon, petroleum jelly gauze strip, urinary catheter
3. *Medications:* 4% lidocaine with epi, Neo-Synephrine, Afrin, Amoxil

B. Assess airway, breathing, and circulation (ABC).
1. If unstable:
a. IV, cardiac monitor with pulse oximetry; note hypotension, tachycardia, extreme HTN
b. Intubation if severe bleeding and unable to protect airway or requires invasive procedure
c. Aggressive resuscitation

C. Control bleeding.
D. Sit upright.
E. Blow nose.
F. Rinse mouth with water.
G. Examine nasopharynx and oropharynx with headlamp and nasal speculum.
H. Pressure
1. Little's area
2. Pinch anterior nose for 10 minutes. Place thumb and index finger to nasal alar area and anterior septal area; sitting leaning forward, spit out blood.
3. If bleeding continues, suction or swab to find bleeding point

I. Local vasoconstrictors
   1. Afrin or Neo-Synephrine
   2. If possible, anesthetize area with cotton pledget soaked in 4% lidocaine with epi. Usually needs 5 to 10 minutes to get vasoconstriction
   3. Gelfoam or other thrombogenic agents
J. Cautery silver nitrate area—no more than 10 seconds
   1. Rolling motion peripherally to centrally, superior to inferior
   2. Only one side of septum–septal necrosis with septal collapse
   3. *Note:* Not to be used on cancerous lesions
K. Nasal packing
   1. Anterior nasal tampon
      a. Insert epistaxis balloon catheter or nasal tampon.
      b. Easier and less distressing to place
   2. Anterior nasal packing
      a. Wear PPE.
      b. Insert pledget with 4% lidocaine with epinephrine.
      c. Use 2 cm petroleum jelly gauze or calcium alginate 2 G pack.
      d. Insert successive layers horizontally along floor using Tilly's dressing forceps.
      e. Adult nose extends 6.5 to 7.5 cm to posterior choanae.
      f. Cephalexin, Augmentin, clindamycin, or trimethoprim/sulfamethoxazole (TMP/SMZ) for 5 days
      g. Refer to ENT for removal of packs within 48 hours.
   3. Severe posterior bleed
      a. Airway management fluid
      b. Fluid resuscitation/blood
      c. Difficult to visualize, noncompressible area; Woodruff's plexus
      d. Anterior and posterior nasal tampons
         i. Place double epistaxis balloon device with separate balloons.
         ii. Tape to cheek.
         iii. Urinary catheter if no nasal tampon available
            (1) Insert far back along floor of nose, inflate balloon, pull forward to occlude back of nose, tape to cheek
            (2) Insert anterior nasal packing as above.
         iv. May need both sides done to stop bleeding
      e. Emergent referral to ENT with admission
L. Pharmacologic therapies
   1. Follow evidence-based guidelines when prescribing.
   2. Lidocaine 4% with epinephrine
   3. Cephalexin, Augmentin, clindamycin, or TMP/SMZ for 5 days
M. Consultation and collaboration
   1. ENT

Patient Disposition

A. Based on bleeding control
B. Observation
   1. *Pressure:* Ensure no rebleeding.
      a. Discharge with nosebleed instructions, humidifier.
      b. Coat nares with petroleum jelly.
   2. *Anterior packing:* Ensure no rebleeding.
      a. Follow up with ENT after 2 to 3 days to have packing removed.
C. Admission or transfer
   1. Multiple recent bleeds, severe anemia, hepatic dysfunction, anticoagulation, and supratherapeutic; requires at least 24-hour observation
      a. Posterior bleeds in monitored setting
      b. Cephalexin, Augmentin, clindamycin, or trimethoprim/sulfamethoxazole for 5 days
D. Age and developmental considerations
   1. Prevention and education
   2. Patient and family education and counseling

Nasal Foreign Body

Medical Screening

A. *Chief complaint:* Foreign body (FB) in nose, nasal drainage, foul odor from nose
B. Signs and symptoms:
   1. Asymptomatic
   2. *Nasal drainage:* Serosanguinous or purulent, foul-smelling, unilateral discharge
   3. Nasal bleeding
   4. Often can be visualized
C. Medication history
   1. None
D. Past medical history (PMH)
   1. *Previous episodes:* Most often in children, witnessed or unwitnessed
E. Physical examination:
   1. *HEENT:* Nasal discharge, foul-smelling drainage, unilateral drainage, visualization of foreign body

Differential Diagnoses

A. Nasal FB
B. Sinusitis
C. Rhinitis

Diagnostic Testing

A. Fiberoptic evaluation may be necessary if in posterior or turbinate area.

Management

A. Gather supplies
   1. Gown, gloves, eye protection
   2. *Equipment:* Bright light, suction, nasal speculum, forceps
B. Sit upright.
C. Have patient aggressively blow nose.
   1. Have parent seal off opposite nares and blow nose.
   2. Have parent seal off opposite nares and have parent blow into mouth.
D. Attempt to suction out; cut tip to flat.
E. Attempt removal with a bent probe or alligator forceps if easily accessible in anterior nose
F. Pharmacological therapies
   1. Pharmacologic therapies should be based on evidence-based recommendations from recognized

sources: for example, the CDC, or guidelines specific to the environment where the clinician practices.

2. Saline drops post removal to moisten nasal passages if needed

3. If purulent drainage, consider course of antibiotics to treat purulent rhinitis or sinusitis.

G. Consultation and collaboration

1. ENT if unable to remove or posterior dislodgement with inhalation of foreign body is of danger

Patient Disposition

A. Discharge home majority of the time.

B. Admission or transfer if unable to remove foreign body during bedside procedure and surgical intervention needed for removal with anesthesia or sedation

C. Age and developmental considerations

1. Prevention and education

2. Patient and family education and counseling

Nasal Fracture

Medical Screening

A. *Chief complaint:* Nasal pain, epistaxis, nasal edema, nasal deformity, obstructed nares, nasal trauma

B. Signs and symptoms:

1. Edema, deformity, ecchymosis, epistaxis following a traumatic event (e.g., direct blow)

2. Difficulty breathing through nose (e.g., obstruction)

3. Pain

4. Crepitus with palpation

5. Septal hematoma (e.g., bulging blue mass, boggy to palpation); can lead to necrosis of nasal cartilage with septal collapse

C. *Medication history:* None

D. *Past medical history:* None

E. Physical examination

1. *Neurologic:* Altered mental status with head injury

2. *Respiratory:* Difficulty breathing

3. *Head, eyes, ears, nose, and throat (HEENT):* Pain, edema, deformity, ecchymosis, epistaxis, crepitus on palpation, septal hematoma, difficulty breathing through nose

Differential Diagnoses

A. Nasal bone or septum fracture

B. Other facial fractures

C. Epistaxis

D. Traumatic brain injury (TBI)

E. Cerebrospinal fluid (CSF) leak

F. Rhinitis

Diagnostic Testing

A. No need for imaging for suspected nasal fractures unless at risk for other injuries that may require imaging (e.g., CT maxillofacial, CT brain)

B. Beta 2 transferrin for CSF as indicated

Management

A. Gather supplies

1. Gown, gloves, eye protection

2. *Equipment:* Bright light, suction, nasal speculum

B. *Minimally displaced:* Pain control alone

C. *Severely displaced with minimal edema:* Immediate closed reduction with local anesthesia can be attempted

D. *Severely displaced with edema:* Refer to ENT or plastic surgery, likely in 5 to 7 days.

E. Control epistaxis.

F. Septal hematoma drainage in ED:

1. Septal necrosis of cartilage causing saddle nose deformity or abscess formation

2. Anesthetize nasal mucosa with topical medication.

3. No. 11 blade; excise inferior portion of hematoma.

4. Suction out clot.

5. Irrigate.

6. Pack nostril, anterior packing.

7. Follow up in 24 hours.

8. Broad-spectrum ATB

G. Pharmacologic therapies

1. Ice pack

2. Analgesia

3. Broad-spectrum antibiotics as needed

H. Consultation and collaboration

1. ENT referral in one week if patient requests operative management for deformity for cosmetic reasons

2. Emergent ENT referral for gross deformity, compound fracture, septal hematoma, laceration with exposed cartilage or bone

3. Emergent OMFS referral when associated with other serious fractures

Patient Disposition

A. Most can be discharged with ENT follow-up.

B. Admission

1. Failure to control epistaxis

2. Other injuries requiring hospitalization

3. CSF leak with deeper fractures (e.g., cribriform plate or ethmoidal fractures)

C. Age and developmental considerations

1. Prevention and education

2. Patient and family education and counseling

Sinusitis

Medical Screening

A. *Chief complaint:* Nasal pain, nasal congestion, nasal discharge, obstructed nares

B. Signs and symptoms:

1. Nasal congestion and obstruction

2. *Nasal discharge:* Green, yellow, white, clear

3. Postnasal drip

4. Altered sense of smell

5. Fever

6. Headache

7. Dental pain

8. Halitosis

9. Acute bacterial rhinosinusitis should be considered when there is no improvement

C. Medical history

1. Recent dental procedure

2. Scuba diver

3. Older diabetic
4. Severe immunosuppression
5. Recent intubation
6. *Primary ciliary dyskinesia:* Recurrent pneumonia; Kartagener syndrome
7. Prior sinus infections

D. Physical examination
1. Observe external surface of the nose.
2. *Observe deformities:* Deviation, obvious fractures
3. *Observe nasal airflow:* Ask patient to breathe in and out.
4. Inspect the nasal passages using a nasal speculum.
5. Inspect the mouth for dental problems or changes such as secondary teeth coming in.
6. Palpate nasal bones for tenderness and irregularity.
7. Palpate the infraorbital ridges.
8. Assess eye movement.

Differential Diagnoses

A. Viral or bacterial upper respiratory infection (URI)
B. Allergies (especially seasonal)
C. Chronic sinusitis
D. Structural deformities
E. Nasopharyngeal cancer
F. Migraine headaches
G. Dental abscesses

Diagnostic Tests

A. Clinical diagnostic criteria (PODS):
1. P: Facial PAIN and PRESSURE or fullness
2. O: Nasal OBSTRUCTION
3. D: Discharge: discolored postnasal, purulent drainage
4. S: SMELL disorder

B. *Laboratory tests:* Complete blood count (CBC), C-reactive protein (CRP)
C. Imaging:
1. CT may be considered for suspicion of a more severe complications related to sinusitis such as an orbital of intracranial infections
2. Radiograph of paranasal sinus
3. MRI may be considered.
4. Ultrasound to evaluate the presence of fluid and the fluid level

Management

A. Differentiate if it is acute or nonacute sinusitis.
B. Supportive treatment for nonacute sinusitis
C. Normal saline irrigation with addition of decongestants
D. Restrict use of nasal decongestant sprays to 3 days to prevent rebound effect. Break is recommended before starting again.
E. Humidification
F. Adequate hydration
G. Recurrent sinusitis should be referred for further evaluation of its cause.
H. *Pharmacological therapies:* Pharmacologic therapies should be based on evidenced-based recommendations from recognized sources, for example, the CDC, or guidelines specific to the environment where the clinician practices
I. Should only be prescribed for patients with clear clinical signs of an acute bacterial sinusitis
1. First line:
   a. Amoxicillin + clavulanic
   b. *PCN allergy:* Doxycycline
      i. Clindamycin + (cefixime or cefpodoxime)
2. Second line:
   a. Amoxicillin + clavulanic (high dose)
   b. Doxycycline
   c. Clindamycin + (cefixime or cefpodoxime)
   d. Levofloxacin or moxifloxacin
   e. *PCN allergy:* Doxycycline
      i. Clindamycin + (cefixime or cefpodoxime)
      ii. Levofloxacin or moxifloxacin
3. Intranasal steroids if not contraindicated by patient's medical problems

Consultation and Collaboration

A. Emergent ENT or Neurology consultation if there are indications of cellulitis or an intracranial infection
B. Referral to ENT for further evaluation when indicated

Patient Disposition

A. Most patients can be discharged from the ED.
B. Admission
   a. Acute infection with fever, headache not responding to initial treatment
   b. Imaging revealing orbital cellulitis or intracranial infection
   c. Patient unable to safely care for themselves

C. Age and developmental characteristics
D. Prevention and education
E. Patient and family education and counseling
F. Discharge care based on patient's age and ability

THROAT CONDITIONS

RENEÉ SEMONIN HOLLERAN

Epiglottitis

A. An inflammation or infection of the epiglottis, vallecula, arytenoids, and aryepiglottic folds
B. Commonly caused by *Haemophilus influenzae* type B, primarily in children and group A streptococci and *H. parainfluenzae* in adults.
C. Unrecognized and untreated epiglottitis can lead to critical airway obstruction and death.

Medical Screening

A. *Chief complaint:* Fever and severe sore throat
B. Signs and symptoms
1. Sudden onset of elevated temperature, severe sore throat, cough, muffled voice, shortness of breath, drooling, stridor, and assuming a posture to be able to breathe, barking cough
2. A tripod posture is more commonly seen in children.

C. *Medication history:* None

D. *Past medical history:* Recent exposure to an upper respiratory infection (URI) and immunization status
E. Physical assessment
  1. Inspect
    a. Level of consciousness
    b. Airway status
    c. Patient position
    d. Drooling
    e. Stridor
  2. Palpation
    a. Cervical lymphadenopathy
    b. Tenderness over the larynx

Differential Diagnosis

A. Acute tonsillitis
B. Peritonsillar abscess
C. Exudative pharyngitis
D. Retropharyngeal abscess
E. Ludwig's angina
F. Infectious mononucleosis
G. Salivary gland infections

Diagnostic Testing

A. Complete blood count (CBC)
B. Blood culture
C. Lateral soft tissue of neck
D. Direct fiber optic visualization in adults
E. Chest radiograph to rule out aspiration and for tube placement

Management

A. Collaboration with ear, nose, and throat (ENT) and ED physician. DO NOT ATTEMPT visualization without emergency equipment available.
B. Airway assessment management is the first priority; need to have skill with intubation and surgical airways
C. High flow oxygen with humidification
D. Antipyretics
E. Fluids for hydration

Patient Disposition

A. Prepare patient for admission or transfer to appropriate facility for care.

Laryngitis

A. Loss of voice generally caused by a viral infection.
B. Other causes may include overuse of one's voice, bacterial infections, inhalation of toxic substances, and allergies.

Medical Screening

A. *Chief complaint:* Sore or dry throat and loss of voice
B. *Signs and symptoms:* Fever and chills, dry throat, dry cough, and minor discomfort
C. *Medication history:* None
D. Past medical history
  1. Recent exposure to an upper respiratory infection (URI), allergies, recent excessive use of one's voice (e.g., attending a concert), and immunization status
E. Physical examination
  1. Inspect
    a. Dysphonia or aphonia
    b. Elevated temperature
    c. Reddened larynx and vocal cords
    d. Swelling of larynx and epiglottis
    e. Postnasal drip
    f. Rhinorrhea
  2. Palpation:
    a. Cervical lymphadenopathy

Differential Diagnoses

A. Acute tonsillitis
B. Peritonsillar abscess
C. Exudative pharyngitis
D. Retropharyngeal abscess
E. Ludwig's angina
F. Infectious mononucleosis
G. Salivary gland infections

Diagnostic Testing

A. Throat culture
B. Strep screen
C. CBC

Management

A. Gather appropriate equipment and supplies, including personal protective equipment (PPE).
B. Evaluation of throat for signs and symptoms of inflammation
C. Rule out more critical diseases.

Patient Disposition

A. Educate patient and family about signs and symptoms of airway obstruction, respiratory distress.
B. Provide patient with a referral for follow-up as needed.
C. Age and developmental considerations
D. Prevention education
E. Patient and family education and counseling

Pharyngitis

A. Pharyngitis is an inflammation of the throat.
B. Most often viral
C. It can be caused by bacterial or viral infections, which may result in peritonsillar and retropharyngeal abscesses.
D. The most common cause abscesses from bacterial infection is Group A beta hemolytic streptococcus (GABHS).

Medical Screening

A. *Chief complaint:* Sore throat, difficulty swallowing
B. *Signs and symptoms:* Difficulty swallowing, drooling, elevated temperature, fatigue, myalgia, arthralgia, swollen tonsils, exudate, halitosis, allergies
C. Centor criteria
  1. Fever greater than 38°C
  2. Tonsillar exudates
  3. Tender anterior cervical lymphadenopathy
  4. Absence of cough
D. *Medication history:* None
E. Past medical history

1. Previous throat infections, poor dental hygiene, lack of preventative vaccinations, exposure to upper airway infections

F. Physical examination
   1. Inspect
      a. Level of consciousness
      b. Status of the airway
      c. Position of patient to maintain an open airway
      d. Elevated temperature
      e. Inability to swallow
      f. Drooling
      g. Stridor
      h. Enlarged tonsils
      i. Halitosis
      j. Erythema
      k. Pharyngeal exudate
      l. Flushed face
      m. Uvula displacement
   2. Palpation
      a. *Enlarged, tender lymph nodes:* Anterior cervical, submandibular
      b. Neck masses
      c. Hot skin

Differential Diagnoses

A. Acute tonsillitis
B. Peritonsillar abscess
C. Exudative pharyngitis
D. Retropharyngeal abscess
E. Ludwig's angina
F. Infectious mononucleosis
G. Salivary gland infections
H. Kawasaki's disease

Diagnostic Testing

A. Rapid *Streptococcus* screen
B. Complete blood count (CBC)
C. Blood cultures
D. Lateral soft tissue neck radiographs
E. Neck CT without contrast
F. Chest radiograph to rule out aspiration

Management

A. Collaboration with ENT and ED physician
B. Airway assessment management is the first priority.
C. Needle aspiration of an abscess
D. Antibiotics when diagnosis indicates that treatment
E. Steroids
F. Antipyretics
G. Warm saline throat irrigations
H. Fluids for hydration
I. Soft foods

Patient Disposition

A. Educate patient and family for critical signs and symptoms and when to call 911 or return to the ED.
B. Provide patient with a referral for follow-up as needed.
C. Prevention for reinfection
D. Patient and family education and counseling
E. Age and developmental considerations

Throat Foreign Body

1. Foreign bodies that are commonly aspirated include hotdogs, peanuts, popcorn, grapes, seeds, other foods and liquids.

Medical Screening

A. *Chief complaint:* Pain, inability to cough or speak
B. *Signs and symptoms:* Vocal changes, coughing, drooling, difficulty talking, difficulty breathing, difficulty swallowing
C. *Medication history:* Large pills for specific medical problems
D. *Past medical history:* CVA, cancer of the throat, other neurological problems that interfere with swallowing
E. Physical examination
   1. Inspect
      a. Ability of patient to maintain their airway
      b. Level of consciousness
      c. Stridor
      d. Drooling
      e. Position of comfort
      f. Foreign body visible in the larynx
      g. Hemoptysis or hematemesis
   2. Auscultation
      a. Wheezes
      b. Decreased breath sounds

Differential Diagnosis

A. Acute tonsillitis
B. Peritonsillar abscess
C. Exudative pharyngitis
D. Retropharyngeal abscess
E. Ludwig's angina
F. Infectious mononucleosis
G. Salivary gland infections

Diagnostic Testing

A. Radiographs of the neck and chest (may need a CT if the substance is not radiopaque)

Management

A. Collaboration with ENT and ED physician
B. Airway assessment management is the first priority; need to have skill with intubation and surgical airways
C. Direct laryngoscope visualization
D. Bronchoscopy

Patient Disposition

A. Prepare patient for admission or transfer to appropriate facility for care.

References and Additional Reading

References and Additional Reading for this chapter are online only and can be found at https://connect.springerpub.com/content/reference-book/978-0-8261-6091-5/part/part02/toc-part/ch12.

13. The Neurologic Patient

NANCY DENKE

Learning Objectives

- Describe the components of a neurologic examination.
- Describe the common neurologic conditions seen in the ED.
- Explain the diagnostic and treatment considerations unique to emergencies involving diseases of the nervous system.
- List the differential diagnosis and diagnostic and therapeutic approach to common neurologic emergencies.
- Formulate a safe transition of care for the neurologic patient.

Neurologic emergencies may be complex and when encountered may cause anxiety in ED clinicians due to the time-sensitive nature of treating these emergencies. When dealing with neurologic emergencies, preservation of as much nervous system tissue as possible is key in reducing devastating long-term disabilities and death. The central nervous system (CNS) is very sensitive to hypoxia and alterations in cerebral blood flow, which destroys tissue that cannot be replaced, thus resulting in loss of function. A rapid and thorough examination exploring for subtle cues can assist in making an accurate diagnosis and providing successful treatment. To complete this examination, it must be divided into two components: the focused examination (chief complaint and history) and the screening element (acquisition of additional cues and neurologic deficits that are built upon your understanding of neuroanatomy).

Important questions to remember

- Is this a neurologic problem (yes/no)? If yes, you then need to decide if the problem is in the central or peripheral nervous system.
  - *Central (CNS):* Brain and/or spinal cord
  - *Peripheral (PNS):* Nerve, neuromuscular junction, or muscle
  - Pathology is usually one or the other, with rare incidence they affect both at the same time.
- As soon as the clinician enters the room, the neurologic exam is beginning. Does the conversation make sense? What does the patient's voice sound like? Do they have a hard time speaking? How do they look, and what do they sound like?
  - This assesses the cranial nerves, coordination, and mental status.
- The two most important components of a neurologic exam are the level of consciousness (LOC) and the reflexes.
- Right side of the brain controls the left side; at some point, everything crosses.
- One side should look like the other. Asymmetry is bad.
- Brainstem malfunction is contralateral. Cross brain findings are always bad (i.e., patient has right facial numbness and something wrong on the other side of the body).
- Psychogenic should never be your first diagnosis.
- Hyperreflexia always indicates some type of CNS problem.
- Spinal cord ends L_1–L_2: Belly button T_{10}; nipple line T_4.
- Spinal cord lesions are often higher than presumed so consider this when ordering radiologic exams.

General Approach to the Neurologic Patient

Medical Screening

A. Identify life-threatening conditions/changes that require intervention during airway, breathing, circulation, disability, exposure (ABCDE).

B. Hypotension and hypoxia are not well-tolerated by the central nervous system (CNS).

1. An increase in the intracranial pressure begins.

C. General questions to ask in the review of systems (ROS)

1. Any headaches
2. Fatigue
3. Fever
4. Blurred vision or double vision
5. Numbness or tingling of arms, face, legs
6. Tremors
7. Decrease in movement/strength of upper or lower extremities
8. Any involuntary movements
9. Changes in speech—garbled, slurred
10. Changes in behavior
11. Any seizure activity

D. History is key! Key elements include

1. Time of onset of changes
   a. Sudden
   b. Paroxysmal
   c. Slow over days/weeks
2. Last time seen normal/well symptoms
3. Medications
4. Prescription, over the counter, herbals, naturopathic
5. Recreational drugs and alcohol use
6. Any recent trauma—especially to the back or neck

General Physical Examination for all Neurologic Emergencies

A. *Mental status/level of consciousness (LOC)*: General state of awareness

1. Result of the integration of various neuronal structures, especially the reticular activating system (RAS)
2. Elements
   a. *Orientation:* "What kind of place is this?" "What is today's date?"
   b. *Memory:* Recall of information
   c. Speech and language (dysarthria or aphasia)
   d. Glasgow Coma Scale (Table 13.1).
3. *Other:* FOUR (Full Outline of UnResponsivenes) Score (Table 13.2) tool with intubated patients.

B. **Gross examination of cranial nerves I–XII** (Table 13.3 and Figure 13.1)

C. *Motor function and balance:* Tone, strength

1. Ask whether patient can stand from a chair alone and walk. Walking assesses multiple systems, almost every system has to work for them to walk down the hall.

TABLE 13.1 GLASGOW COMA SCALE FOR ALL AGE GROUPS

	4 YEARS TO ADULT	CHILD <4 YEARS	INFANT
Eye opening			
4	Spontaneous	Spontaneous	Spontaneous
3	To speech	To speech	To speech
2	To pain	To pain	To pain
1	No response	No response	No response
Verbal response			
5	Alert and oriented	Oriented, social, speaks, interacts	Coos, babbles
4	Disoriented conversation	Confused speech, disoriented, consolable, aware	Irritable cry
3	Speaking but nonsensical	Inappropriate words, inconsolable, unaware	Cries to pain
2	Moans or unintelligible sounds	Incomprehensible, agitated, restless, unaware	Moans to pain
1	No response	No response	No response
Motor response			
6	Follows commands	Normal, spontaneous movements	Normal, spontaneous movements
5	Localizes pain	Localizes pain	Withdraws to touch
4	Moves or withdraws to pain	Withdraws to pain	Withdraws to pain
3	Decorticate flexion	Decorticate flexion	Decorticate flexion
2	Decerebrate extension	Decerebrate extension	Decerebrate extension
1	No response	No response	No response
Total Score			
3–15			

Note: In intubated patients, the Glasgow Coma Scale verbal component is scored as a 1, and total score is marked with a "T"(or tube) denoting intubation (e.g., "8T").
Source: From Festerjian A. Seizures and status epilepticus in children. In: Cydulka RK, Fitch MT, Joing JA, Wang VJ, Cline DM, Ma OJ, eds. *Tintinalli's Emergency Medicine Manual*. 8th ed. McGraw-Hill; 2017:721–725.[1]

TABLE 13.2 SCORING CRITERIA FOR THE FOUR SCORE

EYE RESPONSE	MOTOR RESPONSE	BRAIN STEM REFLEXES	RESPIRATIONS
4: Eyelids open or open/track/blink to command	4: Thumbs-up, fist, or peace sign	4: Pupil and corneal reflexes are present	4: Nonintubated, regular breathing pattern
3: Eyelids open but do not track	3: Localizes to pain	3: One pupil fixed and dilated	3: Nonintubated, Cheyne–Stokes breathing pattern
2: Eyelids closed but open to loud noise or voice	2: Flexion response to pain	2: Pupil or corneal reflexes are absent	2: Nonintubated, irregular breathing pattern
1: Eyelids closed but open to pain	1: Extension response to pain	1: Pupil and corneal reflexes absent; cough present	1: Intubated, but initiates respirations over ventilator rate
0: Eyelids remain closed to pain	0: No response to pain or generalized myoclonus status	0: Absent pupil, corneal, and cough reflex	0: Breathes at ventilator rate or apneic

FOUR, full outline of unresponsiveness.
Source: From McLaughlin D. Neurologic examination of the comatose patient. In: McLaughlin D, ed. *Fast Facts About Neurocritical Care: A Quick Reference for the Advanced Practice Provider*. Springer Publishing Company; 2018. Table 3.2.)[2]

TABLE 13.3 CRANIAL NERVES

CRANIAL NERVE	MNEMONIC	SENSORY (S) MOTOR (M) BOTH (B) AND MNEMONIC
I Olfactory	On	S Some
II Optic	Old	S Say
III Oculomotor	Olympus	M Marry
IV Trochlear	Towering	M Money
V Trigeminal	Tops	B But
VI Abducens	A	M My
VII Facial	Finn	B Brother
VIII Vestibulococclear	And	S Says
IX Glossopharyngeal	German	B Both
X Vagus	Viewed	B Brains
XI Spinal accessory	Some	M Matter
XII Hypoglossal	Hops	M More

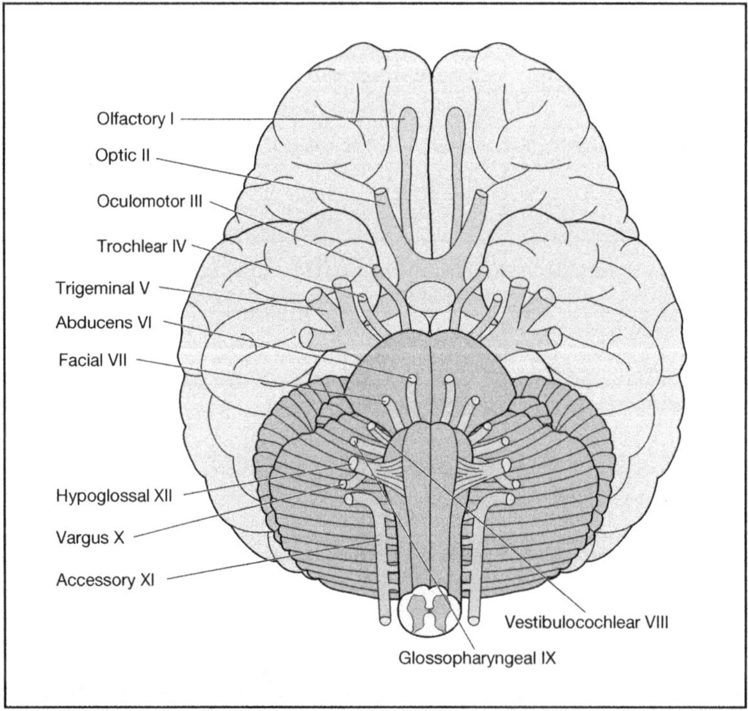

FIGURE 13.1 Location of cranial nerves.
Source: With permission from Armitage A. Advanced health assessment of the neurologic system. In: Myrick KM, Karosas LM, eds. *Advanced Health Assessment and Differential Diagnosis*. Springer Publishing Company; 2021. Figure 11.5.

a. As the patient walks, note hand tremors, spastic gait, foot drop.
b. Ask the patient to turn around. Patients with Parkinson's cannot turn well, and patients with multiple sclerosis (MS) have a hard time turning.
c. One foot in front of the other: assesses balance.

2. One extremity at a time—observe for:
   a. Spasticity, seen when the corticospinal tract is damaged.
   b. Rigidity (resistance to passive range of motion [ROM]) or flaccidity (decreased motor tone)
   c. Posturing (hyperflexion/hyperextension)

d. *Dystonia:* Distorted twisting of body part

D. *Coordination and gait (if able to walk):* Assesses fine and gross movements, balance

1. Perform rapid alternating movements
2. Finger to nose
3. *Heel to shin:* Heel just below the knee and slide down and up
4. *Romberg:* Stand 2 feet together, close eyes, arms either next to body or across chest, count seconds able to stand with eyes closed. Always stand close to the patient in case he/she falls.
5. Tremors and fasciculation

E. *Sensation:* Pain, touch, temperature, sense of position (proprioception), vibration

1. Work bottom-to-top and detect a sensory level.
   a. Sensory levels (numbness into the torso always indicates a spinal cord problem [CNS] problem)
   b. Highest sensory level is C2 at the top of the head.
   c. Observe dermatomes.
2. Check 2-point discrimination.

F. Reflexes (top to bottom)

1. Normal, hyporeflexia, hyperreflexia
2. Clonus suggests upper motor neuron injury
3. Primitive reflexes (moro, rooting, placing) in infants

G. Pupils (size, symmetry, and reaction), eye movements (side-side, up, and down), visual fields to confrontation,

1. Any nystagmus or gaze?

H. Meningeal signs:

1. *Nuchal rigidity:* Passively flex the patient's neck. This test is positive if there is palpable resistance
2. *Kernig's sign:* Position the patients supine with their hips flexed to 90°. This test is positive if the patient expressed pain on passive extension of the knee.
3. *Brudzinski's sign:* Position the patients supine and passively flex their neck. This test is positive if this maneuver causes reflex flexion of the patient's hip and knee.

General Tests for the Neurologic Patient in the ED or Acute Patient

A. Look for cortical symptoms that affect the part of the brain (brainstem, spinal cord, and cerebellum) that influence the patient's experience:

1. Can they understand and have meaningful language? (Aphasia)
2. Does the patient recognize their environment exists? (Neglect)
3. Can they see both halves of the world around them? (Visual field defect?)
4. Do they know how to use object? (Apraxia)

B. *Lab tests*

1. Point-of-care testing (POCT) glucose
2. Complete blood count (CBC) with differential
3. Complete metabolic panel (CMP)
4. Prothrombin time/international normalized ratio (PT/INR)
5. Sedimentation rate
6. Toxicology screen
7. Therapeutic drug levels
8. Urinalysis (UA)

C. X-ray

D. CT scan or MRI of the brain

Pediatric Stroke

Contrary to popular belief, strokes can, will, and do occur in children, infants, and unborn babies. Delays in the diagnosis of childhood stroke limit access to time-critical interventions that improve outcome in adults.[9] Pediatric strokes are classified in different ways when compared to the adult population: age is the major factor.

Anatomy

A. Similar to the adult; see Pathophysiology.

Pathophysiology[4]

A. Classified by age

1. *Perinatal:* 28 weeks gestation to 28 days postnatal
   a. Disruption of either arteries or veins from early gestation through the first month of life
   b. Infarcts in the middle cerebral artery (MCA) territory

B. *Childhood:* 28 days postnatal to 18 years

1. Mode of presentation
   a. Acute perinatal (newborns or close to birth)
      i. Presents with seizures (focal in nature) or encephalopathy
   b. Presumed perinatal (chronic infarcts) and have a delayed diagnosis
      i. There is a pathological early dominance of one hand or seizures. This leads to brain imaging and the diagnosis of a remote infarction.
2. *Classified as in adults:* Ischemic versus hemorrhagic

C. In childhood

1. Thromboembolic
   a. Thrombosis can form with ventricular assist devices, or extracorporeal membrane oxygenation
   b. Arrhythmia
      i. Patient foramen ovale (PFO) role unclear

D. Moyamoya arteriopathy is a syndrome that causes progressive stenosis of the carotid arteries with the formation of collateral vessels.

1. Posterior circulation infarct
   a. See in boys age 6 to 7 years who were otherwise healthy
   b. Common due to vertebral artery dissection

Predisposing Factors[4]

A. *Perinatal:* Can be both maternal or neonatal

1. Activation of coagulation factors in the mother is normal but are low in the infant just before and after delivery
2. Neonatal
   a. Inherited thrombophilia
   b. Cardiac lesions
   c. Infection
   d. Trauma
   e. Coagulopathies
   f. Asphyxia

g. Gene mutations
3. Maternal
a. History of infertility
b. Premature rupture of membranes
c. Preeclampsia
d. Vacuum extraction
e. Emergent C-section
f. Coagulation disorder
4. Childhood
1. *Cardiac:* Congenital disease

Physical Examination

A. Seizure may be a presenting sign.
B. Neurologic examination (as above)
1. Full examination not easy to complete
2. Focal deficits are more common in children with stroke than in adults.
3. Perinatal
a. Seizures
b. A tendency to use only one side of their body
4. Neonatal
a. Lethargy
b. Irritability
c. Seizures
5. *Childhood:* Similar to adults
a. Seizures (especially in <6 years of age)
C. Child with moyamoya
1. Multiple transient ischemic attacks (TIAs) or silent infarcts
2. Hemiparesis
3. Hemisensory deficits
4. Chronic headache (HA)

Differential Diagnoses

A. Mimics are similar to adults.

Diagnostic Testing

A. Routine thrombophilia testing is not required in the perinatal stroke population; this testing has limited clinical value.
B. MRI along with magnetic resonance angiography (MRA) and magnetic resonance venography (MRV; if considering venous thrombosis)
C. Hyperacute therapies of stroke (tissue plasminogen activator [tPA] and endovascular therapeutic procedures) in children with acute stroke are not yet clear and controversial but should be considered in the following cases:
1. Child with confirmed large vessel occlusion (LVO)
2. Pediatric National Institutes of Health NIH Stroke Scale (NIHSS) >6 (https://www.mdcalc.com/pediatric-nih-stroke-scale-nihss)
3. Consult neurology.
D. Transthoracic echocardiogram (TEE) for child with congenital heart disease
E. Labs (as above)

Management

A. There may be a delay in treatment due to delayed consideration of stroke and delay of MRI (most often requires sedation for procedure).
B. Pharmacologic therapies
1. Perinatal stroke
a. Control seizures.
b. Optimize oxygenation.
c. Correct dehydration by administration of IV fluids.
d. Correct anemia.
e. Antiplatelet therapy Is rarely indicated because of the low risk of reoccurrence of acute ischemic stroke (AIS).
f. Vitamin K should be routinely administered to newborns.
2. Childhood
a. Initiate IV fluids.
b. aspirin[5]
C. Blood glucose
1. Treat hyperglycemia and hypoglycemia.
2. Maintain at 140 to 180 mg/dL.
D. Treatment of hypertension is controversial.
1. Increased morbidity noted in first 3 to 4 days of stroke
2. Rivkin et al. (2016)[6]
3. The best approach to blood pressure (BP) management in children with acute stroke has yet to be defined.
a. Treat BP if:
i. Exceeds 15% above the 95th percentile for age for greater than an hour
ii. Anytime BP exceeds 20% above the 95th percentile[5]
E. Treat seizures
F. Thrombolytic agents[4]
1. There is no evidence for hyperacute stroke therapies (thrombolytic agents or embolectomy) for neonates.
2. Use of tPA in children remains limited.
a. IV–tPA may be appropriate in specific children. Consensus on potential eligibility criteria include[7]:
i. Two to 17 years of age
ii. Radiologically confirmed arterial stroke with absence of hemorrhage
iii. Pediatric stroke severity score >4 and <24
iv. Treatment can be administrated within 4.5 hours from known symptom onset
b. Alteplase is most commonly used in pediatrics due to its short half-life (3–5 minutes), and dosing for thrombolysis in children is not standardized.
G. Surgical decompression of space-occupying lesion (hematoma)
1. Rarely indicated in the neonate
2. Decompressive evacuation of a space-occupying lesion should be considered early to prevent herniation and brainstem compression.
H. Ventricular drains and then shunt often appropriate in the neonate and child. Hydrocephalus may result from brain damage caused by a stroke, which may require the use of ventricular drains and then a ventricular shunt in this population.

Patient Disposition

A. Admission to critical care unit with neurology consultation
B. Education

1. Improve stroke awareness and decision support tools to improve diagnosis for clinicians.

Stroke/Transient Ischemic Attack

There are several problems that will fall into this category and discussed in this section:

- Acute ischemic stroke (AIS)
- Acute thrombotic stroke
- Acute intracerebral hemorrhage—subarachnoid hemorrhage (SAH) or intracranial hemorrhage (ICH)

Introduction

Transient ischemic attacks (TIAs) occur in the United States at an approximate rate of 1.1 per 1000 U.S. population.[8]

Risks of adult stroke can usually be predicted based on a distinct set of risk factors. Most pediatric strokes are from some type of congenital anomaly or inborn error of metabolism. The penumbra (viable tissue surrounding ischemic tissue from a thrombus or emboli) has a limited lifespan when receiving limited blood flow. Unless it is reperfused early, damage can progress to an increased infarction size, an increase in irreversibly damaged brain tissue, and increased long-term disability. Thrombolysis and mechanical intra-arterial thrombectomy can reduce long-term disability in appropriately selected patients who have an AIS caused by an occlusion of a large cerebral vessel. Careful screening criteria must be in place to identify the patients to whom these therapies can be initiated to improve optimal treatment benefits.

Pathophysiology

A. Different types of strokes/TIA

1. Pathogenesis of strokes

a. Ischemic 83%

i. Thrombotic

ii. Embolic

iii. Lacunar

iv. Cryptogenic

b. Hemorrhagic 17%

i. Intracerebral (ICH)

ii. Subarachnoid (SAH)

2. TIA

a. Abrupt onset, temporary neurologic deficit with symptoms lasting less than 1 hour. Caused by focal brain, spinal cord, or retinal ischemia without acute infarction.[9]

b. Diagnosis of TIA is based on the patient's history with a rapid decline in symptoms.

3. Middle cerebral artery (MCA)

a. Largest vessel branching off the internal carotid artery (ICA)

b. Most common site for occlusion

c. Feeds a large territory of the brain (frontal, temporal, and parietal lobes along with the deep structures of the brain)

d. Effects of MCA stroke

i. Hemiplegia of contralateral side

ii. Contralateral sensory loss

iii. Contralateral homonymous hemianopia, visual field deficits

iv. Affects face and arm more than the leg but still can affect

e. Right versus left sided

i. If on the left side of the brain: see aphasia. Most people are left side brain dominant so if patient has right-sided weakness with aphasia, consider MCA stroke.

ii. When right hemisphere, the patient may show unilateral neglect. Neglect is often associated with right hemisphere strokes.

4. Cerebellar stroke

a. Anterior cerebral artery (ACA)

i. Branches off the ICA and supplies the anterior and medial portions of the frontal and parietal lobes

ii. Least commonly affected

iii. Look for contralateral leg weakness and sensory loss.

b. Posterior cerebral artery (PCA)

i. Comes off the basilar artery and feeds the medial occipital lobe and inferior and medial temporal lobes

ii. Vision is the primary function of the occipital lobe so visual defects commonly observed, mainly an inability to see out of one eye

iii. If large, it can cause contralateral hemiparesis and hemisensory loss

c. Cerebellar

i. Occur in the cerebellum

ii. Impairs balance and coordination, may also cause vertigo, headache, nystagmus, and slurred speech

d. Brain stem

i. Occurrence in the brain stem and can be devastating

ii. Complex and may be difficult to diagnose

iii. Patients are usually critically ill and may need to be intubated.

5. Lacunar

a. Occur in the deep penetrating small arteries

b. Affects the white matter, basal ganglia, or pons

6. Cryptogenic

a. An unexplained reason for a symptomatic stroke after "adequate" diagnostic evaluation

b. Can occur in about 25% of all strokes

7. Hemorrhagic stroke

a. Caused from bleeding into the subarachnoid space or brain parenchyma

b. The larger the lesion, the higher the mortality rate

c. Deep hemispheric lesions (e.g., brainstem or thalamus) have a poorer prognosis than subcortical or cerebellar hematomas

d. Subarachnoid (SAH)

i. Hemorrhage into the subarachnoid space

e. Intracerebral (ICH)

i. Hemorrhage into the basal ganglia (usually related to uncontrolled hypertension)

ii. Hemorrhage into the thalamus

iii. Hemorrhage into the cerebellum

Predisposing Risk Factors

A. All risk factors found for cardiac disease are the same for cerebrovascular disease.
B. Hypertension (HTN)
C. Diabetes mellitus (DM)
D. Cigarette smoking
E. Heart disease and carotid artery disease
F. Obesity
G. Age (>60) and gender (M>F)
H. Race and ethnicity
  1. African American, Native American, and Alaska Native have higher risk of ischemic stroke
  2. Asian Pacific and African Americans have higher risk of hemorrhagic stroke
I. Personal or family history
  1. Stroke or TIA
  2. Arteriovenous malformation (AVM) or cerebral aneurysms
J. Atrial fibrillation (AF)
K. Alcohol and illicit drug use (cocaine and methamphetamine increase risk of hemorrhagic stroke)
L. Hypercholesterolemia
M. Hypotension after a long surgery that can cause emboli to form

Physical Examination

A. Chief complaint
  1. Sudden onset of numbness, weakness, difficulty speaking, vision changes, or incoordination that are present, improving, or have resolved.
B. Signs and symptoms
  1. BEFAST mnemonic:
    a. *Balance:* Gait, balance issue
    b. *Eyes:* Nystagmus, diplopia
    c. *Face:* Symmetry, facial droop
    d. *Arms:* Any drift
    e. *Speech:* Slurred, aphasia
    f. *Time:*
C. Focused assessment
  1. National Institutes of Health Stroke Scale (NIHSS) is a systematic assessment tool that provides a quantitative measure of stroke-related neurologic deficit. This tool is a 15-item neurologic examination stroke scale used to evaluate the effect of acute cerebral infarction on the levels of consciousness, language, neglect, visual field loss, extraocular movement, motor strength, ataxia, dysarthria, and sensory loss.[16]
  2. Vision, aphasia, neglect (VAN) assessment tool can be utilized to assess for large vessel occlusion (LVO)[10]
  3. Thorough neurologic examination (see above)
  4. Ophthalmologic examination
    a. *Horner's Syndrome:* Ptosis, miosis, and anhidrosis of the affected side
  5. Thorough history, including risk factors
    a. Time of symptom onset (when last normal), duration, present or improving
    b. *History:* Coronary artery disease (CAD), coagulopathy, cardiac dysrhythmias, previous TIA/strokes

Differential Diagnoses

A. Acute ischemic/thrombotic stroke versus intracerebral hemorrhage (SAH or ICH)
B. Stroke mimics[11]
  1. *Seizures:* Todd's paralysis, postictal
  2. *Headache:* Migraine
  3. *Metabolic:* Hypoglycemia
  4. *Infection:* Encephalitis, sepsis
  5. *Space-occupying lesion:* Central nervous system (CNS) tumors, metastasis, SAH
  6. *Psychiatric/functional:* Conversion disorder
  7. *Cerebrovascular:* Vasculitis
  8. Syncope
  9. Toxin/ingestion
  10. *Neurodegenerative disorders:* Guillain-Barré, optic neuritis
  11. Peripheral neuropathy
  12. Bell's palsy

Diagnostic Testing

A. *Point of care testing (POCT) glucose:* Needs to be done prior to infusion of IV alteplase (tPA)
B. *CT brain:* Noncontrast (on arrival to facility)
C. *CT angiography (CTA):* For candidates for mechanical thrombectomy
D. CT perfusion study or MRI: Diffusion
  1. Acute stroke patients within 6 to 24 hours of last known normal or "wake-up stroke," who have evidence of an LVO in the anterior circulation.
  2. These studies will help determine whether the patient is a candidate for mechanical thrombectomy.
E. *EKG:* Look for new onset atrial fibrillation (AF).
F. Lab (see above)
G. Chest x-ray (CXR)

Management

A. Procedures
  1. Rapidly assess ABC and stabilize.
    a. Intubation as needed
  2. Placement of an arterial line for blood pressure (BP) monitoring in patients with a SAH/ICH or receiving tPA
  3. Anticipate potential for operating room (OR) admission with an ICH/SAH.
  4. RN dysphagia screen prior to any oral medications or liquids

Pharmacologic Therapies

A. Aspirin
  1. Recommended in acute stroke patients within 24 to 48 hours after stroke onset if no ICH[8]
  2. Hold for 24 hours if received tPA
B. Alteplase (tPA)
  1. IV tPA should be administered to all eligible acute stroke patients within 3 hours of last known normal and to a more selective group of eligible acute stroke patients (based on ECASS III exclusion criteria) within 4.5 hours of last known normal[8]
  2. Exclusion criteria for administering tPA[12]:
    a. Current ICH
    b. SAH

c. Active internal bleeding
d. Recent (within 3 months) intracranial or intraspinal surgery or serious head trauma
e. Presence of intracranial conditions that may increase the risk of bleeding (e.g., some neoplasms, arteriovenous malformations, or aneurysms)
f. Bleeding diathesis
g. Current severe uncontrolled hypertension (systolic >180 mmHg and diastolic >110 mmHg)
3. Recommended dose is 0.9 mg/kg (not to exceed 90 mg total dose)[12]
a. Ten percent of the total dose administered as an initial intravenous bolus over 1 minute
b. Remainder as an infusion over 60 minutes
c. Vital signs and neurologic assessment (NIHSS/Modified NIHSS Q 15 min for 1 hour)
d. Avoid any new punctures or insertion of urinary catheter
e. OK for patient to be taken to interventional radiology while on tPA

C. Tenecteplase (TNK)
1. Tenecteplase before thrombectomy was associated with a higher incidence of reperfusion and better functional outcome than alteplase among patients with ischemic stroke treated within 4.5 hours after symptom onset.[13]

D. BP control[8]
1. Patients with no ICH or SAH who are candidates to receive tPA will need to have systolic BP (SBP) <180 mmHg and diastolic BP (DBP) <110 mmHg prior to infusion of the medication. The following protocol should be used:
a. Nicardipine (Cardene®)
b. Labetalol
i. Monitor for large drop in BP. Only want to decrease by 15%. DO NOT DROP QUICKLY!
2. Patients with an ICH/SAH and SBP between 150 and 220 mm Hg and without contraindication to acute BP treatment, acute lowering of SBP to 140 mm Hg is safe with either of the above medications.
a. Cautiously lower BP to a mean arterial pressure (MAP) less than 130 mmHg, but avoid excessive hypotension.
3. Patients who are not candidates for thrombolysis and without a ICH/SAH who have SBP of less than 220 mmHg and DBP of less than 120 mm Hg in the absence of evidence of end-organ involvement, no intervention is indicated.
a. BP should be monitored (without acute intervention) and stroke symptoms and complications should be treated.

E. If patient is on anticoagulation and has a SAH/ICH, reversal should be initiated with selected medications.[14]
1. 4-factor prothrombin complex concentrate (4F-PCC)
2. Idarucizumab
3. Andexanet alfa
4. Ciraparantag
5. Fresh frozen plasma (FFP)
6. Vitamin K

F. Antileptics if seizure noted (seen with SAH predominately)

G. Consultation and collaboration
1. Neurologist
2. Endovascular neurosurgeon
3. Therapies: physical, occupational, and speech
4. Acute rehabilitation specialist (physiatrist)
5. Palliative care

Patient Disposition

A. Discharge instructions
1. If a mimic, patient may be discharged home.

B. Transition of care information
1. Admission for workup
a. Admit to ICU post tPA initiation or intracranial bleed (ICH); to a stroke unit for those that did not meet tPA criteria.
b. Continuous EKG monitoring for paroxysmal AF
c. Echocardiogram—to evaluate for patient foramen ovale (PFO)
d. MRI/MRA—to assess vessels for dissection or occlusion

C. Patient and family education and counseling
1. Signs and symptoms of stroke (remind them this is **SUDDEN** onset of symptoms)
2. When to call emergency medical services (EMS)

STRUCTURAL ABNORMALITIES

This section focuses on structural abnormalities that may be either acquired or genetic, addressing aneurysms, cerebral venous thrombosis, carotid/vertebral dissection, and space-occupying lesions.

Cerebral Aneurysm

An aneurysm is an abnormal dilatation of a cerebral artery that results from the weakening of the intima causing a "blister-like" bulge of the vessel wall.[15]

Anatomy

A. Usually found at the base of the brain
B. Thin-walled dilation due to weakening of the intima of the vessel wall

Pathophysiology

A. Aneurysm size and location play a substantial role in determining the risk of rupture.
B. Inflammation plays a critical role in aneurysm pathogenesis.

Predisposing Factors

A. Hypertension (HTN)
B. Smoking
C. Drug use (especially cocaine)
D. Heavy alcohol use
E. Congenital abnormalities
F. Trauma
G. Complications from an infectious process

H. Women >55 years of age
I. African American and Hispanic

Physical Examination

A. Most aneurysms are asymptomatic until they rupture, at which time, subarachnoid hemorrhage (SAH) results (worst headache [HA] of their life or thunderclap HA).
B. Symptoms before rupture or bleeding you may see:
  1. Oculomotor nerve (cranial nerve [CN] III) palsy
  2. Dilated pupil
  3. Possible ptosis
  4. Pain above or behind the eye
  5. Localized HA
  6. Deficits in extraocular movements (EOM)
    a. CN IV (trochlear) and VI (abducens) involvement.
    b. Small intermittent leakage of blood that may result in neck pain, headache, and nausea/vomiting
C. After rupture or bleeding
  1. Nuchal rigidity due to meningeal irritation
  2. CN II, IV, VI deficits
  3. Stroke-like symptoms
    a. Hemiparesis, hemiplegia, aphasia, or cognitive deficits
  4. Numbness of one side of the face
  5. Seizure
  6. HTN, bradycardia, and widening pulse pressure due to increase in intracranial pressure (ICP)
  7. Confusion or loss of consciousness.
D. Ophthalmologic examination may reveal unilateral or bilateral hemorrhages.

Differential Diagnoses

A. AIS
B. Cluster/migraine headache
C. Tumor
D. Meningitis

Diagnostic Testing

A. CT with CT angiogram (CTA)
  1. High sensitivity, specificity, and accuracy and just as good as digital subtraction arteriogram (DSA)
  2. CTA more specific
B. Magnetic resonance angiography (MRA)
C. Digital subtraction arteriogram (DSA)—The "gold standard" for aneurysm diagnosis
  1. Has high radiation risks

Management

A. Medical management
  1. Observation for incidental aneurysms smaller than 10 mm without a previous SAH
  2. **Anemia**
    a. Anemia after aneurysmal SAH is associated with poor long-term neurologic outcome and death.
    b. Transfusion of packed red blood cells (PRBC) is beneficial for patients who were not considerably anemic beforehand.
  3. Blood pressure (BP) management to control hypertension (see BP management with stroke above)
  4. No preventive treatment, but imaging follow-up is indicated in patients with aneurysms that are 3 mm or smaller.
B. Aneurysm surgical treatment is considered if one or more of the following circumstances is met[16,17]:
  1. Size is ≥5 mm.
  2. Location in the posterior circulation or anterior communicating artery (ACA)
  3. Patient has a prior history of cerebral aneurysm rupture.
  4. Aneurysm has an odd, nonsmooth morphology (described as "daughter domes").
  5. Aneurysm changes in shape or size between interval imaging.
C. Coexisting medical problems or factors that favor the need for surgery must be considered (e.g., HTN) to prevent the risk of bleeding.
D. Aneurysms located in the anterior cerebral artery and posterior circulation, including posterior communicating artery aneurysms, are more likely to be initially treated.
E. *Endovascular treatment:* Coiling
  1. Soft metallic coils are inserted within the lumen of the aneurysm with the goal of complete obliteration of the aneurysmal sac.
F. *Surgery:* Clipping[18]
  1. Choosing surgery for patients with an unruptured intracranial aneurysm involves weighing the risk of intracranial rupture against the risks associated with brain surgery.

Patient Disposition

A. Admission with neurosurgical consultation
B. Discuss smoking cessation.
C. Will need monitoring of growth of aneurysm along with BP control as an outpatient

Cervical (Carotid/Vertebral) Artery Dissection

Cervical artery dissection (CAD) refers to the dissection of both the carotid and vertebral arteries. It can occur when there is a tear in the intimal layer of either the carotid or vertebral artery that can then lead to the development of an intramural hematoma.[19]

Anatomy

A. Tear in the carotid or vertebral artery
  1. Dissection of the internal carotid artery can occur intracranially or extracranially.
  2. Tear in the tunica intima or directly within the tunica media
  3. Forms an aneurysm of the arterial wall

Pathophysiology

A. Tears due to
  1. Mechanical forces (e.g., trauma, blunt injury, and stretching)
  2. Underlying arteriopathies or connective tissue disorders
B. Either alone or in combination

Predisposing Factors

A. Chiropractic manipulation of the neck
B. Blunt trauma with hyperextension of the neck due to motor vehicle crash
C. Connective tissue disorders (Marfans or Ehlers-Danlos syndrome)

Physical Examination

A. Signs and symptoms
  1. Severe occipital headache
  2. Posterior nuchal rigidity
  3. Focal symptoms
  4. Ipsilateral numbness and pain of the face
  5. Contralateral loss of pain and temperature sensation in the trunk and limbs
  6. Vertigo
  7. Diplopia or Horner syndrome
  8. Disequilibrium

Differential Diagnoses

A. Migraine
B. Stroke

Diagnostic Testing

A. CT angiogram (CTA)
B. Magnetic resonance angiography (MRA)

Management

A. Antiplatelet therapy
  1. Aspirin
  2. Clopidogrel
  3. Combination of both
B. Anticoagulant
C. Stenting if antiplatelets or anticoagulation do not work

Patient Disposition

A. Admission with neurologic and/endovascular surgery consultation

Space-Occupying Lesion

A space-occupying cranial lesion is a brain (intracranial) tumor that has an abnormal amount of tissue where cells grow and multiply uncontrollably.[16] These lesions can be benign, primary, or metastatic in nature. A glioma is the most common form of metastatic intracranial lesions, with astrocytoma being the most common in this category.

Anatomy

A. Lesion in the extradural space (intracranial) or subdural space

Pathophysiology

A. A lesion that expands in volume to displace normal neural structures
B. Can lead to edema that causes an increase in intracranial pressure (ICP)
C. Mechanisms that lead to symptoms
  1. *Increased ICP:* mass effect and obstruction of cerebrospinal fluid (CSF)
  2. *Seizures:* An irritation of the cortex
  3. *Focal deficits:* Compression, invasion, and circulatory interruption
D. Many different type
  1. *Primary:* Cyst, benign tumor, congenital anomaly
  2. *Trauma:* Subdural, intracranial hemorrhage (ICH)
  3. Metastatic
  4. Parasitic
  5. *Vascular:* Arteriovenous malformation (AVM), aneurysm
  6. *Inflammatory:* Abscess

Predisposing Factors

A. Due to a malignancy elsewhere
B. Dental infection can place patient at risk for abscess.

Physical Examination

A. Signs and symptoms vary depending on the type, location, and growth of the tumor; most symptoms do not develop until the tumor is well advanced.
  1. Progressive focal neurologic deficit, usually motor
  2. Headache
  3. Seizures
  4. Personality changes
  5. Papilledema
  6. Increased ICP
  7. Fever, malaise

Differential Diagnoses

A. Migraine headache
B. Focal lesions that may cause multiple sclerosis

Diagnostic Testing

A. *Important:* Do not rush doing a lumbar puncture (LP) as this can cause a herniation.
B. MRI is the diagnostic test of choice.
C. CT scan can be a helpful screening tool with an atypical headache
D. Cerebral angiography to look at the vessels of the lesion
E. EEG to assess for seizure activity
F. Lab work
  1. Hepatic panel

Management

A. Corticosteroids to decrease vasogenic edema
  1. Dexamethasone (Decadron)
B. Osmotic therapy for rapid reduction of ICP in patients with severe cerebral edema
  1. Mannitol
  2. Hypertonic saline
C. Treat seizures
  1. Can be caused by tumor location, post-operatively and/or edema
  2. Consider use of Levetiracetam (Keppra)
D. May require Burr holes to decrease ICP

Patient Disposition

A. Admission with neurosurgical evaluation
B. Discuss with patient the possible need for surgical and radiation approaches.
C. Palliative care

BRAIN AND CRANIAL NERVE DISORDERS

Acoustic Neuroma/Vestibular Schwannoma (Cranial Nerve VIII)

An intracranial, extra-axial, noncancerous tumor that arises from the Schwann cell sheath involving either the vestibular or cochlear nerve. It is slow growing and displaces some of the structures surrounding this area.[20]

Anatomy

A. Intracranial benign tumor in the internal auditory canal

Pathophysiology

A. Slowly expanding benign tumor in the internal auditory canal, inside the cochlear that can expand to the brainstem

Physical Examination

A. Hearing examination: Positive Rhine and hearing loss
B. Nystagmus
C. Papillary edema
D. Diplopia with lateral gaze

Differential Diagnoses

A. Meningioma
B. Other cranial nerve (CN) disorders
C. Aneurysm

Diagnostic Testing

A. Audiometry and vestibular diagnostics
B. MRI

Management

A. Referral to a neurosurgeon for possible surgery
B. Consider admission and possible surgery if large tumor causing pain, balance issues, hearing loss.[21]

Patient Disposition

A. Home with serial observation by a neurosurgeon
B. Disequilibrium as a presenting symptom may be associated with subsequent tumor growth.

Altered Mental Status

Altered mental status (AMS) or altered levels of consciousness is among the most common and worrisome problems facing clinicians in the ED. The term *altered level of consciousness* (ALOC) describes various disorders including clouded consciousness, confusion, lethargy, stupor, or coma.[22] Patients with an AMS have a problem with the central nervous system (CNS) or, specifically, the brain. When examining these patients, consider the following questions: Can they be awoken? Can they speak? Can they follow a conversation, and are they making sense? Most patients that are altered cannot do these things.

This diagnosis can be difficult. It is essential to identify the underlying cause(s) and treat any emergent conditions. Morgenstern[23] uses this approach when assessing any patient presenting with an altered level of consciousness by asking himself these five questions for rapid medical stabilization:

1. What can kill my patient immediately?
2. What can kill my patient in the next few minutes?
3. What can kill my patient in 10 minutes?
4. What can kill my patient over the next few hours?
5. What am I missing?

AMS can also be confused with delirium and dementia. Each of these disorders is characterized by confusion, impaired memory and judgment, confusion, and some degrees of paranoia and hallucinations.[24] Delirium is an acute process due to an illness or drug toxicity and often reversible. Dementia is usually progressive and chronic but may have a sudden onset at times.

Six Pearls for "Found Down" Patients[25]

A. Do not assume it's (only) ethanol.
B. Thorough examination, full neurologic exam
C. Consider C-spine injury in unclear mechanism.
D. Aggressive airway management
E. Do not delay advanced neuroimaging (CT/ magnetic resonance angiography [MRA]).
F. Thorough approach to toxidromes (pupils, skin)

Anatomy

See specific disorder.

Pathophysiology

A. There are two processes that alter mental status:
  1. Conditions that widely and directly depress the function of the cerebral hemispheres, causing the entire brain to not function well, and may have some brainstem involvement affecting behavior.
  2. Abnormalities that depress or destroy the reticular activating system (RAS) near the central core of the gray matter (diencephalon, midbrain, pons), affects arousal
  3. Can be due to a supratentorial mass lesion (like a hemorrhagic stroke or a tumor with lots of edema); subtentorial mass or destructive lesion; or metabolic disorder

Predisposing Factors

See specific disease state.

Physical Examination

A. Obtain a history.
  1. Some things a clinician may want to know:
    a. Timing (i.e., last known well; hours/days)
    b. Other symptoms (e.g., stiff neck, fever, nausea/vomiting)
    c. Recent illness/hospitalizations/surgeries (may need to talk with other hospitals, nursing home, even pharmacy)
    d. New medications
    e. Living situation
    f. Psychiatric history

B. *Neurologic exam:* Consider sensation, tone, cranial nerves, spinal precautions
  1. *Papilledema:* Consider increased intracranial pressure (ICP)

C. Any odors? (e.g., alcohol, acetone)
D. Check skin for tract marks
E. Approach to the AMS patient along with the order of emergency in caring for this patient, following **SIMPLE**
  1. **S**tructural lesion (massive bleed into the brain)
  2. **I**nfection, inflammation
  3. **M**edication or metabolic
  4. **P**aroxysmal (seizure, migraine, or arrhythmia)
  5. **L**ate-onset decline (dementia)
  6. **E**arly-onset (muscular dystrophy)

Differential Diagnoses

A. Mnemonics to help to rule out causes:
B. **AEIOU Tips**[23]
  1. **A**lcohol, acidosis/anion gap, ammonia, arrhythmias
  2. **E**lectrolytes, endocrinopathies, encephalopathy
  3. **I**nsulin (glucose: hypo/hyper)
  4. **O**verdose (or withdrawal from drug), oxygen (hypoxia), opiates/benzos
  5. **U**remia
  6. **T**rauma (intracranial bleeds), temperature (hyper/hypo), thiamine (Wernicke's), tick-borne disease, toxins (lead, CO poisoning, think toxidromes)
  7. **I**nfection (sepsis, meningitis), ICP
  8. **P**sychiatric, poisonings, porphyria
  9. **S**eizure, stroke, syncope, shunt malfunction, space-occupying lesion, sepsis
C. Anion gap, consider **MUDPILES**[26]
  1. **M**ethanol
  2. **U**remia
  3. **D**KA
  4. **P**araldehyde
  5. **I**buprofen/inborn errors of metabolism/inhalants/iron overdose/ isoniazid,
  6. **L**actic acidosis
  7. **E**thanol/ethylene glycol
  8. **S**alicylates/solvents/starvation

Diagnostic Testing

A. Focal lesions cause focal symptoms, which helps define what diagnostics you will need.
B. Lab
  1. Alcohol level
  2. Therapeutic drug screen (acetaminophen or salicylate). After acetaminophen and salicylate add consider obtaining level of any medications that can cause AMS (i.e., lithium, carbamazepine)
  3. Lactate
  4. Urinalysis (UA)
  5. Blood, urine cultures
  6. Ammonia
  7. Thyroid function
  8. Arterial blood gas (ABG) that has an ionized Ca+
  9. Consider carbon monoxide level
  10. If in metabolic acidosis with an anion gap, consider an ethylene glycol and methanol level.
  11. Lumbar puncture (LP) as indicated
C. CXR
D. EKG, check for prolonged QTc.
E. EEG

Management

A. Supportive care
  1. Maximize oxygenation; intubation if indicated.
  2. IV hydration, isotonic crystalloids
  3. Replace electrolytes.
B. Consider sepsis workup.
C. Pharmacologic therapies[27]
  1. Antibiotics (broad spectrum) as indicated
  2. Antidotes per results of drug screen
  3. Fever/temperature control
  4. Benzodiazepine for seizure and agitation
  5. Antileptics to treat seizure—Keppra is the drug of choice
  6. Consider medications using the **DONT** mnemonic
    b **D**extrose
    c **O**xygen
    d **N**aloxone
    e **T**hiamine

Patient Disposition

A. Admission as indicated to ICU versus medical surgical unit
B. Consultation and collaboration
  1. Social worker to help with history and finding family, friends, etc.
  2. Neurology
  3. Trauma surgeon if trauma related
  4. Neurosurgeon if intracranial hemorrhage (ICH)
  5. Pediatric intensivist or neonatologist for pediatric patients
  6. Anesthesiologist
C. Disposition to detox if able
D. Prevention and education
  1. Drug education
  2. Dispose of unused medication
  3. Simulation-based education (SBE) as an interprofessional education

Bell's Palsy, Facial Nerve Paralysis (Cranial Nerve VII)

A temporary (sometimes permanent) paralysis of cranial nerve (CN) VII that directly affects the muscles of one side of the face, which control eye blinking and closure, and facial expressions. It affects men and women equally. It can occur at any age. Believed to be caused by a viral syndrome.[28]

Anatomy

A. See cranial nerves.

Pathophysiology

A. Viral infection that causes inflammation of CN VII

Predisposing Factors

A. Recent viral infection
B. Trauma
C. Sarcoidosis
D. Herpes simplex

Physical Examination

A. Signs and symptoms
  1. *Ptosis:* Poor eyelid closure
  2. *Facial droop:* Loss of nasolabial fold
  3. Drooping of one brow
  4. Earache
  5. Loss of taste only on one side or changes in taste
  6. Otalgia

B. Ocular exam

C. Otologic exam

Differential Diagnoses

1 Herpes zoster oticus (Ramsay Hunt syndrome)
2 Lyme disease
3 Ischemic stroke
4 Guillen-Barré
5 Acoustic neuroma
6 Otitis media
7 Tumor

Diagnostic Testing

A. MRI if ischemic stroke is being considered

Management

A. Corticosteroids

B. Consider antiviral—No significant benefit noted in the literature

Patient Disposition

A. *Home:* Patient recovery can be 2 weeks to 6 months; warn patient of a permanent facial droop

B. Protect the eye—eye may not completely close—good eye care

C. Follow up with primary care clinician

Dizziness/Vertigo

Distinguishing vertigo from true dizziness can be a challenge. Developing a standardized approach to evaluating dizziness can be helpful and improve outcomes for patients. Dizziness is a nonspecific term that means different things to different people. When people say they are feeling dizzy, it usually means that they have a feeling of being in motion without actually being in motion, like when you get off a boat and still feel like you are on the water.

Vertigo results from a mismatch of the perception of movement by the visual, vestibular, and proprioceptive symptoms.[30] It has a central component to it. It can be differentiated from other forms of dizziness by it being described as a "sense of motion," either subjective (patient is moving) or objective (the room is moving). Once you have decided it is vertigo, you will need to separate peripheral from central vertigo (Table 13.4 and Figure 13.2).

Vertigo and dizziness are not always benign—particularly in the elderly. The ability to perform daily activities can be severely hampered by dizziness or unsteady gait—therefore making the patient more at risk for falls.

Anatomy

A. Vestibular organs include the semicircular canal and cilia.

B. Vestibular organs are a complex set of structures and neural pathways contributing to our sense of proprioception and equilibrium.

C. Otoliths are found in the inner ear and monitor the straight motion of the head and neck.

Pathophysiology

A. Dysfunction of the vestibular system can cause vertigo, nausea, vomiting, visual disturbance, and hearing changes.

B. Can be defined as peripheral or central
  1. Peripheral vertigo is more common than central vertigo.

Predisposing Factors

A. Age >50

B. Female > male (more common in females than males?)

C. Medications—antipsychotics and antidepressants

D. Previous history of vertigo

Physical Examination

A. Signs and symptoms
  1. Nystagmus, an unreliable sign
  2. Gait instability or imbalance
  3. Vertigo, "the room is spinning"[29]

TABLE 13.4 DIFFERENTIATING PERIPHERAL AND CENTRAL VERTIGO

	PERIPHERAL	CENTRAL
Onset	Sudden	Sudden or slow
Severity of vertigo	Intense spinning	Ill defined, less intense
Pattern	Paroxysmal, intermittent	Constant
Aggravated by position/movement	Yes	Variable
Associated nausea/diaphoresis	Frequent	Variable
Nystagmus	Rotary-vertical, horizontal	Vertical
Fatigue of symptoms/signs	Yes	No
Hearing loss/tinnitus	May occur	Does not occur
Abnormal tympanic membrane	May occur	Does not occur
Central nervous system symptoms/signs	Absent	Usually present

Source: From Go S. Vertigo and dizziness. In: Cydulka RK, Fitch MT, Joing JA, Wang VJ, Cline DM, Ma OJ, eds. *Tintinalli's Emergency Medicine Manual*. 8th ed. McGraw-Hill; 2018:784–791.[29]

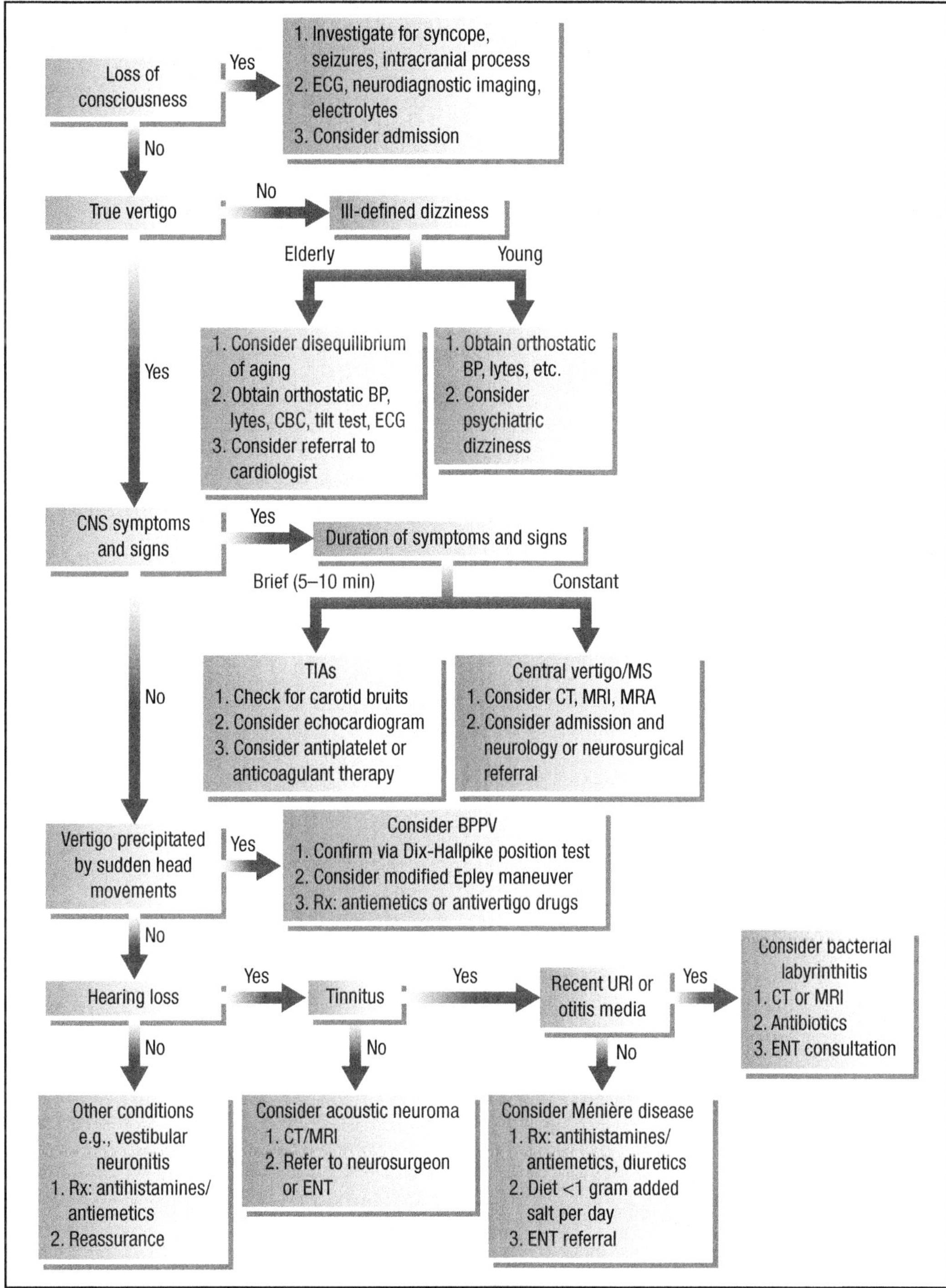

FIGURE 13.2 Assessment algorithm for vertigo and dizziness
Source: From Go S. Vertigo and dizziness. In: Cydulka RK, Fitch MT, Joing JA, Wang VJ, Cline DM, Ma OJ, eds. *Tintinalli's Emergency Medicine Manual*. 8th ed. McGraw-Hill; 2018:784–791.[29]

Focused Assessment

A. Neurologic exam
   1. Any neurologic or auditory disturbance
B. History[30]
   1. Subjective characteristics—which sensation is present
      a. Rotational
      b. Problems with standing and walking
   2. Accompanying symptoms
      a. Tinnitus
      b. Hearing loss
      c. Headache
      d. Visual impairment
   3. Provocation of symptoms
   4. Impact on activities of daily living (ADLs)

Differential Diagnoses

A. Benign paroxysmal positional vertigo (BPPV)
  1. Tiny crystals in the otolith get dislodged and jump around in the semicircular canals
  2. Lasts for seconds to minutes
  3. Dix-Hallpike test associated with reproduction of vertigo and nystagmus
B. Meniere's disease
  1. Can last for hours and can cause symptoms of hearing loss and tinnitus
C. Viral labyrinthitis
  1. Inflammation of the vestibular nerve, secondary to a viral infection
  2. Simultaneous loss of hearing and balance function
D. Medication side effects, ototoxicity
E. Orthostatic hypotension
F. Eighth cranial nerve tumor or brain stem lesion
G. Vertebrobasilar insufficiency (VBI)
H. Vertebral artery dissection
  1. *Presyncope:* Lightheadedness, a sense of impending loss of consciousness
  2. Can be due to hypoperfusion of the brain or some type of metabolic disorder
I. Multiple sclerosis (MS)

Diagnostic Testing

A. Diagnostic evaluations can be inconsistent and should be based on clinical suspicion for the abnormalities.
B. The **STANDING** algorithm can significantly reduce unnecessary neuroimaging[31]
  1. Assessment of the presence and of type of nystagmus (**S**pon**TA**neous, positional, absent)
  2. Assessment of nystagmus direction (**N**ystagmus **D**irection).
  3. Head **I**mpulse test (HIT).
  4. Evaluation of the standing position and gait (sta**N**din**G**).
C. CT does not provide important information; MRI provides more information
D. Dix-Hallpike test, positive in BPPV
E. Epley maneuver, treatment for BPPV

Management[29]

A. IV crystalloids as indicated
B. Pharmacologic
  1. Meclizine
  2. Scopolamine, transdermal—More useful at discharge since it takes about 4 to 8 hours for onset of action
  3. Anxiolytics, benzodiazepines should be used sparingly.
  4. Alpha/beta adrenergic agonists
C. Low salt diet with Meniere's
D. Consultation with
  1. Neurologist
  2. Cardiologist
  3. Physical and occupational therapy

Patient Disposition

A. Discharge instructions
  1. If diagnosed with Meniere's, look at salt restrictions and diuretics.
  2. Patients with peripheral vertigo can be discharged home.
B. Admission as indicated
C. Prevention and education
  1. With BPPV
    a. Avoid sudden jerky head movements and body position changes.
    b. Avoid sleeping on the "bad" side.
    c. Get up slowly and sit on the bed for a minute before getting out of the bed.
    d. Avoid bending down and extending the head.
    e. Avoid driving, working at heights, or with machinery during acute attack.
    f. Home Epley maneuver

Syncope/Near Syncope

Syncope may be due to a decrease in cardiac output, hypovolemia, or a failure of vasomotor tone. Older adult patients' underlying etiology is often challenging to discern.

Anatomy

A. Alterations in blood flow
B. Causes can be
  1. Reflex/neural
    a. Vasovagal
    b. Situational (e.g., coughing and sneezing, micturition, postexercise)
  2. Orthostatic hypotension
    a. Drug induced
    b. Volume depletion
    c. Primary autonomic failure (e.g., Parkinson's, dementia)
    d. Secondary autonomic failure (e.g., diabetes, spinal cord injury)
  3. Cardiac
    a. Brady- or tachycardia
    b. Structural cardiac disease
    c. Pulmonary edema
    d. Cardiomyopathy
    e. Cardiac tamponade
    f. Prosthetic valve disorder

Pathophysiology

A. Table 13.5 summarizes the etiology of syncope.

Predisposing Factors

A. Characteristic of syncope
  1. Occurs during exertion, when supine
  2. Occurs with palpitations
B. Family history
C. History of congestive heart failure (CHF), aortic stenosis, dilated cardiomyopathy
D. Symptoms, signs associated with the syncopal episode
  1. Anemia
  2. Sinus bradycardia
E. History of pulmonary hypertension
F. Prolonged QTc >450

TABLE 13.5 ETIOLOGY OF SYNCOPE

CLASSIFICATION	DEFINITION	CAUSES
Neurocardiogenic	Inappropriate vasodilation ± bradycardia	Increases vagal tone (micturation, defecation); situational (prolonged standing); vagal nerve stimulation (shaving)
Orthostatic	Documented postural hypotension with symptoms	Drop in systolic blood pressure by ≥20 mmHg or tachycardia >20 bpm; example: volume loss, dysfunction of autonomic nervous system, medication side effects
Neurologic	Least common, must return to baseline with no neurologic deficits	Example: transient ischemic attack's, seizure, complex migraine, subclavian steal
Cardiac	Most dangerous form, can be life-threatening, multiple etiologies	Arrhythmias (tachy- or bradycardia), valvular heart disease, myocardial infarction, cardiac tamponade
Unknown	Unexplained despite thorough work-up	Rule out potential life-threatening causes

Source: From Patel PR, Quinn JV. Syncope: A review of emergency department management and disposition. *Clin Exp Emerg Med.* 2015;2(2):67–74, Table 1)[32]

Physical Examination

A. Signs and symptoms
  1. Chest pain/pleuritic chest pain
  2. Abdominal pain
  3. Dyspnea
  4. Syncope on exertion, cardiac in origin
  5. Nausea and vomiting
  6. Prolonged standing or crowded, hot places
  7. Palpitations, cardiac in origin
  8. Syncope with turning head, or while having a bowel movement
B. Focused assessment
  1. Orthostatic blood pressure (BP), supine and standing
  2. Family history of syncope or sudden cardiac death, consider Brugada syndrome

Differential Diagnoses

A. Seizure
B. Stroke
C. Hypoglycemia
D. Subdural/epidural/subarachnoid hemorrhage
E. Hyperventilation
F. Toxins (e.g., drugs/alcohol/environmental)
G. Psychiatric condition
H. Thoracic aortic aneurysm and dissection
I. Pulmonary embolism (PE)
J. Gastrointestinal (GI) bleed
K. Medications

Diagnostic Testing

A. Risk stratification is an important part of decision-making.
B. Diagnostics
  1. EKG to look for dysrhythmias
    a. Presence of arrhythmias associated with cardiac origin
  2. Lab
    a. Cardiac biomarkers
  3. CXR
  4. CT angiogram (CTA) thorax to rule out aneurysm or PE

Management

A. IV isotonic crystalloids (lactated Ringer [LR], normal saline [NS]) as indicated
B. Pharmacologic therapies
  1. Treat arrhythmias as indicated.
C. Consultation and collaboration
  1. Cardiology

Patient Disposition

A. Transition of care
  1. Admission of high-risk patients
B. Discharge instructions
  1. Low-risk patients will not need to be admitted.
  2. Driving and working following syncope must be addressed prior to discharge.
  3. Provide clear direction on when and with whom to follow up.
C. Prevention and education
  1. Ambulatory monitoring device
    a. Holter/event monitor may be applied to low-risk individuals with close follow-up with cardiology.

Age and Developmental Considerations

A. With advancing age, cardiovascular morbidity plays a more frequent and important role in the etiology of syncope.[33]
B. Pediatric syncope is usually benign; approach to diagnosis similar to the adult. Breath holding is common.
C. Geriatric syncope has a higher incidence of cardiovascular causes and other comorbidities, and orthostatic hypotension

Trigeminal Neuralgia (Cranial Nerve V)

Trigeminal neuralgia (TN) is a disorder in which sudden, unilateral, sharp, and severe facial pain is experienced, often in short attacks.[34]

Anatomy

A. Affects the fifth cranial nerve
B. Has three branches that converge on the trigeminal ganglion, which then enters the brainstem at the pons
  1. Ophthalmic nerve (V1)
  2. Maxillary nerve (V2)
  3. Mandibular nerve (V3)

Pathophysiology

A. The function of the fifth cranial nerve is to carry information from the face to the brain related to temperature, light touch, and the motor function of chewing.

Predisposing Factors

A. Injury to the nerve itself
B. Multiple sclerosis (MS)
C. Charcot–Marie–Tooth disease
D. Age—peak onset is between 50 and 60 years of age
E. Hypertension (HTN, especially noted in women)
F. Tumors
G. Stroke

Physical Examination

A. Excruciating paroxysmal pain (sharp in nature—"feels like an electric shock") to the face lasting about 2 minutes
B. Triggers
  1. Eating/drinking
  2. Shaving
  3. Any touching of face
  4. Smiling

Differential Diagnoses

A. TN is essentially a clinical diagnosis based on its characteristic presentation.
B. Paroxysmal attacks of pain lasting from a fraction of a second to 2 minutes, affecting one or more divisions of the trigeminal nerve and fulfilling criteria 1 and 2 below[34]:
  1. Pain has at least one of the following characteristics:
    a. Intense, sharp, superficial, or stabbing
    b. Precipitated from trigger areas or by trigger factors
  2. There is no clinically evident neurologic deficit.
  3. Not attributed to another disorder
C. Headache
D. Dental issues/pain
E. Sinus infection

Diagnostics

A. MRI
B. CT angiogram (CTA)
C. Laboratory work that can identify other causes (Lyme serology)

Management

A. Pharmacological
  1 Anticonvulsants are used to decrease hyperactivity of the nerve. Consider carbamazepine, gabapentin, oxcarbazepine, lamotrigine.
  2 Antispasmodics, consider baclofen.
B. Surgical
C. Local block by anesthesia

Patient Disposition

A. Referral to neurology
B. Referral to surgeon
C. May need admission for pain control

The Pediatric Patient

Signs and Symptoms

A. In young children, altered level of consciousness (ALOC) may manifest as fussiness or irritability.
B. Many of the signs and symptoms, along with the approach to the pediatric patient, are similar to the adult.
C. *Papilledema:* Consider increased intracranial pressure (ICP) as in an adult.
D. *Retinal hemorrhages:* Think of possible nonaccidental trauma ("shaken baby")
E. *Cheyne:* Stokes respirations is an ominous finding, indicating damage to the brain stem. Consider Cushing's triad.
F. "Neurocutaneous stigmata can be associated with certain genetic conditions that predispose individuals to epilepsy (e.g., neurofibromatosis or tuberous sclerosis;" p. 14).[22]

Differential Diagnoses Mnemonic[22]

A. This mnemonic may be used for pediatrics and adults: **MOVESTUPID**
  1. **M**etabolic
  2. **O**xygen insufficiency, carbon monoxide
  3. **V**ascular/cardiac
  4. **E**ndocrine/electrolytes
  5. **S**eizures/sepsis
  6. **T**rauma, toxin, tumor
  7. **U**remia, renal or liver failure
  8. **P**sychiatric/porphyria
  9. **I**nfection/intussusception
  10. **D**rugs, drama

Management in Pediatric Population

A. Seizure
  1. Lorazepam (maximum 4 mg)[22]
  2. Fosphenytoin (Cerebyx®) or intravenous (IV) levetiracetam (Keppra®).[22]
B. DKA
  3. Aggressive IV fluids resuscitation
  4. Early insulin administration
  5. Interventions to improve cerebral edema[22]
  6. Mannitol
  7. Three percent hypertonic saline
C. Hyperglycemic hyperosmolar syndrome (HHS)[22]
  1. Fluid resuscitation, more aggressive and longer and, in contrast to diabetic ketoacidosis (DKA) management
  2. Early insulin administration is unnecessary.
D. Inborn errors of metabolism (IEM)
  1. Ten percent dextrose fluid started empirically to reverse the patient's catabolic state[22]
  2. Keep NPO, no sugars or proteins!
  3. In hyperammonemia crises[22]
    a. Sodium phenylacetate or sodium benzoate
    b. Arginine hydrochloride (10%) is also given in combination with sodium phenylacetate and sodium benzoate

Headache

Headache (HA) is one the most common neurologic complaint presenting to the ED. Goal is to determine if this is an emergency/life-threatening HA or nonemergent and identify the cause. Familiarity with "red flags" is critical to differentiating potentially dangerous, life-/organ-threatening HAs from benign, low-risk HAs. Therefore, it's important to have a systematic approach to evaluating HAs

Difference Between Primary and Secondary HA[35]

A. Primary HA

1. HA not caused by or attributed to another underlying condition or disorder.

B. Secondary HA

1. HA caused by or attributed to another underlying disorder.

Anatomy

A. HAs have different anatomical triggers.
B. The brain cannot generate pain; it comes from a source outside the brain.
C. Migraines tend to occur when the cerebral arteries cause inflammation of the adjacent nerves. These nerve endings are transmitted to the trigeminal ganglion causing the pain.
D. C1, C2, C3 nerve roots irritated
E. Inflammation of the meninges
F. Neck muscle inflammation

Pathophysiology

A. Hypothalamic activation is part of the prodromal phase of HA[36]
B. Potential role of circadian dysregulation in the hypothalamus

Predisposing Factors

Many depend on the type of HA, but may include

A. Stress
B. Anxiety
C. Depression
D. Clenching/grinding teeth
E. Trauma
F. Arthritis in neck
G. Not enough sleep
H. Smoking
I. Hypertension (HTN)
J. Medications

Physical Examination

A. Signs and symptoms

1. Migraine aura is a focal neurologic disturbance that manifests in visual, sensory, or motor symptoms
2. Clinical features of dangerous HA[37]
   - **a.** Subarachnoid hemorrhage (SAH): Use the Ottawa SAH Rule[36](Box 13.1)
     - **i.** "Thunderclap HA"
     - **ii.** Severe/sudden, that is, "worst HA of your life"
     - **iii.** Unable to flex neck
     - **iv.** May have a loss of consciousness, vomiting, seizures, or meningeal irritation
   - **b.** Central nervous system (CNS) infection
     - **i.** Fever
     - **ii.** Meningeal irritation
     - **iii.** Gradual onset—moderate
     - **iv.** Altered mental status (AMS)
     - **v.** Seizures
     - **vi.** Rash
     - **vii.** Photophobia
     - **viii.** Cognitive deficits
     - **ix.** Kernig, Brudzinski sign
   - **c.** Carbon monoxide (CO) poisoning
     - **i.** Waxing and waning HA, cluster of cases
     - **ii.** Dizziness
     - **iii.** Fatigue
     - **iv.** Weakness
     - **v.** Nausea/vomiting (N/V)
     - **vi.** Confusion
     - **vii.** Seizure
   - **d.** Temporal arteritis
     - **i.** *Criteria:* Three of the five that follow
       - **(1)** Age >50 years
       - **(2)** new onset of headache
       - **(3)** tenderness to palpation, decreased pulsation temporal arter tenderness to palpation, decreased pulsation temporal arter
       - **(4)** (ESR) >50 mm/h
       - **(5)** abnormal temporal artery biopsy
     - **ii.** Unilateral frontotemporal HA severe/throbbing
     - **iii.** HA when patient brushes their hair/scalp tenderness
     - **iv.** Jaw claudication
     - **v.** Vision changes/loss of vision
     - **vi.** Polymyalgia rheumatic
   - **e.** Increased intracranial pressure (ICP)
     - **i.** Vision changes

BOX 13.1 OTTAWA SUBARACHNOID HEMORRHAGE (SAH) RULE

To be use on alert >15 year-old-patient, with no new neurologic deficits, previous aneurysm, SAH, tumors, or hx of recurrent HA (≥3 episodes in ≥6 months)
Investigate if ≥1 high-risk variable present:
Age ≥40 years of age
Neck pain or stiffness
Witnessed LOC
Onset during exertion
Thunderclap HA (instantly peaking pain)
Limited neck flexion on examination

HA, headache; LOC, loss of consciousness, SAH, subarachnoid hemorrhage

Source: With permission from Godwin SA, Cherkas DS, Panagos PD, Shih RD, Byyny R, Wolf SJ. Clinical policy: Critical issues in the evaluation and management of adult patients presenting to the ED with acute headache. Ann Emerg Med. 2019;74(4):e41–e74.[38]

f. Cerebral venous thrombosis
   i. HA similar to SAH
   ii. Blurred vision
   iii. Signs of increased ICP
   iv. Optic disc edema
   v. Nausea or vomiting
g. Cervicocranial artery dissection[38]
   i. Classic triad for carotid
      (1) Headache
      (2) Horner's syndrome, usually partial ptosis, meiosis without anhidrosis
      (3) Cerebral ischemia, or transient ischemic attacks (TIAs)
   ii. Carotid you will see cranial nerve palsies
      (1) III: Diplopia
      (2) V: Facial numbness
      (3) VII: Facial paresis,
      (4) XII: Tongue deviation
   iii. Vertebral arterial dissection
      (1) Occipital HA and symptoms suggestive of brain stem or posterior circulation infarction[39]
h. Acute angle closure glaucoma
   i. Sudden severe pain
   ii. Unilateral vision change, eye pain, and redness (more prominent adjacent to limbus)
   iii. Globe is hard
   iv. Unreactive to light
   v. Hazy cornea, dilated pupil
   vi. Tonometry >20 mmHg
i. HA with a seizure
j. Altered level of consciousness

3. Nondangerous signs and symptoms
   a. Cluster
      i. Severe, frequent HA
      ii. Parasympathetic autonomic features including
         (1) Injected sclera
         (2) Lacrimation
         (3) Rhinorrhea
         (4) Facial sweating
         (5) Eyelid swelling
      iii. Unable to lie down and characteristically pace the floor
   b. Tension HA
      i. Bandlike, bilateral
      ii. Nonpulsatile
   c. Migraine
      i. Gradual onset lasting 4 to 72 hours[40]
      ii. Diagnosis of exclusion
   d. Preeclampsia HA
      i. HTN
      ii. Proteinuria
      iii. Nondependent edema
      iv. Pregnancy
   e. Unilateral pain/HA, consider tumor or space-occupying lesion
      i. Progressively worse over time
      ii. Worse in the morning or head-down position
   f. Overuse medication HA
      i. Seen with chronic use (usually months) of over-the-counter (OTC) or prescription headache relievers, such as NSAIDs, narcotics, or triptans
      ii. Symptoms vary with migraine or cluster HA like symptoms

B. Focused assessment
   1. *Mnemonic for secondary cause of a HA:* SNOOP[37]
   a. **S**ystemic (fever, weight loss, other body/muscle pain)
   b. **N**eurologic (any focal signs)
   c. **O**nset
   d. **O**lder age (usually the first onset of a HA in someone older than 40 needs a workup)
   e. **P**attern (any change in frequency or severity)
   2. History of hypercoagulable state, consider clot seen in cerebral venous thrombosis or even dissection.
   3. Headache history
      a. Quality
      b. Onset
      c. Provocation
      d. Radiation
      e. Severity
      f. Temporal
      g. Associated symptoms
   4. Ophthalmologic exam
      a. Visual acuity
      b. Tonometry for intraocular pressure
      c. Fundoscopic exam for papilledema
   5. Head and neck examination
   6. History of HIV or immunocompromised
   7. History of trauma, especially in sentinel headache (SH) and SAH
   8. Alcohol and drug use, consider subdural hematoma (SDH) or SAH
   9. Smoking history
   10. Depression or anxiety
   11. Medication history
      a. Consider SAH or SDH if on anticoagulants.
      b. If patient on antihypertensive, consider stroke.

Differential Diagnoses

A. Emergent
   1. Subarachnoid (SAH) or intracerebral hemorrhage (ICH)
   2. CNS infection: Meningitis, encephalitis, brain abscess
   3. CO poisoning
   4. Temporal arteritis
   5. Increased ICP: Mass, idiopathic intracranial HTN (IIH), shunt failure
   6. Cerebral venous thrombosis
   7. Cervicocranial artery dissection
   8. SDH
   9. Acute angle closure glaucoma
B. Nonemergent
   1. Tension
   2. Migraine
   3. Cluster
   4. Febrile headache
   5. Dental, temporomandibular joint (TMJ)
   6. Trigeminal neuralgia

7. Postlumbar puncture (LP) headache
8. Medication overuse headache

Diagnostic Testing

A. Use the Ottawa SAH Rule as a decision rule[38] (see Box 13.1).
  1. High sensitivity to rule out SAH, but low specificity to rule in SAH
  2. Patients presenting with a normal neurologic examination result and peak HA severity within one hour of onset of pain symptoms.
B. MRI
C. *Magnetic resonance angiography (MRA):* For carotid dissection or arteriovenous malformation (AVM)
D. *Magnetic resonance venography (MRV):* Cerebral sinus thrombosis or AVM
E. Lab
  1. Arterial blood gas (ABG) with carboxyhemoglobin (COHb) level in CO poisoning

Management

A. Procedure
  1. LP if concerned for infection but not indicated for concern of SAH
B. Pharmacologic therapy
  1. Nicardipine or labetalol (IV for HTN related to stroke or SAH)[40]
  2. Acetaminophen, ibuprofen, naproxen sodium, ketoprofen, and diclofenac for primary headaches
  3. Antiplatelet therapy with cervicocranial dissection
    a. Aspirin
  4. Use of the HA management algorithm above if opioid treatment may be considered
  5. Cluster headache[41]
    a. Oxygen
    b. Sumatriptan SQ or intranasal (IN)
    c. Zolmitriptan IN
  6. Migraine[41]
    a. Antidopaminergics
      i. Metoclopramide
      ii. Prochlorperazine
      iii. Chlorpromazine
    b. Anticholinergic
      i. Diphenhydramine for antidopaminergic management
    c. Triptans
      i. Sumatriptan SQ or IN
      ii. Zolmitriptan IN
    d. NSAIDs
      i. Ketorolac IV or intramuscularly (IM)
    e. Corticosteroid
      i. Dexamethasone IV

Patient Disposition

A. Consultation and collaboration
  1. HA specialist
  2. Neurologist
  3. Surgeon for temporal arteritis biopsy
  4. Infectious disease provider
  5. *Therapies:* Physical, occupation, and/or speech
B. Discharge instructions
  1. Describe what was given for HA.
  2. When to return to ED
C. Transition of care information
  1. Consider migraine prophylaxis along with adverse events (especially in women who are pregnant or breastfeeding), contraindications, and drug interactions. May also want to consider effect on comorbidities and using medication that may also treat comorbidity.
  2. Before discharge from the ED, patients with migraine HA should be given an IV dose of dexamethasone, which has been found to reduce rates of migraine recurrence within 72 hours of ED discharge (Peters, 2018)[8]
  3. Admission for HA that is suspicious for an organic process

Pediatric Headache

Approach very similar as to the adult with a headache (HA). Here are some differences in the approach to practice when working with this population.

Medical Screening

A. Search for the so-called red flags. If they have one or more red flags they are at high risk for an underlying intracranial disease.
B. There are factors that may warrant HA neuroimaging in certain clinical contexts, but alone are not absolute red flags.
  1. Changing quality of HA from the usual pattern
  2. HA that occurs in awakening or that awakens the patient from sleep
  3. Lack of family history
  4. Occipital HA
  5. Declining school performance
  6. Functional changes (e.g., vision, gait, coordination, behavior)
C. Most acute, nontraumatic HAs in children are the result of self-limited, medically remediable conditions such as upper respiratory tract infection (URI) with fever or sinusitis

Predisposing Factors

A. Table 13.6 summarizes conditions associated with migraine.

Physical Examination

A. Signs and symptoms—red flags
B. The **SNOOPPPPY** mneumonic[43]
  1. **S**ystemic symptoms, abnormal
  2. **N**eurologic signs, acute
  3. **O**nset
  4. **O**ccipital
  5. **P**recipitated by Valsalva
  6. **P**ositional
  7. **P**rogressive
  8. **P**arents—lack of family history
  9. **Y**ears <6 years old

TABLE 13.6 PEDIATRIC EPISODIC CONDITIONS THAT MAY BE ASSOCIATED WITH MIGRAINE

	AGE	FEATURES	DURATION	ASSOCIATED SYMPTOMS
Cyclic vomiting syndrome	School age (mean onset at 4–9 years)	Episodes of recurrent vomiting	Hours to days	Vomiting up to 4 times/hour Attacks ≥1 hour to 10 days and ≥1 week apart
Abdominal migraine	School age (mean onset at 4–7 years)	Episodes of moderate to severe midline dull pain	Hours to days	Anorexia, nausea, vomiting, pallor
Benign paroxysmal vertigo	Early childhood (mean onset at 2–4 years)	Abrupt onset of vertigo often manifested as ataxia or dizziness	Minutes to hours	Nystagmus, ataxia, vomiting, pallor, fearfulness Normal audiometric and vestibular function between attacks Exclusion of posterior fossa disorder, seizure, and vestibular disorders
Benign paroxysmal torticollis	Early infancy (median onset at 2–5 months)	Episodes of unilateral head tilt occurring at regular intervals	Minutes to days	Irritability, ataxia, pallor, malaise, vomiting Genetic link to CACNA1A
Infantile colic	Infancy (peak at 6 weeks)	Excessive crying	>3 hr/day on >3 d/week	Infants of mothers with migraine 2.6 times as likely to have colic vs. infants of mothers without migraine
Alternating hemiplegia of childhood	Infancy (before 18 months)	Episodes of alternating hemiplegia	Minutes to days	Encephalopathy, paroxysmal spells, dystonic posturing, or choreoathetoid movements, autonomic disturbance Genetic link to ATP1A3

Source: From Greene K, Irwin SL, Gelfand AA. Pediatric migraine: An update. *Neurology Clinics*. 2019;37(4):815–833.[42]

Diagnostic Testing

A. MRI provides superior visualization, but it is more expensive and sometimes requires sedation or general anesthesia, especially in children younger than 6 years.[44]

B. CT scan exposes children to radiation.

1. Each modality must be considered in patients with recent-onset severe HA or change in the type of HA or with associated signs or symptoms suggestive for neurologic dysfunction.
2. If child has a ventriculoperitoneal (VP) shunt, then CT with shunt study.

C. EKG, urinalysis (UA), and electrolytes in acute hypertension (HTN)

D. Lab

1. Toxicology screen
2. Lead screen

E. Procedures

1. Lumbar puncture (LP) done in patient with chronic HA; be sure to obtain an accurate opening pressure to make a diagnosis of idiopathic intracranial HTN (IIH).
2. Opening pressure is higher in children than adults, 28 cm H_2O versus 25 cm H_2O, respectively.[43]

Management

A. Hydration

B. Resting in a dark quiet room

C. Acute medications should be given as early as possible at the onset of HA.

D. Optimize dedication dosing for weight and age as done with all pediatric patients while counseling patient and parents about potential risk/benefits of medications.

E. First-line treatment include NSAIDs and acetaminophen.

F. If there is an inadequate response to acetaminophen or ibuprofen, triptans should be considered.

G. Consider an antiemetic such as prochlorperazine.

Pediatric Seizures

A. Breath-holding spells are most common in the 6- to 18-month age range. Look for an initiating trigger, followed by emotional upset, crying, pallor, and occasionally level of consciousness (LOC). This is highly suggestive of a breath-holding spell.

B. Pseudo-seizures are frequently seen in the adolescent.

C. Migraine can be a mimic

D. Febrile seizure

1. Common in childhood
2. Occurs between 3 months and 6 years of age, typically lasting <15 minutes
3. Have a 1% risk of developing epilepsy[1]

Physical Examination

A. Elements highly suggestive of seizure[45]

1. Lip-smacking
2. Lateralized tongue biting (high specificity)
3. Flickering eyelids, deviation of gaze
4. Dilated pupils with a blank stare
5. Increased heart rate and blood pressure, desaturations in pulse oximetry during event

B. Examine for bulging fontanelle.

C. Examine for papilledema and retinal hemorrhages—suspect maltreatment.

Management

A. Benzodiazepines IV are best. Can also be given via intraosseous (IO), intranasally, intramuscularly, and rectally if you do not have IV access.
B. If an anticonvulsant given, it should be in conjunction with a neurologist.
  1 Pediatrics tend to metabolize tanticonvulsants faster than adults.
  2 Consider phenobarbital, valproic acid, or levetiracetam.[45]

Disposition

A. *Under 6 months of age*: Generally require a full workup and are usually admitted for observation
B. *Six months to 2 years of age*: Disposition will depend on blood work, reassessment, and the ability to have close follow-up.
C. *Over 2 years of age*: Those who have returned to baseline, have a normal neurologic exam with normal workup are often safe to be discharged to close outpatient follow-up. Otherwise, admit.
D. Febrile seizure can be discharged home with close follow-up.

Seizures

Seizures can be challenging. First, seizures must be recognized and managed aggressively. This is easier when seizures have motor component. Second, life-threatening conditions need to be identified. Lastly, a determination on likelihood of recurrence must be made. Seizures account for 5% of calls to 911 and 1% of all ED visits.

Seizures defined as a sudden change in behavior, characterized by an alteration in sensory perception or motor activity.[46] Generalized seizures affect both sides of the brain and include tonic-clonic or absence seizures. Focal seizures—or partial seizures—can start in one area or group of cells on one side of the brain. The terms simple/complex partial and convulsions are no longer used.[47]

Anatomy

A. Neuronal cell membranes are kept stable due to electrochemical gradients across the membranes and regulation of inhibitory mediators such as gamma-aminobutyric acid (GABA).

Pathophysiology

A. Abnormal electrical discharge of cortical neurons caused by a disequilibrium of the neuronal cell membrane
B. Persistent seizure activity results in gradual reduction of $GABA_A$ receptors secondary to receptor internalization and degradation.[46]
C. Physiologic consequences include an increase in body temperature, serum glucose, and lactic acidosis.

Predisposing Factors

A. Hypoglycemia
B. Neurosurgery (e.g., shunt or other hardware)
C. Headaches and tumors
D. Recent fever or infection (especially central nervous system [CNS])
E. Recent trauma
F. Immunosuppression
G. Recent electrolyte abnormality
H. Renal disease
I. Psychiatric disease

Physical Examination

A. Obtain a thorough history.
  1. Observations from witnesses—key to the diagnosis
  2. Circumstances around the event
  3. Some questions that assist in clarifying the type of seizure include the following:
    a. Was there any warning noted before the seizure? If so, what kind of warning occurred?
    b. What did the patient do during the seizure?
    c. Was the patient able to relate to the environment during the seizure, and/or does the patient have recollection of the seizure?
    d. How did the patient feel after the seizure and how long did it take to get back to baseline condition?
    e. How long did the seizure last?
    f. How frequently do the seizures occur?
    g. Is anything known to precipitate the seizures?
    h. Was alcohol or drugs involved?
    i. Is the patient on any medications, and are they compliant?
    j. Any recent travel outside of the United States? Consider malaria or neurocysticercosis.
B. Signs and symptoms
  1. Vital signs
    a. Fever
    b. Hypertension (HTN) with bradycardia
      1. Consider a head injury with an increased intracranial pressure (ICP).
    c. An irregular heart rate can be seen with a seizure accompanying a stroke.
    d. Observe for hypoxia.
  2. While actively seizing, observe motor component.
    a. Focal abnormalities in the hemisphere—opposite the direction of head or eye deviation.
  3. Unexplained bruising must raise suspicion of a bleeding disorder or maltreatment.

Focused Assessment

A. Focal seizures
  1. Very **short-lived**, lasting no more than 1 minute
  2. No change in level of consciousness (LOC). Patient may be awake and aware but may be unable to speak, and may be confused.
  3. Motor symptoms may also include the following:
    a. Jerking (clonic)
    b. Limp or weak muscles (atonic)
    c. Tense or rigid muscles (tonic)
    d. Brief muscle twitching (myoclonus)
    e. Pediatric and adults may see repeated automatic movements, like clapping or rubbing of hands, lip-smacking or chewing, or bicycling movements.
  4. Nonmotor symptoms. You will see changes in
    a. Sensation
    b. Emotions

c. Cognition
d. Autonomic functions (such as gastrointestinal sensations, waves of heat or cold, goosebumps, heart racing, etc.)
5. Absence seizures can cause rapid blinking or a few seconds of staring into space.
a. Brief twitches (myoclonus) that affect specific part of the body or just the eyelids
b. Common in children 6 to 14 years
6. Tonic/clonic
a. May cry out
b. Loss of consciousness
c. Falls to the ground
d. Muscle jerks or spasms/muscle rigidity
e. Respiratory arrest
f. May/may not have urinary incontinence
g. Usually lasts 2 to 5 minutes
7. Key signs or strong markers for seizure[46]
a. Postictal confusion
b. Tongue biting
c. Confirmed unresponsiveness
d. Preceding *déjà vu*/aura
e. Head or eye deviation
f. Pupils are often are dilated during or after a seizure.
g. Rhythmic limb shaking or dystonic posturing
h. Lip-smacking or bicycling movements in neonate and infant

Differential Diagnoses

A. Syncope
B. Dysrhythmia
C. Psychogenic/conversion disorder
D. Breath holding
E. Acute drug or alcohol withdrawal
F. CNS infection
G. Eclampsia, if pregnant

Diagnostic Studies

A. Labs
1. Magnesium
2. Toxicology screen
3. Therapeutic drug levels
4. Alcohol level
B. EKG to evaluate QTc and QRS
C. Lumbar puncture (LP) if an infection is considered
D. EEG
E. Arterial blood gas (ABG) if patient is actively seizing; if anion gap acidosis present, consider other causes.

Patient Management

A. Initial management is supportive and is self-limited.
B. There are three pitfalls to avoid in the management of seizures:
1. Failure to recognize a seizure
2. Failure to treat aggressively
3. Not treating the etiology
C. Protect the patient from injury by padding stretcher.
D. Procedures
1. LP if there is an altered mental status with fever or severe headache
2. Intubation if patient unable to maintain airway
E. *Pharmacologic therapies:* Treat early.
1. Benzodiazepines
a. Lorazepam (Ativan®) most effective and longer seizure half-life than diazepam
2. Fosphenytoin (Cerebyx®)
3. Levetiracetam (Keppra®)
4. Valproic acid
5. Patients with hepatic and renal insufficiency
a. Levetiracetam is excreted mostly by means of renal clearance, and doses adjusted for renal insufficiency. Useful in patients with hepatic failure.
b. Phenytoin and valproic acid have been associated with acute hepatic injury.
6. Glucose for treatment of hypoglycemia (glucose <50 mg/dL)
7. No anticonvulsant for febrile seizure
8. Fever control in the adult and especially pediatric patient
a. Acetaminophen
b. Ibuprofen
F. Consultation and collaboration
1. Neurologist on admission, especially if starting anticonvulsant
2. Depending on the state, may be required to report a seizure
a. Physical and occupational therapy PRN
b. Social work

Disposition/Transition of Care

A. Admit status epilepticus to the ICU.
B. Adult patients with normal neurologic exam can be safely discharged with outpatient follow-up if this is not a first-time seizure.

NEUROMUSCULAR DISORDERS

Neuromuscular disorders are rarely acute and can be managed in out-of-hospital settings. Only a few acute neuromuscular diseases are seen in the ED those being: Guillain–Barré syndrome, acute myasthenia gravis, and amyotrophic lateral sclerosis. However, patients affected with acute and severe manifestations of any of these neuromuscular diseases, treatment in the ED poses major management challenges.[48]

Guillain–Barré

Guillain–Barré (GB) is an autoimmune disorder that often follows a viral illness and is **commonly missed diagnosis** in the ED. The patient's own immune system causes damage to the nerves resulting in ascending numbness and paralysis with a potential to progress to significant morbidity, if not diagnosed. Approximately 3,000 to 6,000 people develop GB each year.[49] Commonly seen in individuals >50 years of age, with gastroenteritis, with some discussion of a link to the flu vaccination and symptoms developing a few days to weeks postvaccination.[49]

Anatomy

A. The peripheral nervous system (PNS) resides outside the spine and the brain.

B. Destruction of the propagation of the nerve fibers causes weakness and paralysis.

Pathophysiology

A. An autoimmune disorder affecting the PNS.
B. Not clear what sets the disorder in motion but a gastroenteritis caused by *Campylobacter jejuni* seen as the most common cause of this neuromuscular disorder.[49]

Predisposing Factors

A. Recent vaccination
B. Recent viral infection

Physical Examination

A. Chief complaint
  1. Acute shortness of breath (SOB)/tachypnea, respiratory distress due to inability to protect airway
  2. Acute weakness or an inability to walk
  3. Joint or muscle pain
  4. Bowel or bladder dysfunction
B. Signs and symptoms
  1. *Typical presenting symptom:* Severe back pain and limb paresthesia, starting in the ankles and wrists, with a "tight band" sensation[48]
  2. Depressed/absent deep tendon reflexes (DTRs)
  3. Only able to speak in short sentences, also known as "staccato speech"
  4. Arrhythmias, especially tachycardia
  5. Diaphoresis
  6. Urinary retention
  7. Labile blood pressure (BP)
  8. Sleep disturbances
C. Focused assessment
  1. Can the patient lift their head off the bed? Usually seen prior to respiratory issues.
  2. Was a traumatic injury involved?
  3. Determine whether the weakness is **focal or nonfocal.**
    a. Muscle weakness, which is worse with **exercise, better at rest, and progressive as the day goes on associated with** myasthenia gravis.
  4. Is it unilateral or bilateral? And is it a single extremity or both?
  5. Does it affect a single nerve or group of nerves?
  6. How does the weakness manifest itself?
  7. Any associated symptoms, including headache (HA)? Sensory involvement?
  8. Any recent infectious processes?
    a. GB disease process occurs **5 to 7 days after an infection illness.**[50]
  9. Medication history and any recent medication change.
  10. Good neurologic exam
    a. Exam proximal and distal muscle groups
    b. Check DTRs.
  11. Watch the patient ambulate if they are able.

Differential Diagnoses

A. Amyotrophic lateral sclerosis (ALS)
B. Myasthenia gravis (MG) crisis
C. Myopathy, West Nile in particular
D. Myositis
E. Spinal muscular atrophy
F. Acute botulism poisoning
G. Organophosphate poisoning
H. Tick paralysis

Diagnostic Testing

A. Magnesium/phosphorus, creatine kinase (CK)
B. Arterial blood gas (ABG)
C. EKG
D. Chest x-ray (CXR)
E. Echocardiogram to look for cardiomyopathy, especially in the pediatric population
F. MRI of the brain and spinal cord
G. Lumbar puncture (LP)
  1. See high protein with a normal white blood cell (WBC)
H. Outpatient
  1. Electromyography (EMG)
  2. Nerve conduction studies
  3. Genetic testing
  4. Muscle biopsy to examine a sample of muscle tissue under a microscope

Patient Management

A. Procedures
B. Bilevel positive airway pressure (BiPAP)
C. Emergency intubation
  1. Avoid succinylcholine.
  2. 20-30-40 Rule for intubation[50]
    a. Forced vital capacity <20 mL/kg
    b. Max inspiratory pressure <30 cm H_2O
    c. Max expiratory pressure <40 cm H_2O
D. Pharmacologic therapies
  1. ***Caution:* Do not administer steroids** as they worsen the problem.
  2. Plasma exchange or intravenous immunoglobulin (IVIG)
  3. Antibiotics if indicated
  4. Neostigmine or Pyridostigmine for secretions
  5. Baclofen for spasticity
  6. Pain management
  7. Deep vein thrombosis (DVT) prophylaxis
E. Consultation and collaboration
  1. Neurology
  2. Surgeon if **thymectomy indicated**
  3. Neurologist or pediatric neurologist
  4. Physical and occupational therapy

Patient Disposition

A. Many times, patient will be admitted to the hospital due to respiratory distress.
  1. ICU if any respiratory depression or insufficiency
B. May be placed on immunosuppressant drugs on discharge.
C. If sent home, be sure to discuss with patient:
  1. Watch for new infections.
  2. This disease process advances quickly, so know when to call emergency medical service (EMS)
D. Age and developmental considerations
  1. Pediatric considerations
    a. Clinical history is very important.
    b. Clinical examination is key.

c. May have deformities of the face, hands, and feet
d. Cannot sit without support (after 6 months of age)
e. GB tends to be less severe in children than adults.

Myasthenia Gravis

Myasthenia gravis (MG) is a chronic autoimmune disorder of the peripheral nerves in which impulses are altered or blocked in some way at the neuromuscular junction by antibodies. This reduction in the number of acetylcholine (ACh) receptors results in a characteristic pattern of progressively reduced muscle strength and muscle weakness that worsens after periods of activity and improves after periods of rest.[51] It affects women more than men in the 20- to 30-year age range.

Anatomy

A. The nerve terminal moves impulses forward to the end plate.

Pathophysiology

A. Autoimmune process
B. Stimulation of the motor nerve released ACh, which depolarizes the motor endplate of the nerve causing the muscle to contract.
C. Antibodies block, alter, or destroy ACh nicotinic postsynaptic receptor.

Predisposing Factors

A. Lesions of the thymus
B. Genetics

Physical Examination

A. Chief complaint
  1. Progressive fluctuating weakness and fatigue
B. Signs and symptoms
  1. Repetitive activity with **ocular symptoms often as the first manifestation**.
  2. Ptosis (seen in 80% of patients)
  3. Diplopia with no pupillary changes (seen in 80% of patients)
  4. Flattened facial expression or change in facial expression
  5. Head droop
  6. Dysarthria or slurred or nasal speech
  7. Dysphonia
  8. Dysphagia (due to fatigable)—Trouble chewing, or swallowing; may have an inability to close jaw after chewing
  9. Progressive weakness (symptoms worsen as the day progresses or sustained activity)
  10. Respiratory depression/failure—Bronchospasm
  11. Triggers
    a. Infections
    b. Trauma
    c. Surgery
C. Focused Assessment
  1. MG crisis may exhibit cholinergic OD symptoms.
    a. Think SLUDGE
      i. Salivation
      ii. Lacrimation
      iii. Urination
      iv. Defecation
      v. Gastrointestinal (GI) upset
      vi. Emesis
  2. Respiratory assessment
  3. Search for triggers (infections)

Differential Diagnoses

Abbott[52] noted, "The NP must include MG in the differential diagnosis with any report of fluctuating muscle weakness or other neurologic, upper GI, respiratory, or ophthalmic complaint. The key diagnostic finding is a specific muscle weakness that can be reproduced and exacerbated with sustained muscle use. These considerations will lead to earlier diagnosis and treatment."
A. Amyotrophic lateral sclerosis (ALS)
B. Stroke
C. Guillain–Barré (GB) syndrome
D. Hyperthyroidism
E. Multiple sclerosis (MS)
F. Cerebral lesion

Diagnostic Testing

A. Chest x-ray (CXR)
B. CT scan or MRI chest (thorax) to detect thymomas
C. Lab
  1. Thyroid function
  2. Serum B12
  3. Anti-MuSK antibody
  4. Acetylcholine receptor antibodies (Anti AChR Ab)

Patient Management

A. Procedures
  1. Airway management
    a. Check a negative inspiratory force (NIF). If less than 20 (some say 30) the patient needs to be intubated.
  2. Intubation
    a. MG is less sensitive to the depolarizing effects of neuromuscular blocking agents and may require two to three times the dose of succinylcholine.[53]
    b. Use etomidate.
    c. DC acetylcholinesterase (AChe) inhibitors while intubated
  3. Edrophonium (Tensilon) test
    a. Short-acting ACh inhibitor that boosts the signal between nerve and muscle.
    b. Injections of edrophonium chloride to briefly relieve weakness.
  4. Plasmapheresis
  5. Electromyography (EMG)
B. Pharmacologic therapies

TABLE 13.7 UNCOMMON NEUROLOGIC CONDITIONS		
CONDITION	**DESCRIPTION**	**KEY POINTS**
ALS: Lou Gehrig's Disease	■ Rare neurogenerative disorder characterized by a spectrum of progressive weakness and atrophy caused by degeneration of both UMN) and LMN or in only one motor neuron area[54]	■ Progressive weakness and atrophy with frequent falls ■ Asymmetrical limb weakness ■ BiPAP ■ Pharmaceutical tx: benzodiazepines, Riluzole ■ End of life discussion
Multiple sclerosis	■ An acquired immune demyelinating disorder of the CNS[55] ■ Focal symptoms—diagnosis largely clinical utilizing McDonald criteria[56]	■ MS flares when they develop a UTI or URI ■ CT brain—"open ring sign"—a crescent-shaped image which is open to the basal ganglia
Parkinson's disease	■ Complex neurodegenerative condition caused by a depletion of "dopaminergic" neurons in the basal ganglia of the brain ■ **Classic triad** ■ Resting tremors ("pill-rolling") ■ Rigidity assessed passively ("cog-wheel") ■ Bradykinesia (e.g., moves slowly with stiffness in a deliberate manner) ■ "End of dose deterioration," seen before the next tablet is due[56] ■ Get a medication history to identify drugs that might cause DIP such as ■ Typical and atypical antipsychotics ■ Antiemetics ■ Calcium channel blockers ■ Classically, DIP presents with: ○ Lack of tremor in comparison to the asymmetric features ○ Resting tremor as seen in Parkinson's	■ **NEVER** miss or delay any Parkinson's medications ■ A few missed doses can be fatal—can affect swallowing or moving ■ Many antiemetics and anti-psychotics are dopamine agonists ■ Check a CK if the patient has been off meds for a period of time or found down
Brain abscess	■ Usually noted in MCA territory of brain ■ Predisposing factors- sinusitis, otitis media, meningitis ■ Classic clinical triad consists of fever, headache, and focal neurologic deficit is present in less than 20% of cases ■ Infants present with irritability or seizure	■ Check the circumference of a child ■ MRI brain with contrast ■ Two key features in workup: Imaging with contrast and avoidance of lumbar puncture[57]
Meningitis	■ **Classic triad of meningitis**: Fever, neck stiffness, and altered mental status ■ Caused by organisms that colonize the nose and pharynx and move into the blood stream, and then to subarachnoid space ■ Two kinds—bacterial and viral ■ Bacterial ■ Most common pathogen *Streptococcus pneumoniae* and *Neisseria meningitidis*[58] ■ *Listeria monocytogenes* more common in older patients (>50 years old), infants (<3 months old), and immunocompromised or pregnant individuals[59]	■ Vaccination against *Haemophilus influenzae*, *S. pneumoniae*, and *N. meningitidis* have lowered their risk ■ Positive Brudzinski's sign ■ LP ■ WBCs found in the CSF indicate bacterial ■ Cloudy in appearance in bacterial, but viral may be clear-cloudy ■ Obtain gram stain and culture ■ Cell count ■ Protein >200 mg/dL ■ Glucose <40 mg/dL ■ Prevention ■ PCV7 and the MCV4

(*continued*)

TABLE 13.7 UNCOMMON NEUROLOGIC CONDITIONS (*CONTINUED*)

CONDITION	DESCRIPTION	KEY POINTS
Encephalitis	■ Encephalitis is an infection of the brain parenchyma causing inflammation within the CNS and often viral in origin[60] ■ Can be viral, bacterial, or fungal—HSV is the most common and curable form ■ Chief complaint ■ Acute confusion ■ Headache and fever—nuchal rigidity ■ New psychiatric symptoms ■ Infants/children may present with poor feeding, lethargy, fever, behavioral changes and seizure	■ Labs ■ CBC mostly lymphocytes ■ Blood and urine culture ■ Toxicology screen for alcohol and drugs ■ IgM, ELISA assay to look for West Nile ■ Antigen assays for: HSV, Toxoplasmosis ■ Lumbar Puncture ■ Protein and glucose normal or slightly elevated ■ RBC normal or may be elevated with HSV ■ Watch for cerebral edema ■ Antibiotic, empiric until cultures return along with antivirals ■ If giving acyclovir monitor for nephrotoxicity ■ Use mosquito repellent—apply on adult's hands and then to child's face ■ Do not use insect repellent on babies younger than 2 months old[62]

ALS, amyotrophic lateral sclerosis; BiPAP, bilevel positive airway pressure; CBC, complete blood count; CNS, central nervous system; CSF, cerebrospinal fluid; DIP, drug-induced Parkinsonism; HSV, herpes simplex virus; LMN, lower motor neuron; LP; lumbar puncture; MCA, middle cerebral artery; meningococcal conjugate vaccine (MCV4); MS, multiple sclerosis; PCV7, pneumococcal seven-valent conjugate vaccine; RBC, red blood cell; UMN, upper motor neurons; URI, upper respiratory tract infection; UTI, urinary tract infections; WBC, white blood cell.

1. Corticosteroids, high dose
   a. Can precipitate a crisis and worsen symptoms
2. Antibiotics if infection noted
   a Possible use of atropine for cholinergic crisis
   b Intravenous **immunoglobulin (IVIG)**

Patient Disposition

A. Neurology consultation
B. Surgeon for possible thymectomy
C. Transition of care to the ICU
   1. Admission for respiratory failure
   2. Worsening of symptoms or new onset of symptoms
D. Neonatal MG usually seen in the first 48 hours but may be present to the ED 10 days postdelivery with weakness and poor feeding.

Uncommon Neurologic Conditions

Table 13.7 summarizes uncommon neurologic conditions for reference.

References and Additional Reading

References and Additional Reading for this chapter are online only and can be found at https://connect.springerpub.com/content/reference-book/978-0-8261-6091-5/part/part02/toc-part/ch13.

14. Thoracic/Respiratory Urgencies and Emergencies

VIRGINIA MANGOLDS | RENEÉ SEMONIN HOLLERAN

Learning Objectives

- Identify common presentations of common respiratory diseases and conditions.
- Determine a differential diagnosis based on a thorough patient history and physical.
- Develop a comprehensive patient evaluation to determine the underlying problem.
- Apply anatomy and pathophysiology concepts to the understanding of the treatment of the disease.
- Implement an actionable treatment plan for the problem.
- Evaluate the treatment process and adjust as needed.
- Provide patient education, including reliable internet resources for ongoing care if appropriate.
- Determine and implement a safe disposition for the patient, whether being discharged to home with education, discharged to home with services, discharged to home with referral to a specialist, or needing inpatient care to work the problem more thoroughly.

This chapter provides the identification, treatment/management, and disposition of patients with common respiratory problems presenting to the ED. These diseases or problems include upper respiratory infection (URI), asthma, chronic obstructive pulmonary disease (COPD), community-acquired pneumonia (CAP), hospital-acquired pneumonia (HAP), aspiration pneumonia (AP), and pleural diseases such as pneumothorax, pleuritis, and pleural effusion. Pertinent background information related to the anatomy/pathophysiology of each problem or disease will be presented and include the recommended treatments and patient dispositions. When publicly available on the Internet, reliable sources of medication administration/dosing will be identified rather than static tables; this information is continuously updated and more accessible during a busy shift. Bookmarking these sites is recommended. Respiratory resuscitation is addressed in Chapter 6.

Approach to the Patient With Respiratory System Disease[1,2]

There are three major categories of disease of the respiratory system:

A. Obstructive
B. Restrictive
C. Vasculature abnormalities

History

A. Cardinal symptoms are dyspnea and cough.
B. Specific questioning should focus on factors that incite as well as resolve the patient's shortness of breath (SOB).
C. Degree of activity resulting in SOB is a gauge of the patient's degree of disability.
D. Dyspnea on exertion (DOE) may be associated with underlying lung or heart disease.
E. Inquire regarding the duration of cough, whether associated with sputum production and any triggers that induce it.
F. Chronic cough (persisting for >8 weeks) is commonly associated with obstructive lung disease (chronic obstructive pulmonary disease [COPD]) as well as gastroesophageal reflux disease (GERD) and postnasal drip.
G. All causes of cough are not respiratory in origin: Broad differential, including gastrointestinal (GI) and cardiac disease as well as psychogenic causes
H. Wheezing is suggestive of airway disease such as asthma
I. Hemoptysis is suggestive of infections of the respiratory tract, pulmonary embolism (PE), or bronchogenic carcinoma.
J. Right strain on the heart because of pulmonary disease may present symptoms such as cor pulmonale, abdominal bloating or distention, and pedal edema.
K. Travel history important to explore specific respiratory tract infections, such as tuberculosis, COVID-19 exposure, and fungi found in specific geographic regions.

Physical

A. *Current vital signs:* Look for tachypnea or hypopnea; pulse oximetry (at rest and with activity—92% or greater).
B. *Inspection:* Use of accessory muscles; kyphoscoliosis may result in restrictive pathophysiology; inability to talk with complete sentences is generally a sign of severe impairment.
C. *Percussion:* Used to establish diaphragm excursion and lung size; can help in differentiating between pneumothorax (hyperresonate) or pleural effusions (dull).
D. *Palpation:* Generally limited in the evaluation of the respiratory system; helpful for demonstrating

subcutaneous air associated with barotrauma; may be used as an adjunctive assessment in determining whether decreased breath sound is due to pleural effusion (decreased tactile fremitus) or consolidation (increased tactile fremitus).

E. *Auscultation:* Most used in assessing the respiratory system; wheezes are a manifestation of airway obstruction, but may not only be heard in asthma but in the setting of congestive heart failure; rhonchi are the result of obstruction in the medium-sized airway, most often associated with secretions and may be associated with viral or bacterial bronchitis, bronchiectasis, or COPD; stridor is usually heard over the neck and indicates an upper airway obstruction.

F. *Other possible related body systems to examine:* Pedal edema, if positive and symmetrical, may indicate cor pulmonale, if asymmetric may be due to deep venous thrombosis (DVT) and associated PE; jugular venous distention may indicate right heart failure and volume overload; pulsus paradoxus is associated with significant negative intrathoracic (pleural) pressures required for ventilation (patients with obstructive lung disease) and is an ominous sign of impending respiratory failure.

Diagnostic Evaluation

A. *Pulmonary function tests:* Generally, not part of the emergency evaluation; refer for outpatient evaluation and follow-up.

B. *Arterial blood gas (ABG) testing:* Further evaluates the pulse oximetry findings of hypoxia and allows the measurement of arterial PCO_2, which may inform compromise from COPD or progressive restrictive physiology as found in neuromuscular disease.

C. *Complete blood count (CBC):* Elevation of the white blood cells (WBCs) as well as a left shift, may indicate an acute infection such as pneumonia

D. *Imaging:* Chest x-ray (CXR) beginning with a plain chest radiograph, but may not provide an appropriate diagnosis. CT of the chest allows better delineation of the parenchymal processes, pleural disease, masses or nodule, PE, and large airways.

Bronchitis (Acute)

Acute bronchitis is an inflammation of the trachea, bronchi, and bronchioles, usually resulting from an upper respiratory tract infection. Cough is the main complaint and can last up to 3 weeks. It is generally self-limited and patients return to their normal level of functioning. Most infections are viral. It affects all ages and equally affects males and females. Results in 10 to 12 million office visits per year.

Pathophysiology/Etiology

A. Acute bronchitis causes an epithelial surface injury, resulting in increased mucus production and thickening of the bronchiole wall.

B. Viral infections, such as adenovirus, influenza A and B, rhinovirus, and herpes simplex virus

C. Bacterial infections, such as *Chlamydia pneumoniae*, Mycoplasma, *Bordetella pertussis*, *Haemophilus influenzae*, *Streptococcus pneumoniae*, *Moraxella catarrhalis*, and *Mycobacterium tuberculosis*

Clinical Presentation

A. Cough for >5 days and no evidence of pneumonia, asthma, or chronic obstructive pulmonary disease (COPD) exacerbation

B. Cough is initially dry and nonproductive, then becomes productive with possible subsequent mucopurulent sputum (may indicate secondary infection)

C. Possible contact with others who have respiratory infections

D. May have dyspnea, wheeze, and fatigue

E. Fever may suggest pneumonia or influenza

Physical Examination

A. Tachypnea

B. Injected pharynx

C. Wheezing or rhonchi

D. Should have no evidence of pulmonary consolidation or rales

E. Fever (uncommon)

Differential Diagnoses

A. Generally, diagnosis is based on history and physical examination

B. *Differential diagnoses:* Common cold, acute sinusitis, bronchopneumonia, influenza, asthma, bacterial tracheitis, allergy, aspiration, retained foreign body, heart failure, gastroesophageal reflux disease (GERD)

Diagnostic Testing

A. If complicated signs and symptoms, the following diagnostic tests may be considered:

1. Complete blood count (CBC) with differential
2. Influenza testing (if appropriate for the time of year)
3. Viral panel
4. Pulse oximetry if an underlying pulmonary disease is present

B. If concerned about pneumonia

1. *Chest x-ray (CXR):* Should be normal
2. Helps to rule out diseases or complications

Management

A. Outpatient treatment unless elderly or complicated by severe underlying disease

B. Antibiotics are not usually recommended unless a treatable pathogen has been identified or there are significant comorbidities.

C. Rest.

D. Refrain from smoking and avoid secondary smoke.

E. Steam inhalation/vaporizers

F. Adequate hydration

G. Antipyretic analgesics such as acetaminophen or ibuprofen

H. Cough suppressant for troublesome cough; honey (1 tbsp every 2–4 hours as needed), benzonatate (Tessalon), guaifenesin, and dextromethorphan

I. Decongestants if associated with a sinus condition

J. Inhaled β agonists (e.g., albuterol inhaler) or in combination with high-dose inhaled corticosteroids for cough with bronchospasm

K. If influenza is highly suspected and symptom onset is <48 hours, oseltamivir (Tamiflu), zanamivir (Relenza)[3]
L. Throat lozenges for pharyngitis
M. Mucolytic agents ARE NOT recommended.
N. Oral corticosteroids probably not indicated, but controversial

Patient Disposition

A. Complications requiring inpatient admission
   1. Hypoxemia—requires supplemental oxygen
   2. Severe bronchospasm
   3. Respiratory failure that may require continuous positive airway pressure/bilevel ventilation
   4. Exacerbation of underlying disease
   5. Frequent bronchodilators if the patient is bronchospastic
   6. Dehydration requiring IV fluid administration
B. Patient education
   1. Explain to patients who likely expect an antibiotic to be prescribed, that antibiotics are not recommended unless a treatable pathogen has been identified or significant comorbidities are present.
   2. Return to the ED for worsening symptoms, including worsening fever or worsening productive cough, chest pain, shortness of breath (SOB), or inability to take adequate oral hydration.

Aspiration Pneumonia[4–6]

Aspiration pneumonia (AP) refers to pulmonary abnormalities following abnormal entry of endogenous or exogenous substances in the lower airways. It is difficult to diagnose and differentiate from other aspiration syndromes, community-acquired pneumonia (CAP) and hospital-acquired pneumonia (HAP). It is linked to a higher mortality rate (29.4%) compared to CAP (11.6%). It is generally classified as (1) aspiration (chemical pneumonitis), (2) primary bacterial AP, and (3) secondary bacterial infection of chemical pneumonitis. Choice of antibiotic depends on where the pneumonia developed (community, hospital, or long-term care facility), risk factors for resistant infections, and the likelihood that anaerobes are involved. It represents 20% to 35% of all pneumonia and has a peak incidence in elderly patients in hospitals or nursing homes.

Etiology

A. Complex interaction of etiologies, ranging from chemical (commonly acid) pneumonitis after aspiration of sterile gastric contents, to bacterial aspiration
   1. Large-volume aspiration of oropharyngeal or upper gastrointestinal (GI) secretions
   2. Microaspiration (small volume aspiration) of oropharyngeal secretions is normal, especially during sleep; however, is involved in the pathogenesis of most types of pneumonia.
   3. AP is different from chemical pneumonitis from aspiration.
      a. AP is a secondary infection that develops over a few days due to the combination of aspirated microorganisms and damaged lung tissue and may not demonstrate infiltrates on chest x-ray (CXR) early on.
      b. Chemical pneumonitis from aspiration leads to inflammation due to aspiration of irritating acidic gastric contents. It may appear like acute respiratory distress syndrome (ARDS) with bronchospasms and frothy sputum with bilateral patchy infiltrates on CXR.
   4. Community-acquired AP generally results from predominantly anaerobic mouth bacteria (anaerobic and microaerophilic streptococci, fusobacteria, gram-positive anaerobic nonspore-forming rods), *Bacteroides* species, *Haemophilus influenzae*, and *Streptococcus pneumoniae*.
   5. Hospital-acquired AP often occurs among elderly patients and others with diminished gag reflex, those with nasogastric tubes, intestinal obstruction ventilator support, and those exposed to contaminated nebulizers.
   6. Causative organisms: Anaerobes listed under community-acquired aspiration pneumonia (AP); *Escherichia coli*, *Pseudomonas aeruginosa*, *Staphylococcus aureus*, methicillin-resistant Staphylococcus aureus (MRSA), *Klebsiella*, *Enterobacter*, *Serratia*, *Proteus* spp., *H. influenzae*, *S. pneumoniae*, *Legionella*, and *Acinetobacter* spp. (rarely *Candida albicans*, but possible)

Predisposing Factors

A. Alcohol use
B. Poor dentition (increases the bacterial load, not necessarily risk of aspiration)
C. Dysphagia and gastroesophageal reflux
D. Head, neck, and esophageal cancer
E. Esophageal strictures
F. Chronic obstructive pulmonary disease (COPD)
G. Seizures
H. Degenerative neurologic disease
I. Impaired consciousness
J. Enteral feeding

History, Physical Examination, Differential Diagnoses, Diagnostic Tests

A. *See "Community-Acquired Pneumonia" section.*

Management

A. Airway management to prevent repeated aspiration
B. Ventilatory support if necessary
C. Chemical pneumonitis may not require antibiotic therapy–initial treatment involves airway maintenance and management of bronchospasm and airway edema.
D. Routine adjunctive treatment with glucocorticoids is not recommended.
E. Consultation with an infectious disease or pulmonary expert is recommended.
F. AP antibiotic selection depends on the site of acquisition (long-term care facility, hospital, community). Consult with your hospital pharmacist for specific institutional recommendations based on local resistance.

Patient Disposition

A. Generally, admission for close monitoring, IV antibiotics, and waiting for culture results

Asthma[7–18]

Asthma is a chronic respiratory disease characterized by periods of variable and recurring symptoms, airflow obstruction, and bronchial hyperresponsiveness that manifests clinically as attacks of impaired breathing. Many cells and cellular elements play a role in the inflammatory process: mast cells, neutrophils, eosinophils, T lymphocytes, macrophages, and epithelial cells. This inflammation causes recurrent episodes of coughing (particularly at night or early in the morning), wheezing, breathlessness, and chest tightness that is usually reversible either spontaneously or with treatment. Status asthmaticus refers to an acute severe asthma that is refractory to standard therapy and may persist for several hours.

Epidemiology and Demographics

A. Asthma has been diagnosed in 7.5% of the U.S. population, and its prevalence is rising among patients older than 65 years, African Americans, women, and persons below the poverty level.
B. Accounts for around 440,000 hospitalizations and 1.8 million ED visits a year
C. Overall asthma mortality rate in the United States has slightly improved to 11 per 1 million persons.

Predisposing Factors for Severe and Fatal Asthma in Adults

A. History of previous nonfatal asthma attack
B. Prior intubation
C. Female gender
D. African American ethnicity
E. Age >65 years
F. Obesity
G. Inhalational drug abuse
H. Tobacco use
I. Poorly controlled disease
J. Steroid dependence
K. Lack of proper use of maintenance medication
L. Lack of access to medical care
M. Psychiatric illness
N. Comorbid heart disease, and/or diabetes

Clinical Presentation

A. History of variable respiratory symptom
- **1.** More than one symptom such as wheeze, SOB, cough, chest tightness
- **2.** Symptoms worse at night, vary in time and intensity, worse with common triggers

Physical Examination

A. Tachycardia, tachypnea
B. Arterial blood gas (ABG) analysis (mmHg)—PaO_2 ≤60 or $PaCO_2$ ≥42 indicates severe asthma
C. Signs of respiratory distress such as use of accessory muscles
D. Upper respiratory tract—rhinitis, swollen nasal turbinate
E. Lower respiratory tract—expiratory wheezing, prolonged expiratory phase (wheezing may be absent in severe exacerbation due to severely reduced airflow)
F. Signs and symptoms of severe asthma
- **1.** "Tripoding"—sitting upright and leaning forward
- **2.** Diaphoresis
- **3.** Use of accessory muscles
- **4.** Asynchronous accessory muscle use
- **5.** Air trapping and hyperinflation manifesting as decreased inspiratory stroke volume and pulsus paradoxus
- **6.** Peak flow <200 L/min and/or <30% predicted
- **7.** Evidence of barotrauma:
  - **a.** Unilateral diminution in breath sounds
  - **b.** Tracheal deviation
  - **c.** Thoracic crepitus

G. Signs of impending respiratory arrest
- **1.** Altered mentation
- **2.** Cyanosis
- **3.** Hypoxia
- **4.** Hypercarbia
- **5.** Hemodynamic instability
- **6.** Silent chest

Differential Diagnoses

A. Chronic obstructive pulmonary disease (COPD), bronchiectasis, heart failure, pulmonary embolism (PE), benign or malignant tumor, pulmonary infiltration with eosinophilia, medication-induced cough (angiotensin-converting enzyme [ACE] inhibitor), vocal cord dysfunction
B. Differentiation of asthma from COPD can be challenging. A history of atopy and intermittent, reactive symptoms points toward a diagnosis of asthma, whereas smoking and advanced age are more indicative of COPD.

Diagnostic Testing

A. Pulmonary function tests (PFTs) are indicated because clinicians often initially tend to underestimate the degree of airway obstruction in acute asthma.
- **1.** Forced expiratory volume in 1 second (FEV_1) from maximal inspiration or the peak expiratory flow rate (PEFR) in liters per second, starting with fully inflated lungs and sustained for at least 10 msec may be used for evaluation.
- **2.** Any patient unable to perform PFTs should be considered to have severe airway obstruction.

B. ABG not usually indicated if pulse oximetry is available or clinician is able to obtain a venous blood gas.
C. *Complete blood count (CBC):* Optional—leukocytosis is common with acute asthma exacerbation but is not of discriminatory value in detecting acute superimposed pulmonary infection.
D. *Serum electrolytes:* Optional—generally normal
E. *Brain natriuretic peptide (BNP):* In older asthmatic patients with cardiovascular comorbidities, it may reveal unrecognized congestive heart failure
F. *Chest x-ray (CXR):* Of little value in most acute asthma exacerbations and should be restricted to patients with a suspected complicating cardiopulmonary process, such as pneumonia, pneumothorax, pneumomediastinum, subcutaneous emphysema, or congestive heart failure)
G. *EKG*: Likely to indicate tachycardia, nonspecific ST-T wave changes; may also show cor pulmonal, right bundle branch block, and right axial deviation

Management

A. Initial treatment of *mild to moderate* asthma exacerbations (*PEV_1 or PEFR [percentage predicted/personal best ≥40%]*)

1. Oxygen therapy—maintain SaO_2 ≥90%

2. Nebulized albuterol solution

a. Levalbuterol (optimal): 1.25 mg every 20 minutes for up to three doses

b. Racemic albuterol: 2.5 mg every 20 minutes for up to three doses

3. Albuterol metered-dose inhaler (MDI) with valved holding chamber (VHC)

a. Levalbuterol (45 μ/puff) (optimal): 6 to 12 puffs every 20 minutes for up to three doses with supervision

b. Racemic albuterol (90 μg/puff): 6 to 12 puffs every 20 minutes for up to three doses with supervision

4. Ipratropium therapy

a. Nebulized solution: If previous response, 0.5 mg every 20 minutes for three doses (may mix with albuterol solution)

b. MDI (18 μg/puff) with VHC: If previous response, eight puffs every 20 minutes for three doses

5. Systemic corticosteroids

a. Oral (preferred): 40 to 80 mg of prednisone or prednisolone per day

b. IV (unable to take orally or absorb): 40 to 80 mg of methylprednisolone per day

B. Initial treatment of *severe* asthma exacerbations (*PEV_1 or PEFR [percentage predicted/personal best <40%]*)

1. Oxygen therapy—maintain SaO_2 ≥90%

2. Nebulized albuterol solution

a. Levalbuterol (optimal): 1.25 mg every 20 minutes for three doses, continuous for 1 hour if severe

b. Racemic albuterol: 2.5 mg every 20 minutes for three doses continuous for 1 hour if severe

3. Albuterol MDI with VHC

a. Levalbuterol (45 μ/puff) (optimal): if able, 6 to 12 puffs every 20 minutes for up to three doses with supervision

b. Racemic albuterol (90 μg/puff): if able, 6 to 12 puffs every 20 minutes for up to three doses with supervision

4. Ipratropium therapy

a. Nebulized solution: If previous response, 0.5 mg every 20 minutes for three doses (may mix with albuterol solution)

b. MDI (18 μg/puff) with VHC: If previous response, eight puffs every 20 minutes for three doses

5. Systemic corticosteroids

a. Oral (preferred): 40 to 80 mg of prednisone or prednisolone per day

b. IV (unable to take orally or absorb): 40 to 80 mg of methylprednisolone per day

c. IV magnesium sulfate: 2 to 3 g over 20 minutes (or at rates of up to 1 g/min) if FEV_1 ≤25% predicted

6. The use of noninvasive ventilation (NIV), bilevel positive airway pressure (BiPAP), or intubation may need to be considered (emcrit.org/wp-content/uploads/2017/01/bond2017.pdf).

Patient Disposition

A. ED disposition decision-making guidelines

1. Good response FEV_1 or PEFR (% predicted/personal best) ≥70%

a. May be discharged from the ED

2. Incomplete response FEV_1 or PEFR (% predicted/personal best) ≥40% but <69%

a. May possibly be discharged but it should be an individualized decision; admission to a short-term ED observation unit (clinical decision unit [CDU]); or hospital ward if no CDU available

3. Poor response FEV_1 or PEFR (% predicted/personal best) <40%

a. May not be discharged—needs continued therapy; may be admitted to the CDU if available and appropriate; may be admitted to the hospital ward; may need critical admission if having respiratory insufficiency or failure

B. Asthmatic patients discharged from the ED have rates of relapse that vary from 11% over 3 days to 45% at 8 weeks.

C. Airway inflammation and peripheral obstruction may take hours to days to resolve.

D. Patients likely to need continued beta-2 agonist rescue therapy (should be able to demonstrate the correct use of their inhalers).

E. If unable to coordinate the canister activation with inhalation, prescribe a breath-activated inhaler or spacer device, or discuss the need for a home nebulizer.

F. Patients receiving ED systemic corticosteroids should continue these orally for 5 to 10 days.

G. Patients should contact their clinician for asthma-related problems within the following 3 to 5 days; should make a follow-up medical appointment within 1 to 4 weeks.

H. Discharged patient education

1. Written education about discharge medications, medication adjustment if the condition is not improving and a peak flow meter for daily measurements.

2. Focused education should address the need for follow-up and for understanding the difference between controller and rescue medication and their use.

3. Smoking cessation needs to be discussed—smoking asthmatics have more respiratory symptoms, lower lung function, and more parenchymal abnormalities.

4. Patients should be instructed to return to the ED for any worsening symptoms, such and worsening SOB, chest pain, or inability to speak in complete sentences due to work of breathing.

I. Online patient resources

1. American Academy of Allergy, Asthma & Immunology: 800-822-2762 or www.aaaai.org/

2. American Lung Association: 800-586-4872 or www.lung.org/

3. Asthma and Allergy Foundation of America: 800-727-8462 or www.aafa.org/

Chronic Obstructive Pulmonary Disease [7,11,19–24]

Chronic obstructive pulmonary disease (COPD) is an umbrella term for various clinical entities with multiple causes that result in airflow limitation that is not fully reversible with treatment. It is an inflammatory disease usually caused by exposure to tobacco smoke. Acute exacerbations and comorbidities contribute to the overall severity and prognosis of the disease. Emphysema and chronic bronchitis are commonly associated with COPD, neither is currently required to make the diagnosis. An overlap syndrome, known as asthma-COPD overlap syndrome (ACOS), characterized by persistent airflow limitation with several features associated with asthma and several features associated with COPD, has been gaining recognition.

Pathophysiology

A. Enhanced respiratory inflammatory response to noxious particles and gases, chronic airway irritation, mucus production, and pulmonary scarring, and changes in the pulmonary vasculature
B. Impaired gas exchange (carbon dioxide and oxygen)
C. Persistent airway obstruction

Etiology and Demographics

A. COPD affects 14% of U.S. adults aged 40 to 79 years.
B. Between 10% and 20% of COPD in the United States is due to occupational or other exposure to chemical vapors, irritants, and fumes; 80% to 90% is due to cigarette smoking.
C. COPD is the third leading cause of death in the United States.
D. Six million office visits, 500,000 hospitalizations, 126,000 deaths annually, and >$18 billion in direct healthcare costs annually.
E. Causes of acute decompensation in the patient with COPD
  1. Viral
     a. Rhinovirus, respiratory syncytial virus, coronavirus, influenza virus
  2. Bacterial
     a. *Haemophilus influenzae, Streptococcus pneumoniae,* Moraxella (Branhamella) catarrhalis, *Pseudomonas aeruginosa*
  3. Atypical bacteria
     a. *Chlamydia pneumoniae, Legionella*

Predisposing Factors

A. *Smoking:* Including passive smoking and water pipe. Marijuana may also contribute.
B. Severe pneumonia early in life including viral
C. Aging
D. Lower level of education and poverty
E. Asthma
F. Indoor pollution
G. Occupational organic or inorganic dusts

Clinical Presentation

A. *Exacerbation:* Increased frequency of sputum production, change in sputum color, frequency and/or amount, fevers, wheezing, chest tightness/pain
B. Discuss patient's use of tobacco and cannabis.
C. Consider indoor pollution and occupational exposures.
D. *Symptoms:* Exertional dyspnea, chronic cough, and sputum production
E. Review possible causes of exacerbation (e.g., cold weather, recent exposure to upper respiratory infection [URI], pneumonia, contact with flu, and noncompliance with medications).

Physical Examination

A. Prolonged expiration, wheezing
B. Barrel chest, diminished breath sounds, distant heart sounds
C. Accessory muscle use, pursed-lip breathing, cyanosis
D. Cachexia
E. Cyanosis chronic cough (usually productive but may be intermittent and may be unproductive), tachypnea, tachycardia
F. Flattening of diaphragm

Differential Diagnoses

A. Heart failure, asthma, tuberculosis (TB) and other respiratory infections, bronchiectasis, anemia, cystic fibrosis, neoplasm, pulmonary embolism, obstructive sleep apnea, hypothyroidism, neuromuscular disease, normal aging of the lungs, chronic sinusitis, reactive airways dysfunction, congestive heart failure (CHF), gastroesophageal reflux disease (GERD)

Diagnostic Testing

A. *Chest x-ray (CXR):* Seldom diagnostic but useful to visualize significant hyperinflation and to exclude alternative diagnosis (e.g., CHF, TB)
B. Decreased vascular markings and bullae in patients with emphysema
C. *CT:* Emphysematous lung, tracheobronchomalacia
D. *Pulmonary function testing (spirometry):* The reference standard for diagnosing and assessing the severity of COPD
E. *Oxygen saturation and arterial blood gases (ABGs):* Useful in selected patients
F. *Complete blood count (CBC):* Generally not useful
G. *Sputum:* Maybe purulent with bacterial respiratory tract infections
H. *EKG:* Peaked P waves in leads V2, V3, VF, low QRS voltage, clockwise rotation, and poor R wave progression in the precordial leads
  1. Continuous EKG monitoring may be helpful, at least for the initial phase of the patient's evaluation and treatment.
I. *Brain natriuretic peptide (BNP):* Limited value, not recommended unless the patient has COPD and CHF
J. *Troponins:* Rarely identify acute cardiac pathology missed by EKG; however, elevations are associated with

patients with increased in-hospital and 30-day mortality and should be considered in the decision-making process for in-hospital disposition

Management

A. General therapeutic guidelines for COPD exacerbations

B. Nonpharmacologic therapy
  1. Smoking cessation and elimination of air pollutants
  2. Vaccination against pneumococcal disease
  3. Supplemental oxygen, usually through a face mask/nasal cannula

C. Mild symptoms
  1. Oxygen to maintain oxygen saturation near 90%
  2. Metered-dose inhaler (MDI) or nebulized beta-agonist
  3. Anticholinergics
  4. Consider oral or IV corticosteroid.
  5. Consider oral antibiotic on discharge.

D. Moderate or severe symptoms
  1. Oxygen to maintain oxygen saturation near 90%
  2. Nebulized beta-agonist, anticholinergic
  3. Intubation with or without rapid sequence technique
  4. Noninvasive ventilation if severe
  5. Inline beta-agonist, (anticholinergic)—IV corticosteroid
  6. IV antibiotics

E. **Pharmaceutical Treatment**
  1. Should be administered in a stepwise approach according to the severity of disease
  2. All three classes of medications most often used in the management of acute COPD exacerbations are short-acting bronchodilators, steroids, and antibiotics.
  3. Minimally symptomatic, low risk of exacerbation
    a. First line: A short-acting bronchodilator to use as a rescue drug
    b. Short-acting β-agonists; albuterol, levalbuterol
    c. Short-acting muscarinic antagonists: ipratropium, oxitropium
  4. More symptomatic, low risk of exacerbation
    a. Regular use of long-acting bronchodilator in addition to as-needed short-acting bronchodilator.
    b. If uncontrolled symptoms with a single long-acting agent, then use combined long-acting β-agonists rather than steroids.
      i. Formoterol, salmeterol

Patient Disposition

A. Significant worsening of symptoms from baseline—admit to in-patient care

B. Inadequate response of symptoms to ED management

C. Significant comorbid condition (e.g., pneumonia, heart failure)

D. Worsening hypoxia or hypercarbia (from baseline)

E. Inability to cope at home or insufficient home resources

Community-Acquired Pneumonia[25–30]

Pneumonia is defined as a new lung infiltrate with suspected infectious origin (although the infectious agent may be nonbacterial). Community-acquired pneumonia (CAP) is classified as an acute infection of the pulmonary parenchyma acquired outside of a healthcare setting or long-term care facility. CAP remains one of the major health problems in the United States and is the eighth leading cause of death, claiming 100,000 Americans per year. Pneumonia is the most common reason for admission to the hospital, costing between $11,000 and $51,000 per admission. National quality measures have been developed over the years to improve the quality of pneumonia care. Once receiving the diagnosis of pneumonia, the patient is usually treated empirically with antibiotics, whether following national or local guidelines. The majority of admitted patients come through the ED, resulting in a major question for the ED clinician to determine patient disposition. Clinical decision aids and biomarkers have been developed to play a role in this determination.

Etiology and Pathophysiology

A. CAP in adults is most frequently associated with (85%): *Streptococcus pneumoniae, Haemophilus influenzae, Staphylococcus aureus*, group A *Streptococcus*, and *Moraxella catarrhalis.*

B. Pathogenicity of the implicated organisms informs the presentation and antibiotic choice.

Predisposing Factors

A. Immunosuppression (e.g., chronic steroid use [>20 mg/day or >2 mg/kg/day prednisone for >14 days], HIV/immunoglobin deficiencies/solid organ transplant/TNF-alpha inhibitor therapy)

B. Chronic health conditions (e.g., asthma, chronic obstructive pulmonary disease [COPD], type 2 diabetes mellitus [DM II], chronic renal failure, congestive heart failure [CHF], liver disease, and tobacco use)

C. Age >65 years

D. Antibiotic therapy in the past 6 months

E. Hospitalization for ≥2 days during the past 90 days

F. Poor functional status

Clinical Presentation

A. Fever, chills, rigors, malaise, fatigue

B. Dyspnea

C. Cough, with/without sputum

D. Pleuritic chest pain

E. Myalgias

F. Gastrointestinal (GI) symptoms

Physical Examination

A. Vitals; fever >100.4°F (38°C)

B. Tachypnea

C. Tachycardia

D. Hypoxemia

E. Severe cases may also present with hypothermia, bradycardia, or hypotension.

F. *Pulmonary examination:* Decreased breath sounds unilaterally or bilaterally with rhonchi, rales, bronchial breath sounds, dullness to percussion, and abdominal tenderness

Differential Diagnoses

A. Differential diagnoses

1. Bronchitis, asthma or COPD exacerbation, pulmonary edema, lung cancer, pulmonary tuberculosis, pneumonitis, and sarcoidosis

Diagnostic Testing

A. Usually can be diagnosed based on clinical findings: Fever, tachypnea, and physical examination findings

B. In the outpatient setting of significant symptoms

1. Pulse oximetry or arterial blood gas (ABG)

2. Complete blood count (CBC)

3. Chest x-ray

4. Chest CT (should not be used routinely but helpful to identify cavitation and loculated pleural fluid; recommended in the evaluation of nonresponding patients)

5. Blood cultures (recommended in patients with severe CAP, particularly if not on antibiotic therapy at the time of testing); usually shows pneumococcus, 50% to 80% of positive samples; defines antibiotic susceptibility

Management

A. Hospital systems may have their own guidelines based on local epidemiology. It is important to know the guidelines for management in the system that one practiced in.

B. Provide oxygen to maintain partial oxygen pressure in arterial blood > mmHg or oxygen saturation >88% in COPD patients and >92% in non-COPD patients.

C. General guidelines for previously healthy adults in the community with no antibiotic use in the past 3 months include the following:

1. Amoxicillin now recommended for first-line due to increased resistance

2. Azithromycin, clarithromycin, or erythromycin should be used in areas where resistance to macrolides are <25%.

3. An alternative is doxycycline.

D. Comorbid conditions, immunosuppressed, antibiotic use in the past 3 months:

1. Levofloxacin, moxifloxacin, amoxicillin, or amoxicillin-clavulanate + macrolide/doxycycline

Patient Disposition

A. Clinical judgment and use of a validated severity of illness score are recommended to determine inpatient management as indicated.

B. Indications for hospital admission

1. Hypoxemia (oxygen saturation <90% while on room air)

2. Hemodynamic instability

3. Inability to tolerate medications

4. Active coexisting condition requiring hospitalization

C. *Pneumonia Severity Index (PSI):* Used to calculate the probability of morbidity and mortality among patients with CAP.[31] PSI is risk stratified from I–V. PSI risk class from I–II can be treated as outpatients and class IV to V should be hospitalized. Calculation support can be found at: www.mdcalc.com/psi-port-sccore-pneumonia-severity-index-cap

D. *CURB-65 or CRB 65:* A severity of illness score for stratifying adults with CAP into different management groups (www.mdcalc.com/curb-65-severity-severity-score-community-acquired-pneumonia)

E. *SMART-COP:* Systolic BP, multilobar chest radiography, albumin, RR, tachycardia, confusion, oxygen level, and arterial pH—a newer method to predict which patients will require intensive respiratory/vasopressor support. A score of ≥3 has a sensitivity of 92% to identify patients who may require intensive treatment.

F. Patients with CHF or COPD are more likely to require ICU admission.

G. Clinical judgment may be more accurate than following conflicting clinical decision tools.

H. Basic treatment considerations

1. Analgesia and antipyretics

2. IV fluids (and conversely, diuretics) may be indicated.

3. Pulse oximetry

4. Oxygen supplementation

5. Positioning to minimize aspiration risk

I. Patient education upon discharge

1. Return for worsening symptoms such as increased SOB, fever not resolving with antipyretics or chest pain

2. Refrain from smoking or vaping.

3. Maintain good oral hydration.

4. Yearly immunizations for influenza

5. 23-valent pneumococcal polysaccharides vaccine in the appropriate setting

Healthcare-Associated Pneumonia/ Hospital-Acquired Pneumonia

Nosocomial pneumonia is an acute infection of the pulmonary parenchyma acquired in healthcare settings. Healthcare-associated pneumonia (HCAP) occurs in a nonhospitalized patient with extensive healthcare contact such as residing in a long-term care facility, hospitalization in an acute care hospital for ≤2 days within the past 90 days, or has been in a hemodialysis clinic for the past 30 days. Hospital-acquired pneumonia (HAP) occurs ≥48 hours after admission and did not appear to be incubating at the time of admission. HAP is the leading cause of death among nosocomial infections and is one of the leading causes of death in the ICU.

Etiology and Pathophysiology

A. Aerobic gram-negative bacilli; *Pseudomonas aeruginosa*, Escherichia coli, *Klebsiella pneumoniae*, and *Acinetobacter* sp.

B. Gram-positive cocci; *Streptococcus* sp., and *Staphylococcus aureus* (including methicillin-resistant *Staphylococcus aureus* [MRSA])

Risk Factors, History, Physical Exam, Differential Diagnoses, Diagnostic Tests

A. *See "Community-Acquired Pneumonia" section.*

Management

A. Use IV antibiotics, treat for 7 days minimum
B. Early-onset (<5 days) and no risk factors for multidrug-resistant pathogens
  1. Piperacillin-tazobactam, Cefepime, levofloxacin, imipenem, or meropenem
C. Late-onset (≥5 days) or risk factors for multidrug-resistant pathogens (antibiotic therapy in preceding 90 days, high frequency of antibiotic resistance in community/hospital immunosuppressive disease/therapy (risk factors for HCAP)
D. MRSA coverage: Linezolid or vancomycin + one drug from each group noted below:
  1. Cefepime, ceftazidime, imipenem, meropenem, or piperacillin-tazobactam
  2. Levofloxacin, ciprofloxacin, aztreonam, or aminoglycosides (amikacin, gentamicin, or tobramycin)
E. Drug-resistant *Streptococcus pneumoniae* should be treated with high-dose amoxicillin, amoxicillin/clavulanate, or cefpodoxime with a macrolide, or a respiratory fluoroquinolone
F. Basic treatment considerations
  1. *See "Community-Acquired Pneumonia" section.*

Patient Disposition

A. Requires admission for IV antibiotic administration and close monitoring

PLEURAL DISEASE

The pleural cavity is considered a potential space. It can become a true space when it is affected by air, fluid, or a tumor. These can lead to critical life-threatening emergencies. The pleural anatomy consists of two membranous components that include the parietal pleura and visceral pleura. The parietal pleura lines the chest wall, the diaphragm, and the mediastinum. The visceral pleura covers the lung surface and goes into the fissures of the lobes. The pleural space and the fluid within it allow the lungs to move within the chest wall. Only a minimal amount of pleural fluid is needed for adequate function. The parietal pleura is innervated by somatic intercostal nerves except for the central diaphragm, which is innervated by the phrenic nerve. Pain complaints are related to the partial pleura, not the visceral pleura. Pleural pain is generally referred to the same shoulder side.[32] Three specific pleural emergencies will be discussed.[32–36]

Pleural Effusion[32,34–37]

Pleural effusion, which is a common problem, is caused by an accumulation of excessive fluid between the pleural spaces that cover the lungs. There is a small amount of fluid (approximately 15 mL) normally within these spaces; however, an increase of excessive fluid is a pleural effusion. There are multiple causes that require a systematic assessment of the potential cause of the effusion. This will help direct the management of pleural effusion in the emergency care environment.

Pathophysiology[35]

A. The underlying mechanisms that may cause a pleural effusion include the following:
  1. Obstructed lymphatic flow
  2. Reduced tissue osmotic pressure
  3. Excessive negative intrapleural pressure
  4. Increased permeability of the pleural membrane
  5. Reduced tissue oncotic pressure
  6. Fluid movement from the peritoneum
B. The effusion can be caused by transudate or exudate fluid. [*See "Pleuritis (Pleurisy)" section for definitions.*]

Etiologies of Pleural Effusion

A. Transudates
  1. Trapped lung
  2. Nephrotic syndrome
  3. Congestive heart failure (CHF)
  4. Cirrhosis of the liver
  5. Hypoalbuminemia
  6. Pulmonary embolism (PE)
B. Exudates
  1. Malignancy
  2. Pneumonia
  3. Post coronary artery bypass grafting (CABG)
  4. Viral pneumonia
  5. PE
  6. Collagen vascular disease

Predisposing Factors[35]

A. Chronic illnesses such as cirrhosis or renal disease
B. Tuberculosis
C. CHF
D. Malignancy
E. Medications
  1. Amiodarone
  2. Nitrofurantoin
  3. Phenytoin
  4. Methotrexate
  5. Cabergoline
  6. Pergolide
  7. Dasatinib

Clinical Presentation

A. Dependent upon the patient's respiratory status and the volume of the accumulation of fluid
B. Shortness of breath
C. Tachypnea
D. Hypoxemia
E. Tachycardia
F. Sharp chest pain
G. Fever (if infectious origin)

Physical Examination

A. Dependent on the amount of accumulated fluid
B. Generally, no physical findings in effusions of less than 300 mL
C. Asymmetrical chest expansion
D. Mediastinal shift away from the side of the effusion

E. Decreased or absent breath sounds
F. Decreased or absent tactile fremitus
G. Dullness to percussion on the affected side
H. Bronchial breath sounds can be auscultated above the effusion
I. Egophony changes
J. Pleural friction rub

Differential Diagnoses

A. Pneumothorax
B. CHF
C. PE
D. Cystic fibrosis
E. Lung cancer
F. Neuromuscular disease
G. Pulmonary infection
H. Drug-induced
I. Connective tissue disease (rheumatoid arthritis, lupus pleuritis)
J. Central venous catheter migration

Diagnostic Testing

A. Chest radiograph
B. Thoracic ultrasound (TUS) examination
C. CT of the chest may be needed depending on the complexity of the disease
D. Thoracentesis (*See previous procedure*). This procedure can be used for diagnosis as well as management.
E. CBC, BNP, renal and liver function, gram stain, and culture of fluid
F. Pleural fluid should be evaluated using *Light's Criteria* for pleural effusion (healthjade.net). Criteria include the following:
   1. Effusion protein/serum protein ratio greater than 0.5
   2. Effusion lactate dehydrogenase (LDH)/serum LDH ratio greater than 0.6
   3. Effusion LDH level greater than two-thirds the upper limit of the laboratory's reference range of serum LDH

Management

A. Assist with patient's breathing as indicated by the patient's presentation (see Chapter 6).
B. If the effusion is asymptomatic and has no indication for drainage, patient should be observed, and conservative management can be considered.
C. Thoracentesis (see *Thoracentesis)* to identify the cause of the effusion
   1. Pus indication of infection
   2. Blood indication of a hemothorax
   3. Determine if effusion is transudate or exudate fluid. [See the "Pleuritis (Pleurisy)" section.]
D. Chest tube drainage is indicated in patients with pleural fluid pH <7.2; positive pleural fluid microbiology; or purulent pleural fluid (*see Primary Spontaneous Pneumothorax*).
E. Possible insertion of a pleural catheter for symptoms relieved by thoracentesis.
F. Consult with appropriate medical support depending on the cause of the effusion. Surgery may be required in some situations.
G. Pharmacological treatment
   1. Intrapleural fibrinolytics may be used to treat loculated infected effusions, the presence of septae, and fibrinous pleural rind formation. Patients who are not candidates for surgery may also benefit from this treatment.
   2. Amoxicillin for first-line treatment for community-acquired pleural infection. May require longer courses for effective treatment. Culture and sensitivity will assist in identifying appropriate antibiotics especially if a broader cover may be required.

Patient Disposition

A. Depending on the size and the cause of the effusion, patient may be able to be observed in the ED if treatment is successful.
B. Patient with a large effusion requiring a chest tube will need admission.
C. Referral for follow-up is needed depending on the cause of the effusion.

Pleuritis (Pleurisy)[32,33,37]

Pleuritis results from inflammation from a bacterium, virus, or parasite, which affects the pleural layers of the lung. It is often associated with pleural effusion.

Pathophysiology

A. Causes of pleuritis include the following:
   1. Infection from bacteria, virus, or parasites
   2. Tumor or cancer of the lungs
   3. Inhaling toxic substances
   4. Pulmonary embolus
   5. Autoimmune diseases such as rheumatoid arthritis or lupus
   6. Trauma to the chest

Clinical Presentation

A. Chest pain aggravated by breathing
B. Pain will decrease with breath-holding
C. Shortness of breath
D. Chest wall tenderness
E. May have back and shoulder pain
F. Cough and fever may be present at times.

Physical Examination

A. Pain with inspiration
B. Chest wall tenderness with palpation
C. Cough
D. Fever
E. Shortness of breath
F. Pulmonary friction rub

Differential Diagnoses

A. Pleural effusion
B. Traumatic chest injury
C. Pulmonary tumor

Diagnostic Testing

A. Chest radiograph
B. CT of the chest

C. Ultrasound of the chest
D. Complete blood count (CBC) to rule out infection
E. EKG to rule out a cardiac source
F. Thoracentesis to obtain fluid for evaluation and treatment (*see Needle Aspiration Procedure under Primary Spontaneous Pneumothorax*):
  1. *Exudate fluid:* High in protein, sugar, LDH enzyme, and white blood cells (WBCs), which can indicate an infection, tuberculosis, cancer
  2. *Transudate fluid:* Normal fluid that can indicate congestive heart failure (CHF), liver, and renal failure

Management

A. Splinting of the chest wall to help breathing and decrease pain
B. Take medications as directed.
C. Stop smoking or inhaling substances.
D. Get rest.
E. Drink fluids.
F. Attend follow-up appointments as directed (that is, pulmonologist, rheumatologist, oncologist) to determine and manage the cause of the symptoms.
G. **Pharmacological treatment**
  1. Anti-inflammatory drugs for pain and to decrease inflammation
    a. Steroids
    b. Ibuprofen or naproxen
  2. Cough syrup to help manage cough that will also help manage the chest pain
  3. Antibiotics if an infection is found

Patient Disposition

A. Depending on the severity of the symptoms, patient may need to be admitted or placed in the observation area.
B. Indications for return to the ED include increasing shortness of breath, coughing, fever, and chills
C. Follow-up plan developed and reviewed with patient depending on the findings

Primary Spontaneous Pneumothorax[32–34]

Primary spontaneous pneumothorax has been defined as a pneumothorax that occurs in individuals without a history of lung disease. However, technology has found that many patients do have underlying lung abnormalities. Smoking has been found to be one of the greatest risk factors.[33]

Pathophysiology[32,33]

A. Break in the parietal pleura
B. Air accumulates in the intrapleural space.
C. Air pressure achieves equilibrium, which will result in either partial or complete collapse of the lung.
D. Results in hypoxemia related to the shunting and a lower ventilation/perfusion ratio
E. Amount of shunting will determine the size of the pneumothorax.

Etiology and Demographics

A. Statistics have shown that 7.4 to 18 cases per 100,000 in males and 1.2 to 6 per 100,000 in females.
B. Smoking contributes to a high risk for the development of a spontaneous pneumothorax.
C. May be related to other specific disease processes such as Marfan's syndrome

Predisposing Factors

A. Smoking—research has found the number of cigarettes smoked daily increases the overall risk.
B. Inherited factors such as Marfan's syndrome and homocystinuria.
C. Anorexia nervosa probably related to malnutrition damaging the pulmonary parenchyma
D. Thoracic endometriosis
E. Chronic obstructive pulmonary disease (COPD)
F. Endemic tuberculosis
G. Pulmonary infections including Pneumocystis pneumonia
H. Ehrler's-Danlos syndrome
I. Cystic fibrosis
J. Esophageal rupture

Clinical Presentation

A. Chest pain
B. Dry cough
C. Hyperpnea
D. Fatigue
E. Dyspnea

Physical Examination

A. Shortness of breath (SOB)
B. Tachycardia
C. Decreased breath sounds on affected side
D. Hyperresonance
E. *Severe symptoms:* Respiratory distress, tachycardia, hypotension, tracheal deviation, cyanosis, possible tension pneumothorax

Differential Diagnoses

A. Traumatic chest injury
B. Pneumonia
C. Asthma
D. COPD
E. Pulmonary embolus

Diagnostic Testing

A. Chest radiograph
  1. The American College of Chest Physicians (ACCP) defines the size of a pneumothorax by the distance measured from the apex of the lung to the ipsilateral thoracic cupola at the parietal surface. A small pneumothorax is defined as less than 3 cm and a large pneumothorax one as greater than 3 cm.[33]
  2. Ultrasonography
  3. CT of the chest

Management

A. *Observation:* Less than 20% without causing any respiratory compromise.[34] Use of oxygen is recommended.

It can help accelerate the rate of pleural air absorption. It works by causing a significant partial pressure gradient for nitrogen across the tissue capillary bed from the pneumothorax space increasing the absorption rate of the pneumothorax.[34]

B. Needle aspiration (thoracentesis) with a 14 to 16 G IV, usually done with a cannula than a needle to prevent injury to the lungs.[34,37]

1. Equipment
   a. Antiseptic swab
   b. Large bore over the needle catheter
   c. Syringe
   d. Stopcock
   e. Drain
   f. Extension kit
   g. Connection tubing
2. Procedure
   a. Assemble and organize the equipment.
   b. Cleanse the site with antiseptic swabs.
   c. Select anatomic landmark.
      i. Second intercostal space over the top of the rib in the midclavicular line
      ii. Fourth or fifth intercostal space on the anterior midaxillary line of the affected side
   d. Insert needle over the superior aspect of the rib at a 90° angle and push into the intercostal space.
   e. Attach the syringe and aspirate to confirm placement.
   f. Advance catheter to the hub.
   g. Remove needle or if using a catheter, leave it in.
   h. Attach the extension set.
   i. Attach the drainage tube.

C. If a needle aspiration does not improve the patient's symptoms, a chest tube is recommended.[37]

1. Equipment
   a. Antiseptic swabs
   b. Sterile drape and towels
   c. Sterile gloves
   d. Lidocaine or another appropriate anesthetic
   e. No. 10 scalpel
   f. Large, curved clamp
   g. Large straight clamp
   h. 28 to 32 French tubes (adults)
   i. Water seal drainage equipment
   j. Needle holder
   k. 0-silk suture
   l. Sterile gauze and tape
2. Procedure
   a. Procedural sedation may be necessary.
   b. Assemble and organize equipment.
   c. Place patient's arm over the head, in females displace breast tissue.
   d. Surgically prepare the area for insertion.
   e. Anesthetize the subcutaneous tissue and the periosteum of underlying rib.
   f. After anesthetizing the underlying rib, gently advance the needle and alternately aspirate and inject lidocaine into the pleural fluid.
   g. Identify the insertion site at the fourth or fifth intercostal space on the affected side. Insertion site is one rib below the insertion site. Making the incision below the insertion allows for a subcutaneous tunnel to be formed to aid in tract sealing.
   h. Clamp the proximal end of the chest tube.
   i. Make a 2 to 4 cm vertical incision along the fifth or sixth rib just anterior to the midaxillary line through the skin and subcutaneous tissue.
   j. Insert a curved clamp and advance toward the superior aspect of the rib. Strong controlled force is needed with the intention of not causing any iatrogenic injury.
   k. Enter the thorax at the fourth or fifth intercostal space between the lateral border of the pectoralis major and the medial border of the latissimus dorsi.
   l. Enter the pleural cavity by penetrating the intercostal muscles and parietal pleura superiorly over the rib to avoid damage to the neurovascular bundle below each rib.
   m. Insert a gloved finger into the thoracic cavity to perform a digital examination.
   n. Using a finger or curved clamp as a guide, insert the chest tube past the last hole into the thoracic cavity in a posterior and superior direction.
   o. Attach the chest tube to a suction device or one-way flutter valve.
   p. Secure the tube to the skin, preferably with a purse-string suture.
   q. Place a sterile dressing over the area.
   r. Ensure that all the tube connection sites are secure as well as the chest tube itself to prevent dislodgement.
   s. Chest radiograph should be obtained to confirm tube placement.
   t. Monitor tube function.

Complications

A. Extrapleural placement
B. Infection
C. Pulmonary vessel laceration
D. Intercostal vessel laceration
E. Incorrect placement such as in the subcutaneous tissue
F. Injury to the abdominal organs, that is, liver or spleen

Patient Disposition

A. Patient will require observation.
B. Discharge or admission will be based on the procedure required to manage the pneumothorax.
C. If discharged, the patient and family will require education about procedure management as well as indications to return to the ED.

Upper Respiratory Tract Infections[38–42]

A mild upper respiratory tract infection is frequently referred to as "the common cold." It is generally a benign self-limited illness caused by several families of viruses. The common cold is one of the most frequent acute illnesses throughout the industrialized world and the United States, with two to three episodes of illness per year in adults. It is not possible to identify the likely viral pathogen based on clinical symptoms, due to the over 200 subtypes of viruses associated with the disease. The majority of URIs are transmitted by hand contact and may remain viable on human skin for up to 2 hours.

Pathophysiology

A. Symptoms of the common cold are primarily due to the immune response to infection, rather than viral damage to the respiratory tract. Fever is rare in adults. Host factors including age, prior immunological experience, and underlying illnesses influence the intensity and type of symptoms experienced. Symptoms vary from person to person the most common being:

1. Rhinitis
2. Nasal congestion
3. Sore throat
4. Cough
5. Malaise

Physical Examination

A. Awake, alert, and oriented to person, place, and time (AAO × 3)

B. Normal heart sounds, S1, S2, no murmurs, rubs, or gallops (MRG)

C. Breathing should be nonlabored, breath sounds normal, good air exchange. Pulse oxygenation should be greater than 92% on room air. Respiratory rate should be less than 20 breaths per minute.

D. Mucous membranes should be moist, throat clear (maybe mildly injected), uvula midline

E. Skin warm, dry, well-perfused

Differential Diagnoses

A. Diagnosis is generally based on clinical exam and reported symptoms and/or observed signs. Patients should appear only mildly ill, taking adequate PO and in no true respiratory distress. If any of their signs and symptoms are outside of the expected norm, then further evaluation is warranted

1. Differential: URI (viral), influenza, pneumonia, pharyngitis, acute bronchitis allergic rhinitis, pertussis, and acute bacterial rhinosinusitis

Diagnostic Testing

A. Based on physical examination. If normal, no further testing is necessary.

Management

A. Symptomatic treatment, rest, oral hydration, NSAIDs such as naproxen or ibuprofen.

Patient Disposition

A. Outpatient treatment based on the patient's diagnosis.

B. *Patient education:* Rest, drink plenty of fluids, NSAIDs for muscle aches and pains. Return to the ED for worsening symptoms, such as SOB, chest pain, inability to take adequate oral fluids, fever, or productive cough.

Additional Resources

Pneumonia Severity Index (PSI): http://www.mdcalc.com/psi-port-sccore-pneumonia-severity-index-cap

CURB-65 or CRB 65: http://www.mdcalc.com/curb-65-severity-severity-score-community-acquired-pneumonia

References

References for this chapter are online only and can be found at https://connect.springerpub.com/content/reference-book/978-0-8261-6091-5/part/part02/toc-part/ch14.

15. Cardiovascular Medical Emergencies

COLLEEN ANDREONI | LORI HULL-GROMMESH

Learning Objectives

Chest Pain and Acute Coronary Syndrome

- Identify common differential diagnoses for patients presenting with chest pain.
- Identify EKG findings consistent with cardiovascular conditions.
- Discuss emergent diagnostic studies and management of patients presenting with acute coronary syndrome (ACS).

Heart Failure and Atrial Fibrillation

- Define congestive heart failure and the common presenting signs/symptoms of ED presentation.
- Describe the pharmacological and nonpharmacological approaches to the emergent treatment of congestive heart failure.
- Examine the common arrhythmias patients present to the ED with and the associated signs/symptoms and emergent treatments.

Acute Coronary Syndrome

COLLEEN ANDREONI

Acute coronary syndrome (ACS) is a collection of clinical conditions, including non-ST-elevation myocardial infarction (NSTEMI), unstable angina (UA), ST-elevation myocardial infarction (STEMI), and cardiac death. Plaque erosions and ruptures in the coronary arteries are the pathophysiologic causes of ACS. Intervention for ACS includes both interventional percutaneous revascularization and also antithrombotic treatment. The role of the emergency clinician is to rapidly identify whether the patient is experiencing an acute myocardial infarction (AMI) and implement early interventions. However, the patient may not be experiencing an AMI but continues to have an ACS, manifesting as UA. The patient with UA will benefit from early coronary intervention to decrease the risk of major adverse cardiac events (MACE). Thus, the role of the ED clinician is to rule out ACS, not only the AMI.

Medical Screening

A. *Chief complaint:* Chest pain

1. History, EKG, cardiac biomarkers, and chest x-ray (CXR) are the primary components of evaluating a patient presenting to the ED with chest pain.
2. History alone is an unreliable predictor of AMI.
3. Atypical symptoms cannot rule out ACS and typical symptoms cannot rule in ACS.
4. Women may present with no chest discomfort or with other symptoms. Chest pain at presentation to the ED is less likely in women ≤45 years of age with an AMI. Women often have atypical symptoms such as fatigue, dyspnea, indigestion, weakness, anxiety, sleep disturbances, or palpitations. Women >65 years with ACS have less chest pain and more dyspnea.

B. Signs and symptoms

1. Chest pain described as tightness, pressure, squeezing, or heavy
2. Pain may radiate to the jaw, neck, shoulder, back, arms, or epigastrium.
3. Acute onset most likely worse with exertion
4. Nausea, vomiting, diaphoresis, dyspnea, lightheadedness, fatigue, indigestion
5. Hypotension

C. *Focused assessment:* Priority is given to immediate life threats.

1. History
   a. Prior history of coronary artery disease (CAD) or myocardial infarction (MI), smoking, hypertension (HTN), hyperlipidemia (HL), diabetes mellitus (DM), peripheral arterial disease (PAD)
   b. Family history of CAD, sudden cardiac deaths, MI before age 60
   c. Recent physical exertion or psychological stress
2. Focused physical exam
   a. *General:* Diaphoresis, behavior, color, temperature
   b. *Cardiac:* Peripheral pulse quality, rate and rhythm, heart sounds, jugular vein distention (JVD), edema, blood pressure (BP)
   c. *Pulmonary:* Respiratory rate, quality, use of accessory muscles, breath sounds, pulse oximetry

Medical Decision-Making and Differential Diagnoses

A. Decision-making tools are used in the evaluation of patients presenting with chest pain to support risk stratification and safe disposition. The emphasis is often on early discharge of patients after risk stratification using an objective tool. The success of decision-making tools used in the risk stratification of chest pain is measured by the incidence of MACE for a certain period.

B. Knowledge and familiarity with the troponin assay used will assist in choosing the best medical decision aid. Formal risk stratification tools such as Thrombolysis in Myocardial Infarction (TIMI) consider all components of ACS.

C. TIMI score

1. The primary purpose is to identify patients at low risk for an ACS although they have a history of previous ACS.

2. The TIMI score assists with decision-making by ruling out NSTEMI or UA.

3. The TIMI score combines age, presence of ≥3 risk factors for CAD (family history, HTN, HL, DM, and/or active smoker), known CAD with stenosis >50%, aspirin use within the past 7 days, angina within the past 24 hrs, elevated cardiac markers (cTn), and ST deviation ≥0.5 mm.

4. The clinical threshold for identification of patients who are considered low risk is a TIMI score = 0 with a 99% sensitivity.

5. When the threshold is increased to a score of 1, the sensitivity is decreased to 98% and decreased to < 98% with a TIMI score of 2.

6. Although 98% sensitivity appears favorable and would place more patients in the low-risk group, allowing for earlier disposition, the risk for MACE is increased.

D. HEART score[1,2,3]

1. Designed in 2015 for risk stratification of ED patients with chest pain

2. Combines history, EKG, age, risk factors, and cTn at 0 and 3-hour intervals

3. Both high-sensitivity cardiac troponin hs-cTn and contemporary cTn have been used. Each component is assigned a score of 0, 1, or 2 points.

4. Patients are categorized as low risk if scoring 0 to 3, and as intermediate–high risk if scoring ≥4. A score of 4 is predictive of worse cardiac outcomes at 6 weeks and 1 year.

5. Men have a higher 6-week risk of MACE across all HEART risk categories; consider this when determining a disposition for low-risk HEART score patients.[4]

E. ED Assessment of Chest Pain Score (EDACS)

1. Accelerated Diagnostic Protocol (EDACS-ADP)

2. Designed to identify patients with chest pain who may be safely discharged. Patients are assigned positive or negative values based on clinical characteristics including age, sex, age between 18 and 50 years with either known CAD or ≥3 risk factors, signs/symptoms of diaphoresis, radiation of pain, pain worse with inspiration, and pain reproduced by palpation.

3. Early discharge is considered for patients with a score of ≤16, no new ischemia on EKG, and negative cTn at 0 and 2 hours after presentation to ED.

F. The EDACS-ADP did not achieve a 99% negative predictive value (NPV) for MACE, which many experts believe is the acceptable level.[5]

G. Manchester Acute Coronary Syndromes (MACS) decision aid[1,2]

1. Combines clinical symptoms, EKG findings, heart-type fatty acid-binding protein (h-FABP), and troponin T (hs-cTnT) concentration at time of arrival.

2. Based on a <2% probability, patients can be ruled out for ACS, or on a >95% probability, ruled in immediately for ACS.

3. Patients are then categorized to be low risk or moderate risk and await serial troponins. (Studied extensively in the United Kingdom).

H. Troponin-only Manchester Acute Coronary Syndromes (T-MACS)[1,2]

1. Clinical rule to assess risk in patients presenting to ED with chest pain, as above, except that h-FABP is not measured.

2. Patients are very low risk if their probability is <2%, low risk if 2% to 5%, moderate risk if 5% to 95%, and high risk if >95%.

3. These probabilities of a MACE within 30 days are used to determine disposition from the ED (studied extensively in the UK).

I. ADAPT ADP (2-hour ADP)[1,2]

1. Combines TIMI score with troponin at 0 and 2 hours.

2. Consider discharge if hs-cTnT, 14 ng/L at 0 and 2 hours and TIMI score <1 and normal EKG. If using hs-cTnI, consider discharge if hs-cTnI <26 ng/L at 0 and 2 hours and TIMI <1 and normal EKG.

Diagnostic Testing

A. Cardiac biomarkers[6]

1. Cardiac biomarkers (cTnI or cTnT or hs-TnI). Cardiac troponin (cTn) requires serial troponin testing over 3 to 12 hours.

2. The Fourth Universal Definition of Myocardial Infarction for both STEMI and NSTEMI includes the use of myocardial necrosis biomarkers, preferably cTnI or cTnT.[7]

3. High-sensitivity troponin (hs-cTn) can identify low-risk patients in single test (recommended 2–3 hours after initial onset of symptoms) or serial testing if presentation to ED is less than 3 hours.

4. Most low-risk patients with a normal EKG undergoing evaluation for ACS may be safely discharged with a single hs-cTn value of less than the level of detection (LOD) after 3 hours.[7]

5. The use of a changing pattern, rising and/or falling, can help differentiate between chronic hs-cTn elevation and an AMI. Chronic conditions that may result in hs-cTn elevations include congestive heart failure and end-stage renal disease. The serial hs-cTn values will remain elevated and unchanging.[7]

B. EKG

1. ~14% of patients have a diagnostic EKG.

2. See Table 15.1 EKG Findings in ACS

3. The presence of a left bundle branch block (LBBB) alone does not indicate an acute coronary occlusion.[9]

a. Use the weighted Sgarbossa score to evaluate EKG with LBBB.

TABLE 15.1 EKG FINDINGS IN ACUTE CORONARY SYNDROME

	STEMI LEADS OF INJURY AND INFARCTION: INJURY: ST ELEVATION ≥1 MM ABOVE BASELINE INFARCTION: Q WAVE ≥0.03 SECONDS WIDE AND >1 MM BELOW BASELINE	NSTEMI CONSIDERATIONS: INJURY: TRANSIENT ST SEGMENT ELEVATION ≥0.5 MM ISCHEMIA: ST SEGMENT DEPRESSION ≥0.5 MM OR DYNAMIC T WAVE INVERSION	RECIPROCAL LEADS: AMI MAY PRODUCE ST-SEGMENT DEPRESSION OR INVERTED T WAVES IN LEADS OPPOSITE OF THOSE INDICATING ACUTE INJURY	CORONARY ARTERY
Inferior wall	II, III, aVF	II, III, aVF	I, aVL	Right coronary artery
Anterior wall	V2, V3, V4	V2, V3, V4	None	Left circumflex
Lateral wall	I, aVL, V5, V6	I, aVL, V5, V6	II, III, aVF	Left circumflex
Septal wall	V1 and V2	V1 and V2	None	Left coronary artery—septal branch
Anteroseptal	V1, V2, V3, V4	V1, V2, V3, V4	None	Left circumflex or right coronary artery (RCA) posterior branch
Anterolateral	I, aVL, V3, V4, V5, V6	I, aVL, V3, V4, V5, V6	II, III, aVF	Left circumflex
Posterior	None	None	V1, V2, V3, V4	

Source: Yiadom, M.Y.A.B. (2018). Acute coronary syndromes: Myocardial infarction and unstable angina. In Cydulka RK, Fitch MT, Joing SA, Wang VJ, Cline DM, Ma OJ. (Eds.), Tintinalli's emergency medicine manual. (8th ed.). McGraw-Hill; Green, GB, Hill, PM. (2011). Chest pain: Cardiac or not. In Tintinalli JE, Stapczynski J, Ma OJ, Cline DM, Cydulka RK, Meckler GD. Cardiovascular disease. In: Tintinalli's Emergency Medicine: a comprehensive study guide. (7th ed.). McGraw-Hill[6,8]

SGARBOSSA SCORE

CRITERIA	SCORE
ST elevation ≥1 mm concordant with QRS complex	5 points
ST depression ≥1 mm in leads V1, V2, or V3	3 points
ST elevation ≥5 mm discordant with QRS complex*	2 points

b. A Sgarbossa score of ≥3 indicates acute coronary occlusion.

c. A modified Sgarbossa score improves the sensitivity and specificity. The third criteria of a weighted Sgarbossa score is replaced by evaluation of the ST/S ratio (ST elevation/S wave amplitude): the ratio of ST segment elevation measured at J point to the R or S wave, whichever is most prominent and in discordance of the ST segment in the opposite direction of QRS complex.[10] A score of < -0.25 indicates acute coronary occlusion.

4. *Nonspecific ST segment and T wave changes (NSSTTW):* ≤1 mm ST elevation or depression with or without reciprocal changes. This condition may be indicative of a later cardiac event.[11,12]

5. *Consider augmented Vector Right (aVR) lead:* aVR elevation of ST with concomitant diffuse ST depression is associated with diffuse subendocardial ischemia and an indication of acute coronary occlusion.

6. T wave inversion in augmented Vector Left (aVL) lead not seen in other leads should not be considered insignificant or normal. It may indicate right ventricular involvement and/or imminent inferior AMI.[11,12]

7. Wellens' syndrome is suggestive of stenosis of the left anterior descending (LAD) coronary artery, which can progress to an anterior AMI.

a. *Type A:* Deeply inverted T waves in V2 and V3

b. *Type B:* Biphasic T waves in V2 and V3

Management: STEMI[8,13]

Acute STEMI indicates irreversible myocardial injury resulting in necrosis of the myocardium. The goal is immediate reperfusion and limitation of infarct size. Reperfusion may be achieved by percutaneous coronary intervention (PCI) or by fibrinolysis with antiplatelet and antithrombin therapy. See Figure 15.1 for management considerations for the patient with ACS.

A. Procedures STEMI

1. Advanced cardiac life support (ACLS) measures as necessary

2. *Pharmacologic therapies:* STEMI

a. Follow evidence-based guidelines when prescribing.

b. *Oxygen:* 2 L by cannula or higher flow to maintain pulse oximetry above 90% to 92%.

c. *Nitroglycerine (NTG):* Has direct vasodilator effects on coronary vessels and can increase myocardial blood flow.

i. NTG 0.4 mg SL every 5 minutes × 3 prn pain

ii. NTG infusion start at 10 mcg/min, titrate to between 10% and 30% decrease in mean arterial pressure (MAP)

d. *Morphine*

e. *Beta-blockers:* Antiarrhythmic, anti-ischemic, and antihypertensive properties. Recommended for all STEMI patients unless contraindicated. Potentially harmful when risk factors for cardiogenic shock are present.

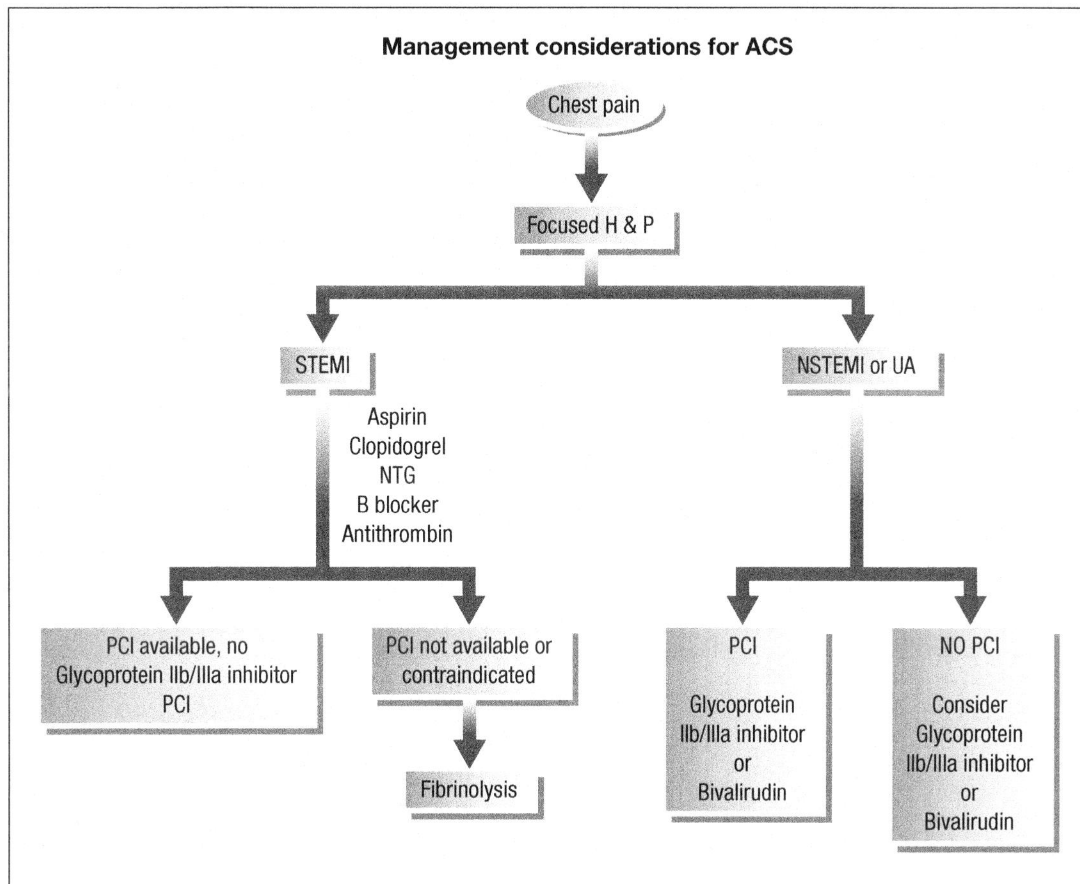

FIGURE 15.1 Management considerations for acute coronary syndrome (ACS).
NSTEMI, non-ST-segment elevation myocardial infarction; NTG, nitroglycerine; PCI, percutaneous coronary intervention; UA, unstable angina.

- **i.** Metoprolol
- **ii.** Atenolol

f. Antiplatelets

- **i.** Aspirin
- **ii.** Clopidogrel

g. Antithrombins, until PCI is performed

- **i.** Heparin
- **ii.** Enoxaparin
- **iii.** Fondaparinux

h. *Fibrinolytics:* Indicated as reperfusion option if time to treatment is <6 to 12 hours from symptom onset. The goal of fibrinolytic therapy administration (door to needle time) is ≤30 minutes. The risk of fibrinolytic therapy is hemorrhage. Absolute contraindications to fibrinolytics are prior intracerebral hemorrhage (ICH), known structural cerebral vascular lesion, known intracranial neoplasm, ischemic stroke <3 months ago, active internal bleeding, suspected aortic dissection, or pericarditis. Relative contraindications are also considered. Use of a standard fibrinolytic checklist to identify contraindications, both absolute and relative, is recommended.

- **i.** *Streptokinase:* If previously treated with streptokinase, patient should not receive it again.
- **ii.** Anistreplase
- **iii.** Alteplase (tPA)
- **iv.** Reteplase (rtPA)
- **v.** *Tenecteplase (TNK):* Weight-based dosing
- **vi.** Glycoprotein IIb/IIIa inhibitors inhibit platelet aggregation
  - **(1)** Abciximab
  - **(2)** Eptifibatide
  - **(3)** Tirofiban

B. *Consultation and collaboration:* STEMI

1. Cardiologist
2. Interventional cardiologist

C. *Disposition/transition of care:* STEMI

1. *PCI:* Immediate transfer to cath lab for coronary angiography and PCI for revascularization if door to balloon time is ≤90 minutes
2. Fibrinolysis for limited PCI availability, if the patient is >120 minutes from a PCI facility, or increased patient risk of complications from PCI

Management: NSTEMI[8]

A. *Procedures:* NSTEMI

1. ACLS measures as necessary

B. *Pharmacologic therapies:* NSTEMI

1. Follow evidence-based guidelines when prescribing.
2. *Oxygen:* 2 L by cannula or higher flow to maintain pulse oximetry above 90% to 92%

3. *NTG:* Has direct vasodilator effects on coronary vessels and can increase myocardial blood flow.
   a. NTG
   b. *NTG infusion:* Start at 10 mcg/min, titrate to between 10% and 30% decrease in MAP.
4. *Morphine*
5. *Betablockers:* Have antiarrhythmic, anti-ischemic and antihypertensive properties.
   a. Metoprolol
   b. Atenolol
6. Antiplatelets
   a. Aspirin
   b. Clopidogrel
7. Antithrombins
   a. Heparin
   b. Enoxaparin
   c. Fondaparinux
8. Direct thrombin inhibitor
   a. Bivalirudin
9. *Glycoprotein IIb/IIIa inhibitors:* Inhibit platelet aggregation
   a. Abciximab
   b. Eptifibatide
   c. Tirofiban

C. *Consultation and collaboration:* NSTEMI
   1. Cardiologist
   2. Interventional cardiologist

D. Patient disposition and transition of care for NSTEMI
   1. Transfer to cath lab after adequate evaluation of clinical indications, EKG and cTn, for coronary angiography and PCI for revascularization.

Management: Unstable Angina[8]

A. *Procedures:* UA
   1. ACLS measures as necessary

B. *Pharmacologic therapies:* UA
   1. Follow evidence-based guidelines when prescribing.
   2. *Oxygen*
   3. *NTG:* Has direct vasodilator effects on coronary vessels and can increase myocardial blood flow.
      a. NTG
      b. *NTG infusion:* Start at 10 mcg/min, titrate to between 10% to 30% decrease in MAP.
   4. *Morphine*
   5. *Beta-blockers:* Have antiarrhythmic, anti-ischemic and antihypertensive properties.
      a. Metoprolol
      b. Atenolol

C. *Consultation and collaboration:* UA
   1. Cardiologist

D. Patient disposition and transition of care for UA
   1. Consider admission to monitored bed, chest pain unit, or ED observation area. Further management may include coronary angiography with or without PCI.

Age and Developmental Considerations

A. Prevention and education
   1. Behaviors to decrease the risk of ACS
   2. No smoking
   3. Maintain good control of HTN and DM
   4. Compliance with medications
   5. Prompt evaluation of symptoms such as chest pain or shortness of breath (SOB)
   6. Regular primary care physician (PCP) and/or cardiology outpatient visits

B. Patient and family education and counseling
   1. End of life discussion and decisions, including Do Not Resuscitate (DNR) status and physician orders for life-sustaining treatment (POLST)

Documentation

A. Initial presentation and findings
B. Reassessments
C. Include the use of decision-making/risk stratification tools used.
D. Inclusion of family or friends present during discussions
E. Consultation with ED physician, cardiologist, radiologist, case manager, or others

Atrial Fibrillation

LORI HULL-GROMMESH

Arrhythmias are a common presenting condition in the ED. The emergency nurse practitioner (ENP) must be alert to arrhythmias and prepared to provide rapid diagnosis and intervention. The ENP must be aware that the arrhythmia is commonly a result of another underlying condition that must be treated, or it is the result of a chronic condition such as heart failure (HF). Arrhythmias can be divided into bradycardia arrhythmias and tachycardia arrhythmias, which include supraventricular, ventricular, and atrial tachycardias. The most commonly presenting arrhythmia is atrial fibrillation (AF). The ENP must accurately differentiate the arrhythmias from one another; for example, differentiating supraventricular arrhythmias from ventricular arrhythmias is critical to providing appropriate treatment as the treatment modalities are different. The ENP must be aware that sinus bradycardia and tachycardia can result from other conditions, and that anxiety, sleep, and exercise may be a compensatory response (e.g., hypotension with resultant tachycardia). The physical examination and 12-lead EKG can provide clues to diagnose the arrhythmia. The bradycardia arrhythmias include conduction delays and heart blocks. A common finding in the elderly is sick sinus syndrome.

Medical Screening

A. Chief complaint
   1. Palpitations
   2. Shortness of breath (SOB)
   3. Chest pain/discomfort
   4. Dizziness
   5. Syncope/fainting

B. Signs and symptoms
   1. Palpitations
   2. SOB

3. Chest pain/discomfort
4. Dizziness
5. Syncope/fainting
6. Hypotension
7. Diaphoresis
8. Signs of HF
9. Edema
10. Anxiety

C. Focused assessment
1. Priority is given to immediate life threats.
2. Be aware of the underlying causes of AF and atrial flutter. Atrial flutter is often precipitated by hyperthyroidism or catecholamine response, and is usually paroxysmal.
3. Focused history
a. Presence and description of symptoms associated with the AF
b. Assess whether the AF is a first-time episode, paroxysmal, or permanent.
c. Onset date of first occurrence
d. Precipitating factors and what helped or terminated the AF, including medications (e.g., digoxin, diltiazem)
e. Assess noncompliance to treatment regimen for AF and/or conditions that may have caused AF
f. Assess for the presence of underlying heart disease and reversible causes.
g. Prior history of known or family history of HF, CAD, HTN, DM, PAD, syncope, irregular or fast heartbeat
h. History of heart valve abnormalities or surgery
i. Recent hospitalization, especially for cardiac surgery or cardiac procedure
j. Recent illness, viral or bacterial infections
k. Recent or past use of illicit drugs or alcohol
l. Recent or past use of herbal or nonapproved FDA drugs
m. History of obstructive sleep apnea
n. Recent or ongoing stress, extreme fatigue, or exertion
4. Focused examination
a. The focused exam can give the ENP critical information quickly and help the ENP determine whether the patient is hemodynamically tolerating the AF.
b. *General:* Orientation, diaphoresis, behavior, color, temperature
c. *Cardiac:* Peripheral pulse quality, rate and rhythm, heart sounds, murmurs, jugular vein distension (JVD), edema, blood pressure (BP) in both arms
d. *Pulmonary:* Respiratory rate, quality, use of accessory muscles, splinting respirations, stridor, breath sounds, pulse oximetry, subcutaneous emphysema, presence of edema

Differential Diagnoses

A. Other atrial arrhythmias (e.g., atrial tachycardia, atrial flutter, atrioventricular nodal reentry tachycardia, multifocal atrial tachycardia, paroxysmal supraventricular tachycardia, and Wolff–Parkinson–White syndrome)

Diagnostic Testing

A. EKG
1. EKG should document a strip of greater than or equal to at least 30 seconds and document a rhythm with no P waves, or no discernable P waves, and is irregular.
2. Flutter waves are identified in atrial flutter. A 1:1 flutter may be regular. In greater than 1:1 conduction the rhythm may be regular or irregular.

B. Chest x-ray (CXR)
1. The CXR gives the ENP critical information as to possible contributing factors to the AF, especially CXR signs of fluid overload and/or HF.
2. Presence of vascular congestion, enlarged cardiac silhouette, infiltrates, pneumonia, pneumothorax, and other abnormalities, such as nodules or displaced trachea

C. Echocardiogram
1. Common abnormalities found on the echocardiogram can lead the ENP to suspect the patient is at high risk for AF.
2. Decreased left ventricular function and increased left ventricular size
3. Increased left/right atrial size
4. *Valvular heart abnormalities:* Regurgitation, stenosis, prolapse, bicuspid aortic valve, identification of vegetation on valve
5. Left ventricular hypertrophy (LVH)
6. Presence of left atrial thrombus (low sensitivity)
7. Pericardial effusion
8. Pulmonary HTN

D. Labs
1. Comprehensive metabolic profile, including renal and hepatic values
2. Troponin(s)
3. Brain natriuretic peptide (BNP)
4. Complete blood count (CBC)
5. Thyroid (thyroid-stimulating hormone [TSH])

Management

A. Management initially focuses on rate control of the atrial fibrillation (AF) or flutter.
1. Follow evidence-based guidelines when prescribing.
2. Control with beta-blockers; metoprolol tartrate is commonly used or nondihydropyridine calcium channel antagonists, such as diltiazem.
3. Rate control versus rhythm conversion can be controversial. Elective cardioversion is indicated in the hemodynamically unstable patient. Assessment of risk of stroke is paramount, and if elective cardioversion is determined to be needed, anticoagulation should be started with heparin if not contraindicated. Beta-blockers, nondihydropyridine calcium channel blockers, and antiarrhythmic medications may be used to manage AF.

B. Pharmacological cardioversion of AF is indicated in a hemodynamically stable patient, after consideration of the thromboembolic risk (genetic predisposition, history of previous thromboembolism, and increasing age).

C. In patients with a QTc interval >500 ms, arteriovenous (AV) conduction conditions, and/or sick sinus syndrome, pharmacological cardioversion attempts should not be done unless all risks for proarrhythmias and bradycardia are considered.[14]

D. In patients with AF, except with moderate-to-severe mitral stenosis or a mechanical heart valve), the CHA_2DS_2-VASc score is recommended for assessment of stroke risk. See Table 15.2.

E. Nonvitamin K antagonist oral anticoagulants (NOACs) are recommended in preference to vitamin K antagonists (VKAs), excluding patients with mechanical heart valves or moderate-to-severe mitral stenosis. In AF patients with acute coronary syndrome (ACS) undergoing an uncomplicated percutaneous coronary intervention, early cessation (≤1 week) of aspirin and continuation of dual therapy with an oral anticoagulation (OAC) and a P2Y12 inhibitor (preferably clopidogrel) for up to 12 months is recommended. Triple therapy with aspirin, clopidogrel, and an OAC for >1 week after an ACS should be considered when risk of stent thrombosis outweighs the bleeding risk, with the total duration (≤1 month).

F. Long-term OAC therapy to prevent thromboembolic events should be considered in patients at risk for stroke with postoperative AF after noncardiac surgery, taking into consideration the anticipated net clinical benefit of OAC and informed patient preferences. Beta-blockers should not be used routinely for the prevention of postoperative AF in patients undergoing noncardiac surgery (Class III).

G. Lenient rate control (heart rate <110 bpm on EKG) is often sufficient to improve AF-related symptoms. The primary indication for rhythm control is reduction in AF-related symptoms and improvement of quality of life. Catheter ablation is a well-established, safe, and superior alternative to antiarrhythmic drugs for maintenance of sinus rhythm.

H. CHA_2DS_2-VASc clinical stroke risk score should be used to identify patients at low risk (CHA_2DS_2-VASc score = 0 in men, or 1 in women), who should not be offered antithrombotic therapy. Antiplatelet therapy alone is not recommended for stroke prevention in AF (class III). Oral anticoagulation (OAC) is recommended for stroke prevention in AF patients with CHA_2DS_2-VASc score ≥2 in men or ≥3 in women, and it should be considered in patients with a CHA_2DS_2-VASc score of 1 in men or 2 in women, with treatment individualized based on net clinical benefit and patient values/preferences.

I. A bleeding risk assessment (HAS-BLED) is recommended to help identify patients at high risk of

TABLE 15.2 STROKE RISK STRATIFICATION WITH CHA_2DS_2-VASC SCORING

	CONDITION	SCORE
C	Congestive heart failure (or left ventricular systolic dysfunction)	1
H	*Hypertension*: Blood pressure consistently above 140/90 mmHg (or treated hypertension on medication)	1
A_2	Age ≥75 years	2
D	Diabetes mellitus	1
S_2	Prior *stroke* or *TIA* or *thromboembolism*	2
V	Vascular disease (e.g., peripheral artery disease, myocardial infarction, aortic plaque)	1
A	Age 65–74 years	1
Sc	Sex category (i.e., female sex)	1
		9

TIA, transient ischemic attacks.
Source: Lip GY, Nieuwlaat R, Pisters R, Lane DA, Crijns HJ. Refining clinical risk stratification for predicting stroke and thromboembolism in atrial fibrillation using a novel risk factor-based approach: the Euro Heart Survey on Atrial Fibrillation. *Chest.* 2010;137:263–272.[15]

TABLE 15.3 STROKE AND BLEEDING RISK STRATIFICATION WITH THE HAS-BLED SCHEMA

CONDITION	SCORE
Hypertension (i.e., uncontrolled BP)	1
Abnormal renal/liver function	1 or 2
Stroke	2
Bleeding tendency or predisposition	1
Labile INR	1
Age > 65	1
Drugs (e.g., concomitant aspirin or NSAIDs) or alcohol	1
	9

BP, blood pressure; INR, international normalized ratio; NSAIDs, nonsteroidal anti-inflammatory drugs.
Source: Pisters R, Lane DA, Nieuwlaat R, de Vos CB, Crijns HJ, Lip GY. A novel user-friendly score (HAS-BLED) to assess 1-year risk of major bleeding in patients with atrial fibrillation: the Euro Heart Survey on Atrial Fibrillation. *Chest.* 2010;138:1093–1100.[16]

bleeding who should be scheduled for more frequent clinical follow-up (see Table 15.3).

J. Consultation and collaboration
   1. Cardiology
      a. Need for management/angiography
      b. Uncertain EKG findings
      c. Assist with disposition decision
      d. Arrange for follow-up

Patient Disposition

A. Discharge
   1. Goals:
      a. Regain normal sinus rhythm, control heart rate, and prevent stroke.
      b. Prevent unnecessary hospital admissions and testing; identify and intervene appropriately for those at risk for major cardiac events.
      c. Use risk stratification tools for early discharge of low-risk patients.
      d. Give clear instructions for patient follow-up.
      e. Hemodynamically stable patients may be discharged with outpatient follow-up with primary care physician, cardiologist, and/or other clinician (e.g., the nurse clinician in the arrhythmia clinic).
      f. Patients should be given prescriptions of the same class as used in the ED for rate control and/or rhythm control.
      g. Aggressive education and treatment of obesity, cardiac risk factors, smoking, alcohol abuse, and sleep apnea will greatly improve outcomes. Provide education in a team- and patient-centered approach for all personnel (e.g., nurse practitioner [NP], pharmacist, MD, others).
      h. The patient's risk for stroke MUST be assessed and appropriate anticoagulation treatment be initiated based on the patient's CHA_2DS_2-VASc score. The risk of stroke is the same for the patient with paroxysmal and persistent atrial fibrillation. The retrospective study by Kea et al.[17] of 138 patients discharged from the ED with a diagnosis of atrial fibrillation found that the majority (80.7%) of high-risk patients were not discharged on oral anticoagulants. Of the high-risk patients discharged with OAC, female gender and cardiology consultation were key findings.
      i. Stable patients may be discharged with outpatient follow-up if rate-controlled and absence of structural heart disease.
         i. If patient required medications for rate control during ED stay, prescribe same class of medications when discharged.
         ii. Risk of stroke is equal for paroxysmal and persistent AF, and so anticoagulation should always be considered based on CHA_2DS_2-VASc score.

B. Admission
   1. Indicated for patients who are unstable, require increasing oxygen to maintain O_2 sat 93%, and have identified ischemia, infection, HF, difficulty controlling ventricular rate of the atrial fibrillation/flutter, severe left ventricle (LV) dysfunction.
   2. Patients may be admitted to the observation unit who are stable and need observation to ensure patient is tolerating medications and to search for underlying causes, such as ischemia, hyperthyroidism, and to assess the need for anticoagulation.

C. Documentation
   1. Presentation, history, and findings
   2. Reassessments
   3. Include the decision-making/risk stratification tools used.
   4. Patient acknowledgment of discharge instructions
   5. Inclusion of family or friends present during discussions
   6. Plans for follow-up
   7. Consultation with ED physician, cardiologist, EP physician, specialist, radiologist, case manager, or others

D. Prevention and education
   1. Patient behaviors to decrease risk
   2. Smoking cessation
   3. Increase activity
   4. Weight reduction
   5. Maintain control of HTN and DM.
   6. Compliance with medications
   7. Prompt evaluation of symptoms such as chest pain or SOB
   8. Regular PCP and/or cardiology outpatient visits

E. Patient and family education and counseling
   1. Discussion of signs and symptoms which would require a return to the ED and/or an urgent visit to their primary care clinician. Include when emergency medical services (EMS) should be activated.
   2. Medications to be continued or discontinued
   3. New medications and potential adverse effects discussed
   4. Activity restrictions, if any

Age and Developmental Considerations

A. Pediatric considerations[18]
   1. Atrial arrhythmias may be seen in children and a search for underlying congenital heart disease should be done. Follow pediatric advanced life support for management of atrial fibrillation/flutter in the pediatric population.

Chest Pain

COLLEEN ANDREONI

Chest pain accounts for six to eight million ED visits annually, as the second most frequent cause of adult ED visits.[19,20] Chest pain may be from somatic or visceral pain fibers. Visceral fibers are found in internal organs, while somatic fibers are mainly from the dermis and parietal pleura. Somatic pain is easily localized and described as sharp. Visceral pain is more difficult to describe and may be diffusely located and/or referred to other body areas.

Coronary artery disease (CAD) is the leading cause of death in the United States.[7] Risk factors for CAD include age >40 years, male or postmenopausal female, history of

TABLE 15.4 DIFFERENTIAL DIAGNOSES OF NONTRAUMATIC CHEST PAIN

	PAIN	ASSOCIATED SYMPTOMS	SELECTED ASSESSMENT FINDINGS	SELECTED DIAGNOSTIC FINDINGS	IMAGING	COMMENTS
Cardiovascular						
STEMI	Acute dull, ache, pressure, tight, heavy. Retrosternal, may radiate to jaw, neck, shoulder, arms. Lasts >15–30 minutes.	SOB, nausea, vomiting, diaphoresis, fatigue, palpitations	Anxious, VS often wnl, may have pulmonary rales, S3, S4	EKG: ST segment elevation ≥ 1 mm in 2 contiguous leads, new LBBB Elevated cTn	CXR often wnl	Prepare for emergency PCI or thrombolysis
NSTEMI	Acute dull, ache, pressure, tight, heavy. May radiate to jaw, neck, shoulder, arms. Lasts >15–30 minutes.	SOB, nausea, vomiting, diaphoresis, fatigue, palpitations	Anxious, VS often wnl, may have pulmonary rales, S3, S4	EKG: ST segment depression or T wave inversion in multiple precordial leads Elevated cTn	CXR often wnl	Prepare for PCI or thrombolysis
UA	Acute dull, ache, pressure, heavy. Change in pattern of preexisting angina. Angina at rest	Mild SOB, nausea, vomiting, diaphoresis	VS often wnl may be anxious	EKG: Normal or nonspecific changes, cTn wnl	CXR often wnl	Prinzmetal's (or variant) angina has ST segment elevation
Pericarditis	Sharp anterior precordial, constant. Positional pain may be relieved when leaning forward, worse with inspiration, coughing, supine position.	HO recent viral illness. Systemic symptoms: fever, headache, myalgias	Pericardial friction rub, distant heart sounds and/or pulses paradoxus with effusion	EKG: Diffuse concave upward ST segs, PR segment depression without T wave inversion, ESR: Elevated Hs-CRP: elevated cTn: May be elevated without coronary ischemia	CXR: Possible cardiomegaly	May also have myocarditis. Cardiac tamponade is rare complication.
Myocarditis	Chest pain Dyspnea	HO recent viral infection, fever, myalgia, headache	Tachycardia, tachypnea, muffled heart sounds	EKG: Changes seen in pericarditis, prolonged QRS interval and possible AV blocks. ESR: Elevated cTn: May be elevated without coronary ischemia	CXR: wnl in mild to moderate disease. Cardiomegaly and pulmonary edema with severe disease	

(continued)

TABLE 15.4 DIFFERENTIAL DIAGNOSIS OF NONTRAUMATIC CHEST PAIN (*CONTINUED*)

	PAIN	ASSOCIATED SYMPTOMS	SELECTED ASSESSMENT FINDINGS	SELECTED DIAGNOSTIC FINDINGS	IMAGING	COMMENTS
Aortic dissection	Acute midline substernal tearing sensation, sharp pain. Radiation to interscapular area or abdomen	HO HTN, atherosclerosis, Marfan's syndrome, smoking. Feeling of impending doom	BP/radial pulses discrepancy New aortic murmur or pericardial friction rub	D-dimer often elevated cTn: May be elevated without coronary ischemia.	CTA is gold standard: Obvious defect, CXR and US less diagnostic CXR: Abnormal aortic contour TEE is dependent upon operator expertise.	Secondary symptoms may arise from arterial occlusions: stroke, AMI, limb ischemia
Pulmonary						
Spontaneous pneumothorax	Acute, unilateral, sharp pleuritic pain	Dyspnea	Localized decreased or absent BS on affected side if > 15% hyperresonance, tactile fremitus, hypoxia, hypotension		CXR: Air in pleural space, possible subcutaneous air. Bedside ultrasound is more sensitive than CXR.	Tall, thin body habitus, younger adult, or older adult with COPD. Risk of tension pneumothorax
Pneumonia	Pleuritic pain, sharp	Fever, cough, productive sputa, dyspnea, fatigue	Tachypnea, hypoxia, rhonchi, crackles, decreased breath sounds, pleural rub, dullness to percussion, leukocytosis		CXR: Infiltrate, consolidation	Appears ill Determine whether community-acquired pneumonia or hospital-acquired. Fever may be absent in elderly or immunocompromised. Refer to CURB-65 and pneumonia severity index to assist with medical decision-making.
Pulmonary embolism	Acute, sharp, worse with inspiration	Dyspnea	Hypoxia, tachycardia, cough, hemoptysis, hypotension	D-dimer: Elevated, not necessary if patient is determined to be intermediate or high risk	CXR: May see abrupt hilar cut off. CTA: Filling defect	Risk factors: Deep vein thrombosis, HO malignancy, clotting disorder, recent surgery, immobility, estrogen therapy, pregnancy. Refer to Wells score and if low risk, use PERC criteria.
Pleurisy/Pleuritis	Pleuritic pain (as defined in text)	Dyspnea, fever. May be worse with cough, sneeze, deep inspiration.	Tachycardia may be present due to pain or fever		CXR may be wnl or show pleural effusion.	May have infectious or autoimmune etiology.

(*continued*)

TABLE 15.4 DIFFERENTIAL DIAGNOSIS OF NONTRAUMATIC CHEST PAIN (*CONTINUED*)

	PAIN	ASSOCIATED SYMPTOMS	SELECTED ASSESSMENT FINDINGS	SELECTED DIAGNOSTIC FINDINGS	IMAGING	COMMENTS
Gastrointestinal						
Esophageal rupture (Boerhaave syndrome)	Acute, sharp substernal. Follows an episode of forceful vomiting.	Dyspnea	Tachycardic, diaphoretic		CXR may be wnl or show pleural effusion, pneumothorax, pneumomediastinum, or subcutaneous air. Esophagogram with water soluble contrast or endoscopy for definitive diagnosis	
PUD, gastritis	May be acute onset. Epigastric dull, ache, gnawing	Dyspepsia. Often postprandial	May have epigastric TTP.	CBC: Evaluate for anemia. Stool for occult blood		May be relieved with food, antacids. Associated with stress, NSAID use, alcohol
Esophagitis	Substernal, sharp, associated with swallowing	Odynophagia				Referral for EGD
FB ingestion	Acute midsternal	Dysphagia, HO choking episode	Drooling			May require urgent endoscopy to remove FB.
GERD	Substernal or epigastric, burning	Regurgitation of a bitter taste or acid in mouth	May have epigastric TTP.			May be exacerbated by certain foods, supine position.
Hiatal hernia	May be acute onset. Midsternal, dull, sharp positional					May be exacerbated by certain foods, supine position.
Esophageal spasm/ dysmotility	Acute midsternal, sharp, constricting, spasmodic	Recent ingestion of hot or cold liquids or food bolus				Often recurrent, may have HO EoE.
Cholecystitis	May be acute onset. Epigastric, RUQ, dull, sharp, spasmodic	Nausea, vomiting,	+ Murphy sign			May be exacerbated by certain foods.
Pancreatitis	May be acute onset. Epigastric, sharp, burning	Nausea, vomiting,	Epigastric TTP			Often associated with alcohol use

(*continued*)

TABLE 15.4 DIFFERENTIAL DIAGNOSIS OF NONTRAUMATIC CHEST PAIN (*CONTINUED*)

	PAIN	ASSOCIATED SYMPTOMS	SELECTED ASSESSMENT FINDINGS	SELECTED DIAGNOSTIC FINDINGS	IMAGING	COMMENTS
Musculoskeletal						
Costochondritis	Localized ache or sharp anterior pain over multiple costochondral junctions. Worse with movement	HO recent physical strain: pushing, pulling, lifting, exercise	Exacerbated or reproduced with palpation of area		CXR: wnl	May benefit from trigger point injection.
Muscle strain	Localized dull, aching	HO recent physical strain: pushing, pulling, lifting, exercise	Exacerbated or reproduced with palpation of thoracic musculature or ROM		CXR: wnl	
Slipping rib syndrome	Localized under anterior 8th–10th ribs Sharp		Exacerbated by sudden upward movement, plus popping sensation		CXR: wnl	May reproduce pain by hooking technique over involved ribs.
Tietze syndrome	Localized sharp pain at one costosternal or costochondral junction		Exacerbated or reproduced with palpation of costochondral junction, most often 2nd or 3rd, plus swelling and erythema of the isolated costochondral junction		CXR: wnl	
Precordial catch syndrome (Texidor twinge)	Acute sharp Lasting 1–2 minutes, occurs in episodic bunches near cardiac apex. Associated with deep breath at rest	Often recurrent HO poor posture and inactivity	Normal exam		CXR: wnl	

(*continued*)

TABLE 15.4 DIFFERENTIAL DIAGNOSIS OF NONTRAUMATIC CHEST PAIN (*CONTINUED*)

	PAIN	ASSOCIATED SYMPTOMS	SELECTED ASSESSMENT FINDINGS	SELECTED DIAGNOSTIC FINDINGS	IMAGING	COMMENTS
Psychogenic						
Panic attack	Acute	May have other somatic complaints, SOB, palpitations, nausea, dizziness, paresthesias, chills, hot flushes, fear they are dying.	Tachycardia, tachypnea, diaphoresis, tremor	EKG: Sinus tachycardia		Acknowledgmnt of stressor(s) HO anxiety, panic, hyperventilation
Hyperventilation syndrome	Acute	Circumoral and distal extremity tingling	Tachypnea, abnormal affect, mood	EKG may have T wave inversion that reverses after resolution of hyperventilation.		HO anxiety, stress
Heme/Oncologic						
Sickle cell crisis	Chronic, recurrent, usual pain pattern	Recent illness, stress	Tachycardia, hypoxia,	CBC Retic count	CXR: May not be necessary if this is typical pain pattern.	HO SCD
Acute chest Syndrome	Acute change in quality or severity of usual pain pattern		Tachycardia, tachypnea, hypoxia, wheezing, fever, hypotension	CBC cTn Retic count CMP	Thoracic CT	HO SCD
Tumorthoracic, metastatic	Dull	May have weight loss.		CBC CMP	CXR, Thoracic CT	HO cancer or new finding

AMI, transthoracic echocardiogram; BP, blood pressure; CBC, complete blood count; CMP, comprehensive metabolic panel; COPD, chronic obstructive pulmonary disease; CTA, CT of abdomen; CXR, chest x-ray; EGD, esophagogastroduodenoscopy; EoE, eosinophilic esophagitis; ESR, erythrocyte sedimentation rate; FB, foreign body; HO, history of; HTN, hypertension; NSAIDs, nonsteroidal anti-inflammatory drugs; NSTEMI, non-ST-segment elevation myocardial infarction; PCI, percutaneous coronary intervention; PERC, pulmonary embolism rule-out criteria; PUD, peptic ulcer disease; ROM, range of motion; RUQ, right upper quadrant; SCD, sudden cardiac death; SOB, shortness of breath; STEMI, ST-elevation myocardial infarction; TEE, transthoracic echocardiogram; TTP, thrombotic thrombocytopenic purpura; VS, vital sign; UA, unstable angina; US, ultrasound; wnl, within normal limits.

Source: Briggs LA. Deciphering chest pain in women. *Nurse Pract.* 2018;4:25–33. https://doi.org/10.1097/01.NPR.0000531071.96311.9f; Moran B, Bryan S, Farrar T, et al. Diagnostic evaluation of nontraumatic chest pain in athletes. *Curr. Sports Med. Rep.* 2017;16(2):84–94. https://doi.org/10.1249/JSR.0000000000000342; Abid S, Shuaib W, Ali S, et al. Chest pain assessment and imaging practices for nurse practitioners in the emergency department. *Adv Emerg Nurs J.* 2015;37(1):12–22. https://doi.org/10.1097/TME.0000000000000048; Acra P, Perez MT. The evaluation of adolescent chest pain: a screening ECG or PSC-17? *Curr Opin Pediatr.* 2017;29(4):414–419. https://doi.org/10.1097/MOP.0000000000000503; Carlton EW, Pickering JW, Greenslade J, et al. Assessment of the 2016 National Institute for Health and Care Excellence high-sensitivity troponin rule-out strategy. *Heart.* 2017;104:665–672. https://doi.org/10.1136/heartjnl-2017-311983; Hamilton GC, Sanders AB, Strange GR, Trott AT, eds. Chest pain. In: Hamilton GC, Malone S, Janz TG, eds. *Emergency Medicine: An Approach to Clinical Problem-Solving.* 2nd ed. W. B. Saunders; 2003; Hsia RY, Hale Z, Tabas JA. A national study of the prevalence of life-threatening diagnoses in patients with chest pain. *JAMA Internal Med.* 2016;176(7):1029–1032. https://doi.org/10.1001/jamainternmed.2016.2498; Jordan KS, Mennle SE. An unusual case of chest pain in an adolescent male. Important cues to differential diagnosis. *Adv Emerg Nurs J.* 2017;39(1):10–17. https://doi.org/10.1097/TME.0000000000000135; Manthey DE. Aortic aneurysms and aortic dissection. In: Cydulka RK, Fitch MT, Joing SA, Wang VJ, Cline DM, Ma OJ, eds. *Tintinalli's Emergency Medicine Manual.* 8th ed. McGraw-Hill; 2018; Niemann JT. The cardiomyopathies, myocarditis, and pericardial disease. In: *Tintinalli's Emergency Medicine: A Comprehensive Study Guide.* 7th ed. McGraw-Hill; 2011; Nyce N. Chest pain: Cardiac or not. In: Cydulka RK, Fitch MT, Joing SA, Wang VJ, Cline DM, Ma OJ, eds. *Tintinalli's Emergency Medicine Manual.* 8th ed. McGraw-Hill; 2018; Thibodeau L. The cardiomyopathies, myocarditis, and pericardial disease. In: Cydulka RK, Fitch MT, Joing SA, Wang VJ, Cline DM, Ma OJ, eds. *Tintinalli's Emergency Medicine Manual.* 8th ed. McGraw-Hill; 2018.[20,22–32]

hypertension (HTN), smoking, hypercholesterolemia, diabetes, truncal obesity, family history, alcohol use, sedentary lifestyle, and cocaine use. Heredity can also play a role.

Six life-threatening conditions are traditionally considered in all patients who present with nontraumatic chest pain to the ED. These are acute coronary syndrome (ACS), aortic dissection, pulmonary embolism, tension pneumothorax, esophageal rupture, and perforated peptic ulcer. Of these, ACS is the most common and the ENP must be mindful of the risks involved in excessive diagnostic testing when considering differential diagnoses. However, the ENP is tasked with quickly ruling out all life-threatening causes of chest pain. A rapid, accurate, focused history and physical examination will guide the diagnostic evaluation and ensure diagnostic accuracy. The prevalence of serious diagnoses increases with the patient's age.

Medical Screening

A. Chief complaint
  1. Nonanginal pain
    a. *Pleuritic pain:* Sudden, sharp pain associated with inspiration or exhalation
      i. Associated with inflammation of parietal pleura
      ii. May have referred pain to ipsilateral shoulder or neck
      iii. Worse with coughing, sneezing, laughing
      iv. Pulmonary embolism is the most common life-threatening cause.[21]
      v. Other serious etiologies include pneumonia, pericarditis, pneumothorax, aortic dissection, and acute myocardial infarction (AMI).
      vi. Viruses/infectious causes of pleuritic pain are less serious and develop more slowly.
    b. Other causes of chest pain include pulmonary, gastrointestinal, musculoskeletal, psychogenic, or hematologic/oncologic origins.
    c. See Table 15.4 for differential diagnosis of nontraumatic chest pain.
  2. Anginal pain
    a. Typical anginal pain is substernal or left anterior chest and epigastric pain, which often occurs with physical exertion or emotional stress and relieved by rest or nitroglycerin.
    b. The pain is described as heavy, pressure, tightness, crushing, or squeezing.
      i. Pain may last 2 to 20 minutes.
  3. Infarction pain
    a. AMI, ST-elevation myocardial infarction (STEMI), and non-ST-elevation myocardial infarction (NSTEMI) pain is more severe and prolonged, lasting up to 2 hours.
    b. Pain is described as heavy, pressure, tightness, crushing, or squeezing.
    c. Associated symptoms include radiation to hand, jaw, shoulders, arms, and neck, as well as dyspnea, diaphoresis, and nausea.
  4. Atypical pain
    a. Atypical cardiac chest pain occurs more frequently in women, elderly, and diabetic patients.
    b. Signs and symptoms
      i. Heart rate, respiratory rate, blood pressure (BP), pulse oximetry, and temperature may be normal or may be deranged above or below normal limits.
        (a) Breath sounds
        (b) Decreased with pneumonia; rales or crackles with heart failure (HF), pneumonia; hyperresonance with pneumothorax; wheezing with bronchoconstriction; pleural friction rub with pleurisy
        (c) Heart sounds
          (i) S3 or S4 with new-onset HF, large AMI; pericardial friction rub with pericarditis, new onset of irregular rhythm (i.e., AF, atrial or ventricular premature beats)

B. Focused assessment
  1. Priority is given to immediate life threats
    a. Focused history
      i. Prior history of CAD, myocardial infarction (MI), smoking, HTN, hyperlipidemia (HL), diabetes mellitus (DM), peripheral arterial disease (PAD)
      ii. Family history of CAD, sudden cardiac deaths, MI before age 60
      iii. Recent viral or bacterial illness, invasive procedure, choking episode, or vomiting
      iv. Recent physical exertion or psychological stress
      v. *History of chronic conditions:* Sickle cell disease, collagen disorders (Marfan), rheumatic disorders (systemic lupus erythematous), pancreatitis, cholecystitis, peptic ulcer disease (PUD), alcohol abuse, cocaine or amphetamine abuse, eosinophilic esophagitis (EoE), anxiety, panic attacks, cancer
      vi. ACS risk assessment tools (see section Acute Coronary Syndrome)
    b. Focused exam
      i. *General:* Diaphoresis, behavior, color, temperature
      ii. *Cardiac:* Peripheral pulse quality, rate and rhythm, heart sounds (murmur or rubs), jugular vein distention (JVD), edema, BP in both arms
      iii. *Pulmonary:* Respiratory rate, quality, use of accessory muscles, splinting respirations, stridor, breath sounds, pulse oximetry, subcutaneous emphysema
      iv. *Musculoskeletal:* Chest wall tenderness, erythema, swelling
      v. *Gastrointestinal:* Epigastric or abdominal tenderness, nausea, vomiting

Differential Diagnoses

A. Refer to section on Acute Coronary Syndrome for chest pain decision-making tools.

Diagnostic Testing

A. *EKG:* Recommended to have EKG done and reviewed by ED clinician within 10 minutes after arrival. EKG changes may be specific or nonspecific. Serial EKGs may be necessary to assess for evolving ischemia. The EKG changes are best interpreted when correlated with the patient's history and clinical examination. Whenever possible, compare current EKG with previous EKG to determine the presence of changes.

1. *ACS/AMI:* ST segment deviations, pathologic Q waves, new left bundle branch block (LBBB), T wave inversions (see Acute Coronary Syndrome section).
2. *Pericarditis:* Widespread concave ST segment elevation, PR segment depression without T wave inversion
3. *Prinzmetal angina:* Dramatic elevations of ST segments, similarly seen in an AMI

B. Labs

1. Cardiac biomarkers
    a. *Troponin:* Troponins (cTnI, cTnT, and a calcium-binding unit cTnC) are released in the presence of myocardial ischemia. Various troponin analyses, cTnI or cTnT or hs-TnI, are available.
        i. cTn may be normal, depending on how soon after the onset of pain the patient presents to the ED.
        ii. hs-cTnI can detect levels of troponin at 2 hours; however, a single troponin at a minimum of 3 hours or serial troponin analysis are used most commonly.
        iii. Troponin levels reach their peak at 12 hours and remain elevated for 7 to 10 days. The ENP must be familiar with the troponin analysis used and the implications for practice, as levels of detection (LoD) may vary.
        iv. Left ventricular hypertrophy (LVH), pericarditis, myocarditis, HF, pulmonary embolism, and sepsis may result in a false positive elevation of cTn.
2. *CBC:* Assess for leukocytosis, leukopenia, anemia.
3. *Metabolic panel:* Assess renal function, glucose, electrolytes, hepatic function.
4. *Coagulation studies (prothrombin time/partial thromboplastin time [PT/PTT], international normalized ratio [INR]):* Useful if patient is currently taking anticoagulants (warfarin or nonvitamin K antagonist oral anticoagulants [NOACs]), and in anticipation of need for percutaneous coronary intervention (PCI)
5. *Cultures:* Including blood, sputum, strep, pleural fluid, as indicated by history and physical exam
6. *D-dimer:* Used to determine risk for pulmonary embolism. D-dimer is a product of coagulation breakdown. False positive results are common, as the positive predictive value (PPV) is low, despite a high negative predictive value (NPV).

C. *CXR:* Useful in identifying pneumonia, pneumothorax, mass, cardiomegaly, aortic dissection. A CXR is easily obtained and costeffective in the ED.

D. *Echocardiogram:* To assess cardiac structure and hemodynamic function. Can identify abnormal wall motion, ejection fraction, valve function. Can identify pericarditis, cardiac tumors.

E. *CT coronary angiography (CTCA) 64-slice (or above):* Useful for typical or atypical pain in low- to intermediate-riskpatientswithoutknownheartdiseaseand nondiagnostic EKG and cardiac biomarkers[33,34]

1. The CTCA is a quick (~20 min), widely available, cost-effective 3D visualization of coronary arteries. It is most useful in low- and intermediate-risk patients to detect obstructive CAD. It can replace the up to 12-hour serial EKGs and biomarker analyses and stress testing, while decreasing ED length of stay (LOS) and reducing hospital admissions.
2. A CTCA can also rule out a pulmonary embolism and aortic dissection ("triple rule-out") using a special contrast protocol.

F. *Ventilation-perfusion (VQ) scan:* Able to identify pulmonary embolism when CTCA is not readily available or contraindicated.

G. *Thoracic CT scan:* Useful to identify pericarditis and pneumonia

H. *Functional (stress) testing:* Considered if CTCA is inconclusive or if patient has history of CAD with uncertainty if chest pain is due to myocardial ischemia

I. *MRI:* Useful in identifying various cardiac and noncardiac abnormalities with difficult differential of chest pain. Not easily obtained in the ED due to time required out of the ED for unstable patients, resulting in increased risks, limited availability in some settings.

J. *Coronary angiography:* Gold standard for diagnosis of cardiac pathology

1. PCI is based on the angiography findings.
2. Revascularization with stenting is recommended for STEMI and NSTEMI and selected unstable angina (UA) patients.
3. The time frame from presentation to the ED and to PCI balloon inflation is closely monitored to ensure quality standards.
4. For STEMI patients, it is most beneficial if performed ≤90 minutes of presentation to the ED, for unstable NSTEMI patients ≤2 hours, and for stable NSTEMI within 72 hours.

Management

A. Procedures

1. Emergent procedures are guided by the use of ACLS protocols.
    a. Pharmacologic and nonpharmacologic therapies
        i. Follow evidence-based guidelines when prescribing.
        ii. *ACS:* See Acute Coronary Syndrome section.
        iii. *Pericarditis:* Management depends on the etiology of the pericarditis.
            (1) NSAIDs are prescribed for 1 to 3 weeks for an idiopathic or viral etiology.
            (2) Follow-up may include a repeat echocardiogram.
            (3) Patients with a large pericardial effusion are usually admitted for monitoring hemodynamic compromise.
        iv. *Myocarditis (inflammatory cardiomyopathy):* NSAIDs are prescribed for 1 to 3 weeks for

an idiopathic or viral etiology and supportive therapy.

(1) Severe disease with congestive heart failure (CHF) symptoms requires admission.

v. *Aortic dissection:* Administration of antihypertensive agents to a systolic blood pressure (SBP) goal of 120 to 130 mmHg. Most commonly used are beta-blockers.

vi. Beta-blockers most commonly used

(1) Metoprolol

(2) Esmolol

(3) Labetalol

(4) Following beta-blockade or calcium channel blockade, the goal BP may be maintained with nitroprusside at 0.3 mcg/kg/min.

(5) Blood and blood products may be required, and urgent surgical referral is necessary.

vii. *Other:* Refer to Pulmonary, Gastrointestinal, Musculoskeletal, Psychiatric, and Hematology/Oncology chapters for detailed management of selected conditions which may present with chest pain.

B. Consultation and collaboration

a. Cardiology

i. Need for invasive management/angiography/PCI

ii. Uncertain EKG findings

iii. Assist with disposition decision.

iv. Assist with ED management as requested.

v. Arrange for follow-up.

b. *Cardiothoracic surgeon:* Surgical repair of aortic dissection

Patient Disposition

A. Goal is to prevent unnecessary hospital admissions and testing, and to identify and intervene appropriately for those at risk for major adverse cardiac events (MACE).[35]

1. Discharge

a. Use risk stratification tools for early discharge of low-risk patients (see section "Acute Coronary Syndrome").

b. Patients with known cardiac disease must have close follow-up if sent home from the ED; they remain at higher risk than patients without known disease, but admission or observation will not yield any benefit.

B. *Cath Lab:* Coronary angiography with PCI

1. Emergently upon identification of STEMI or unstable NSTEMI

2. *Goal:* Door to balloon time ≤90 minutes

C. *Surgery:* Unstable aortic dissection

D. Admission

1. Following PCI or surgery

2. Stable NSTEMI, or for patients in whom PCI is contraindicated, UA

3. Severe pericarditis or myocarditis

4. Administration of thrombolytics

E. *Observation unit:* Observation status admissions are decreasing as technology and medical decision-making tools are validated for discharge of low-risk patients directly from the ED.

F. Patient may require transfer to a higher level of care for additional interventions not available at the primary care setting.

G. Documentation

1. Presentation, history, findings

2. Reassessments

3. Include the decision-making/risk stratification tools used.

4. Patient acknowledgment of discharge instructions

5. Inclusion of family or friends present during discussions

6. Plans for follow-up

7. Consultation with ED physician, specialist, radiologist, case manager, or others

H. Prevention and education

1. Patient behaviors to decrease risk

a. Smoking cessation

b. Increase activity

c. Weight reduction

d. Maintain control of hypertension (HTN) and diabetes mellitus (DM)

e. Compliance with medications

f. Prompt evaluation of symptoms such as chest pain or shortness of breath (SOB)

g. Regular PCP and/or cardiology outpatient visits

I. Patient and family education and counseling

1. Discussion of signs and symptoms that would require a return to the ED and/or an urgent visit to their PCP. Include when emergency medical services (EMS) should be activated.

2. Medications to be continued or discontinued

3. New medications and potential adverse effects discussed

4. Activity restrictions, if any

Age and Developmental Considerations

A. Pediatric considerations[18]

1. The child or adolescent with chest pain

a. A common presentation, although rarely life-threatening or pertaining to a cardiac etiology

b. A thorough history and physical exam are essential to determine the need for further diagnostic studies, consultation, or referrals.

c. An acute onset may be associated with blunt trauma, spontaneous pneumothorax, rib fractures, pneumonia, asthma exacerbation, acute chest syndrome in children with sickle cell disease, or esophageal foreign body.

d. Consider musculoskeletal or psychological etiologies for chest pain with a gradual onset or repeated nonacute episodes of chest pain.

e. A child with a history of syncope, known congenital or acquired heart disease, or Kawasaki disease, will require a more detailed evaluation of their chest pain, as will the child with abnormal physical findings such as an irregular heart rate or rhythm, abnormal heart sounds, or an abnormal EKG.

f. The focused family history identifies family members with early heart disease, sudden cardiac death, and prolonged QT syndrome.

B. Sex

1. Women have a greater risk for CAD and CAD mortality with a personal history of DM or a family history of MI before age 60, as compared to same risk factors in men.

2. Women with a history of preeclampsia, eclampsia, and gestational HTN are at greater risk for CAD and lifetime risk for MI, stroke, venous thromboembolism (VTE), or sudden cardiac death.

3. Especially true in younger women presenting with chest pain

C. Athletes

1. Chest pain in athletes may be cardiac or noncardiac. At the forefront of medical decision-making is the knowledge that chest pain in an athlete may be an early warning sign of sudden cardiac death. The risk for cardiac disease rises with the age of the athlete; in those >35 years old CAD, hypertrophic cardiomyopathy (HCM), and cardiac anomalies may be identified. Most often in young athletes, the causes of nontraumatic chest pain are noncardiac and benign. Consider gastroesophageal reflux disease (GERD), costochondritis, pleurisy, and anxiety as possible noncardiac etiologies.

2. History should note any chest pain, syncope, palpitations during exercise, along with recent illnesses (consider pericarditis or myocarditis).

3. Family history includes sudden cardiac death (SCD) <50 years old. Consider congenital or genetic causes of chest pain: anomalous coronary arteries, aortic stenosis, arrhythmogenic right ventricular dysplasia (ARVD), Marfan syndrome with aortic dissection or sickle cell trait.

4. Use of supplements and prescription meds, especially those acting on the sympathetic nervous system. Use of illicit drugs

5. Common training-related EKG changes in athletes include sinus bradycardia, sinus arrhythmia, ectopic atrial rhythm, junctional escape rhythm, first-degree AV block, Mobitz type 1 second-degree AV block, incomplete right bundle branch block (RBBB), early repolarization, QRS voltage criteria for LVH, prolonged QT.[22]

6. Further diagnostic testing is determined by the history and physical findings. When the chest pain is determined to be noncardiac in origin, consider musculoskeletal, gastrointestinal, pulmonary, or psychiatric etiologies.

Heart Failure

LORI HULL-GROMMESH

Patients present to the ED with varying degrees of heart failure (HF). Expert task forces have defined HF classifications based on severity of symptoms limiting activities (functional class or New York Heart Association class I–IV) and objective assessment of symptoms and their effect on the patient's activities of daily living (Class A–D) (Table 15.5).

HF can be systolic or diastolic and is referred to as either HF with reduced ejection fraction (HFrEF; or systolic HF) or HF with preserved ejection fraction (HFpEF; or diastolic HF). In HFrEF, there is impairment of the left ventricle affecting the pumping action or contractility of the heart with resultant enlargement of the left ventricle as the systolic HF progresses. In HFpEF, there is stiffening of the left ventricle affecting the filling, while maintaining contractility of the left ventricle. Acute transmural myocardial infarction (MI) is a common cause of HFrEF,

TABLE 15.5 HEART FAILURE CLASSIFICATIONS

NEW YORK HEART ASSOCIATION CLASS	
I.	No limitation of physical activity. Ordinary physical activity does not cause undue fatigue, palpitation, dyspnea (shortness of breath).
II.	Slight limitation of physical activity. Comfortable at rest. Ordinary physical activity results in fatigue, palpitation, dyspnea (shortness of breath).
III.	Marked limitation of physical activity. Comfortable at rest. Less than ordinary activity causes fatigue, palpitation, or dyspnea.
IV.	Unable to carry on any physical activity without discomfort. Symptoms of heart failure at rest. If any physical activity is undertaken, discomfort increases.
OBJECTIVE ASSESSMENT CLASSIFICATION	
A.	No objective evidence of cardiovascular disease. No symptoms and no limitation in ordinary physical activity.
B.	Objective evidence of minimal cardiovascular disease. Mild symptoms and slight limitation during ordinary activity. Comfortable at rest.
C.	Objective evidence of moderately severe cardiovascular disease. Marked limitation in activity due to symptoms, even during less-than-ordinary activity. Comfortable only at rest.
D.	Objective evidence of severe cardiovascular disease. Severe limitations. Experiences symptoms even while at rest.

Source: Adapted from Yancy CW, Jessup M, Bozkurt B, et al. ACCF/AHA Guideline for the Management of Heart Failure: A Report of the American College of Cardiology Foundation/American Heart Association Task Force on Practice Guidelines. *J Am Coll Cardiol.* 2013;62(16):e147–e239.[36]

and the most common cause of HFpEF is uncontrolled or long-term hypertension.

The common and most severe consequence of HF is pulmonary edema. While pulmonary edema has other or noncardiac causes (e.g., acute respiratory distress syndrome from altered capillary permeability, high altitude pulmonary edema), the increased pulmonary capillary pressure seen in pulmonary edema from congestive HF is the most common cause of pulmonary edema.[37] The terms congestive heart failure (CHF) and HF are used interchangeably. This section focuses on CHF, with the primary emphasis on cardiac causes. Although there are noncardiac causes of CHF, the treatment varies in the sense that the underlying cause must be treated and if the CHF persists the treatment medications, lifestyle changes, and health monitoring are the same.

Medical Screening

A. Chief complaint
  1. Shortness of breath
    a. The shortness of breath should be questioned fully to help determine the severity of the HF. Often patients adjust their lifestyle to their symptoms and limit their activities. It is important to find out the extent of their activities of daily living. Patients may have no shortness of breath, or only, for example, when climbing one flight of stairs, or they may need to sit up to sleep or sleep on more than one pillow (see Table 15.5).
  2. Swelling/edema
  3. Cough
  4. Weight gain
  5. Chest tightness or chest pain
  6. Palpitation

B. Signs and symptoms
  1. Shortness of breath
  2. Edema
  3. Jugular venous distention (JVD)
  4. S3 heart sound, often a S3 gallop
  5. Lung crackles
  6. Vascular congestion on CXR
  7. Enlarged heart on CXR
  8. Displaced apical impulse or point of maximum intensity (PMI)
  9. Tachycardia may present with AF or new-onset AF.
  10. Positive hepatojugular reflux
  11. Murmur of mitral regurgitation (systolic murmur)
  12. Other murmurs such as aortic regurgitation (diastolic murmur)
  13. Chest tightness or chest pain
  14. Cough
  15. Weight gain
  16. Palpitations
  17. *Arrhythmias:* AF, ventricular arrhythmias, including ventricular tachycardia, premature ventricular contractions, and ventricular fibrillation
  18. Hypoxia
  19. Hypotension may present in a shock state.
  20. Hypertensive as a compensatory mechanism or common in HFpEF

C. Focused assessment
  1. Priority is given in identifying and treating life-threatening conditions.

D. Focused history
  1. Focus on symptoms, especially the shortness of breath. When did it start, has the patient had this before? Is it different? Does it hurt to breathe? Do you use oxygen? Continuous positive airway pressure (CPAP)? Are there associated symptoms of chest pain, palpitations, dizziness, and diaphoresis? Was onset sudden or gradual? When does the shortness of breath occur, and what relieves the shortness of breath? When was the patient's last hospitalization?
  2. Has the patient gained weight without an increase in sodium, food, or fluid intake?
  3. Does the patient have a history of HF or a low left ventricular ejection fraction? Often the patient will say they have a "weak heart."
  4. Does the patient have an automatic internal cardiac defibrillator (AICD)? Has it delivered any shocks? And when was the last time the AICD fired?
  5. Is there a prior history of CAD or myocardial infarction (MI), cardiac procedures (cardiac stenting, cardioversion, coronary artery bypass grafting [CABG]), smoking, HTN, hyperlipidemia (HL), DM, PAD, thyroid disease?
  6. Question female patients on past and current pregnancy. Research shows that female patients present differently in acute coronary syndromes and may exhibit HF as the only sign of an acute coronary event.
  7. Is there a family history of CAD, sudden cardiac deaths, MI?
  8. Is there a recent viral or bacterial illness?
  9. Is there recent anemia?
  10. Is there recent physical exertion or psychological stress?
  11. Has the patient had any dizziness, palpitations, or syncopal episodes, giving clues to possible arrhythmias associated with decreased left ventricular function and associated ventricular arrhythmias or AF?
  12. Does the patient use alcohol in excess or other drugs?
  13. Has the patient been compliant with their medications for HF? for HTN?

E. Focused examination
  1. The physical examination in determining HF is invaluable as HF at times can be determined by physical examination alone.
  2. Patients may be anxious and scared but are often alert and oriented; however, in severe cases patients will be confused from hypoxia and or hypercapnia.
  3. Depending on the degree of compensation, patients often present with tachycardia and hypotension. Patients presenting with HTN often have preserved left ventricular function or normal left ventricular

ejection fraction with echocardiogram evidence of diastolic dysfunction.

4. The respiratory rate of hypertensive patients is high with use of accessory muscles and JVD. The patients are hypoxic, requiring oxygen at varying levels of support from nasal cannula to intubation.

5. AF is common, as well as ventricular arrhythmias. Patients with a decrease in their left ventricular (LV) ejection fraction will have ventricular arrhythmias from unifocal premature ventricular complexes (PVCs) to multifocal ventricular tachycardia progressing to ventricular fibrillation.

6. Examine for the presence of pacemaker and/or AICD.

7. The patient's skin may be pale and cool or warm and dry. Skin appearance is dependent on the degree of the HF and if a shock state is present. Patients with class IV HF often present in a shock state, especially if undiagnosed or noncompliant with treatment management plan.

8. Pulmonary rales or crackles may be present. In right sided HF, there may not be pulmonary congestion but rather signs of right HF (e.g., positive hepatojugular reflux and edema). Left-sided HF can cause right-sided HF. The absence of rales or crackles does not rule out HF. Do the rales or crackles clear with coughing? Examine the sputum of any productive cough.

9. Patients with HF may present with abnormal heart sounds. An S3 gallop is common and may be present without the finding of rales or crackles in the lungs. An S4, common in patients with ischemia and always pathological of ischemic CAD, may be found as acute MI; coronary ischemia is a cause of HF. A sequela of MI is the rupture of mitral valve chordae, resulting in HF and pulmonary edema. Pay close attention to findings of new murmurs, especially the systolic murmur of mitral regurgitation.

10. Patients may or may not have edema. The edema may be present in the legs, around the abdomen, and even the sacral and back. Patients with severe right-sided HF may have ascites.

11. Patients may have decreased peripheral and extremity pulses. Palpation of pulses can give the ENP insight to the perfusion state and if there is irregularity in the heartbeat.

12. Decreased peripheral pulses

13. Other findings on the examination may include decreased bowel sounds and neurologic findings secondary to hypoxia, hypercapnia, arrhythmia anemia, and/or abnormal electrolytes.

Differential Diagnoses

A. Patients may present with signs and symptoms of CHF but do not have evidence of HFrEF or HFpEF. The following can result in pulmonary edema, peripheral edema, and other signs of CHF. These conditions can lead HFrEF and HFpEF if not recognized and treated.

1. ACS
2. Acute valvular dysfunction
3. Acute respiratory distress syndrome
4. Anaphylaxis
5. Aortic dissection
6. Bacterial or viral pneumonia
7. Renal failure
8. Myocardial infarction (MI)
9. Nephrotic syndrome
10. Pulmonary embolism
11. Pneumothorax
12. Venous insufficiency
13. Pulmonary fibrosis
14. Chronic obstructive lung disease (COPD)

Diagnostic Testing

A. Chest x-ray (CXR)

B. EKG

C. Echocardiogram

D. Labs

1. Comprehensive metabolic profile, including hepatic studies
2. Brain natriuretic peptide (BNP) or ProBNP
3. Arterial blood gas (ABG)
4. Complete blood count (CBC)
5. Thyroid stimulating hormone (TSH)
6. Coagulation studies
7. Other labs if suspect underlying cause such as infection (draw blood cultures)

Management

A. Procedures

1. Emergent procedures are guided by the advanced cardiac life support (ACLS) protocols.
2. Pharmacologic and nonpharmacologic therapies
   - **a.** Follow evidence-based guidelines when prescribing
   - **b.** *Oxygen support:* BiPAP or intubation
   - **c.** Diuretics, Lasix for fluid overload
   - **d.** Milrinone and dobutamine for cardiogenic shock states
   - **e.** Inotropes are not indicated in HFpEF.
   - **f.** Nitrates
   - **g.** Nitroprusside for HTN
   - **h.** Angiotensin-converting enzyme (ACE) inhibitor
   - **i.** Calcium channel blockers and beta-blockers should be avoided in severe HF and with hypotension.
   - **j.** No NSAIDs
   - **k.** Morphine for symptom control in stable HF
   - **l.** Entrestro
   - **m.** Other medications that may be considered
     - i. Lisinopril
     - ii. Captopril
     - iii. Benazepril
     - iv. Losartan
     - v. Valsartan
     - vi. Carvedilol
     - vii. Metoprolol
     - viii. Hydralazine/isosorbide
     - ix. Spironolactone

B. Consultation and collaboration

1. Cardiology
   - **a.** Need for invasive management/angiography/percutaneous coronary intervention (PCI)/left ventricular support devices

b. Uncertain EKG findings
c. Assist with disposition decision.
d. Assist with ED management as requested.
e. Arrange for follow-up.

Patient Disposition

A. Goal is to prevent unnecessary hospital admissions and testing, and to identify and intervene appropriately for those at risk for major adverse cardiac events (MACE).

1. Discharge

a. Clear instructions on medications and follow-up appointments. Appointment should be made for patient to see a provider within 1 to 2 days of ED visit. Collaborative teams of nurse practitioner (NP), MD, pharmacist, dietician, and others should see the patient. Ideally, the patient would be seen in a HF clinic.

b. Patients with known cardiac disease must have close follow-up if sent home from the ED; they remain at higher risk than patients without known disease, but admission or observation may not yield any benefit.

2. Admission

a. Hypoxic
b. Altered mental status (AMS)
c. To treat underlying cause
d. Maximize goal-directed medical therapy (GDMT)

3. *Observation:* Observation status admissions are decreasing as technology and medical decision-making tools are validated for discharge of low-risk patients directly from the ED. The goal is to prevent readmission, and if patients are managed by an outpatient HF clinic and followed closely with guidelines and protocols, readmissions are reduced. Observation may be needed to ensure patient has diuresis and returned to goal weight.

B. Documentation

1. Presentation, history, findings
2. Reassessments
3. Include decision-making/risk stratification tools used
4. Patient acknowledgment of discharge instructions
5. Inclusion of family or friends present during discussions
6. Plans for follow-up
7. Consultation with ED physician, specialist, radiologist, case manager, or others

C. Prevention and education

1. Patient behaviors to decrease risk

a. Smoking cessation
b. Importance of compliance with medications, appointments, and treatments. Telemedicine should be offered for patients who have difficulty traveling to see providers.
c. Increase activity
d. Weight reduction
e. Maintain control of HTN and DM
f. Prompt evaluation of symptoms, weight gain, shortness of breath, palpitations, chest pain, or discomfort
g. Primary care clinician and/or cardiology outpatient visits

D. Patient and family education and counseling

1. Discussion of signs and symptoms that would require a return to the ED and/or an urgent visit to their primary care clinician. Include when emergency medical services (EMS) should be activated.
2. Medications to be continued or discontinued
3. New medications and potential adverse effects
4. Activity restrictions, if any
5. Dietary restrictions
6. Importance of compliance with medications, appointments, and treatments, including daily weight and reporting of increased weight gain, even if no symptoms

Age and Developmental Considerations

A. Pediatric considerations

1. A thorough history and physical exam are essential to determine the need for further diagnostic studies, consultation, or referrals.

B. Sex

1. Women may present differently to the ED (e.g., fatigue, pain or chest discomfort, shortness of breath, nausea, and palpitations) than men.

C. Athletes

1. May present with HF or sudden cardiac death (SCD) as a result of undiagnosed systolic HF, hypertrophic cardiomyopathy.

Additional Arrhythmias (2020 AHA Advanced Cardiac Life Support [ACLS] Guidelines—Saving American Hearts Inc.)

Follow advanced cardiac life support (ACLS) and pediatric advanced life support (PALS) algorithms for:

A. Supraventricular arrhythmias
B. Ventricular arrhythmias
C. Bradycardia arrhythmias

References and Additional Reading

References and Additional Reading for this chapter are online only and can be found at https://connect.springerpub.com/content/reference-book/978-0-8261-6091-5/part/part02/toc-part/ch15.

16. Vascular Medical Emergencies

COLLEEN ANDREONI | RENEÉ SEMONIN HOLLERAN

Learning Objectives

- Identify vascular emergencies seen in the ED, including hypertension (HTN), abdominal aortic aneurysms (AAA), aortic dissection, deep vein thrombosis (DVT), and pulmonary embolism (PE).
- Develop and implement a plan of care for the management of HTN, AAA, aortic dissection, DVT, and PE.
- Consider the disposition of patients with HTN, AAA, aortic dissection, DVT, and PE.

Vascular disease affects millions of Americans every year. Vascular emergencies are not an uncommon occurrence. It has been estimated that over 40% of patients seen in the ED have hypertension (HTN).[1] About 19 million cases of thromboembolism resulting in deep vein thrombosis (DVT) or pulmonary embolism (PE) occur worldwide annually. Abdominal pain may be the result of an AAA or an aortic dissection. This chapter addresses some of the conditions that may be seen in the ED by the emergency nurse practitioner (ENP).

Abdominal Aortic Aneurysm

An aneurysm is most often associated with atherosclerosis. Risk factors include smoking, diabetes mellitus (DM), CAD, hypertension (HTN), age >50 years, and family history. The intimal layer of the aorta dissects creating a false lumen and dilation of the vessel. AAA is >3 cm in diameter; the larger the aneurysm the greater the risk of rupture. Patients may be asymptomatic until leakage or rupture of the aneurysm occurs. Elderly males are most at risk.

Medical Screening

A. *Chief complaint*
  1. *Pain:* May be epigastric or abdominal pain, back pain, or groin pain
  2. Sudden onset of pain
  3. Described as shearing, tearing, sharp, and severe
  4. Nausea and vomiting
  5. Syncopal episode, weakness from hypovolemia
  6. May present unresponsive and unable to provide a chief complaint or history when in hypovolemic shock from acute blood loss

B. *Signs and symptoms*
  1. Vital signs may be normal or tachycardia, hypotension, or tachypnea.

C. *Focused assessment*
  1. Priority is given to immediate life threats.
  2. Abdominal examination may reveal a pulsatile mass, usually >5 cm when palpable.
  3. Abdominal rigidity, guarding, and rebound due to the intra-abdominal hemorrhage.
  4. Cullen's sign or Grey Turner's sign due to retroperitoneal hemorrhage.
  5. Scrotal or labial hematomas.
  6. Abdominal examination/palpation of the aneurysmal mass is often difficult on obese patients.
  7. Asymmetric or unequal femoral pulses are not a reliable finding.

Differential Diagnoses

A. Renal colic
B. Low back strain
C. Gastrointestinal (GI) bleed

Diagnostic Testing

A. *EKG:* Assists in ruling in or out differential diagnoses; valuable preoperatively

B. *Laboratory studies*
  1. Complete blood count (CBC)
  2. Coagulation studies
  3. Type and crossmatch
  4. Comprehensive metabolic panel (CMP)
  5. Cardiac troponin (cTn)

C. *Plain radiographs:* Anteroposterior (AP) and lateral views
  1. Look for a calcified bulging outline of the aorta.
  2. Abnormal in 50% of patients with AAA

D. *Bedside ultrasound:* Done quickly at the bedside for unstable patient. Obesity and bowel may decrease the accuracy. Pain may interfere with ability to get adequate visualization.

E. *Abdominal CT with contrast:* Indicated for stable patients to provide details of the aneurysm as well as any associated bleeding

Management

A. *Procedures*
  1. Vascular access
    a. Minimum two large-bore IV lines; use IV crystalloids cautiously—the amount and rate of fluid resuscitation remains controversial while awaiting blood. Target systolic blood pressure (SBP) is 90 mmHg.

2. Blood and blood product transfusion
   a. May need to implement hospital's massive transfusion protocol

B. *Pharmacologic therapies*
   1. Follow the evidence-based guidelines when prescribing.
   2. Beta-blockers
      a. Reduce significantly elevated blood pressure (BP)
      b. Esmolol
         i. Esmolol is short acting.
         ii. Monitor BP closely. If active bleeding is present, the BP will fall quickly.
   3. Opioid pain medication
      a. Administer cautiously; avoid hypotension.

C. *Consultation/collaboration*
   1. Vascular or endovascular surgeon

Patient Disposition

A. *Unstable patient*
   1. Requires emergent surgical repair of ruptured aneurysm

B. *Stable patient*
   2. Outpatient referral to vascular surgeon; control BP

C. *Documentation*
   1. Initial presentation and findings
   2. Reassessments
   3. Inclusion of family or friends present during discussions
   4. Consultation with ED physician, vascular surgeon, radiologist, or others

Age and Developmental Considerations

A. *Prevention and education*
   1. Behaviors to decrease the risk of atherosclerosis
   2. No smoking. The U.S. Preventive Services Task Force (USPSTF) recommends that men ages 65 to 75 who have ever smoked should have a one-time screening for AAA by abdominal ultrasound.
   3. Maintain good control of HTN.
   4. Compliance with medications
   5. Regular preventative and wellness visits with primary care physician (PCP)

B. *Patient and family education and counseling*
   1. Support for family during emergent situation
   2. Discussion of patient's wishes for resuscitation

Aortic Dissection

Aortic dissection is more frequent in men than women. Hypertension (HTN) and smoking are the most common risk factors. Other risk factors include Marfan syndrome, collagen vascular disease, atherosclerosis, ≥60 years of age, family history, trauma, cocaine use, or prior cardiac surgical procedures. A tear in the intimal layer of the aorta allows blood to seep between the intimal and the medial layers of the aorta. This process creates a false lumen and may affect perfusion of other vessels. There are two classification systems for aortic dissections. They are classified by anatomical location of the dissection: Stanford and DeBakey. Stanford classification type A dissections involve the ascending aorta; type B comprises those of the descending aorta. Type I of the DeBakey classification involves the ascending and descending aorta, type II is only of the ascending aorta, and type III is only of the descending aorta.

Associated conditions include aortic valve insufficiency, acute coronary syndrome (ACS), stroke symptoms, paraplegia due to occlusion of vertebral circulation, laryngeal nerve compression, and superior cervical sympathetic ganglion compression resulting in Horner's syndrome.

Medical Screening

A. *Chief complaint:* Sudden onset of sharp, tearing chest pain, often with radiation to between scapulae
   1. Dissection of ascending aorta is associated with anterior chest pain.
   2. Dissection of descending aorta is associated with abdominal or back pain.
   3. Syncope

B. *Signs and symptoms*
   1. Cardiovascular
      a. Tachycardia
      b. Hypertension (HTN), normal blood pressure (BP), or hypotension
      c. *Widened pulse pressure:* A difference of >15 mmHg difference in BP in each upper extremity, or difference in pulse quality between upper extremities
   2. Anxious, restless
   3. Nausea, vomiting, diaphoresis
   4. Poor peripheral perfusion
   5. Sense of impending doom
   6. Hemoptysis

C. *Focused assessment*
   1. Unequal BP or pulse deficit or ischemia in two sites
   2. Diastolic murmur due to aortic insufficiency
   3. New-onset aortic regurgitation
   4. Pericardial friction rub, muffled heart sounds
   5. Jugular vein distention (JVD)

Differential Diagnoses

A. ACS, pericarditis
B. Stroke, spinal cord disorder
C. Pulmonary embolus, pneumothorax

Diagnostic Testing

A. *EKG*
   1. Ischemia, nonspecific changes
   2. May see left ventricular hypertrophy (LVH), nonspecific ST- and T-wave changes, or be normal

B. *Chest x-ray (CXR)*
   1. Abnormal aortic silhouette, widening of the mediastinum
   2. May see tracheal or esophageal deviation, apical capping, pleural effusion
   3. CXR may be normal.

C. *Laboratory studies*
   1. Complete blood count (CBC), comprehensive metabolic panel (CMP), prothrombin time/international normalized ratio (PT/INR), coagulation studies, cardiac troponin (cTn)
   2. Consider brain natriuretic peptide (BNP), d-dimer, based on history and clinical examination.

D. *CT angiography (CTA):* Will identify a false lumen, extent of dissection, and extension into other vessels.
   1. Obtain CT chest before aortography, if time allows.
E. *Transesophageal echocardiogram (TEE)*
   1. Availability may be limited in some facilities.
   2. 97% to 100% sensitive and 97% to 99% specific.
F. *Coronary CT angiography (CCTA)*
   1. "Triple-rule-out" can diagnose coronary artery disease (CAD), pulmonary embolism (PE), and acute aortic dissection.
   2. Not yet widely available.
   3. Requires specialized contrast protocol.

Management

A. *Procedures*
   1. IV Large bore IV access, IV crystalloids cautiously for hypotension, the amount and rate of fluid resuscitation remains controversial.
   2. *Blood and blood product transfusion:* May need to implement hospital's massive transfusion protocol.
B. *Pharmacologic therapies*
   1. Follow evidence-based guidelines when prescribing.
   2. Opioids
      a. Administer for pain
   3. Beta-blockers:
      a. Target systolic blood pressure (SBP) is 100 to 120 mmHg: target heart rate (HR) is 60 to 70 bpm.
         i. Metoprolol, or
         ii. Labetalol, or
         iii. Esmolol infusion
   4. *Sodium nitroprusside:* Goal is controlled hypotension; lower SBP to 100 to 120 mmHg.
C. *Consultation/collaboration*
   1. Thoracic surgeon
   2. Endovascular surgeon

Patient Disposition

A. *Admission or outpatient referral*
   1. Descending dissections may be managed medically.
B. *Emergent surgical intervention:* Ascending dissections are generally managed surgically.
C. *Documentation*
   1. Initial presentation and findings
   2. Reassessments
   3. Inclusion of family or friends during discussions
   4. Consultation with ED physician, vascular surgeon, radiologist, or others

Age and Developmental Considerations

A. *Prevention and education*
   1. No smoking
   2. Maintain good control of HTN.
   3. Compliance with medications
   4. Regular preventative and wellness visits with PCP
B. *Patient and family education and counseling*
   1. Support for family during emergent situation
   2. Discussion of patient's wishes for resuscitation

Deep Vein Thrombosis

Deep vein thrombosis (DVT) is the formation of a blood clot within a deep vein. It is part of venous thromboembolism, which also includes pulmonary embolism. A DVT may occur within the upper or lower limbs, deep veins, visceral veins, and even a larger vein such as the vena cava.[2,3] Venous embolisms are associated with significant morbidity and mortality.[3] It is estimated that about 60,000 to 100,000 people die from venous thrombosis annually.[3] It is important to note that the patient may be at risk for developing another clot. Women are at greater risk than men to develop a DVT during childbearing years, especially during pregnancy. Predisposing factors that can cause hypercoagulability and provoke the development of a DVT include increasing age; postsurgical procedures, particularly orthopedic surgeries; immobilization; obesity; fractures; extended travel; cancer; and heritable risk factors such as Factor V Leiden. Unfortunately, many DVTs may not have an identifiable cause.[3]

Medical Screening

A. *Chief complaint*
   1. Extremity pain
   2. Redness in an extremity
   3. Swelling in an extremity
B. *Signs and symptoms*
   1. Edema greater in one extremity than another
   2. Erythema
   3. Fever
   4. Affected extremity tenderness
   5. *Rare cases:* Affected extremity pulseless in massive DVT
C. *Focused assessment*
   1. Evaluation of risk factors
   2. Homans' sign (forced dorsiflexion of the foot) is not a reliable sign; not recommended because it may dislodge a clot
   3. *Cardiac assessment:* Tachycardia
   4. *Pulmonary:* Decreased breath sounds may be related to a pulmonary embolism.
   5. Peripheral perfusion to the affected area
   6. Presence of pain, tenderness with palpation
   7. Increase in circumference or diameter of the calf

Differential Diagnoses

A. Cellulitis
B. Varicose veins
C. Laceration

Diagnostic Testing

A. *Prediction scores:* Well's score composed of specific patient factors, with 1 point for each factor (www.mdcalc.com/wells-criteria-dvt). Patient scores are stratified into low, intermediate, and high risk.
B. *Laboratory tests*
   1. D-dimer
   2. International normalized ratio (INR)
   3. Activated partial thromboplastin time (aPTT)
   4. Chemistry including electrolytes, liver, and renal function
   5. Complete blood count (CBC)

C. Radiology
  1. Doppler venous flow testing
  2. Venography
D. EKG

Management

A. *Procedures*
  1. Compression stockings
  2. Early ambulation
B. *Pharmacological*
  1. Anticoagulation agents for 3 months. The choice of agent to use is dependent upon hepatic and renal function; cancer; pregnancy; current medications, drug to drug interactions; and risk of bleeding.
  2. Follow evidence-based guidelines for prescribing.
    a. Direct acting oral anticoagulants (DOACs)
    b. Warfarin
    c. Low-molecular-weight heparin (LWMH)
    d. Intravenous unfractionated heparin

Patient Disposition

A. Unstable patient with risk factors, such as age or inability to initially manage their medications, or DVT of unclear etiology will require inpatient admission. DVT above the knee may require admission as well.
B. Stable patient may be treated on an outpatient basis with appropriate education and follow-up arranged before discharge.
C. Documentation
  1. Initial presentation and findings
  2. Reassessments
  3. Inclusion of family and friends in discussions, particularly related to medication use
  4. Consultation with ED physician, radiologist, primary or medical specialist caring for the patient

Age and Developmental Considerations

A. *Prevention and education*
  1. Education related to compression stocking use
  2. Education of medication use, including signs and symptoms of adverse effects related to medication use
  3. Medication management generally used for 3 months
  4. Importance of follow-up with medical care
  5. Importance of ambulation
B. *Patient and family education*
  1. Support for family during time in the ED
  2. Discussion with family about sources of support related to the diagnosis

Hypertension

Hypertension (HTN) or high blood pressure (BP) afflicts about 1.3 billion people all over the world. It is a serious disease because it can affect the heart, brain, and kidneys, thus contributing to end organ diseases. The American Heart Association (AHA) recognizes these high BP stages: hypertension stage 1—130–139 systolic and 80–89 diastolic; hypertension stage 2—140 or higher systolic and 90 or higher diastolic; hypertensive crisis—a BP of ≥180/≥120 mmHg.

In the ED, unless the patient is experiencing a hypertensive crisis, HTN can be harder to diagnose because of stress, injury, or illnesses. "White coat syndrome," a change in BP levels due to the presence of a clinician, is not uncommon and something that should be considered when evaluating the causes of a patient's HTN.[4]

Recognition of HTN and appropriate referral can reduce the risk of end organ damage such as angina, left ventricular hypertrophy (LVH), myocardial infraction (MI), cerebrovascular accident (CVA), and renal failure.[1,4–7]

Management of HTN provides an opportunity for the emergency nurse practitioner (ENP) to not only pharmacologically manage a patient's HTN but also offer education to prevent future problems.[1,5]

Medical Screening

A. *Chief complaint*
  1. Chest pain
  2. Abdominal pain
  3. Headache
  4. Vision changes
  5. Dyspnea
  6. Sleep disturbances
B. *History*
  1. Current diagnosis of hypertension
  2. Current medications for BP management
  3. Lack of following plan of care, including taking prescribed medications
  4. History of end organ failure disease
  5. *Comorbid conditions:* Obesity, diabetes, atherosclerosis, cardiovascular disease
C. *Focused assessment*
  1. BP assessment in supine and upright positions on both sides
  2. *Funduscopy:* Evidence of end organ disease, including hemorrhages, exudate, and papilledema
  3. Heart
    a. S_4 gallop
    b. New murmurs
  4. Pulmonary
    a. Increased respiratory effort
    b. Rales
    c. Anxious and uncomfortable
  5. Abdominal
    a. Palpable mass
    b. Pulsation
  6. Peripheral edema

Differential Diagnoses

A. Pheochromocytoma (PCC)
B. Hyperthyroidism
C. Myocardial infarction (MI)
D. Congestive heart failure (CHF)
E. Abdominal aortic aneurysm (AAA)

Diagnostic Testing

A. *EKG*
  1. Arrhythmia
  2. Left ventricular hypertrophy (LVH)
  3. Ischemic changes
B. *Chest radiograph*
  1. Enlarged cardiac silhouette
  2. Widened mediastinum
  3. Signs of heart failure

4. May be normal

C. *Laboratory studies*

1. Complete blood count (CBC), comprehensive metabolic panel (CMP), prothrombin time/international normalized ratio (PT/INR), coagulation studies, cardiac troponin (cTn)
2. Consider brain natriuretic peptid (BNP), d-dimer, based on history and clinical examination.
3. Urinalysis may reveal proteinuria or hematuria related to renal damage.

Management

A. Measure BP using properly sized cuff, correct position, both arms, and at least two separate times, which should include the patient resting in a comfortable position.

B. *Pharmacologic therapies*

1. Follow the evidence-based guidelines when prescribing drugs used in a hypertensive crisis.[7]
   a. Sodium nitroprusside
   b. Labetalol
   c. Esmolol
   d. Nitroglycerine
   e. Enalapril
   f. Furosemide
   g. Fenoldopam
   h. Nicardipine
   i. Clevidipine
   j. Verapamil
   k. Hydralazine
   l. Phentolamine
2. Drugs for used for high BP stages 1 and 2 (as described by the AHA [www.heart.org/-/media/files/health-topics/high-blood-pressure/hbp-rainbow-chart-english-pdf-ucm_499220.pdf]) should be prescribed by the patient's primary care physician (PCP). However, the ENP may consider starting treatment in the ED, especially if patient does not have a PCP. Pharmacological treatment is based on the stage of the disease, and the ENP should follow evidence-based guidelines.
   a. Thiazide diuretic
   b. ACE inhibitor
   c. Angiotensin-II receptor antagonist
   d. Calcium channel blocker
   e. Beta-blocker
   f. Combination medications

C. *Lifestyle changes*

1. Exercise
2. Weight loss
3. Low sodium diet
4. Smoking cessation
5. Monitoring alcohol use

Patient Disposition

A. *Admission or outpatient referral*

1. Hypertensive crisis may require admission for stabilization.
2. Hypertension urgency, which is described as a BP of >180/>110 mmHg; has no symptoms or indications of acute organ damage. Patient should be referred for outpatient follow-up once BP has been managed.

B. *Documentation*

1. Initial presentation and findings
2. Reassessments
3. Inclusion of family or friends during discussions
4. Consultation with ED physician, cardiologist, hospitalist, PCP, or others

Age and Developmental Considerations

A. *Prevention and education*

1. Start or continue lifestyle modifications
2. Maintain good control of HTN
3. Compliance with medications
4. Regular preventive and wellness visits with PCP

B. *Patient and family education and counseling*

1. Support for family during emergent situation
2. Review medication and lifestyle changes with patient and family.

Pulmonary Embolism

Pulmonary embolism (PE) is another form of venous thromboembolism that causes mechanical obstruction in the pulmonary vasculature.[8] Pulmonary emboli have been classified as acute, subacute, and chronic. A hemodynamically unstable PE, associated with hypotension, is known as a massive PE. Men are more likely to develop a PE than women. Risk factors for a PE are similar to the risk factors for DVT and include increasing age; postsurgical procedures, particularly orthopedic surgeries; immobilization; obesity; fractures; extended travel; cancer; and heritable risk factors such as Factor V Leiden.[3] It has also been found that, like a DVT, 50% of patients who have a PE may not have an obvious reason why it occurred.[3] In the United States, death from a PE has been estimated at about 100,000 patients per year.[8]

Treatment for a diagnosed PE is based upon the stability of the patient. Treatment with systemic fibrinolysis is recommended for high-risk unstable patients. Low-risk stable patients diagnosed with a PE may be treated with medications in the ED and, after monitoring, may be released to be followed up by their healthcare clinician.

The emergency nurse practitioner (ENP) must always assess the risk factors for the use of any anticoagulation medications, including: history of active major bleeding, pregnancy, history of bleeding risk, thrombocytopenia, and hemorrhage.

Medical Screening

A. *Chief complaint*

1. Shortness of breath
2. Pleuritic pain
3. Hemoptysis

B. *Signs and symptoms*

1. Tachypnea
2. Orthopnea
3. Tachycardia
4. Hypotension (HTN)
5. Jugular vein distention (JVD)
6. Rales
7. Decreased breath sounds
8. Fever
9. Swelling and erythema in calf or thigh
10. Agitation and "feelings of impending doom"

C. *Focused assessment*[9]

D. Assessment of hemodynamic stability: signs of circulatory collapse
E. Cardiac rhythm
F. Breath sounds
G. Edema in calf or thigh
H. Erythema in calf or thigh
I. Evaluation of risk factors

Differential Diagnoses

A. Pneumonia
B. Acute myocardial infarction (AMI)
C. Cardiogenic shock

Diagnostic Testing

A. Clinical experience with focus on high index of suspicion, particularly in patients who present with hemodynamic instability. Clinical assessment has been found to be non-inferior to clinical assessment performed by experienced clinicians.[9]
B. *Prediction scores*
   1. Well's score composed of specific patient factors, with 1 point for each factor (www.mdcalc.com/wells-criteria-pulmonary-embolism). Patient scores are stratified into low, intermediate, and high risk.
   2. Geneva score (www.mdcalc.com/geneva-score-revised-pulmonary-embolism) has a different point system for patient risk determination.
C. *Laboratory tests*
   1. D-dimer
   2. International normalized ratio (INR)
   3. Activated partial thromboplastin time (aPTT)
   4. Chemistry including electrolytes, liver, and renal function
   5. Complete blood count (CBC)
   6. Arterial blood gases
   7. Troponin
D. *EKG*
E. *Radiology*
   1. Chest radiograph
   2. Multidetector computed tomographic pulmonary angiography (MDCTPA)
   3. Ventilation–perfusion (VQ) scan
   4. Point-of-care ultrasound

Management

A. *Procedures*
   1. Unstable patient will require immediate resuscitation and treatment with IV thrombolytic agents *following evidence-based guidelines.*
   2. Other interventions for the unstable patient include catheter-directed thrombolysis and caval filters when anticoagulation is contraindicated.
   3. Stable patient with confirmed PE should receive an additional risk assessment score. Examples include Pulmonary Embolism Severity Index (PESI) and simplified Pulmonary Embolism Severity Index (sPESI).
B. *Pharmacologic*[10]
   1. Follow evidence-based guidelines when prescribing.
   2. *Unstable patient:* Systemic thrombolysis, tissue plasma activator is initiated.
   3. *Stable patient:* Patients considered low risk may be treated with the following:
      a. Low-dose molecular heparin
      b. Apixaban
      c. Rivaroxaban
      d. Patients need to be monitored in ED before discharge.

Patient Disposition

A. Unstable patient will require critical care admission or transfer for appropriate care.
B. Stable patient may be treated on an outpatient basis with appropriate education and follow-up arranged before discharge.
C. Documentation
   1. Initial presentation and findings
   2. Reassessments
   3. Inclusion of family and friends, particularly related to medication use
   4. Consultation with ED physician, radiologist, primary or medical specialist caring for the patient

Age and Developmental Considerations

A. *Prevention and education*
   1. Education of medication use, including signs and symptoms of adverse effects related to medication use
   2. Medication management: can be for several months or longer
   3. Importance of follow-up with medical care
   4. *Signs and symptoms of bleeding:* blood in stool, urine, excessive bruising
   5. Education related to compression stocking use, if prescribed
B. *Patient and family education*
   1. Support for family during time in the ED
   2. Discussion of patient's wishes for resuscitation if patient requires resuscitation
   3. Discussion with family about sources of support related to the diagnosis

Resources

- Pulmonary Embolism Severity Index (PESI) www.mdcalc.com/pulmonary-embolism-severity-index-pesi
- Simplified Pulmonary Embolism Severity Index (sPESI) www.mdcalc.com/simplified-pesi-pulmonary-embolism-severity-index

References

References for this chapter are online only and can be found at https://connect.springerpub.com/content/reference-book/978-0-8261-6091-5/part/part02/toc-part/ch16.

17. Medical Emergencies of the Stomach, Esophagus, and Duodenum

TIFFANY ANDREWS

Learning Objectives

- Describe clinical features, diagnosis, and acute management of common disorders of the esophagus, duodenum, and stomach.
- Identify red flag symptoms in patients with acute abdominal pain that indicate emergent or urgent conditions that require surgical consult.
- Determine appropriate diagnostic and imaging studies based on the location of the pain and the presentation of the patient.
- Discuss the treatment and disposition for common disorders of the esophagus, duodenum, and stomach.

Disorders of Esophagus, Stomach, and Duodenum

Abdominal pain complaints comprise 5% to 10% of ED visits per year, and undifferentiated abdominal pain remains the diagnosis for approximately 25% of patients discharged from the ED (80% pain-free within 2 weeks of presentation). Between 35% and 41% of those admitted to the hospital have undifferentiated abdominal pain. The terms "acute abdomen" and "abdominal emergency" signify the need for prompt diagnosis and early treatment but does not always mean surgery. The U.S. National Center for Health Statistics data indicate that abdominal pain was the most frequently mentioned reason for patients visiting the ED in 2006. Admission rates for abdominal pain vary markedly, ranging from 18% to 42%, with rates as high as 63% in patients >65.

Appendicitis is one of the most common abdominal emergencies. In appendicitis, an acute obstruction of the appendiceal lumen results in distention followed by organ ischemia, bacterial overgrowth, and eventual perforation of the viscus. Misdiagnosis remains an important cause of successful malpractice claims against emergency clinicians. Mesenteric ischemia is a common nonspecific abdominal complaint that needs to be considered early in the patient's ED presentation, otherwise the intestines will rapidly become gangrenous and infarct, leading to multisystem organ failure, sepsis, and eventual death.

Nausea and vomiting (N/V) are a common and distressing presenting complaint in the ED related to GI disorders, but for systemic causes as well. Common conditions presenting as N/V include cyclic vomiting syndrome (CVS), hyperemesis gravidarum, and gastroparesis. Diarrhea is defined as three or more watery stools per day. Common conditions presenting as diarrhea include *Clostridium difficile* or pseudomembranous colitis, indeterminate colitis, and gastroenteritis.

Inflammatory bowel diseases (IBD) include ulcerative colitis (UC), Crohn's disease, and diverticulitis. These conditions have unique pathophysiologic elements, but each involves inflammation of the bowel wall with risk for episodic inflammation, perforation, infection, or bleeding. IBD may be related to autoimmune and/or genetic factors and may involve the entire bowel from duodenum to rectum (Crohn's disease) or be isolated to the colon and rectum (ulcerative colitis, diverticulitis).

Constipation is the one of the most common digestive complaints in the United States and ED. It is a symptom, rather than a disease, and represents an interpretation of real or imagined disturbance of bowel function. Constipation is characterized by the presence of two or more of the following complaints: straining, hard stools, sensation of incomplete evacuation, and fewer than three bowel movements per week. Constipation is chronic in patients with symptoms for 3 months consecutive or nonconsecutive for 12 months. Approximately 300,000 patients are hospitalized annually with acute small bowel obstruction (SBO) and typically admitted from the ED after imaging and stabilization. Hernias are a protrusion of any viscus from its normal cavity, are the leading cause of intestinal obstruction in the world, and a common surgical problem.

Hepatic disorders may present as manifestations of hepatocellular dysfunction, including jaundice, RUQ pain, hepatomegaly, abdominal distention, and ascites secondary to worsening cirrhosis due to infectious, toxic/allergic, immunopathological/autoimmune, or vascular processes. Diseases of the biliary tract are common and result in significant morbidity and mortality. Pancreatitis is an inflammation of the pancreas. Acute liver failure (ALF) is a rare clinical presentation in the ED, although it carries a high mortality, morbidity, and resource cost. It differs clinically, therapeutically, and prognostically from hepatic cirrhosis, but priorities in management are the same. ALF definition includes international normalized ratio (INR) ≥1.5, neurologic dysfunction with any degree of hepatic encephalopathy, no preexisting cirrhosis, and disease course of 26 weeks or less. Coagulopathies and GI bleeding are associated with the loss of protein synthesis and vascular congestion associated with portal hypertension. GI bleeding, alone without liver failure, is a common presentation to the ED, which involves bleeding anywhere from the mouth to the anus.

Esophageal disorders include perforation of the esophagus, foreign object ingestions, dysphagia, GERD, and peptic ulcer disease (PUD). Perforation of the esophagus is associated with high mortality rate regardless of cause. Foreign objects can be located anywhere along the GI tract and may be caused by ingestion, insertion via the rectum or ostomy opening, or secondary to trauma. Dysphagia is an alarm symptom or subjective sensation that may be due to a structural or motility abnormality. GERD is a highly variable chronic condition characterized by periodic episodes of backward flow of gastric contents into the esophagus. PUD is a chronic illness of recurrent ulcerations in the stomach and proximal duodenum.

Gastritis is the acute or chronic inflammation of the gastric mucosa. Dyspepsia is continuous or recurrent upper abdominal pain or discomfort with or without other symptoms.

Disorders of the esophagus, duodenum, and stomach are the common ED complaints that can range from benign, undifferentiated conditions to life-threatening. It is important for the emergency nurse practitioner to start with a timely, systematic approach with a focused history and physical examination to identify and manage these conditions.

Biliary Disease and Pancreatitis

Prevalence

A. 20% of people in the United States will suffer from symptomatic gallstones, and if untreated, 20% to 30% of these patients will develop serious complications, such as choledocholithiasis, cholecystitis, cholangitis, or pancreatitis.
B. Overall mortality of pancreatitis is 5%, and in severe disease can reach 25% to 35%.
C. Pancreatitis affects between 12.4 and 31.2 per 100,000 in all age groups; 3.5 per 100,000 in children.

Anatomy

A. Biliary tract refers to the liver, gallbladder, and bile ducts.
B. The tract is referred to as a tree because of its many small branches that end in the common bile duct. The duct, the branches of the hepatic artery, and the portal vein form the central axis of the portal triad.
C. The biliary tract flows from the bile canaliculi → canals of Hering → intrahepatic bile ductile (in portal tracts) → interlobular bile ducts → left and right hepatic ducts that merge to form the common hepatic duct.
D. The tract exits to the liver and joins with the cystic duct from the gallbladder, and together they form the common bile duct that joins the pancreatic duct, which passes through the ampulla of Vater and enters the duodenum.
E. The pancreas is about 6 inches long across the back of the abdomen, behind the stomach, passes to the right of the abdomen, and is connected to the duodenum through the pancreatic duct.

Pathophysiology

A. *Cholelithiasis*
  1. Stones occur because of supersaturation of bile with cholesterol, fragments such as bilirubin, or both combined with delayed emptying of the gallbladder. Gallstones remain in the gallbladder.
  2. Fatty meals exacerbate the painful episodes secondary to the secretion of hormones that cause the gallbladder to contract and bile to release into the digestive tract to aid in the breakdown of fats in the intestines.
B. *Choledocholithiasis*
  1. Stone moves out of the gallbladder and is obstructing the common bile duct, then the stone obstructs flow from contributing ducts—the cystic and hepatic ducts.
  2. With significant obstruction comes congestion of the biliary tree, which causes backflow into the liver and eventually into the blood, leading to bilirubinemia.
C. *Cholecystitis*
  1. Inflammation of the gallbladder and is related to the presence of gallstones in 90% to 95% of cases. Acalculous cholecystitis occurs in <10% of cases and is seen more in older adults, postoperative, or critically ill.
  2. The cystic duct is blocked by a gallstone, causing obstruction, pain, and inflammation in calculus cholecystitis.
    a. If untreated, cholecystitis can progress to necrosis, gangrene, and perforation.
D. *Cholangitis*
  1. Inflammation of the bile ducts that is most often caused by a polymicrobial infection.
  2. Biliary obstruction, from a stone or neoplasm, is a major factor pathology.
E. *Pancreatitis*
  1. Classified as mild (no organ failure or necrosis), moderately severe (<48 hours of organ failure or local complication), or severe (>48 hours of organ failure).
  2. *Toxic causes:* Alcohol (most common), methanol, drugs (angiotensin-converting enzyme [ACE], azathioprine, calcium, cisplatin, steroids, estrogen, erythromycin, furosemide, mercaptopurine, metronidazole, nitrofurantoin, propofol, octreotide, ranitidine, salicylates, sulfa, tamoxifen, tetracycline, thiazide, and valproate)
  3. *Metabolic causes:* Hypercalcemia, hyperlipidemia, diabetic ketoacidosis (DKA)
  4. *Obstructive causes:* Gallstones (most common), ampullary tumors, pancreas divisum, endoscopic retrograde cholangiopancreatography (ERCP), post-pancreatography, neuroendocrine tumors, pancreatic cancer, stricture, fibrosis of sphincter of Oddi
  5. *Infectious causes:* Viral (adenovirus, coxsackievirus, cytomegalovirus [CMV], EBV (Epstein Barr virus), HIV (human immunodeficiency virus), hepatatis A, B, or C,

varicella, rubella, echovirus) or other (aspergillus, campylobacter, cryptococcus, mumps, tuberculosis [TB] salmonella, streptococcus, legionella)

6. *Other causes:* Crohn's, cystic fibrosis, emboli hemochromatosis, hypothermia, vasculitis, lupus, ischemia, pregnancy, Reye's syndrome, trauma, uremia, scorpion bites, idiopathic

Predisposing Factors

A. Biliary disease, alcohol abuse, high cholesterol, acetaminophen use, certain medications, female gender, older age, obesity, rapid weight loss, parity, family history, total parenteral nutrition (TPN), diabetes, squamous cell carcinoma (SCC)

Medical Screening

A. *Chief complaint:* Dull, boring, achy epigastric, or right upper quadrant (RUQ) pain that may radiate to right shoulder and is associated with eating a large meal of fatty foods. Patient may also have nausea and vomiting (N/V).

B. *High yield history*

1. *Risk factors for cholecystitis:* 4F's—obese (fat), female, pregnant (fertile), forty; recent weight loss or history of gallstones
2. Classic pain is in RUQ and exacerbated by eating meals with high fat content.
   a. Pain may radiate to the right shoulder (Collins' sign).
   b. Rapid onset of epigastric or upper quadrant pain radiating to back that is severe in nature with N/V is more consistent with pancreatitis.
3. Most patients will complain of intermittent RUQ pain after meals for several weeks or months before they present to the ED with severe pain.
   a. In uncomplicated symptomatic cholelithiasis, the pain may last 4 to 6 hours before it spontaneously resolves.
   b. Pain lasting over 6 hours or with other associated features, such as fever, jaundice, or confusion, suggest more serious complications.
4. N/V are common.

C. *Signs and symptoms*

1. Fever occurs in cholecystitis or cholangitis.
2. Episodic RUQ or epigastric pain associated with N/V (caused by intermittently obstructing the neck of the gallbladder).
3. Pain may radiate to back, right flank, tip of the right scapula, and right shoulder.
4. Patients with pancreatitis may present with fever, tachycardia and hypoxia, epigastric tenderness, and jaundice. Pain is worse when supine.
5. Hemorrhagic pancreatitis will have Cullen's sign (periumbilical ecchymosis) or Grey Turner's sign (flank ecchymosis).

D. *Past medical history (PMH)*

1. Heavy alcohol use (can cause cirrhosis and fatty liver, mimicking cholecystitis, Inflammatory bowel disease, cirrhosis, and diabetes increase risk of cholecystitis. History of pancreatitis may suggest prior gallstones, alcohol abuse, diabetes, and pancreatic cancer.

Physical Examination

A. *General*

1. *Charcot's triad:* Fever, RUQ pain, and jaundice (cholangitis)
2. *Reynold's pentad:* Fever, RUQ pain, jaundice, shock, and altered mental status (AMS; severe cholangitis)
3. Patients with asymptomatic gallstones or biliary colic appear to be well.
4. Patients with pancreatitis will be in moderate distress.

B. *Vital signs*

1. May have fever, tachycardia, or hypotension if severe or sepsis

C. *Skin*

1. Jaundice of the skin in obstructive jaundice. May appear pale
2. Erythematous skin nodules may be seen due to fat necrosis.
3. May exhibit muscle spasms due to hypocalcemia

D. *Head, eyes, ears, nose, and throat (HEENT)*: Scleral icterus or mucous icterus can be seen with hyperbilirubinemia.

E. *Cardiac*: Normal, regular pulse

F. *Pulmonary*: Typically normal

1. Hypoxia or tachypnea pleural effusions may be seen or heard as diminished breath sounds or rales if severe pancreatitis.

G. Abdominal

1. RUQ, epigastric tenderness, rebound tenderness, and guarding may be present.
2. *Murphy's sign*: Patient stops inhaling when the RUQ is being palpated.
3. *Blumberg sign*: Rebound tenderness
4. *Courvoisier's sign*: Palpable abdominal mass in right upper quadrant
5. *Grey Turner's sign*: Hemorrhagic discoloration of flanks
6. *Cullen's sign*: Hemorrhagic discoloration of umbilicus
7. *Grunwald sign*: Appearance of ecchymosis around the umbilicus due to local toxic lesion of the vessels
8. *Korte's sign*: Pain or resistance 6 to 7 cm above umbilicus
9. *Kamenchik's sign*: Pain with pressure under xiphoid process
10. *Mayo-Robson's sign*: Pain while pressing at top of the angle lateral to erector spinae muscles or below left 12th rib (cerebrovascular accident [CVA])
11. Bowel sounds may be diminished.
12. Abdominal distention secondary to ileus
13. Rectal examination should be normal. A positive hemoccult or blood on examination suggests alternative diagnosis.

H. Neurologic*:* AMS if septic; may appear anxious

Differential Diagnoses

A. *Acute cholecystitis*

1. Acute inflammation and obstruction of the gallbladder resulting in >6 hours of pain
2. May occur with or without bacterial infection. RUQ pain, fever, N/V, plus Murphy's sign

B. *Cholelithiasis*

1. Gallstones without evidence of obstruction or inflammation
2. Biliary colic is the intermittent obstruction of the cystic or common bile ducts (CBD) resulting in pain. Precursor for cholecystitis
3. Epigastric or RUQ pain that can be intermittent or constant. Pain can radiate to left shoulder, although examination generally benign.
4. Associated with eating fatty foods, N/V

C. *Choledocholithiasis*
1. Obstruction of CBD
2. If uncomplicated a similar presentation and exam can be seen in cholelithiasis

D. *Cholangitis*
1. An obstruction and ascending infection of the common bile duct
2. Charcot's triad (RUQ pain, jaundice +/-fever)

E. *Pancreatitis*
1. Diagnosis established by presence of 2/3 criteria, such as abdominal pain consistent with disease, lipase, or amylase >3x upper limit of normal and characteristic findings from abdominal imaging

F. Gallstone pancreatitis, abdominal aortic aneurysm, peptic ulcer disease, pancreatitis, appendicitis, pyelonephritis, renal colic, small bowel obstruction, hepatitis, emphysema, pneumonia, diverticulitis, hepatitis, esophagitis, pulmonary embolism, acute coronary syndrome (ACS)

Diagnostic Testing

A. *Labs*
1. Urinalysis (UA), human chorionic gonadotropin (hCG) to look for urinary tract infection (UTI) or pregnancy as alternative diagnosis
2. Complete blood count (CBC) may show leukocytosis in cholecystitis or cholangitis.
3. *Liver function tests (LFTs):* Alkaline phosphatase and bilirubin elevated in choledocholithiasis and may be elevated in cholecystitis. Alanine aminotransferase (ALT) >150 iU suggests biliary pancreatitis.
4. Amylase/lipase elevated in pancreatitis. Lipase is more sensitive. Patients with recurrent or chronic pancreatitis may have normal or minimally elevated lipase level.
5. *Biliary colic:* Generally normal
6. *Acute cholecystitis:* White blood cells (WBC) (normal or elevated), aspartate aminotransferase/alanine aminotransferase (AST)/(ALT), T-bili, and alk phos (normal or elevated)
7. *Choledocholithiasis:* Alkaline phosphatase (increased), total bilirubin (increased), AST/ALT (increased), lipase (increased), WBC (increased)
8. *Cholangitis:* WBC (increased), bili (increased), alk phos (increased), AST/ALT (increased)
9. *Pancreatitis:* Ranson criteria
   a. The Ranson criteria form is a clinical prediction rule for predicting the prognosis and mortality risk based on initial ad 48-hour lab values.
   b. For non-gallstone pancreatitis, the criteria on admission:
      i. Age >55 years; glucose >200 mg/dL; WBC count >16 × 10^3/microliter; serum AST (serum glutamic-oxaloacetic transaminase [SGOT]) >250 units/L; and serum lactate dehydrogenase (LDH) >350 units/L
   c. Criteria after 48 hours of admission:
      i. Hct fall >10%; estimated fluid sequestration >6 L; base deficit >4 mEq/L; blood urea nitrogen rise >5 mg/dL; serum calcium <8 mg/dL; PO_2 <60 mmHg. Number of criteria and approximate mortality (%): 0 to 2 = 0%, 3 to 4 = 15%, 5 to 6 = 50%, above 6 = 100%
   d. For gallstone-associated pancreatitis:
      i. *Criteria on admission:* Aage >70 years; glucose >220 mg/dL; WBC count >18 × 10^3/ microliter; serum AST (SGOT) >250 units/L; and serum LDH >400 units/L. Criteria after 48 hours of admission: Hct fall >10%; estimated fluid sequestration >4 L; base deficit >5 mEq/L; blood urea nitrogen rise >2 mg/dL; serum calcium <8 mg/dL

B. *Consider EKG.*

C. *Imaging*
1. *RUQ ultrasound (US):* Identify gallstones, dilated CBD (3 mm at 30 years old and add 1 mm for each 10 years), gallbladder wall thickening, pericholecystic fluid
   a. *Biliary colic:* Gallstones
   b. *Acute cholecystitis:* Pericolic fluid, gallbladder wall thickness >3 mm, and sonographic Murphy's sign
   c. *Choledocholithiasis:* CBD >6 mm
   d. *Cholangitis:* Ductal dilatation, stones
   e. Gold standard
      i. Visualization of gallbladder can be affected by colonic gas. Patients should be NPO for 12 hours prior to study if possible.
2. *CT with contrast:* Not normally needed, although can help if diagnosis uncertain or concern for complication. Does not visualize gallbladder well. Use for evaluation of necrosis, masses, other cause, persistent fever, systemic inflammatory response syndrome (SIRS), organ dysfunction 48 to 72 hours after admission.
3. Chest x-ray (CXR) if concern for effusion/infiltrates
4. *Endoscopic retrograde cholangiopancreatography (ERCP):* Diagnostic to characterize a biliary duct obstruction as well as to intervene
5. *Magnetic resonance cholangiopancreatography (MRCP):* To further characterize biliary duct obstructions, if no signs of obstruction on US, to screen for choledocholithiasis
6. Hepatobiliary iminodiacetic (HIDA) scan
   a. If high suspicion but indeterminate US
   b. Shows uptake of radioactive isotope in the gallbladder if there is no obstruction but delayed filling or no filling in cholecystitis.

Management

A. Start IV fluids (IVF) if needed; aggressive hydration of 250 to 500 mL/hour or 5 to 10 mL/kg/hour in pancreatitis (LR over NS).

B. Keep patient from taking anything by mouth (NPO, esp. if N/V present) until symptoms resolve.
C. Reassess resuscitation within 6 hours and the next 24 to 48 hours and monitor for complications such as volume overload, pulmonary edema, or abdominal compartment syndrome.
D. Replace electrolytes as needed, especially calcium in pancreatitis secondary to saponification.
E. Vasopressors are indicated if hypotension not responsive to fluids.
F. *Provide pain relief:* NSAIDs are effective in treating biliary colic. Narcotic for pancreatitis is usually needed.
G. Antiemetics (ondansetron, metoclopramide, prochlorperazine) as needed
H. Cholelithiasis requires no treatment but increases the risk of acute cholecystitis.
I. Biliary colic with impacted stone symptoms less likely to resolve and will need surgery consult.
J. Acute cholecystitis
  1. Consult surgery for cholecystectomy.
    a. May be delayed several days to allow inflammation to decrease and prevent operative complications.
  2. Start antibiotics to prevent complications.
    a. Zosyn, ampicillin + gentamicin, third-generation cephalosporin, imepenem-cilastin (penetrates pancreatic necrosis), meropenem, ciprofloxacin plus metronidazole
K. Cholangitis
  1. Requires aggressive treatment to prevent sepsis and hemodynamic collapse.
  2. Start broad-spectrum antibiotics with anerobic coverage.
    a. Pipercillin-tazobactram, imipenem, unasyn + metronidazole
  3. ERCP with gastrointestinal (GI) consult versus surgery consult
  4. Arrange for emergent biliary drainage if abscess.
    a. May require percutaneous cholecystectomy tube if patient is too unstable for surgery.
L. *Choledocholithiasis:* Symptom control, ERCP for high risk, MRCP for low or intermediate risk, GI consult
M. If pancreatitis is severe, causing systemic disease, patient may require intubation, ICU, or transfusion.

Age and Developmental Considerations

A. Acalculous cholecystitis is more common in older adults and critically ill patients, especially those on TPN, as well as AIDS patients because of CMV.
  1. Associated with long-term TPN. Fever may be only symptom. Higher acuity and mortality than calculous cholecystitis
  2. Emphysematous cholecystitis is characterized by gas in the gallbladder wall thought to be invasion of mucosa by gas-producing organisms.
  3. Common in diabetic patients, males, and 50% of acalculous cholecystitis cases
B. Patients who have had a cholecystectomy can still develop choledocholithiasis.
C. Normally CBD is 6 mm and can increase 2 mm every decade after 60 years old and is usually dilated after cholecystectomy.
D. Consider gallstone pancreatitis in patients who present with pancreatitis (lipase >3x normal).
E. Postoperative pain after laparoscopic surgery can have retained stone or bile leak.

Patient Disposition (Referrals, Follow-Up, Education)

A. Patients with biliary colic with improving symptoms may be discharged with outpatient follow-up with general surgeon for possible elective cholecystectomy.
B. Advise patients to return to ED if prolonged symptoms >6 hours or associated with fever or jaundice.
C. Patients with choledocholithiasis should be admitted for definitive treatment secondary to risk of associated complications.
D. Acute cholecystitis and cholangitis should be admitted for IV antibiotics and possible surgical intervention.
E. ICU admission if signs of sepsis, end organ dysfunction, or hypotension

Constipation and Obstruction

Prevalence

A. Constipation represents 2.5 million healthcare visits per year
B. Incidence increases with age, with 30% to 40% of patients >65 years old citing constipation, 3% of preschool-age children and 1% to 2% of school-age children, and is more common in boys.
C. Constipation affects as many as 80% of critically ill patients and is directly associated with patient mortality in older adults.
D. Incidence of small bowel obstruction (SBO) is 1.47 per 100,000 per year in the United States.
E. Patients with large bowel obstruction (LBO) is approximately 0.15 to 0.29 per 100,000. In patients with Crohn's disease may be as high as 250 per 100,000.
F. Approximately 100 to 500 per 100,000 patients with no prior abdominal surgery and 600 per 100,000 in patients who have.
G. Abdominal wall hernias are common, with a prevalence of 1.7% for all ages and 4% for those over 45 years. Inguinal hernias account for 75% of abdominal wall hernias.

Anatomy

A. Intestines are a long, continuous tube running from the stomach to the anus, including the small intestine (20 feet long, 1 inch diameter), large intestine (5 feet long, 3 inch diameter), and rectum.
B. Colon terminates in the rectum, which, in turn passes through the levator ani muscles and becomes the anal canal.
C. The internal anal sphincter (involuntary) and external anal sphincter (voluntary)
D. A nearly 90-degree angle is formed at the junction of the rectum and the anal canal, which straightens with flexion of the hips.
E. Hernias are classified by location, contents, and status of the contents (reducible, incarcerated, or strangulated).
  1. *Reducible*: When contents can easily be returned to the original cavity by manipulation.

2. *Incarcerated*: When contents are not reducible.
3. *Strangulation:* Vascular compromise of the incarcerated contents; condition is a surgical emergency. Can lead to gangrene, peritonitis, and septic shock.

F. Inguinal hernia
1. Protrusion through Hesselbach's triangle medially to the inferior epigastric vessels or through the internal inguinal ring, transverses the inguinal canal to external ring and may extend into the scrotum.
2. Common causes are increased pressure within the abdomen and preexisting weak spot in the abdominal wall, chronic coughing/sneezing, abdominal wall defects, and advanced age.

G. Femoral hernia
1. Protrusion below the inguinal ligament through the femoral canal
2. High risk for incarceration or strangulation

H. Umbilical hernia
1. Congenital malformation common in infants, can be acquired as well.
2. Weakness of the abdominal fascia or failure to fully form the fascia, which may lead to a herniation after increased abdominal pressure caused by obesity, lifting, coughing, or multiple pregnancies.
3. Strangulation and incarceration are rare.

I. Diaphragmatic hernia
1. Congenital anomaly that occurs due to a failure of the diaphragm to close, leading to herniation of the abdominal contents into the thoracic cavity
2. Presents in neonates as respiratory distress.

J. Incisional hernia
1. Caused by an incompletely healed surgical wound (median incisions in the linea alba are frequently used in laparotomy, ventral hernias are common)

K. Hiatal hernia
1. Sliding (most common)
   a. Herniation of the distal esophagus and gastric cardia into the thoracic space (type I)
2. Paraesophageal
   a. Herniation of the gastric fundus but not the gastroesophageal junction (type II)
   b. Type III is a combination of types I and II through the diaphragm.
   c. Type IV is the most severe and when other abdominal organs along with the stomach and distal esophagus herniate into the thoracic cavity.

L. Epigastric hernia
1. Caused by weakness or defect in the upper abdominal muscles or tendons
2. Herniated contents are mostly compromised of vascular, peritoneal fat or abdominal viscera.

M. Spigelian hernia is caused by a defect in the anterior abdominal wall.

N. Amyand's hernia is an inguinal hernia containing the appendix vermiformis.

O. Parastomal hernia is a complication of colostomy or ileostomy, a type of incisional hernia.

Pathophysiology

A. The process of defecation involves the propulsion of stool through the colon to the rectum, the recognition of stool within the rectum, and the conscious act of defecation.

B. Within 3 to 4 hours after ingestion, food enters the cecum, and then after several more hours reaches the rectum.

C. When the rectal wall is distended by stool, reflex contraction of the rectum occurs, the internal anal sphincters relax, and fecal material pushes into the anal canal.

D. The stool stretches the receptors, and a conscious decision is made to push the stool out by relaxing the external anal sphincter, squatting, or increasing abdominal pressure with the Valsalva maneuver or to postpose defecation by contracting the external anal sphincter and gluteal muscles.

E. Gut motility is affected by diet, activity level, fluid intake, fiber intake, exercise, medications, toxins, anatomic lesions, gut flora, hormone levels, and a host of medical and psychiatric conditions.

F. Functional constipation includes changes in medications, dietary supplements, decrease in fluid or fiber intake, change in activity level, illness, or injury.
1. *Dietary:* Low fiber, excessive alcohol, excessive caffeine, dehydration
2. *Medications:* Opioids, antihistamines, chronic laxative use, antidiarrheal
3. *Metabolic and endocrine:* Hypercalcemia, hyperparathyroidism, hypothyroidism
4. *Neuromuscular:* Parkinson's, cauda equina syndrome, autonomic neuropathy
5. *Congenital:* Hirschsprung's, cystic fibrosis, meconium ileus

G. Organic constipation is typically from obstruction or carcinoma, hernia, appendicitis, intussusception, or pregnancy.

H. Consider intussusception, foreign bodies, or congenital abnormalities as causes of obstruction in children.

I. Intestinal obstruction results from mechanical blockage of forward flow or the loss of normal peristalsis.

J. *Two types of obstructions:* SBO and LBO
1. *SBO:* Adhesions from prior surgery, malignancy, Crohn's disease, incarcerated hernia, inflammatory diseases, diverticulitis with stricture
2. *LBO:* Volvulus, malignancy, diverticular abscess, pseudo-obstruction, ulcerative colitis/Crohns

K. Diarrhea may occur with constipation/obstruction symptoms, as liquid stool can pass around impaction or obstructive source.

Predisposing Factors

A. Family history of colon, ovarian or uterine cancer, hypothyroidism, diverticulitis, inflammatory stricture, nephrolithiasis, hyperparathyroidism, low fiber diet, diabetes mellitus, Down syndrome, spinal cord abnormalities, infant botulism, Chagas disease, lupus, scleroderma, past medical history (PMH) of prior abdominal surgeries, hernia repair, malignancy, IBD, immunocompromised state, lack of developmental maturity, undescended testes, genitourinary abnormalities, conditions that increase intra-abdominal pressure, ascites, pregnancy, chronic obstructive pulmonary disease (COPD), surgical incision sites, heavy lifting, straining to defecate or urinate

Medical Screening

A. *Chief complaint:* Constipation, abdominal bloating, abdominal pain characterized as crampy, intermittent (often poorly localized), distention, nausea, and vomiting (N/V) with the absence of flatus or bowel movements (if obstruction present), bulging of the abdominal wall or groin

B. *High yield history*

1. Pain may be intermittent and colicky in nature or constant and crampy.
2. May have bilious or fecal vomiting (if obstruction).
3. Any abdominal surgery increases the risk of adhesion formation and secondary bowel obstruction; can also be associated with ileus.
4. Asymptomatic hernias have swelling or fullness at hernia site, aching sensation that radiates into hernia (no pain or tenderness on exam), enlarges with increasing intra-abdominal pressure or standing.
5. Incarcerated hernias are a painful enlargement of a previous hernia or defect that cannot be manipulated through the fascial defect. Patients commonly have N/V, symptoms of bowel obstruction.
6. Strangulated hernias have symptoms like incarceration, with systemic toxicity due to ischemic bowel possible. Pain and tenderness of an incarcerated hernia persists after reduction.
7. Ask about the patient's last bowel movement. Constipation and lack of flatus are signs of complete obstruction, but a patient may still pass flatus with a partial obstruction.
8. Ask patient about new medications or dietary supplements, a decrease in fluid or fiber intake, or a change in activity level.
9. A history of unexplained weight loss, rectal bleeding, change in stool caliber, or unexplained iron deficiency anemia suggests colon cancer.
10. A family history of colon cancer would escalate your suspicion of obstruction.
11. *Associated illnesses:* Cold intolerance (hypothyroidism), or nephrolithiasis (hyperparathyroidism)

C. *Signs and symptoms*

1. Most hernias are detected on routine physical exam or accidentally by the patient and may have pain that is worse with standing, straining, and lifting something heavy.
2. Straining, hard stools, incomplete evacuation, and fewer than three bowel movements per week
3. In SBO, crampy, colicky, or intermittent progressive abdominal pain and inability to have a bowel movement or inability to pass flatus
   a. LLQ pain and longer spasms in LBO
   b. Patients with partial bowel obstructions can still pass flatus.
4. Nausea, vomiting (N/V), and biliousness occurs in proximal obstructions or strangulated hernias, and feculence in distal obstructions.
5. Constant severe pain indicates peritoneal irritation; sudden severe pain indicates bowel perforation.

D. *Past medical history*

1. Medication use (anticholinergics, tricyclics, narcotics, alcohol, caffeine); Parkinson's, cystic fibrosis, Hirschsprung's, metabolic or endocrine disorders, pregnancy, diabetes mellitus, Down syndrome, spinal cord abnormalities, infant botulism, Chagas disease, lupus, scleroderma, abdominal surgeries, cancer increases the risk of peritoneal metastasis and adhesion formation, ulcerative colitis and Crohn's disease, intestinal pseudo obstruction (mimic LBO), diverticulitis, hernias, volvulus, colorectal resection, adhesive bowel disease.
2. *Conditions that increase risk:* Parkinson's and so on.

Physical Examination

A. *General*

1. Check patient weight, overall nutritional status.
2. Generally, patient is well-appearing and stable unless strangulation, obstruction, perforation have occurred.
3. Perform hernia exam both supine and standing, with and without Valsalva maneuver.

B. *Vital signs:* Fever, tachycardia, tachypnea, hypotension (sepsis or perforation)

C. ***Skin:*** Pallor, signs of hypothyroidism (reduced body hair, skin dryness, fixed edema), dry mucous membranes, or decreased turgor in dehydration

D. *Head, eyes, ears, nose, and throat (HEENT):* Commonly normal

E. *Cardiac:* Commonly normal

F. *Pulmonary:* Commonly normal; tachypnea if distention severe

G. *Abdominal*

1. Look for evidence of hernias (tenderness, reducibility, and appearance of skin) or abdominal masses (volvulus, hernia, tumor, and impacted feces), surgical scars, and ascites.
   a. Attempt to identify hernia sac as well as the fascial defect through which it is protruding (allows for proper direction of pressure for reduction).
   b. Look for swelling or mass in area of fascial defect.
   c. Inguinal hernias
      i. Coughing may be necessary to expose hernia.
      ii. May feel a thickened cord in the scrotal sac.
      iii. Place fingertip into scrotal sac and advance upward into the inguinal canal.
      iv. If the inguinal hernia comes from superolateral to inferomedial and strikes the distal tip of the finger, most likely indirect—an indirect hernia (or a hernia into the scrotum).
      v. If the inguinal hernia strikes the pad of the finger from deep to superficial, most likely direct—A direct hernia (or a hernia that forms on one side of the groin but not in the scrotum).
   d. If felt below the inguinal ligament, the type of hernia is more consistent with a femoral hernia.

e. Peritoneal signs and intestinal obstruction suggest incarceration.

f. Pain out of proportion to exam or pain that persists after reduction suggests strangulation

2. *Abdominal distention*: Mild in ileus; moderate if severe obstruction.

3. Bowel sounds will be decreased in the setting of slow gut transit but increased in the setting of obstruction. Tympanic to percussion.

4. Assess for tenderness

a. Diffuse in ileus, may localize to upper quadrants in obstruction

b. Peritoneal signs (guarding, tenderness or rebound tenderness) are concerning for strangulation or perforation.

5. Rectal examination will detect tenderness, masses, foreign bodies, hemorrhoids, abscesses, fecal impaction, anal fissures, or fecal blood (peptic ulcer disease [PUD], ischemic bowel, strangulation, incarceration, malignancy, diverticular bleed).

a. Blood accompanied by weight loss or decreasing stool caliber may confirm the presence of cancer. Fecal impaction itself can cause rectal bleeding from stercoral ulcers.

6. Ascites in postmenopausal women raises suspicion of ovarian or uterine carcinoma.

H. *Neurologic*

1. Look for any signs of focal deficits or a delayed relaxation of the deep tendon reflex.

2. Anxious, altered mental state (AMS) if perforation or sepsis

Differential Diagnoses

A. *Acute causes*

1. Quickly growing tumors, strictures, hernias, adhesions, inflammatory conditions and volvulus, narcotics, antipsychotics, anticholinergics, antacids, antihistamines, decreased exercise, fiber intake, fluid intake, anal fissure, hemorrhoids, anorectal abscesses, proctitis

B. *Chronic causes:*

1. Slowly growing tumor, colonic dysmotility, chronic anal pathology, chronic laxative abuse, narcotics, antipsychotics, anticholinergics, antacids, antihistamines, neuropathies, Parkinson's disease, cerebral palsy, paraplegia, hypothyroidism, hyperparathyroidism, diabetes, electrolyte abnormalities, hypomagnesemia, hypocalcemia, hypokalemia, amyloidosis, scleroderma, lead, iron

C. *Other differential diagnoses:*

1. Gastroenteritis, pancreatitis, fecal impaction, PUD, diverticulitis, pelvic inflammatory disease (PID), appendicitis, mesenteric ischemia, ascites, perforated viscous, intra-abdominal sepsis, postoperative ileus, cholecystitis, hernia with incarceration, volvulus, intussusception, adhesions, foreign body insertion, constipation, obstruction, ascites, obstructive uropathy, pseudoaneurysm, spermatocele, varicocele, epididymitis, hydrocele testicular torsion, groin abscess, lipoma, hematoma (hernias)

Diagnostic Testing

A. EKG in patients if concern for myocardial infarction (MI) as cause of abdominal pain, nausea

B. *Labs*

1. Complete blood count (CBC) to look for anemia, hemoconcentration of hematocrit or leukocytosis (may indicate translocation of intestinal bacterial).

a. Suspect abscess, gangrene, or peritonitis if >20,000 or left shift (strangulation as well).

2. Thyroid-stimulating hormone (TSH) if hypothyroidism suspected

3. Basic metabolic panel (BMP) to evaluate for electrolyte disturbance, renal injury

4. Lipase if concern for pancreatitis

5. HCG if concern for pregnancy; UA for infectious cause

6. Coagulation studies if concern for end-stage liver disease, coagulopathy, or GI bleed

7. Lactic acid if concern for mesenteric ischemia or pain out of proportion to exam

8. Stool should be tested for occult blood.

C. *Imaging*

1. Flat and erect abdominal XR if concern for obstruction, pseudo obstruction, or assessing stool burden

a. Diagnostic in 60% of cases; order if high pretest probability or suspect perforation. If negative, but still high suspicion, obtain CT.

b. Assess for free air under diaphragm (perforation), air fluid levels (obstruction), or dilated loops of bowel proximal to site of obstruction with a lack of air distal to obstruction.

c. Can localize obstruction as colon has haustra that appear as lines that only partially cross the lumen of the colon and the small bowel has plicae circulares that completely cross the lumen.

2. CT scan abdomen/pelvis with contrast to identify organic causes.

a. The CT scan 90% sensitive and can identify location of obstruction by presence of transition point.

b. Absence of contrast in rectum is a sign of complete obstruction.

c. May show alternative diagnosis, detect elusive hernias by demonstrating location of bowel, bladder, or uterus, and can help guide operative repair if needed.

3. Ultrasound is 88% sensitive and can assess for dilated loops of fluid-filled bowel with back and forth peristalsis or for blood flow through a hernia.

4. Flexible sigmoidoscopy and colonoscopy to identify lesions that narrow or occlude the bowel (typically done outpatient)

a. Colonoscopy is the examination of choice in patients with iron deficiency anemia, a positive guaiac stool test, or a first degree relative with colon cancer.

b. Barium enema and flexible sigmoidoscopy can demonstrate colonic dilatation and strictures.

Management

A. Treatment of functional constipation is directed at symptomatic relief as well as addressing lifestyle issues.

B. Most important prescription is a dietary and exercise regimen that includes 1.5 L fluids daily, 10 g of daily fiber, and exercise.

1. Fiber in the form of bran (1 cup/day) or psyllium (1 tsp three times a day) increases stool volume and gut motility.

C. Medications can provide temporary relief (stimulants, milk of magnesia in the absence of renal failure, hyperosmolar agents).

1. Docusate sodium facilitates the mixture of stool fat and water, improving symptoms of discomfort.

2. Docusate sodium/sennosides bisacodyl in adults or children, milk of magnesia, magnesium citrate, lactulose or sorbitol, polyethylene glycol

3. In children, glycerin rectal suppositories or mineral oil

D. Enemas of soapsuds or phosphate is generally reserved for severe cases.

1. Use care to avoid rectal trauma or rectal perforation.

E. Fecal impaction should be removed manually using local anesthetic lubricant and parenteral analgesia or sedation as required.

1. In female patients, transvaginal pressure with the other hand is helpful.

2. An enema or suppositories to complete evacuation can follow.

3. Following disimpaction, medications should be prescribed to reestablish fecal flow.

F. In palliative care, chronic opioid use or abuse, there is no definitive regimen.

G. If above is unsuccessful, use methylnaltrexone.

H. The temporary use of binders or corsets can be useful in patients with large-necked hernias, during the preoperative period, or in situations where there is a high risk of operation on a long-term basis.

I. Hernia reduction

1. Provide adequate sedation and analgesia to prevent straining or pain (reduce intraabdominal pressure). cold packs can be used to reduce swelling and blood flow while analgesia takes effect.

2. Patient should be supine with pillow under the knees.

a. *Inguinal hernias:* Place patient in Trendelenburg position at about 15 to 20 degrees. The ipsilateral leg is placed in an externally rotated and flexed position (unilateral frog leg).

b. Simple pressure over distal sac is usually ineffective.

c. Place two fingers at the edge of the hernial ring and apply firm, steady pressure to the side of the hernia closest to the hernia opening and maintain this pressure for several minutes while hernia is being guided back through defect.

J. If bowel obstruction:

1. Make patient NPO for bowel rest.

2. Start IV fluids as generally hypovolemic.

a. Large fluid deficits may be present because of prolonged vomiting or third spacing.

3. Pain and nausea control (ondansetron or metoclopramide)

a. If nausea is persistent and there is a large amount of abdominal distention, consider placing a nasogastric tube to decompress the stomach.

4. If ileus is suspected, use conservative measures such as IV fluids (IVF), NPO, and observation without surgical intervention.

5. Consider urinary catheter to monitor urine output in response to resuscitation.

6. Correct metabolic derangement, especially hypokalemia from vomiting.

7. Consider antibiotics.

a. Follow evidence-based guidelines when prescribing.

b. Antibiotics are only indicated if concern for bowel strangulation or perforation.

i. Consider ciprofloxacin and metronidazole, piperacillin/tazobactam, ticarcillin-clavulanate ampicillin/sulbactam.

ii. Double coverage with cefotaxime or ceftriaxone plus clindamycin or metronidazole or a carbapenem such as meropenem.

8. Note that hypertonic CT contrast agents (gastrografin) may be somewhat therapeutic by reducing bowel edema and promoting peristalsis.

9. In patients with pseudo obstruction, colonoscopy may be both diagnostic and therapeutic.

Age and Developmental Considerations

A. Constipation is more prevalent in children and older adults.

B. In children, few benign medical conditions are as distressing as constipation.

1. Commonly have symptoms of scybalous, pebble-like hard stools for most stools or firm stools two or fewer times per week for at least 2 weeks.

2. Frequently begins with the transition from breast milk to formula or from strained foods to table foods.

3. School-age kids may have an increase in constipation with consequent loss of privacy.

4. May have fecal mass on exam of the suprapubic area in many children.

C. In children, hernia pressure should be applied from the posterior and directed lateral and superior through the internal ring, as it is more medial than adults.

D. In adults, chronic constipation diminishes perceived quality of life and may signal more serious underlying problems such as colonic dysmotility or mass lesions.

E. In children, colonic intussusception can be diagnosed and treated with a barium or air enema.

F. SBO in patient without history of abdominal surgeries is concerning for malignancy.

G. Always have a high degree of suspicion for cardiac process in older adult patients who present with abdominal pain.

H. The absence of flatus or bowel movement is not always present in partial/early obstruction.

Patient Disposition (Referrals, Follow-Up, Education)

A. Reduction can often be carried out in the ED, but a surgeon should be consulted if unable to reduce the hernia

after one or two attempts, due to concern for a strangulated bowel or toxic appearance.
B. Easily reducible hernias, umbilical hernias <2 cm in diameter, or with hernias found upon physical examination, schedule a follow-up visit with the general surgeon within 1 to 2 weeks following the procedure.
C. All incarcerated or strangulated hernias demand admission and immediate surgical evaluation.
   1. Comorbid risks for sedation; patients with such risks should have a surgeon present for the initial reduction attempt.
   2. Surgical options depend on the type and location of the hernia.
D. Chronic constipation is usually a functional disorder that can be worked up as an outpatient with early follow-up.
E. Complications of chronic constipation, such as fecal impaction and intestinal pseudo-obstruction, require either manual, colonoscopy, or surgical intervention.
F. Consider admission with chronic constipation associated with systemic symptoms such as weight loss, anemia, change in stool caliber, refractory constipation, and constipation requiring chronic laxative use.
G. Intestinal pseudo-obstruction and sigmoid volvulus can sometimes be corrected colonoscopically.
H. Surgical consultation
   1. Surgical consultation for conservative versus operative management
   2. If mesenteric ischemia, organic constipation, pseudo-obstruction, complete bowel obstruction, or strangulated hernia is suspected
I. Admit for trial of bowel decompression with nasogastric (NG) tube, followed by surgical intervention if no resolution of symptoms.
J. Some patients with history of recurrent SBO may present with partial obstruction that resolves. Partial obstruction or ileus can be admitted or observed; treat cause.
K. Strict return precautions should be discussed with and given to the patient.
L. Return if symptoms return, persistent vomiting, severe pain, fever or any other new or concerning symptoms.

Dysphagia and Foreign Object Ingestion

Prevalence

A. Estimated that 25 per 1,000 persons/year present to the ED with food impaction, foreign body (FB) ingestion, or dysphagia.
B. Children from 18 to 48 months account for 80% of all cases of ingested FB.
C. Seen in adults with esophageal disease, prisoners, and psychiatric patients.

Anatomy

A. In adults, the esophagus is approximately 20 to 25 cm in length.
   1. Extends from the hypopharynx, tongue, hard and soft palate, pharyngeal muscles, and esophagus to the stomach at the gastroesophageal junction.
   2. The esophagus has an inner mucosa layer and a muscle layer made up of inner circular muscles and outer longitudinal muscles.
   3. The upper third of the esophagus is made up of voluntary striated muscles that allow initiation of swallowing, while muscles of the lower third are involuntary smooth muscles.
   4. Coordination of swallowing is controlled by the trigeminal (cranial nerve [CN] V), facial (CN VII), glossopharyngeal (CN IX), vagus (X), and hypoglossal (CN XII).
   5. The most common site for FB ingestion is in the esophagus.
   6. 80% to 90% of swallowed objects that reach the stomach will eventually pass without intervention.
B. In children, the most common site for obstruction is at the thoracic inlet, the area between the clavicles.
   1. The cricopharyngeal sling located at C6 is at this level and known to be a common site for FBs.
   2. About 10% to 15% of FBs get trapped in the mid esophagus, where the carina and aortic arch goes over the esophagus.
   3. The rest get entrapped at the lower esophageal junction.

Pathophysiology

A. Dysphagia can result from propulsive failure, structural disorders, or intrinsic or extrinsic compression of the oropharynx or esophagus.
B. *Physiologic:* Due to aging, reduced lingual movement, delayed onset of the pharyngeal swallow, delayed upper esophageal sphincter relaxation during swallowing, decreased nerve function, decreased muscle mass, or diminished pharyngolaryngeal response
C. *Pathologic:* Esophageal narrowing of strictures inflammation, malignancy or esophageal webs, or nonobstructing gastro-esophageal disorders (motility, rheumatic, neurologic, medication)
D. *Transfer dysphagia:* Difficulty transferring from the mouth to the proximal esophagus caused by a neuromuscular disorder resulting in bulbar muscle weakness or impaired coordination
E. *Transport dysphagia:* Failure of normal transit through the esophagus due to obstruction or motility disorder
F. *Functional dysphagia:* Diagnosis of exclusion caused by infections, medication-induced, and inflammatory conditions
G. *Other associated conditions:* Peptic stricture, esophageal cancer, spasm
H. Small objects typically lodge in the narrow proximal esophagus (coins, toys, crayons); in adults, most foreign objects are distal. Irregular, sharp, wide (>2.5 cm), or long objects may become lodged distal to pylorus.
I. Esophageal impaction can cause airway obstruction, stricture, or perforation.
J. Esophageal mucosal irritation can be perceived as a FB sensation.

Predisposing Factors

A. Peptic strictures, alcohol abuse, scleroderma, smoking, caffeine abuse, older age, pregnancy, obesity, radiation therapy, certain medications, psychiatric disorders, learning difficulties, preexisting digestive tract abnormalities, boy, intoxication, stroke, esophageal cancer, dysphagia

Medical Screening

A. *Chief complaint:* Ingested FB, FB sensation in throat, dysphagia

B. High yield history

1. Oropharyngeal or transfer dysphagia is characterized by initiating a swallow accompanied by nasopharyngeal regurgitation, aspiration, or sensation of food in pharynx.

2. Esophageal dysphagia is characterized by difficulty swallowing several seconds after initiating a swallow and a sensation of food getting stuck (solids worse than liquids with neurologic disorders).

3. Globus sensation is defined as persistent intermittent nonpainful sensation of a lump or FB in the throat between meals with the absence of dysphagia, odynophagia, or gastroesophageal reflux.

a. May point to neck to identify site and may reposition body to optimize alignment of the bolus for presentation of the pharynx and turn head or neck to swallow.

4. Ask what the patient ingested.

a. Small button batteries are the most worrisome because they can cause an alkaline burn and erode through the esophagus in as little as 2 hours after ingestion, with more severe damage after 8 to 12 hours, and require emergent removal if they become lodged in the esophagus.

5. Object may cause airway obstruction or press on the trachea.

6. Obstruction in the esophagus can cause odynophagia or dysphagia.

7. Chest pain may be seen with esophageal perforation or after retching.

8. If dysphagia develops late in a meal, may be due to myasthenia gravis.

C. Signs and symptoms

1. In adults

a. Retrosternal pain, dysphagia, vomiting, choking, inability to tolerate pooled secretions, coughing, gagging, anxiety

b. Hoarseness (neuromuscular dysfunction), vocal cord paralysis (weak cough), slurred speech, dysarthria, nasal speech, hematemesis, heartburn, anemia, weight loss

c. Food regurgitation, sensation of neck fullness, halitosis (may be Zenker's diverticulum)

2. In children

a. Refusal or inability to eat, vomiting, gagging, choking, neck or throat pain, drooling, or stridor

D. Past medical history (PMH)

1. *History of FB ingestion:* Psychiatric patients, prisoners, and children most common

2. Gastric banding increases the risk of impaction by food bolus.

3. History of alcohol abuse (esophageal spasm, GERD, peptic ulcer disease [PUD]), weight loss, dry mouth, radiation therapy, smoking, blood in mouth (concern for malignancy), aspiration pneumonia, prolonged intubation, Sjogren's syndrome, lupus, multiple sclerosis, hiatal hernia, Parkinson's disease, rheumatoid arthritis (RA), muscular dystrophy

Physical Examination

A. *General:* Varies from well-appearing, appearing uncomfortable, to moderate distress

B. *Vital signs:* Typically, normal. Fever and hemodynamic instability may be seen with esophageal rupture.

C. *Skin:* Typically, normal

D. Head, eyes, ears, nose, and throat (HEENT)

1. Perform thorough inspection of the oral cavity, head, neck, nose, mouth, and supraclavicular region for lymphadenopathy, masses, facial muscle weakness, poor dentition, gagging, drooling, or other abnormalities.

2. Hoarseness of voice may indicate vocal cord paresis or paralysis.

3. Bilateral ptosis may indicate muscle disease.

4. Unilateral nasal discharge can be seen with nasal FBs.

5. Listen over the trachea for stridor.

E. *Pulmonary:* Listen for egophony, wheezing, or decreased breath sounds that may be seen with bronchial obstruction.

F. *Abdominal:* Generally normal

G. Neurological

1. Altered mental status (AMS) if hypoxia is present

2. CN examination

3. Presence of cogwheeling, rigidity, or shuffling gate may indicate Parkinson's disease.

4. Motor and sensory deficits should raise suspicion for multiple sclerosis.

Differential Diagnoses

A. Structural or obstructive dysphagia causes, such as neoplasms, esophageal strictures, webs, Schatzki ring, diverticula

B. Motor lesions include stroke, achalasia, diffuse esophageal spasm.

C. Most common objects ingested are coins.

D. Objects tend to lodge at one of three levels.

1. Cricopharyngeal level is the narrowest in children and can cause complete airway obstruction.

2. T4 level at the aortic arch and carina is the most common in adults.

3. Proximal to the gastroesophageal junction

E. *Other causes of dysphagia:* Peptic stricture, food bolus, esophagitis, esophagogastric junction outflow obstruction, caustic ingestion, epiglottis, retropharyngeal abscess, CNS infection, botulism, diphtheria, head injury, or esophageal perforation, croup

Diagnostic Testing

A. EKG and cardiac work-up if associated chest pain

B. *Labs:* Not generally indicated unless suspect perforation; basic metabolic panel (BMP) if need for contrasted CT

C. Imaging:

1. Chest x-ray (CXR)

a. Assess for esophageal FBs, aspiration pneumonia, masses, or lack of air in the stomach.

b. Will show radiopaque objects (e.g., button batteries, coins, dense plastic).

i. Coins will be seen on edge if in the trachea or face on if in the esophagus on posteroanterior CXR.

2. Anteroposterior (AP)/lateral neck XR
   a. Can show objects in the posterior pharynx, which are concern for transport or transfer dysphagia.
3. Gastrografin or barium swallow (outpatient) for non-radiopaque objects
4. Direct laryngoscopy allows for direct visualization and removal.
   a. Often, FB sensation results from a small laceration or abrasion of the posterior pharynx caused by the FB (e.g., chicken bone).
5. Chest and abdominal CT
   a. Very sensitive and can evaluate surrounding structures and may show alternative diagnosis.

Management

A. Aspiration is a major concern for causes of dysphagia.
B. Treat underlying cause. Many structural lesions require esophageal dilatation.
C. IV hydration and pain control if needed
D. Most objects that have passed in the stomach and small intestine can be observed and treated expectantly.
E. Food boluses
   1. IV or IM glucagon can increase peristalsis, reflex contraction of the esophagus, and expel the bolus.
   2. Nitroglycerin/calcium channel blockers relax the smooth muscle of the esophagus and proximal gastroesophageal sphincter, allowing FB to pass to the stomach.
   3. Do not treat with meat tenderizer because it may cause esophageal perforation.

Age and Developmental Considerations

A. Higher risk associated with extremes of age
B. Decreased functional swallowing motility as people age
C. Causes of pediatric dysphagia in infants and newborns include prematurity, congenital malformations, neuromuscular disease, infection, congenital malformation, inflammation, or FB ingestion.

Patient Disposition (Referrals, Follow-Up, Education)

A. Arrange for emergent endoscopy removal of any FB causing airway obstruction or airway compromise
   1. All button batteries in the esophagus need to be removed immediately as can cause a tracheoesophageal fistula.
   2. If the battery has passed into the stomach and intestine, they can be managed expectantly.
   3. Sharp objects (knives, glass) should be removed ASAP.
B. Schedule elective endoscopy with gastroenterology if:
   1. Smooth objects in the esophagus have not passed into the stomach within 24 hours.
   2. Button batteries have remained in the stomach after 48 hours.
C. Discharge patients
   1. Objects have been removed in the ED or objects have passed into small intestine and can tolerate by mouth (PO). Instruct patients to monitor their stools.
   2. With button batteries in the stomach, patients need to return in 48 hours to ensure they have passed into the intestines.
D. Admit patients
   1. Esophageal FBs or food bolus that cannot be treated in ED
   2. If unable to drink liquids or at high risk for aspiration

Esophageal Perforation

Prevalence

A. Boerhaave syndrome accounts for 15% of all cases of spontaneous perforations of the esophagus, typically seen among patients 50 to 70 years old.

Pathophysiology

A. Iatrogenic injury is most common cause.
B. Other causes are Boerhaave syndrome (full thickness perforation of the esophagus caused by sudden rise in intraesophageal pressures due to forceful emesis), trauma, and foreign body ingestion.

Predisposing Factors

A. Overindulgence of food, alcohol use, iatrogenic activity, esophagitis, infectious ulcers

Medical Screening

A. *Chief complaint:* Acute, severe, unrelenting, diffuse pain in the chest, neck, and abdomen
B. High yield history
   1. Note onset, duration, and progression of symptoms.
   2. *Location of pain:* Retrosternal chest pain, neck pain, and epigastric pain can help localize area of perforation.
C. Signs and symptoms
   1. Pain can radiate to back and shoulders or back pain can be predominant symptom; neck pain, dysphagia, dysphonia, odynophagia (swallowing makes pain worse) are other symptoms.
   2. Fever, tachycardia, dyspnea, cyanosis, hypotension

Physical Examination

A. *General:* Varies on the severity of the rupture and time between rupture and presentation.
B. *Vital signs:* Tachycardia, weak pulse, hypotension, fever, and tachypnea are common.
C. *Skin:* Pallor
D. *Head, eyes, ears, nose, and throat (HEENT):* May be normal, no blood in oropharynx
E. Cardiac
   1. Low jugular venous pressure
   2. Mediastinal emphysema (Hamman's crunch) caused by air in the mediastinum being moved by the beating heart
F. *Pulmonary:* Pleural effusions develop in about half of patients.
G. *Abdominal:* May have abdominal rigidity.
H. *Neurological:* Normal, anxious to altered mental status

Differential Diagnoses

A. Myocardial infarction, pulmonary embolus, aortic catastrophe, peptic ulcer disease, acute abdomen

Diagnostics

A. Labs are often nonspecific.
  1. Complete blood count (CBC) for evaluation of anemia (can be masked if acute) or leukocytosis.

B. Imaging
  1. Chest XR
    a. Most useful in early diagnosis
    b. Naclerio V-sign is seen as radiolucent streaks of air in the retro cardiac region in a V shape.
    c. May also see pneumomediastinum, pneumopericardium, subcutaneous emphysema, pneumothorax, mediastinal widening, hydropneumothorax.
  2. CT of the chest and abdomen
    a. Can see esophageal wall edema and thickening, periesophageal fluid, mediastinal widening, evidence of extravasation of food particles or bile from the esophageal lumen into the pleural space, or mediastinum air and fluid in the pleural spaces, retroperitoneum, or lesser sac.
  3. Endoscopy
    a. Contrast gastrographin or barium esophogram can show the location and extent of perforation.

Management

A. Rapid and aggressive management of shock

B. Broad-spectrum antibiotics
  1. Follow evidence-based guidelines when prescribing.
  2. Piperacillin-tazobactam or double coverage with cefotaxime or ceftriaxone plus clindamycin or metronidazole

Patient Disposition (Referrals, Follow-Up, Education)

A. Differentials for Foreign Body Ingestion:
  1. Disk Battery Ingestion, Esophageal Rupture, Mediastinitis, Retropharyngeal Abscess, Small Bowel Obstruction, Tracheal Foreign Body, Esophageal Foreign Body, Failure to Thrive, Dysphagia, Esophagitis, Pharyngitis, Peptic Ulcer Disease, and Pyloric Stenosis

Gastroesophageal Reflux Disease, Peptic Ulcer Disease, and Gastritis

Prevalence

A. Gastroesophageal reflux disease (GERD) affects about 20% of the population, and incidence is higher in older adults.

B. Incidence of esophageal disease with chest pain ranges from 20% to 60%.

C. Peptic ulcer disease (PUD) is acquired during childhood and incidence increases with age, with median age at diagnosis of 18 to 30 years. Affects men more frequently than women and has an incidence of 23.1/100,000 individuals per year.

Anatomy

A. The esophagus is divided into three parts, cervical, thoracic, and abdominal. The proximal third of the esophagus is striated muscle which transitions to smooth muscle in the distal 2/3.

B. Proximal esophagus contains the upper esophageal sphincter.

C. Distal thoracic esophagus is left of midline and enters the abdomen through esophageal hiatus.

D. The hiatus is formed by the right crus of the diaphragm, forming a sling around the esophagus with a right and left pillar, which allows for the esophagus to narrow when the diaphragm contracts.

E. Peptic ulcers are defects in the gastric or duodenal mucosa that extend through the muscularis mucosa.

Pathophysiology

A. GERD is a syndrome caused by the reflux of gastric contents into the esophagus, causing local irritation and inflammation.

B. Transient relaxation of the lower esophageal sphincter (LES) complex is the primary cause of GERD.

C. Epithelial cells of the stomach and duodenum secrete mucous in response to irritation secondary to cholinergic stimulation.

D. Normally, a physiologic balance exists between gastric acid secretion and gastroduodenal mucosal defense (bicarbonate and prostaglandins). Reflux and ulcers occur when this balance is disrupted.

E. Most cases of PUD are related to *H. pylori* infection or chronic NSAID use (inhibit prostaglandin synthesis and decrease blood flow, bicarbonate, or mucosal secretion).

F. Acute gastritis is usually caused by ischemia due to severe illness, *H. pylori* infection, or toxic effects.

G. Dyspepsia is usually caused by esophagitis, PUD, or GERD.

Predisposing Factors

A. Symptoms may be present and progressive for months to years before patients seek medical treatment.

B. High fat food, nicotine, ethanol, caffeine, medications, pregnancy, psychological stress, mechanical ventilation, Zollinger-Ellison syndrome, decreased esophageal motility (achalasia, scleroderma, diabetes), prolonged gastric emptying (outlet obstruction, gastroparesis), or hiatal hernia

Medical Screening

A. *Chief complaint:* Burning epigastric pain that often radiates into the chest

B. High yield history
  1. Given that many patients report a chief complaint of chest pain, the ENP should obtain information on any patterns or radiation of pain, especially related to food (timing, amount, specific foods) and location.
  2. Associated with foods high in fat content or acidity that tend to increase symptoms.
    a. GERD is worse after meals.
    b. PUD is often relieved with milk, food, or antacids.
  3. Bending over or lying down tend to increase symptoms with GERD.
  4. Intake of large amounts of food in one sitting or tight/restrictive clothing can increase gastric pressures and exacerbate symptoms.
  5. Recurs at night with duodenal ulcers daily for weeks, resolves, and then comes back in weeks to months.
  6. Alcohol, tobacco, chocolate, or caffeine overuse can cause LES stimulation, increasing symptoms.

7. If patient has tried over-the-counter (OTC) antacids, document their response to that treatment.
8. Dysphagia is suggestive of esophageal spasm or stricture.
9. Odynophagia is suggestive of ulcerative esophagitis.
10. Opiates, calcium channel blockers, nitrates, theophylline, and anticholinergics can increase symptoms by relaxing the lower esophageal sphincter.
11. Elevated stress levels can be a contributing factor.
12. Change in character of the pain may indicate a complication.
   a. Abrupt onset of severe pain in perforation with peritonitis
   b. Rapid onset of back pain associated with posterior perforation or pancreatitis
   c. Nausea and vomiting (N/V) from gastric outlet obstruction
   d. Vomiting blood or blood per rectum with GI bleeding

C. Signs and symptoms
1. Burning sensation in the chest, epigastric tenderness, N/V, foul taste or odor in mouth, hoarseness, shortness of breath, chronic cough, asthma
2. Can be associated with N/V and acidic reflux, especially at night and with lying recumbent.
3. Severe pain, bleeding (hematemesis, melena, or hematochezia), changes in voice, or shortness of breath may be indicative of pathological changes in tissue morphology and may also be a sign of perforation or ulcerations.
4. Gastric ulcer pain usually occurs 1 to 2 hours after eating, worse with eating, and not common to have night pain, whereas duodenal ulcer pain occurs 2 to 5 hours after eating, decreases with food, and commonly causes pain at night.
5. Acute gastritis patients may have epigastric pain, N/V, or GI bleeding.
6. Can cause complications such as strictures, inflammatory esophagitis (chest pain, odynophagia), and Barrett's esophagus.
7. Atypical symptoms
   a. Chest pain with exertion, associated with diaphoresis, shortness of breath, or radiation to the jaw, upper extremities (myocardial infarction [MI])
   b. Coughing and/or wheezing (asthma, pneumonia, hoarseness, aspiration), otitis media, enamel erosion or other dental manifestations
   c. N/V, or regurgitation (delayed gastric emptying)
   d. Pain radiation directly into the back (pancreatitis or dissecting aortic aneurysms)
8. Pediatric
   a. Reflux is physiologic in infants but pathologic if it causes complications such as failure to thrive, weight loss, esophagitis, respiratory symptoms.

D. Past medical history (PMH)
1. Coronary atherosclerotic disease (CAD) or risk factors for CAD (similar symptoms), prior history of reflux, pregnancy, NSAID use, *H. pylori* infection, family history of PUD, short gut syndrome, leukemia, gastrectomy, abdominal aortic aneurysm (AAA), gastroparesis, gastric cancer.

Physical Examination

A. General
1. Typically, normal examination unless perforation has occurred
2. Look for indications of respiratory distress, discomfort, active vomiting.

B. *Vital signs:* Normal initially; with perforation, patient will have tachycardia, thready pulse, low BP, and high-grade fever.
C. *Skin:* Mucus membranes and skin color should be inspected for pallor, icterus/jaundice, and dehydration.
D. *Head, eyes, ears, nose, and throat (HEENT):* Dental erosions, vocal cord ulcers and granulomas, laryngitis with hoarseness, chronic sinusitis, chronic cough, lower conjunctiva pallor
E. *Cardiac:* Normal
F. *Pulmonary:* The presence of stridor is highly unlikely, but upper airway patency is important. Breath sounds should be clear in the diagnosis of GERD.
G. *Abdominal:* Epigastric tenderness; assess for distention or rigidity if perforation. Rectal examination can rule out occult GI blood loss.
H. *Neurological:* Quality of speech should be assessed.

Differential Diagnoses

A. Myocardial ischemia, cholelithiasis, gastroenteritis, PUD, gastritis, esophageal foreign body, functional dyspepsia, GERD, pericarditis, pneumonia, pyelonephritis, bowel obstruction, gastritis, PE, splenic infarction, hepatitis, aortic dissection, gastric cancer, gastroparesis, hepatitis, pancreatitis, or biliary disease

Diagnostic Testing

A. EKG for concern of myocardial ischemia
B. Labs
1. Laboratory testing is not needed for diagnosis but should be ordered if acute coronary syndrome (ACS), perforation, infection, bleeding, or airway compromise are a concern.
2. CBC may see chronic anemia caused by esophagitis or peptic ulcer disease.
3. Cardiac enzymes if suspect myocardial disease or damage
4. LFTs if concern for hepatitis or biliary disease; lipase for pancreatitis
5. Stool if concern for *H. pylori* infection

C. Imaging
1. Chest XR
   a. May demonstrate hiatal hernia, although not all hiatal hernias cause symptoms.
   b. Free air or pleural effusion may be seen with esophageal perforation.
   c. May see an esophageal foreign body.
2. *Abdominal XR:* If concern for perforation (free air under diaphragm)
3. Abdominal ultrasound if concern for gallbladder disease or AAA
4. Esophagogastroduodenoscopy (EGD) has evolved as the standard of care for evaluation of patients with suspected GERD or for visualization of ulcer in patients with PUD.

5. pH probe testing has become increasingly easy and cost-effective to obtain (not emergent and can be done outpatient).

Management

A. Follow evidence-based guidelines when prescribing.
B. Goals are to control symptoms and heal esophagitis or other complications.
C. Give a trial of antacid.
 1. GI cocktail consisting of viscous lidocaine, aluminum hydroxide/magnesium hydroxide, and donnatal can provide almost immediate pain relief and improvement. Some places add lidocaine to the cocktail.
D. Goal of PUD treatment is healing the ulcer while relieving pain and preventing complications or recurrence.
E. H2 receptor antagonists (cimetidine or ranitidine)
 1. Ongoing therapy to promote healing
F. Proton pump inhibitors (omeprazole, lansoprazole)
 1. Generally, proton pump inhibitors heal ulcers faster that H2 receptor antagonists.
G. If acute *H. pylori* infection, antimicrobial and antisecretory therapy should be started with PPI, clarithromycin, and amoxicillin or metronidazole for 14 days.

Age and Developmental Considerations

A. Management of ulcer disease in older adults is like that in the younger population.
B. Consideration must be given to the potential for increased incidence of side effects and medication interactions in older adults.
C. GERD is physiologic in infants.
D. Older adults have more esophageal and extraesophageal complications that may be potentially life-threatening.
 1. *Esophageal complications:* Erosive esophagitis, esophageal stricture, Barrett's esophagus, adenocarcinoma
 2. *Extraesophageal complications:* Atypical chest pain, globus sensation, laryngitis, dental problems, chronic cough, asthma, pulmonary aspiration

Patient Disposition (Referrals, Follow-Up, Education)

A. Complications require consultation or admission based on diagnosis and stability.
B. Many patients with epigastric pain do not receive definitive diagnosis in the ED, but if a critical diagnosis (AAA or MI) is still in the differential, then admission should be considered.
C. Educate patient on lifestyle modifications.
 1. Elevate head of bed 4 inches.
 2. Do not eat within 2 hours of lying down.
 3. Eat small meals and avoid overeating.
 4. Avoid late-night meals or snacks.
 5. Avoid foods or medications that lower the LES tone (NSAIDs, alcohol, tobacco, caffeine).
D. Arrange outpatient evaluation
 1. If diagnosis is unclear or patient has failed antacid treatment
 2. *Endoscopic referral:* Age >55 years, unexplained weight loss, early satiety, persistent vomiting, dysphagia, anemia or GI bleeding, abdominal masses, persistent anorexia, jaundice
E. Most patients can be discharged home.
F. Consider admission if severe reactive airway disease, dehydration, evidence of esophageal perforation, or evidence of gastrointestinal bleed.

Gastrointestinal Bleeding

Prevalence

A. Upper gastrointestinal (GI) bleeding incidence of acute upper GI bleed is approximately 50 to 100 per 100,000 worldwide (75% have upper source).
B. Lower GI bleeding occurs in about 20 per 100,000 people in the United States, with approximately 540,000 hospitalizations.
C. More common in males and older adults.

Anatomy

A. Categorized into upper or lower GI bleeds, based on whether the bleeding occurs anatomically above or below the ligament of Treitz.

Pathophysiology

A. Hemorrhoids
 1. Develop due to a combination of genetic predisposition, weak rectal veins, surrounding connective tissue, diet, and defecation habits.
 2. Internal hemorrhoids are above the dentate line and occur because of dilatation of the superior hemorrhoidal plexus.
 3. External hemorrhoids are below the dentate line and occur because of dilatation to the inferior hemorrhoidal plexus.
 4. Occur in pregnancy, old age, portal hypertension (HTN).
 5. Increased tone of the internal anal sphincter causes the feces to press the hemorrhoid against the muscle, causing symptoms.
 6. Usually symptom seen as bright red blood on tissue or in the toilet.
B. Anal fissures
 1. Hard stool passes and "cuts" a linear tear from dentate line to anoderm.
  a. Posterior midline 95%
  b. Anterior midline 5%
  c. Externally forms skin tag or sentinel pile.
  d. Internally forms hypertrophied anal papilla.
  e. Chronic fissure may reveal fibers of internal sphincter with sentinel pile.
 2. Stress or an overly tight anal sphincter leads to local ischemia of posterior anoderm.
 3. Local trauma from anal intercourse or sexual abuse
 4. Lateral fissures indicate underlying systemic disease such as Crohn's disease, anal cancer, leukemia, syphilis, previous anal surgery.
C. Upper GI bleed (UGIB)
 1. Originates proximal to the ligament of Treitz.

2. Peptic ulcer disease is the most common cause followed by gastritis, esophagitis, varices, and Mallory-Weiss tears.
3. Other causes to consider include anthrax, Ebola, duodenal ulcer, esophagitis, gastric tumors, gastric ulcer, Mallory-Weiss syndrome.

D. Lower GI bleed (LGIB)
1. Most common cause is diverticular disease followed by colitis, polyps, and malignancies.
2. Other common causes include vascular ectasias, ischemic colitis, hemorrhoids, anal fissures, ulcerative colitis, Crohn's disease, infectious colitis, radiation proctitis, rectal varices, stercoral ulceration, Meckel diverticulum, intussusception, Henoch-Schoenlein purpura (HSP).
3. Due to an upper source about 10% to 14% of the time. 80% resolve spontaneously.

Predisposing Factors

A. Alcohol, salicylate and NSAID use, pregnancy, older age, infectious process, peptic ulcer disease (PUD), cancer

Medical Screening

A. *Chief complaint:* Acute or chronic bleeding from the upper or lower GI tract (hematemesis or red stool per rectum) or vague symptoms indicative of slow blood loss

B. High yield history
1. Bleeding
   a. May not be noticed, may only present with generalized weakness, fatigue, syncope, dyspnea on exertion or lightheadedness.
   b. Black, tarry stools or melena are common with UGIB.
   c. Hematochezia can be seen with a brisk UGIB or more commonly, with a LGIB.
   d. Bright red blood on normal brown stool or on the toilet paper is common with anal fissures or hemorrhoids.
2. Vomiting or retching
   a. Coffee ground emesis may be seen with an UGIB.
   b. If bleeding follows the vomiting or retching (Mallory-Weis Tear).
3. Medication use
   a. Heavy NSAID or steroid use increases the risk for PUD and gastritis as cause of an UGIB.
   b. Iron, bismuth, and charcoal can turn the stool black; beets can stimulate hematochezia.
4. Recent endoscopy or colonoscopy
   a. Concern for postprocedural bleeding for polypectomy
5. Weight loss or change in bowel habits may be signs of malignancy.
6. Alcohol use history suggests possibility of cirrhosis and secondary variceal as etiology of blood loss.

C. Signs and symptoms
1. Fatigue, dizziness, palpitations, shortness of breath, coffee ground emesis, dark or tarry stools, hematochezia, melena, abdominal pain, bright red blood seen in the toilet or on tissue paper
2. More subtle presentations of hypotension, tachycardia, angina, syncope, weakness, or confusion

D. Past medical history (PMH)
1. PUD or gastritis (UGIB)
2. Diverticulosis (LGIB), painless hematochezia (diverticular bleed)
3. Coronary atherosclerotic disease can put the patient for risk of MI with severe anemia.

Physical Examination

A. *Vital signs:* Tachycardia or hypotension if severe bleeding

B. *Skin:* Spider angiomata, palmar erythema, jaundice (liver disease)

C. *Head, eyes, ear, nose, throat (HEENT):* Look for scleral icterus or evidence of swallowed blood.

D. *Cardiac/chest:* Spider hemangioma, gynecomastia (liver disease)

E. *Pulmonary:* Tachypneic if perforation from retching or aspiration of blood

F. Abdominal
1. May have tenderness to palpation anywhere in the abdomen.
   a. Epigastric pain may indicate gastritis, PUD.
   b. Diffuse pain
      i. May indicate PUD, gastrointestinal perforation, inflammatory bowel disease (IBD), infective colitis, colon carcinoma, ischemic colitis, ruptured abdominal aortic aneurysm (AAA), intra-abdominal or retroperitoneal hemorrhage.
   c. Periumbilical pain (mesenteric ischemia, appendicitis)
   d. RUQ pain (Budd-Chiari syndrome, hemochromatosis, cirrhosis)
   e. LLQ pain (diverticulitis or UC)
2. Look for signs of guarding or rebound tenderness.
3. Note liver size to suggest cirrhosis.
4. Rectal examination
   a. May note frank blood on rectal exam, hemoccult positive stool or melena, abscess, or masses. Use anoscope to visualize internal hemorrhoids or fissures.
   b. Gently retract buttocks and have patient bear down to visualize the fissure.
   c. Severe pain usually prevents a manual or digital exam with hemorrhoids or fissures. Use lidocaine jelly or ELA-Max5, a topical lidocaine ointment, before attempting.
   d. External hemorrhoids appear on inspection of anal verge as skin tags, strangulated or free prolapsed veins.
   e. Internal hemorrhoids appear as bluish bulging of the veins in the mucosa.

G. *Neurological:* Altered mental status (AMS) or confusion (anemia, dehydration)

Differential Diagnoses

A. Crohn's disease, chronic ulcerative colitis, anorectal carcinoma, perirectal abscess, thrombosed hemorrhoid, sexual abuse, acute abdomen, GERD, TB, syphilis, lymphoma, leukemia, previous anal surgery

B. *Upper sources:* PUD, esophageal varices, angiodysplasia, gastritis, Mallory-Weiss tear, esophagitis

C. *Lower sources:* Angiodysplasia, polyp or cancer, anal fissure, diverticular bleed, hemorrhoids
D. *Pediatrics:* Consider Meckel's diverticulum or intussusception.

Diagnostic Testing

A. EKG to exclude cardiac ischemia with severe bowel ischemia
B. Labs
  1. CBC to evaluate the degree of anemia, leukocytosis
    a. In an acute bleed, the hemoglobin may not equilibrate for several hours and is not indicative of actual blood loss.
  2. Note platelets and any thrombocytopenia.
  3. Prothombin time/international normalized ratio/partial thromboplastin time (PT/INR/PTT) to exclude coagulopathy as a confounding factor of bleeding
  4. Type and cross for packed red blood cells (PRBCs) or clotting factors as needed.
  5. Electrolytes, BUN, creatinine to exclude metabolic disturbance or renal insufficiency or injury
  6. LFTs to evaluate for evidence of liver dysfunction
  7. Guaiac testing of NG aspirate can yield both false positive and false negative results.
    a. Direct visualization of coffee ground emesis or bloody, maroon aspirate the most reliable confirmation of bleeding.
C. Imaging
  1. Upper GI endoscopy is study of choice in evaluating UGIB.
  2. Angiography should be considered to detect site of bleeding and management with embolization or infusion of vasoactive substances in LGIB.
  3. Scintigraphy localizes site of bleeding in obscure hemorrhage.
  4. Endoscopy is more accurate than angiography or scintigraphy.
  5. CT scan abdomen/pelvis for emergent evaluation.

Management

A. Emergency stabilization of airway, breathing and circulation
B. Start IV fluids (crystalloid) with 2 large-bore IVs to replace volume loss and maintain BP.
C. Nasogastric (NG) tube
  1. Diagnostic (show occult UGI source and assess for ongoing gastric bleeding)
  2. Therapeutic (gastric lavage with room temperature water and prep for endoscopy)
  3. A negative NG aspirate does not exclude UGI source.
  4. Concern for NG tube passage may provoke bleeding in patients with varices should be considered, but typically unwarranted.
D. Oxygen via nasal cannula to improve oxygen delivery and prevent ischemia
E. Follow serial hemoglobin (Hgb) and transfuse PRBCs as needed.
  1. If nonresponsive to fluids (up to 2L), actively bleeding, and Hgb <8 or <10 with history of CAD
F. Consider starting the following medications:
  1. *IV/IM/PO pain medications:* Tylenol, muscle relaxants to relieve sphincter spasm in anal fissures, topical anesthetics
  2. *Proton pump inhibitor:* Pantoprazole, esomeprazole, lansoprazole bolus followed by infusion
  3. H2 blocker decreases acid secretion and may prevent rebleeding with PUD and gastritis. Not beneficial in acute UGIB.
  4. Octreotide bolus followed by infusion if patient has uncontrolled UGIB awaiting endoscopy, or when unsuccessful, contraindicated, or unavailable can decrease recurrent variceal bleeding
  5. Vasopressin may help decrease bleeding by vasoconstriction in variceal or ulcer bleeding.
  6. Sitz baths (with warm water) to relieve sphincter spasm
  7. Balloon tamponade with the Sengstaken-Blakemore tube can control documented variceal hemorrhage as only a temporizing measure.
  8. Emergent surgical intervention may be necessary in patients who do not respond to medical or endoscopic therapy.

Patient Disposition (Referrals, Follow-Up, Education)

A. For anal fissures
  1. *High-fiber diet instruction:* Fiber/bran: 21 to 25 g/day in women and 30 to 38 g/day in men. Psyllium seeds (Metamucil or onsyl): 1–2 tsp (peds: 0.25–1 tsp/day) PO q24h
  2. Encourage consumption of 10 to 12 oz glasses of water per day.
B. Consult gastroenterology for emergent endoscopy to localize and control bleeding.
C. Consider surgery if severe bleeding (consider CT before to localize bleeding).
D. Admission
  1. Ongoing blood loss, borderline vitals, or clinical features predicting adverse outcomes
    a. Initial hematocrit <30%, initial systolic BP <100 mmHg, red blood in NG lavage, history of cirrhosis or ascites on exam, and a history of vomiting red blood
E. Discharge
  1. Stable vital signs, Hgb >10, no evidence of active bleeding, and normal coagulation studies

Hepatic Disorders and Liver Failure

Prevalence

A. Acute hepatic failure occurs in only about 2,000 patients per in the United States, but carries a high mortality rate.
B. Hepatic cirrhosis is a common condition in the United States and associated with a high mortality rate. It is commonly caused by alcoholism or hepatitis C.

Anatomy

A. The liver is in the upper right-hand quadrant of the abdomen, beneath the diaphragm, and on top of the stomach, right kidney, and intestines.

B. Shaped like a cone, the liver is a dark reddish-brown organ that weighs about 3 pounds and consists of two lobes with eight segments and 1,000 lobules.
C. *Two sources of blood supply:* Hepatic artery supplies oxygenated blood and hepatic portal vein takes nutrient-rich blood in (holds about one pint (13%) of the blood supply).
D. The lobules are connected to small ducts (tubes) that connect with larger ducts to form the common hepatic duct.
E. The common hepatic duct transports the bile made by the liver cells to the gallbladder and duodenum (the first part of the small intestine) via the common bile duct.

Pathophysiology

A. Acute liver failure (ALF) is the clinical manifestation of sudden and severe hepatic injury.
B. Etiologies vary and can include drug toxicity, viral infections, autoimmune and genetic disorders, thrombosis, malignancy, heat injury, ischemia, Wilson disease, hemolysis, elevated liver enzymes, low platelet count (HELLP) syndrome, Reye's syndrome, galactosemia, hereditary fructose intolerance, hemochromatosis, alpha-1 antitrypsin deficiency, and tyrosinemia.
C. As serum ammonia levels increase, asterixis is seen on the neurologic exam.
D. Dysfunctions in glucose regulation may cause hypoglycemia, which can become severe as disease progresses.
E. Early elevations in serum bilirubin can be seen in icterus on the underside of the tongue as well as the conjunctiva and sclera, followed by jaundice of the skin. Discoloration of urine and stool is a late sign; urinalysis should be examined for hyper bilirubin.
F. Peripheral edema and the development of spider angiomas or varicose veins may correspond with the accumulation of ascites in the peritoneal cavity, a reflection of both abnormal fluid shifts and mechanical compression of the vessels.
G. Loss of hepatocyte function results in liver necrosis, which releases toxins and cytokines leading to severe systemic inflammation and secondary bacterial infection from decreased immunity.
H. Hepatic necrosis causes rapid loss and severe metabolic dysfunction leading to decreased gluconeogenesis, lactate clearance, ammonia clearance presenting as hypoglycemia, lactic acidosis, coagulopathy, hyperammonemia (resembles septic shock).
I. Acute renal failure and hepatorenal syndrome can occur secondary to hypovolemia.
J. Encephalopathy is thought to be caused by excess inflammatory mediators and circulatory neurotoxins altering blood flow and blood–brain barrier permeability.

Predisposing Factors

A. Hepatitis, gallbladder disease, alcohol abuse, age >40, female gender, poor nutritional status, pregnancy, Tylenol use

Medical Screening

A. *Chief complaint:* Varies
B. High yield history
  1. Careful risk assessment for alcohol use disorder, acute exposure to toxins or overdose (including acetaminophen, vitamin or herbal supplements) should be included.
  2. Exposure to pathogens via foodborne or fecal-oral routes (hepatitis A); sexual or body fluid exposures (hepatitis B, C)
C. Signs and symptoms
  1. The hallmark signs include coagulopathy, encephalopathy, abnormal fluid shifts because of increased capillary permeability leading to distributive shock, and hepatorenal syndrome.
  2. Often present with altered mental status (AMS), shortness of breath (due to ascites and osmotic shifts), or bleeding (severe thrombocytopenia, disseminated intravascular coagulation, or vascular lesions). Generalized malaise, anorexia, fatigue, nausea/vomiting (N/V), and abdominal pain may be present.
  3. Patients developing hepatic encephalopathy may present with mild confusion but progress to delirium.
D. *Past medical history:* Alcohol use, acetaminophen use, pregnancy, hepatitis, fatty liver disease

Physical Examination

A. *General:* Appears weak due to weight loss, anorexia, muscle atrophy.
B. Vital signs: Normal to low blood pressure may be present.
C. Skin
  1. Jaundice, scleral icterus, spider angiomata, palmar erythema, pallor, bruising, telangiectasis, edema of the lower extremities, gynecomastia, inversion of normal pubic hair in men
  2. Nail changes such as Muehrcke nails (paired horizontal white band separated by normal color), terry nails (proximal 2/3 of the nail plate appears white and the rest red, clubbing
  3. Muscle atrophy or Dupuytren's contracture causing flexion deformities of the fingers
D. HEENT
  1. Thinning of the hair
  2. Kayser-Fleischer rings (dark rings encircling the iris in Wilson disease)
  3. Parotid gland enlargement
  4. Fetor hepaticus or sweet pungent smell in the breath
E. *Cardiac:* May have signs of congestive heart failure (CHF) from secondary hepatic congestion.
F. *Pulmonary*: Tachypnea, pleural effusions, rales, signs of CHF
G. Abdominal
  a. Hepatomegaly or splenomegaly may be present with portal hypertension.
  b. Abdominal distention may be due to ascites and may have a "fluid wave."
  c. Flank dullness (ascites)
  d. Cruveilhier–Baumgarten murmur or a venous hum may be heard in patients with portal hypertension at the epigastrium, which is exacerbated by Valsalva maneuver and diminished by pressure above the umbilicus.
  e. Rectal examination may show occult or frank blood.

H. Neurological

1. Encephalopathy can range from drowsiness, slowed mentation, cognitive impairment, confusion, and euphoria to deep coma.

2. May have decreased attention span, anxiety, disorientation asterixis, slurred speech.

Differential Diagnoses

A. Fatty liver disease may be asymptomatic and an incidental finding.

B. Acute hepatitis is rapid onset of jaundice, hepatomegaly with significant tenderness, and hyperbilirubinemia, often in the presence of high fever.

C. Chronic hepatitis is the presence of cirrhosis and portal hypertension with structural changes and vascular congestion. Present with abdominal pain or distension, severe pruritis, peripheral edema, anorexia, shortness of breath, or constitutional complaints of generalized weakness or fatigue. Coagulopathy with bleeding from the gums, stool, or hemorrhoids, as well as potentially life-threatening bleeding from esophageal varices.

D. Diffuse abdominal pain, especially with fever, should raise concern for spontaneous bacterial peritonitis.

Diagnostic Testing

A. Labs

1. *CBC with differential:* Anemia, thrombocytopenia, or leukocytosis (infection)

2. Complete metabolic panel (CMP)

a. Elevated transaminases in early or acute liver disease

i. These may normalize or become low with end stage liver disease, as hepatocytes become necrotic and nonfunctional.

b. Elevation of ALT/AST

i. AST/ALT > occurs with chronic exposure to alcohol

3. Elevated ammonia

4. Prolonged PT/INR

5. *Urinalysis:* Elevated specific gravity, protein, bilirubin

6. Serum albumin, prealbumin

7. Hepatitis A, B, C serologies (anti-IgM hep A antibody; hep B surface antigen and antibody; anti-hep C antibody)

8. *Consider:* Serum ETOH and urine drug testing, acetaminophen, and salicylates

9. Fecal pathogen panel

10. Pregnancy test if at risk for HELLP syndrome

11. ABG with subsequent serial VBGs should be used to guide therapy for metabolic/lactic acidosis, and any other acid–base imbalances which arise.

B. EKG should be considered for patients exhibiting electrolyte dysregulation.

C. Paracentesis for cell count, protein, culture and sensitivity, and cytology, as indicated.

D. Imaging

1. Both ultrasonography and CT scan can be useful in detection and quantifying of ascites, as well as neoplasm, free air, portal hypertension, or abscess.

2. CT scan of the brain should be ordered for patients with altered mentation, especially with thrombocytopenia, to investigate for potential cerebral bleeding.

Management

A. Individuals exhibiting signs of infection or pending sepsis should receive adequate fluid resuscitation, with the caveat that increased permeability may lead to worsening fluid overload.

B. Albumin may temporarily provide expansion of intravascular volume.

C. Broad-spectrum antibiotics, following collection of blood, urine, and peritoneal fluid cultures, if possible

D. Fluid overload and hyperosmolar hyponatremia are commonly seen with fulminant liver failure and ascites and may be treated with spironolactone (first line), amiloride, or loop diuretics.

E. Electrolyte derangements, including hyponatremia, hypokalemia, and hypomagnesemia, should be corrected per institutional protocols.

F. Large volume ascites may require paracentesis. If risk for rapid reaccumulation is a concern, consult GI or interventional radiology.

G. If hepatic encephalopathy, administer lactulose with serial ammonia measurements and monitoring for clinical effect.

H. Severe thrombocytopenia or anemia from GI bleeding may require transfusion of blood products.

I. Individuals with acute viral hepatitis A receive supportive care and may require admission for dehydration and symptom management.

Age and Developmental Considerations

A. In children, causes of liver disease

1. Hepatitis B, hepatitis C, autoimmune hepatitis, inherited diseases (glycogen storage, tyrosinemia, Wilson disease, alpha1-antitrypsin deficiency, cystic fibrosis), bile duct diseases (biliary atresia, sclerosing cholangitis, hepatitis fibrosis, choledochal cysts), drugs and toxins (isoniazid, methotrexate, excessive vitamin A), fatty liver disease

Patient Disposition (Referrals, Follow-Up, Education)

A. Consult with the patient's primary care physician and consider early GI consult.

B. Model for End Stage Liver Disease (MELD) scoring may be useful in decision-making regarding patient disposition, appropriateness for placement on an emergent transjugular intrahepatic shunt (TIPS), and for discussion with patient and family on their preferences for care.

C. Consider if patient is candidate for liver transplantation.

D. Disposition should consider the patient's risk profile.

E. Pregnant patients, the very young, or older frail adults should increase the tendency for admission.

F. GI bleeding, inability to tolerate oral intake, high serum bilirubin (>20 mg/dL), brittle glycemic regulation, or prolonged bleeding times >50% above normal are criteria for admission.

G. Those with hemodynamic instability should receive critical care consultation and admission to the ICU.

Inflammatory Bowel Disease

A. Crohn's disease

1. A chronic, idiopathic, granulomatous inflammatory disease characterized by segmental ulceration of the gastrointestinal tract anywhere from the mouth to the anus.

2. Patients present with complications of the disease, such as intestinal obstruction, intra-abdominal abscess, or a variety of extraintestinal manifestations. One third of patients develop perianal fissures, fistulas, abscesses, or rectal prolapse.

a. Fistulas occur between the ileum and sigmoid colon, the cecum or other ileal segment or the skin, or between the colon and vagina.

b. Abscesses can be intraperitoneal, retroperitoneal, interloop, or intramesenteric.

c. Obstruction, hemorrhage, and toxic megacolon also occur. Toxic megacolon can be associated with massive GI bleeding.

3. Extraintestinal manifestations (50% of patients) include arthritis, uveitis, nephrolithiasis, and skin disease (erythema nodosum, pyoderma gangrenosum); hepatobiliary disease, including gallstones, peri cholangitis, and chronic active hepatitis: and as in pancreatitis, thromboembolic disease because of hypercoagulable state.

4. Malabsorption, malnutrition, and chronic anemia develop in long-standing disease and high incidence of GI tract carcinoma.

5. The recurrence rate for those treated medically is 25% to 50% and higher when treated surgically.

6. Definitive diagnosis of ulcerative colitis (UC) or Crohn's is usually established months or years after the onset of symptoms.

B. Ulcerative colitis

1. An idiopathic chronic inflammatory and ulcerative disease of the colon and rectum, characterized by intermittent episodes of crampy abdominal pain and bloody diarrhea, with complete remission between bouts.

2. Complications include GI hemorrhage, abscess and fistula formation, obstruction secondary to stricture formation, acute perforation and a 10- to 30-fold increase in the risk of developing colon carcinoma.

C. Diverticulitis

1. Common GI disorder that occurs when small herniations through the wall of the colon (diverticula) become acutely inflamed and infected, with micro abscesses of one or more diverticula.

2. Third most common inpatient gastrointestinal diagnosis in the United States, at an annual cost of $2.1 billion, it is the most frequently listed gastrointestinal diagnosis in outpatient clinics and the ED.

3. Diverticulosis is the asymptomatic herniation of the colonic mucosa into the muscularis layer. Approximately 50% of patients with diverticulosis will develop diverticulitis in their lifetime.

4. Incidence increases in older adults and in societies that eat a low-fiber diet.

5. Diverticular bleeds are the acute hemorrhage of a diverticulum. More common in the left colon

Anatomy of IBD

A. In Crohn's disease, any part of the digestive tract from the mouth to the anus can be involved, but most commonly affects the end of the small intestine called the terminal ileum and the beginning of the large intestine called the cecum.

B. In ulcerative colitis, inflammation extends proximally from the anal verge in an uninterrupted pattern to involve part or the entire colon. The rectum is involved in >95% of cases of ulcerative colitis even when the rest of colon is spared. Occasionally UC involves the terminal ileum (up to 30 cm), due to an incompetent ileocecal valve. The reflux of noxious inflammatory mediators from the colon results in superficial mucosal inflammation of the terminal ileum, called backwash ileitis.

C. *Diverticulitis:* See Figure 17.1

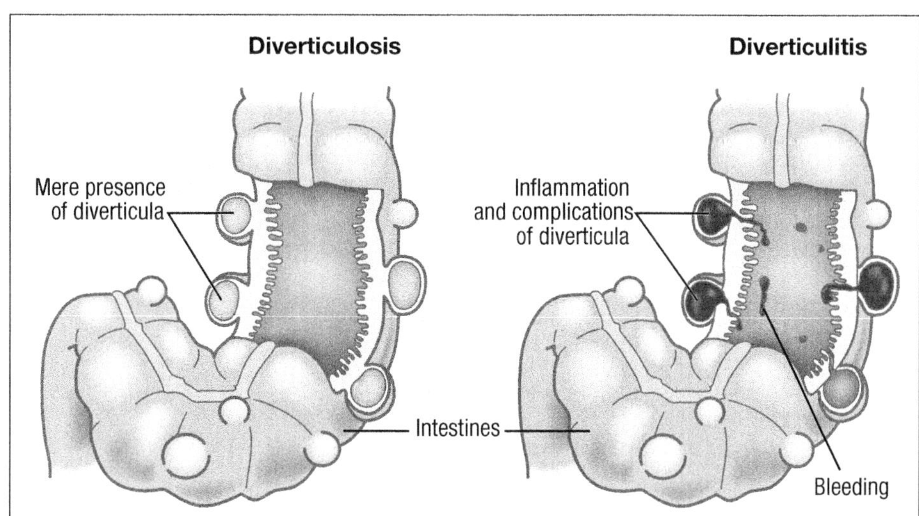

FIGURE 17.1 Diverticulosis and diverticulitis

Pathophysiology of IBD

A. Genetic and environmental influences are involved in the pathogenesis.
B. A condition of visceral hypersensitivity (leading to abdominal discomfort or pain) and gastrointestinal motor disturbances (leading to diarrhea or constipation)
C. Crohn's disease is variable, unpredictable with multiple remissions, and exacerbations typically located throughout the small and/or large intestine, but can be found anywhere along the GI tract.

1. Characterized by focal lesions or ulcerations resulting in fistulas that may communicate with other structures, including other sections of bowel, bladder, skin, or vagina
2. The incidence of gallstones and kidney stones is increased in Crohn's disease because of malabsorption that occurs in the small bowel due to loss of functional mucosal absorptive surface.

a. Dietary calcium binds to malabsorbed fatty acids in the colonic lumen, absorbing free oxalate and resulting in hyperoxaluria and stones.
b. Involvement of the terminal ileum can result in malabsorption of bile acids, leading to steatorrhea, fat-soluble vitamin deficiency, and gallstone formation (due to increased cholesterol concentration in the bile caused by a reduced bile salt pool).
c. Malabsorption can lead to malnutrition, dehydration, multiple nutrient deficiencies.
d. Steatorrhea and fat-soluble vitamin deficiency may lead to clotting abnormalities, calcium deficiency, osteomalacia.

3. Extraintestinal diseases associated with Crohn's disease

a. Osteopenia, osteoporosis, iron deficiency anemia, vitamin B12 anemia, folate deficiency, anemia of chronic disease, autoimmune hemolytic anemia, thrombocytosis, thrombosis, nephrolithiasis, obstructive uropathy, glomerulonephritis, amyloidosis, granulomatous lung disease, fibrosing alveolitis, pulmonary vasculitis, pericarditis, myocarditis, vasculitis

D. Ulcerative colitis is usually confined to the large intestine and characterized by a contiguous sheet of mucosal inflammation, with the formation of crypt abscesses, epithelial necrosis, and mucosal ulceration characterized by bloody diarrheal stool of up to 11 to 20 episodes daily.

1. Predisposes patients to significant fluid losses, anemia, malnutrition, infection/sepsis, and dehydration.
2. The disease increases in severity more distally, deeper layers of bowel typically spared, with rectal involvement in nearly every case.

E. Diverticulitis is an acute inflammation of the intestinal mucosa of the colon associated with small out-pouches or mucosal protrusion through the intestinal wall in areas of muscle weakness (diverticula) located anywhere along the large intestine. It is most common in the left colon (descending or sigmoid colon).

1. As individuals age, the colonic wall collagen develops more cross-linking, leading to decreased elasticity and an increased risk of mucosal herniation and more prone to submucosal tears.
2. With inflammation, infection, or fecal material collecting in the diverticula, regions of the colon can become friable or prone to micro (pericolonic fat and mesentery wall off the perforation) or macro abscess formation.
3. Increased intraluminal pressure or inspissated food particles cause erosion of the diverticular wall, resulting in obstruction, distention of the diverticula, overgrowth of bacteria, mucous secretion, perforation, intestinal rupture vascular compromise, peritonitis, focal necrosis, or bleeding.
4. Complications of disease

a. Colovesicular fistulas more common in men; ureteral or colovaginal fistulas common in women. Other complications include abscess, intestinal fistula, perforation, obstruction, generalized peritonitis, sepsis, stricture disease.

Prevalence

A. 25% of cases of inflammatory bowel disease occur during childhood and adolescence, initially in teens and twenties, with another peak occurring ages 50 to 70 years.
B. Risk of irritable bowel disease in family members increases childhood risk.
C. IBS affects between 400,000 to 600,000 people in North America per year.
D. Whites and European Ashkenazi Jews (2–4 times higher incidence rate) account for most cases in the United States and other industrialized countries without association with social class or occupation.
E. The annual incidence of ulcerative colitis is 10.4 to 12 cases per 100,000 people, and the prevalence rate is 35 to 100 cases per 100,000 people. It is three times more common than Crohn's disease and affects about 1 million people in the United States.
F. Ulcerative colitis is more common in women than men, peaks at 15 to 25 years old, peaks again at 55 to 65 years old, and is uncommon in children under 10 years old.
G. Incidence of diverticulitis has increased over the past 20 years due to low fiber diets and ranges from 20% at age 40 and 60% by age 60. Incidence increases with age with equal sex distribution, although increasing more in women.
H. Diverticulitis affects 180/100,000 persons per year. 15% to 20% of patients with diverticulosis will develop diverticulitis; 20% have one or more recurrent episodes within 10 years. It is the leading indication for elective colectomy.
I. Diverticulitis may be more severe in those who are immunocompromised, older adults, those with comorbid conditions, or those taking anti-inflammatory medications.

Predisposing Factors

A. If new diagnosis of IBD, consider genetic factors, obesity, age 15 to 40 years or 60 to 80 years, family history of IBD, smoking, diet rich in sugars, long-term NSAID use, low fiber diet, high fat diet, industrialized country, infectious disease exposure.

Medical Screening

A. *Chief complaint:* Altered bowel habit, focal or diffuse abdominal pain, abdominal bloating/distention, recurring fever, frequent diarrhea (can be bloody in UC or diverticulitis), mucoid stools (UC)

B. *High yield history:* Intermittent recurring fever, diffuse abdominal cramping or localized pain, and diarrhea over several years.

1. Detailed history of bowel symptoms.
2. Pregnancy status (ectopic can mimic IBS or diverticulitis).
3. Location of pain (diffuse, RLQ, LLQ), Radiation of pain (typically nonradiating), increased with movement but not positional.
4. Any associated symptoms.

C. Signs and symptoms

1. Altered bowel habit
   a. *Constipation:* Hard stools of narrow caliber, painful or infrequent defecation, and intractability to laxatives
   b. *Diarrhea:* Small volumes of loose stool (in UC), large volumes in UC or diverticulitis, with evacuation preceded by urgency or frequent defecation
   c. Postprandial urgency is common (esp. Crohn's), as is alternation between constipation and diarrhea.
   d. One feature generally predominates in a patient, but significant variability exists among patients (Crohn's or UC).
2. Abdominal pain
   a. Pain is frequently diffuse without radiation and episodes of sharp pain intermittent between the dull aches. Meals may exacerbate pain.
   b. Common sites are lower abdomen, specifically RLQ (Crohn's) and LLQ (UC and diverticulitis).
   c. Gas pockets in the splenic flexure may manifest itself as anterior chest pain or LUQ abdominal pain.
3. Abdominal bloating/distention
   a. Patients with mild UC (limited to rectum) can have fewer than four bowel movements per day, Severe UC (pancolitis) is associated to systemic complaints, and few extraintestinal manifestations.
   b. Moderate disease (colitis to splenic flexure)
   c. Severe UC (pancolitis) is associated with frequent daily bowel movements, weight loss, fever, tachycardia, anemia, frequent extraintestinal manifestations.
4. *Other symptoms:* Anorexia, weight loss, dyspepsia, heartburn, nausea/vomiting (N/V), sexual dysfunction, urinary frequency/urgency/dysuria (UTI), comorbid fibromyalgia, clear or white mucorrhea, vitamin deficiencies, fatigue, bone loss, rectal bleeding, psychosocial issues, pain worse before period
5. Painless rectal bleeding is the hallmark of a diverticular bleed and common cause of GI bleeding in older adults.
6. May present with complications of the disease.
   a. Intestinal obstruction, intra-abdominal abscess, perianal fistulas, rectal prolapse, abscesses, toxic megacolon, GI bleeding, vaginal–rectal fistulas, thromboembolic disease because of hypercoagulable state, malabsorption, malnutrition, chronic anemia
   b. Extraintestinal manifestations
      i. Arthritis, uveitis, nephrolithiasis, skin disease, hepatobiliary disease, pancreatitis, ankylosing spondylitis, episcleritis, uveitis, pyoderma gangrenosum, erythema nodosum, thromboembolic disease, renal stones, malnutrition
7. Symptoms that should alert to other pathology
   a. Acute symptoms, onset in middle age or older, steatorrhea, gluten intolerance, fever, nocturnal symptoms, progressive symptoms

D. Past medical history (PMH)

1. Family history of similar symptoms, stress, use of laxatives/antacids, foreign travel, recent antibiotic use, gastric cancer, *H. pylori* infection, history of peripheral vascular disease (suggests alternative diagnosis of mesenteric ischemia and increased sensitivity to blood loss), diabetes (higher rate of complications), diverticulosis (higher risk for diverticulitis)

Physical Examination

A. General

1. Overall healthy appearance but may be tense or anxious. Symptoms reflect severity of illness.
2. May have arthritis or arthralgia of the large joints, ankylosing spondylitis, sacroiliitis (Crohn's or UC).

B. *Vital signs:* Fever (if infection present), tachycardia, low BP, or orthostatic hypotension if dehydration, sepsis, or anemia

C. *Skin (typically normal):* Pallor, jaundice, erythema nodosum, pyoderma gangrenosuum in Crohn's or UC. Clubbing of fingers (UC)

D. HEENT (typically normal)

1. Dryness of tongue and oral mucosa due to decreased salivary secretions
2. May reveal episcleritis or uveitis, mucocutaneous or aphthous ulcers in Crohn's disease or UC. Scleral icterus in UC

E. *Cardiac:* Typically, normal; tachycardia or orthostatic hypotension if dehydrated

F. *Pulmonary:* Typically, normal

G. *Abdominal:* Varies from normal to acute abdomen

1. Tenderness to the RLQ with ileal involvement in Crohn's or with right-sided diverticulitis
2. Sigmoid tenderness (LLQ) or a palpable sigmoid cord, but can have abdominal tenderness anywhere (UC or diverticulitis)
3. Masses may be felt due to thickened or matted loops of inflamed bowel.
4. Distention may indicate obstruction or toxic megacolon. Tympanic abdomen and normal bowel sounds.
5. Rectal examination to look for tenderness (colitis or abscess), mucosal abnormalities (UC), strictures, skin tags, masses, prolapse, fistulas (especially of the skin, bladder, or vagina), hemorrhoids, abscesses, fissures,

impaired sphincter function due to neurologic disorder, stool characteristics, hematochezia

H. *Neurological:* Typically, normal

Differential Diagnoses

A. Bacterial or viral etiology, including traveler's diarrhea, exacerbations of inflammatory bowel disease, GI bleeding, thyrotoxicosis, high fiber intake, poisonings or drug related (e.g., antibiotics, polystyrene, sorbitol), UTI, appendicitis, neoplasm, trauma, pregnancy/threatened abortion/ectopic pregnancy, ovarian cyst or torsion, nephrolithiasis, sarcoidosis, lymphoma, chronic mycotic infections, TB, Kaposi sarcoma, celiac disease, Behçet's disease, NSAID enteropathy, giardiasis, mesenteric ischemia, hemolytic uremic syndrome, pseudomembranous colitis, allergic colitis, Henoch-Schoenlein purpura (HSP), parasitic colitis, necrotizing colitis, appendicitis, pediatric malabsorption syndrome, radiation antineoplastic agent induced, pelvic inflammatory disease (PID), epiploic appendagitis, gallbladder disease, vascular disease, sarcoidosis, pancreatic disease, pyelonephritis

B. When confined to the colon, ischemic colitis, infectious colitis, pseudomembranous enterocolitis, IBS, and ulcerative colitis should be considered.

C. If limited to the rectum, consider sexually acquired diseases such as rectal syphilis, gonococcal proctitis, lymphogranuloma venereum, herpes simplex virus (HSV), *Entamoeba histolytica*, *Shigella*, and *Campylobacter*.

D. The most feared complication is toxic megacolon (fever, tachycardia, dehydration, and a tender distended abdomen). Perforation and peritonitis are life-threatening.

E. *Criteria for diagnosis for Crohn's/UC in IBS:* Rome IV criteria

1. Requires that patients have had recurrent abdominal pain on average at least 1 day per week during the previous 3 months that is associated with two or more of the following:
   a. Related to defecation, change in stool frequency, stool form and appearance
2. Supporting symptoms
   a. Altered stool frequency, form, passage (straining/urgency), mucorrhea, abdominal bloating, or subjective distention

Diagnostic Testing

A. Decision-making should include identification of acute versus chronic illness, presence of dehydration, and the severity of colitis.

B. *Labs:* Typically, nonspecific

1. CBC may show leukocytosis or anemia, CMP for renal function or electrolyte imbalance, LFTs for liver involvement, lipase (if upper abdominal involvement).
2. Stool studies, type and crossmatch, inflammatory markers (ESR, CRP), lactate, and urinalysis, as indicated
3. Patients who are febrile or on immunosuppressant drugs should have blood cultures drawn.

C. Imaging

1. *Abdominal XR:* May show obstruction, macro perforation, toxic megacolon (appears as long, continuous segment of air-filled colon >6 cm in diameter).
   a. Generally not helpful, lack of sensitivity for perforation/micro perforation, abscess, and inflammation
2. Contrasted CT of the abdomen and pelvis
   a. If localized pain, nonspecific acute abdominal pain
   b. May show bowel wall thickening, segmental narrowing, destruction of normal mucosal pattern, mesenteric edema, abscess formation, fistulas or extraintestinal complications in Crohn's or UC.
   c. In diverticulitis, shows pericolonic inflammation, colonic diverticula, soft tissue inflammatory masses, phlegmon, bowel wall thickening, abscess perforation, or alternative diagnosis.
   d. *Uncomplicated diverticulitis:* Inflammation only. *Complicated diverticulitis* is associated with obstruction, perforation, bleeding, fistula, or abscess.
   e. Can help guide percutaneous drainage of abscesses, if indicated (>4 cm diameter).
3. *Ultrasound:* Identification of perianal or rectovaginal fistulas in patients with Crohn's disease.
4. Colonoscopy can detect early mucosal lesions, define the extent of colonic involvement, identify colon cancer in Crohn's or UC, but contraindicated in acute diverticulitis.
5. Barium enema will show diverticula but contraindicated in acute disease because of risk of colonic overdistention and perforation.

Management

A. IV fluid (IVF; crystalloid) resuscitation in severe cases.

B. Parenteral analgesics for pain control; narcotics preferred as NSAIDs can increase risk of colonic perforation.

C. Bowel rest, then advance to clear liquids only as tolerated, then slowly incorporate solid foods (over 2–3 days). Once symptoms resolve, can begin adding fiber back into diet.

D. Correction of electrolyte abnormalities

E. Nasogastric (NG) suction if obstruction, ileus, or toxic megacolon

F. Empiric broad-spectrum antibiotics should be prescribed for suspected infection.

1. In Crohn's and UC, can help induce remission and can be used with perianal disease, including ciprofloxacin and metronidazole for anaerobic coverage.
2. In uncomplicated diverticulitis, use ciprofloxacin, trimethoprim-sulfamethoxazole (TMP/SMZ) plus metronidazole, or amoxicillin/clavulanic acid.
3. In complicated diverticulitis, use metronidazole plus a third-generation cephalosporin or fluoroquinolone, piperacillin/tazobactam, ampicillin/sulbactam, ticarcillin/clavulanic acid, imipenem, or meropenem (preferred if immunocompromised).

G. Sulfasalazine is effective for mild or moderate Crohn's disease but has multiple toxic side effects. Mesalamine has less.

H. High-dose IV corticosteroids (hydrocortisone, methyl prednisone, prednisolone) are indicated for acute severe exacerbations of Crohn's disease or UC and should be included in the management of infection as well.

1. Hydrocortisone is indicated for those who are immunosuppressed or on chronic steroids to avoid adrenal insufficiency and crisis.

I. Immunosuppressive drugs are used as steroid sparing agents in healing fistulas and in patients with serious surgical contraindications (6-mercapropurine).

J. Medically resistant, moderate to severe Crohn's may benefit from antitumor necrosis factor antibody infliximab.

K. Amino salicylates and immunomodulating therapies should be initiated by gastroenterology and are not in the purview of emergency care.

L. Diarrhea can be controlled by loperamide, diphenoxylate, or cholestyramine, but should be avoided in UC secondary to increased risk of toxic megacolon.

M. Supportive measures include nutritious diet (high fiber in diverticulosis, low fiber in acute flares), psychical and psychological rest, replenishment of iron stores, elimination of lactose.

Age and Developmental Considerations

A. Careful assessment of growth and development is important in pediatrics, looking for decreased growth velocity or pubertal delay.

B. Initial presentation for IBS is typically in adolescents age 15 to 25 years of age, with 20% to 40% of patients diagnosed during childhood.

C. Fulminant disease (UC) occurs more often in children than adults.

D. Children with UC often present with lethargy, fatigue, arthritis, failure to gain weight, delayed puberty.

E. Diverticulitis has traditionally been considered a condition in older adults, but is starting to be seen earlier in the industrialized world secondary to low fiber diets.

Patient Disposition (Referrals, Follow-Up, Education)

A. Disposition is determined by the patient's hemodynamic stability, pain control, severity of infection, ability to maintain oral hydration, and risk assessment in terms of immunologic compromise.

B. Most patients who are deemed appropriate for discharge should have a plan for reevaluation by PCP in 24 to 48 hours, and should have another follow-up with GI in 6 to 8 weeks once symptom free to undergo colonoscopy to rule out malignancy. Provide education regarding antibiotic and steroid prescriptions (as indicated).

C. Consider complications of IBD, including inflammation (exacerbation), infection (abscess vs. diffuse infection), perforation, and hemorrhage. Surgical complications should prompt immediate consultation.

D. Hospital admission is recommended for patients with demonstrated fulminant colitis, peritonitis, obstruction, significant hemorrhage, severe dehydration, or electrolyte imbalance or have failed outpatient management.

E. Consultation/collaboration with gastroenterologist for alterations in therapy, should be initiated early in admission and upon discharge. Patients may be observed or admitted for endoscopy to evaluate the status of their underlying disease.

F. Patients with IBD are often maintained on immunosuppressive agents, biologic similar agents, or chronic anti-inflammatory agents (5-ASA, prednisone), increasing the risk for infection, sepsis, and septic shock.

G. Consider emergent surgical consultation as indicated for obstruction, significant hemorrhage, toxic megacolon, perianal disease, abscess or fistula formation, findings of peritonitis or acute abdomen, or radiological or clinical indications of perforation. Elective resection after three or more episodes of uncomplicated diverticulitis.

H. Patients should be aware of an increased thromboembolic risk and the signs for which to seek medical care, as well as indications of treatment failure or worsening infection.

I. Immunosuppressed patients should be counseled on atypical presentations of infection and regular infection control after the exacerbation has subsided.

J. Some patients with UC will use fiber supplements to add bulk to stool, reducing the volume of diarrhea. They should dilute such products (i.e., Metamucil) with adequate volumes of water to prevent toxic megacolon.

Nonspecific Abdominal Pain, Appendicitis, and Mesenteric Ischemia

Prevalence

A. Appendicitis peaks between ages 10 to 30 years and is one of the most frequent diagnoses for ED visits among children aged 5 to 17 years old in the United States.

B. Approximately 100/100,000 people will develop appendicitis in their lifetime. Occurs more often in Caucasians and in males more often than females.

C. Ischemia due to superior mesenteric artery occlusion is 8.6/100,000 per year.

1. Annual incidence is about 5.5%/100,000 individuals; increases with age.

D. Nonocclusive mesenteric ischemia affects 6,000/100,000 individuals worldwide.

Anatomy (Figure 17.2)

A. Diffuse pain

B. *Epigastric pain:* Stomach, duodenum, pancreas

C. *Right upper quadrant (RUQ) pain:* Liver, gallbladder, pancreas

D. *Right lower quadrant (RLQ) pain:* Terminal ileum, cecum, appendix

1. The appendix sits at the junction of the small intestine and large intestine, is thin and about 4 inches long.

2. Carcinoid tumors (rare) secrete chemicals that cause periodic flushing, wheezing, and diarrhea.

E. *Left upper quadrant (LUQ) pain:* Spleen, pancreas (tip), stomach

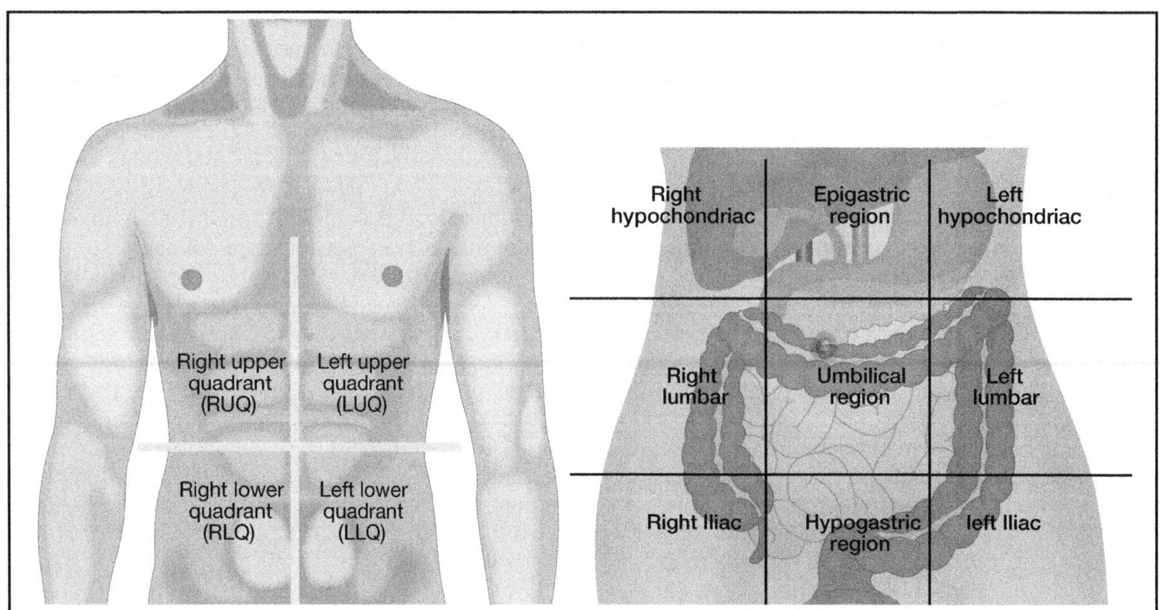

FIGURE 17.2 Quadrants of the abdomen to describe the location and symptoms of pain. (A) Four quadrants. (B) Nine quadrants.

Source: Small L, Spencer T, Medina R, Reed KZ, Dudley S, Gawlik K. Evidence-based assessment of the abdominal, gastrointestinal, and urological systems. In: Gawlik, KS, Melnyk, BM, Teall, AM, eds. *Evidence-Based Physical Examination: Best Practices for Health and Well-Being Assessment.* Springer Publishing Company; 2021. Fig. 16.4

F. *Left lower quadrant (LLQ) pain:* Descending colon
G. *Flank pain:* Large bowel, kidney
H. *Hypogastric:* Small bowel
I. *Umbilical:* Transverse colon, small bowel
J. Vasculature
  1. *Celiac artery:* Esophagus, stomach, proximal duodenum, liver, gallbladder, pancreas, spleen
  2. *Superior mesenteric artery:* Distal duodenum, jejunum, ilium, colon up to splenic flexure.
  3. *Inferior mesenteric artery:* Descending colon, sigmoid colon, rectum

Pathophysiology

A. Visceral abdominal pain is caused by the stretching of fibers innervating the walls or capsules of the hollows of solid organs, respectively and less commonly caused by early ischemia and inflammation.

B. Foregut organs (stomach, duodenum, and biliary tract) produce pain in the epigastric region; midgut organs (small bowel and appendix) cause periumbilical pain; and hindgut organs (colon, sigmoid, and organs of the genitourinary system) produce pain in the suprapubic or hypogastric area.

C. Appendicitis results when the appendiceal lumen is obstructed Increased luminal pressure leads to vascular compromise, bacterial invasion, inflammatory response, and resultant tissue necrosis with possible perforation and tissue necrosis or peritoneal contamination.

D. Pain migration in appendicitis

  1. Atypical presentations with variability of the anatomic location (retrocecal, retroileal)

  2. Appendiceal distention stimulates stretch receptors which relay pain via visceral afferent pain fibers to the 10th thoracic ganglion, which inhibits lymphatic and venous drainage.

  3. Bacterial invasion of the wall, with edema and blockage of arterial blood flow, perforation, and spillage of contents into peritoneal cavity, causing peritonitis (24–36 hours from onset) or abscess (gram-negative rods and aerobic organisms)

  4. RLQ pain occurs as inflammation extends to surrounding tissues. Pain occurs owing to stimulation of parietal nerve fibers and localizes to the position of the appendix.

E. Parietal or somatic abdominal pain is caused by irritation of fibers that innervate the parietal peritoneum, usually the portion covering the anterior abdominal wall.

F. In contrast to visceral pain, parietal pain can be localized to a dermatome directly above the stimulus.

G. As underlying disease progresses, the symptoms of visceral pain give way to parietal pain, with tenderness and guarding.

H. As localized peritonitis progresses further, rigidity and rebound appear.

I. Referred pain can be felt in a location distant from the diseased organ.

J. Narrowing of the arteries that supply blood to the intestine can cause ischemia.

  1. Arterial embolism (40%–50%) from the heart and associated with risk factors of coronary artery disease (CAD) post PCI, valvular disease, atrial fibrillation

2. Nonocclusive (20%) caused by mesenteric vasoconstriction or low flow states leading to decreased perfusion to watershed areas associated with hypotension, splanchnic vasoconstriction from pressors, or cocaine use.
3. Venous thrombosis (5%–10%) caused by venous stasis, hypercoagulable states, trauma, polycythemia vera, and inflammatory states.

Predisposing Factors

A. Older age, prior abdominal surgery, history of bowel disorders, exposure to stomach virus, steroid use, diabetes, chronic obstructive pulmonary disease (COPD), family history of appendicitis, cystic fibrosis, atrial fibrillation (AF), low cardiac output states, trauma, smoking, immobility, PVD, valvular disorders

Medical Screening

A. *Chief complaint:* Abdominal pain, "pain out of proportion to clinical examination" (ischemia), RLQ pain evolving over minutes to hours (appendicitis)
B. High yield history
1. Previous surgeries, alcohol (ETOH) or drug history, pancreatitis history or hepatitis history, pregnancy status and gynecologic (GYN) history, relationship to food, recent antibiotic history, gastrointestinal (GI) bleed, trauma history, last bowel movement and renal complaints, what makes it better or worse, radiated or referred pain, chest pain, dyspnea, cough, genitourinary (GU) symptoms, any similar prior episodes
2. Last oral intake, including what was eaten and relation of pain to that oral intake
3. Onset, provocation, quality, radiation, severity, and time questions about pain
a. Appendicitis starts in the epigastric/periumbilical region and migrates towards RLQ, may radiate to groin or flank, and be worse with walking, hopping, or hitting bumps on the way to the hospital (prefers not to move). Shuffling gait, "appy" walk. Many patients prefer to have their knees in a flexed position for comfort.
b. Migratory pain in appendicitis
i. Initially periumbilical pain, followed by anorexia (95%) and nausea followed by vomiting and fever, which may be low grade
ii. Normal location of pain RLQ 1 to 12 hours after onset
iii. Retrocecal appendix (28%–68%) presents with back, flank, testicular pain.
iv. Pelvic appendix (27%–53%) presents as suprapubic pain, urinary or rectal symptoms.
v. Long appendix (<0.2%) may cause pain in RUQ or LLQ, anorexia, vomiting, change in bowel habits (diarrhea 33%, constipation 9%–33%).
vi. Factors that increase likelihood of appendicitis are RLQ pain, rebound tenderness and/or rigidity, migration of pain to RLQ, pain before vomiting, positive psoas sign, fever, and guarding, although nonspecific.
c. Mesenteric ischemia presents as acute onset abdominal pain that is persistent, poorly localized, vague, variable, colicky, and severe, with associated nausea/vomiting (N/V), and diarrhea.
C. Signs and symptoms
1. Absence of flatus, absence of bowel movement (small bowel obstruction [SBO]), anorexia (pancreatitis, appendicitis), diarrhea (*C. diff*), bloody diarrhea (inflammatory bowel disease [IBD], infection or mesenteric ischemia), N/V (hyperemesis, gastroparesis, cyclic vomiting, gastroenteritis), shortness of breath (pneumonia, perforation), vaginal bleeding (ectopic pregnancy, abortion), worse with meals (biliary colic, peptic ulcer disease [PUD]), pain radiation to back (pancreatitis, abdominal aortic aneurysm [AAA]), pain diffuse, severe, or colicky (SBO), bloating, pain out of proportion (mesenteric ischemia), pain radiation to groin (renal colic), pelvic discomfort (pelvic inflammatory disease [PID], sexually transmitted diseases [STD]), heartburn (gastroesophageal reflux [GERD], PUD), indigestion, gas, fever (may or may not be present, late finding in appendicitis), chest pain or back pain (acute coronary syndrome [ACS], AAA, PNA), urinary symptoms (UTI, renal colic), LMP (ectopic), antibiotic use (may mask symptoms)
2. Classic triad of appendicitis is anorexia, N/V with pain often described as dull, aching, or throbbing, migrating. Onset is insidious or gradual.
3. In mesenteric ischemia, pain out of proportion to exam, associated with nausea (56%–93%), vomiting (38%–80%), diarrhea (18%–48%), pain with eating and food avoidance, may have low-grade fever, tachycardia, often "writhing in pain"
D. *Medication history:* Steroids, antibiotics, NSAIDs, cocaine use, digoxin, alpha-adrenergic agonists, beta-blockers
E. *Past medical history:* Myocardial infarction (MI), dysrhythmias, coagulopathies, vasculopathies, GYN history (missed periods, vaginal bleeding, discharge), diverticulitis, pregnancy, prior abdominal surgeries, valvular heart disease, infective endocarditis, ventricular aneurysm, atherosclerosis, peripheral artery disease, heart failure, aortic insufficiency, hyperlipidemia, HTN, diabetes, end-stage renal disease (ESRD), hepatitis

Physical Examination

A. General
1. Etiology of abdominal pain may arise from various body systems and can be distant from the abdominal cavity.
2. Before even talking to the patient, watch them walk and sit down on the stretcher, assess general discomfort, and mental status.
a. *Appendicitis:* Patients remain very still, shuffling gait; kidney stones or ovarian torsion: usually writhing and cannot get comfortable

3. Visceral pain by nature can be difficult for patients to describe in terms of localization and vague complaint.
   a. Pneumonia in children often presents with abdominal pain.
   b. Vascular lesions such as abdominal aneurysm produces abdominal pain and bleeding, while the nausea and sensation of indigestion or abdominal discomfort may represent coronary ischemia.
   c. With acute occlusive ischemia, patients are in acute distress.
4. Include genitourinary symptoms and examination.
5. Patients with peritonitis tend to look ill and complain of intense pain with only light palpation of the abdomen.

B. Vital signs
1. Low-grade fever (normal to mild elevation initially and increases with perforation or infection). Absence of fever does not rule out infection, especially in older adults.
2. Tachycardia, hypotension, tachypnea if sepsis or shock

C. *Skin and mucous membranes:* Observed for pallor, icterus, jaundice, diaphoresis, and dehydration. Cyanosis may be present in late ischemia.

D. *Eyes:* Scleral icterus

E. Cardiac
1. Tachycardia from hypovolemia due to blood loss or volume depletion or infection. Irregular rhythm if atrial fibrillation
2. Carotid bruits may be auscultated unilaterally or bilaterally, jugular vein distention (JVD) if congestive heart failure (CHF), loud S1/S2, may hear S3 if CHF (mesenteric ischemia).
3. Due to medications or the physiology of aging, tachycardia may not always occur.

F. *Pulmonary:* May be tachypneic if septic, diminished in the bases or crackles if pneumonia, but typically normal.

G. Abdominal
1. Inspection
2. Bowel sounds
   a. Should be assessed, prior to palpation or percussion, in all four quadrants for presence, frequency, and tone.
   b. Bowel sounds (hyperactive, high pitched, tinkling, or absent in small bowel obstruction [SBO], absent in ileus)
3. Palpation (most important part)
   a. Start pressing opposite where patient is having pain; if patient has trouble relaxing, bend knees to 45 degrees.
   b. *Assess location of tenderness:* Should be performed in a rotation that includes the area of reported last pain to facilitate assessment.
   c. Light palpation should precede deep palpation in each quadrant.
      i. Look for focal tenderness, masses, organomegaly, hernias or rebound tenderness.
      ii. Rebound/guarding (surgical abdomen/perforation)
         (1) Rebound tenderness is often regarded as clinical criteria for peritonitis, but has limitations.
         (2) Pain with heel tap, pelvic shake, or any rapid movement of peritoneum.
         (3) In patients with peritonitis, combination of rigidity, referred tenderness, and "cough pain" usually provides enough diagnostic confirmation (esp. with appendicitis).
         (4) Guarding (voluntary due to muscular resistance to palpation or involuntary or rigidity in perforation or inflammation)
      iii. Distention (SBO)
      iv. Fluid wave (ascites)
      v. Abdominal examination is generally benign unless significant ischemia has occurred or has peritoneal signs.
   d. Special signs
      i. *Peritoneal:* Lightly shake the stretcher or, for kids, have patient jump up and down. Pain in RLQ is a positive sign.
      ii. *Carnett sign:* Sit-up test, after identification of the site of maximum abdominal tenderness; fold patient's arms across the chest and have sit up halfway. Maintain finger on tender area, and if palpation in the semi-sitting position produces same tenderness, then is positive for abdominal wall syndrome.
      iii. *Murphy's sign:* Patient ceases inspiration while you palpate RUQ at midclavicular costal margin (gallbladder disease).
      iv. *McBurney's point:* Tenderness to palpation two-thirds between umbilicus and anterior superior iliac spine (appendicitis)
      v. *Obturator:* Pain with flexion and internal rotation of right leg (appendicitis)
      vi. *Psoas:* Patient on left side, pain with hyperextension of right hip (appendicitis)
      vii. *Rovsing:* Pain in RLQ with palpation of LLQ (appendicitis)
4. Percussion
   a. Used to assess tone (tympany or dullness), organ borders, and potential fluid levels or consolidation within the abdominal cavity.
   b. Testing for costovertebral angle tenderness
5. Pelvic examination in postpubertal females with pelvic pain (adnexal tenderness with ovarian cyst, torsion, ectopic, TOA or appendicitis)
6. Testicular examination in all males
7. Rectal examination with guaiac (GI bleed, diverticulitis, colitis), subcutaneous air/mediastinal air (esophageal rupture)

Differential Diagnoses

A. Diffuse pain
1. Aortic aneurysm (leaking, ruptured), aortic dissection, early appendicitis, bowel obstruction, diabetic gastroparesis, familial Mediterranean fever, gastroenteritis, heavy metal poisoning, hereditary angioedema, malaria, mesenteric ischemia,

metabolic disorder, narcotic withdrawal, pancreatitis, perforated bowel, peritonitis, sickle cell crisis, volvulus

B. Epigastric pain

1. Gastritis, PUD, duodenitis, pancreatitis, cardiac ischemia, biliary colic, cholecystitis, cholangitis, AAA, dissection, early appendicitis, epigastric hernia

C. RUQ pain

1. Biliary colic, cholangitis, cholecystitis, Fitz-Hugh-Curtis syndrome, hepatitis, hepatic abscess, herpes zoster, myocardial ischemia, perforated duodenal ulcer, pneumonia, pulmonary embolism, common bile duct stone, duodenitis, PUD, pleural effusion, retrocecal appendicitis

D. RLQ pain

1. Aortic aneurysm (leaking, ruptured), appendicitis, Crohn's disease, diverticulitis (cecal), ectopic pregnancy, endometriosis, epiploic appendagitis, herpes zoster, inguinal hernia (incarcerated, strangulated), ischemic colitis, Meckel diverticulum, mittelschmerz, ovarian cyst (ruptured), PID, psoas abscess, regional enteritis, testicular torsion, ureteral calculi

E. LUQ pain

1. Gastric ulcer, gastritis, herpes zoster, myocardial ischemia, pancreatitis, pneumonia, pulmonary embolism, splenic rupture/distention

F. LLQ pain

1. Aortic aneurysm (ruptured, leaking), diverticulitis (sigmoid), ectopic pregnancy, endometriosis, herpes zoster, inguinal hernia (incarcerated, strangulated), ischemic colitis, mittelschmerz, ovarian cyst (ruptured), PIDe, psoas abscess, regional enteritis, testicular torsion, ureteral calculi

Diagnostic Testing

A. *Labs:* UA (infection, blood), HCG (pregnancy), CBC (leukocytosis, anemia, thrombocytopenia), BMP (electrolytes, dehydration, endocrine or metabolic disorder, acute renal failure, renal insufficiency), LFTs (cholecystitis, hepatitis, increased Aspartate transaminase/Alkaline phosphatase [AST/ALK phos] in ischemia), lipase (pancreatitis), lactate (if sick or concern about sepsis, mesenteric ischemia), EKG (women, diabetics rule out cardiac cause or arrhythmias with mesenteric ischemia), coagulation studies (GI bleeding, end-stage liver disease [ESLD], coagulopathy), CPK, troponin (cardiac concern)

B. Diagnosis of appendicitis is primarily clinical. Labs are most helpful in female patients of childbearing age with unclear diagnosis.

C. Imaging

1. Patients with epigastric or LUQ rarely require imaging unless rigid abdomen or suspect bowel obstruction.

2. X-ray

a. Nonspecific, to assess for free air in perforated viscous, evaluate for dilated loops of bowel or bowel obstruction or a renal stone with a KUB (kidneys, ureters, and bladder).

b. May see appendiceal fecalith, appendiceal gas, localized paralytic ileus, blurred right psoas muscle and free air in appendicitis.

3. CT without contrast useful in identifying urolithiasis

4. CT with IV contrast

a. Help visualize vasculature, abscesses, masses, inflammatory conditions.

b. In appendicitis, will see appendix wall thickening, fat stranding, cecal apical thickening, appendiceal masses. Diagnostic if appendix >6 mm in diameter

c. Preferred imaging for mesenteric ischemia, pancreatitis, biliary obstruction, aortic aneurysm, appendicitis

i. Will show edema of bowel wall, intramural gas, ascites. If negative and high suspicion, CTA recommended.

d. Difficult to interpret in thin individuals due to minimal separation between loops of bowel.

5. CT with oral contrast

a. Aids in the diagnosis of bowel obstruction, mesenteric ischemia, or appendicitis, but otherwise less useful.

6. MRI

a. Diagnostic in appendicitis with >7 mm in diameter, shows appendiceal fat stranding.

b. Useful in pregnant patients due to lack of ionizing radiation, but high cost, limited availability, lengthy exam, and lack of radiologist familiarity with appendicitis

7. Ultrasound (US)

a. Imaging of choice for the biliary system (RUQ pain)

b. RLQ US limited in evaluating ruptured appendix or abnormally located appendix of obese patient, but is preferred for females or children to limit radiation exposure. Helpful if positive, not if negative

c. In appendicitis without rupture, may see noncompressible appendix (6 mm AP diameter), presence of appendicolith, peri appendiceal fluid/mass.

d. Useful in diagnosis of cholelithiasis, choledocholithiasis, cholecystitis, biliary duct dilatation, pancreatic masses, hydroureter, aortic aneurysm

8. Pelvic US

a. If concern for GYN pathology, including ectopic pregnancy, ovarian cysts, torsion, or TOA

D. *Diagnostic procedures/surgery:* Laparoscopy (diagnostic and therapeutic), open exploration and repair, percutaneous drainage

Management

A. Keep patient NPO initially.

B. Unstable patients should be resuscitated immediately, then diagnosed clinically with emergent surgical consultation.

C. Pain control

1. Judicious use of analgesics is appropriate and may facilitate a better history and more accurate physical exam.

2. Morphine can be used if necessary, but avoid if suspected cholecystitis as this can contract the gallbladder, leading to an inaccurate diagnostic study. Can mask appendicitis.
3. NSAIDs are useful in renal colic, but use in other conditions is controversial and may mask peritoneal inflammation.

D. Treat N/V
1. Ondansetron or metoclopramide can increase comfort and facilitate assessment.

E. Hydration with normal saline or lactated ringers

F. Correct electrolytes as needed.

G. Start antibiotics as indicated.

For appendicitis: Use a third-generation cephalosporin or penicillin/B-lactamase inhibitor to start and add anaerobic coverage if perforation suspected.

1. Ampicillin/sulbactam, cefoxitin, ceftriaxone, ciprofloxacin, ertapenem, metronidazole, piperacillin/tazobactam if severe sepsis or perforation

H. The mainstay of treatment of mesenteric ischemia is surgery if bowel necrosis or gangrene has occurred.

I. Medical therapy in ischemia is considered initially if hemodynamically stable.
1. Depends on duration, nature, and severity of ischemia.
2. Anticoagulation with heparin
3. Hypovolemia or hypotension (fluid +/- pressors, although avoid alpha agonists)
4. Control arrhythmias (avoid digoxin, beta-blockers)
5. Stop vasoconstrictive medications if possible.
6. Nasogastric (NG) tube for enteral decompression
7. Consider interventional radiology (IR) for angiography and catheter-directed antithrombotic therapy.
8. Broad-spectrum antibiotics (piperacillin-tazobactam or third generation cephalosporin plus metronidazole)

Age and Developmental Considerations

A. Pediatrics
1. Appendicitis misdiagnosis in patients <12 years is 28% to 57% (nearly 100% in patients <2 years). 70% to 90% appendiceal perforation rate in children <4 years correlates strongly with delayed diagnosis.
2. Presentations often nonspecific and difficult to localize. Anorexia, vomiting, and diarrhea most common (half-eaten meal hours before complaints of pain may more accurately indicate duration of symptoms of appendicitis).
3. Observe child before examination for subtle indicators of local inflammation, such as limping gait, hesitation to move or climb, flexed right hip in appendicitis.

B. Geriatric considerations
1. Decreased inflammatory response
2. Three times more likely to have appendiceal perforation owing to anatomic changes
3. Older adult patients may present with mental status change or vague symptoms; therefore, diagnosis of acute process or appendicitis can be delayed.
4. Older patients with abdominal pain have a six- to eightfold increase in mortality compared to younger adults.
5. Older adults account for 20% of ED visits, of which 3% to 4% are for abdominal pain and about half to two-thirds require hospitalization.
6. Consider EKG, especially in older adult patients, women, and diabetics, as abdominal pain can be anginal equivalent.
7. Have lower threshold for imaging in older adults, immunosuppressed, and patients with previous surgery, especially gastric bypass which puts patients at risk for internal hernia.
8. Older adult patients often fail to manifest the same signs and symptoms as younger patients, with decreased pain perception and decreased febrile or muscular response to infection or inflammation.
9. Biliary disease, bowel obstruction, diverticulitis, cancer, and hernia are more common in patients >50 years old.
10. Hypotension from volume contraction, hemorrhage, or sepsis can be missed if a normally hypertensive person appears normotensive.
11. Conditions somewhat less frequent but proportionately higher in older adults include sigmoid volvulus, diverticulitis, acute mesenteric ischemia, and AAA.
12. Mesenteric ischemia should be considered in the patient >50 years old with abdominal pain out of proportion with exam.

C. Pregnancy considerations
1. Most common extrauterine surgical emergency in pregnancy is appendicitis. Enlarging uterus displaces the appendix upward and laterally.
2. Increased risk of fetal mortality (7–10% to 24%) if rupture occurs, slightly higher rate in second semester compared to first, third, and postpartum periods, increased perforation rate (25% to 40%) highest in third trimester.
3. Hyperemesis gravidarum should not cause abdominal tenderness.

Patient Disposition (Referrals, Follow-Up, Education)

A. Surgical or OB/GYN consultation should be obtained in patients with suspected acute abdominal, mesenteric ischemia, or pelvic pathology requiring immediate intervention. Appendicitis does not need diagnostic study prior to consult if high suspicion.

B. Indications for admission include serial abdominal exams, toxic appearance, unclear diagnosis in older adults or immunocompromised patients, inability to reasonably exclude serious etiology, intractable pain or vomiting, altered mental status, inability to follow discharge or follow-up instructions or surgical intervention.

C. Many patients with nonspecific abdominal pain can be discharged safely with 24 hours of follow-up and instructions to return immediately with increased pain, vomiting, fever, or failure of symptoms to resolve.

D. Discharge of an early appendicitis can occur if there are no peritoneal signs, patient can tolerate food and liquids, and has close follow-up within 24 to 48 hours. Do not discharge on antibiotics.

Nonspecific Diarrhea

A. *Clostridioides difficile*

1. *Clostridioides difficile* (*C. diff.*) is the most common cause of infectious diarrhea in hospitalized patients. Transmission can occur with humans and fomites.
2. Clinical manifestations may appear any time from 4 days to 10 weeks (typically 7–10 days) following initiation of antibiotic therapy, but may occur up to several weeks later.
3. Caused by a toxin-producing Gram-positive bacillus, typically associated with the healthcare environment and/or antibiotic use.
4. Increased morbidity and mortality related to enterocolitis, which is characterized by voluminous diarrheal stool with or without hemorrhage.

B. Indeterminate colitis

1. Inflammatory condition of the colon, which may be caused by infectious or noninfectious etiologies, associated with enteritis (inflammation of the small intestine), proctitis (inflammation of the rectum), or both

C. Gastroenteritis

1. An acute inflammation of the mucous membranes of the gastrointestinal (GI) tract, the condition may be referred to as "food poisoning" or "stomach flu" and can be viral, bacterial, or noninfectious in etiology.
2. One of the most common reasons patients seek medical care in the developing world.

Prevalence

A. There are approximately 178 million cases of acute gastroenteritis annually in the United States, resulting in 473,000 hospitalizations and 5,000 deaths.

B. Most are of viral etiology, self-limited, and require only supportive care.

C. *Norovirus* causes 50% to 80% of all infectious diarrheas in the United States, followed by non-Shiga toxin-producing *Escherichia coli*, *C. difficile*, invasive bacteria (*Campylobacter*, *Shigella*, and *Salmonella*), and Shiga toxin–producing *E. coli* and protozoa.

D. A history of foreign travel with consumption of contaminated food or drink is associated with an 80% probability of bacterial diarrhea, primarily toxin and nontoxin producing strains of *E. coli*.

E. Necrotizing enterocolitis affects 1% to 5% of patients admitted to the neonatal ICUs. Occurs in 2% to 5% of infants with birth weights lower than 1,500 g and up to 10% of infants with birth weights lower than 1,000 g.

F. Parasitic colitis in high-risk groups is reported to be 1% to 4%.

Pathophysiology

A. Increased intestinal secretion (cholera) occurs through the crypts and decreased intestinal absorption (enterotoxins, inflammation, and ischemia) through the villi.

1. Fluids are absorbed passively with the transport of sodium and actively with the absorption of glucose.

B. Increased osmotic load (laxatives, lactose intolerance)

C. Abnormal intestinal motility (irritable bowel syndrome [IBS], neuropathy)

D. Pathophysiology of *C. diff*

1. Broad-spectrum antibiotics (clindamycin, cephalosporins, ampicillin, amoxicillin, and fluoroquinolones) alter gut flora in such a way that *C. diff* can flourish within the colon, causing enteropathy.
2. Inflammation is the result of toxins produced by the organism and the formation of a biofilm along the intestinal lining as byproducts of the toxin lead to formation of discrete nodules, which coalesce into a contiguous sheath, or pseudomembrane. When caused by *C. diff*, the membrane-like yellowish plaques of exudate overlay and replace necrotic intestinal mucosa.

E. Pathophysiology of gastroenteritis

1. Inflammation results in an imbalance between fluid ingestion/secretion and absorption, produces increased intraluminal fluid, resulting in fluid losses through diarrhea leading to dehydration, volume contraction, and electrolyte deficiencies.
2. Preformed toxins (*Staphylococcus aureus* or *Bacillus cereus*) may cause symptoms in 1 hour following exposure. Viral (70% norovirus) and bacterial pathogens have incubation periods in the range of a few days.

F. Pathophysiology of indeterminate colitis

1. Can be caused by infection, hypersensitivity to allergens, ischemia, vasculitis, or several drugs.
2. Necrotizing enterocolitis
   a. Common cause of colitis in newborns, low and very low birth weight preterm infants, affecting the distal ileum and proximal colon. In severe cases, gangrene may involve the whole bowel.
   b. Produce inflammatory mediators and other cytokines, decreased epidermal growth factor, and progressive mucosal damage (mucosal edema, hemorrhage, coagulation necrosis, and mucosal ulceration) by free radical production.
   c. Associated with hypoxic ischemia and aggressive enteral feedings.
   d. Presents with gas accumulation in the submucosa of the bowel wall and progresses to necrosis, leading to perforation of the bowel, peritonitis, and sepsis.
3. Allergic colitis
   a. Children age 2 weeks to 1 year resulting from hypersensitivity, commonly to cow's milk (from breast milk or bottles) and soy milk.
   b. Immunologic responses may range from classic allergic mast cell activation to immune complex formation.
4. Pseudomembranous colitis
   a. Inflammatory colitis caused by *C. diff.*
5. Ischemic colitis
   a. Occurs in school-age children and young adults, common in males, common in Henoch-Schonlein purpura (HSP).
   b. Form of vasculitis that results from inflammation and ischemia of colonic mucosa, causing rectal bleeding and abdominal pain.
6. Congenital immune deficiency

a. Several primary immunodeficiency syndromes (common variable immunodeficiency, chronic granulomatous disease, Wiskott-Aldrich syndrome, and IPEX (immunodysregulation, polyendocrinopathy, enteropathy, and X-linked)
b. Indistinguishable from IBS

Predisposing Factors

A. *General diarrhea, colitis:* Celiac disease, food intolerance/allergy, milk/soy protein intolerance, medications, IBS, Crohn's disease, ulcerative colitis, antibiotic use, family history of IBS, immunosuppression, inadequate vaccinations, anal sex
B. *In* C. diff: Frequent and/or recent antibiotic use, advanced age, contact with infected patients and with their healthcare clinicians, immunosuppression, proton pump inhibitor use, post pyloric tube feeding
C. *In gastroenteritis:* Domestic or international travel to areas with poor sanitation practices; exposure to zoonoses; work in healthcare, prisons, long-term care facilities, childcare; consumption of raw, unpasteurized, or undercooked dairy, meat, poultry, eggs, fruit, or vegetables.

Medical Screening

A. *Chief complaint:* Nausea and vomiting (N/V, in gastroenteritis), diarrhea (defined as three or more watery stools per day), typically in large volumes, can be bloody or nonbloody, abdominal cramping
B. High yield history
1. Ask about fever, pain, pattern of onset, bloody vomit or stool, timing (time of day, associated with eating or drinking), evolution of symptoms, last bowel movement, and how many episodes per day, including the characteristic of the bowel.
a. Functional diarrhea is not typically associated with nocturnal symptoms. Suggests an infectious etiology.
2. Acute diarrhea (<3 weeks duration) is more likely to represent a serious problem such as infection, mesenteric ischemia, intoxication, or inflammation. Chronic diarrhea is described as >3 weeks.
3. In C. *diff,* onset is typically 7 to 10 days after initiating antibiotic use, but may occur several weeks following treatment.
4. Ask the patient to describe the appearance of the stool.
a. Watery diarrhea associated with viral disease (Norwalk) and noninvasive (toxin-mediated) disease (*Staphylococcus aureus, Bacillus cereus,* and *Clostridium perfringens*)
b. Bloody diarrhea associated with invasive disease that is typically seen with *Shigella* and *E. coli*
5. Ask the patient about recent travel, including foreign travel (suggestive of giardiasis and traveler's diarrhea).
6. Ask the patient about recent antibiotic use (risk for C. *diff*).
7. Ask about suspicious foods, food association, other sick contacts, or others who may have eaten same food.
8. *Associated symptoms:* N/V, crampy abdominal pain, dehydration, fever, pain, presence of blood, or type of food ingested may help in the diagnosis of infectious gastroenteritis, food poisoning, diverticulitis, or IBS.
C. Signs and symptoms
1. Wide spectrum ranging from guaiac-positive stools to disease with peritonitis, perforation, shock, coagulopathy, and death.
2. Frequent loose, watery stools, abdominal cramps or pain, fever, chills, vomiting, bleeding, lightheadedness or dizziness, mucous of blood in stool, nausea, urgent need to have a bowel movement, bloating
3. In *C. diff* or pseudomembranous colitis, ranges from frequent, watery, mucoid stools to a toxic picture, including profuse diarrhea, crampy abdominal pain, fever, leukocytosis, and dehydration within 1 week of antibiotic therapy.
4. First sign is abdominal distention with gastric retention, emesis, and discomfort in indeterminate colitis.
5. Infants with allergic colitis present with blood and mucus in the stool, vomiting, and diarrhea; may be indistinguishable from esophageal reflux.
6. Onset of irritable bowel syndrome (IBS) is usually insidious, consisting of growth failure, weight loss, diarrhea, and occult rectal bleeding.
7. Perianal disease, including fissures, skin tags, fistulae, abscesses, arthralgias, arthritis, renal caliculi, aphthous stomatitis, uveitis, iritis, episcleritis
8. A child may experience abdominal cramps, nausea after about 8 to 48 hours from exposure to foodborne illness from *Salmonella*
9. With *Shigella,* stools can be frequent (10–12 times/day) and contain mucus and blood, as well as symptoms of fever and seizures.
10. *Campylobacter* enteritis from ingestion of raw meat, poultry, fish, and contaminated water presents with abrupt onset of fever and abdominal pain, shortly followed by diarrhea (2–20 times/day and bloody). Vomiting is uncommon.
11. *Yersinia enterocolitica* presents with abdominal pain and the abrupt onset of watery diarrhea that may contain blood. Often mistaken for appendicitis
12. Parasitic colitis usually presents with dysenteric colitis, bloody diarrhea, abdominal pain, and fever.
13. HSP is usually proceeded by upper respiratory infection followed by colicky abdominal pain, migratory arthritis affecting larger joints, and symmetric purpuric rash.
D. Past medical history (PMH)
1. Ask about pregnancy, comorbid conditions, recent antibiotic use, GI surgery or manipulation, severe underlying illness, chemotherapy, family history of IBS, exposure to cow's milk or soy milk, ingestion of contaminated food or water.
2. Bulimia and anorexia are associated with factitious diarrhea.
3. Inflammatory bowel disease (IBD; Crohn's or ulcerative colitis) may present with diarrhea during an acute flare but can also be associated with constipation.

4. Malabsorption from pancreatic insufficiency or HIV-related bowel disorders need not be considered in a healthy host.
5. Dietary practices, including frequent restaurant meals, exposure to day-care centers, consumption of street vendor food or raw seafood, overseas travel, and camping with ingestion of lake or stream water
   a. Lakes and streams (*Giardia*), oysters (*Vibrio*), rice (*Bacillus cereus*), eggs (Salmonella), and meat (*Campylobacter, Staphylococcus, Yersinia, E. coli, Clostridium*)
6. Certain medications, particularly antibiotics, colchicine, lithium, and laxatives can contribute to diarrhea.
7. Social history, such as sexual preference, drug use, and occupation, may suggest diagnoses of HIV-related illness or organophosphate poisoning.

Physical Examination

A. General (ranges from normal to toxic appearing)
   1. *Assess hydration status:* Vital signs, mental status, skin, and mucus membranes
   2. Allergic colitis may present with failure to thrive.

B. *Vital signs:* Fever, tachycardia, orthostatic hypotension (dehydrated, necrotizing colitis, or sepsis)

C. *Skin:* Check skin turgor, sunken eyes, and mucous membranes (dehydration)

D. *Head, eyes, ears, nose, and throat (HEENT)*: Evaluate icterus, jaundice, jugular venous distention, or flattening for signs of hepatic involvement, dehydration, or right heart strain.

E. Cardiac/pulmonary (generally normal)
   1. Tachycardia and hypotension (dehydration, sepsis)
   2. Can progress to disseminated intravascular coagulation (DIC) or even cardiopulmonary arrest if severe.
   3. Tachypnea if significant distention or septic shock present

F. Abdominal
   1. Inspect and palpate for tenderness, ascites, hypo/hyperactive bowel sounds, distention, and correlate with severity of diarrhea.
   2. A rigid board-like abdomen, significant tenderness, focal tenderness, abdominal distention, and/or fever can indicate complications including toxic megacolon, obstruction, or intestinal perforation.
   3. Hyperactive bowel sounds (*C. diff*); decreased or absent bowel sounds (obstruction, complications)
   4. Appendicitis can present with diarrhea in up to 20% of cases.
   5. *Rectal examination:* Look for gross blood or hemoccult positive, rectal tenderness, especially in pseudomembranous colitis, IBS, or necrotizing colitis
      a. Can rule out impaction or presence of blood, the latter suggesting inflammation, infection, or mesenteric ischemia.

G. *Neurological:* Lethargy and altered mental status can be a sign of dehydration or sepsis.

Differential Diagnoses

A. Infectious diarrhea
   1. Parasitic conditions, bacterial infections (*Salmonella, Shigella*), traveler's diarrhea, GI bleeding, thyrotoxicosis, bacterial gastroenteritis, inflammatory bowel conditions, *C. diff*, viral infections (primarily rotavirus, norovirus)

B. Factitious diarrhea
   1. Self-induced diarrhea by laxative or factitious reporting, high fiber intake

C. Functional diarrhea
   1. Associated with irritable bowel disease and psychiatric disorders not caused by structural or chemical abnormality.

D. Others
   1. Malabsorption syndrome, hyperthyroidism, ischemic bowel, HIV, pregnancy, biliary colic, or obstruction, partial small or large bowel obstruction, upper urinary tract infections, nephrolithiasis, appendicitis, hepatitis, poisoning, drug-related, hemolytic uremic syndrome, allergic colitis, pseudomembranous colitis, HSP, necrotizing colitis, pediatric malabsorption syndrome

E. Temporal associations of nausea followed by vomiting, especially with resolution in the reverse order may aid in diagnosis.

Diagnostic Testing

A. Most diarrhea is viral or self-limiting; lab testing in routine cases is not indicated.

B. Labs
   1. Complete blood count (CBC) may see leukocytosis with invasive disease, allergic colitis, pseudomembranous colitis, but normal in HSP.
   2. Check platelets or coagulation profile if concern for DIC.
   3. Comprehensive metabolic panel (CMP) to evaluate for dehydration, electrolyte imbalance, kidney injury, or identify hemolytic-uremic syndrome (*E. coli*) characterized by acute kidney injury (AKI) and hemolytic anemia, especially in the children and older adults
   4. LFTs (hepatic involvement)
   5. Lactic acid (mesenteric ischemia, sepsis, or severe dehydration, to monitor effectiveness of treatment)
   6. *Stool culture:* May isolate the causative agent.
      a. Should be limited to severely dehydrated or toxic patients, blood or pus in their stool, immunocompromised patients. and those with diarrhea lasting >3 days.
      b. Fecal fat and leukocytes
         i. Fecal fat (malabsorption syndrome)
         ii. Leukocytes (intestinal inflammation or invasive disease), such as infectious diarrhea from foods, travel, or ill contacts
      c. Consider testing for *Salmonella, Shigella, Campylobacter*, Shiga toxin–producing *E. coli, Entamoeba histolytica* antigen, *Giardia intestinalis,* and *Cryptosporidium parvum* or amoebic infection.
      d. Ova and parasites (patients with diarrhea >7 days, traveled abroad, or consumed untreated water, rule out giardia or cryptosporidium)

e. C. difficile *toxin:* Confirmation of disease, useful in ill patients with antibiotic-associated diarrhea or recent hospitalization.

i. Also can be confirmed by nucleic acid amplification or polymerase chain reaction (PCR) testing, enzyme immunoassay for *C. diff* antigen, or enzyme immunoassay for *C. diff* toxins A and B.

C. Imaging

1. Imaging typically unnecessary for patients with gastroenteritis unless concern for alternative diagnosis

2. *Chest x-ray (CXR)*: Reserved for ruling out intestinal obstruction, or pneumonia (particularly legionella), toxic megacolon, perforation.

3. CT scan or angiography may be useful if focal tenderness or acute mesenteric ischemia suspected to evaluate for other causes of illness.

a. PO +/- IV contrast if concern for perforation or abscess. If unable to tolerate PO, IV only.

4. Colonoscopy not needed for diagnosis *C. diff* or other forms of diarrhea.

Management

A. Dependent on etiology of diarrheal illness and in general consists of correcting fluid and electrolyte imbalances.

B. Initiate specific therapy for any life-threatening cause identified in the initial workup.

C. Ensure contact isolation, use of personal protective equipment, and appropriate hand hygiene with soap and water (alcohol-based rubs are ineffective with *C. diff*).

D. Treatment of moderately severe infectious diarrhea (including viral causes) includes antibiotics, antimotility agents, fluid resuscitation (oral or parenteral), and dietary modification (BRAT diet [banana, rice, applesauce, and toast]).

E. Provide supportive care.

F. Replace fluids and electrolytes.

1. Mildly dehydrated patient without vomiting may tolerate an oral rehydration solution (or coconut water) containing sodium as well as glucose to enhance fluid absorption.

2. IV hydration may be needed with extreme N/V diluting with severe dehydration, hypovolemic, or septic shock or if oral hydration has failed.

3. If needed, start IV fluids (IVF) (NS [normal saline] or LR [lactated Ringer's]) with boluses of 500 mL IV in adults and 20 mg/kg in children.

G. Start antidiarrheal agent.

1. Antidiarrheal agents, especially in combination with antibiotics, can shorten the course of diarrhea, especially in chronic disease.

a. Avoid antimotility agents in patients with bloody, suspected inflammatory, or infectious diarrhea and prolonged fever because of the potential for toxic megacolon, relapse in *C. diff* and hemolytic uremic syndrome in children with Shiga toxin–producing *E. coli.*

2. Bismuth subsalicylate reduces secretions, binds bacterial toxins, and possess antimicrobial effects.

3. Loperamide or atropine/diphenoxylate inhibits peristalsis.

H. Antiemetics (ondansetron or metoclopramide) as needed

1. Isopropyl alcohol pad held 2.5 cm from nose, twice, 2 minutes apart can provide some relief.

I. Antibiotic-associated diarrhea often responds to withdrawal of the offending drug (mild cases of *C. diff*), and is confirmation of organism and clinical monitoring.

J. Probiotics may help with management of gastroenteritis.

K. Consider starting an antibiotic.

1. Follow evidence-based guidelines when prescribing.

2. Recommended for adults with severe or prolonged diarrhea >72 hours or immunocompromised, but reserved for severe or invasive causes as it may prolong the carrier state.

3. Trimethoprim-sulfamethoxazole or a fluoroquinolone plus azithromycin are generally recommended for empiric treatment because they have been shown to shorten the duration of diarrhea in some cases. Recommended for children or nursing moms.

4. Ciprofloxacin shortens duration of illness by about 24 hours.

a. Avoid in cases of Shiga toxin–producing *E. coli.*

5. Metronidazole is recommended for the empiric or initial treatment of suspected *Giardia* or *C. diff.*

a. Add iodoquinol or paromomycin for *Entamoeba* infection.

6. Vancomycin PO is drug of choice for *C. diff* with severe persistent infection, or if outpatient treatment failed, IV vancomycin and admission may be needed.

7. If *Salmonella* is suspected, IV cefotaxime or alternative therapies, including chloramphenicol or fluoroquinolones.

8. If *Yersinia enterocolitica* is likely, IV gentamicin, especially in patients with persistent diarrhea or sepsis.

9. Allergic colitis requires dietary modifications.

Age and Developmental Considerations

A. Older adult patients are at very high risk for mortality, independent of causative organism, with 83% of deaths occurring in patients 65 years or older.

B. Parents should be educated on the effectiveness of rotavirus vaccinations, given at 2, 4, and 6 months of life.

C. Patients at high risk due to extremes of age, pregnancy, or immunosuppression often require specific therapy, aggressive workup to ensure resolution of symptoms, and prevention of hypovolemia or acute kidney injury.

D. Gastroenteritis frequently is seen in early childhood (rotaviruses), but mortality has risen in older patients (*C. diff* and norovirus infections).

E. Children <2 years of age are at increased risk of being asymptomatic carriers of *C. diff.*

Patient Disposition (Referrals, Follow-Up, and Education)

A. Disposition should be based on the patient's ability to maintain hydration at home, need for anti-inflammatory medications (autoimmune) and antibiotics (infectious).

B. Admit

1. Patients with hemodynamic instability or inability to tolerate oral liquids/foods, toxic or severely dehydrated patients, particularly older adults and infants

2. True diarrheal emergencies (GI bleed, adrenal insufficiency, thyroid storm, toxicologic exposures, acute radiation syndrome, and mesenteric ischemia) are of noninfectious origin requiring intensive treatment and hospitalization.

C. Most patients can be discharged home after treatment, even with unclear diagnosis but favorable examination.

D. Educate patients regarding the need for frequent hand washing to minimize transmission, oral hydration, and the BRAT diet, and avoiding raw fruit, caffeine, lactose, and sorbitol-containing products.

E. Provide work excuses for those employed in food, daycare, or healthcare industries.

F. Patients should be counseled about the proper selection of food and beverages consumed abroad, as well as water for drinking, brushing teeth, and preparation of food and formula.

G. If allergic colitis, eliminate offending protein from both mother's and infant's diet.

1. Surgical consultation may be indicated if concern for perforation, intestinal obstruction, fulminant colitis, significant GI bleeding, appendicitis, or toxic megacolon.

Nonspecific Nausea and Vomiting

Introduction of the Problem

A. Cyclic vomiting syndrome (CVS)

1. Recurrent, discrete, and stereotypical episodes of rapid-fire vomiting between varying periods of completely normal health first described in 1800s.

2. In children, the average age of diagnosis is 9.6 years with, the onset of symptoms at 5.3 years.

3. In adults, the average age of first symptom onset is 21 years, but most are not diagnosed until age 34.

4. Female > male, Caucasian

5. CVS is disabling (32%) for patients as they may have up to 10 ED visits per year, with over five ED visits before actual diagnosis, and 93% will not be diagnosed in the ED.

6. Diagnostic criteria for CVS

a. Pediatrics

i. *Rome IV diagnostic criteria* (both must be met): At least two periods of unremitting vomiting with or without retching, lasting hours to days within a 6-month period and a return to the usual state of health that lasts weeks to months

ii. *NASPGHAN criteria* (all must be met): At least five episodes, or a minimum of three over a 6-month period, of intense nausea and vomiting (N/V) lasting 1 hour to 10 days, occurring at least 1 week apart; stereotypical pattern and symptoms in the individual patient; vomiting during episodes occurs at least 4 times an hour for at least 1 hour, a return to baseline health during episodes; symptoms cannot be attributed to another disorder

b. Adults

i. *Rome III criteria:* Stereotypical episodes of vomiting regarding onset (acute) and duration (<1 week), a minimum of three discrete episodes in the preceding year, absence of N/V between episodes, and no metabolic, gastrointestinal (GI), or central nervous system (CNS) structural or biochemical disorders

ii. *Rome IV criteria:* Stereotypical episodes of vomiting regarding onset (acute) and duration (less than 1 week), three or more discrete episodes in the prior year and two episodes in the past 6 months, occurring at least 1 week apart; absence of vomiting between episodes, but other milder symptoms can be present between cycles; history or family history of migraine helps support diagnosis

7. Cannabis hyperemesis syndrome

a. Chronic marijuana use in large quantities, endures daily vomiting episodes, and has improvement of symptoms with bathing/showering using hot water

b. Differentiate CVS and cannabis hyperemesis; the patient must stop using marijuana for at least 1 week. If symptoms resolve, cannabis hyperemesis is likely.

B. Hyperemesis gravidarum

1. Morning sickness describes the mild or moderate disease, whereas hyperemesis gravidarum is the term to describe the severe end of the symptom spectrum.

2. Hyperemesis is a severe and intractable form of nausea and vomiting in pregnancy that does not respond to simple measures (dietary changes, reassurance) that affects 0.8% to 2.3% of pregnant women.

3. Peaks at 8 to 12 weeks of pregnancy, and symptoms usually resolve by week 20 in all but 10% of patients. If it begins after 9 weeks' gestation, other causes should be investigated.

4. Uncomplicated N/V of pregnancy are generally associated with a lower rate of miscarriage, but hyperemesis gravidarum may affect the health and well-being of both the pregnant woman and the fetus.

5. Diagnosis of exclusion. Condition may result in weight loss, nutritional deficiencies, abnormalities in fluids, electrolyte levels, and acid–base balance.

C. Gastroparesis

1. A symptom of objectively delayed gastric emptying in the absence of a mechanical obstruction. Type

I (4.6%) or type II (1.3%) diabetics can have complications associated with gastroparesis.

Pathophysiology of Nausea and Vomiting

A. Typically caused by GI tract (visceral afferent neurons) disorders, but must consider systemic causes as well. Neurologic, infectious, cardiac, endocrine, renal, obstetric, pharmacologic, toxicologic, and psychiatric disorders may all cause N/V.
B. Complex, highly coordinated process involving the GI tract, central and autonomic nervous system, and vestibular system
C. Associated with stimulation of gut receptors (usually by toxins) and stretch receptors involving serotonin, acetylcholine, and histamine.
D. Chemoreceptor trigger zone (CTZ) senses toxins in the blood and induces N/V before more toxin absorbed involving dopamine and serotonin.
E. Vestibular apparatus senses motion and body position (i.e., motion sickness) involving histamine and acetylcholine.
F. Cerebral cortex stimulates nausea associated with taste, sight, smell, memory, and emotion through unknown neurotransmitters.
G. Three stages of vomiting have been described: nausea, retching, and emesis.
   1. With nausea comes hypersalivation and tachycardia.
   2. Retching occurs with gastric relaxation and repetitive simultaneous contraction of the diaphragm and abdominal muscles.
   3. In response to changes in the intra-abdominal and intrathoracic pressure, emesis occurs, expelling gastric contents from the stomach.
H. Pathophysiology of CVS
   1. Several proposed brain–gut mechanisms associated with migraine headaches, sympathetic hyperresponsiveness, and autoimmune dysfunction, the stress response mediated by the hypothalamic–pituitary–adrenal axis, mutations in mitochondrial DNA (pediatrics), chronic cannabis use (CVS), gastroparesis, food sensitivities (like migraines), and estrogen sensitivity
I. Pathophysiology of hyperemesis gravidarum
   1. Hormonal changes, abnormal GI motility, *H. pylori*, genetic factors, nutrient deficiencies, alterations in lipid levels, changes in autonomic nervous system, immunologic dysregulation
J. Pathophysiology of gastroparesis
   1. Normal GI motor function is complex and requires coordination with the sympathetic and parasympathetic nervous systems, neurons, interstitial cells of Cajal within the stomach and intestines (pacemaker cells), and the smooth muscle in the gut and abnormalities can lead to a delay in gastric emptying.
   2. Causes
      a. Idiopathic (most common)
      b. Diabetic
         i. Type I > type II, more complications in patients >5 years
         ii. Abnormalities of the process of gastric emptying, including abnormal postprandial proximal gastric accommodation and contraction, reduced frequency of antral contractions, primarily due to autonomic dysfunction or abnormal intrinsic nervous system, possible role of oxidative stress
         iii. Hyperglycemia contributes to delayed gastric emptying.
      c. Viral
         i. Norwalk virus, rotavirus, Epstein-Barr virus (EBV), cytomegalovirus (CMV), varicella zoster virus (VZV)
         ii. May lead to severe dysautonomia or even selective cholinergic dysautonomia leading to persistent symptoms.
      d. Iatrogenic
         i. *Medications:* Narcotics, alpha-2 adrenergic agonist, tricyclic antidepressants, calcium channel blockers, dopamine agonists, muscarinic cholinergic receptor agonists, octreotide, glucagon-like peptides, phenothiazines, cyclosporine, immune checkpoint inhibitor therapy
      e. Postsurgical
         i. Previous gastric or thoracic surgery, esophageal variceal sclerotherapy, botulinum toxin injection, radiofrequency ablation resulting in gastric stasis due to intended or accidental injury to the vagus nerves, extrinsic vagal denervation, or loss of the antrum reduces the capacity of the stomach to empty nondigestible solid foods during fasting, resulting in bezoar formation and to triturate and only empty food postprandially.
      f. Neurologic
         i. Extrinsic neural control may be affected in cases of multiple sclerosis, brainstem stroke or tumor, parkinsonism, diabetic or amyloid neuropathy, or primary dysautonomia.
      g. Autoimmune disease
         i. Autoimmune GI dysmotility is a dysautonomia affecting the GI tract that occurs idiopathically or in association with an anatomically remote neoplasm, most commonly small cell lung cancer.
      h. *Other causes:* Mesenteric ischemia, scleroderma

Predisposing Factors for Nausea and Vomiting

A. Female gender, postpuberty, nonsmoker, history of postoperative N/V (PONV) or motion sickness, childhood after infancy and younger adults, increasing duration of illness, volatile anesthetic use, nitrous oxide, large dose neostigmine or intraoperative/postoperative opioids, history of migraines, intense anxiety, increased duration of analgesia, long-acting opioids, marijuana or other drug use, alcohol use, gastroparesis, diabetes
B. *For CVS:* Infection, sinusitis, psychological stress, foods (chocolate, cheese, monosodium glutamate [MSG]), physical exhaustion, lack of sleep, motion sickness, menses, marijuana use

C. *For hyperemesis gravidarum:* Hyperemesis in prior pregnancy, female gestation, multiple gestation, triploid, trisomy 21, current or prior molar pregnancy, hydrops fetalis, nausea with estrogen-based medications, underweight pregestational, hyperthyroidism, pyridoxine deficiency, GI disorders, nonuse of prenatal vitamins before 6 weeks' gestation or during preconception, gastroesophageal reflux disease (GERD)

D. *For gastroparesis:* Diabetes, multiple sclerosis, gastric or thoracic surgery, Parkinson's disease, autoimmune disease, viral illness

Medical Screening

A. A comprehensive history and physical (H&P) as well as the use of various diagnostics are needed to determine cause and complications.

B. *Chief complaint:* N/V, occasionally generalized crampy abdominal pain, early satiety, flatulence, and bloating (in gastroparesis)

C. High yield history

1. Predominant symptom is dependent on underlying cause.

2. Onset/duration, frequency and timing of episodes, content of the vomitus (undigested food, bile-tinged, feculent), age at onset of symptoms if chronic, triggers, improvement with hot showers, associated symptoms (fever, abdominal pain, and diarrhea), exposure to foodborne pathogens, sick contacts, surgical history

3. *Acute causes:* Gastroenteritis, postoperative, vestibular neuritis secondary to herpes simplex virus (HSV), chemotherapy, drugs

4. *Chronic causes:* Pregnancy, gastroparesis, gastroesophageal reflux, gastric outlet obstruction, CVS

5. *In CVS:*

a. Peak rate of emesis is usually 6 episodes per hour; in peds >4 episodes per hour is highly sensitive; episodes typically decline within 8 hours.

b. Begin early in a.m. upon waking, with a prodrome of N/V within an hour.

c. Nonbloody emesis, no biliary findings

d. Generalized abdominal pain described as crampy, improves between episodes although initially can be severe enough to mimic an "acute abdomen."

e. May have epigastric pain secondary to peptic injury of esophagus.

f. Unrelenting nausea, unrelieved by vomiting, disappears when asleep or episode is done. Fever, diarrhea, or both in one-third of patients.

g. *Behavioral symptoms:* Fetal positioning, social withdrawal, turning off lights/television

h. Lethargy and pallor are common (may appear comatose or unable to walk).

i. Excessive salivation and neurologic symptoms (headache, photophobia, phonophobia, vertigo) may be present.

6. *In hyperemesis gravidarum:* Symptoms typically start at 5 to 6 weeks' gestation, peak at 9 weeks, and subside by 16 to 20 weeks; prior history of hyperemesis.

7. *In gastroparesis:* Early satiety, belching, bloating and/or upper abdominal pain, weight loss in severe cases

D. General signs and symptoms

1. Hypotension, tachycardia, lethargy, poor skin turgor, dry mucous membranes, delayed capillary refill, extreme thirst, and abdominal pain suggest dehydration.

E. Past medical history (PMH)

1. Liver failure, alcohol use disorder, anorexia, benign paroxysmal positional vertigo, brain tumor, bulimia, depression, diabetes, GERD, heart failure, hepatitis, hiatal hernia, hyperparathyroidism, intussusception, irritable bowel syndrome, Meniere's disease, radiation therapy, pyloric stenosis, pseudotumor cerebri, peptic ulcer disease, pancreatitis, recent infection, migraines, medications patient is taking (side effects)

2. *For CVS:* History of cyclic vomiting, anxiety, postural orthostatic tachycardia syndrome (POTS), chronic marijuana use, migraines, gastroparesis

3. *For hyperemesis gravidarum:* Prior history of hyperemesis

4. *For gastroparesis:* Diabetes, gastric or thoracic surgery, multiple sclerosis, Parkinson's disease, medication use, autoimmune disease, viral illness

Physical Examination

A. General

1. Examination findings are often nonspecific. Generalized weakness (chronic malnutrition), weight loss (malignancy), night sweats, toxic appearing, tachycardia, hypotension, lethargy, poor skin turgor, dry mucous membranes (dehydration)

2. Patients with CVS and gastroparesis may be in moderate distress.

3. *Red flag features:* GI bleeding, unilateral abdominal pain, bilious vomiting, weight loss (if severe), metabolic abnormalities, neurologic changes, gait disturbance

B. Vital signs

1. Fever likely indicates another process (infection, appendicitis, gastroenteritis, cholecystitis).

2. Tachycardia, hypotension, postural hypotension (bowel perforation, peritonitis, dehydration), hypertension (intracranial hemorrhage, stroke)

C. Skin

1. Scarring on dorsal surface of the hands from purging (bulimia)

2. Jaundice (hepatobiliary disease, hepatitis, choledocholithiasis, liver failure), poor skin turgor (dehydration), hyperpigmentation (Addison disease), decreased elasticity (scleroderma), track marks (drug abuse/withdrawal)

3. Taut skin in the hands, chest telangiectasia, small joint arthropathy in systemic sclerosis and Raynaud's phenomenon (in gastroparesis)

D. Head, eyes, ears, nose, throat (HEENT)

1. Nystagmus (peripheral vs. central cause), exophthalmos, goiter (thyroid disease), pinpoint pupils (opioid abuse), fixed-dilated pupils (glaucoma), dry mucous membranes (dehydration), poor dental enamel (bulimia), parotid gland enlargement, and lymphadenopathy may indicate another disease process as cause.

2. Absence of pupillary reaction to light with persistence of the accommodation response (tonic pupil) can be present in gastroparesis.

E. Pulmonary

1. Typically, normal but can have increased respiratory rate (RR) or shallow respirations.

2. If autoimmune incompetent, may have crackles in the lower lung fields.

F. Abdominal

1. Possible generalized or epigastric tenderness, but if localized tenderness, should raise suspicion for other cause.

2. Assess for distention, decreased bowel sound (BS) (small bowel obstruction [SBO], gastroparesis, gastric outlet obstruction, ileus), surgical scars, hernias (incarceration or strangulation) or palpable masses (tumor), and abdominal rigidity (peritonitis).

G. Neurological

1. Altered mental status, lethargy (dehydration, sepsis), CN findings or neurologic deficits (intracranial lesion), papilledema (elevated ICP)

Differential Diagnoses

A. Vomiting with blood (bright red in color or coffee-grounds emesis) could represent gastritis, peptic ulcer disease, or carcinoma.

B. Aggressive nonbloody vomiting followed by hematemesis is more consistent with Mallory-Weiss tear.

C. Vomiting bile rules out gastric outlet obstruction from pyloric stenosis or strictures.

D. The presence of abdominal distention, surgical scars, or an incarcerated hernia suggest a SBO.

E. The presence of fever suggests an infectious or inflammatory cause such as gastroenteritis, appendicitis, or cholecystitis.

F. Vomiting with chest pain suggests a myocardial infarction. Post-tussive vomiting suggests pneumonia.

G. Vomiting with back or flank pain can be seen with aortic aneurysm or dissection, pancreatitis, pyelonephritis, or renal colic.

H. Headache with vomiting suggests increased intracranial pressure (ICP), such as with subarachnoid hemorrhage (SAH), tumor, migraine, or head injury.

I. The presence of vertigo and nystagmus suggest vestibular or CNS cause.

J. Vomiting in a pregnant patient is consistent with hyperemesis gravidarum in the first trimester, but in the third trimester can represent preeclampsia if accompanied by hypertension and severe headache.

K. *Associated medical conditions:* Diabetes mellitus suggests diabetic ketoacidosis (DKA) or gastroparesis; peripheral vascular disease suggests mesenteric ischemia; and medication use or overdose (lithium, digoxin) suggests toxicity.

L. *Other differential diagnoses:* Pyelonephritis, molar pregnancy, pseudotumor cerebri, acute fatty liver of pregnancy, appendicitis, cholecystitis and biliary colic, urinary tract infection (UTI), cystitis (bladder infection), DKA, pancreatitis, gastroenteritis, ovarian torsion, peptic ulcer disease, pregnancy, preeclampsia, SBO, mechanical obstruction, viral hepatitis, psychiatric disease (depression, anxiety, bulimia, anorexia), rumination syndrome, functional dyspepsia, CVS, cholecystitis or cholangitis, gastritis, gastroenteritis, DKA, medication side effect

Diagnostic Testing

A. Indicated with persistent N/V to determine severity of disease, assess volume/metabolic status, or identify/exclude other cause of symptoms.

B. *Alarm signs absent* (no abnormal labs, imaging, or response to trial of prophylactic therapy): Only need limited screening to exclude other conditions

C. *Alarm signs present* (acute onset unilateral/flank pain, metabolic warning signs, neurologic signs, upper GI bleeding, concern for Mallory-Weiss tear, prolapse gastropathy, or upper GI symptoms between episodes): Needs further investigation

D. Labs

1. All women of childbearing age warrant a pregnancy test.
2. No diagnostic markers for CVS; lab tests are typically normal but can see mild metabolic acidosis, hypoglycemia, and ketosis.
3. Hemoglobin a1c if diabetic
4. ANA titer if concern for autoimmune disease (can be done outpatient)
5. Complete blood count (CBC) to look for leukocytosis, anemia if bleeding, or hemoconcentration of hematocrit due to volume depletion
   a. White blood cells (WBC) may be higher in pregnant patient with hyperemesis.
6. CMP
   a. If severe dehydration and prolonged vomiting, suspect electrolyte imbalance. Test can confirm Addison crisis (hyperkalemia and hyponatremia) and help rule out other conditions.
   b. Hypoglycemia, hypokalemia, hypochloremia metabolic alkalosis, ketosis, hypomagnesemia, hypocalcemia (marked dietary deprivation)
7. Liver function tests (LFTs), lipase
   a. Increased in 50% of patients with hyperemesis (ALT>AST)
   b. If concerned for pancreatitis or hepatitis
      i. Lipase elevated in 10% to 15% of patients with hyperemesis, as much as five to tenfold in patients with pancreatitis.
8. Urinalysis (UA) may reveal ketones suggesting dehydration or DKA; nitrates, leukocyte esterase, bacteria, or WBCs may suggest urinary tract infection (UTI); red blood cells (RBCs) may suggest a kidney stone or cystitis.
9. Drug levels for acetaminophen, salicylates, digoxin when toxicity suspected, urine and serum toxicology when ethanol or illicit drug use suspected
10. Lactate if suspicion of ischemia, sepsis, or severe acidosis
11. Thyroid studies

a. High serum concentrations of human chorionic gonadotropin (hCG) can have thyroid-stimulating activity.
b. T3/T4 level if concern for hyperthyroidism. Thyroid-stimulating hormone (TSH) can be suppressed in hyperemesis gravidarum.
12. If concerned for possible inborn error of metabolism in children or metabolic disorders associated with presentation <2 years, vomiting with other illness/fasting/increased protein intake, neurologic findings
a. Venous blood gas (VBG), ammonia, amino acids, ketones, lactate

E. EKG and chest x-ray (CXR) can be reserved for patients with suspected cardiac ischemia or pulmonary infection

F. Imaging
1. If the patient is having a "typical" exacerbation of chronic condition without other red flags, imaging may be deferred.
2. Abdominal XR can be used to confirm the presence of an obstruction.
3. RUQ ultrasound if localized pain or concern for gallbladder disease
4. RLQ ultrasound if localized pain or concern for appendicitis
5. Pelvic or transvaginal ultrasound if concern for molar pregnancy, ectopic pregnancy, or multiple gestations
6. Fetal heart tones with a handheld device or by ultrasound to confirm viability of pregnancy and gestational age
7. CT scan of the abdomen with IV +/- PO contrast (if able to tolerate PO) to reveal evidence of or the location of a mechanical obstruction in patients without prior diagnosis of CVS or gastroparesis with abdominal pain may clarify alternative explanations for the patient's symptoms.
a. If symptoms are "typical" for patient or in patients with hyperemesis, CT can be deferred.
8. CT of the brain if CNS lesion is suspected.
9. Measuring intraocular pressure is useful if glaucoma suspected.
10. Upper GI series to the ligament of Treitz should be performed in all children with CVS to exclude intestinal malrotation or nonfixation with possible intermittent volvulus.
11. *Upper GI endoscopy:* Can assess gastric motility in patients with persistent symptoms and no evidence of mechanical obstruction.
12. Scintigraphy gastric emptying study as outpatient

Management

A. Initiate specific therapy for any life-threatening cause identified in initial workup.

B. Follow evidence-based guidelines when prescribing.

C. Correct any fluid and electrolyte problems.
1. Hypokalemia, dehydration, and metabolic alkalosis common
2. Continue treatment until little or no ketones in urine or patient can tolerate PO.

D. Start nutritional supplementation orally as soon as symptoms subside. Consider adding glucose, multivitamins, magnesium, pyridoxine, folate, and thiamine as needed.
1. Susceptible to deficiencies of iron, vitamin B12, fat-soluble vitamins, thiamine (prior to dextrose), and folate

E. Resuscitation of seriously ill patients requires IV boluses of normal saline (NS) 20 kg/mL, repeated as needed to target euvolemia.
1. Caution should be used in older adults and those with compromised left ventricular function (LVF).

F. Mildly dehydrated patients may tolerate oral rehydration solutions (ORS) containing sodium as well as glucose to enhance fluid absorption.
1. Quickly advance from clear liquids to solids, such as rice and bread.

G. Optimize glycemic control in patients with diabetes or gastroparesis.

H. NSAIDs for pain unless GI bleed suspected. Narcotics as indicated

I. Antiemetic agents in actively vomiting patients with dehydration
1. The combination of doxylamine and pyridoxine should be considered first-line therapy in hyperemesis gravidarum.
2. Pyridoxine alone (vitamin B6) can improve nausea, has a good safety profile, and has minimal side effects.
3. Serotonin antagonist
a. Ondansetron, dolasteron, granisetron
b. Can cause headaches, especially if it is not used properly.
c. Ondansetron with a benzodiazepine or diphenhydramine works better than ondansetron alone in patients with CVS.
d. Use of ondansetron in pregnancy is controversial secondary to small risk of cardiovascular abnormalities; use alternative measures before 10 weeks of pregnancy.
4. Phenothiazines in patients with vertigo, motion sickness, postoperative vomiting, chemotherapy
a. Promethazine, prochlorperazine
b. Can cause sedation, orthostatic hypotension, extrapyramidal symptoms. Can assist with GI motility.
5. Benzamides
a. Metoclopramide (dopamine 2 receptor antagonist, 5-HT4 agonist and weak 5-HT4 antagonist)
b. First-line therapy in gastroparesis due to antiemetic and prokinetic effects, assists in gastric motility, improves gastric emptying by enhancing gastric antral contractions and decreasing postprandial fundus relaxation.
c. Adverse effects include fatigue, extrapyramidal symptoms, hyperprolactinemia, anxiety, restlessness, dystonia, parkinsonian reactions, and prolonged QT interval.
6. Macrolide antibiotics (gastroparesis, delayed gastric emptying)

a. Erythromycin or azithromycin, which are motilin agonists, that produce high-amplitude gastric propulsive contractions increasing gastric emptying, stimulate fundic contractility, or inhibits the accommodation response of the proximal stomach after food ingestion.

7. Antihistamines

a. Meclizine

b. Benadryl can block histamine receptors in patients with vertigo, motion sickness, and migraines, but are associated with drowsiness, hypotension, and urinary retention.

c. Butyrophenones (chemotherapy-related vomiting, postoperative vomiting, and CVS)

d. Haldol, droperidol blocks dopamine effects but can prolong QT interval, movement disorders, sedation, and hypotension

8. *Cannabinoids* (dronabinol; chemotherapy related): Sedation, tachycardia, confusion, and euphoria are common

9. *Anticholinergics:* Scopolamine blocks histamine, acetylcholine, and serotonin activity, but can cause drowsiness, blurred vision, and hypotension.

10. Others

a. Triptans (CVS), (sumatriptan) with recurrent episodes (migraine)

b. Dexamethasone (severe or refractory cases) should be last resort in pregnancy.

c. Benzodiazepines (anxiety associated with N/V)

i. Work through GABA receptors agonism, thus neurotransmitter inhibition, causing sedation, anxiolysis, and muscle relaxation.

d. Tricyclic antidepressants, zonisamide, cyproheptadine, levetiracetam, coenzyme Q10, propranolol, phenobarbital, and erythromycin have shown some success in intractable cases of CVS.

e. *Antihypertensives:* Most do not require therapy as blood pressure (BP) resolves with pain relief. With persistently high BP, small doses of short-acting medications can be used.

f. Capsaicin cream or haloperidol (D2 receptor antagonist) in cannabis-associated CVS

i. No randomized or controlled studies performed, but IM haloperidol can assist with a reduction in opioids and anxiety.

g. Prokinetic agents (gastroparesis, GERD) such as erythromycin, bethanechol

h. Ginger, acupuncture, acupressure, hypnosis, marijuana use, and psychotherapy may also be helpful.

i. In refractory cases, chlorpromazine, tube feeding, NGT to decompress stomach, parenteral nutrition, or surgery may be needed.

11. Domperidone and cisapride

a. In patients with gastroparesis who do not respond to metoclopramide. Only prescribed through Food and Drug Administration (FDA) approval of investigational drug secondary to increased risk of cardiac arrythmias.

b. Cisapride stimulates antral and duodenal motility and accelerates gastric emptying.

Age and Developmental Considerations

A. Pediatrics

1. In children and adolescents with CVS, pattern of vomiting episodes is variable, but usually stereotypical to patient, beginning in early morning (2 a.m.–7 a.m.), last the same duration, and can last anywhere from 24 to 48 hours to 10 days.

2. CVS in children has a prodromal period of pallor, anorexia, nausea, abdominal pain, and/or lethargy and usually associated with psychological stress or infectious events.

3. With CVS, recurring vomiting is often accompanied by conditions including anxiety, POTS, and coalescent CVS.

B. Pregnancy

1. If preexisting diabetes, beware of hypoglycemic crisis, especially after taking insulin.

a. Prescribe glucose tablets, juice, or other glucose-containing liquids, and adjust insulin as needed.

Patient Disposition (Referrals, Follow-Up, and Education)

A. Life-threatening causes of vomiting, toxic or severely dehydrated patients, especially infants and older adults, or those still intolerant of oral fluids following hydration warrant admission.

B. Patients with an unclear diagnosis, but favorable examination findings following hydration, can be discharged home safely with antiemetics.

C. Work excuses are indicated for patients in the food, day-care, and healthcare industries.

D. If anxiety plays a role, cognitive behavioral therapy plus anxiolytic agents.

E. Dietary considerations

1. Meals and snacks

a. Should eat before or as soon as they feel hungry to avoid empty stomach, including snacks before getting out of bed or during the night in hyperemesis.

b. Eat meals slowly and in small amounts; frequent, small, carbohydrate-predominate meals/snacks, protein-rich foods

c. If symptoms are related to delayed gastric emptying, low-fat solids are recommended.

d. Avoid foods such as raw fruit, caffeine, lactose, and sorbitol-containing products; fatty, acidic, spicy, or roughage-based food; carbonated beverages; alcohol; and smoking.

2. Fluids

a. Consume 30 minutes prior to or after solid food to minimize effect of full stomach.

b. Cold, clear, and carbonated or sour fluids in small amounts are better tolerated. Lemon, ginger or mint tea, electrolyte replacement drinks if tolerated

F. Trigger avoidance

1. *CVS:* Patients usually know their causes (diet, drugs, psychological).

a. Sleep deprivation, infection, cannabis (counsel for decreased use). Avoid fasting or long-acting caloric snacks. Avoid chocolate, cheese, cow's milk.

b. In children, excessive excitement, such as birthdays, holidays, vacations, school outings, appear to trigger CVS more often than negative stress.

2. Hyperemesis

a. Avoid stuffy rooms, odors, heat, humidity, noise, visual or physical motion, lying down too soon after eating and lying on left side (delays gastric emptying), iron-containing supplements (gastric irritation).

b. Cold, solid foods better tolerated (less prep time and odors)

c. Frequently brushing teeth or washing out mouth can be helpful unless mint toothpaste aversion.

Additional Reading

Additional Reading for this chapter are online only and can be found at https://connect.springerpub.com/content/reference-book/978-0-8261-6091-5/part/part02/toc-part/ch17.

18. Renal, Genitourinary, and Reproductive Conditions

TRACY BROWN | TRACIE GADLER

Learning Objectives

- Identify and treat genitourinary emergencies in either male or female patients.
- Identify genitourinary emergencies in male or female patients requiring specialist involvement and consult or refer when appropriate.
- Identify and treat reproductive system and breast emergencies.
- Identify reproductive system or breast emergencies requiring specialist involvement and consult or refer when appropriate.
- Identify and begin treatment of renal failure.
- Evaluate and treat complications associated with chronic renal failure treatments.

RENAL, GENITOURINARY, AND REPRODUCTIVE CONDITIONS

Renal emergencies discussed in this chapter focus on acute renal failure and the emergencies associated with chronic renal failure treatment. While a clinician's institution may not provide dialysis care, this does not mean emergencies associated with specific types of dialysis will not present to the given institution. Treatment of genitourinary and reproductive emergencies is based on the sex of the individual patient. Male and female genitourinary systems are the same regarding the internal organs of the system. Similarities end there; treatment is thus individualized to the sex of the patient despite the emergency. Reproductive system emergencies and treatments of both sexes are discussed.

Acute Renal Failure

Medical Screening

A. *Signs and symptoms*[1, 2]
   1. Range as widely as the causes of the injury/failure of the kidney. Focus is on identification of cause based on the signs and symptoms of the diagnosis being seen. Identification of injury/failure occurs during the identification of the causative diagnosis.

B. *Focused assessment*
   1. The focused assessment for the patient is based on the causative diagnosis.

Diagnostic Testing

A. *Labs*
   1. Complete blood count (CBC)
   2. Chemistry
   3. Qualitative b-hCG
   4. Urinalysis (UA)
   5. Urine culture
   6. Urine electrolytes

B. *Imaging*
   1. CT renal
   2. CT abdominal/pelvis with and/or without contrast pending suspected diagnosis
   3. Ultrasound (US) renal
   4. EKG

Medical Decision-Making, Differential Diagnoses, and Treatment

A. *Prerenal causes*
   1. *Volume depletion:* Vomiting and diarrhea, diuretic use, hemorrhage, and shock
   2. *Decreased cardiac output causes:* Myocardial infarction, cardiomyopathy, and pericardial tamponade
   3. *Renal artery and small vessel causes:* Sepsis, transplant rejection, and sickle cell crises

B. *Post-renal causes*
   1. Urethral and bladder outlet blockages
   2. Ureteral atresia, phimosis, ureterocele, and meatal stenosis
   3. *Ureteral obstructions:* Stone, clot
   4. Neurogenic bladder

C. *Intrarenal causes seen in ED*
   1. *Tubulointerstitial disease:* Overdose of heavy metal toxins, ethylene glycol
   2. Acute tubular necrosis
      a. Volume loss, shock, sepsis
      b. Nephrotoxins, contrast dye, antibiotics
      c. *Endogenous pigments:* Myoglobinurea (seen in rhabdomyolysis from multiple causes)
   3. Other causes include severe liver disease, allergic reactions, NSAID use, HIV.

D. *Peritoneal dialysis complications (PDC), ambulatory or cycling*
   1. Superficial skin infections at the catheter exit site need to be taken seriously. Normal skin flora is usually the cause of the infection. Exit site infections,

however, can progress to tunnel infections. Tunnel infections can be tricky in diagnosing. Patients may not get diagnosed until they have had several peritoneal infections found to be for the same bacteria.[3]

2. Hernias
   a. Because of increased peritoneal pressures from the dialysis process, patients are at greater risk of developing hernias. Development is usually seen at sites of prior abdominal surgeries.
3. Peritonitis
   a. *Primary:* Infection directly associated with the intraabdominal dialysis catheter. On occasion, bacteria can contaminate the fluid and thus the peritoneum. This infectious process is not as severe as peritonitis from other causes. The patient is usually able to make the diagnosis based on the appearance of the dialysate. These cases are often handled outpatient. An initial loading antibiotic dose is put through the catheter with a follow-up 10 days' to 2 weeks' course of antibiotics via the same route. ED presentation of this type of peritonitis may be a result of failed antibiotic therapy. Specialist consultation is necessary for antibiotic recommendations since there is no one best regimen. Need for catheter removal is determined by the specialist.[4,5]
   b. *Secondary:* A result of infection associated with normal causes not associated with the dialysis (e.g., cholecystitis, pancreatitis, appendicitis, and diverticulitis). Treat the cause of the infection. Consultation with specialist to aid in ongoing dialysis is necessary.
4. Misleading findings in evaluating a PDC patient
   a. Abdominal imaging may identify pneumoperitoneum. This finding, however, may simply be a result of a fluid exchange that had air involvement.[6]
   b. Gross blood identified in dialysate in female patients can be seen during menstruation as a result of retrograde menstruation.

E. *Emergent hemodialysis*
1. Criteria for emergent dialysis[7]
   a. Hyperkalemia above 6.5 mmol/L or an elevating K with EKG changes
   b. Sodium changes <115 or >165 mEq/L
   c. Fluid overload not responding to therapy with ongoing hypoxia
   d. Uremic pericarditis
   e. Encephalopathy, asterixis, or seizure activity associated with worsening uremia/metabolic changes
   f. Severe metabolic acidosis with acute kidney injury (AKI) (source of acidosis must be treated)
   g. Potentially lethal poisonings (salicylate, methanol, ethylene glycol, isopropanol, lithium)
   h. Bleeding dyscrasias that are a result of uremia
   i. Extremely elevated blood urea nitrogen (BUN) or creatinine levels (no absolute parameters—should be patient-specific)
2. Diagnostic testing considerations[7]
   a. Glomerular filtration rate (GFR) must be calculated using a steady-state creatinine level, thus value not very useful in ED setting.
   b. Urine output for AKI requires 6 hours of observation with urinary catheter placement, which is not helpful in the ED.
   c. BUN/creatinine ration is not helpful with AKI diagnosis that resolves with fluid resuscitation. This type of AKI is commonly seen in the ED.
   d. Renal US is the imaging of choice for identifying obstruction-related injury. 90% specificity and sensitivity noted for hydronephrosis.
3. Treatment algorithms for determining emergent versus urgent hyperkalemia
   a. Most facilities have a specific step-by-step plan for treating hyperkalemia. The most current data breaks down the correction process into emergent reduction, urgent reduction, and slow reduction over time.[8]
   b. *Emergent reduction:* Treatment therapies such as IV calcium, insulin, and glucose in combination with dialysis, diuretics, and gastrointestinal (GI) exchangers
      1. *Any of the following:* K over 6.5 meq/L, EKG changes, muscle weakness, or paralysis
      2. *Have all of the following:* K over 5.5 meq/L, significant impaired renal status including end stage renal disease (ESRD), and ongoing tissue breakdown seen with tissue injuries or ongoing absorption of K seen with GI bleeding.
   c. *Urgent reduction:* Reduction should be within 6 to 12 hours. Treatment therapies include dialysis treatment for ESRD patients, reversing the cause of the hyperkalemia by employing bicarbonate therapy, diuretics, and GI exchangers.
      1. K over 5.5 meq/L and dx of ESRD or current oliguria
      2. Patient needs quick correction prior to surgical intervention.
   d. *Slow replacement over time:* Treatment therapies include dietary changes, medication adjustments and discontinuations, diuretics, bicarbonate therapy, and GI exchangers.
      1. K over 5.5 meq/L without significant renal impairment
4. Types of accesses used for hemodialysis
   a. *Arteriovenous (AV) fistula*: Preferred type for dialysis, must mature over time—at least 6 months.[9] Good long-term patency, low infection rates
   b. *AV graft*: A graft placed between the artery and vein. Most common product used for this is polytetrafluoroethylene (PTFE), especially when patient doesn't have good vasculature to support a fistula. Can be used as soon as 2 weeks after placement; 3 to 6 weeks is noted in guidelines. There is an increased risk in thrombosis and infections.
   c. Tunneled hemodialysis catheters can be used immediately and are a type of central access

usually used short term. May be used long term when all AV access sites have been exhausted or AV access is contraindicated in the patient.

d. Patient education review in AV fistulas and grafts[9]

1. Routine checking for ongoing thrill
2. No blood draws in extremity with site
3. No blood pressure checks in extremity with site
4. No carrying anything over 5 pounds in arm with site
5. No tight clothing should be worn over area
6. No sleeping on the area with site

e. *Dermal flare:* Erythematous-appearing skin without induration, isolated to skin overlying a newly placed graft. Will not spread like with cellulitis.[10]

5. Step-by-step approach to fistula/graft evaluation[10]

a. *Inspection of graft:* Evaluate region just over the graft for typical skin appearance changes (erythema, swelling, induration, fluctuance, pustules), constriction, and bulging (evidence of pseudoaneurysm), and changes in skin over bulging areas to look for thinned skin.

b. *Extremity:* Evaluation of skin color changes (compare to other side), size of entire extremity up into chest for swelling (suggesting venous outflow obstruction)

c. *Palpation:*

i. Tissue should be soft overlying site, slightly warmer in relation to the surrounding tissue.

ii. Overused areas of cannulization can be felt—lack of graft material is left and the sides of graft are felt (called railroad track deformity).

iii. Pulse evaluation best done with fingers

(1) Palpate entire length of graft

(2) Pulse is mild

(3) Pulse with an AV site is more prominent—graft material is not palpable

iv. Arterial flow evaluation

(1) Occlude outflow vein a few centimeters (cm) from the arterial anastomosis

(2) Pulse between the two will become more prominent

(3) The change (known as pulse augmentation) is directly related to the quality of arterial flow

v. Thrill palpation—sensation over AV site

(1) Use palm of hand

(2) Two components—systolic and diastolic

d. *Auscultation:* Either by stethoscope or with handheld Doppler to evaluate bruit (sound of the thrill). With very low flow Doppler, extremely low flow from occlusion can be identified.

6. Specific graft problem evaluation[10]

a. Any of the stenotic problems noted in the following, if identifiable on exam are severe enough to warrant diagnostic evaluation. Ultrasound better identifies the problem and thus may be used for initial evaluation. The gold standard is angiography; it is used in preparation for treatment of the problem.

b. *Stenotic vascular lesion:* Most common complication. Not easily seen since patient usually develops a thrombus before urine flow drops during dialysis. No intervention for the ED clinician.

c. *Venous outflow stenosis:* Noted with a hyperpulsatility because of increased pressure downstream from the graft. An audible increase in bruit pitch can be heard that progresses to the point of a whistle. Most severe outflow stenosis cases will see the absence of the thrill and bruit. No intervention for ED clinician.

d. *Arterial stenosis:* Results from a stenosis prior to inflow into the AV site. Examination identifies a reduced pulse in the site.

e. *Central vein stenosis:* Examination identifies diffuse upper extremity edema. Sometimes very severe, along with prominent visible subcutaneous vasculature in both upper extremities and on the anterior chest.

f. *Thrombosed graft:* The only unique exam finding is the absence of any bruit.

g. *Infected graft:* Infections can be either superficial or deep in nature. Superficial infections are usually related to prior sites of cannulation. With deep infections, the exam findings will include erythema, swelling, areas of induration or fluctuance, and pain. Abnormalities such as perigraft hematomas, abscesses, or aneurysms may be seen with a deep infection.

h. *Pseudoaneurysms:* A result of a defect in the graft along with a pressure change through the graft. Examination findings include bulging in a localized area. New pseudoaneurysms need emergent evaluation to prevent any additional enlargement. Spontaneous bleeding or severe thinning of skin over the site are grounds for emergent surgical intervention. The specialty uses the "pinch test" to evaluate the thinness of the tissue. If the skin can't be pinched over the site, rupture is of high concern.

i. *Extremity ischemia:* Caused by AV graft placements. There are two prominent types. Dialysis access steal syndrome (DASS) is ischemia of the hand. DASS is seen more often with AV fistula versus a graft. Development of DASS is immediately following the graft placement. Exam findings range in relationship to the severity of the problem. Evaluation with opposite extremity is most effective. Expect pale to cyanotic skin color in the hand, with diminished to absent radial pulse. The other ischemic problem is ischemic monomelic neuropathy (IMN), associated with the use of the brachial artery for AV site. This problem is seen most often with diabetics. The problem is as the name implies, a neuropathy involving all three forearm nerves: ulnar, radial, and medial. The examination findings involve weakness and altered sensation in the three distributions. Each distribution deficit may vary in severity, but all are involved and required to make the diagnosis.

MALE GENITOURINARY AND REPRODUCTION CONDITIONS

Internal Genitourinary System

Complicated Cystitis and Pyelonephritis in Adults

Complicated cystitis is defined as a lower urinary tract infection (UTI) in patients with concomitant medical conditions which predispose them to bacterial colonization and reduced treatment efficacy. These conditions include anatomic abnormalities of the urinary tract, urinary tract dysfunction, drug resistance, and immunosuppression.[11] Patients will have evidence of pyuria (white blood cell [WBC] >10) with symptomology clinically supporting an UTI.[12]

Pyelonephritis is an upper UTI. Patients with pyelonephritis demonstrate with symptoms of a lower UTI with the addition of flank pain, costovertebral angle (CVA) tenderness, and may or may not have associated fever, nausea, and vomiting.[13]

Medical Screening

A. *Chief complaint:* Dysuria

B. *Signs and symptoms*

1. Urinary burning
2. Dysuria
3. Urinary frequency
4. Suprapubic pain, pressure
5. Occasionally hematuria, cloudy or malodorous urine

C. *Focused assessment*

1. Abdominal assessment
2. Focused suprapubic palpation and CVA tenderness

Diagnostic Testing

A. *Urinalysis and culture and sensitivity*

Medical Decision-Making and Differential Diagnoses

See Uncomplicated Cystitis section of this chapter. Differential diagnoses include sexually transmitted infection, nephrolithiasis or bladder calculi, overactive bladder, trauma, prostatitis, and neoplasm.[11] Parental verses oral antibiotic course is based on the degree of illness (e.g., toxic appearance) and ability to tolerate oral medications. If a previous culture with sensitivities exists, clinicians should use these results to direct initial antimicrobial management. Infections isolated to the bladder should not produce CVA tenderness on palpation, as this is indicative of an upper UTI such as pyelonephritis. Special consideration should be used in patients with chronic indwelling catheterization; these patients tend to be colonized with microbes, and antibiotic treatment should be limited to those with associated symptoms (hematuria, fever, suprapubic pressure, malaise, and altered mental status), as all will have evidence of pyuria. The prevalence of bacteria after 30 days of catheter use is 100%.[14] Patients who are unable to tolerate oral medications, or those toxic-appearing, warrant hospital admission.

Management

A. Collect midstream clean catch urine, or straight catheterization or sterile urine specimen from urinary catheter port

B. *Pharmacologic therapies:* Antimicrobial treatment should be determined by local resistance patterns, insurance coverage, allergies, and tolerability. Follow evidence-based guidelines when prescribing.

1. Antibiotics[11,13]
   - a. Ciprofloxacin
   - b. Levofloxacin
   - c. Cefpodoxime
   - d. Alternative treatment, initiate parenteral therapy
     - i. Ciprofloxacin
     - ii. Ceftriaxone
     - iii. Gentamicin or tobramycin
     - iv. Piperacillin-tazobactam
   - e. Only if susceptibilities are known, consider:
     - i. Trimethoprim-sulfamethoxazole DS (not enterococcus or pseudomonas)
     - ii. Amoxicillin-clavulanate
2. Analgesics and antipyretic
   - a. Pyridium
   - b. Tylenol or NSAIDs for fever

Patient Disposition

A. *Consultation/collaboration*

1. Unresponsive to appropriate antibiotic therapy (per culture and sensitivities) after 48 to 72 hours warrants further imaging of the urinary tract.
   - a. Ultrasound (US) or CT scan
   - b. Evaluate for structural abnormalities, abscess, or presence of stones.[12]
2. Complications of pyelonephritis can lead to septic shock, renal or perinephric abscess, urinary tract obstruction, or emphysematous pyelonephritis.[15]
3. Transition of care information
   - a. Consider urologic referral for patients with recurrent infections or those that anatomic abnormality cannot be ruled out.

Age and Developmental Considerations

Please see UTI in pregnancy and pediatric populations, Chapters 52 and 53.

A. *Prevention and education*

1. Practice postcoital urination.
2. Proper perineal skin hygiene
3. Females should be reminded to wipe front to back.
4. Avoid spermicides.

B. *Patient and family education and counseling*
1. Increase hydration.
2. Return for symptoms not improving within 48 hours.
3. Pyridium stains the urine orange.

Hematuria

Asymptomatic microhematuria (AMH) is the evidence of blood, via microscopy or laboratory confirmation, that is not visible to the eye. Specifically, ≥3 red blood cells (RBC) per high-powered field.[16] Macroscopic or gross hematuria is defined as the ability to visibly recognize blood within the urine without microscopy.

Medical Screening

A. *Chief complaint:* Hematuria
B. *Signs and symptoms*
1. Gross blood in the urine (macroscopic)
2. Blood noted via microscopy but not visible (microscopic)
C. *Focused assessment*
1. Genitourinary and renal system
a. Palpate bladder for pain, masses, distention
b. Palpate for costovertebral angle (CVA) tenderness
c. Evaluate urinary meatus for evidence of blood, lesions, or trauma.

Diagnostic Testing

A. UA evaluating for infection and hematuria
B. Consider imaging if no obvious urinary infection.
1. Evaluate for renal calculi or urogenital neoplasms in at-risk individuals.

Medical Decision-Making and Differential Diagnoses

Known causes of microscopic hematuria include conditions such as glomerular disease, menstruation, or urinary tract infections, or those patients who exercise in excess.[16] Patients who demonstrate with gross hematuria that is painless have a higher likelihood of urinary tract neoplasm, vascular or hyperplastic cause.[13] A thorough history evaluates for any signs and symptoms associated with infection or renal or bladder calculi, and recent urogenital instrumentation, procedures, or sexual behaviors that may cause trauma and result in hematuria. Other differentials include benign prostatic hyperplasia (BPH), glomerulonephritis, pyelonephritis, radiation cystitis, hydronephrosis, vascular disease, hematologic disease, anticoagulation therapy, medications, congenital and idiopathic causes.[17]

Management

A. *Procedures:* Midstream clean catch urine, or straight catheterization, or sterile urine specimen from urinary catheter port
B. *Pharmacologic therapies:* Depends on underlying cause

Patient Disposition

A. *Consultation/collaboration*
1. Urologic referral
a. Patients with gross hematuria without benign disease
b. Recommended[18]
i. Patients at increased risk for bladder neoplasm
(1) Over the age of 40
(2) History of smoking/chemical exposure
(3) Have nonglomerular hematuria
ii. Patients with microscopic hematuria, without neoplasm risk factors

Prostatitis

Prostatitis is defined as an inflamed, edematous, and painful prostate. Prostatitis can be due to a bacterial infection or secondary reaction from an environmental stimulus, such as recent urologic instrumentation, bicycle riding, or sexual abuse.[19]

Medical Screening

A. *Chief complaint:* Urinary urgency, dysuria, nocturia, difficulty emptying bladder
B. *Signs and symptoms*
1. Perineum pain
2. Testicle pain
3. Penis pain
4. Pain during ejaculation
5. Pain in lower abdomen, bladder
6. Bladder outlet obstruction (BOO)
7. Blood in semen
8. Urinary symptoms
C. *Focused assessment*
1. Abdominal assessment
2. Focused suprapubic palpation and costovertebral angle (CVA) tenderness
3. Prostate exam (avoid prostate massage as it may induce bacterial shed). Prostate will be edematous.

Diagnostic Testing

A. *Labs*
1. Complete blood count (CBC)
2. Basic metabolic panel (BMP)
3. Prostate-specific antigen (PSA)
4. Urinalysis (UA) with Gram stain and culture
5. Sexually transmitted infection (STI) testing (see Medical Decision-Making and Differential Diagnoses)

Medical Decision-Making and Differential Diagnoses

A. *Differentials to consider:* Cystitis, benign prostatic hyperplasia (BPH), urethritis
B. Men under 35, who are sexually active, and all ages who engage in high-risk sexual behaviors should be tested for *Neisseria gonorrhea* and *Chlamydia trachomatis*.

Management

A. *Procedures:* Midstream clean catch urine, or straight catheterization. See STI testing.

B. *Pharmacologic therapies*

1. Follow evidence-based guidelines when prescribing.
   a. Trimethoprim-sulfamethoxazole (TMP/SMZ)[20]
   b. Ciprofloxacin (Cipro) [20]
   c. Severely ill or urosepsis
      i. Ampicillin, IV every 6 hours, plus gentamicin, every day or every 8 hours, until afebrile[20]
   d. Treatment courses are a minimum of 6 weeks, but often need to be extended for bacterial eradication.
   e. Treatment considerations need to be made based on local resistance rates.

Age and Developmental Considerations

A. *Prevention and education*

1. Left untreated, it can lead to overwhelming sepsis or the development of a prostate abscess.
2. Prostatic massage is not recommended in patients with acute prostatitis as this may cause bacterial spread.
3. Prostatitis can be caused by an STI and this should be considered in at-risk patients when making treatment decisions.
4. If fever persists or fails to demonstrate a decline after 36 hours, a prostatic abscess should be considered. Urology consultation should be obtained.

B. *Patient and family education and counseling*

1. Take antibiotic medication as recommended. Return for any new, worsening, or recurrent symptoms. Treatment courses are a minimum of 6 weeks, but often need to be extended for bacterial eradication.

Uncomplicated Cystitis

Uncomplicated cystitis is defined as a lower urinary tract infection affecting the bladder. An uncomplicated urinary infection is one that occurs in an otherwise healthy individual without any known anatomic abnormality of the urinary tract.[11]

Medical Screening

A. *Chief complaint:* Dysuria

B. *Signs and symptoms*

1. Urinary burning
2. Dysuria
3. Urinary frequency
4. Suprapubic pain, pressure
5. Occasionally hematuria, cloudy, or malodorous urine

C. *Focused assessment*

1. Abdominal assessment
2. Focused suprapubic palpation and costovertebral angle (CVA) tenderness

Medical Decision-Making and Differential Diagnoses

Patients with classic symptoms (urinary burning, dysuria, and frequency) of an isolated lower urinary tract infection, without health risk factors, pregnancy, anatomic urinary structural concerns, or vaginal discharge may be diagnosed from presentation; however, it is common practice to perform urinalysis. A positive urinalysis is indicated by evidence of bacteriuria (5+), pyuria (+leukocyte esterase or white blood cells [WBC]>10), or positive for nitrite.[21] Most common pathogen is *Escherichia coli* (86%). Patients with dysuria without evidence of acute urinary infection on UA should be evaluated for STI. Suprapubic tenderness occurs in 80% to 90% of female patients with urinary tract infections (UTIs).[22] Females are at greater risk of developing a UTI over males, 35:1 in patients between 15 and 64 years old, partially due to the close approximation of the urethra to the rectum and potential exposure to gastrointestinal flora. Sexual history should be obtained in all patients, specifically addressing if there is a history of anal insertive practice as the likelihood of enteric organisms causing the infection is greater in this population. Men with UTIs are often associated with structural abnormalities, such as bladder outlet obstruction, or prostatitis. At the age of 66, the risk for developing a UTI in women compared to men is 2:1.[13]

A. *Differential diagnosis*

1. STI
2. Nephrolithiasis
3. Overactive bladder
4. Prostatitis
5. Neoplasm

Diagnostic Testing

A. UA, culture if indicated

Management

A. Mid-stream clean catch urine, or straight catheterization

B. *Pharmacologic therapies:* Antimicrobial treatment should be determined by local resistance patterns, insurance coverage, allergies, and tolerability. Follow evidence-based guidelines when prescribing.

1. Antibiotics[22,23]
   a. Nitrofurantoin
   b. Trimethoprim/sulfamethoxazole
   c. Fosfomycin
2. Analgesics and antipyretics
   a. Pyridium
   b. Tylenol or NSAIDs for fever
3. According to the American Urological Association (AUA),[18] treatment should be extended to 7 to 10 days in patients with concomitant diabetes, symptoms lasting longer than 7 days, pregnancy, over the age of 65, or a significant history of drug-resistant cultures of pyelonephritis.

Patient Disposition

A. *Discharge instructions*
   1. Patients should start demonstrating improvement of symptoms within 48 to 72 hours postantibiotic treatment.
   2. Those patients who do not improve, develop a fever, or have worsening symptoms should change antimicrobial regimens and consider reevaluation.

B. *Transition of care information*
   1. Consider urologic referral for patients with recurrent infections or those that anatomic abnormality cannot be ruled out.

Age and Developmental Considerations

Please see urinary tract infection in pregnancy and pediatric populations, Chapters 52 and 53.

A. *Prevention and education*
   1. Practice postcoital urination.
   2. Proper perineal skin hygiene
   3. Females should be reminded to wipe front to back.
   4. Avoid spermicides.

B. *Patient and family education and counseling*
   1. Increase hydration.
   2. Pyridium stains the urine orange.

Urolithiasis

Renal calculi are typically found in the calyx and renal pelvis (nephrolithiasis). Calculi within the ureter is termed ureterolithiasis.[24] Pain is normally associated with the blockage of urine flow from the renal system ascending down the upper urinary tract.

Medical Screening

A. *Chief complaint:* Flank pain

B. *Signs and symptoms*
   1. Can be asymptomatic
   2. Colicky
   3. Agonizing back pain, radiating to groin, testicles/labia and suprapubic region, abrupt onset
   4. Hematuria
   5. Urinary tract infection (UTI) symptoms
   6. Fever, chills, nausea, vomiting
   7. Costovertebral angle (CVA) tenderness
   8. Severe pain causing tachycardia, tachypnea, or diaphoretic[24]

C. *Focused assessment*
   1. CVA tenderness
   2. Genitourinary (GU) examination

Diagnostic Testing

A. *Labs*
   1. Urinalysis (UA)
   2. Complete blood count (CBC)
   3. Basic metabolic panel (BMP)

B. *Imaging*
   1. Kidney, ureter, and bladder x-ray (KUB)
   2. Noncontrast CT, ultrasound (US)

Medical Decision-Making and Differential Diagnoses[24]

A. Pyelonephritis

B. Musculoskeletal pain

C. Abdominal aortic aneurysm (AAA), appendicitis

D. Cholecystitis

E. Gastric disease

Management

A. *Strain urine:* Stones greater than 6 mm, or those with associated moderate to severe hydronephrosis, require referral and possible surgical stone ablation; 4 to 6 mm generally pass on own, others consult urology.[25]

B. *Pharmacologic therapies*
   1. Follow evidence-based guidelines when prescribing.
   2. Tamsulosin 4 weeks then reimage if symptoms present
   3. NSAIDs (recommendation, most require narcotics)

Patient Disposition

A. *Consultation and collaboration*
   1. Urology referral and follow-up

Age and Developmental Considerations

A. Renal calculi in the pediatric population are most commonly caused by increased levels of phosphorus, calcium, and oxalate. These levels can increase by the consumption of certain foods and beverages. Sedentary lifestyles also increase the risk of calcium release from the bones and secondary calcium stone formation.[26]

B. *Prevention and education*
   1. Strain urine for stone analysis.
   2. Hydration
   3. Consider secondary cause of stone formation, such as parathyroid dysfunction, vitamin C over consumption, dehydration, and excessive protein intake.

EXTERNAL GENITOURINARY SYSTEM

Balanitis, Phimosis, and Paraphimosis

Balanitis is inflammation of the distal end or the penis, known as the glans penis, and is seen commonly in patients with concomitant diabetes. Balanitis can cause phimosis or paraphimosis. Phimosis occurs when the foreskin of the penis is inflamed and edematous causing difficulty retracting the tissue. Whereas paraphimosis occurs when the foreskin tissue of an uncircumcised individual is retracted and unable to be manipulated forward over the glans penis, this is a urologic emergency.[27]

Medical Screening

A. *Chief complaint:* Penile pain

B. *Signs and symptoms*

1. Penile pain, with or without odor, puritis, dysuria

C. *Focused assessment*

1. Evaluate the foreskin for suppleness.

2. Penile examination evaluating for any signs of infection, tissue induration or exudate, lesions, or masses

Diagnostic Testing

For balanitis, do a skin culture if exudate present or unclear presentation, evaluating for viral, bacterial, and fungal pathogens. Consider blood glucose in diabetic patients, or those with diabetic risk factors. Phimosis and paraphimosis are diagnosed on clinical presentation.

Medical Decision-Making and Differential Diagnoses

A. Differential diagnoses include contact dermatitis, sexual abuse, cancer, and STIs. Also consider underlying immunosuppression, such as HIV, in recurrent cases. Patients who are uncircumcised who have recurrent infection may consider circumcision.

Management

A. *Procedures*

1. Paraphimosis requires immediate surgical intervention if manual reduction cannot be achieved, and often requires sedation for pain, to avoid tissue necrosis of the glans penis.[28]

a. Place ice on penis to reduce swelling.

b. Pain management, local anesthetic

c. Possible sedation

d. To further reduce swelling gently apply squeezing pressure with hand to the foreskin for 5 to 10 minutes.

e. Place both thumbs at the glans while pulling the foreskin outward and forward with fingers.

f. If unsuccessful, repeat applying manual squeezing pressure to the foreskin for a longer duration.

g. If unsuccessful, contact urology for emergent surgical procedure and placement if a dorsal foreskin slit.

2. Phimosis

a. Treatment indicated if patient unable to void or if unable to perform a catheterization, contact urology for dorsal slit incision. Treat underlying cause of inflammation. Do not forcefully retract foreskin.

b. Pharmacologic therapies

i. Follow evidence-based guidelines when prescribing.

ii. Treatment depends on cause.

(1) *Balanitis:* Candidal infection is most common cause[29]:

(2) Clotrimazole cream 1% or Miconazole cream 2% BID until symptoms resolve

(3) Fluconazole (for those with diabetes-mellitus [D] or refractory cases)

(4) Topical steroids, hydrocortisone cream 1% apply to BID

B. *Prevention and education*

1. Proper hygiene, try to keep area dry, and blood sugar control

Epididymitis

An acute or chronic inflammation of the epididymis most often caused by bacterial infection.

Medical Screening

A. *Chief complaint:* Unilateral scrotal pain

B. *Signs and symptoms*

1. Acute (<6 weeks) or chronic (≥6 weeks)

2. Severe edema and pain of scrotum

3. Fever, rigors, and urinary frequency, urgency, or dysuria

C. *Focused assessment*

1. *Acute:* Induration and edema of the involved epididymis with severe scrotal tenderness, and possibly erythema, and a secondary reactive hydrocele

2. Prehn sign, relief of pain with elevation of the affected testis

3. *Chronic:* Subtle epididymal induration and unilateral scrotal tenderness, with or without edema. Inflammatory nodule may be palpated.

Diagnostic Testing

A. Based on physical examination and confirmed with urine studies.

B. Sexually transmitted infection (STI) cultures for patients with urethral discharge or history supporting increased risk of STI

C. Ultrasound if any concerns with testicular torsion

Medical Decision-Making and Differential Diagnoses

A review of systems should include sexual activity and high-risk sexual behaviors, history of intense physical exertion, and perineum irritation from activities such as bicycle and motorcycle riding, without a known history of urinary dysfunction.[30]

A. *Common pathogens*

1. Men <35 years old *Chlamydia trachomatis* and *Neisseria gonorrhoeae*

2. Men >35 years old *Escherichia coli* and *Pseudomonas* most common

B. *Differentials*

1. Testicular torsion, urethritis, testicular neoplasm, trauma, hydrocele, spermatocele, varicocele

Management

A. Ice, scrotal elevation, and NSAIDs

B. STI

1. Ceftriaxone *plus* doxycycline

C. STI in men who practice insertive anal sex

1. Ceftriaxone *plus* levofloxacin *or* ofloxacin

D. Enteric organisms (negative Gram stain/STI testing)

1. Ofloxacin *or* levofloxacin[31]

E. Severe epididymitis and testicular pain

1. Referral to urology for potential surgical exploration. Septic patients, refer to ED for IV antibiotics, hydration.

Age and Developmental Considerations

In the pediatric population, infection from *Haemophilus influenzae* with bacteremia may go on to develop secondary epididymitis and secondary to other causes such as adenovirus or enterovirus.[30]

Fournier's Gangrene

Fournier's gangrene is a form of necrotizing fasciitis, which is an acute, potentially lethal, infection occurring within the tissue of the anus, genital, and perineal locations, with subsequent abdominal tissue involvement. Rapid disease identification, diagnosis, and emergent surgical intervention is paramount to reduce morbidity and mortality.

Medical Screening

A. *Chief complaint:* Perineal, rectal, or scrotal pain
B. *Signs and symptoms*
  1. Genital, peritoneal, or anorectal edema, erythema, and cellulitis, which progresses rapidly into vesicles. Vesicles may further advance into bullae formation, ischemia, and necrotic lesions.
C. *Focused assessment*
  1. Genitourinary dermatologic assessment
  2. Rectal examination

Diagnostic Testing

A. *Labs*
  1. Complete blood count (CBC)
  2. Basic metabolic panel (BMP)
  3. C-reactive protein
B. *Imaging (not at the cost of delaying surgical intervention)*
  1. Abdominal pelvic radiograph, CT, or ultrasound
  2. Specifically assessing for the evidence of gas bubbles within the tissue planes of the peritoneal and abdominal cavities[32]

Medical Decision-Making and Differential Diagnoses

A. Gangrene vulvitis or balanitis should be considered, especially in patients with diabetes. Ulcerations or chancre.[33] Other differentials include those for acute scrotal pain. Patient management, rapid infusion for septic patients, broad-spectrum antibiotics, and surgical preparation

Management

A. Emergent surgical referral
B. Pharmacologic therapies
  1. Broad-spectrum antibiotic
C. Aggressive management for septicemia
D. Consultation and collaboration
  1. After disease recognition, immediate referral to urology or general surgery for surgical debridement

Age and Developmental Considerations

A. *Prevention and education*
  1. Maintaining good blood glucose control for diabetics. Performing thorough skin assessments on patients with concomitant disease processes such as diabetes mellitus (DM), immunocompromised, alcohol abuse, traumatic genitourinary injuries, or urologic or rectal surgeries.

Hydrocele

A hydrocele is excess serous fluid within the scrotum; this may occur secondary to inflammation, injury, or anatomical leakage from the peritoneal cavity along the inguinal canal. Conditions that can cause an inflammatory hydrocele include, but are not limited to, epididymitis and testicular torsion. A hydrocele that communicates with the peritoneal cavity is one that enlarges throughout the day or with increased intraabdominal pressure, such as the Valsalva maneuver. A hydrocele that is noncommunicating is one that does not change in volume or shape with increased intraabdominal pressure, such as crying or the Valsalva maneuver.[34]

Medical Screening

A. *Chief complaint:* Enlarged scrotum
B. *Signs and symptoms*
  1. Typically painless, depending on underlying cause
  2. Fluid-filled scrotum
C. *Focused assessment*
  1. Scrotal assessment
  2. Transillumination of the scrotum to rule out any masses

Diagnostic Testing

A. *Duplex or color Doppler*
  1. Helps evaluate for any neoplastic lesions or torsion as underlying cause of hydrocele.
B. Follow-up CT scan without contrast if unable to identify cause from ultrasound.[34]

Medical Decision-Making and Differential Diagnoses

A. *Differentials include:*
  1. Testicular neoplasm
  2. Testicular torsion
  3. Mumps
  4. Inguinal hernia
  5. Scrotal trauma

Management

A. *Procedure and treatments*
  1. Based on primary cause of hydrocele. Once emergent primary conditions are ruled, an outpatient urology referral may be warranted.

Age and Developmental Considerations

A. Up to 95% of hydroceles noted in children under 1 year of age are congenital. If present after 1 year, outpatient urology referral should be obtained.

Priapism

A prolonged abnormal erection of the penis, unrelated to sexual desire, causing pain. After 6 to 8 hours, there is a risk of tissue ischemia.[35] The timing of the diagnosis and identification of priapism is essential to tissue survival if ischemic changes are identified.

Medical Screening

A. *Chief complaints:* Prolonged erection
B. *Signs and symptoms*
  1. Penile pain and tenderness
C. *Focused assessment*
  1. Assessment should be focused on the penis, and the ability to differentiate between early stages of tissue ischemia verse nonischemic priapism.[36]

Diagnostic Testing

A. *Labs*
  1. Complete blood count (CBC) and reticulocyte count if concerns with sickle cell disease
  2. May consider drug screen to evaluate cause.

Medical Decision-Making and Differential Diagnoses

A. A thorough history, including street drugs, medications, cancer history, trauma (see spinal cord injury), clotting disorders, or sickle cell anemia, should be obtained.

Management

A. ***Procedures***
  1. Ischemic priapism should be managed with the treatment of an intracavernous injection, with phenylephrine, and/or therapeutic aspiration, most often performed by a urologist. If the priapism continues, a secondary round of the same treatment should be initiated, followed by surgical intervention.[36]
  2. Nonischemic priapism is typically caused by arterial flow deficiencies and typically requires observation only.
B. *Pharmacologic therapies*
  1. *For clinicians trained in IV injections:* Phenylephrine, follow evidence-based guidelines when prescribing. Lower concentration in patients with known cardiovascular disease or children. Secondary side effects include reflex bradycardia, headache, hypertension, tachycardia, cardiac arrhythmia, and palpitations.[36]
C. *Consultation/collaboration*
  1. Urology consultation

Age and Developmental Considerations

A. Children with a history of sickle cell disease are at risk for the development of priapism.[37]

Testicular Torsion

Testicular torsion is the rotation of the testicle and twisting of the spermatic cord, which results in reduced blood flow and ischemia of the testicle. Acute identification and surgical intervention is necessary to salvage the testicle.[38]

Medical Screening

A. *Chief complaint:* Acute onset of unilateral testicular pain
B. *Signs and symptoms*
  1. Severe scrotal pain affecting one side of the scrotum
  2. Nausea and vomiting
C. *Focused assessment*
  1. Physical examination findings may demonstrate an absent cremasteric reflex and a high-riding testicle with an abnormal transverse position.

Diagnostic Testing

A. If physical examination findings support testicular torsion, the patient should be prepped for immediate surgery without delay from imaging. If immediate surgical intervention is not an option, or there is diagnosis uncertainty, a scrotal Doppler ultrasound should be performed.

Medical Decision-Making and Differential Diagnoses

A. *Differential diagnoses include*
  1. Epididymo-orchitis
  2. Infection
  3. Idiopathic scrotal edema
  4. Inguinal hernia
  5. Torsion of the appendix testis (Box 18.1)
  6. Trauma
  7. Testicular neoplasm
  8. Varicocele
B. *The viability of the testicle decreases with time.*

TIME SINCE SYMPTOM ONSET	TESTICLE SALVAGE RATES
6 hours	90%–100%
12 hours	50%
>24 hours	10%

Management

A. *Procedures:* Surgical preparation
B. *Pharmacologic therapies:* None

Patient Disposition

A. ***Consultation/collaboration***
  1. Emergent urology referral
B. *Documentation*
  1. Documentation should include exact time urologic referral was obtained and time to the operating room.

Age and Developmental Considerations

A. Most often occurs in males under the age of 18
B. *Prevention and education*
  1. Bilateral testicular fixation (orchiopexy) will be performed on both testicles as the incidence of torsion on the contralateral side is 80% in some patients.[38]

BOX 18.1 APPENDAGE TORSION

Torsion of the appendix testis is caused from twisting of a vestigial appendage that is situated along the testicle. Patients with this condition may display a tender protuberance with blue discoloration (blue dot sign) on the upper end of the testis. Torsion of the testicular appendices is a benign condition. Necrotic tissue is reabsorbed without any secondary effect in almost all cases. The clinical presentation appendix testis torsion is difficult for most clinicians to discern from testicular torsion. Torsion of the appendix testis usually occurs in boys aged between 7 and 12 years.

FEMALE GENITOURINARY AND REPRODUCTION CONDITIONS

Given their role within emergency medicine, some emergency nurse practitioners (ENPs) will find themselves caring for many diverse populations, some in very remote areas. It is important to be able to provide initial care for these unique problems until the patient can follow up with a specialist for definitive care.

Breast Pain

Medical Screening

A. *Chief complaint:* Breast pain[39]

B. *Signs and symptoms*

1. Pain in area
2. Areolar discharge
3. Erythema
4. Wound and drainage from site
5. Fever in some cases
6. Malaise

C. *Focused assessment*

1. Appearance of area that is painful
2. Assessment of area compared to the other breast
3. Erythematous changes to skin
4. Induration and fluctuant areas in region of pain

Diagnostic Testing

A. *Labs*

1. Complete blood count (CBC)
2. Chemistry
3. Qualitative b-hCG.

B. ***Imaging***

1. Ultrasound (US) of site; all other imaging is nonemergent

Medical Decision-Making, Differential Diagnoses, and Treatment

A. *Breast mass*

1. The differentiation between infectious and noninfectious processes needs to initially be determined. Once infection is ruled out, consult breast specialist for further evaluation of the problem.

B. *Cellulitis in nonbreastfeeding patients*

1. Treat like any cellulitis. Evaluation for fluid collection should occur to ensure appropriate treatment. Antibiotic therapy should take into consideration methicillin-resistant *Staphylococcus aureus* (MRSA) (see following).

C. *Abscess*

1. Can stem from a primary abscess or from breastfeeding complication. Treatment of an abscess can start with US-guided needle aspiration of site when overlying tissue is normal. Surgical drainage is necessary if overlying skin is concerning for ischemia or pressure-induced necrosis, or if patient has failed any type of antibiotic therapy.[40,41]Incision and drainage (I&D) is not typically used for cosmetic reasons, as well as for complications associated with the procedure in the area of milk ducts (e.g., mammary duct fistulas). Surgical intervention is also associated with cosmetic complications as well as milk fistula, seen with large incisions or when drain placement is required. Antibiotic therapy is added to the treatment.
2. Treatment
   - **a.** Needle aspirate
     - **i.** Surface tissue should be normal in appearance. Aspirated material should be sent for culture. Because of thickness of drainage, thinning it by an injection of anesthetic can make withdrawing the drainage via needle aspirate easier.[42] Confirmation of abscess is important, as to not cause trauma to milk ducts with a needle aspirate procedure that would yield breast milk.
   - **b.** Antibiotic therapy
     - **i.** Follow evidence-based guidelines when prescribing.
     - **ii.** *Mild infections not associated with MRSA:* Dicloxacillin, for 10 to 14 days *or* cephalexin, for 10 to 14 days
     - **iii.** *Concern for MRSA:* Clindamycin, for 10 to 14 days *or* trimethoprim-sulfamethoxazole, for 10 to 14 days
     - **iv.** *Severe infection requiring initial IV therapy:* Vancomycin, q8–12h[42]; culture-driven antibiotic therapy should then follow.
     - **v.** In cases of suspected anaerobic infection (hidradenitis suppurativa or nipple retracted infections), amoxicillin-clavulanic acid with MRSA, clindamycin or dicloxacillin with metronidazole[42,43]

D. *Breastfeeding-related complications*

1. Mastitis
   - **a.** Cellulitis mimicking changes, which if caught early, will not require antibiotic therapy. Breastfeeding in the early stages to unclog a milk duct can frequency resolve the problem within 12 to 24 hours.[42,44] Anti-inflammatories and cold compresses can be used for pain and swelling.[42] Antibiotic therapy should be considered in extreme cases. Treatment should cover *Staphylococcus aureus*. Trimethoprim-sulfamethoxazole (TMP/SMZ) can be used when the infant is healthy and at least 1 month of age and a full-term delivery. Do not use with infants under 1 month of age or those with glucose-6-phosphate dehydrogenase deficiency.[42] Referring to a breastfeeding educator will help with the resolution process. Antibiotic therapy is decided based on severity of problem, accounting for need to "pump and dump" milk. Severe infection or antibiotic failure requires inpatient therapy with vancomycin IV until culture results can tailor therapy.[40] Length of therapy is dependent on patient response to treatment.
2. Milk duct problems
   - **a.** Milk fistulas and galactocele problems need to be referred to a breast specialist. Antibiotic therapy is not indicated unless cellulitis changes are identified on exam. Needle aspirate can cause other complications, including fistulas, and should be avoided unless the fluid collection is

BOX 18.2 PELVIC PAIN IDENTIFICATION BY LOCATION

RIGHT LOWER QUADRANT	MIDLINE/SUPER PUBIC	LEFT LOWER QUADRANT
Appendicitis	Urinary retention	Diverticulitis
Crohn's disease	Cystitis	Ulcerative colitis
Ovarian cyst	Uterine fibroids	Constipation
Ovarian torsion	Pelvic inflammatory disease	Ovarian cyst
Ectopic pregnancy		Ovarian torsion
Tubo-ovarian abscess		Ectopic pregnancy
Pelvic inflammatory disease		Tubo-ovarian abscess
Renal calculi		Pelvic inflammatory disease
Hernia		Renal calculi
		Hernia

definitively identified as purulent material and not breast milk.

E. *Breast implant complications*
   1. Infection
      a. Normal bacteria involved in skin infections, coagulase-negative *Staphylococcus* as well as Gram-negative bacteria, must be considered when deciding treatment. Admission for IV antibiotics to include vancomycin and piperacillin/tazobactam is necessary.[45] Specialist consultation should be included. Breast implant removal is often necessary to resolve infection. Clinical features of an infectious process are seen as expected to make diagnosis. If aspirate of fluid collection is performed, US guidance is a must to prevent puncture of implant.[15]
   2. Implant rupture
      a. *Background:* There remain two types of implants on the market: saline and silicone. Both products can have leakage/failure/rupture. Damage or failure can result from product malfunction, valve defect, fatigue of the product over time, damage to product during filling, or damage as a result of blunt trauma to region.
      b. *Saline considerations:* The presentation of problems with this type is the loss of breast size either abruptly or over several days. Diagnosis of implant rupture is easily made without the need for any imaging or testing.[46] Referral to a specialist is needed for repair.
      c. *Silicone considerations:* Presentation of the problem, other than gross blunt trauma-related pain, is pain in an area of the breast, signs of granuloma development, or localized inflammation. These changes are only seen with extracapsular rupture. "Silent ruptures" are those within the capsule, providing no symptoms and most often identified during an ongoing routine imaging of the implant via MRI.[46] There is no emergent intervention for this type of implant either; specialist referral is needed.

Pelvic Pain

Medical Screening

A. *Chief complaint:* Pelvic pain[47–49]
B. *Signs and symptoms*
   1. Pain in pelvic region
   2. Referred pain to shoulder
   3. Fever case dependent
   4. Hypotension case dependent
   5. Tachycardia case dependent
   6. Nausea and/or vomiting
   7. Dysuria, frequency, hematuria
   8. Vaginal complaints
C. *Focused assessment*
   1. *Location of pain:* Adnexal, midline, cervical motion tenderness. Differentiating the diagnosis by location is one of the options for more thorough diagnosis considerations (Box 18.2).
   2. *Quality and pain pattern:* Dysuria, cervical motion tenderness, severity of pain, focal versus diffuse
   3. *Speculum examination findings:* Vaginal discharge characteristics, cervical friability
      a. Onset of symptoms in relation to menstrual cycle

Diagnostic Testing

A. *Labs*
   1. Complete blood count (CBC)
   2. Chemistry
   3. Qualitative b-hCG
   4. Urinalysis (UA)
   5. Urine culture
   6. Gonorrhea and chlamydia cultures

B. *Imaging*
 1. Transvaginal or transdermal, pending suspected diagnosis
 2. CT abdominal/pelvis with and/or without contrast, pending suspected diagnosis[50]

Medical Decision-Making, Differential Diagnoses, and Treatment

A. *Pelvic mass*
 1. *Background:* Differentiation of cause can be either benign or malignant. If malignancy is suspected, urgent referral to a gynecological specialist is necessary. The nonemergent causes can be divided into gynecological and nongynecological causes.
 2. Gynecological diagnoses to consider include multiple types of cysts, ectopic pregnancy, hydrosalpinx, and tubo-ovarian abscess, to name a few.
 3. Nongynecological diagnoses to consider include constipation, appendiceal abscess, diverticular abscess, and pelvic abscess.

B. *Ovarian cyst*
 1. *Background:* In general, a cyst less than 8 cm in size, unilocular and unilateral, resolves within two menstrual cycles. If the cyst is larger than 8 cm, multilocular or solid in composition, the diagnoses of neoplasm, dermoid cyst, and endometrioma should be considered.
 2. Types
  a. *Follicular:* A mature ovum that ruptures at the time of ovulation
  b. *Corpus luteum:* Cyst left after ovulation that after implantation will enlarge and begin secreting estrogen and progesterone to maintain pregnancy.
  c. *Hemorrhagic:* Rupture of a blood vessel within the wall of a cyst
  d. *Dermoid cyst:* Contains sebaceous fluid, bone or cartilage, fat, and so on. This type of cyst results in peritonitis and requires surgical intervention.[51]
 3. *Treatment of rupture*: Hemodynamic stability is the focus of care, preparation for surgical intervention as indicated. Rupture of a cyst is typically uncomplicated and thus observation only is needed.[51]

C. *Ovarian torsion*
 1. *Background:* Diagnosis is a result of ovarian enlargement from large cysts and masses. Twisting initially blocks venous return, causing congestion that subsequently progresses to decreased arterial flow resulting in ischemia. The problem usually includes the ovary and the oviduct together.
 2. *Presentation:* Traditionally, symptoms are usually sudden in onset, severe, and unilateral, 50%, however, have been found to present with intermittent, gradual onset of pain.[24] Bilateral adnexal pain is seen in 30% of cases. Blood flow reduction seen on ultrasound is not seen till late in the process.[52]
 3. *Treatment:* Emergent gynecology consultation for surgical intervention is necessary to preserve ovary function.

D. *Tubo-ovarian abscess*
 1. *Background:* Patients may be asymptomatic for the presentation, especially older patients. [53] The development of an abscess meets admission criteria for parenteral therapy.[54]
 2. Treatment options involve both antibiotic and surgical interventions[54,55]
  a. Antibiotics therapy alone is for candidates who show no signs of rupture, size is less than 7 cm in diameter, and patient is premenopausal. Multiple antibiotic regimen options are available, as seen in Table 18.1. The regimens vary slightly from pelvic inflammatory disease (PID) as a result of abscess development.
  b. Surgical intervention can include minimally invasive drainage (sono-guided aspiration) or open invasive surgery. Severity of the problem will determine best surgical course of action.[55]
  c. Surgical interventions before broad-spectrum antibiotics include hysterectomy and oophorectomy.[56]
 3. Antibiotic therapy failure identification includes new or worsening fever, elevated white blood cell (WBC) count, increased abnormal pain, symptoms of developing sepsis, and enlargement of mass. Prior to broad-spectrum antibiotic invention there was a 50% mortality rate.[55]
 4. Suspected rupture is seen in 15% of cases. If patient presentation is suggestive of a rupture or sepsis, surgical intervention is emergent for evaluation and treatment.[55]
 5. Postmenopausal patients are at higher than normal risk for malignancy when they develop a tubo-ovarian abscess.[57] If surgical intervention is performed, frozen section analysis and abdominopelvic exploration should be included to evaluate for malignancy and metastasis. If there is low risk of malignancy, serial imaging can be performed to confirm resolution.[55]

E. PID
 1. *Background:* The ascent of infection above the endocervix up through the upper reproductive tract, resulting in endometritis, salpingitis, and peritonitis. Negative cervical cultures do not rule out sexually transmitted disease (STD)–related bacteria as the cause of infection.[58]
 2. *Antibiotic treatment:* Regimen dependent upon outpatient or inpatient treatment as noted in Table 18.1
 3. Indications for hospitalization[54]
  a. Severe illness or sepsis
  b. PID complication of abscess development
  c. Differential diagnosis rule-out not completed
  d. Pregnancy
  e. Antibiotic failure outpatient
  f. Potential noncompliance with treatment

F. Nongynecologic diagnosis and treatments can be found in Chapter 17.

TABLE 18.1 ANTIBIOTIC TREATMENT IN PELVIC INFLAMMATORY DISEASE AND TUBO-OVARIAN ABSCESS

OUTPATIENT TREATMENT		
	PID	TOA
Ceftriaxone syringe *plus* Doxycycline	**X**	–
Add If trichomonas, bacterial vaginosis, or gynecologic procedure within 3 weeks Metronidazole	**X**	–
INPATIENT TREATMENT		
First-line	**PID**	**TOA**
Cefoxitin *plus* Doxycyline *plus* Gentamycin	**X**	**X**
Ampicillin *plus* Clindamycin *plus* Gentamycin	**X**	**X**
Secondline (allergy or unavailability of first-line regimen)	**PID**	**TOA**
Ampicillin-sulbactam *plus* Doxycycline	**X**	**X**
Ampicillin *plus* Clindamycin *plus* Gentamycin	-	**X**
Levofloxacin *plus* Metronidazole	-	**X**
Imipenem cilastatin	-	**X**

Note: Follow evidence-based guidelines when prescribing.

IM, intramuscularly; IV, intravenous; PID, pelvic inflammatory disease; PO, orally; q, every; TOA, tubo-ovarian abscess.

Source: Wiesenfield H. Pelvic inflammatory disease: treatment in adult and adolescents. In: Bloom A, ed. *UpToDate*. UpToDate; 2019. www.uptodate.com.; Beigi R. Management and complications of tubo-ovarian abscess. In: Eckler K, ed. *UpToDate*. UpToDate; 2019. www.uptodate.com.[54,55]

Vaginal Bleeding

Medical Screening

A. *Chief complaint:* Vaginal bleeding[59,60]

B. *Signs and symptoms*

1. Bleeding history, including quality and quantity
2. Any pain or lack of pain in the abdomen associated with onset of bleeding
3. Weakness and fatigue
4. Hypotension
5. Tachycardia

C. ***Focused assessment***

1. Appearance, quality, and quantity of bleeding on examination (history best obtained by identifying the number of pads used)
2. Hemodynamic stability
3. History surrounding onset
4. Speculum examination

Diagnostic Testing

A. *Labs*

1. Complete blood count (CBC)
2. Chemistry
3. Qualitative b-hCG
4. Type and cross
5. Coagulation Panelp
6. UA
7. Urine culture
8. Gonorrhea and chlamydia cultures

B. *Imaging*

1. Transvaginal or transdermal, pending suspected diagnosis

2. CT abdominal/pelvis with and/or without contrast, pending suspected diagnosis

Medical Decision-Making, Differential Diagnoses, and Treatment

A. *Endometriosis*[61]

1. NSAIDs are the first-line choice of treatment; avoid COX2 inhibitors, however, in patients who are trying to get pregnant because the group of drugs can delay or prevent ovulation. Hormone therapy is also an option in treatment. Estrogen–progesterone combination therapy is a first-line therapy, but progesterone-only options are preferred in women not wanting to take estrogen. Multiple other hormone options exist, but for ED purposes, these other combinations should be prescribed by a specialist.

B. *Leiomyomata*[62]

1. Surgery is the predominant treatment for this problem. The options include hysterectomy and endometrial ablation for those who have completed childbearing. Myomectomy is the option for those who still want the choice of having children. Nonsurgical therapy involves hormone therapy. Since these patients frequently present with vaginal bleeding issues, it is reasonable to begin with hormone treatment from the ED with referral to gynecology.

C. *Malignancies (cervical or endometrial)*

1. The ED setting is not where diagnosing and staging of these problems takes place; however, identifying possible malignancies should prompt urgent referral and follow-up with a specialist for definitive diagnosis and treatment.

D. *Endocrine causes*[59]

1. Polycystic ovary disease, excessive estrogen usage/production/storage, thyroid disorder, hyperprolactinemia
2. Consult specialist.

E. *Systemic causes*[59]

1. Hemolytic disease (hemophilia, von Willebrand), anticoagulation, thrombocytopenia, leukemia, pancytopenia from immunosuppressants
2. Consult specialist.

F. *Special considerations*

1. Female circumcisions[63]

a. *Overview:* The cutting of female genitals is a cultural practice, the results of which are now seen around the world. The practice is seen in areas of the Middle East, Asia, and Africa.[64] The practice involves manipulation or removal of parts of the female external genitalia. Some cultures associate this procedure with a celebration that takes place between the ages of 5 to 12. Sometimes the procedure is performed in the middle of the night after the young girl is abducted. Details of how this procedure is performed range from the use of anesthetics, antibiotics, and sterile instruments, by a trained professional, down to unclean, very old instruments, without the use of medications by an untrained person. Hemostasis in the more primitive cases is done with local practices including topical mixtures of egg and sugar or even animal feces. Catgut suture and thorns are used in other cases. The care of women having undergone the practice will require unique long-term help from providers handling ED care when faced with this special patient group. The World Health Organization classifies the changes into four types.

b. *Type I:* Removal of the prepuce along with part or all of the clitoris

c. *Type II:* Complete removal of the clitoris with all or part of the labia majora and minora

d. *Type III:* All or the majority of the external genitalia is removed, and what remains of the labia majora is sewn together, covering the urethral introitus and vaginal introitus.

e. *Type IV:* Any other injury to the external genitalia, such as piercing, pricking, or burning

f. Long-term implications

i. Women develop what is known as an infibulation scar over the region, which covers the urethral meatus. The scar results in several complications that may be confronted in the ED.

ii. Urinary tract complications

(1) Meatal strictures and obstructions
(2) Urinary retention problems
(3) Increase in chronic urinary tract infections and urinary stones

iii. Reproductive tract complications

(1) Increase in vulvar abscesses
(2) Labial majora and labial minora fusions—partial and complete
(3) Increased vaginal infections

g. Additional long-term issues

i. Other complications not directly addressed in the ED include infertility, sexual dysfunction, and childbirth issues. Some women will undergo a procedure to open the scar tissue to avert the complications it has created.[65] The procedure is known as defibulation.

2. Urinary catheters

a. *Overview:* Many ED visits are seen in conjunction with urinary catheters, either complications requiring a visit, or an ED discharge diagnosis that requires the patient to go home with a catheter in place.

b. Complications[66]

i. *Catheter malfunctions:* May not directly affect the patient's health but will complicate lifestyle and living conditions. Replacement of the device is often required, but other complications need to be assessed since the age of the device may impact the malfunction(s) occurring.

ii. Urethral obstruction from retained balloon fragments from ruptured balloon

iii. Urinary tract infections—increased rates of infection begin as early as 1 week after placement.

iv. *Bladder trauma:* Can include fistula formation and perforation

v. Bladder stone formation

c. *Considerations of catheter type:* Information on complications to look for or consider when deciding on catheter placement. General problems like leakage can be seen with any of the catheters.

i. *Women's external* (e.g., PureWick™): Still new in the market, thus long-term complication research is not prevalent in the literature. Skin-related irritation may still be present, but is less than that of other noncatheter options for incontinence.

ii. *Urethral:* Trauma with placement of catheter, catheter rejection problems, patient discomfort, increased urinary tract infections

iii. *Suprapubic:* Complications with surgical placement, skin erosion at surface skin insertion site

d. Catheter care teaching should occur when patient is going home with a device. Review of care with any encounter is encouraged.

Vulvovaginal Pain, Irritation, Vaginal Discharge

Medical Screening

A. *Chief complaint:* Vulvovaginal pain, irritation, vaginal discharge[67–69]

B. *Signs and symptoms*

1. Vaginal pain
2. Skin irritation with or without urination
3. Lesions or wounds
4. Rash
5. Vaginal discharge
6. Foul odor
7. Fever and/or chills

C. *Focused assessment*

1. Visual perineal findings
2. Speculum examination

Diagnostic Testing

A. *Labs*

1. Urinalysis (UA)
2. Vaginal cultures
3. Wet prep

Medical Decision-Making, Differential Diagnoses, and Treatment

A. Follow evidence-based guidelines when prescribing

B. *Gonorrhea*

1. Antibiotic treatment

a. Ceftriaxone *with* azithromycin (current recommendations based on potential resistance issues associated with doxycycline)[70]

C. *Chlamydia*

1. Antibiotic treatment

a. Azithromycin *or* doxycycline, 100 mg[71]

D. *Bacterial vaginosis*

1. Antibiotic treatment

a. Metronidazole, single-dose treatment is no longer recommended,[72] *or* metronidazole gel, vaginally[73]

b. Clindamycin

c. Clindamycin, 2% cream

E. *Trichomonas vaginalis*

1. Antibiotic treatment

a. Metronidazole *or* metronidazole×dose. Tinidazole is an alternative but more expensive treatment.[74]

F. *Candidiasis*

1. Antifungal treatment

a. Fluconazole. Uncomplicated infections do not require a repeat dose. Complicated and recurrent infections may require two to three doses, each dose being 72 hours apart.[75] Fluconazole has been found to remain at effective levels in vaginal secretions for up to 72 hours. Topical treatment is also an option but tends to be less utilized because of the mess. Cure rates of the two approaches are very similar. Sexual partner treatment is not necessary.

G. *Bartholin's cyst*

1. Incision and drainage (I&D) of site with placement of Word catheter to facilitate ongoing drainage of site. Follow-up for Word catheter removal is required.

2. *Antibiotic therapy:* Pharmacologic therapies should be based on evidence-based recommendations from recognized sources, such as the Centers for Disease Control and Prevention (CDC) or guidelines specific to the environment where the clinician practices.

a. Previously, up to one-third of bacterial cultures identified were found to be sexually transmitted diseases (STIs). This finding has since declined and methicillin-resistant *Staphylococcus aureus* has become more prominent with skin infections.[76,77] Antibiotic dosing needs to reflect change in bacterial involvement.[76]

H. *Uterine prolapse*

1. *Reduction:* Positioning in either lithotomy or knee-chest may be used. The knee-chest position decreases any abdominal pressure experienced during the procedure.[78] Catheterization of the bladder prior to the procedure is needed to aid in the reduction.[79] Gentle pressure is applied, reverting the uterus back into the abdominal cavity. Pessary placement can be used to prevent reprolapse till follow-up with a gynecological specialist. If one is not available, the vaginal vault needs to be packed to retain the position of the uterus.

2. *Complications:* Swelling may need to be reduced to ease in reduction. Dressings soaked with hypertonic saline can be wrapped around the exposed uterus, and then the uterus can be gently squeezed to reduce the size.[79] Do this procedure in the appropriate positions, as noted above. If visible tissue denotes any concerning erosions or ulcers, biopsy samples should be sent for pathology.

a. *Admission criteria:* Inability to reduce the prolapse that is obstructing ureteral urine flow, resulting in acute renal injury/failure.[80,81] The lower portion of one or both ureters get twisted, as a result of the prolapse, causing the problem.

I. *Pessary neglect*

1. *Background:* There are two general types of pessaries: supportive and space occupying. Individual pessaries are specifically designed for different problems, including pelvic organ prolapse from stages I to IV and for urinary incontinence. The devices are frequency offered as first-line therapy. The popularity of pessaries is growing with the aging population, especially when patients are poor candidates for surgery. They are used for those not done having children and anyone not wanting to undergo surgery.[82] Pessary care requires removal and cleansing with soap and water from daily to once a month, depending on the type and the recommendation of the specialist.

2. *Complications:* While very safe, problems associated with foul discharge, vaginal wall erosions, and necrosis, as well as vaginal bleeding may occur. The typical ED presentation centers around vaginal discharge or bleeding, in extreme cases, urosepsis, and any stage of erosion. Erosions can be seen with any extended time a foreign body is in the vaginal vault, not just a pessary.[83,84] Extreme erosion can result in veicovaginal and rectovaginal fistulas.[79] The removal of the device is essential in the ED, along with thorough assessment of the vaginal wall lining.

a. Treatments

i. *Vaginal infection without erosion:* Vaginal antimicrobial creams may be used and with severe infection antibiotic creams.[79,84]

ii. *Erosions of the vaginal wall and necrosis:* Initial debridement of necrotic tissue is necessary before treatment. Topical estrogen creams can be used for superficial erosions but will require several weeks of therapy.

iii. *Fistulas:* Emergency care includes urinary catheter placement for vesicovaginal fistulas.[79] Both vesicovaginal and rectovaginal need specialist consultation urgently for surgical repair.

iv. Keep other vaginal infectious processes in consideration and treat accordingly. There is no data recommendations available for any one specific drug therapy when pessary usage in involved.[84]

J. *Fournier's gangrene* (see Male section)

References

References for this chapter are online only and can be found at https://connect.springerpub.com/content/reference-book/978-0-8261-6091-5/part/part02/toc-part/ch18.

19. Metabolic and Endocrine Conditions

MICHAEL D. GOOCH | DARLIE SIMERSON

Learning Objectives

Adrenal Disorders

- Identify adrenal conditions that may be encountered in the emergency care setting.
- Identify clinical manifestations associated with adrenal dysfunction requiring emergency management.
- Formulate a list of differential diagnoses considering all assessment findings and predisposing factors.
- Identify diagnostic tests/tools that will aid in determining the final diagnosis.
- Utilize practice guidelines to develop a management and patient education plan.
- Utilize evidence-based practices to develop a plan for referral, consultation, or transition of care.

Diabetes Mellitus

- Identify pancreatic conditions that may be encountered in the emergency care setting.
- Identify clinical manifestations associated with diabetes mellitus requiring emergency management.
- Formulate a list of differential diagnoses considering all assessment findings and predisposing factors.
- Identify diagnostic tests/tools that will aid in determining the final diagnosis.
- Utilize practice guidelines to develop a management and patient education plan.
- Utilize evidence-based practices to develop a plan for referral, consultation, or transition of care.

Thyroid Conditions

- Identify thyroid conditions that may be encountered in the emergency care setting.
- Identify clinical manifestations associated with thyroid dysfunction requiring emergency management.
- Formulate a list of differential diagnosis considering all assessment findings and predisposing factors.
- Identify diagnostic tests/tools that will aid in determining the final diagnosis.
- Utilize practice guidelines to develop a management and patient education plan.
- Utilize evidence-based practices to develop a plan for referral, consultation, or transition of care.

Pituitary Conditions

- Identify pituitary conditions that may be encountered in the emergency care setting.
- Identify clinical manifestations associated with pituitary dysfunction requiring emergency management.
- Formulate a list of differential diagnosis considering all assessment findings and predisposing factors.
- Identify diagnostic tests/tools that will aid in determining the final diagnosis.
- Utilize practice guidelines to develop a management and patient education plan.
- Utilize evidence-based practices to develop a plan for referral, consultation, or transition of care.

ADRENAL GLAND FUNCTION

The adrenal glands contribute to several aspects of homeostasis, and are influenced by the mean arterial pressure, the kidneys, extracellular fluid and electrolyte concentrations, and exogenous and endogenous steroids and hormones. The glands are divided into the medulla and cortex. The adrenal medulla is responsible for the release of epinephrine and norepinephrine and is regulated by the sympathetic nervous system. The cortex is regulated by the hypothalamic–pituitary–adrenal (HPA) axis through the release of ACTH, which regulates the secretion of mineralocorticoids, glucocorticoids, and androgens. Mineralocorticoids help regulate sodium and potassium balance. Glucocorticoids regulate glucose as well as lipid and protein metabolism.

Cortisol is the primary glucocorticoid, and aldosterone is the main mineralocorticoid produced by the adrenal cortex. Aldosterone increases the reabsorption of sodium and increases the excretion of potassium in the kidneys, significantly influencing sodium and water balance. Secretion of aldosterone is influenced by renin released from the kidneys as well as extracellular fluid and electrolyte concentrations. Cortisol has many effects including increasing gluconeogenesis, reducing cellular uptake of glucose, suppressing the immune response, and slowing the activity of white blood cells. Cortisol release is often stimulated by some type of physiological stress, including infection, trauma, or surgery.

Addison's Disease (Hypoadrenalism) and Cushing's Syndrome (Hyperadrenalism)

Pathophysiology: Addison's Disease (Hypoadrenalism)

Adrenal insufficiency occurs when the adrenal cortex is unable to secrete adequate amounts of hormones to meet the body's demand. Primary dysfunction is related to some type of injury to the adrenal glands, usually from an autoimmune process. Secondary dysfunction is related to dysfunction of the HPA axis, resulting in a decrease in ACTH secretion. Without adequate aldosterone release, sodium as well as water loss is increased through the renal tubules leading to volume depletion and hyponatremia. Potassium excretion is slowed, increasing the risk for hyperkalemia. With the reduced secretion of cortisol, glucose metabolism and regulation are altered, leading to hypoglycemia, and poor energy production. In patients taking exogenous glucocorticoids for prolonged periods of time, the HPA axis is suppressed and during acute physiological stress or abrupt cessation of the exogenous steroid, crisis can occur. Addisonian crisis refers to an extreme state of dysfunction resulting in the body's inability to regulate perfusion and other physiological functions. Death will soon occur without replacement.

Pathophysiology: Cushing's Syndrome (Hyperadrenalism)

Cushing's syndrome results from the over stimulation of the adrenal cortex. Cushing's disease refers to dysfunction due to excess release of ACTH from the pituitary gland, often from an adenoma. Other causes of this syndrome include hypothalamic dysfunction leading to pituitary dysfunction, ectopic secretion of ACTH from a tumor or an adrenal adenoma. This syndrome may be due to prolonged use of exogenous steroids to treat inflammatory or autoimmune conditions. Overstimulation leads to increased sodium and water reabsorption, leading to volume overload and hypertension. Increased excretion of potassium leads to hypokalemia, and increased mobilization of glucose causes hyperglycemia. One of the classic signs of hyperadrenalism is the redistribution of body fat, leading to the classic moon face and buffalo hump appearance. Cushing's syndrome is usually not life-threatening, unlike Addison's disease. Cushing's disease is rarely the primary reason patients seek emergency medical care.

Physical Examination

A. *Chief complaint:* Weakness, dizziness, fatigue
B. Signs and symptoms
   1. Addison's disease
      a. Hyperpigmentation of the skin and mucous membranes
      b. Hyperkalemia
      c. Hypoglycemia
      d. Hyponatremia
      e. Hypotension
      f. Weight loss
   2. Cushing's syndrome
      a. Moon face
      b. Buffalo hump
      c. Hirsutism
      d. Hypokalemia
      e. Hyperglycemia
      f. Hypernatremia
      g. Hypertension
C. *Focused assessment*
   1. Airway, breathing, circulation (ABC)
   2. Neurologic exam
   3. Cardiovascular and respiratory exam

Differential Diagnoses

A. Monitor mental status and perfusion.
B. Consider Addisonian crisis in any hypotensive patient not responding to traditional therapy.
C. Sepsis
D. Look for the trigger in adrenal crisis.

Diagnostic Testing

A. Complete blood count (CBC)
B. Comprehensive metabolic panel (CMP)
C. Venous blood gas (VBG)
D. Lactate
E. Urinalysis
F. Cortisol level with ACTH stimulation test (diagnostic test for Addison's)
G. Electrocardiogram
H. Pregnancy test, if indicated

Management

A. *Procedures*
   1. Manage airway and ventilation, if indicated.
   2. If rapid sequence intubation is needed, consider avoiding etomidate for induction in patients with Addison's disease as it has the potential to suppress cortisol formation.
B. *Pharmacologic therapies*
   1. Follow evidence-based guidelines when prescribing.
   2. Support perfusion and urine output with crystalloids, then vasopressors if needed.
      a. Consider use of D_5NS, if hypoglycemia is present.
   3. Administer hydrocortisone for adrenal crisis.
      a. Alternative is dexamethasone.
C. *Consultation/collaboration*
   1. Consult hospitalist, intensivist, endocrinologist.

Patient Disposition

A. *Transition of care information*
   1. Admit or transfer for inpatient or intensive care if in Addisonian crisis.
      a. If stable, then may be discharged home with close follow-up.
   2. Monitor mental status, vital signs, urine output, labs—glucose and potassium.
B. *Age and development considerations*
   1. Prevention and education
      a. Proper use of medications

b. For those with Addison's, stress the importance of taking replacement hormone as scheduled and notifying their clinician of any acute illness.
c. For those on chronic corticosteroids, stress the importance of not abruptly stopping the medication.

NORMAL PANCREATIC FUNCTION

The pancreas is mainly an exocrine gland and plays a significant role in digestion. Though only a small percent of its mass consists of the islets of Langerhans, its endocrine function has a significant influence on the metabolism of glucose, as well as lipids and proteins. There are four types of endocrine cells in the pancreas. Alpha cells release glucagon, beta cells secrete insulin and amylin, delta cells secrete somatostatin and gastrin, and gamma cells secrete pancreatic polypeptide. Glucagon is released in response to a drop in the serum glucose. Glucagon causes glycogenolysis, leading to the breakdown of glycogen and the release of glucose stores. Glucagon also increases gluconeogenesis in the liver, where proteins are converted to amino acids and then glucose. Lastly, glucagon activates lipase to increase the release of fatty acids from adipose stores and suppresses the storage of triglycerides.

Insulin is constantly released into the portal vein at a basal rate, and this rate changes to correspond to glucose levels. As glucose levels increase, so does the release of insulin; as the levels lower, so does the release of insulin. Insulin increases the activity of GLUT4, which increases the uptake of glucose by cells, especially skeletal muscles, adipose tissue, and the liver. Insulin inhibits gluconeogenesis by inhibiting the release of glucagon. Insulin also increases glycogenesis and lipogenesis and inhibits protein catabolism. Insulin is rapidly degraded by insulinase, which leads to a short half-life of only a few minutes. Amylin also inhibits the release of glucagon and slows gastrointestinal motility. Lastly, somatostatin and pancreatic polypeptide both regulate overall pancreatic function. Somatostatin suppresses the release of insulin, glucagon, pancreatic polypeptide, and other gastric hormones, along with reducing the blood supply to the gastrointestinal tract.

Lastly, there are two other hormones that play a role with glucose metabolism. They are often referred to as gut hormones or incretins. Glucagon-like peptide-1 (GLP-1) is released by cells in the small intestines and enhances insulin release in response to food intake. This gut hormone also decreases glucagon secretion, increases beta cell mass, promotes insulin sensitivity, and slows gastric emptying. GLP-1 is degraded by dipeptidyl peptidase-4 (DPP-4). Several newer medications either mimic GLP-1 or inhibit DPP-4 to augment this aspect of pancreatic function.

Diabetes Mellitus

Pathophysiology

Diabetes is separated into several types based on the accepted cause. Type 1 diabetes, formerly known as juvenile diabetes, has several theories as to why it exists, including genetic influences, autoimmune conditions, germ exposure or the lack thereof, and exposure to cow's milk. The common understanding is that with type 1, there is an autoimmune-type process, which leads to islet cell antibody production and cellular dysfunction, mainly beta cell atrophy. This often occurs during school age or adolescent years. Without beta cells, insulin secretion stops; without insulin, glucagon secretion increases and lipase increases the conversion of adipose tissue into fatty acids. Fatty acids now become the primary source of energy and lead to an increased production of ketone bodies; this accumulation reduces the body's pH. Without insulin, amino acids cannot enter cells as easily, and cell growth is reduced. This overall process leads to uncontrolled hyperglycemia, resulting from glycogenolysis and gluconeogenesis, which results from catabolism of proteins and adipose stores.

Without insulin replacement, patients with type 1 diabetes will develop diabetic ketoacidosis (DKA). There are four problems that occur with DKA: hyperglycemia, volume depletion, acidosis, and potassium depletion. The hyperglycemia causes osmotic diuresis leading to polyuria and eventual volume depletion. As volume is lost, perfusion is altered, and eventually a lactic acidosis may develop. Acidosis causes electrolyte shifts, leading to potassium being displaced from the intracellular space, which increases potassium loss during osmotic diuresis. Patients often develop a metabolic gap acidosis due to elevated ketone and lactate levels.

As with type 1 diabetes, some patients may develop type 1.5 diabetes, better known as latent autoimmune diabetes in adults (LADA). Unlike type 1, patients with LADA are usually adults whose beta cell function is so reduced they display indications of diabetes. The remainder of the pathophysiology is the same for patients with type 1, though it often progresses slower.

Type 2 diabetes is the most common form of diabetes seen today, accounting for roughly 90% of cases. Unlike type 1, patients with type 2 still produce insulin, but they either do not produce enough or have developed significant insulin resistance at the cellular level. There is no evidence of an autoimmune progress or antibody production. There may be a genetic connection, though. Most patients are adults when they develop type 2. Type 2 was previously referred to as adult-onset diabetes; however, it is now seen in pediatrics as well. Obesity is highly associated with the development of type 2 diabetes and is the main cause of insulin resistance and the reduced release of insulin. Resistance is associated with elevated levels of free fatty acids, which reduces glucose uptake at the cellular levels and stimulates the release of insulin. Over time, patients may have reduced insulin release as beta cells are exhausted from attempting to regulate the blood glucose as well as increased fatty acids levels.

Patients with type 2 usually do not develop DKA since they still produce some insulin, which suppresses ketosis and catabolism. These patients develop what is often referred to as hyperosmolar hyperglycemic syndrome or state (HHS). This syndrome is very similar to DKA, though it develops and progresses slower and usually does not involve a metabolic acidosis. Patients usually have a higher glucose level, more volume loss, a higher osmolality, and less potassium loss.

The fourth type of diabetes is gestational diabetes, sometimes labeled type 4. It is estimated that roughly 7% of pregnancies are affected by gestational diabetes. It is thought that some placental hormones increase insulin resistance or may reduce insulin production. Risk factors include those with a family history of diabetes, those who are obese, and women with increased maternal age. It is recommended that all pregnancies are screened for diabetes between 24 and 28 weeks. Gestational diabetes usually resolves after delivery, but it increases the risk for type 2 diabetes later.

There are several reasons a patient may experience hyperglycemia in addition to being a diabetic. This could be simply from a loss of insulin, such as a new onset of diabetes, noncompliance, or lack of access to medications. Corticosteroids, ischemia, and infection are other triggers that can lead to hyperglycemia and exacerbate diabetes.

Lastly, hypoglycemia is sometimes encountered with diabetics. It is more common in type 1 patients and those who take insulin or medications that increase insulin release. Patients usually develop hypoglycemia due to inadequate food intake, improperly timed insulin administration, or too much insulin administration. In rare cases, this can be caused by an insulinoma, hepatic, adrenal, or pituitary dysfunction.

Physical Examination

A. *Chief complaint:* Abnormal glucose reading, weakness, altered mental status (AMS), abdominal pain

B. *Signs and symptoms*

1. Polyuria, polydipsia, polyphagia (hyperglycemia)
2. Nausea, vomiting
3. Blurred vision (hyperglycemia)
4. Tachycardia
5. Hypotension
6. Tachypnea (DKA)
7. Altered mental status (AMS)
8. Seizures (hypoglycemia)
9. Fruity ketone breath (DKA)

C. *Focused assessment*

1. Airway, breathing, circulation (ABC)
2. Neurologic examination
3. Cardiovascular and respiratory examination
4. Abdominal examination

Differential Diagnoses

A. Always consider infection.

B. Monitor mental status and perfusion.

C. Too-rapid correction of hyperglycemia can lead to cerebral edema.

D. Hyponatremia will correct itself once perfusion is restored and the glucose normalizes.

E. Alcoholic ketoacidosis (DKA)

F. Other causes of a metabolic gap acidosis (DKA)

G. Overdose of a sulfonylurea (hypoglycemia)

Diagnostic Testing

A. Complete blood count (CBC)

B. Comprehensive metabolic panel (CMP)

C. Venous blood gas (VBG)

D. Lactate

E. Serum ketones

F. Urinalysis

G. Pregnancy test, if indicated

Management

A. *Procedures*

1. Manage airway and ventilations, if indicated.
   - **a.** If intubation is required, it must match the patient's preintubation minute volume.
   - **b.** Secure vascular access.

B. *Pharmacologic therapies*

1. Follow evidence-based guidelines when prescribing.
2. Support perfusion and urine output.
   - **a.** 0.9% normal saline (NS) or lactated Ringer (LR) to restore perfusion
   - **b.** 0.45% NS once perfusion is restored
   - **c.** D5 ½ NS once glucose is <250 to 300 mg/dL
3. Correcting hypoglycemia
   - **a.** If alert and protecting airway—give oral glucose.
   - **b.** Otherwise, administer dextrose.
   - **c.** If dextrose is not an option, consider glucagon.
   - **d.** Consider thiamine in malnourished patients and alcoholics.
4. Correcting hyperglycemia
   - **a.** Volume replacement as above
   - **b.** Initiate insulin replacement.
     - **i.** Evaluate glucose and potassium first.
     - **ii.** IV regular insulin bolus of 0.1 unit/kg
       - **(1)** Avoid in pediatrics.
       - **(2)** Often avoided in adults now, consider risk and benefits.
     - **iii.** IV regular insulin infusion at 0.1 unit/kg/hour
       - **(1)** Titrate to goal of 75 to 100 mg/dL/hour reduction.
       - **(2)** Slow reduction rate once glucose <250 mg/dL.
       - **(3)** Continue insulin until glucose is normalized and acidosis or gap is resolved.
     - **iv.** Replace potassium.
       - **(1)** If K^+ <3.3, must replace K^+ before insulin therapy.
       - **(2)** If K^+ <4, initiate IV K^+ replacement at 20 to 30 mEq/L with insulin.
       - **(3)** If K^+ 4 to 5, initiate IV K^+ replacement at 10 to 20 mEq/L with insulin.
       - **(4)** If K >5, no K replacement needed at this time.
     - **v.** Sodium bicarbonate therapy
       - **(1)** Bolus only to manage a hyperkalemic emergency
         - **(a)** 1 to 2 mEq/kg IV
5. *Consultation and collaboration:* Consult hospitalist, intensivist, endocrinologist.

Patient Disposition

A. *Transition of care information*

1. Admit or transfer for inpatient or intensive care if in DKA or HHS.

2. Hypoglycemia easily resolved and not on a sulfonylurea may be safe to discharge home, consider admission otherwise.
3. Monitor mental status, vital signs, urine output, labs—glucose, and potassium.

B. *Age and development considerations*
1. Prevention and education
a. Proper use of medications
b. Proper timing of insulin and meals
c. Consider if the patient on insulin has access to injectable glucagon.

THYROID CONDITIONS

The thyroid gland is integral to the metabolic processes of the body. Any disruption in thyroid function can result in a multitude of symptoms and sequela. Abnormal thyroid conditions often result in over or under production of important thyroid hormones. Some of these conditions can lead to the need for emergency treatment. It is important for the emergency nurse practitioner (ENP) to recognize the presentation of thyroid conditions and to manage appropriately.

The thyroid gland is in the anterior neck and controls the body's energy utilization, heat production, and growth, affecting multiple organ systems. It is controlled hormonally by the hypothalamus transmission of thyrotropin-releasing hormone (TRH) to the anterior pituitary gland. This in turn stimulates the pituitary gland to produce and secrete thyroid-stimulating hormone (TSH). When TSH reaches the thyroid gland, it triggers the production of thyroxine (T4) and triiodothyronine (T3). In a normally functioning thyroid, normal blood levels of T3 exert negative feedback to inhibit TRH and TSH release. When this feedback system or gland are not functioning normally, there is an over or under production of thyroid hormones resulting in hyper or hypothyroidism and the accompanying signs and symptoms. Severe conditions of both hyper and hypothyroidism may occur requiring access to immediate and lifesaving treatment.

Hyperthyroidism (Thyrotoxicosis)

Pathophysiology

Hyperthyroidism, also known as thyrotoxicosis, is a disorder caused by elevation of thyroid hormones thyroxine (T4) and triiodothyronine (T3). This can be the result of dysfunction of the thyroid gland (primary), or excess production of thyroid-releasing hormones (TRH) or thyroid-stimulating hormones (TSH) in the hypothalamus or pituitary, respectively (secondary). Thyrotoxicosis is defined as elevated thyroid hormones by any cause, including thyroid hormone drug overuse or overdose. The clinical signs and symptoms are caused by the increased sensitivity to catecholamines. Hyperthyroidism affects all organs but most specifically raises the basal metabolic rate and causes an increased adrenergic effect on the cardiovascular system. The most common form of primary hyperthyroidism is Grave's disease, which is an autoimmune disease. Grave's disease is distinguished by three common features, including goiter, ophthalmopathy, for example, exophthalmos, and dermopathy, for example, pretibial myxedema. Older adult patients may exhibit few symptoms of hyperthyroidism (apathetic hyperthyroidism) and, as a result, develop single organ failure or thyroid storm from lack of diagnosis and treatment.

Predisposing Factors

Primary hyperthyroidism is caused by Grave's disease in 85% of all cases and is most commonly found in females ages 20 to 40 years.

Physical Examination

A. *Common chief complaints:* Palpitations, nervousness

B. *Signs and symptoms*
1. Labile emotions, anxiety
2. Shortness of breath
3. Heat intolerance, sweating
4. Fatigue, weakness
5. Increased appetite but poor weight gain
6. Oligomenorrhea
7. Hair loss
8. Diarrhea

C. *Medication history for drug-induced hyperthyroidism*
1. Thyroid medications—including thyroid hormones not prescribed to patient
2. Amiodarone
3. Lithium
4. Iodine—after treatment or use of contrast agents
5. Interleukin-2, alpha-interferon

D. *Past medical history pertinent to condition*
1. Thyroid conditions
2. Pregnancy, current or recent

E. *Focused physical assessment*
1. *General:* Nervousness, agitation, flat affect, weight loss
2. *Skin:* Warm, moist, hair loss, palmar erythema, pretibial myxedema (skin thickening, nonpitting edema), onycholysis, thyroid acropachy (soft tissue edema and bone changes in fingers and toes)
3. *Eyes:* Lid lag, dry eye, chemosis (conjunctival edema), visual impairment, paralysis of extraocular movements, periorbital edema, proptosis
4. *Neck:* Thyroid bruit, thyroid enlargement or nodules, goiter, thyroid tenderness, cervical lymphadenopathy
5. *Cardiac:* Tachycardia, systolic hypertension, atrial fibrillation, wide pulse pressure, high-output congestive heart failure (CHF)
6. *Pulmonary:* Dyspnea
7. *Neurological:* Hyperreflexia, fine tremor, muscle wasting

Differential Diagnoses

A. Grave's disease
B. Toxic multinodular goiter
C. Toxic nodular goiter
D. Transient hyperthyroid phase of Hashimoto's thyroiditis
E. Thyroiditis (subacute, silent, and postpartum)
F. Hydatidiform mole secreting chorionic gonadotrophin, which has TSH-like effects

G. Ovarian teratoma containing thyroid tissue
H. Pituitary tumor, thyroid cancer
I. *Thyrotoxicosis factitia:* Ingestion of excessive amounts of T3; often to lose weight
J. *Thyroid medication misuse or abuse:* Abuse of thyroid hormone medications and underuse of prescribed antithyroid medication

Diagnostic Testing

A. *Thyrotropin (TSH):* Subnormal (usually undetectable)—TSH is recommended initial screening test as high levels of T3 and T4 inhibit production of TSH
B. *Triiodothyronine (T3) and/or free thyroxine (free T4):* Elevated
  1. Free thyroid hormone levels are preferable for diagnosis in patients taking protein binding drugs such as NSAIDs, estrogen, heparin, furosemides, salicylates, and so on.

Management

A. Pharmacologic therapies
  1. Follow the evidence-based guidelines when prescribing.
  2. Thiouracils (propylthiouracil [PTU]) and thiamazoles (methimazole and carbimazole) block production of thyroid hormones.
    a. Methimazole has less hepatic toxicity than PTU and is preferred in hyperthyroidism.
      i. PTU is recommended during the first trimester of pregnancy.
      ii. Take medication with food.
    b. Administered over 1 to 3 years and then tapered off while monitoring T3 and T4 levels
    c. Drug can be resumed if relapse occurs.
    d. *Side effects:* Rash, pruritus, elevated liver function, arthralgia, agranulocytosis (rare)
  3. Propranolol to block B-adrenergic receptors
    a. Use to treat tachycardia, hypertension, atrial fibrillation, fine tremor.
    b. Metoprolol or esmolol may be substituted for patients with asthma.

Patient Disposition

A. *Referral*
  1. Emergency nurse practitioner (ENP) consultation with internal medicine or endocrinologist should occur during ED visit to assure follow-up.
  2. Endocrinologist
    a. Monitor thyroid levels and adjust medication.
    b. Referral for radioactive iodine therapy or thyroid surgery if indicated
  3. Ophthalmology for any eye pathology noted
  4. Refer all patients with a palpable thyroid nodule for a fine needle aspiration biopsy to rule out carcinoma.
B. *Patient education*
  1. Follow-up with endocrinologist is a must for monitoring thyroid levels, medication adjustments, and for any adjunctive therapies needs.
  2. Stress importance of medication compliance to prevent thyroid storm.
  3. Hyperthyroid medications must be tapered and cannot be stopped abruptly unless directed by healthcare clinician.
  4. Hyperthyroidism may go into remission but advise patient that a relapse can occur.
  5. Keep thyroid medication in childproof container to prevent accidental ingestion.

Hypothyroidism (Primary and Secondary)

Pathophysiology

A. Hypothyroidism is a syndrome of inadequate thyroid hormone production causing a slowing of cellular metabolism. Primary hypothyroidism is the most common and is the result of thyroid gland failure. In adults, autoimmune thyroiditis (Hashimoto's thyroiditis) is the most common form, but primary hypothyroidism can also be the result of removal/ablation of the thyroid or treatment with certain medications. Dietary iodine is necessary for production of thyroid hormones, but deficiency in the diet is rarely a cause of hypothyroidism in the United States. Secondary hypothyroidism is the result of a lack of thyrotropin-releasing hormone (TRH) or thyroid-stimulating hormone (TSH) production by the hypothalamus or pituitary glands, respectively. All newborns are screened for hypothyroidism in the United States. Treatment must begin at birth to avoid permanent loss of growth potential and mental ability.

Predisposing Factors

Hypothyroidism is more prevalent in females and the risk increases with age. Management includes lifelong thyroid hormone replacement in most cases. Cessation of this hormone places the patient at risk for exacerbation of symptoms and myxedema crisis.

Physical Examination

A. *Common chief complaint:* Fatigue, weight gain
B. *Signs and symptoms*
  1. Fatigue, lethargy, cold intolerance
  2. Dry skin and hair
  3. Arthralgias, myalgias
  4. Gradual weight gain, facial, or extremity swelling
  5. Constipation
  6. Menstrual irregularities (menorrhagia)
  7. Depression
  8. *Newborn assessment:* Decreased activity, increased sleep, feeding difficulty, constipation, and prolonged jaundice
C. *Medication history for drug-induced hypothyroidism*
  1. Lithium
  2. Amiodarone
  3. Thyroid medications
D. *Past medical history pertinent to condition*
  1. Pregnancy, current or recent
  2. Iodine deficiency
  3. Neoplasms—brain, pituitary, lymphoma
  4. Tuberculosis
  5. Sarcoidosis
  6. Radiation therapy to neck, surgical removal of or ablation to thyroid gland

E. *Focused physical assessment*

1. *General:* Coarse voice, hypothermia, depressed mood
2. *Skin:* Dry skin/hair, hair loss, loss of outer half of eyebrows, pallor, nonpitting edema of extremities (myxedema), facial edema
3. *Eyes:* Periorbital edema
4. *Ears, nose, and throat (ENT):* Macroglossia, dysphagia
5. *Neck:* Thyroid nodules, goiter, or enlargement; thyroid tenderness, surgical scar, cervical lymphadenopathy
6. *Cardiac:* Bradycardia, angina, pericardial effusion, cardiomyopathy
7. *Pulmonary:* Shortness of breath, hypoventilation, pleural effusion
8. *Neurological:* Delayed reflexes, peripheral neuropathy

Differential Diagnoses

A. Hashimoto's thyroiditis (autoimmune)
B. Thyroiditis (subacute, silent, and postpartum)
C. *Thyroid medication–induced hypothyroidism:* Overuse of antithyroid or underuse of thyroid hormone medication
D. Thyroid cancer
E. Myxedema crisis
F. Pituitary or brain tumor

Diagnostic Testing

A. *Primary hypothyroidism:* TSH is elevated, total and free T4 and T3 are low.
B. *Secondary hypothyroidism:* TSH is low, total and free T4 and T3 are low.
C. TSH is a recommended initial screening test as low levels of T3 and T4 stimulate increased production of TSH.

Management

A. *Pharmacologic therapy*

1. Follow evidence-based guidelines when prescribing.
2. Levothyroxine: Synthetic thyroxine (T4)

Patient Disposition

A. *Patient education*

1. Primary hypothyroidism usually requires lifelong treatment.
2. Take oral levothyroxine 30 to 60 minutes before breakfast with full glass of water.
3. Levothyroxine is safe in pregnancy (Class A) and during breastfeeding.
   a. Important to continue levothyroxine during pregnancy to avoid adverse maternal and neonatal outcomes. Hypothyroidism must be followed closely in pregnancy as the thyroid hormone requirement increases due to the increased metabolic demands of the fetus. Levothyroxine dosage is adjusted as needed based on thyroid function tests performed regularly throughout the pregnancy.
4. Keep thyroid medication in childproof container to prevent accidental ingestion.
5. Thyroid medication should not be used for weight loss and can cause life-threatening toxicity.

B. *Follow-up and referral*

1. Instruct the patient to follow up with their primary care clinician for monitoring and further dose adjustments in 4 to 6 weeks.
2. Refer all patients with a palpable thyroid nodule for a fine needle aspiration biopsy to rule out carcinoma.

Myxedema Crisis

Pathophysiology

Myxedema crisis is a multiorgan response to untreated hypothyroidism resulting in decreased mental status (myxedema coma), hypothermia, and myxedema. Myxedema's nonpitting edema is caused by protein deposits in intradermal areas. Myxedema crisis has a high mortality rate and requires rapid management and intensive care admission.

Predisposing Factors

This crisis can be precipitated by thyroid medication noncompliance as well as many acute disorders and stressors such as surgery, certain medications, infection, cardiovascular events, cold exposure, and trauma.

Physical Examination

A. *Signs and symptoms*

1. Extreme weakness
2. Swelling to face and extremities
3. Lethargy, mental status change
4. Shortness of breath

B. *Focused physical assessment*

1. *General:* Hypothermia (<35.5°C), absence of shivering, normal temperature may indicate infection
2. *Skin:* Cool, pallor, facial edema, myxedema of lower extremities
3. *Cardiac:* Bradycardia, hypotension, pericardial effusion
4. *Pulmonary:* Hypoventilation, pleural effusion, upper airway obstruction due to glottic edema
5. *Neurological:* Altered mental status (AMS), prolonged relaxation phase of deep tendon reflex—twice the length of contraction phase

C. *Medication history for drug-induced myxedema crisis*

1. Thyroid medications
2. Beta-blockers
3. Sedatives, opioids
4. Phenothiazine
5. Amiodarone

D. *Past medical history pertinent to condition:* Thyroid disease

Differential Diagnoses

A. Sepsis
B. Hypoglycemia
C. Adrenal crisis
D. Toxin exposure

E. Drug overdose
F. Cerebral vascular event
G. CHF

Diagnostic Testing

A. Clinical diagnosis once hypothyroidism has been established.
B. Adjunctive diagnostics depend on suspected or known precipitating factors:
1. *Arterial blood gas (ABG):* Hypoxia
2. *EKG:* Cardiac event
3. *Blood chemistry, complete blood count (CBC):* Evaluating for anemia, infection, hyponatremia, hypoglycemia, elevated creatinine

Management

A. *Pharmacologic therapies*
1. Follow evidence-based guidelines when prescribing.
2. Thyroxine (T4)
OR
3. Triiodothyronine (T3)
a. Although T3 has a more rapid onset of action, it can cause cardiac arrhythmias and must be given with caution in patients with cardiac disease or if elderly.
4. If patient remains hemodynamically unstable, give both thyroxine and triiodothyronine.
5. Hydrocortisone, given to compensate for increased metabolic demand
6. Dextrose 50% IV if hypoglycemic
7. Vasopressors, if needed, must be started along with thyroid hormone replacement.

B. **Nonpharmacologic therapies**
1. Identify and treat precipitating factor.
2. Supportive treatment of cardiovascular and pulmonary systems
a. Airway management, oxygen, IV access, cardiac monitoring
3. Passive rewarming
4. Consider water restrictions if hyponatremic.

Patient Disposition

A. *Transition of care*
1. Requires admission to ICU with endocrine consult.
2. Precipitating factors may require additional consultation.

B. *Role of emergency nurse practitioner (ENP)*
1. Hemodynamic/mental status assessment and thyroid hormone replacement plan must be carefully recorded and communicated to clinician assuming care in ICU or other transfer unit.
2. Record and report any consultation that occurred in the ED to facilitate continuity of care.

C. ***Patient education***
1. Medication compliance with thyroid hormone replacement is important in preventing myxedema crisis.
2. Primary hypothyroidism usually requires lifelong treatment.

Thyroid Storm (Thyrotoxic Crisis)

Pathophysiology

Thyroid storm is a severe case of thyrotoxicosis. Although rare, this life-threatening thyrotoxic crisis usually occurs in those with Grave's disease and carries a high mortality rate (8%–25%) if not treated quickly and appropriately. Thyroid storm can be precipitated by many conditions including surgery, vigorous manipulation of thyroid gland, trauma, burns, infection, certain drugs, myocardial infarction (MI), cerebrovascular accidents, pulmonary emboli, diabetic ketoacidosis, childbirth, and eclampsia. The rapid rise in free hormone levels may be responsible for the crisis as often the resulting thyroid hormone levels are not higher than is seen in uncomplicated hyperthyroidism. The extreme response to catecholamines in thyroid storm is responsible for the severe symptoms associated. Clinical diagnosis of this condition is often complex due to the multisystem involvement including thermoregulatory, cardiovascular, gastrointestinal, and central nervous system.

Predisposing Factors

Most common predisposing factor is Grave's disease.

Physical Examination

A. *Chief complaint:* Palpitations, vomiting, diarrhea
B. *Signs and symptoms*
1. Fever
2. Palpitations
3. Agitation, impaired mental status
4. Vomiting, diarrhea

C. *Medications that may precipitate thyroid storm*
1. Amiodarone
2. Iodine
3. Thyroid hormone medication—overuse or overdose
4. Antithyroid medication withdrawal
5. Pseudoephedrine
6. Illicit drug use—sympathomimetics

D. *Past medical history pertinent to condition*
1. Hyperthyroidism, Grave's disease
2. Radioactive iodine therapy
3. Alcohol or drug abuse

E. *Focused physical assessment*
1. *General:* High fever, agitation, extreme lethargy (elderly)
2. *Skin:* Profuse sweating, jaundice
3. *Cardiac:* Tachycardia, pedal edema, atrial fibrillation, cardiac ischemia, widened pulse pressure, congestive heart failure (CHF), shock
4. *Pulmonary:* Shortness of breath, pulmonary edema
5. *Gastrointestinal:* Profuse vomiting and diarrhea, abdominal pain
6. *Neurologic:* Stupor, delirium, seizures, coma

Differential Diagnoses

A. Infection, sepsis
B. *Sympathomimetic ingestion:* Cocaine, amphetamines, ketamine, and so on
C. Heat exhaustion, heat stroke
D. Delirium tremens
E. Malignant hyperthermia

F. Hypothalamic stroke
G. Pheochromocytoma
H. *Drug withdrawal:* Cocaine, opioids
I. Psychosis
J. Organophosphate poisoning

Diagnostic Testing

A. Clinical diagnosis once hyperthyroidism has been established as underlying condition

B. *Scoring system:* Burch–Wartofsky Point Scale (BWPS) diagnostic criteria to distinguish likelihood of thyroid storm versus uncomplicated hyperthyroidism. Scoring is determined by the presence of elevated body temperature, tachycardia, atrial fibrillation, CHF, agitation, delirium, psychosis, stupor, seizure, and coma, as well as nausea, vomiting, diarrhea, hepatic failure (jaundice), and the presence of an identified precipitant. Treatment should be initiated with a diagnosis of thyroid storm if the score is greater than or equal to 45. Scores of 25 to 45 are diagnostic of impending storm and scores <25 are indicative of low likelihood of thyroid storm (Table 19.1).

C. Adjunctive diagnostics depending on suspected or known precipitating factors

1. *EKG:* MI, atrial fibrillation
2. *Electrolytes:* Fluid depletion, hyperglycemia
3. *Complete blood count (CBC), chest x-ray (CXR):* Infection
4. *Thyroid hormone levels:* Not diagnostic but helpful as baseline

Management

A. *Pharmacologic therapies*

1. Follow evidence-based guidelines when prescribing.
2. Thiouracil to inhibit new thyroxine (T4) production
   a. Propylthiouracil (PTU) is favored in treatment of thyroid storm because it also decreases conversion of T4 to triiodothyronine (T3). Available orally or rectally but not intravenously (IV).
3. Nonradioactive iodine administration to decrease new thyroid hormone synthesis

   Saturated solution potassium iodide (SSKI) to inhibit thyroid hormone release

   a. Must be administered at least 60 minutes after administration of PTU and PTU must be continued during iodine (SSKI) therapy

   OR

   b. Lugol's solution
      i. Must be administered at least 60 minutes after administration of PTU and PTU must be continued during iodine (Lugol) therapy
4. Propranolol to block beta-adrenergic receptors and decrease conversion of T4 to T3
5. Hydrocortisone to prevent adrenal insufficiency
6. Treat fever with acetaminophen as salicylates may increase free thyroid hormone.
7. Inotropic agent, diuretics, sympatholytics as needed for CHF, atrial fibrillation, and so on

B. *Nonpharmacologic therapies*

1. Supportive treatment of cardiovascular and pulmonary systems

TABLE 19.1 BURCH AND WARTOFSKY POINT SCALE (BWPS) DIAGNOSTIC CRITERIA FOR THYROID STORM

THERMOREGULATORY DYSFUNCTION	POINTS	CARDIOVASCULAR DYSFUNCTION	POINTS
Temperature:	5	**Tachycardia:**	5
99–99.9	10	90–109	10
100–100.9	15	110–119	15
101–101.9	20	120–129	20
102–102.9	25	130–139	25
103–103.9	30	≥140	0
≥104.0		**Congestive Heart Failure:**	5
		Absent	10
		Mild (pedal edema)	15
		Moderate (bibasilar rales)	0
		Severe (pulmonary edema)	10
CENTRAL NERVOUS SYSTEM EFFECTS		**Atrial Fibrillation:**	
		Absent	
Absent	0	Present	
Mild (agitation)	10		
Moderate (delirium, psychosis, extreme lethargy)	20		
Severe (seizure, coma)	30		
GASTROINTESTINAL-HEPATIC DYSFUNCTION		**PRECIPITANT HISTORY**	
Absent	0	Negative	0
Moderate (diarrhea, nausea/vomiting, abdominal pain)	10	Positive	10
Severe (unexplained jaundice)	20		

Scoring: 45 or greater is highly suggestive of thyroid storm; 25–44 is suggestive of thyroid storm; <25 is unlikely to represent thyroid storm.

Source: Burch HB, Wartofsky L. Life-threatening thyrotoxicosis: Thyroid storm. *Endocrinol Metab Clin North Am.* 1993; 22 (2) 263–277. https://doi.org/10.1016/S0889-8529(18)30165-8.

a. Airway management, oxygen, IV access, cardiac monitoring
2. Aggressive IV fluid replacement including dextrose if low serum glucose
3. *External cooling:* Cooling blankets, ice packs
4. Treat precipitating factor.

Patient Disposition

A. *Referral and transition of care*
1. Requires admission to ICU with endocrine consult
2. Precipitating factors may require additional consultation.
3. Severe, refractory thyroid storm may require alternative treatments:
a. Therapeutic plasma exchange to remove thyroid hormone
b. Emergency surgical intervention to remove all or part of the thyroid gland

B. *Emergency nurse practitioner (ENP) role*
1. Hemodynamic assessment and antihyperthyroidism treatment plan must be carefully recorded and communicated to clinician assuming care in ICU or other transfer unit.
2. Record and report any consultation that occurred in the ED to facilitate continuity of care.

C. *Patient education*
1. Compliance with hyperthyroidism medication prescribed dosing can help prevent thyroid storm.
2. Keep thyroid medication in childproof container to prevent accidental ingestion.
3. Continued treatment for hyperthyroidism is needed once thyroid storm resolves.
4. Patients taking Amiodarone require regular monitoring of thyroid levels as the high iodine content, when taken chronically, can precipitate thyroid storm.
5. Thyroid hormone medication should not be used for weight loss and can cause life-threatening toxicity.

PITUITARY CONDITIONS

Diabetes Insipidus (Central)

Pathophysiology

Central diabetes insipidus (DI) is a deficiency of antidiuretic hormone (ADH), otherwise known as arginine vasopressin (AVP), which is produced by the posterior pituitary. The function of ADH is to promote water reabsorption in the distal renal tubules. The lack of ADH results in excretion of large volumes of dilute urine. A less severe type of DI is nephrogenic and is caused by end-organ resistance to ADH, which will not be discussed in this section. Central DI can be inherited as an autosomal dominant mutation, or it can be secondary to other disorders. Some of the causes of central DI include infections such as meningitis, pituitary tumors, traumatic brain injury, neurosurgery, autoimmune conditions, or anorexic encephalopathy. Because the primary presentation of DI includes polyuria and polydipsia, the concern is whether the patient can take in enough fluid to counter the increased urine output. This balance is needed to prevent hyponatremia and decreased serum osmolality.

Predisposing Factors

Central DI can be a genetic condition in which the AVP producing neurons do not function normally. Secondary causes include traumatic brain injury, anoxic encephalopathy, meningitis, and as a result of brain death.

Physical Examination

A. *Chief complaint:* Increased urination, increased thirst

B. *Signs and symptoms*
1. Nocturia (often first sign)
2. Abrupt onset increased, dilute "like water" urine
3. Dry mouth
4. *Dehydration indicators:* Fatigue, tachycardia, dry skin, headache

C. *Medication history*
1. Phenothiazine (dry mouth)
2. Diuretic misuse or abuse

D. *Past medical history*
1. Diabetes mellitus
2. Family history of central DI
3. Recent head trauma or neurosurgery
4. *Sarcoidosis:* Infiltration of pituitary
5. Anorexia nervosa
6. Brain tumor
7. *Current pregnancy:* Central DI may first appear during pregnancy.
8. Psychiatric illness

E. *Focused physical assessment*
1. *General:* Fatigue, altered mental status, extreme weight loss
2. *Skin:* Dry oral mucosa, poor skin turgor
3. *Cardiac:* Tachycardia
4. *Genitourinary (GU):* Enlarged prostate; clear, large volume urine

Differential Diagnoses

A. Idiopathic central DI
B. *Primary polydipsia (psychogenic polydipsia):* Intentional increase in water intake
C. Uncontrolled or new-onset diabetes mellitus
D. Resolution of urinary tract obstruction
E. *Prostate hypertrophy:* Nocturia
F. Familial central DI (rare)

Diagnostic Testing

A. *Electrolytes/glucose:* Rule out hyponatremia, hyperglycemia
1. Polyuria is defined as urine output exceeding 3 L/day in adults and 2 L/m^2 in children.

B. Urine osmolarity <200 mosm/L is indicative of DI.

C. *Water deprivation test:* Complete fluid restriction will indicate a diagnosis of DI if serum sodium and osmolality increase in response.

D. Vasopressin 5 units IV is administered to determine central versus nephrogenic DI.
1. *Central DI:* Urine osmolality increases by 50% immediately.
2. *Nephrogenic DI:* Urine osmolality is unchanged.

Management

A. *Pharmacologic therapies*

1. Follow evidence-based guidelines when prescribing.
2. Vasopressin 2 to 5 units subcutaneously every 4 to 6 hours to prevent water loss
   a. Monitor serum sodium to avoid hyponatremia, water intoxication.
3. IV fluid replacement may be necessary until vasopressin takes effect.

Patient Disposition

A. *Consultation/collaboration*

1. Requires ICU admission with immediate consultation by endocrinology and neurology to find cause of central DI.

B. *Transition of care information*

1. Hemodynamic assessment, urine output, and vasopressin treatment plan must be carefully recorded and communicated to clinician assuming care in ICU or other transfer unit.
2. Record and report any consultation that occurred in the ED to facilitate continuity of care.

C. ***Patient education***

1. ADH replacement therapy may be required for life.
2. Genetic testing is recommended for suspected familial central DI.

NORMAL PITUITARY FUNCTION

The pituitary gland has wide-reaching effects on body functions. It is regulated by the hypothalamus and, when stimulated, secretes hormones that regulate the function of other glands or organs. This relationship is called the hypothalamic–pituitary axis (HPA).

Anatomy

The pituitary gland is located in the brain at the base of the skull and has two distinct functioning areas. The anterior pituitary secretes the adrenocorticotropic hormone (ACTH), follicle-stimulating hormone (FSH), luteinizing hormone (LH), growth hormone (GH), prolactin, and thyroid-stimulating hormone (TSH). The posterior pituitary secretes two hormones including vasopressin, also named antidiuretic hormone (ADH), and oxytocin. Any condition that interferes with the pituitary release of these hormones has far-reaching effects on the body. Thyroid, adrenal, and renal disorders related to the pituitary function will be discussed in the respective chapters.

Pituitary Apoplexy (Acute Hypopituitarism)

Pathophysiology

Pituitary apoplexy is the destruction of pituitary tissue leading to acute dysfunction and resulting in hormone deficiency and lack of regulation of the many organs and glands that the pituitary controls. The specific hormone deficiency can vary dependent on the cause of the destruction and location within the hypothalamic–pituitary–adrenal (HPA). The most common causes of pituitary apoplexy are pituitary adenoma, traumatic brain injury, aneurysmal subarachnoid hemorrhage (SAH), and Sheehan's syndrome. These result in inflammation, infarct, or hemorrhage into the pituitary gland causing it to be dysfunctional and creating accompanying signs and symptoms. Although the condition is rare, risk of mortality is high secondary to the loss of these regulatory hormones, especially adrenocorticotropic hormone (ACTH).

Predisposing Factors

Acute pituitary apoplexy is rare but occurs most often in ages 50 to 60 years. In most cases, an undiagnosed pituitary tumor is the cause.

Physical Examination

A. *Chief complaint:* Severe headache, sudden onset

B. *Signs and symptoms*

1. Retro-orbital, bifrontal, or suboccipital headache; may be described as thunderclap headache
2. *Visual changes or loss:* Optic nerve compression
3. Nausea, vomiting
4. *Symptoms of acute lack of ACTH:* Vomiting, hypotension, hyponatremia, polyuria, polydipsia

C. *Medications that may precipitate pituitary apoplexy*

1. Immunotherapy for cancer
2. Anticoagulant therapy

D. *Past medical history pertinent to condition*

1. Pituitary surgery or brain radiation therapy
2. Brain tumor—primary or metastatic
3. Recent head trauma or low-intensity repeated head trauma
4. *Pregnancy:* Pituitary gland increases in size during pregnancy
5. Recent cerebral angiography

E. *Focused physical assessment*

1. *General:* altered mental status (AMS)
2. *Eyes:* Reduced visual acuity or visual loss, ophthalmoplegia, visual field defects (bitemporal hemianopsia), ocular palsy (third cranial nerve—ptosis, limited eye movements in adduction, mydriasis), photophobia
3. *Cardiac:* Hypotension
4. *Neurological:* Cranial nerve palsies, meningismus (meningeal signs not caused by meningitis)

Differential Diagnoses

A. Hemorrhage or infarct caused by pituitary adenoma

B. Traumatic brain injury

C. Subarachnoid hemorrhage

D. Sheehan's syndrome—pituitary infarct secondary to postpartum hemorrhage and resulting hypoperfusion of pituitary gland

E. Meningitis

F. Migraine headache

G. Lymphocytic hypophysitis—inflammation of pituitary in pregnancy/postpartum or in those receiving immunotherapy for cancer

Diagnostic Testing

A. *Serum cortisol level:* Low

B. *Serum ACTH level:* Low

C. Electrolytes, thyroid function: hyponatremia, low triiodothyronine (T3), thyroxine (T4)
D. *CT scan (noncontrast):* Most available and will rule out subarachnoid hemorrhage (SAH), intrasellar mass
E. *MRI:* Imaging of choice to detect new bleeding

Management

A. *Pharmacologic therapies*
- **1.** Follow evidence-based guidelines when prescribing
- **2.** *ACTH replacement:* Critical hormone deficiency and should be addressed without waiting for diagnostic confirmation

Patient Disposition

A. *Consultation/collaboration*
- **1.** Requires ICU admission with immediate consultation by endocrinology, ophthalmology, and neurology
- **2.** May require urgent neurosurgical consultation and intervention

B. *Transition of care information*
- **1.** Hemodynamic assessment and hydrocortisone replacement treatment plan must be carefully recorded and communicated to clinician assuming care in ICU or other transfer unit.
- **2.** Record and report any consultation that occurred in the ED to facilitate continuity of care.

C. *Patient education*
- **1.** Hormone replacement therapy may be required for life.
- **2.** Permanent vision impairment may result from optic nerve atrophy.
- **3.** Advise helmet use in high-risk activities for all ages.

Additional Reading

Additional Reading for this chapter are online only and can be found at https://connect.springerpub.com/content/reference-book/978-0-8261-6091-5/part/part02/toc-part/ch19.

20. Inflammatory and Immunologic Conditions

TRACY BROWN

Learning Objectives

- Identify and treat isolated joint conditions.
- Identify and treat multiple joint conditions.
- Identify risks and benefits of joint injections and the medications to be used.
- Identify information obtained from a joint aspirate and utilize the information to determine treatment.
- Identify systemic lupus erythematosus specific risks associated with a patient's chief complaint, evaluate the additional differential diagnoses, and treat.
- Identify systemic lupus erythematosus complications and treat.
- Identify presentations in the systemic lupus erythematosus patient requiring consultation or referral to a specialist for further care.
- Identify allergic reactions and anaphylaxis and treat the conditions.
- Identify dermatologic disorders utilizing the algorithm.

The topics of inflammation and immunology encompass a vast expanse of information associated with most organ systems within the human body. Each area of discussion in and of itself contains enough information to consume an entire book. The focus here is to provide the clinician with general knowledge of topics, which may not be considered mainstream emergency medicine. Additionally, this chapter looks at the ED visit as it relates to the topic, including how best to initiate treatment and incorporate consultation and/or referral to a specialist for further evaluation, definitive diagnosis, and long-term patient treatment. While some procedures are discussed in the section on invasive evaluation and treatment, the ENP needs to reference a procedure text (e.g., *Essential Procedures for Emergency, Urgent, and Primary Care Settings*, 3rd Ed. [Campo T, Lafferty K, Eds.])[1] and watch a procedural video before performing any procedure. It is important for ENPs to be aware of the procedures they have been credentialed to perform at their facility.

Pain to an Isolated Joint[2]

Signs and Symptoms—Noted to One Joint

A. Swelling to joint area
B. Erythema to joint area
C. Warm to the touch
D. Clicking or popping sounds or sensations with movement
E. Crepitus with passive movement of the joint
F. Radiation of pain from joint
G. Decreased range of motion (ROM), inability to fully extend or flex
H. Joint deviation/subluxation of joint
I. Changes in surrounding tissues

Diagnostic Laboratory Testing and Imaging

A. Labs
  1. Complete blood count (CBC)
  2. Erythrocyte sedimentation rate (ESR)
  3. C-reactive protein (CRP)
  4. Prolactin level
  5. Complete metabolic panel as needed
  6. Coagulation studies as needed
  7. Additional studies specific to disease process noted below

B. Imaging
  1. *Radiographs:* Evaluate for acute injury. Acute nontraumatic problems will show no changes. Chronic conditions will show changes that have occurred over a period of time.
  2. *CT/MRI:* Early bone changes are more easily identified with these forms of imaging.

C. Synovial fluid evaluation
  1. Cell counts and differentials including polymorphonucleocytes
  2. Aerobic and anaerobic cultures
  3. Gram stain
  4. Monosodium urate (MSU) crystals
  5. Lactate
  6. Lactate dehydrogenase

Diagnosis and Treatment

A. Specialist consultation should be considered; orthopedics, rheumatology, and infectious disease as indicated. Information specific to a particular diagnosis is below.
  1. Acute articular problems
    a. Septic arthritis[2,3]
      i. 75% to 90% of organisms associated with diagnosis are gram-positive, such as methicillin-resistant *Staphylococcus aureus* (MRSA). 10% to

20% of organisms are gram-negative. The rest of the cases are associated with fungal, anerobic bacteria, and other atypical organisms.

ii. Special population organism considerations

(1) *Sickle cell patients: Salmonella*

(2) *Intravenous drug users: Staphylococcus aureus (Staph a), Streptococcus*, gram-negative organisms

(3) *Infants*: *Staph a*, group B *Streptococcus*, gram-negative organisms

(4) *Children: Staph a, Haemophilus influenza*

(5) *Adolescence and adults: Neisseria gonorrhoeae, Chlamydia trachomatis*

(6) *Geriatrics: Staph a, Streptococcus*, Gram-negative organisms

iii. Laboratory and radiographic study findings

(1) *CBC:* Expected elevated white blood cells (WBC)

(2) *CRP:* Expected elevation

(3) *ESR:* Expected elevation

(4) *Polymorphonucleocyte levels:* Expected elevation

(5) *Lactate:* >5.6 mmol/L

(6) *Lactate dehydrogenase (LDH):* >250 U/L

(7) *Radiographs:* Osteomyelitis evaluation

(8) *Synovial fluid WBC:* Levels from 50,000 to 150,000 micro/L

iv. Treatment[2,4]

(1) Follow evidence-based guidelines when prescribing.

(2) Admission for IV antibiotic therapy

(3) While testing is pending, starting vancomycin 15 mg/kg BID is acceptable.

(4) *Gram-positive organisms:* Vancomycin[5]

(5) *Gram-negative organisms:* Ceftriaxone or cefotaxime

(6) *Pseudomonas:* Ceftazidime or cefepime *and* ciprofloxacin or gentamycin[5]

(7) *Vancomycin allergy alternatives:* Daptomycin or clindamycin

(8) *Immunocompromised patients and intravenous drug users:* Vancomycin *and* ceftazidime or cefepime for Pseudomonas coverage

(9) IV treatment lasts 2 to 4 weeks followed by oral therapy for 2 to 6 weeks.

v. Open arthrotomy (specialist intervention)

(1) Failed antibiotic therapy

(2) Osteomyelitis

(3) Hip or shoulder joint involvement

(4) Prosthesis associated with infection

Disseminated Gonococcal Infection[6]

A. Types of infection

1. *Purulent arthritis:* Septic arthritis form of the problem

2. *Arthritis-dermatitis syndrome:* Symptoms of dermatitis over joint, tenosynovitis, and isolated join pain or polyarthralgia

B. Predisposing factors

1. A mucosal infection that is asymptomatic, resulting in delayed diagnosis and beginning antibiotic treatment[7,8]

2. Recent menstruation that can alter the bacteria's cell membranes;[9] these changes in the membrane allow the bacteria to avoid adhering to neutrophils,[10] while having a greater adherence for the fallopian tubes.[11]

3. Normal pregnancy changes are suspected in the increased risk of the disease between pregnancy and postpartum.[12,13]

4. Research on increased risk in lupus patients is still conflicting.

Signs and Symptoms

A. Arthralgias in multiple joints that may migrate

1. Arthritis in one or more joints

2. Tenosynovitis—hallmark distinction between other septic arthritis types[14]

3. Dermatitis to skin over joint

4. Fever

5. Genitourinary symptoms

Laboratory Studies

A. Blood cultures, typically negative

B. Skin lesion scraping (if done), typically negative

C. Synovial fluid culture is positive only about 50% of the time. Lab notification of disseminated gonococcal infection (DGI) evaluation is necessary to assure specimen is prepared correctly.

D. Mucosal site specimens typically test positive for *Neisseria gonorrhoeae*, while patient remains asymptomatic for disease in the location.

Treatment

A. *Initial therapy (preferred regimen):* Ceftriaxone and azithromycin[15]

B. Doxycycline may be substituted for azithromycin.

C. Length of treatment

1. *Arthritis (dermatitis syndrome):* Ceftriaxone until patient begins improving; 24 to 48 hours after improvement begins, the patient can be switched over to ceftriaxone intramuscularly.[15]

2. *Purulent arthritis:* Ceftriaxone should continue for 7 to 14 days.

D. Ceftriaxone allergy[6]

1. Skin testing is required to confirm allergy and severity.

2. Patient will require desensitization for administration of the medication.

3. Patient who has developed Stevens–Johnson syndrome will need a specialist who is highly specialized in the disease process for treatment.

Special Considerations

A. *Coinfection of chlamydia:* Azithromycin will cover infection.

B. *Partner treatment:* Anyone with sexual contact within the last 60 days prior to a patient's diagnosis treat with ceftriaxone (intramuscularly) and azithromycin.

SPECIFIC DIFFERENTIAL DIAGNOSES TO CONSIDER WITH DISSEMINATED GONOCOCCAL INFECTION: HEPATITIS B VIRAL INFECTIONS, HIV, SYPHILIS, AND HERPES SIMPLEX VIRUS

Gout[2,16]

Diagnosis-Specific Information

A. *Population:* Middle age and postmenopausal
B. *Risk factors:* Diabetes, hypertension, obesity, use of thiazide diuretics and cyclosporins
C. Increased risk with high-purine diets, high-fructose syrup, and soft drinks[17]
D. Decreased risk with increased coffee intake and dairy intake[16]
E. *Pathophysiology:* Inflammation as a result of excess uric acid from oversaturated fluid outside of cells
F. 90% of patients will end up having a classic presentation in the great toe.
G. Other joints involved include ankle and foot bones.
H. Polyarticular gout flares are possible but rare.

Diagnostic Tests

A. Laboratory studies
- **1.** Gold standard is synovial fluid test for (monosodium urate [MSU]) crystals
- **2.** Synovial fluid white blood cells (WBC) count may be elevated.
- **3.** C-reactive protein (CRP) and erythrocyte sedimentation rate (ESR) will show general inflammation only if elevated.
- **4.** Serum uric acid may or may not be elevated.

B. Radiographic changes
- **1.** Acute onset will not have any changes aside from soft tissue swelling.
- **2.** Chronic ongoing disease, radiographic changes will appear as bone erosions in the bone surrounding joints affected with the disease.
- **3.** MRI will denote erosions on the bones or gouty tophi.
- **4.** Ultrasound (US) used for early evaluation of the disease process. A hyperechoic linear density is seen on the joint cartilage (double contour sign).[18,19]

Treatment[16]

A. Follow evidence-based guidelines when prescribing.
B. Glucocorticoids
- **1.** Contraindicated when perceived flare is accompanied by a fever; further evaluation is needed to identify diagnosis.
- **2.** Taper as needed to prevent rebound flare to start when the flare resolves.
- **3.** Intraarticular route is an option with gout flares involving only one joint.

C. NSAIDs
- **1.** Treatment recommendations include potent options in drug class (e.g., naproxen, indomethacin).
- **2.** Multiple options exist in the drug class. Use maximum dose for pain control during flare unless contraindicated.

D. Colchicine[20]
- **1.** Good alternative to glucocorticoids or NSAIDs
- **2.** Best when started within the first 24 hours of the flare
- **3.** Good option for flare-ups when the patient is on prophylactic therapy
- **4.** Warning when using with renal or hepatic dysfunction patients
- **5.** The drug goes through cytochrome p450 system.

Pseudogout or Calcium Pyrophosphate Dihydrate Deposition Disease[21]

Diagnosis-Specific Information

A. The majority of patients are asymptomatic with the respect of calcium deposits within joints.
B. Symptoms can range from mild pain and stiffness to an acute attack mimicking gout, where the name pseudogout comes from. There is now a classification system to encompass all the types of calcium pyrophosphate dihydrate (CPPD) seen. The disease can mimic other arthritis types, thus leading to classification names such as pseudo-rheumatoid arthritis (pseudo-RA) and pseudo-osteoarthritis (pseudo-OA).[22]
C. *Complication:* Acute calcified periarthritis is where the crystals leak into the surrounding tissue. Anti-inflammatory therapy aids in resolution of symptoms, which usually occurs within a week.[2]

Diagnostic Studies

A. Labs
- **1.** Synovial fluid evaluation of the affected joint
  - **a.** Identification of calcium pyrophosphate crystals requires special microscopic identification.
  - **b.** Fluid leukocytosis from 15,000 to 30,000/mm[33] and as high as 100,000/mm[33]

B. Radiographs
- **1.** Calcium pyrophosphate deposits are noted on plain films, CT, and ultrasound (US).
- **2.** MRI is not as effective in identifying deposits.
- **3.** US images show double contour sign as in gout.
- **4.** Plain film images that better show diagnosis include
  - **a.** *Knee:* Anterior to posterior
  - **b.** *Pelvis/symphysis pubis:* Anterior to posterior
  - **c.** *Wrist:* Posterior to anterior

Treatment[23]

A. *Multiple joint treatment:* Follow gout flare treatment recommendations as above.
B. *Single joint treatment:* When joint aspirate is done, joint injection recommended. Symptoms expected to resolve in 48 to 72 hours.

Hemarthrosis[24]

Signs and Symptoms

Severity and onset of each symptom varies based on the reason for the development of the hemarthrosis, and while typically seen in knee joints, it may also be seen in other joints of the body.

A. Pain
B. Swelling
C. Decreased range of motion (ROM)
D. Stiffness
E. Warm to the touch
 1. Traditional traumatic onset of hemarthrosis is the most common cause of the diagnosis.
F. The trauma is a twisting motion or loading injury to the knee joint.[25,26]
G. Anterior cruciate ligament tear is found in 70% of traumatic cases.[25] Positive drawer test will be identified on exam.
H. Treatment involves aspiration of the tense effusion, consultation to a specialist for urgent arthroscopy.
I. Pediatric patients will frequently present with a patellar subluxation injury.[26]
J. Pediatric patients will need rapid intervention. It has been identified that a pediatric patient's growing joint cartilage is damaged when the cartilage is exposed to blood.[18]

Diagnosis in Patients With Bleeding Disorders

A. Most common diagnosis associated with the musculoskeletal system in patients with hemophilia.[24] The diagnosis can be chronic, subacute, or acute.
B. Minimal trauma or no trauma at all can cause the diagnosis in the hemophilia population.
C. Damage of cartilage tissue in hemophilia patients can come from the tissue being exposed to blood in as little as 2 days.[27,28]
D. Hemarthrosis is not usually seen with platelet problems, but more often with coagulation factor deficiencies.
E. Elbow and ankle joints are affected as well.
F. Patients with chronic hemarthrosis are noted to complain of tingling in the joint shortly prior to new swelling from a new bleed.[29]
G. Specialist consultation should include hematology as well as orthopedics.
 1. Atypical causes of hemarthrosis
H. *Postoperative:* Uncommon problem postarthroplasty, but can occur up to a year postsurgery. Thus, diagnosis should be considered in nontraumatic pain in a joint that has had prior surgical procedure. Specialist consultation needed for treatment.
I. *Osteoarthritis:* Mild bleeding only; the problem is uncommon but possible.
J. *Vascular causes:* Aneurisms to the peripheral arteries, usually postprocedure in nature, and vitamin C deficiency can make vascular walls fragile, leading to the problem.[30] Vitamin deficiency can add to any other predisposing factors. Specialist consultation needed for treatment. Patient may require surgical revision or a vascular specialist for possible embolization therapy.[31,32]
K. *Septic arthritis:* Bacterial-associated infection can, on a rare occasion, lead to hemarthrosis without prior trauma.[31]
L. Tumors
 1. *Synovial hemangiomas:* Type of vascular tumor usually associated with knee joints. This tumor is more common in children. Should be considered when patient has multiple episodes of isolated joint hemarthrosis.[33]
 2. *Tenosynovial giant cell tumor (TGCT):* Previously referred to as pigment villonodular synovitis (PVNS), affects the ankle, knee, hip, and elbow joints. The patient has history of atraumatic joint swelling episodes. Specialist's outpatient follow-up is needed on patients with repeat visits of this nature. MRI will identify the diagnosis, as well as special synovial fluid testing.
M. *Neurologic disorders:*[34] Charcot's arthropathy, also known as neuropathic arthropathy, previously associated with syphilis, now associated with diabetes,[35] predisposes patients to developing a hemarthrosis. The disease process in the joint involves the buildup of debris in the joint space that includes bone and cartilage.

Laboratory and Radiographic Studies

A. Synovial fluid testing
 1. Color ranging from pink, red, to brown
 2. *Lipohemarthrosis:* The presence of fat deposits in the fluid associated with capsule disruption and extensive soft tissue injury within the joint
 3. True hemarthrosis, blood will not clot upon obtaining via needle aspirate because of the chronic fibrinolysis. Blood associated with a traumatic tap will clot.[31]
 4. Special population with bleeding disorders requires additional blood work to include prothrombin time, partial thromboplastin time, and specific test associated with specific disorder diagnosis.
B. Radiographs
 1. Imaging identifies acute injury associated with the potential diagnosis of hemarthrosis.
 2. Fluid layers can be seen in imaging and can identify particulates within the fluid. If two layers are seen, the diagnosis of lipohemarthrosis can be made.[36] Easier seen with CT or MRI.

Treatment of Hemarthrosis

A. General acute treatment includes immobilization, compression, and ice.
B. Tense effusions may require evacuation.
C. Cyclooxygenase (COX) 2 inhibitor for
 1. Anti-inflammatory properties and pain relief
 2. Traditional NSAIDs should be avoided for the first 48 to 72 hours post-injury.
D. Pain control should be individually evaluated for choice in medications.
E. Postacute treatment
 1. Traditional NSAIDs may be used.
 2. Continue compression and ice therapy.
F. Other treatment options have been noted in the individual sections.

Special Considerations

Anticoagulation therapy

A. Major hemarthrosis in these patients is rare.
B. Patients can undergo arthrocentesis for therapeutic or simple diagnostic purposes without reversing therapy.[37,38]
C. If repeat hemarthrosis diagnosis continues, another reason for the diagnosis needs to be looked for.

CHRONIC ARTICULAR PROBLEMS

Osteoarthritis or Degenerative Joint Disease[39,40]

Diagnosis-Specific Information

A. Risk factors associated with degenerative joint disease (DJD) include age, gender, genetics, joint alignment, joint injury history, and obesity.[41]
B. Inflammatory mediators and how they affect the breakdown of the joints have been researched extensively, and thus treatments are now being developed based on the individual markers.
C. Disease is now viewed as a chronic disease state and thus care is based on this premise.
D. Affects older generations
E. Crepitus is noted on passive range of motion evaluation frequently.
F. Multiple assessment tools are used for evaluation of treatment. The tools are used mainly in research only; however, there are a few clinicians who are beginning to use them to evaluate outcomes.

Diagnostic Testing

A. There are no laboratory studies or radiographic studies that are used to assess the disease process.
B. Radiographic imaging is used in the ED to rule out any organic problems.
C. Osteoarthritis is sometimes seen measured on radiographs by a radiologist. One type of scoring system is the Kellgren–Lawrence classification system. It grades the severity of osteoarthritis on a scale from 0 to 4. Osteophyte presentation, size, and quantity are considered along with joint space narrowing.[42]

Treatment

A. Focused on minimizing pain, minimizing joint damage, and optimizing joint function. The specific joint along with the number of joints plays a role in treatment plan.
B. Lifestyle changes
  1. Self-management programs are done in a variety of ways and have been shown to be more beneficial than traditional treatment.[43,44] The key to this type of program involves patient input.
  2. Realistic expectations should be included in patient education.
  3. Exercise has found to improve pain and function as well as NSAIDs.[45] A combination of strength training and aerobic exercise is recommended.
  4. A weight reduction in obese patient of as little as 10% of their body weight will show improvement in pain and joint function in both hips and knees.[46,47]
  5. Prosthetic devices for malalignment correction will improve function and decrease pain.[43]
C. Topical preparations
  1. Used in initiation of NSAID therapy because topical safety profile looking better than oral regimens.[48]
  2. Other topical preparations include capsaicin, which is a transient receptor potential vanilloid 1 receptor (TRPV1) agonist/antagonist. The pain relief comes from 2 mechanisms, stimulation of receptor in the skin, and suppression of the receptor at the nerve ends.
D. Oral preparations
  1. NSAIDs in their oral form have a range of dosages. COX2 inhibitors may be chosen instead of traditional NSAIDs. It is now recommended to use a proton pump inhibitor when using NSAID therapy,[39] because contraindications include gastrointestinal bleeding history as well as renal failure.
  2. Acetaminophen is no longer a first-line therapy drug given research identifying no clinically significant relief of pain.[49]
  3. Duloxetine (Cymbalta) can be used when comorbid result in NSAIDs in their oral preparation are contraindicated.[39]
E. Nutritional supplementation[39] details are not discussed here.
  1. Glucosamine and chondroitin are the most commonly known on the market.
  2. Vitamin D and fish oil are also used.
F. Alternative medicine to consider[39] details are not discussed here.
  1. Acupuncture associated with Chinese medicine
  2. Transcutaneous electrical nerve stimulation (TENS)
G. Surgical options are available, but referral to specialist for evaluation is required. Surgical intervention is not emergent in osteoarthritis.

Joint Effusions[50]

A. Effusion types
  1. Noninfectious/noninflammatory
    a. Joint fluid findings
      i. Transparent clarity
      ii. Yellow in color
      iii. High viscosity
      iv. White blood cells (WBC) 2,000 cells/microL
      v. Polymorphonuclear leukocytes (PMN) 5%
    b. *Examples:* Osteoarthritis, avascular necrosis, trauma
  2. Hemorrhagic
    a. Joint fluid findings
      i. Bloody in clarity
      ii. Red in color
      iii. PMN 50% to 75%
      iv. Cultures negative
    b. *Examples:* Hemorrhagic diathesis, anticoagulation therapy, hemophilia, trauma to joint, tumors, neuropathic arthropathy

3. Inflammatory
   a. Joint fluid findings
      i. Translucent to mildly opaque in clarity
      ii. Yellow in color
      iii. Low viscosity
      iv. WBC >2,000 cells/microL
      v. PMN >50%
   b. *Examples:* Crystal-induced arthritis (pseudogout and gout), septic arthritis, spondylarthritis, rheumatoid arthritis or juvenile idiopathic arthritis, lupus, Lyme
4. Septic
   a. Joint fluid information
      i. Opaque in clarity
      ii. Yellow in color
      iii. WBC >20,000 cells/microL
      iv. PMN over 75%
      v. Cultures frequently positive
   b. Physical examination findings identifying infection in joint
   c. Infections can be from bacteria or fungus.

B. Treatment should follow guidelines for the diagnosis responsible for the effusion.

4. Tendinopathies[51]
   a. Diagnosis-specific information
      i. Most commonly associated with repetitive motion activities and overuse injuries
      ii. Pain with palpation or pain with stress loading on the tendon are the typical clinical findings on exam.
      iii. Delay in pain is commonly seen in tendinopathies. This is termed as latency in the literature and is seen more often with Achilles and patellar tendons.
      iv. During activity patients notice an increase in pain from the stress loading on the tendon. This pain temporarily improves once at rest. Issues arise with a significant increase in the pain the following day.
      v. Patient presentation for care related to a tendinopathy usually occurs once the problem has become chronic.
      vi. Only on fourth of patients with tendinopathies get any improvement beyond 4 months without treatment.

Diagnostic Imaging

A. Ultrasound (US)
   1. Ability to identify blood flow to deep regions of the tendon
   2. Identify hypoechoic area.
   3. Visualize thickened tendons.
   4. While this modality is useful, determining prognosis definitively with it is limited.[52]

B. MRI
   1. This modality can better identify small tears that can affect treatment and bring up surgical options.
   2. An MRI allows visualization of surrounding structures to determine their involvement.

Treatment[51,53]

A. Physiotherapy that focuses on active exercise treatments have shown very high improvement rates when compared with other treatment options.[54] Although ED clinicians are in most cases unable to order therapy, this fact should prompt taking the time to add the exercise education information to an ED patient's discharge plan.

B. Patient education on how using the injured tendon region stimulates repair has been found to improve success.[55] It is also important to educate on the time it will take in the healing process and to expect a mild worsening of symptoms at the onset of rehabilitation exercises.

C. ED care should surround an actual or perceived acute phase. This should include:
   1. NSAID therapy with standard dosing but short-term therapy only ~7 days. Long-term therapy is not recommended. It has been found there is minimal inflammation at the cellular level.[56]
   2. Glucocorticoid treatment may be found useful in an acute phase for pain control. There has been no long-term benefit identified.
   3. RICE care (rest, ice, compression, elevate)
   4. Ice and heat therapy have been found beneficial in the acute phase of tendinopathy problems; in the chronic phase neither have shown any significant direct benefit. Heat has been found to have patient satisfaction, but this is felt to be associated with reduction in muscle spasms.[57,58]

D. Use of topical patch nitrites as adjunct to rehabilitation has been studied with Achilles injuries and elbow injuries and found to show reduced pain over time and improved outcomes after 6-month course of therapy.[59,60] For patients in areas where the ED is the closest available care and thus keep returning multiple times regarding an ongoing tendinopathy, the clinician may want to consider this adjunct. Patient's past medical history and compliance with other therapies should be considered before opting to try this adjunct.

Bursitis[61]

A. Diagnosis-specific information
   1. Over 150 bursa sacs are found in the human body.
   2. Inflammatory changes usually result from trauma associated with the area, resulting in an acute process.
   3. Repetitive movement or arthropathies involving inflammation of an area will create the same inflammatory changes, resulting in a chronic bursitis.
   4. The diagnosis may also be from infection or disease associated with microcrystals.
   5. Pain is brought on by active range of motion (ROM). Passive ROM pain only occurs when it elicits an increase in the bursa pressure.

Diagnostics

A. Labs
   1. Elevated C-reactive protein (CRP) (acute phase)
   2. Elevated erythrocyte sedimentation rate (ESR) (acute phase)
   3. Aspirate studies
      a. Monosodium urate (MSU) crystals
      b. White blood cells (WBC) count with differential
      c. Culture
      d. Gram stain

B. Bursa aspiration
 1. Used to identify infection or microcrystalline diseases
 2. Superficial bursa sac aspirations increase the risk of sepsis when superficial skin infections are present.[62]
 3. See *Essential Procedures for Emergency, Urgent, and Primary Care Settings*, 3rd ed. (Campano T, Lafferty K, Eds.)[1] for specific information on how to perform the procedure.

C. Imaging is not indicated unless needed for differential rule out.

Treatment[61]

A. NSAIDs (e.g., ibuprofen, naproxen)
 1. Patients with gastric contraindications
  a. Cyclooxygenase inhibitor (e.g., celecoxib)
  b. Use of any NSAID in conjunction with usage of a proton pump inhibitor

B. Glucocorticoid intrabursal injection
 1. Treatment used for deep bursa only
 2. Combination of local anesthetic and the glucocorticoid are used (see section specific to medications used for injection for details).
 3. Superficial bursa sites are a contraindication to this form of treatment related to development of tissue infection from the side effects of the steroids on the tissue.[63]

Septic Bursitis[64]

A. Signs and symptoms
 1. Erythema
 2. Pain
 3. Swelling
 4. Fullness sensation
 5. Warm to touch
 6. Fever
 7. Puncture wound history
 8. Possible foreign body association
 9. Signs of decreased blood perfusion
 10. Signs of nerve compression

Diagnostics

A. Labs
 1. Complete blood count (CBC): Noted leukocytosis and bandemia (elevated immature white blood cells [WBCs])
 2. Elevated C-reactive protein (CRP) (acute phase)
 3. Elevated erythrocyte sedimentation rate (ESR) (acute phase)
 4. *Blood cultures:* One third of septic bursitis cases have bacteremia.[65,66]

Treatment[64]

A. Follow evidence-based guidelines when prescribing.

B. Outpatient
 1. Outpatient antibiotic therapy options
  a. Dicloxacillin
  b. Amoxicillin
  c. Cephalexin
  d. Cefadroxil
  e. Clindamycin
 2. Outpatient antibiotic therapy options for methicillin-resistant *Staphylococcus aureus* (MRSA)–associated infection
  a. Trimethoprim-sulfamethoxazole (TMP/SMZ)
  b. Doxycycline PLUS amoxicillin
  c. Minocycline PLUS amoxicillin
  d. Clindamycin

C. Inpatient
 1. Admission criteria
  a. Clinical presentation
  b. Comorbid conditions
 2. IV antibiotic therapy options
  a. Cefazolin
  b. Nafcillin
  c. Oxacillin
  d. Vancomycin, dosing adjusted based on blood levels
 3. IV antibiotic therapy options for MRSA-associated infection
  a. Vancomycin, dosing adjusted based on blood levels
  b. Daptomycin

Differential Diagnoses

A. Other diagnoses noted in the sections

B. Early onset of polyarticular diagnosis

Special Considerations

A. Infection in prosthetic joint[67,68]
 1. Early onset
  a. Symptoms begin less than 3 months postoperative.
  b. Signs and symptoms
   i. Joint pain
   ii. Warm
   iii. Erythema
   iv. Induration/edema at incision site
   v. Wound drainage
   vi. Dehiscence
   vii. Joint effusion
   viii. Fever
 2. Delayed onset
  a. Symptoms begin 3 to 12 months postoperative.
  b. Frequently mistaken for aseptic failure
  c. Signs and symptoms
   i. Persistent joint pain with or without loosening of hardware
   ii. Possible sinus track formation with or without drainage intermittent
 3. Late onset
  a. Symptoms begin over 12 months postoperative.
  b. Usually from hematogenous seeding from another infection
  c. Signs and symptoms
   i. Acute onset of systemic symptoms associated with bacteremia
   ii. Previously well joint that is now painful, warm, indurated, and/or swollen
   iii. Joint effusion
   iv. Fever
   v. Dislocation of joint is possible.

Skeletal Tuberculosis[69]

A. Background
1. Diagnosis seen higher in immigrant populations in endemic countries or who have migrated from those parts of the world.[69]
2. Extrapulmonary tuberculosis (TB) is seen most often in the first year after a lung infection. In nonendemic regions of the world, it is from reactivation of the disease.
3. Immunosuppressed patients are more susceptible to extrapulmonary TB. HIV patients have not been studied with great frequency concerning extrapulmonary TB. The current data shows no significant difference in cases with or without HIV.[70,71] Additional research is needed.
4. The difficulty in diagnosing the disease stems from thinking of it in the differential. Past medical history should include country of origin of the patient and any prior TB history.

Types of Skeletal Tuberculosis[69]

A. *Spondylitis (Pott disease):* Vertebral osteomyelitis
1. Infection to the lumbar and lower thoracic regions of the spine. Primary symptom is localized pain. Patients' gait is distinct, avoiding bouncing or movement of the spine with small steps. Fever and weight loss in some cases. Cord compression is seen 40% to 70% of the time with the initial diagnosis of the disease.[72]
2. Disease attacks the anterior portion of the vertebral body first as inflammatory process changes.
3. Disc space involvement is later in the disease process once two adjacent discs have been infected.
4. Soft tissue masses (cold abscesses), osteophytes, and other degenerative changes can lead to paraplegia.

B. TB-associated infectious arthritis
1. TB infection of an isolated joint is typical, primarily the hip and secondly the knee. Symptoms include pain, swelling, and loss of function in just weeks to months. Weight loss and fever are only seen in a small number of cases.
2. Multiple joint involvement of patients is seen in endemic countries or in those who have migrated from these locations.
3. Progressive disease involving damage to the hip joint can be treated with hip replacement.[73] Debridement and drug therapy must accompany the replacement.

C. TB-associated inflammatory arthritis (Poncet's disease)
1. Symmetric polyarthritis during active TB anywhere in the body. No active TB evidence is seen within the joints.
2. Resolution of the inflammatory process takes only a few weeks once on TB multidrug therapy.

D. TB-associated osteomyelitis
1. Any bone in the body can be infected with TB. Usually, only one site is involved.
2. Presentations vary based on location and can have unusual onset signs and symptoms. Prior trauma or surgery to the area is common and can cloud the evaluation picture.
3. Unusual presentation examples include
   a. Rib involvement beginning as a chest wall mass or even a breast mass
   b. Mastoid involvement can cause a facial nerve palsy.
   c. Unusual bone sites can appear as lytic lesions concerning for some type of metastatic disease form a malignancy.

Diagnostics

A. Labs
1. Definitive TB diagnosis is made with culture and microscopic examination of infected tissue.
2. Rifampin-resistant TB strains now exist, and thus drug susceptibility testing needs to be completed.
3. Synovial fluid evaluation results are found to be nonspecific.

Radiographic Imaging

A. Radiographs are helpful in establishing the location of the disease.

B. Chest x-ray (CXR) should be completed to confirm no active pulmonary TB, which is rarely seen at the time of musculoskeletal TB diagnosis.

C. CT and MRI are extremely helpful in evaluating extension of the disease into the soft tissue and adjacent joints.

Treatment

Standard pulmonary TB medication regimens are the initial therapy recommendations for musculoskeletal TB.

A. Follow evidence-based guidelines when prescribing.

B. Drug regimens based on stage 76
1. Intensive phase for pulmonary TB: Newly diagnosed preferred regimen
   a. Isoniazid (INH)
   b. Rifampin (RIF)
   c. Pyrazinamide (PZA)
   d. Ethambutol (EMB)
   e. Pyridoxine (vitamin B6) to be given with INH for high-risk patients susceptible to neuropathy. Risk population includes diabetes, elderly, chronic renal failure, HIV, pregnant or breastfeeding women.
2. Continuation phase for pulmonary TB involves the same drugs as noted above in the same dosing schedule but for an additional 4.5 months.
3. Musculoskeletal TB utilizes the same drugs but for a 6- to 9-month regimen.[74]
4. There are several alternative medication regimens for TB. Consultation with infectious disease is recommended when adjustments to the initial regimen needs to be made for onset of therapy.
5. From an emergency medicine treatment perspective, beginning traditional medications for intensive phase pulmonary TB for the treatment of musculoskeletal TB is prudent, with consultation or referral to infectious disease specialist and orthopedics for ongoing care and any adjustments to medication regimens.

C. Surgical intervention
1. Orthopedic, spine, or general surgery consultation is needed in the ED for cases meeting surgical intervention criteria. The specific service that handles care is institution-specific and site of infection-specific.
2. Criteria for surgical intervention[75,76]
a. Neuro deficits in spinal infection patients
b. Worsening neuro symptoms on drug therapy
c. Abscess noted on chest wall
d. Patients who have kyphosis with an angle larger than 40 degrees
3. Surgical treatment options include abscess drainage, surgical debridement, decompression of involved site for neurologic deficit improvement, and hardware placement to stabilize site.

Candida Osteoarticular Infection[77]

Background

A. The diagnosis of candida osteoarticular infection is usually seen in patients who have had indwelling catheters, street drug injection history, have been on broad-spectrum antibiotics, or are in some way immunosuppressed.
B. Seeding of the infection mostly occurs when the patient has developed the infection in the bloodstream, at either bone or joint-specific sites.
C. Exogenous development of candidiasis infections includes intraarticular injection, prosthetic implantation, trauma, or postsurgical procedures.
D. Candidiasis infection can present as a septic arthritis or even an osteomyelitis.
E. Most common areas associated with septic arthritis presentation include knee joints and intervertebral discs.[78,79]
F. Osteomyelitis presenting site is age focused. Adult site is vertebral. Pediatric site is long bones of any extremity.[80]

Diagnosis

A. High index of suspicion required to identify the diagnosis.
B. History of risk factors along with a recent candidiasis infection should be looked for.[79]
C. Include past medical history risk factors and any recent central line catheter placements and broad-spectrum antibiotic usage.

Treatment

A. Follow evidence-based guidelines when prescribing.
B. Candida-associated septic arthritis
1. Candida infections that are susceptible to fluconazole
a. *First-line therapy:* Oral fluconazole[81]
b. *First-line therapy:* IV echinocandin can be given × 2 weeks, converting to oral fluconazole for the last 4 weeks. Options include anidulafungin, caspofungin, and micafungin.[81]
c. Previous use of amphotericin B continues to be a viable alternative; no longer first-line choice because of nephrotoxic effects.
i. Previous discussion on joint injection of amphotericin B exists; not recommended because of tissue irritation. Affective levels of the drug in synovial fluid can be obtained with IV therapy.[77]
C. Candida-associated osteomyelitis
1. Candidiasis infections susceptible to fluconazole
a. Oral fluconazole
b. IV echinocandin can be given as above for 2 weeks and then transition to fluconazole oral dosing for 6 to 12 months.
c. Amphotericin B remains a viable alternative. Dosing is the same as above × 2 weeks, followed by oral fluconazole × 6 to 12 months. Nephrotoxicity remains the deciding factor in this medication not being first-line therapy.
D. Orthopedic specialty consultation is recommended. Consider infectious disease consultation.
E. Ongoing care of these infections can be tailored based on identification of the specific species of candida on culture.
F. Special considerations
1. Prosthetic joint infections from a fungal etiology mostly require removal of the prosthesis, thus orthopedic consultation will be necessary.

Pain to Multiple Joints[2]

Signs and Symptoms

A. Swelling to joint areas
B. Erythema to joint areas
C. Warm to the touch
D. Clicking or popping sounds or sensations with movement
E. Crepitus with passive movement of the joint
F. Radiation of pain from joint
G. Decreased range of motion (ROM), lack of ability to fully extend or flex
H. Joint deviation/subluxation of joint
I. Changes in surrounding tissues
J. Pattern of symptoms relative to joints involved

Diagnostic Laboratory Testing and Imaging

A. Labs
1. Complete blood count (CBC)
2. Erythrocyte sedimentation rate (ESR)
3. C-reactive protein (CRP)
4. Prolactin level
5. Comprehensive metabolic panel (CMP) as needed
6. Coagulation studies as needed
7. Additional studies specific to disease process noted below
B. Imaging
1. *Radiographs:* Evaluating for any acute injury; acute nontraumatic problems will show no changes. Chronic conditions will show changes that have occurred over a period of time.
2. *CT/MRI:* Early bone changes are easily identified.
C. Synovial fluid evaluation

1. Cell counts and differentials including polymorphonucleocytes
2. Aerobic and anaerobic cultures
3. Gram stain
4. Monosodium urate (MSU) crystals
5. Lactate
6. Lactate dehydrogenase

Diagnosis and Treatment

A. Acute polyarticular problems
 1. Symmetrical polyarticular problems are all chronic in nature.
 2. Asymmetrical polyarticular problems
  a. Gonococcal arthritis
   i. See information noted with acute monoarticular therapy.
   ii. The presentation of multiple joint involvement is rare but still a possibility.
  b. Lyme arthritis[82]
   i. General information
    (1) Associated with infection from *Borrelia burgdorferi*, affecting multiple organ systems
    (2) Most common illness in the Western world that is vector borne; Ixodes tick[83]
   ii. Disease process
    (1) Symptoms include nontraditional arthralgias and migratory myalgias.
    (2) Early disease identified weeks to months following tick bite.
    (3) Late disease lasts from months to years.
    (4) Episodes of flare-ups gradually decrease in frequency and intensity over time.
   iii. Treatment[84]
    (1) Follow evidence-based guidelines when prescribing.
    (2) *Doxycycline:* Prophylaxis for time spent longer than 36 hours in regions with ticks; traditional treatment when diagnosed.
    (3) Pregnant or breastfeeding patients require amoxicillin and cefuroxime.
  c. Acute rheumatic fever (ARF)[84]
   i. General information
    (1) Acute illness starts within a few weeks of having a posterior pharynx/tonsillar group A strep infection.
    (2) 75% of cases present as an acute febrile illness with joint pain and frequently carditis complaints.
    (3) A very small percentage present with central nervous system problems.
   ii. Disease process
    (1) *Major findings*[84]*:* Pericarditis with endocardium, epicardium, myocardium, pericardium, or valvular involvement
    (2) Minor findings
     (a) *Arthralgias:* Diffuse and sometimes migrating
     (b) EKG findings note prolonged PR interval
     (c) Elevated inflammatory markers
     (d) Fever
    (3) American Heart Association (AHA) criteria to diagnose ARF includes two major findings or one major and two minor findings.[84]
    (4) Exam findings will note a murmur most prominent at the apex during mid-diastole.
    (5) Differential diagnosis includes post-streptococcal reactive arthritis.
    (6) Development of rheumatic heart disease occurs 10 to 20 years after the original disease.

Treatment[85, 86]

A. Follow evidence-based guidelines when prescribing.
B. Group A *Streptococcus* eradication options
 1. Penicillin G benzathine
 2. Penicillin V
 3. Cephalexin
 4. Azithromycin
C. Arthritis relief management
 1. NSAIDs) Utilize maximum dosing a day for 1 to 2 weeks.
 2. Extended treatment course from 6 to 12 weeks is used while CRP and ESR lab values remain elevated.
D. Cardiac management needs to follow traditional treatments for congestive heart failure, any third-degree heart blocks, or severe heart enlargement.
E. Prevention treatment based on severity of ARF
 1. Carditis involvement with ongoing heart disease: 10 years or until the age of 40, whichever is longer
 2. Carditis without ongoing heart disease: 10 years or until the age of 21, whichever is longer
 3. ARF without cardiac involvement: 5 years or to the age of 21, whichever is longer
 4. Lifelong prevention therapy is only needed if the patient has ongoing valvular disease.
F. Prevention medication options include penicillin G benzathine, penicillin V, and azithromycin.

CHRONIC POLYARTICULAR PROBLEMS

Symmetrical Chronic Polyarticular Problems

Rheumatoid Arthritis (RA) Flare[87]

General Information

A. The disease is gradual in onset with multiple joints involved.
B. Destruction of joints—bone and cartilage— occurs if the disease is not kept under control.
C. More frequently seen in the hands

Disease Process

A. Primary presentation involves joint swelling, pain, and stiffness.

B. Morning stiffness with RA lasts over an hour minimum.
C. Reduction in grip strength is noted on exam with whole hand swelling, pitting in nature.
D. Each joint presents with variations to pain and swelling.
E. Generalized symptoms not directly associated with joint problems include generalized body aches and stiffness, weight loss, depression, and fatigue (suggestive of chronic fatigue syndrome).

Diagnosis and Treatment[88]

A. Laboratory studies include the standard complete blood count (CBC) and chemistry, with addition of inflammatory markers. Inflammatory markers will be elevated in acute disease but may be normal in chronic disease.
B. Prolactin levels have been found to be elevated in both serum and synovial tissue within RA patients.[89]
C. Radiographic imaging identifies narrowing of the joint space and erosions. MRI and ultrasound (US) is more sensitive in identifying these changes.
D. Initial symptomatic control from the ED includes NSAID (at full strength) and glucocorticoids.
E. With NSAID usage consider proton pump inhibitor usage in patients with history of gastrointestinal (GI) complications with NSAIDs. The patient should stay on the regimen for 10 to 14 days.
F. Glucocorticoid usage in addition to NSAIDs is recommended given their rapid onset and effectiveness in symptom control in RA patients.[49]
G. Put the patient on disease-modifying antirheumatic drugs (DMARDs). Methotrexate is usually the initial drug therapy choice.
H. Referral to rheumatologist is required to establish DMARDs treatment. This classification of drugs is typically not started in the ED.

Psoriatic Arthritis[90]

General information

1. Disease is loosely associated with skin psoriasis, originally an RA variant.
2. Rates of psoriatic arthritis in those with the skin disease have only been as high as 30%.[91]

Disease Process

1. Symptoms involve pain and stiffness, noted more prevalent in the morning. A small number of patients experience fatigue.
2. Activity alleviates the symptoms; thus, patient's presenting complaint is frequently related to the deformity development in the joint and less about pain. Distribution of disease varies in number of joints, but is most often asymmetrical.
3. Periarticular disease findings associated with psoriatic arthritis include a pitting effect noted to the fingernails, diffuse swelling to an entire toe or finger referred to as "sausage digit," medically termed dactylitis.
4. There may be ocular involvement up to 20% of the time, presenting as conjunctivitis or uveitis. The ocular presentation can be seen with other inflammatory arthritis disease processes.
5. Laboratory study findings will note elevated inflammatory markers and one third of the cases will see leukocytosis. There are disease-specific markers evaluated for in the clinic setting, but not needed in the ED.
6. Prolactin levels have been found to be elevated in both serum and synovial tissue within psoriatic arthritis patients.[89]
7. Distinctive radiographic findings are seen with this type of arthritis. They include terminal phalange bone lysis, with new bone formation in the same digit, and fluffy periostitis. New bone growth appears over the joint (ankylosis).[92] MRI may be of value in the outpatient setting for further evaluating disease process.

Treatment[93]

A. Mild peripheral form of this arthritis can be tried on NSAID therapy, remembering to use standard precautions regarding risk factors to include adding a proton pump inhibitor.
B. The key element of care from the ED is early referral to a rheumatologist for further evaluation to definitively determine the type of arthritis present.[94] Diagnosis and treatment should involve a multidisciplinary approach with rheumatology, dermatology, and the patient's primary care clinician. The next step in pharmacologic therapy involves DMARDs.
C. Physical and occupational therapy is recommended for these patients; thus, encouragement of exercise should be included in the ED discharge process.
D. Encouragement of weight reduction in obese patients should also be included in discharge planning because of the general increased problems with overwweight in any arthritis disease process

Polymyalgia Rheumatica[95]

General information

A. 1. Disease is seen in patients over the age of 50, with a peak in those aged 70 to 80.
    2. Disease is associated with 50% of giant cell arteritis patients.

Disease Process Signs and Symptoms

A. Stiffness in the neck, torso, pelvis, and shoulders
B. Systemic symptoms can also be seen such as anorexia, depression, fatigue, fever (low grade), malaise, and weight loss.
C. Onset of symptoms is abrupt and severe enough to prompt patient to seek medical evaluation.
D. Symptoms worse in the mornig
E. Labs
    1. C-reactive protein (CRP) almost always elevated
    2. Erythrocyte sedimentation rate (ESR) sometimes elevated
    3. Rheumatoid studies will be negative.
    4. Additional laboratory studies should be added to exclude other disease processes with similar

symptoms. These include liver studies, calcium level, thyroid-stimulating hormone (TSH) level, rheumatoid studies, vitamin D level, and creatinine kinase.

F. When the shoulders involved (up to 90% of the time), tenosynovitis and bursitis are noted on radiographs and US.

Treatment[96]

A. Follow evidence-based guidelines when prescribing.
B. Initial treatment is with glucocorticoids–prednisone. Dose can be adjusted as needed with diabetes, heart disease, or hypertension.
C. NSAID usage will not relieve symptoms, thus NSAID failure in arthralgia patients who return to the ED should have symptomology further investigated to see if polymyalgia rheumatica needs to be considered so medication regimen can be changed.
D. Rapid follow-up within a week is needed to evaluate effectiveness of initial treatment dose to determine the need for an increase in the dose.
E. Follow-up with primary care is frequently adequate; referral to rheumatology is needed when signs and symptoms are atypical.
F. Carefully assess the patient for signs of giant cell arteritis.

Enteric Arthritis[97]

General information

A. Arthritis is associated with multiple GI disorders in various degrees.
B. Examples include inflammatory bowel disease, pseudomembranous colitis, celiac disease, Whipple's disease, Behcet syndrome.
C. Bacterial and parasite infections can have joint pain involvement.
D. A side effect of GI bypass surgery includes joint pain involvement.
    1. Disease processes are not individually discussed here given the variety. When reviewing past medical history in ED patients who present with joint pain not associated with an injury, consider GI diseases processes as being associated with the problem.

Treatment

A. Symptoms relief is usually the first step in treatment.
B. Pay close attention to prior NSAID complications when starting pain control from the ED.
C. Disease specialist consultation/referral should be included in the ED discharge plan.
D. GI specialist consultation/referral should be included as well for those patients with prior NSAID complications.
E. Reinforcement of compliance with patient's GI disease process treatment should also be included in the ED discharge plan.

Asymmetrical Chronic Polyarticular Problems

A. Reactive arthritis or formerly Reiter's syndrome[98]
  1. General information
    a. Associated with a recent infection elsewhere in the body. Common bacteria include *Campylobacter*, *Chlamydia* (both *Trachomatis* and *Pneumoniae*), *Clostridium difficile*, *Escherichia coli*, *Salmonella*, *Shigella*, and *Yersinia*
    b. Reiter's syndrome is associated with the triad of infections that include arthritis, conjunctivitis, and urethritis. Reactive arthritis covers much more than just this triad.

Disease Process

A. Presentation is acute in onset 1 to 4 weeks after the infectious process.[99,100]
B. Symptoms resolution is from several days to several weeks. 50% of patient see resolution of symptoms by 6 months, most by 1 year.[101]
C. There are four major components to the presentation.
  1. *Arthritis:* Knees and lower extremities being most prominent
  2. *Back pain:* Inflammation of the sacroiliac joints and the lower spine
  3. *Dactylitis:* "Sausage digits"
  4. *Enthesitis*: Inflammation at tendon, ligament, and joint capsule attachment sites.
D. Laboratory study findings note classic inflammatory markers may or may not be elevated. Synovial fluid counts note a white blood cell (WBC) elevation.
E. No specific radiographic findings will be seen.
F. Definitive diagnosing centers on the four predominant findings, rule out other possible arthritis diagnosis, and find evidence of the precursor infection. For precursor identification, stool, urine, and other testing is indicated.

Treatment

A. Treatment with antibiotics is associated with the underlying infection, not for treatment of the arthritis. Specific antibiotic therapy is tailored to the specific organ system and infection thought to be the cause.
B. Follow evidence-based guidelines when prescribing.
C. The acute phase of the arthritis is treated like other arthritis disease process.
D. Recommendations include naproxen, diclofenac, and indomethacin. [100,102]
E. Inadequate NSAID response leads to the usage of glucocorticoids.
F. ED referral is needed early in the process in preparation for chronic treatment since DMARDs are used.

Viral-Associated Arthralgias

A. The topic is mentioned here since the source of the problem is associated with a virus, but the emergent complaint involves joint pain. Briefly getting historic information related to development of a specific virus can avoid missing a systemic issue requiring specific ED care and/or specific outpatient follow-up.

B. Specific viruses involved

1. HIV
2. Hepatitis A
3. Hepatitis B
4. Rubella virus or vaccine
5. Parvovirus
6. Alphaviruses (e.g., Ross River, chikungunya, Mayaro)

INVASIVE EVALUATION AND TREATMENT OF JOINTS

Arthrocentesis Procedure Tips by Joint

Indications for Procedure

A. Arthrocentesis

1. Evaluation of a joint to determine sepsis
2. Conformation of diagnosis of gout

B. Joint injection

1. Steroid use for inflammatory arthritis
2. Isolated soft tissue structure pain control

Technique[103]

A. Needle size is usually 22 gauge. For smaller joints, smaller gauge. For larger joints, 20 gauge or larger. If 20 gauge or larger is used, a pressure dressing needs to be applied after procedure.

B. Typically, a 5-mL syringe should be used to obtain specimen. Large syringes have too much suction. If dealing with a large effusion to a joint, such as a knee or shoulder, in which excess fluid is being removed a 20-mL syringe may be used.

C. The site should be prepped in a sterile manner using three chlorohexidine preps, making progressively larger circles from the site to be used outward, or with iodine, again prepping site three times. It is the practice not to touch the site after sterile preparation to minimize iatrogenic joint infection.

D. Anticoagulation therapy patients may undergo the procedure if taking warfarin and in a therapeutic range or those on aspirin and clopidogrel.[37,104] A 22 gauge or smaller needle should be used no matter the size of the joint.

E. Ultrasound-guided joint aspirates are becoming more common. This practice is site-dependent, since improved results have not been found with ultrasound in some joints.

1. Joint-specific approaches are in procedure-specific references. Consider reviewing a video of the procedure online before proceeding.

Synovial Fluid Studies[50]

A. *Goss appearance:* Clarity, color, and viscosity

B. *Cell count and differential:* White blood cells (WBCs) and specific types, such as polymorphonuclear leukocytes, and red blood cells (RBCs)

C. *Crystals:* Monosodium urate (MSU), calcium pyrophosphate dihydrate (CPPD), other crystals including lipids/cholesterol crystals and hydroxyapatite crystals

D. Lactate and lactate dehydrogenase levels

E. *Gram stain and culture:* Gram stain identifies quickly the presence of bacteria while waiting for cultures to grow bacteria.

Joint Injections[105]

A. Medications

1. Glucocorticoids

a. Examples include methylprednisolone, triamcinolone hexacetonide (outside the United States), and triamcinolone acetonide.

b. Specific drug choices are based on the area of the country practiced within.

c. Doses are site-specific based on size of joint. There is no set dosage in the literature.[105]

i. Methylprednisolone; drug effectiveness lasts up to 2 ½ months.

ii. Triamcinolone acetonide; drug effectiveness lasts up to 2 weeks

2. Lidocaine[105]

a. 1:1 combination with the steroid for immediate pain relief, decrease in atrophy in the area from the steroid,[106] and decrease damage from crystal formation. 1% or 2% may be used.

b. Lidocaine/epinephrine combination not used given problems with vasospasms in digital arteries.

3. Hyaluronic acid injections are used in isolated knee conditions; however, not used in mainstream emergency medicine.

4. Platelet-rich plasma injections have been used for treatment of tendonitis, plantar fasciitis, and osteoarthritis. In the ED setting, emergent treatment of the conditions should be addressed first.

B. Frequency of injections to a given site is dependent on the effects on the cartilage within the joint since cartilage damage occurs at a varying rate depending on diagnosis.[105] If an injection in the ED is considered, prior injection information should be reviewed.

Contraindications[107]

A. Joint instability from weakening of ligaments and joint capsule and possible subchondral osteonecrosis[108]

B. Juxta-articular osteoporosis because of worsening bone density with steroid use

C. Periarticular fractures can show decrease in healing with the steroid usage.[109,110]

D. Periarticular infection from introducing bacteria into the joint

E. Septic arthritis infections are an absolute contraindication for glucocorticoid usage, further worsening the infection.

F. Anticoagulants *are not* generally contraindication for injections; smaller needles should be used. Timing of injection and temporary holding are outpatient options.

1. Joint injections for pain control in the ED are now being evaluated. Current literature discusses the use of pain control via joint injection in acromioclavicular separations. An ultrasound-guided approach is used.[106] If this approach to pain control proves long term to be affective, pain control in additional joints can be considered.

a. Complications associated with joint injections or aspirations[111]

i. Noninfectious complications

(1) Tendon rupture
(2) Cartilage damage
(3) Neurovascular damage
(4) Joint or site bleeding
(5) Postinjection flare
(6) Glucocorticoid-associated toxicity
(7) Osteonecrosis
(8) Transient hyperglycemia

ii. Infectious complications

(1) Septic arthritis
(2) Septic bursitis

Systemic Lupus Erythematosus[112,113]

Pathophysiology[114]

A. At the end of a cell's life, intracellular substances are released into the bloodstream. The immune system of a patient with lupus identifies the cellular debris as foreign and thus mounts an immunologic response against the debris. The initial response includes T cells and antigen-presenting cells. As the cascade continues, the appearance of plasma cells and B cells begins.

Diagnosis[114]

A. The diagnosing of lupus is usually seen after multiple outpatient appointments and multiple rounds of blood work. The diagnosis is rarely made in the ED.

B. Blood work may be sent with outpatient referral for follow-up to a specialist, if diagnosis is suspected. Blood testing includes antinuclear antibody, anti-DNA, anti-Smith (Sm) antibody, and aPL antibody.

C. Specialist consultation and testing may occur after admission for emergent condition identified in the ED.

D. For those patients with known lupus, the disease process must be considered when treating any emergent condition in the ED.

Diagnostic Studies Relative to ED Care

A. Labs

1. Complete blood count (CBC)
2. Metabolic panel
3. Liver function studies
4. Prothrombin time (PT)
5. Partial thromboplastin time (PTT)
6. International normalized ration (INR)

B. Other tests

1. Urinalysis
2. EKG

C. Imaging

1. *Chest x-ray (CXR):* For identification of pneumonia, pleural effusion, pericarditis, atypical infections, cardiomegaly, and pulmonary emboli
2. *CT of the chest:* For identification of pulmonary emboli and diagnosis suspected but unable to confirm via CXR (mention lupus nephritis and contrast)
3. *CT of the abdomen (contrast info as above):* Lupus enteritis (LE)
4. *Echocardiogram:* Bedside exam to evaluate for pericardial fluid
5. *Nuclear medicine testing:* Ventilation-perfusion (VQ) scan for pulmonary emboli evaluation

Presentation Based on Chief Complaint[114,115]

A. *Abdominal pain*[114,115]*:* Systemic lupus erythematosus (SLE) patient's symptoms are usually vague. Remember immunosuppressants and corticosteroids mask severity of problem.

1. Diagnosis to consider

a. *LE:* Name to encompass the severe gastrointestinal (GI) manifestation associated with SLE

i. Diagnosis included

(1) Mesenteric arteritis or vasculitis
(2) GI vasculitis, intestinal vasculitis
(3) Acute GI distress syndrome
(4) Reversible acute GI syndrome

ii. Vasculitis within the mesentery can develop with chronic ischemic problems as what is believed to be an immune response. The superior mesenteric artery is most commonly affected.[116,117]

iii. CT needed for definitive diagnosis; radiographs, in the early stages, mimic pseudo-obstruction findings.

iv. Treatment is high-dose corticoids transitioning to a tapered dose with bowel rest[116,117]; admission and specialty consultation drive ongoing treatment should steroids fail and/or surgical intervention be needed.[116,117]

v. Cyclophosphamide has been used in treatment as well. Effectiveness is not well established, but reducing reoccurrence has been noted.[116]

b. Progressive complications of ischemic enteritis to bowel infarct to peritonitis to bowel perforation

i. Acute peritonitis presents traditionally with flare-ups of lupus. Immunosuppressants can mask symptoms.

ii. Chronic peritonitis in SLE patients may present with no pain but ascites development.[118]

c. *Pancreatitis:* Etiology of the problem in an SLE patient is the same as non-SLE patient. Treatment is also unchanged—intravenous fluids with no oral intake for intestinal rest, pain medications, and electrolyte correction. There is no indication that glucocorticoids play a role in pancreatitis in SLE patients.[119] Earlier literature has cited elevated amylase without symptoms of pancreatitis, including absence of abdominal pain. It has been thought the elevation was associated with the SLE disease process. More recent studies have identified pancreatitis on imaging with elevated amylase, but without abdominal pain. This condition is referred to as silent pancreatitis. Thus, further evaluation for pancreatitis should be considered in patients with elevated amylase without abdominal pain.[120,121]

d. *Peptic ulcer disease (PUD):* Glucocorticoids worsen ulcerative effects of NSAID use; alone there is no increased risk of problems.[115] Proton pump inhibitors should be added to medication regimen if the SLE patient requires extended NSAID therapy.

e. *Pseudo-obstruction:* Presentation of obstruction without having structural obstruction. Seen in SLE patients and can be an initial presentation of the disease.[122] Pathology of process is unknown. Treatment of SLE is with high-dose steroids alone or with an immunosuppressant drug. For ED care, specialist consultation is recommended if immunosuppressants will be used. Prokinetic agents are used specifically for this problem; consultant recommendations should be followed regarding usage.

2. SLE-specific facts
   a. Splenomegaly is common in up to almost half of all SLE patients. This fact should be taken into account when abdominal pain is associated with any type of trauma.[123]
3. ED evaluation
   a. *Abdominal radiographs:* Will show free air within the peritoneum, ileus, pseudo-obstruction, pneumatosis cystoids intestinalis. These findings may be caused form electrolyte problems, sepsis, or ischemia.
   b. CT is best imaging for SLE abdominal complaints.[124] Along with findings seen with radiographs, abscess and pseudocysts can also be identified.
   c. Anticipated CT findings in SLE patients: Bowel wall thickening, dilated bowel, enhancement of the bowel wall (known as target sign), ascites, mesenteric vessel engorgement, or mesenteric edema[125]
   d. Laboratory studies should include liver function studies; commonly elevated in SLE. Liver disease of any clinical significance is rare.[126,127]
   e. Amylase can be elevated in SLE patients without pancreatitis or with pancreatitis without symptoms.[128] Definitive evaluation of pancreatitis should take place in the ED if amylase is elevated.
   f. Paracentesis for diagnostic purposes should be considered in patients with ascites. Laboratory testing on fluid collection is discussed in Chapter 3, "Diagnostic and Therapeutic Procedures."

Arthritis[129]

A. Diagnosis to consider
   1. Arthralgias with a known lupus flare
   2. Fibromyalgia
   3. Gout
   4. Osteoarthritis
   5. Septic arthritis
   6. Avascular necrosis
   7. Medication-induced myopathy
B. SLE-specific facts
   1. The pattern is traditionally migratory and focused on knees, hands, and fingers.
   2. Morning stiffness resolves in minutes compared with rheumatoid arthritis (RA) morning pain and stiffness.
   3. Radiographs do not show erosions as noted in other arthritis diseases.
   4. Glucocorticoids and antimalarial drugs can cause myalgias. Elevated creatinine kinase levels will be noted.
C. ED evaluation
   1. Ultrasound (US) may be used for ruling out other diagnosis.
   2. ED care focuses on symptom control and outpatient follow-up.
   3. Medications for pain relief
      a. Hydroxychloroquine and NSAIDs (typical dosing) combined. SLE patients are frequently on an antimalarial agent which help to minimize joint symptoms.
      b. If the patient is actively having an SLE flare, a short dose of glucocorticoids may be used.
      c. Referral to the rheumatologist for ongoing care and adjustment to immunosuppressants as needed. Increasing immunosuppressant dosages can also help in ongoing arthritis symptoms.

Altered Mental Status[130,131]

A. Diagnosis to consider
   1. *Stroke:* Rule out organic causes
   2. Psychiatric etiology
   3. Infectious processes
B. SLE-specific facts
   1. Traditional risk factors associated with coronary artery disease are the same for cerebral vascular disease and found to be more prevalent in SLE patients on glucocorticoids, as noted in the chest pain section to follow.[132–134]
   2. Average onset of strokes in SLE patients is age 35.[135]
C. ED evaluation unchanged from standard altered mental status (AMS) work-up, see Chapter 13 for specific work-up considerations.
   1. Age should not play a part in ruling in or out a specific differential diagnosis.
   2. CT imaging identifies traditional organ processes only.
   3. MRI may identify neuropsychiatric lupus abnormalities, such as periventricular hyperintensities in brain white matter. These can be present even without symptoms of neuropsychiatric SLE.[136]
   4. Cerebrospinal fluid (CSF) evaluation tests for traditional infectious processes. There are several disease-specific tests on cerebral spinal fluid to evaluate for neuropsychiatric SLE. While these tests will not be ordered by an ED clinician, it is helpful to ensure additional specimen tubes are sent to the lab in anticipation of specialist orders.
   5. Psychiatric consultation will be needed to rule out psychiatric etiology causing altered mental state, after emergent organic processes have been eliminated from the differential.

Chest Pain[114]

A. Diagnoses to consider
   1. Musculoskeletal pain
   2. Pericarditis
   3. Pleuritis
   4. Pneumonia
   5. Pulmonary emboli
   6. Endocarditis
   7. Arrhythmias
   8. Cardiac tamponade

B. SLE-specific facts
   1. Coronary artery disease (CAD) is a significant risk as a result of the disease process of SLE due to early plaque formation from several mechanisms, such as high-density lipid malfunction, inflammatory increase from oxidative stress, increased risk of clot formation from antiphospholipid antibodies, as well as others.[137] Traditional SLE treatment with corticosteroids increases traditional risk factors at any age.[138]
   2. Age is no factor in the evaluation of acute coronary conditions.
   3. Initial lupus presentations of cardiac in nature to include cardiac tamponade.[139]

C. ED evaluation
   1. Evaluation of emergent cardiac problem should be implemented without regard for the age of an SLE patient.
   2. Work-up for any of the potential diagnoses listed above should be considered, based on additional complaints the patient is experiencing along with chest pain.
   3. Patient will need referral for definitive cardiac evaluation by a specialist. Calcification of coronary arteries is much higher than the same population without SLE.[140]
   4. Outpatient referral to SLE specialist is needed for potential medication regimen modification. Current recommendation is to use corticosteroids at the lowest possible dose to keep SLE inflammation halted. Beginning early statin therapy in this population is also recommended.[141]
   5. Hydroxychloroquine, an antimalarial drug, has been found to help offset increased heart disease risk factors in patients on glucocorticoids.[132,142]

Delirium[130,131]

A. Diagnoses to consider
   1. Neuropsychiatric lupus
   2. Steroid psychosis

B. SLE-specific facts
   1. Glucocorticoids are the primary treatment for SLE. Steroid-induced problems are dose dependent, but most often seen in doses over 40 mg/day. Resolution of symptoms resolve after stopping steroid therapy.[143]
   2. Information about test findings and recommendations regarding neuropsychiatric SLE is found in AMS section.

C. ED evaluation
   1. Emergent organic causes should be ruled out.
   2. Psychiatric consultation to evaluate for psychiatric etiology to the presenting complaint
   3. CT and MRI considerations noted above in AMS.
   4. Cerebrospinal fluid (CSF) evaluation considerations noted above in AMS.
   5. Specialist consultation regarding medication adjustments when drug-induced problem is suspected

Fever[113]

A. Diagnoses to consider
   1. Infectious processes typical and atypical
   2. Atypical infections to consider
      a. *Listeria monocytogenes*: A foodborne pathogen
      b. *Pneumocystis carinii:* Fungal-based pneumonia
      c. *Cryptococcal meningitis:* Fungal-based meningitis
   3. Spread of SLE to additional organ systems

B. SLE-specific facts
   1. Fever while taking glucocorticoids and immunosuppressants should be evaluated thoroughly for new infection, despite patient not having any significant symptoms.
   2. Fever associated to SLE medication regimen frequently responds quickly to antipyretic medications. When fever does not resolve, further investigation should take place to identify source of new infection.
   3. SLE flare-up itself can result in a febrile state. This fever responds well to traditional antipyretic treatment.

C. ED evaluation
   1. Current use of immunosuppressant therapy or prednisone, predisposing patient to infection
   2. Atypical infections should be considered in differential diagnosis for a new infection given the immunosuppressed state.

Headache[114]

A. No additional diagnosis to consider outside of standard headache workup differentials

B. ED evaluation should follow recommendations in Chapter 13.

Leg Swelling

A. Diagnoses to consider
   1. Deep vein thrombosis (DVT)
   2. Heart failure; right-sided, developed from a pulmonary emboli or pulmonary hypertension. Presentation can be isolated to abdominal ascites.
   3. Protein-losing enteropathy[116,121]
      a. Presents as profound swelling accompanied by hypoalbuminemia without proteinuria. Diarrhea noted in half of all presentations. Clinically mimics

nephrotic syndrome. Diagnosis is rare and typically seen in young women and those of Asian descent.
   4. Protein-losing enteropathy is a diagnosis of exception when other hypoalbuminemia causes have been ruled out.
   5. Renal failure—see special considerations.

B. SLE-specific facts
   1. Age does not play a role in the evaluation of an SLE patient with leg swelling.
   2. Management of protein-losing enteropathy centers around SLE treatment, thus specialist consultation is necessary.

C. ED evaluation
   1. Work-up should follow traditional evaluation for lower extremity edema causes.
   2. Additional differential diagnosis should be added to the work-up for SLE patients.

Localized Motor Weakness

A. Diagnoses to consider
   1. Stroke
   2. Guillain–Barré
   3. Demyelination disorders

B. SLE-specific facts
   1. Specifics regarding SLE and strokes is found in AMS section.
   2. Inflammatory polyradiculoneuroathy disease is seen in SLE patients. The changes are associated with the patient's SLE disease. The clinical presentation, however, will mimic Guillain–Barré and demyelination diseases such as chronic inflammatory demyelinating polyradiculoneuropathy (CIPD).[144,145]

C. ED evaluation
   1. Significant increased risk of stroke in patients with the diagnosis
   2. Age is not associated with complications; patient does not have traditional risk factors.
   3. Work-up is the same as for non-SLE patients; however, because of very specific disease mimicking SLE problems, specialist consultation should include SLE specialist.

Mood Changes and Anxiety[130,131]

A. Diagnoses to consider
   1. Neuropsychiatric SLE
   2. Psychiatric pathology

B. SLE- specific facts
   1. Information of test findings and recommendations regarding neuropsychiatric SLE is found in AMS section.

C. ED evaluation
   1. Rule-out of organic causes is necessary.
   2. Poisonings/ingestions/toxins should be ruled out as well.
   3. After medical possibilities have been ruled out, psychiatric consultation for evaluation.
   4. Should the patient have a known history of SLE, consultation with patient's rheumatologist could be helpful.

Rash and Skin Discoloration[114,146]

A. Diagnoses to consider
   1. Discoid SLE
      a. Circular, raised, erythematous lesions
      b. Lesions found on the scalp and face of patients
      c. Hair loss and pigment changes in the skin followed by scarring
   2. Drug-induced subcutaneous cutaneous erythematosus[147]
      a. Can present in isolation from a systemic drug response leading to SLE, but can play a part in a drug-induced SLE.
      b. Drugs that can trigger the cutaneous reaction include NSAIDs, calcium channel blockers, proton pump inhibitors, angiotensin-converting enzyme (ACE) inhibitors, and antiepileptics.
   3. Raynaud's
      a. Blanching of tissue from a vasospastic process
      b. Problem usually seen on fingers and toes
      c. Less commonly seen on ears, nose, and nipples
      d. Treatment of this specific rash[148]
         i. Nonpharmacologic care includes smoking cessation, cold avoidance, and avoidance of vasoconstricting drugs.
         ii. First-line oral therapy is long-acting calcium channel blockers.
         iii. Topical nitrate usage
            (1) Used with small areas of disease lasting short lengths of time.
            (2) Avoid in patients with dehydration, hypotension, pulmonary hypertension, and acute congestive heart failure.
            (3) Avoid in patients requiring oral treatment with phosphodiesterase type 5 inhibitors for refractory Raynaud's.
   4. Malar rash
      a. Best known as the butterfly rash
      b. Erythematous rash across the cheeks and bridge of nose in a butterfly appearing distribution
      c. The nasolabial folds are spared.
   5. Toxic epidermal necrolysis (TEN) is a rarer type appearance of acute cutaneous lupus erythematosus.[146]
      a. On rare occasions, the response is severe enough to create blisters and bulla creating a much more severe rash.
      b. TEN can mimic the look of Stevens–Johnson syndrome.
      c. Consultation for treatment and admission is needed.
   6. Lupus vasculitis—see vasculitis section.
   7. There are a vast number of cutaneous presentations both urgent and chronic in nature. Those discussed above are a representation of what to consider during evaluation of the patient.

B. ED evaluation/treatment[146]
   1. First-line treatment for problems
      a. Education of sun exposure and implementation of preventive therapy with topical protection.
      b. Topical 1% hydrocortisone

c. Topical calcineurin inhibitors
d. Extensive cutaneous involvement may require oral corticosteroids or antimalarial medications. Consider consultation with specialist if patient has not been treated previously for these problems.
2. Secondary therapy
a. Immunosuppressants and glucocorticoid sparing agents are used.
b. Consultation with specialist is needed for establishment of treatment.

Seizures

A. Diagnoses to consider
1. *Lupus-related seizure activity:* Found to present as status epilepticus without having convulsive movement.
2. Stroke
B. SLE-specific facts
1. Seizure development in SLE patients occurs in the first year postdiagnosis half of the time. It can even be the initial presenting complaint.[149,150]
2. Stoke specific information as it is associated with SLE is noted in AMS section.
3. Antimalarial drugs used in decreasing arteriosclerotic risk factors are used for seizure prevention as well.[151]
C. ED evaluation
1. Unchanged from traditional seizure work-up, see Chapter 13 for specifics.
2. Age should not eliminate differential diagnoses.
3. Treatment of seizures is no different in the SLE patient. While some neuroleptic drugs (carbamazepine, phenytoin) have been associated with drug-induced SLE, the use should not be avoided.[131]
4. Since there is probably an inflammatory component to seizure activity in SLE patients, prednisone at 1 mg/kg/day may be given in a short course. It is thought to prevent development of permanent foci in the brain for epileptic activity.[152] IV dosing has been shown to reduce refractory seizures.[153]

Shortness of Breath[113,154]

A. Diagnoses to consider
1. *Anemia:* See hematologic disorders in special consideration section below.
2. *Interstitial lung disease:* Multiple types of this disease exist; presentation of dry cough with shortness of breath (SOB) and activity intolerance.
3. Pericardial effusion
4. Pericarditis
5. Pleural effusion
6. Pleuritis
7. Pneumonia
8. Pulmonary emboli
9. Pulmonary hypertension
10. *Shrinking lung syndrome:* Presentation of SOB and chest pain that is pleuritic in nature with decreasing lung volumes. Minimal disease findings noted on CT.[155]
B. SLE-specific facts
1. Interstitial lung disease evaluation should take into account drug toxicity involvement and environmental factors. Heart failure needs to be considered in the differential diagnosis, thus add a brain natriuretic peptide to the work-up.
2. Shrinking lung syndrome pathology has varying thoughts. One is that myopathy affects the diaphragm, resulting in decreased function. Others believe that chronic inflammatory process results in decrease in deep inspiration.
3. Anticipated onset of shrinking lung disease is about 4 years after SLE diagnosis.[156]
4. CT imaging is the standard for diagnosis of lung disease in SLE. CT imaging is sometimes performed in both the supine and prone positions to differentiate dependent atelectasis from true disease.[154]
C. ED evaluation
1. Work-up needs to include both pulmonary and cardiac causes of SOB.
2. Referral to specialist for further testing, such as pulmonary functions studies, bronchoscopy, bronchoscopy with biopsy, echocardiogram, and heart catheterization.
3. Emergent treatment of any of these conditions is the same as non-SLE patients.
4. Disposition with supplemental oxygen is needed for an oxygenation saturation of 89% or less at rest or with exercise.

SPECIAL CONSIDERATIONS

Antiphospholipid Syndrome[114]

A. *Definition:* Immunologic disorder resulting in the body attacking its own proteins in the blood
B. Facts
1. Hepatic complications contribute to complications of the disease[131]
2. Transient ischemic attacks are the most common neurologic problem associated with antiphopholipid syndrome (APLS).[124]
3. Preventive stroke treatment in patients with APLS involves ongoing anticoagulation therapy. Both warfarin and aspirin are used, depending on the specific type of stroke and the patient's ongoing risk.[131]

Hemolytic Disorders

A. *Anemia:* Most common hematologic disorder
1. Types to consider in SLE
a. Anemia of inflammation (anemia of chronic disease)
b. Aplastic anemia
c. Autoimmune hemolysis
d. Hypersplenism associated anemia
e. Iron deficiency anemia
f. Medication induced
g. Renal insufficiency
2. Anemia evaluation in the ED should focus initially on reversible causes such as bleeding.[123]

3. Consultations and referrals for ongoing work-up of the problem needs to include SLE specialist along with hematology.
4. It is common for SLE patients to have anemia associated with more than one problem.

B. Lymphocytopenia
1. Infection-associated, increased SLE disease–associated, asymptomatic problem[157]
2. Treatment of infectious process is necessary. If not infection-associated, the treatment of SLE is needed to regulate the problem.

C. Thrombocytopenia[123]
1. Platelet counts can be mildly low in the 100 to 150 range for 25% to 50% of all SLE patients.
2. Most common type associated with SLE patients is idiopathic thrombocytopenic purpura (ITP).
3. Other types include drug-induced thrombocytopenia, splenomegaly, and APLS.
4. When thrombocytopenia is noted in the ED on a work-up of an SLE patient, ITP evaluation and treatment need to be considered.
5. Treatment of platelet count for emergent situations such as surgery involves IV gamma globulin (IVIg), which is used in SLE patients as well.

D. Pancytopenia[123]
1. Emergent evaluation related to severe infections, sepsis, and the development of disseminated intervascular coagulopathy should follow traditional non-SLE patient work-ups.
2. SLE specific pancytopenia causes require specialist consultation to determine hospitalization requirement for further evaluation or outpatient testing for disposition home.

E. Lymphadenopathy
1. Problem is seen in 50% of SLE patients. Treatment for the problem is related to treating SLE.
2. ED evaluation focus needs to remain associated with possible causes in non-SLE patients.
3. Traditional treatment for the problem should be considered for disposition from the ED, with referral to SLE specialist for adjustments to treatment.

F. Thrombocytosis
1. Traditional causes for platelet counts over 400 in SLE patients should be considered.
2. Hyposplenism, also referred to as autosplenectomy, is also seen in SLE patients, frequently those with APLS.
3. Treatment of thrombocytosis is not necessary, but other causes of the problem require specialist evaluation to identify.

Renal Disease in SLE[158]

A. *Renal Pathology Society/International Society of Nephrology (RPS/ISN) classification system*[158]: Diagnosis is made by biopsy. For ED purposes, signs and symptoms seen are listed below.
1. *Class I:* Minimal mesangial lupus nephritis (rarely diagnosed). Usual findings include a normal urinalysis and creatinine; occasionally very low protein level may be seen.
2. *Class II:* Mesangial proliferative lupus nephritis; microscopic evidence of proteinuria and/or hematuria may be seen, rare incidences of hypertension.
3. Class III: Focal lupus nephritis; hematuria and proteinuria are usually apparent with a decreased glomerular filtration rate, increased prevalence of hypertension compared with class II.
4. *Class IV:* Diffuse lupus nephritis; worse case of lupus nephritis, evidence of nephrotic syndrome, hypertension noted, further decrease in glomerular filtration rate. Almost all patients present with hematuria and proteinuria.
5. *Class V:* Lupus membranous nephropathy; classic presentation of a nephrotic syndrome with the extensive diffuse edema, fatigue, and weight gain. Hypertension may be present; creatinine may be slightly elevated.
6. *Class VI:* Advanced sclerosing lupus nephritis. This condition is a slow progression of renal dysfunction as a result of global sclerosis of the glomeruli, appears as chronic ongoing presentation of prior classes.

B. Nonimmunosuppressant treatment[159]
1. Aggressive antihypertensive therapy; drug dependent on proteinuria history
2. Minimizing proteinuria with aggressively blocking the renin–angiotensin system. Drug options:
   - **a.** ACE inhibitors
   - **b.** Angiotensin II receptor blocker (ARB)
3. Lowering cholesterol levels
   - **a.** Statin drug therapy is recommended.
   - **b.** Small selection of studies has suggested that there might be a slowing of renal disease by using lipid lowering agents.[160]

C. Immunosuppressant treatment[159]
1. Aggressive type therapy for patients with any type of glomerulonephritis. Immunosuppressant therapy is handled outpatient with specialists.
2. Preventive care with immunosuppressant and glucocorticoid regimens
   - **a.** Pneumocystis *pneumonia:* SLE patients may be on antibiotic therapy as HIV patients. Recommendation is trimethoprim-sulfamethoxazole (TMP/SMZ) single strength dose tablet daily.[161] Taking the antibiotic daily should be taken into consideration when choosing antibiotic therapy for infectious processes identified in the ED that require treatment.
   - **b.** Drug-induced cystitis associated with the immunosuppressant therapy
     - **i.** Problem can progress to hemorrhagic cystitis.
     - **ii.** Recommended preventive therapy is increased oral hydration daily, with input and output monitoring daily.[161]

D. ED considerations
1. New-onset renal insufficiency of any kind in the ED in patients with SLE should be consulted/referred to their SLE specialist and the renal specialist who handles complex renal patients in the region.

2. Any acute-onset renal insufficiency versus renal failure needs consultation with SLE specialist for recommendations on admission.

Drug-Induced Lupus[162]

A. Some medications can trigger an autoimmune response involving the patient's histone proteins.
B. Identifying lupus versus drug-induced lupus: Malar rash will rarely be seen if presentation is drug-related. Rarely are any major organs involved.
C. *Drug examples:* Chlorpromazine, hydralazine, isoniazid, methyldopa, minocycline, procainamide, and quinidine
D. Treatment surrounds controlling symptoms—NSAIDs and steroids.

Treatment

A. Traditional treatment of emergent diagnosis should be implemented.
B. Special considerations given lupus diagnosis for individual presentations are noted above.
C. Treatment of worsening lupus disease process
D. Long-term steroid therapy considerations included in treatment of any ED complaint
E. Treatment of inflammatory conditions in the lupus patien.
F. Specialist consultation and referral as necessary

Vasculitis[114,163]

A. The history of this topic and attempts at classification have been many. The topic is traditionally taught by grouping disease processes by the vessel size. This section presents the basics associated with evaluating the patient and viewing types of vasculitis based on the system it is affecting.

Keys to Diagnosing

A. History of complaints
B. Symptoms involved
C. Organ system involved with the chief complaint
D. Demographics of the patient

Signs and Symptoms of Vasculitis

A. Malaise
B. Fever
C. Arthralgias
D. Weight loss

Specific Types of Vasculitis

A. See Table 20.1 for the general presentation findings, signs and symptoms, prevalent demographic information, and generalized treatment.
B. ED evaluation
  1. Labs
    a. ED testing
      i. Complete blood count (CBC)
      ii. Comprehensive metabolic panel (CMP)
      iii. Blood cultures
      iv. Erythrocyte sedimentation rate (ESR)
      v. C-reactive protein (CRP)
      vi. Creatine phosphokinase (CPK)
      vii. Coagulation studies
      viii. HIV
      ix. Urinalysis (UA)
    b. Admission testing
      i. Antiglomerular basement membrane
      ii. Antinuclear antibody (ANA)
      iii. Complement levels
      iv. Antineutrophil cytoplasmic antibodies (ANCA) pattern
      v. Hepatitis B and C serology
      vi. Rheumatoid factor
      vii. Rapid plasma reagin (RPR)/VDRL
  2. Radiographic diagnostics
    i. Chest x-ray (CXR)
    ii. CT of specific area
    iii. Arteriography of specific area
  3. *Admission studies:* Biopsy of specific tissues done inpatient; arteriography and echocardiogram needed for diagnosis not done in ED; bronchoalveolar lavage and/or biopsy

Differential Diagnoses

A. Antiphospholipid antibody syndrome
B. Disseminated intravascular coagulopathy
C. Drug-induced vasospasm (cocaine, ergots)
D. Embolic disease
E. Endocarditis
F. Heparin- or warfarin-induced thrombosis
G. Systemic infection
H. Thrombotic thrombocytopenic purpura (TTP)
I. Vessel thrombosis, stenosis, or spasm

Treatment

A. Primary treatment includes treatment of infectious processes until rule-out is complete.
B. Secondary treatment is associated with any emergent condition to be addressed in the ED (see associated chapter for recommendations).
C. Consultation for admission or referral for ongoing outpatient care to specialist

Allergy, Hypersensitivity, and Anaphylaxis [173]

The Body's Defense System

A. First-line defense system in the human body includes resident cells, infiltrative cells, and proteins, giving a fast, nonspecific response.
B. Once sensitization has taken place, the adapted system uses B cells and T cells, which are antigen specific, mounting a response specific to the offender.

TABLE 20.1 SYSTEMS-BASED DIAGNOSTIC APPROACH TO VASCULITIS AND TREATMENT INITIATION[113,114,163–172,]

GENERAL PRESENTATION	EMERGENT INTERVENTION POTENTIAL—SEE SPECIFIC CHAPTER FOR TESTING AND TREATMENT	BEHCET'S DISEASE	CHURG-STAUSS VASCULITIS	COGAN'S SYNDROME	CRYOGLOBULINEMIA	GIANT CELL ARTERITIS	GOODPASTURE SYNDROME	LEUKOCYTOCLASTIC ANGIITIS	MICROSCOPIC POLYANGITIS	POLYARTERITIS NODOSA	SLE-ASSOCIATED VASCULITIS	TAKAYASU'S ARTERITIS	WEGENER'S GRANULOMATOSIS
Prominent demographics													
Age		YA	MA			E				MA		YA	Ma
Gender		=	M			F				M		F	M
Ethnicity		Me				Ca						A	
Cutaneous	X												
Extremity claudication to gangrene of extremity	Necrotic tissue sepsis	X	X							X	X	X	X
Palpable purpura		X	X	X	X		X	X	X	X	X		X
Skin ulcers		X	X					X	X	X	X		X
Tongue claudication						X							
Cardiovascular	X												
Chest pain	MI		X				X				X		
Aortic involvement											X	X	
ENT													
Allergic rhinitis			X										
Epistaxis													X
Hearing loss				X									
Tinnitus				X									
Gastrointestinal tract	X												
Abdominal pain /mesenteric ischemia	Sepsis		X					X		X	X		
Gastrointestinal bleeding	Hemorrhagic shock		X							X	X		
Musculoskeletal													
Myalgias/ arthralgias			X		X	X		X		X	X	X	X
Neurologic	X												
Peripheral neuropathy										X			
Mononeuritis multiplex			X		X				X	X			X
Headache/stroke	Stroke	X				X		X			X		
Dizziness/vertigo				X							X		

(continued)

TABLE 20.1 SYSTEMS BASED DIAGNOSTIC APPROACH TO VASCULITIS AND TREATMENT INITIATION (*CONTINUED*)

GENERAL PRESENTATION	EMERGENT INTERVENTION POTENTIAL—SEE SPECIFIC CHAPTER FOR TESTING AND TREATMENT	BEHCET'S DISEASE	CHURG-STAUSS VASCULITIS	COGAN'S SYNDROME	CRYOGLOBULINEMIA	GIANT CELL ARTERITIS	GOODPASTURE SYNDROME	LEUKOCYTOCLASTIC ANGIITIS	MICROSCOPIC POLYANGITIS	POLYARTERITIS NODOSA	SLE-ASSOCIATED VASCULITIS	TAKAYASU'S ARTERITIS	WEGENER'S GRANULOMATOSIS
Ophthalmic	X												
Conjunctivitis/ keratitis/ uveitis		X		X					X				X
Vision changes or loss	Vision loss	X		X		X					X		
Pulmonary	X												
Alveolar hemorrhage	Hypoxia PE						X		X		X		
Pulmonary infiltrates / cavities	Hypoxia		X										X
Renal	X Acute renal failure												
Glomerulonephritis					X		X		X		X		X
Ischemia/ Ischemic renal failure			XX							X	X	X	XX
ASSOCIATED MEDICAL CONDITIONS & HALLMARK FINDINGS				Onset after infection/ isolated to eyes or ears/ systemic -polyarteritis nodosa appearance	Raynaud's/ Nondestructive oligoarthritis	Polymyalgia rheumatica/ Fever of unknown etiology in E				CLASH		Nondestructive oligoarthritis/ asymmetric pulses/ uneven BPs	
		Behcet's disease	Churg-Stauss vasculitis	Cogan's syndrome	Cryoglobulinemia	Giant Cell Arteritis	Goodpasture syndrome	Leukocytoclastic angiitis	Microscopic polyangitis	Polyarteritis nodosa	SLE associated vasculitis	Takayasu's arteritis	Wegener's granulomatosis

=, female and male equal; ?, cause to consider; A, Asian; Ca, Caucasian; CLASH, cryoglobulinemia, leukemia, arthritis, Sjogren's syndrome, hepatitis; E, elderly; F, female more prominent; M, male more prominent; MA, middle age; Me, Middle Eastern; X, applies; XX, applies but less common; YA, young adult.

To utilize the table:

1. Identify the presentations seen in the patient during the initial evaluation.
2. Narrow down the potential vasculitis types based on initial patient physical. The most common presentation findings are noted in the chart, but rare presentation findings may be identified in an individual patient's exam.
3. Return to the patient, if needed, to evaluate for any presentation findings not obvious on the initial evaluation to narrow possible diagnoses.
4. Consider any further testing needed based on diagnoses, with or without current presentation findings, and associated medical conditions.
5. When dealing with vasculitis problems, the emergent condition that could result from the associated vasculitis is of top importance. The emergent concern is what is addressed from an EM perspective.
6. Formal diagnosis confirmation is not done in the ED. The vast majority of vasculitis diagnoses involve long-term treatment requiring specialist involvement.

Coombs and Gell's Classification of Immune Responses[2]

A. Type 1
  1. Prior sensitization has taken place.
  2. Rapid response reaction of both IgE-dependent and IgE-independent pathways with immediate release of mediators (e.g., basophils and mast cells)
  3. Examples include allergic asthma, anaphylaxis, angioedema, hay fever, and urticaria.

B. Type 2
  1. Cytotoxic antibody reaction where IgM and IgG antibodies bind with antigens
  2. There is a resulting lysis of cells.
  3. An example is blood transfusion reactions, as with Rh factors.

C. Type 3
  1. Antibodies (IgM and IgG) bind with antigens, and then adhere to vascular walls or migrate outside the vascular system to create an anaphylactic reaction, as seen with blood transfusions.

D. Type 4
  1. Prior sensitization of immune cells (T cells) releasing a delayed response, no anaphylaxis pathways
  2. Antigen recognition prompts recruitment of lymphocyte and mononuclear cells to create an inflammatory response to the antigen.
  3. Examples include contact dermatitis, Steven–Johnson syndrome, toxic epidermal necrosis, and erythema multiform.

E. Allergic responses in the human body based on organ system
  1. *Cardiac:* Weakness, syncope, lightheadedness, chest pain, tachycardia, hypotension, palpitations, dysrhythmias, cardiac arrest
  2. *Central nervous system (CNS):* Impending doom sensation, anxiety, headache, confusion, seizure, coma
  3. *Eye:* Itching, erythema, inflammation
  4. *Gastrointestinal/genitourinary (GI/GU):* Dysphagia, abdominal cramping and pain, nausea and vomiting, diarrhea, pelvic pain, urinary incontinence
  5. *Hematologic:* Abnormal bleeding and bruising, progressive bleeding problems up to and including disseminated intravascular coagulation
  6. *Upper respiratory:* Congestion, runny nose, sneezing, itching nares, hoarse voice, throat tightness, hypersalivation
  7. *Lower respiratory:* Cough, wheezing, rhonchi, tachypnea
  8. *Skin:* Pruritis, urticaria, diffuse flushing/erythema/hives, perioral swelling, nonpitting peripheral edema (frequently not symmetrical)

F. Risk factors associated with anaphylaxis and severity
  1. Age
  2. Comorbid disease processes
  3. Seasonal involvement
  4. Route of exposure
  5. Emotional and physical stressors
  6. Use of specific medications (e.g., antihypertensives or cognition-impairing drugs)

G. Laboratory studies for the purpose of ruling out differential or concomitant problems

H. Treatment of basic allergic responses
  1. Medications[174]
    a. Follow evidence-based guidelines when prescribing.
    b. Antihistamines
      i. Not for use in airway obstruction or shock states
      ii. Examples
        (1) H1 antihistamines (e.g., diphenhydramine, cetirizine)
        (2) H2 antihistamines (e.g., famotidine)
    c. Bronchodilators
      i. Epinephrine
      ii. Inhaled bronchodilators (e.g., albuterol)
    d. Glucocorticoids
      i. Methylprednisolone

Treatment of Anaphylaxis[173]

A. Emergent interventions
  1. Remove caustic agent and call for emergent help.
  2. Airway assessment, patient positioning, oxygen administration
  3. Initial epinephrine dose (intramuscularly [IM]) delay in dosing has been associated with fatalities.[174,175]
  4. Establishment of IV access for additional epinephrine doses and IV fluid resuscitation as indicated

B. Initial assessment and ongoing management
  1. Thorough evaluation of airway, breathing, and circulation; oral cavity evaluation for swelling including lips, face, angioedema, and pharyngeal edema
  2. If airway is intact, the patient should be positioned in the supine position with the legs slightly elevated. The early positioning of the patient in this manner prevents a phenomenon known as empty ventricular syndrome that results in sudden death associated with hypoperfusion.[176]
  3. Airway
    a. Upper airway compromise or stridor requires emergent intubation.
    b. Emergent assessment findings for intubation include rapid tongue swelling, uvula swelling, other oral and pharyngeal tissue swelling, voice changes.
    c. Alternative airway capability to be available
  4. Breathing: Initial oxygen administration should be traditional 15 L via nonrebreather.
  5. Circulation
    a. IV access should include two large-bore catheters for IV fluid administration and ongoing IV-administered medications.
    b. IV fluid infusion should be maintained at 125 mL/hour unless bolus infusions required for hypotension/hypoperfusion.
    c. Aggressive fluid resuscitation to start with a minimum of 2 L normal saline. The arguments of normal saline versus lactated ringers are ongoing, thus many clinicians alternate the two fluids in large fluid resuscitation situations.
    d. Colloid usage for the distributive shock affect has shown no benefit.
  6. Ongoing monitoring
    a. Frequent vital signs

b. Continuous cardiac monitoring
c. Continuous pulse oximetry

C. Epinephrine usage in anaphylaxis
1. Epinephrine IM.
2. IM dosing is preferred over subcutaneous route because of better absorption and IV dosing to prevent cardiac complications of arrhythmias and hypertension.
3. If the patient is not responding to IM dosing, continuous IV infusion is recommended over intermittent IV boluses because of errors related to dosing concentrations used and cardiac complications associated with the medication.[177,178]

D. Additional medications
1. Patients on beta-blockers may not respond to epinephrine and thus glucagon is recommended.
a. Glucagon can be used because it works outside the beta receptor channels and has both ionotropic and chronotropic effects.
b. Continuous infusion can be started after initial dose.
2. Antihistamines as noted above
3. Bronchodilators as noted above

Refractory Anaphylaxis[173]

A. Alternative vasopressors[179]
1. Vasopressin
2. Norepinephrine (Levophed)
3. Dopamine
4. Other vasopressors may be used at the recommended dosages per manufacturers guidelines.

B. Alternative therapy: Methylene blue[173]
1. Used in the operative setting, usually cardiac surgeries
2. Contraindicated in patient with lung damage, pulmonary hypertension
3. Caution in patients on serotonergic medications

Admission Criteria

A. Significant anaphylaxis response
B. Hypotension and airway involvement
C. IV epinephrine used or two or more doses of IM epinephrine
D. Lack of outpatient social support

Discharge Plan

A. Emergent action plan for anaphylaxis
B. Epinephrine auto-injector at home
C. Follow up with allergist specialist
D. Written discharge information
E. Use of the "SAFE" program for anaphylaxis
1. Seek support
2. Allergen identification
3. Follow up with specialist
4. Epinephrine for emergencies

Dermatologic Presentations

A. Terminology review—see Table 20.2[180]

B. History of present illness (HPI) considerations
1. Onset/history of problem
2. Distribution/beginning location
3. Progressive macular hypomelanosis (PMH) which are areas of hypopigmentation in a circle pattern seen more so on the trunk.

C. Patient assessment—see Figure 20.1 and Figure 20.2. The charts are designed to help in the identification of the rash aside from any additional signs or symptoms the patient may have associated with the diagnosis. Treatment of the condition associated with the rash finding is in the chapter associated with diagnosis.

D. Steps in rash identification and treatment[181,182]
1. Febrile versus afebrile
2. Appearance of rash (e.g., petechiae, purpura, vesicles, bulla, papules, macules, diffuse erythema)
3. Additional physical examination findings
a. *Palpation:* Palpable (raised), not palpable (flat)
b. *Distribution of the rash:* Central, peripheral, diffuse, localized
c. Nikolsky's sign presence or absence
4. Treatment: Found in the chapter discussing the individual diagnosis in detail, unless stated below.

TABLE 20.2 DERMATOLOGY TERMINOLOGY

TERM	DEFINITION
Papule	Solid lesion that is <1 cm in diameter that is elevated
Macule	Lesion that is <1 cm in diameter that is flat
Vesicle	Lesion that is fluid filled, <1 cm in diameter, and elevated
Pustule	Lesion that is pus filled, <1 cm in diameter, and elevated
Bulla	Lesion that is fluid filled, >1 cm in diameter, and elevated
Patch	Lesion that is >1 cm in diameter that is flat
Plaque	Lesion that is >1 cm that is flat but elevated
Nodule	Solid lesion that is >1 cm in diameter that is elevated
Purpura	Blood appearance under skin 4–10 mm in diameter from leaking blood vessels
Petechiae	Pinpoint, red, round spots from blood
Diffuse erythema	Red appearance of tissue
Nikolsky's sign	Visible sliding of top layer of skin from other layers when tissue is rubbed

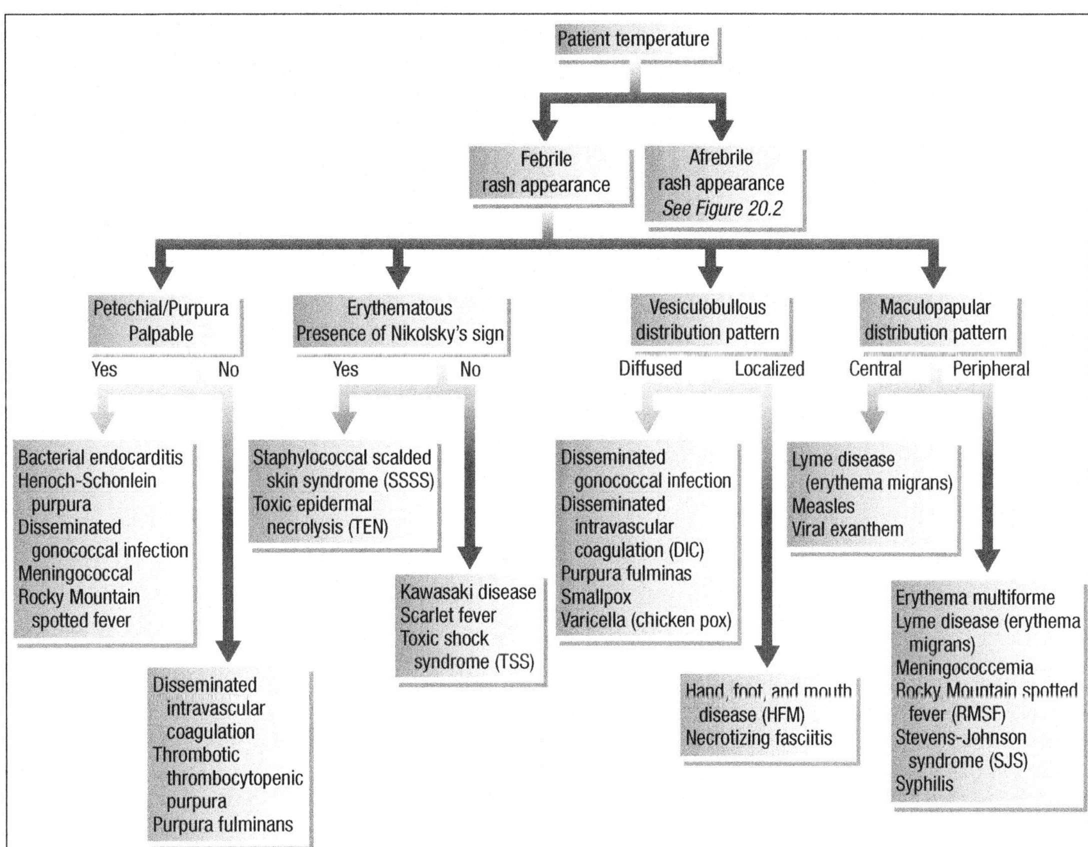

FIGURE 20.1 Evaluation of emergent rashes in febrile patients.

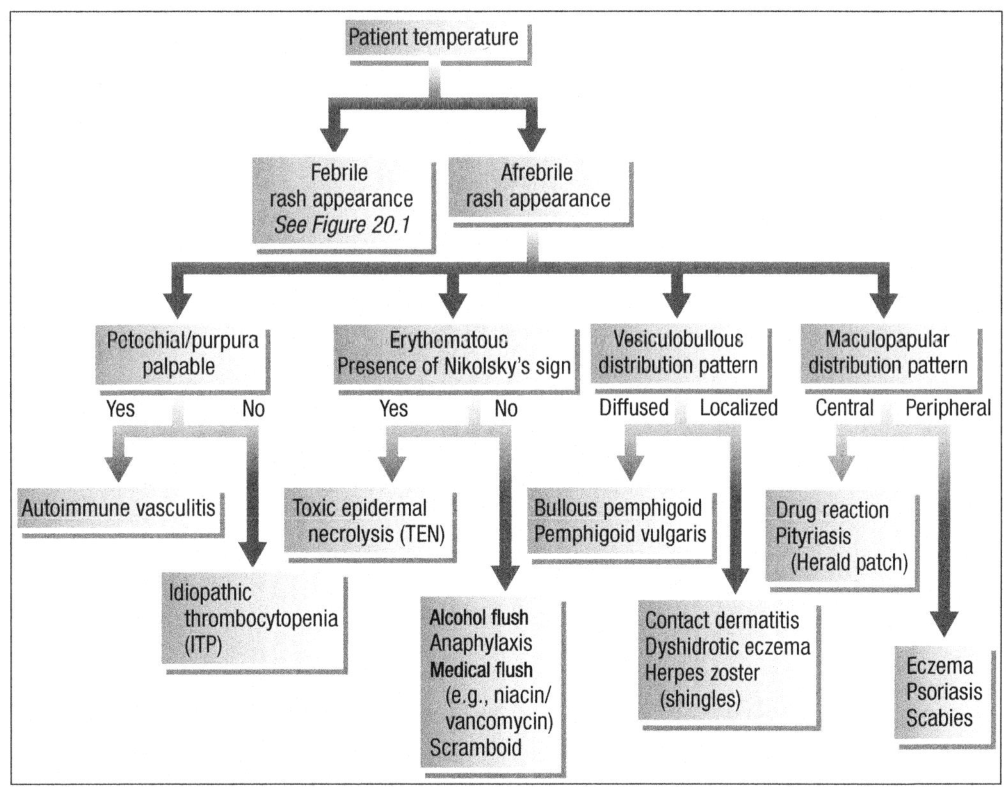

FIGURE 20.2 Evaluation of emergent rashes in afebrile patients.

E. Itching of the skin can be found in isolation from a number of causes.[183]

1. Blood disorders such as anemia (iron deficiency), leukemia, lymphoma (Hodgkin's), myeloma, polycythemia
2. Cholestasis from jaundice changes
3. HIV patients in the initial stages
4. Senile itching in patients over the age of 70 thought to be related to dry skin
5. Tumors that are solid in nature associated with specific cancers, that is, brain tumors and nasal itching, cervical tumors and vulval itching, prostate tumor, and scrotal itching
6. Uremia associated with chronic renal patients on hemodialysis

F. Nonemergent rashes[184,185]

1. Geriatric-specific rashes
a. Asteatotic eczema
i. Seen in the lower extremities with appearance in the skin of shallow cracks, like severe dry skin that has been untreated
ii. Treatment consists of topical corticosteroids and emollient therapy.
iii. Consideration of other possible underlying causes: Drug hypersensitivity, prebullous pemphigoid, or paraneoplastic disease
b. Mycosis fungoides
i. Most frequently seen form of cutaneous T-cell lymphoma
ii. Average age of onset is 55
iii. Seen as worsening of fine-scaled, erythematous patches with mild itching
iv. Referral to specialist is needed for definitive diagnosis

2. Traveler's rashes
a. Swimmer's rash (cercarial dermatitis)
i. Diffuse rash, extremely itchy, to exposed skin
ii. It is a reaction to parasite-infected snails in either freshwater or saltwater. The parasite burrows into human skin if it comes in contact with people.
iii. Prevalent areas include ponds, lakes, and marshy areas
iv. Prevention is the key.
(1) Swim in areas to avoid contact with snails
(2) Avoid putting feet down in high-risk areas.
(3) Rinse and wash well after swimming.
b. Seabather's eruption/sea lice
i. From certain jellyfish larval stings
ii. Skin covered by swimsuits is the area affected.
iii. Seen more in summertime/warmer saltwater
iv. Eruptions develop shortly after getting out of the ocean.
v. Treatment involves applying rubbing alcohol or diluted vinegar to the skin so the toxins on the skin are neutralized. Hydrocortisone 1% topical lotion should then be applied BID-TID x 1 to 2 weeks.
vi. Avoid wearing wet suit for extended period of time; wash suit or use a vinegar rinse to kill the larvae.
c. Cutaneous larva migrans
i. The hookworm parasite infection of the skin seen in pets and other animals
ii. The larvae are known for traveling under the skin leaving red tracts, usually involving only one extremity, and found to be both uncomfortable and itchy.
iii. Usually acquired from walking outside barefoot in contaminated areas.
iv. Antiparasitic medication regimen for up to 3 days. Specific medications may differ pending availability.
d. Phytophotodermatitis
i. Skin response due to being sensitive to certain fruits and plants. The skin involved is exposed to the chemical and then exposed to the sun, causing the condition. The pattern denotes areas of skin directly touched by the chemical, for example, a contaminated hand touching an area of skin drops agents on skin that leave run marks.
ii. Citrus juice is the most common cause as a result of getting juice on the skin from a tropical drink.
iii. This condition is not seen often and not well known. The pattern is confusing unless you are aware of this skin condition.

References and Additional Reading

References and Additional Reading for this chapter are online only and can be found at https://connect.springerpub.com/content/reference-book/978-0-8261-6091-5/part/part02/toc-part/ch20.

21. Hematologic and Oncologic Emergencies

WESLEY DAVIS | RENEÉ SEMONIN HOLLERAN

Learning Objectives

- Analyze the major abnormalities of hemostasis.
- Differentiate the disorders of blood coagulation.
- Compare/contrast the effects of electrolytes.
- Design a treatment plan for electrolyte and acid–base abnormalities.
- Explain the effects of oncological disorders on hemostasis and homeostasis.
- Identify some of the most common oncologic emergencies in the ED.
- Describe the management of febrile neutropenia, spinal cord compression, superior vena cava syndrome, and tumor lysis syndrome.

HEMATOLOGY AND ONCOLOGY IN THE EMERGENCY DEPARTMENT

Hemostasis is the mechanism that controls blood coagulation and stops bleeding. Disorders of hemostasis can lead to abnormal bleeding and abnormal blood coagulation. Abnormal bleeding may present as a common complaint, such as hematuria or bleeding gums. These disorders include thrombotic thrombocytopenic purpura, disseminated intravascular coagulation, and hemophilia. Abnormal coagulation most often presents as a type of thrombosis, such as a deep vein thrombosis.

The distribution of body fluids, intake and output, fluid pressures, and osmolality contribute to homeostasis. Disruptions in the sophisticated interaction between fluids and electrolytes are a common cause of medical problems that often present as nonspecific complaints. A thorough understanding of the homeostatic mechanisms that regulate fluid and electrolyte balance is essential to diagnosing and treating these disorders. Deregulation of the body's hemostasis and homeostasis mechanisms is commonly seen in patients with neoplastic diseases.

Anemia[1–3]

Pathophysiology

Anemia is a less than normal mass of red blood cells (RBCs) as measured by the hemoglobin (Hgb), hematocrit (Hct), or RBC count. Anemia decreases the oxygen-carrying capacity of the blood. The normal Hgb and Hct varies with age. Anemia in adult females is defined as a Hgb <12 g/dL or Hct <35%. Anemia in adult males is defined as a Hgb <14 g/dL or Hct <40%. While anemia can be acute or chronic, it is always an indication of disease and may be the initial manifestation of a health problem. Table 21.1 summarizes normal Hgb and Hct values by age.[3]

A. *Etiology*
   1. Anemia results from one of three causes:
      a. Blood loss (most common cause)
         i. Heavy menstruation
         ii. Gastrointestinal bleeding
         iii. Trauma
      b. Decreased production of RBCs
         i. Hypochromic and microcytic
            (1) Iron deficiency
            (2) Chronic disease states
            (3) Sideroblastic anemia
            (4) Lead poisoning
            (5) Thalassemia
         ii. Normochromic and macrocytic
            (1) Liver diseases
            (2) Folate deficiency
            (3) Vitamin B12 deficiency
            (4) Hypothyroidism
            (5) Myelodysplasia
            (6) Certain types of leukemia
         iii. Normochromic and normocytic
            (1) Aplastic anemia
            (2) Renal disease
            (3) Cancer
            (4) Hyperparathyroidism
            (5) Adrenal insufficiency
            (6) Alcohol abuse
            (7) Acute blood loss

TABLE 21.1 NORMAL HEMOGLOBIN AND HEMATOCRIT VALUES BY AGE

Age	Hemoglobin	Hematocrit
Birth	16.5	51
3 months	10.4–12.2	30–36
3–7 years	11.7–13.5	34–40
Adult male	14–18	40–52
Adult female	12–16	35–47

c. Destruction of RBCs

i. The most useful method to classify hemolytic anemias is by processes that are either intrinsic or extrinsic to the cell membrane.

ii. Intrinsic

(1) Enzyme defects

(a) Pyruvate kinase deficiency

(b) Glucose-6-phosphate dehydrogenase (G6PD) deficiency

(2) Membrane abnormality

(a) Spherocytosis

(b) Paroxysmal nocturnal hemoglobinuria

(3) Hgb abnormality

(a) Hemoglobinopathies

(b) Thalassemias

(c) Hgb M

(d) Sickle cell disease

iii. Extrinsic

(1) *Immunologic*

(a) Alloantibodies (blood transfusion reaction)

(b) Autoantibodies

(2) *Mechanical:* Prosthetic heart valve

(3) Environmental

(a) Toxic substances

(b) Infections (malaria)

Medical Screening

A. *Chief complaint:* Generalized weakness, exertional dyspnea, and/or chest pain

B. *Signs and symptoms*

1. Depends on speed of onset

a. Acute onset may cause signs and symptoms of hypovolemia.

b. Chronic or mild anemia may be asymptomatic.

2. Fatigue and/or decreased energy level, exercise intolerance

3. Dyspnea

4. Worsening heart failure or angina, syncope

5. Dizziness

6. Heavy or irregular menses, blood in stools, easy bruising, pallor

7. Poor nutrition

8. Non-nutritive cravings (ice)

C. *Past medical history*

1. Diet history including vegetarianism and alcohol intake

2. Drugs such as hydroxyurea and chemotherapeutic agents may cause anemia.

3. Approximately 10% to 14% of African American males have G6PD deficiency.

D. *Focused assessment*

1. *Skin:* Cool and pale skin, purpura, petechiae, ecchymosis, jaundice, telangiectasia, alopecia

2. *Eyes:* Pale conjunctiva

3. *Ears, nose, and throat (ENT):* Glossitis, angular stomatitis, loss of tongue papillae

4. *Cardiac:* Tachycardia, orthostatic hypotension

5. *Neurological:* Altered mental status

6. *Gastrointestinal:* Hepatosplenomegaly

Differential Diagnoses

A. Blood loss

B. Congestive heart failure

C. Anemia of chronic disease

D. Hemolysis

E. Malignancy

F. Dilutional anemia

G. Nutritional deficiency

H. Bone marrow suppression

I. G6PD deficiency

Diagnostic Testing

A. *Labs*

1. Complete blood count (CBC) with peripheral smear. The RBC indices are useful for determining the cause of anemias.

2. Prothrombin time (PT) and international normalized ratio (INR) may be prolonged if there is an underlying disease state.

3. Partial thromboplastin time (PTT) may be prolonged if there is an underlying disease state.

4. Type and screen with crossmatch

5. Stool for occult blood

B. *Vital signs, orthostatic vital signs*

Management

A. *Pharmacologic therapies*

1. Iron

2. Vitamin B12

3. Vitamin B9 (folic acid)

4. Corticosteroids for autoimmune-related anemia

5. Recombinant erythropoietin for anemia related to chronic kidney disease

6. Stop offending drug if drug-induced hemolytic anemia

B. *Nonpharmacologic therapies*

1. Airway, breathing, circulation (ABCs)

2. Oxygen

3. Control bleeding (pressure, tourniquets)

4. Large bore intravenous (IV) lines

5. IV crystalloid resuscitation for hypotension

6. Transfusion of packed RBCs for abnormal vital signs not responsive to IV crystalloids

C. *Consultation/collaboration*

1. Hematologist consult

2. Oncologist consult for anemias related to cancer and chemotherapeutic agents

3. Surgical consult for trauma

4. Gastroenterology consult for anemia related to gastrointestinal bleeding

Patient Disposition

A. *Admit*

1. Unstable vital signs

2. Anemia with cardiac or neurologic symptoms, such as dyspnea or chest pain

3. Need for blood product transfusion

4. Anemia with comorbid disease states (coronary artery disease)

5. Initial unexplained Hgb less than 10 g/dL or a Hct <30%

Age and Developmental Considerations

A. *Pediatric*
   1. Consider hemolytic anemia of the newborn in the neonatal period.
   2. The physiologic nadir, or physiologic anemia of infancy, occurs at age 8 to 12 weeks for full-term infants and age 3 to 6 weeks for preterm infants.

B. *Pregnancy*
   1. Physiologic or dilutional anemia of pregnancy is attributed to a 25% increase in mass of RBCs and 50% increase of plasma volume during the third trimester.

C. *Geriatric*
   1. Hgb and Hct values in healthy geriatric population will likely be lower than in younger adults.

Deep Vein Thrombosis[1,2,4]

Pathophysiology

A deep vein thrombosis (DVT) results when fibrin production exceeds its breakdown. According to Virchow's triad, DVT is caused by vessel wall injury, blood stasis, and hypercoagulability. Catalysts for DVT include trauma, systemic inflammation, cancer, pregnancy, and slow blood flow. After an inciting event, DVT begins in the calf and extends proximally through the deep venous system.[3]

Medical Screening

A. *Chief complaint:* Unilateral extremity pain

B. *Signs and symptoms*
   1. Unilateral extremity pain and/or swelling
   2. Muscle cramping

C. *Past medical history*
   1. Screen for risk factors including age greater than or equal to 40 years, prior DVT, malignancy, prolonged immobilization, major surgery, trauma, pregnancy, hormone replacement therapy, and oral contraceptive use.

D. *Focused assessment*
   1. *Skin:* Erythema of the affected extremity
   2. *Cardiovascular:* Tenderness along the deep venous system, extremity warmth, leg swelling >1 cm compared to the opposite leg, palpable venous cord, arm swelling on the same side as an indwelling catheter

Differential Diagnoses

A. Superficial thrombophlebitis
B. Cellulitis
C. Lymphedema
D. Venous insufficiency
E. Post-thrombotic syndrome
F. Thoracic outlet syndrome
G. Muscle strain or tear or unrecognized trauma
H. Baker's cyst
I. Phlegmasia cerulea dolens (may mimic arterial occlusion)

Diagnostic Testing

A. *Risk stratification based on pretest probability:* Well's score for DVT

B. *Labs:* D-dimer elevated

C. *Imaging:* Venous duplex ultrasound in combination with d-dimer has nearly a 100% negative predictive value.

Management

A. *Pharmacologic therapies*
   1. For isolated DVT, direct oral anticoagulants (DOACs), such as rivaroxaban or apixaban, with close follow-up are recommended.
   2. In patients with active cancer and DVT, low-molecular-weight heparin (LMWH) is preferable.
   3. If vitamin K antagonist therapy is chosen, it must be overlapped with parenteral unfractionated heparin or LMWH.
   4. For patients with limb-threatening thrombosis, such as iliofemoral venous obstruction, or patients with a creatinine clearance <30 mL/min, weight-based IV heparin is preferred.

B. *Nonpharmacologic therapies:* Compression stockings are no longer warranted for routine treatment of DVT.

C. *Consultation/collaboration*
   1. Consult vascular surgery for severe cases requiring thrombolysis or thrombectomy, such as iliofemoral venous obstruction, and for cases of septic thrombophlebitis. Also, consult vascular surgery for DVTs of the upper extremities.

Patient Disposition

A. Patients with a negative ultrasound (US) but a medium to high clinical suspicion of DVT should have a repeat US in approximately 1 week.

B. Use modified Hestia criteria to select patients with DVT for home therapy.

Age and Developmental Considerations

A. *Pediatric considerations*[3]
   1. DVT in children is rare. When DVT does occur in the pediatric age group, look for an underlying cause of hypercoagulability.
   2. In consultation with a hematologist, DVT in pediatric patients (newborn to adolescence) should be treated with unfractionated heparin or LMWH while initiating warfarin.

B. *Pregnancy:* Pregnancy is a risk factor for DVT.

Disseminated Intravascular Coagulation[1,4,5]

Pathophysiology

Disseminated intravascular coagulation (DIC) is a life-threatening coagulopathy resulting from a disruption in the balance between thrombus formation and lysis. The cascade of events leading to DIC is always the result of an inciting event, such as trauma, a major surgical procedure, sepsis, massive blood transfusions, pregnancy complications, allergic reactions, and snakebites.[3]

Medical Screening

A. *Chief complaint:* Related to excessive bleeding

B. *Signs and symptoms*
   1. *Gastrointestinal:* Bleeding, menorrhagia, epistaxis, hemoptysis, wound bleeding

2. Weakness, dizziness, headache
3. Shortness of breath
4. Bruising
5. Joint pain from hemorrhage into synovial space

C. *Past medical history*
1. Recent major trauma or surgical procedure
2. Recent pregnancy complications, such as septic abortion

D. *Focused assessment*
1. *Skin:* Petechiae, purpura, jaundice, cyanosis, bleeding at invasive line sites
2. *Cardiac:* Hypotension, tachycardia, diminished peripheral pulses
3. *Pulmonary:* Tachypnea
4. *Neurological:* Altered mental status, seizure, coma
5. *GI:* Abdominal distention for intra-abdominal hemorrhage
6. *Genitourinary:* Hematuria, oliguria, anuria

Diagnostic Testing

A. *Labs*
1. Complete blood count (CBC)
   a. Thrombocytopenia
   b. Anemia
   c. Hemoglobin and hematocrit decreased
2. Coagulation profile
   a. Prothrombin time (PT) and partial thromboplastin time (PTT) prolonged
   b. Presence of fibrinogen degradation products (FDPs)
   c. Fibrinogen decreased
   d. D-dimer increased
   e. Antithrombin III level decreased
   f. Bleeding time prolonged
3. Blood urea nitrogen (BUN) and creatinine elevated
4. *Urinalysis:* Hematuria
5. Stool for occult blood
6. Pregnancy test

B. *Imaging*
1. CT scan and ultrasound (US) as necessary to rule out sites of bleeding
   a. Intracranial hemorrhage
   b. Hemoptysis
   c. Hemorrhage associated with pregnancy or obstetric complication

Differential Diagnoses

A. Genetic coagulation disorders
B. Immune thrombocytopenic purpura (ITP)
C. Thrombotic thrombocytopenic purpura (TTP)
D. Bleeding related to anticoagulant prescriptions
E. Liver disease

Management

A. *Pharmacologic therapies*
1. Treat underlying cause
   a. Antibiotics for bacteremia
   b. Heparin if thrombotic events are more dominant
2. Recombinant human activated protein C (rhAPC)
3. Tranexamic acid
4. Avoid NSAIDs and aspirin.

B. *Nonpharmacologic therapies*
1. Transfusions to replace depleted blood and clotting factors
   a. Packed red blood cells (PRBCs), washed
   b. Platelet concentrates
   c. Cryoprecipitate
   d. Fresh frozen plasma (FFP)
2. Limit invasive procedures that may cause bleeding.
3. Pressure dressings to sites of bleeding

C. *Consultation/collaboration*
1. Hematologist or intensivist for assistance with determining treatment options
2. Obstetrics for DIC associated with an obstetrical complication

Disposition

A. All cases of DIC should be admitted to the ICU.

Age and Developmental Considerations

A. Successful treatment leads to a decrease in fibrin degradation products and a rise in platelet counts and fibrinogen levels.

Hemophilia[1–3]

Pathophysiology

Hemophilia is the result of a congenital coagulation disorder resulting in the deficiency of factor VIII, IX, or XI, hemophilia A, B, or C, respectively. The severity of the disease is directly related to the percentage of factor activity. Hemophilia is a sex-linked disease that primarily affects males.[2]

Medical Screening

A. *Chief complaint:* Related to excessive bleeding

B. *Signs and symptoms*
1. Excessive bleeding after minor trauma, gingival bleeding, blood in stool, hematuria, epistaxis
2. Headache, neurologic dysfunction
3. Abdominal pain
4. Joint pain and swelling from hemarthrosis
5. Pale skin

C. *Past medical history:* Family history of a bleeding diathesis

D. *Focused assessment*
1. *Skin:* Ecchymosis, pallor, hematoma, uncontrolled bleeding
2. *Ears, nose, and throat (ENT):* Examine oral and nasal mucosa for bleeding.
3. *Cardiac:* Signs of shock from hemorrhage
4. *Neurological:* Neurologic deficits if associated with intracranial hemorrhage
5. *Gastrointestinal:* Abdominal tenderness if intra-abdominal hemorrhage; evaluate for splenomegaly.
6. *Musculoskeletal:* Joint tenderness, swelling, and limited range of motion due to hemorrhage into synovial spaces, compartment syndrome

Differential Diagnoses

A. Von Willebrand disease
B. Thrombocytopenia

C. Vitamin K deficiency and warfarin-associated bleeding
D. Anticoagulant and antiplatelet drugs
E. Liver disease
F. Disseminated intravascular coagulation (DIC)
G. Compartment syndrome from large hematomas

Diagnostic Testing

A. *Labs*
  1. Complete blood count (CBC)
  2. Coagulation profile
    a. Prothrombin time (PT) and partial thromboplastin time (PTT)
    b. Factor VIII, IX, XI levels
  3. Type and screen
  4. Urinalysis for hematuria

B. *Imaging*
  1. Head CT if any neurologic symptoms
  2. Renal ultrasound (US) or CT for excessive hematuria
  3. Abdominal CT to evaluate for suspected intra-abdominal hemorrhage

Management

A. *Pharmacologic therapies*
  1. Replace factors immediately with factor concentrate.
  2. Desmopressin (DDAVP) may be used to stimulate the release of factor VIII.
  3. Topical thrombin for epistaxis

B. *Nonpharmacologic therapies*
  1. Avoid all invasive procedures until factors have been replaced.
  2. Topical collagen, fibrin, or thrombin for bleeding associated with tooth extraction
  3. Splint and ice joints with suspected hemarthrosis

C. *Consultation/collaboration*
  1. Collaborate with patients' hematologist to facilitate ED care.
  2. Consult neurosurgery for intracranial bleeding.
  3. Consult general surgery for suspected compartment syndrome.
  4. Consult GI for associated GI bleeding.

Patient Disposition

A. Patients with minor bleeding can be discharged home after receiving factor concentrate and the bleeding is controlled.
B. Admit patients with bleeding involving the central nervous system (CNS), abdomen, and muscles where compartment syndrome may develop.
C. Admit patients who are refractory to treatment and may require multiple transfusions.

Age and Developmental Considerations

A. Initiate factor replacement early and prior to performing diagnostic procedures.

Polycythemia[1,3,5]

Pathophysiology

Polycythemia is an increase in the number of red blood cells (RBCs) above the normal range. Polycythemia is commonly encountered in the ED, but it rarely requires emergency treatment. The majority of the signs and symptoms of polycythemia are directly related to increased blood viscosity. As a result of hyperviscosity, thrombosis is the leading cause of death in patients with polycythemia vera.

Medical Screening

A. *Chief complaint:* Headache, epistaxis, dizziness, vertigo, changes in vision

B. *Signs and symptoms*
  1. Spontaneous bruising, pruritus
  2. Generalized weakness and fatigue
  3. Visual disturbances, tinnitus, paresthesias
  4. *Gastrointestinal:* Bleeding, gingival bleeding

C. *Focused assessment*
  1. *General:* Diaphoresis
  2. *Skin:* Erythema of hands, feet, and nail beds; excoriations from pruritus; ecchymosis
  3. *Eyes:* Conjunctival suffusion, venous engorgement of the fundus
  4. *Ears, nose, and throat (ENT):* Gingival bleeding
  5. *Cardiac:* Edema
  6. *Pulmonary:* Crackles and signs of fluid overload

Differential Diagnoses

A. Dehydration
B. Polycythemia vera
C. Kidney disease
D. Cocaine abuse
E. Viral hepatitis
F. AIDS
G. Smoking
H. Chronic pulmonary disease

Diagnostic Testing

A. *Labs*
  1. *Complete blood count CBC with platelets:* Men hemoglobin >17.5 g/dL, hematocrit >52%; women hemoglobin >16 g/dL, hematocrit >48%; often associated with thrombocytosis and leukocytosis

Management

A. *Pharmacologic therapies*
  1. 0.9% normal saline bolus for hemodilution and in the absence of fluid overload
  2. Aspirin
  3. Diphenhydramine for pruritus

B. *Nonpharmacologic therapies*
  1. Emergency phlebotomy of 500 mL of blood over 2 hours
  2. Replace blood with equal amount of 0.9% normal saline.
  3. Goal hematocrit is <60%.

C. *Consultation/collaboration:* Consult hematologist.

Patient Disposition

A. Admit for hematocrit >60%, hemodynamic instability, or signs and symptoms of hyperviscosity.
B. Asymptomatic patients with a hematocrit <60% can be discharged.

Sickle Cell Disease[1,4,5]

Pathophysiology

Sickle cell disease (SCD), the most common genetic disorder in the United States, is responsible for many ED visits due to the often severe, acute pain associated with vaso-occlusive crisis (VOC). VOCs are often precipitated by stressors, such as an infectious process, hypoxia, cold temperature, or dehydration.

Medical Screening

A. *Chief complaint:* Muscle, joint, and back pain
B. *Signs and symptoms*
  1. Severe pain, fever, joint swelling
  2. Pain in extremities, joints, and back
  3. Tachypnea, hypoxemia, chest pain
  4. Abdominal pain, nausea, vomiting
  5. Fatigue and pallor
  6. Focal neurologic deficit, headache
C. *Past medical history*
  1. Family or personal history of sickle cell trait or SCD
D. *Focused assessment*
  1. *General:* Pain in the bones and joints
  2. *Skin:* Jaundice, pallor, chronic skin ulcers
  3. *Eyes:* Jaundice
  4. *Cardiac:* Tachycardia, jugular vein distention (JVD), peripheral edema, murmurs
  5. *Pulmonary:* Tachypnea, hypoxia, wheezing, rales
  6. *Neurological:* Focal such as cranial nerve palsy
  7. *Gastrointestinal:* Hepatomegaly, splenomegaly
  8. *Musculoskeletal:* Edema of hands and feet in children

Diagnostic Testing

No diagnostic test is available to confirm or rule out VOC.
A. *Labs*
  1. Complete blood count (CBC) with differential
    a. Peripheral smear may show sickled erythrocytes.
    b. Leukocytosis
    c. Thrombocytosis
    d. Compare results with previous values.
  2. Reticulocyte count elevated
  3. Lactate dehydrogenase (LDH) and total bilirubin elevated due to hemolysis
  4. Cultures with gram stain for fever
    a. Indwelling lines or catheters
    b. Blood
    c. Urine
    d. Sputum
    e. Wound
    f. Cerebrospinal fluid (CSF)
  5. Type and screen for anemia
B. *Imaging*
  1. Chest x-ray (CXR) for any signs of pulmonary complication, such as acute chest syndrome
  2. Head CT for neurologic deficits suggestive of cerebrovascular accident (CVA)
  3. Ultrasound (US) for hepatosplenomegaly and abdominal tenderness

Differential Diagnoses

A. Consider VOC mimics.
  1. Myocardial ischemia/infarction
  2. Pulmonary embolism
B. Consider complications of SCD.
  1. Aplastic crisis
  2. CVA
  3. Acute chest syndrome
  4. Splenic infarction or acute sequestration
  5. Osteomyelitis
  6. Bone infarcts and avascular necrosis of femoral or humeral head
  7. Retinal hemorrhage

Management

A. *Pharmacologic therapies*
  1. IV opioids are the mainstay of treatment for acute VOC.
    a. Reassess pain level frequently.
    b. Due to often coexistent renal and hepatic dysfunction, NSAIDs and acetaminophen should be used cautiously.
    c. IV rehydration if not tolerating PO or for signs of shock
    d. Supplemental oxygen if there is hypoxia
    e. Antibiotics for infectious etiologies
B. *Nonpharmacologic therapies*
  1. Transfusion for aplastic or splenic sequestration crisis
  2. Exchange transfusions are indicated in some cases.
  3. Lumbar puncture to rule out infection or subarachnoid hemorrhage
C. *Consultation/collaboration*
  1. Consult hematology for cases associated with complications of SCD.
  2. Consult neurology for acute changes in central or focal neurologic status.
  3. Emergent urological consult for priapism lasting more than 2 hours.

Patient Disposition

A. Discharge home if pain is resolved.
B. Follow up with hematologist.
C. Hospital admission if pain is not controlled, if unable to tolerate PO intake, or if there is any associated complication, such as acute chest syndrome or aplastic crisis
D. ICU admission for any neurologic or hemodynamic instability

Age and Developmental Considerations

A. *Pediatric*
  1. Complications of SCD have a high morbidity rate.
  2. VOC is often precipitated by an infectious process.
  3. Verify immunization status.
  4. Ask if the patient is taking prophylactic penicillin.
  5. Infants may present with hand–foot syndrome with swelling of the hands and feet and painful ambulation.
B. *Pregnancy*
  1. Pregnancy may cause increased frequency of vaso-occlusive episodes.

2. Higher risk for complications during pregnancy, including hypertensive disorders of pregnancy, spontaneous abortions, premature rupture of membranes, preterm labor, and low birth weight
3. Anemia can be more profound during pregnancy.

C. *Prevention and education*
1. Primary care is essential.
2. All patients with SCD should be evaluated by a hematologist regularly.

Thrombotic Thrombocytopenic Purpura[3,4]

Pathophysiology

Thrombotic thrombocytopenic purpura (TTP) is an acquired or congenital thrombotic microangiopathy that causes thrombi formation in small vessels leading to organ damage. Thrombus formation results from an accumulation of von Willebrand factor multimers.

Medical Screening

A. *Chief complaint:* Neurologic symptoms are usually the presenting complaint.
B. *Signs and symptoms*
1. Headache, confusion, weakness, seizure, sensory and motor deficits
2. Fever
3. Ecchymosis, epistaxis, menorrhagia, GI bleeding, hematuria
4. Abdominal pain

C. *Past medical history*
1. Recent infectious illness
2. Coagulation disease

Physical Examination

A. *General:* Distress or discomfort depending on etiology of TTP
B. *Skin:* Ecchymosis, jaundice, petechiae, generalized purpura
C. *Eyes:* Retinal hemorrhage
D. *Ears, nose, and throat (ENT):* Epistaxis, bleeding gums
E. *Cardiac:* Signs of shock, hypotension, edema
F. *Pulmonary:* Tachypnea
G. *Neurological:* Focal neurologic deficits consistent with stroke, confusion, paresthesias
H. *Gastrointestinal:* Rectal bleeding, hematemesis, abdominal tenderness

Differential Diagnoses

A. Shiga toxin-mediated hemolytic uremic syndrome
B. Hemolysis, elevated liver enzymes, low platelet count (HELLP)
C. Idiopathic thrombocytopenic purpura
D. Disseminated intravascular coagulation
E. Sepsis
F. Heparin-induced thrombocytopenia
G. Systemic lupus erythematosus

Diagnostic Testing

A. *Labs*
1. Complete blood count (CBC)
a. Anemia
b. Hemoglobin and hematocrit may be normal without overt hemorrhage.
c. Thrombocytopenia
2. Urinalysis
a. Hematuria
b. Proteinuria
3. Creatinine
a. Elevated indicating acute renal failure
4. Prothrombin time (PT), partial thromboplastin time (PTT), and bleeding time are not useful and will likely be normal.
5. D-dimer
6. Lactate dehydrogenase (LDH) and bilirubin elevated

B. *Imaging*
1. X-ray and CT focused to possible areas of ischemia based on signs/symptoms

Management

A. *Pharmacologic therapies*
1. Follow evidence-based guidelines when prescribing.
2. Prednisone
3. Aspirin

B. *Nonpharmacologic therapies*
1. Large bore intravenous (IV) lines
2. Plasma exchange
3. Transfuse blood products as indicated.
a. Fresh frozen plasma (FFP) is a temporizing measure until plasma exchange transfusions can occur.
b. Red blood cells (RBCs) for anemia
c. Platelet transfusion should be avoided.
4. Dialysis for renal failure

C. *Consultation/collaboration:* Emergent hematologist consult

Patient Disposition

A. Emergent transfer to facility with plasma exchange capability
B. Admit to ICU if active bleeding or any neurologic dysfunction.

Age and Developmental Considerations

A. Patient and family education/counseling
1. May be associated with ticlopidine and clopidogrel therapy

ELECTROLYTE DISTURBANCES[6]

Fluid and electrolyte imbalances are a common finding in the acute care setting. Electrolytes have many duties in the body. They help with electrical impulses along cell membranes, regulate acid base balance so that an effective transport of fluids and water can occur in different areas of the body, and control or regulate neuromuscular function or irritability. Clinicians must consider these imbalances in many disease processes. The kidneys, antidiuretic hormone (ADH), aldosterone, and atrial natriuretic peptide all play a vital role in the excretion and retention of fluid and electrolytes.[6] These electrolytes can be positively or negatively charged. The positively charged electrolytes (cations) are sodium (Na^+), potassium (K^+), magnesium (Mg++), and calcium (Ca++). The negatively electrolytes (anion) are chloride (Cl-), bicarbonate (HCO_3-), sulfate (SO_4^{2-}), and phosphate (PO_4-). When electrolytes fall below normal range this condition can affect the delicate balance of organ function. The normal ranges are sodium 135 to 146 mEq/L, potassium 3.5 to 5.5 mEq/L, calcium 8.5 to 10.5 mg/dL, magnesium 1.5 to 2.5 mEq/L, phosphate 1.7 to 2.6 mEq/L, chloride 96 to 109 mEq/L, and bicarbonate 22 to 26 mEq/L. The hyper- hypostates of sodium, magnesium, calcium, and potassium are the most prevalent imbalances.[6]

Calcium: Hypercalcemia[7]

Medical Screening

A. *Chief complaint:* Headache, nausea and vomiting, flank pain

B. *Signs and symptoms*

1. Confusion, fatigue, generalized weakness, depression, anxiety
2. Weight loss, generalized bone pain
3. Abdominal pain, anorexia, polydipsia, constipation, polyuria
4. Prolonged immobilization

C. *Past medical history*

1. Medications such as thiazide diuretics and vitamin D may cause hypercalcemia
2. Recent radiation therapy or chemotherapy for malignancy may cause hypercalcemia

D. *Focused assessment*

1. *Cardiac:* Bradycardia, AV block, hypotension
2. *Neurological:* Irritability, lethargy, depressed reflexes

Differential Diagnoses

A. Hyperparathyroidism disease
B. Malignancy
C. Paget disease
D. Renal failure
E. Thiazide diuretic use
F. Excessive calcium and/or vitamin D use

Diagnostic Testing

A. *Labs*

1. Basic metabolic panel
2. Serum albumin level
3. Calcium, serum: >10.5 mg/dL
   a. Serum level must be corrected for albumin level.
4. Calcium, ionized is not useful in the diagnosis and treatment of hypercalcemia.
5. *Urinalysis:* may be oliguric

B. *EKG:* QT shortening, widened T wave, bundle branch blocks, AV blocks

Management

A. *Pharmacologic therapies*

1. Diuresis is the treatment of choice for hypercalcemia.
2. Frequently monitor serum electrolytes during diuresis.
3. Administer0.9% normal saline bolus until hypotension has been corrected then 200 to 300 mL/hr.
4. Furosemide can be used to avoid volume overload, but it is no longer recommended to treat hypercalcemia.
5. Calcitonin 4 units/kg IM or SC Q12h
6. Bisphosphonates

B. *Nonpharmacologic therapies*

1. Maintain airway, breathing, circulation.
2. Continuous cardiac monitoring
3. Establish IV or intraosseous (IO) access

C. *Consultation/collaboration*

1. Consult endocrinologist if hyperparathyroidism is suspected.
2. Consult nephrologist if hypercalcemia occurs in the setting of chronic renal failure.
3. Consult oncologist if hypercalcemia is related to malignancy.

Patient Disposition

A. *Admit*

1. Patients with a corrected total calcium level >13 mg/dL
2. Patients with any signs or symptoms from hypercalcemia

Age and Developmental Considerations

A. *Pediatric considerations*

1. Infantile hypercalcemia
2. May present with hypotonia.

Calcium: Hypocalcemia[8]

Medical Screening

A. *Chief complaint:* Weakness, irritability, muscle cramps

B. *Signs and symptoms*

1. Circumoral, hands and feet paresthesias
2. Carpopedal spasm or tetany
3. Anxiety and hyperventilation
4. Seizures
5. Abdominal cramping

C. *Past medical history*

1. Bisphosphonate therapy may cause hypocalcemia.

D. *Focused assessment*

1. *Cardiac:* Hemodynamic instability
2. *Pulmonary:* Wheezing due to bronchospasm, stridor due to laryngospasm
3. *Neurological:* Skeletal muscle fasciculations, Chvostek and Trousseau signs, and hyperreflexia

Differential Diagnoses

A. Hyperventilation from anxiety or stimulants
B. Severe pancreatitis
C. Toxins and drugs
D. Tumor lysis syndrome
E. Hypomagnesemia
F. Hyperphosphatemia

Diagnostic Testing

A. *Labs*
1. Calcium, ionized: <2 mEq/L
2. Calcium, serum: <8.5 mg/dL
a. Serum level must be corrected for hypoalbuminemia.
3. *Phosphate:* Hyperphosphatemia often coexists with hypocalcemia. The serum phosphate level should be measured before replacing calcium intravenous (IV).
4. *Magnesium:* Hypomagnesemia often coexists with hypocalcemia.
5. *Albumin:* Hypoalbuminemia is the most common cause of hypocalcemia.

B. *EKG:* QTc prolongation without morphological changes

Management

A. *Pharmacologic therapies*
1. Hypocalcemia rarely presents as a life-threatening condition requiring emergent intervention.
2. Calcium carbonate orally
3. Calcium gluconate IV
4. For life-threatening hypocalcemia, calcium chloride through a central line is preferred.

B. *Nonpharmacologic therapies*
1. Maintain airway, breathing, circulation
2. Continuous cardiac monitoring
3. Establish IV or IO access
4. Seizure precautions

C. *Consultation/collaboration:* Consult intensivist for symptomatic hypocalcemia.

Patient Disposition

A. Admit if symptomatic hypocalcemia
B. Discharge with oral calcium carbonate if hypocalcemia is chronic and asymptomatic.

Magnesium: Hypermagnesemia[5,9]

Medical Screening

A. *Chief complaint:* Neurologic symptoms
1. Signs and symptoms
a. Muscle weakness, mental obtundation, confusion
2. Past medical history
a. Hypermagnesemia is almost always caused by chronic renal failure.
3. Focused assessment
a. *Cardiac:* Hypotension, cardiac arrest with magnesium levels >10 mg/dL
b. *Pulmonary:* Respiratory muscle paralysis with severe hypermagnesemia
c. *Neurological:* Decreased deep tendon reflexes, flaccid paralysis
d. *Gastrointestinal:* Signs of ileus including hypoactive bowel sounds
e. *Genitourinary:* Distended bladder and other signs of urinary retention

Differential Diagnoses

A. Lithium overdose
B. Iatrogenic sources of magnesium
C. Renal failure
D. Diabetic ketoacidosis (DKA)
E. Addison disease
F. Bowel obstruction, chronic constipation
G. Tumor lysis syndrome

Diagnostic Testing

A. *Labs*
1. Magnesium >2.2 mg/dL (symptoms usually appear at levels >4 mg/dL)
2. *Basic metabolic panel (BMP):* Hyperkalemia and hypocalcemia often coexist with hypomagnesemia.
3. Creatinine elevated

B. *EKG:* Broad QRS complexes, peaked T waves, increased PR interval

Management

A. *Pharmacologic therapies*
1. Calcium antagonizes the effects of magnesium.
2. Calcium chloride IV
3. Calcium gluconate IV for life-threatening hypermagnesemia
4. For mild symptoms, IV 0.9% normal saline can be used in combination with diuretics to promote renal elimination of magnesium.
5. Asymptomatic patients can usually be managed by restricting magnesium intake.

B. *Nonpharmacologic therapies*
1. Maintain airway, breathing, circulation
2. Continuous cardiac monitoring
3. Establish IV or IO access.

C. *Consultation/collaboration*
1. Consult nephrology for hypermagnesemia related to severe kidney disease. These patients may require emergent dialysis.

Patient Disposition

A. Admit all patients with signs or symptoms of hypermagnesemia.

Age and Developmental Considerations

A. *Prevention and education:* Avoid hidden sources of magnesium, such as antacids and laxatives.

Magnesium: Hypomagnesemia[2,3,10]

Medical Screening

A. *Chief complaint:* Neurologic symptoms
B. *Signs and symptoms*
1. Delirium, coma, convulsions, tremor, apathy, ataxia
2. Muscle cramps, seizures, tetany, weakness
3. Palpitations

C. *Past medical history*
1. Hypomagnesemia is common in patients with poor diets or malnutrition, including chronic alcoholics.
2. Loop and thiazide diuretics can cause mild hypomagnesemia.

D. *Focused assessment*

1. *Cardiac:* Cardiac dysrhythmia, hypotension/hypertension
2. *Neurological:* Trousseau's and Chvostek's signs, dysarthria, dysphagia, hyperreflexia

Differential Diagnoses

A. Malnutrition
B. Alcoholism
C. Proton pump inhibitor (PPI) therapy
D. Diuretic therapy

Diagnostic Testing

A. *Labs*
   1. Magnesium <1.5 mEq/L
   2. *Basic metabolic panel (BMP):* Hypokalemia, hypocalcemia, and hyponatremia often coexist with hypomagnesemia.

B. *EKG:* PR and QT interval prolongation, ST segment depression, T wave changes, torsades de pointes

Management

A. *Pharmacologic therapies*
   1. For life-threatening hypomagnesemia in patients with normal renal function, give magnesium sulfate 1 to 2 g IV over 10 to 20 minutes.
   2. For patients in cardiac arrest, 1 to 2 g of magnesium sulfate should be given IV push.
   3. For mild and asymptomatic hypomagnesemia in patients with normal renal function, give magnesium gluconate 400 mg orally twice a day.

B. *Nonpharmacologic therapies*
   1. Maintain airway, breathing, circulation
   2. Continuous cardiac monitoring
   3. Establish IV or intraosseous (IO) access.
   4. Seizure precautions

C. *Consultation/collaboration:* Consult nephrology for hypomagnesemia in the setting of renal failure.

Patient Disposition

A. Admit all patients with signs or symptoms of hypomagnesemia.

Age and Developmental Considerations

A. *Prevention and education:* Encourage adequate dietary magnesium intake.

Phosphorus: Hyperphosphatemia[3,4]

Medical Screening

A. *Chief complaint:* Neurologic symptoms or nonspecific

B. *Signs and symptoms*
   1. Muscle cramping, muscle weakness
   2. Pruritus
   3. Anorexia, nausea, vomiting

C. *Past medical history*
   1. Common in patients with renal failure

D. *Focused assessment*
   1. *Cardiac:* Arrhythmias, hypotension or hypertension, bradycardia, or tachycardia
   2. *Pulmonary:* Respiratory failure
   3. *Neurological:* Seizures, Trousseau sign, hyperreflexia

Differential Diagnoses

A. Renal failure
B. Missed dialysis
C. Thyrotoxicosis
D. Diabetic ketoacidosis (DKA)
E. Tumor lysis syndrome
F. Rhabdomyolysis

Diagnostic Testing

A. *Labs*
   1. Phosphorus >2.5 mg/dL
   2. *Basic metabolic panel (BMP):* Hyperkalemia, creatinine may show evidence of concomitant kidney injury.
   3. Calcium low
   4. *Creatinine kinase:* Severe hyperphosphatemia can be caused by rhabdomyolysis.
   5. Urinalysis
   6. *Complete blood count (CBC):* Hemolytic anemia, platelet dysfunction

Management

A. *Pharmacologic therapies*
   1. Phosphate binders such as calcium carbonate

B. *Nonpharmacologic therapies*
   1. Maintain airway, breathing, circulation
   2. Continuous cardiac monitoring
   3. Establish intravenous (IV) or intraosseous (IO) access
   4. Seizure precautions
   5. Prepare for emergent dialysis if life-threatening signs and symptoms are associated with renal failure.

C. *Consultation/collaboration*
   1. Consult nephrology for patients with hyperphosphatemia related to kidney disease.

Patient Disposition

A. Admit if severe hyperphosphatemia requires emergent dialysis or for concomitant disease, such as acute renal failure.

Age and Developmental Considerations

A. Restrict exogenous sources of phosphate.
B. Hyperbilirubinemia, hemolysis, and hyperlipidemia may cause spurious elevations in phosphorus.

Phosphorus: Hypophosphatemia[3,4]

I. Medical Screening

A. *Chief complaint:* Neurologic symptoms or nonspecific

B. *Signs and symptoms*
   1. Paresthesias, irritability, confusion, seizures
   2. Anorexia
   3. Pain in muscles and bones, fractures

C. *Past medical history*
   1. Severe hypophosphatemia is common in chronic alcoholics.
   2. Patients with chronic obstructive pulmonary disease (COPD) and asthma who take xanthine derivative drugs may have hypophosphatemia.

D. *Focused assessment*
  1. *Skin:* Petechial hemorrhages
  2. *Cardiac:* Arrhythmias, hypotension or hypertension, bradycardia, or tachycardia
  3. *Pulmonary:* Respiratory failure
  4. *Neurological:* Dysarthria, altered mental status

Differential Diagnoses

A. Alcohol withdrawal or alcoholic ketoacidosis
B. Sepsis
C. Diuretic use
D. Hyperparathyroidism
E. Hyperthyroidism
F. Hyperventilation
G. Hypercalcemia
H. Hypomagnesemia

Diagnostic Testing

A. *Labs*
  1. *Phosphorus:* Hypophosphatemia level mild (2–2.5 mg/dL), moderate (1–2 mg /dL), severe (<1 mg/dL)
  2. Basic metabolic panel (BMP): Hyperkalemia, creatinine may show evidence of concomitant kidney injury.
  3. Calcium low
  4. *Creatinine kinase:* Severe hypophosphatemia can cause rhabdomyolysis.
  5. Urinalysis
  6. *Complete blood count (CBC):* Hemolytic anemia, platelet dysfunction

Management

A. *Pharmacologic therapies*
  1. Oral phosphate replacement is preferable for patients with a phosphorus level 1 to 2 mg/dL. Give sodium phosphate or potassium phosphate
  2. IV phosphorus should be reserved for phosphorus levels <0.5 mEq/L or for life-threatening signs.
B. *Nonpharmacologic therapies*
  1. Maintain airway, breathing, circulation
  2. Continuous cardiac monitoring
  3. Establish IV or intraosseous (IO) access.
  4. Seizure precautions
C. *Consultation/collaboration*
  1. Consult gastroenterology for patients with hypophosphatemia from decreased gastrointestinal absorption.
  2. Consult endocrinology for patients with hypophosphatemia related to hyperparathyroidism.
  3. Consult nephrology for patients with hypophosphatemia related to kidney disease, such as renal tubular defects.

Patient Disposition

A. Patients with severe signs or symptoms of hypophosphatemia should be admitted.

Age and Developmental Considerations

A. *Prevention and education:* Transient hypophosphatemia is common after treatment of hyperglycemia and diabetic ketoacidosis (DKA).

Potassium: Hyperkalemia[3,11]

Medical Screening

A. *Chief complaint:* Weakness, fatigue, palpitations
B. *Signs and symptoms*
  1. Abdominal cramping and diarrhea
  2. Muscle weakness and numbness
  3. Crush or burn injury
C. *Past medical history*
  1. Medication history
    a. Digitalis toxicity can cause an intracellular to extracellular potassium shift.
    b. Beta-blockers
    c. Angiotensin-converting enzyme (ACE) inhibitors and angiotensin receptor blockers (ARBs)
    d. Potassium-sparing diuretics
D. *Focused assessment*
  1. *Cardiac:* Cardiac dysrhythmias and hemodynamic instability with severe hyperkalemia
  2. *Neurological:* Muscular weakness progressing to paralysis, depressed deep tendon reflexes
  3. *Gastrointestinal:* Hyperactive bowel sounds

Differential Diagnoses

A. *Pseudohyperkalemia:* Hemolysis of erythrocytes is the most common cause of hyperkalemia.
B. Renal failure
C. Diabetic ketoacidosis
D. Rhabdomyolysis
E. Tumor lysis syndrome
F. *Toxicological causes:* Acute digitalis overdose

Diagnostic Testing

A. *Labs*
  1. Serum potassium level
    a. *Mild:* 5.5 to 6 mEq/L
    b. *Moderate:* 6.1 to 6.9 mEq/L
    c. *Severe:* >7 mEq/L
  2. Creatinine kinase: Rhabdomyolysis may cause hyperkalemia.
  3. Arterial or venous pH
  4. Lithium or digitalis levels if currently taking these medications
B. *EKG*
  1. *Mild hyperkalemia:* Large-amplitude T waves, QT interval shortening
  2. *Moderate hyperkalemia:* PR interval prolongation, QRS widening
  3. *Severe hyperkalemia:* AV block, sine-wave pattern, ventricular fibrillation, asystole

Management

A. *Pharmacologic therapies:* Pharmacologic therapy is needed for serum potassium levels >6 mEq/L or any EKG changes consistent with hyperkalemia.
  1. Membrane stabilization
    a. Calcium chloride 10 to 20 mL IV push, or
    b. Calcium gluconate 10 to 30 mL IV push
  2. Intracellular shift

a. Regular insulin 10 units IV push combined with 100 mL of 50% dextrose IV push
b. Albuterol nebulized by face mask, 15 to 25 mg
c. Sodium bicarbonate 50 to 100 mL
3. Potassium elimination
a. Sodium polystyrene sulfonate 25 to 50 g orally or by enema
b. Normal saline infusion with furosemide

B. *Nonpharmacologic therapies*
1. Maintain airway, breathing, circulation
2. Continuous cardiac monitoring
3. Establish IV or intraosseous (IO) access

C. *Consultation/collaboration*
1. *Nephrology:* Hemodialysis should be considered for hemodynamically unstable patients and patients in renal failure.

Patient Disposition

A. All patients with hyperkalemia require admission except in rare instances.

Age and Developmental Considerations

A. *Prevention and education*
1. Hyperkalemia is asymptomatic until late in the course.
2. Hyperkalemia should be suspected in patients with renal disease, diabetes, and those taking potassium supplements.

Potassium: Hypokalemia[11]

Medical Screening

A. *Chief complaint:* Muscle cramps and spasms, palpitations, paresthesias, fatigue

B. *Signs and symptoms*
1. Anorexia, nausea, vomiting, constipation
2. Shortness of breath
3. Urinary frequency
4. Polydipsia

C. *Past medical history*
1. Assess for diuretic use.

D. *Focused assessment*
1. *Cardiac:* Hypotension, orthostasis, irregular heart rhythm
2. *Pulmonary:* Depressed respirations in severe hypokalemia
3. *Neurological:* Hyporeflexia, muscle tenderness, weakness may range from mild to complete paralysis

Differential Diagnoses

A. Neuromuscular disease

B. Cardiac dysrhythmias associated with cardiac disease

C. Toxicological causes

Diagnostic Testing

A. *Labs*
1. Basic metabolic panel
a. Serum potassium level
i. *Mild:* 3 to 3.5 mEq/L
ii. *Moderate:* 2.5 to 3 mEq/L
iii. *Severe:* <2.5 mEq/L
2. *Magnesium:* Depletion often coexists with potassium depletion.
3. *Arterial or venous pH:* Acidotic patients should be considered severely potassium depleted.

B. *EKG:* T-wave depression, flattened T waves, AV block, premature ventricular contractions, prolongation of the QT interval, torsades de pointes, ventricular fibrillation

Management

A. *Pharmacologic therapies*
1. Potassium chloride oral replacement is preferred: 40 to 60 mEq PO every 2 to 4 hours.
2. Potassium chloride IV is recommended for severe hypokalemia and hypokalemia associated with neuromuscular symptoms or EKG changes.
a. Potassium chloride can be infused through a peripheral line at 10 to 20 mEq/hour.
b. For sustained life-threatening cardiac dysrhythmias, potassium chloride may be given through a central line at 20 to 40 mEq/hour.
c. Do not treat acidosis until hypokalemia has been corrected.
d. Recheck potassium after every 40 mEq IV.

B. *Nonpharmacologic therapies*
1. Maintain airway, breathing, circulation
2. Continuous cardiac monitoring
3. Establish IV or intraosseous (IO) access.

C. *Consultation/collaboration*

Patient Disposition

A. Admit if the serum potassium level is <2.5 mEq/L or the patient requires IV replacement.

B. May discharge home if asymptomatic and able to take potassium replacement orally at home.

Age and Developmental Considerations

A. *Prevention and education:* Follow up with primary care for repeat potassium level in 2 to 3 days.

Sodium: Hypernatremia[1,3,4]

Medical Screening

A. *Chief complaint:* Confusion, seizure, headache

B. *Signs and symptoms*
1. Anorexia, thirst, fatigue
2. Muscle cramps
3. Dizziness
4. Diarrhea, nausea, vomiting

C. *Past medical history*
1. Use of phenytoin, lithium, aminoglycosides

D. *Focused assessment*
1. *General:* Acute weight change
2. *Skin:* Poor skin turgor
3. *Cardiac:* Tachycardia, hypotension
4. *Pulmonary:* Assess airway patency

5. *Neurological:* Altered level of consciousness, confusion, hyperreflexia, asterixis, coma

Differential Diagnoses

A. Diabetic ketoacidosis (DKA)
B. Diabetes insipidus
C. Heatstroke
D. Cushing's syndrome
E. Renal failure
F. Drug side effect (phenytoin, lithium, aminoglycosides)

Diagnostic Testing

A. *Labs*
   1. Point of care glucose for altered mental status
   2. Comprehensive metabolic panel
      a. *Mild hypernatremia:* Sodium 146 to 155 mEq/L
      b. *Severe hypernatremia:* Sodium >155 mEq/L
      c. Chloride may be increased or decreased.
      d. Blood urea nitrogen (BUN) elevated in dehydration
   3. Serum osmolality increased
   4. Urine osmolality
   5. Urinalysis
B. *Imaging*
   1. Chest x-ray (CXR)
   2. May have signs of fluid overload
   3. Head CT for neurologic signs and symptoms
      a. Rule out other differentials associated with the neurologic signs and symptoms that often accompany hypernatremia.
C. *EKG*

Management

A. *Pharmacologic therapies*
   1. Volume resuscitation with 0.9% normal saline for hemodynamic instability
      a. Change to D5W or hypotonic saline when hemodynamically stable.
   2. Desmopressin (DDAVP) if hypernatremia caused by diabetes insipidus
   3. Diuretics to remove excess fluid in hypervolemic hypernatremia
   4. D5W or hypotonic saline for isovolemic hypernatremia
   5. Limit sodium correction to 0.5 mEq/hour.
   6. Frequent serum sodium level checks are needed to guide treatment.
B. *Nonpharmacologic therapies*
   1. Maintain airway, breathing, circulation
   2. Establish IV or intraosseous (IO) access
   3. Rapid sequence intubation (RSI) to maintain airway and breathing
   4. Seizure precautions
   5. Continuous cardiac monitor
   6. Calculate water deficit.
C. *Consultation/collaboration*
   1. Consult neurology for neurologic deficits and seizure.
   2. Consult pharmacist to assist with calculation of sodium correction rate.

Patient Disposition

A. *Admit if:*
   1. Sodium >150 mEq/L
   2. Any symptomatic hypernatremia will likely need ICU admission
B. *Discharge if:*
   1. Sodium <150 mEq/L
   2. Chronic sodium levels >150 mEq/L are at baseline
   3. Intact thirst mechanism

Age and Developmental Considerations

A. *Geriatric considerations:* Hypernatremia is more common in the elderly population.

Sodium: Hyponatremia[12]

Medical Screening

A. *Chief complaint:* Confusion, excessive water consumption, recent trauma, large surface area burn, or surgery
B. Signs and symptoms
   1. Nausea and vomiting, diarrhea, thirst
   2. Seizures, coma, headache, hyperthermia, altered mental status, dizziness
   3. Weight gain/loss
   4. Ascites
   5. Muscle spasms and cramps
C. *Past medical history:* Diuretic use
D. *Focused assessment*
   1. *Skin:* Poor skin turgor
   2. *Eyes:* Sunken eyes
   3. *Ears, nose, and throat (ENT):* Dry mucous membranes
   4. *Cardiac:* Mild to moderate: tachycardia Severe: bradycardia. Other signs are positive orthostatic vital signs, peripheral edema.
   5. *Pulmonary:* Compromised airway due to altered level of consciousness or coma
   6. *Neurological:* Altered level of consciousness, diminished deep tendon reflexes
   7. *Psychiatric:* Hallucinations

Differential Diagnoses

A. Elevated sodium due to hyperglycemia
B. Radiocontrast dye
C. Hyperproteinemia
D. Hyperlipidemia
E. Syndrome of inappropriate antidiuretic hormone secretion (SIADH)
F. Hypothyroidism
G. Psychogenic polydipsia

Diagnostic Testing

A. *Labs*
   1. Comprehensive metabolic panel (CMP)
      a. Chloride low
      b. Sodium <135 mEq/L

c. Bicarbonate may be increased or decreased.
d. Hyperproteinemia and hyperglycemia may cause factitious hyponatremia.
2. *Lipids:* Hyperlipidemia may cause factitious hyponatremia.
3. Serum osmolarity low
a. Volume status and serum osmolarity are essential to diagnose hyponatremia and the corresponding etiology.

B. *Imaging*
1. *Chest x-ray (CXR):* May have signs of fluid overload
2. Head CT for neurologic signs and symptoms
a. Signs of herniation due to cerebral edema
b. Rule out other differentials associated with the neurologic signs and symptoms that often accompany hyponatremia.
3. *EKG:* Bradycardia with severe hyponatremia

Management

A. *Pharmacologic therapies*
1. Severe neurologic symptoms, seizures, signs of herniation
a. Raise sodium level by 4 to 6 mEq/L within 6 hours.
b. 100 mL of 3% hypertonic saline over 10 minutes
c. May repeat 100 mL of 3% hypertonic saline over 50 minutes
d. Use caution in patients who may have a chronic hyponatremia.
2. Hypovolemic hyponatremia
a. Volume resuscitation with 0.9% normal saline to treat hypotension
b. Limit sodium correction to 0.5 mEq/hour to avoid central pontine myelinolysis.
3. Hypervolemic or euvolemic hyponatremia
a. Increase sodium in diet.
b. Restrict fluids.
c. Limit sodium correction to 0.5 mEq/hour.

B. *Nonpharmacologic therapies*
1. Maintain airway, breathing, circulation.
2. Establish IV or intraosseous (IO) access.
3. Rapid sequence intubation (RSI) to maintain airway and breathing
4. Seizure precautions
5. Continuous cardiac monitor

C. *Consultation/collaboration*
1. Consult neurology for neurologic deficits, coma, and seizure.
2. Consult pharmacist to assist with calculation of sodium correction rate.

Patient Disposition

A. *Admit if:*
1. Symptomatic hyponatremia
2. Sodium <120
3. Mild hyponatremia with comorbidities

B. *Discharge home if:*
1. Hyponatremia is chronic and asymptomatic.
2. No comorbidities
3. Has close follow-up as an outpatient

Age and Developmental Considerations

A. *Pediatric considerations*
1. Educate parents about proper dilution of formula.
2. Avoid hydration with water.

B. *Geriatric considerations*
1. Hyponatremia is common secondary to ineffective water regulation mechanisms.
2. Low sodium diets for cardiovascular disease may be contributory.

ACID–BASE DISTURBANCES

Acid–base balance is maintained by the pulmonary excretion of carbon dioxide and renal excretion of nonvolatile acids. Detection of a patient's acid–base imbalance requires measurement of pH, carbon dioxide partial pressure (PCO_2), and plasma bicarbonate from an arterial blood sample (Table 21.2). The human body creates acids in generous amounts daily. It is the body's job to metabolize and excrete these acids to function normally. A small change in this delicate balance can set off a cascade effect of damage to multiple organ systems. When this disturbance has been produced, an array of acid–base derangements are constructed.

Acids are substances that provide hydrogen ions (H+). Bases provide hydroxide ions (OH–). Acids will lower the pH, and bases will raise the pH. The pH scale measures from 0 to 14 from acidic to alkaline. A pH below 7 is acidic, and a pH above 7 is alkaline. The normal serum pH range is 7.35 to 7.45. The pH of blood is slightly alkaline. Acidemia refers to an arterial pH lower than 7.35, and alkalemia is an arterial pH above 7.45. Acidosis is the

TABLE 21.2 ACID–BASE ABNORMALITIES

	pH	$PaCO_2$	HCO_3
Normal values	7.35–7.45	35–45	22–26
Respiratory acidosis	Decreased	Increased	Normal
Respiratory alkalosis	Increased	Decreased	Normal
Respiratory acidosis with metabolic compensation	Decreased	Increased	Increased
Metabolic acidosis	Decreased	Normal	Decreased
Metabolic alkalosis	Increased	Normal	Increased
Metabolic alkalosis with respiratory compensation	Increased	Increased	Increased

process that lowers extracellular fluid pH, and alkalosis is the rise of extracellular fluid pH.[13]

The delicate balance of acid and bases is maintained by different buffering systems in the body. Chemical buffers in the blood, such as plasm proteins, bicarbonate, and phosphate, help work inside the cell to keep this equilibrium. The major plasm protein is hemoglobin. Hemoglobin buffers hydrogen, which is released by the conversion of CO_2 into bicarbonate. These sequences of actions help maintain a normal pH. The carbonic acid–bicarbonate buffer system helps maintain normal pH by converting strong bases to a weak base and strong acids to a weak acid. The renal systems help maintain a normal pH by excreting hydrogen ions into the urine and reabsorbing bicarbonate from the urine. Carbon dioxide plays a large factor in the lung's role in regulating acid and base in the body—the balanced is maintained by the change in tidal volume and respiratory rate.[13] Arterial chemoreceptors notice a difference in pH and will either increase or decrease tidal volume and respiratory rate. This process can take up to minutes or hours.

Simple acid–base disorders are metabolic acidosis, respiratory acidosis, metabolic alkalosis, and respiratory alkalosis. Metabolic acidosis is the result of a decrease in serum bicarbonate and pH below 7.35. The presence of a normal or abnormal anion gap will help with the differential diagnosis of this acid–base imbalance. The anion gap is the difference between the number of cations versus anions. Cations are positive (base), and anions are negative (acid). An elevated anion gap in metabolic acidosis can be caused by ketoacidosis (e.g., diabetic, alcoholic, and starvation), lactic acidosis, renal failure, toxins metabolized to acids, and severe rhabdomyolysis.[14] Causes of an elevated anion gap can be remembered by the mnemonic MUDPILES:

A. Methanol toxicity
B. Uremia
C. Diabetic ketoacidosis
D. Paraldehyde
E. Isoniazid or iron toxicity
F. Lactic acidosis
G. Ethylene glycol toxicity
H. Salicylate toxicity

Metabolic Acidosis

Metabolic acidosis with a normal anion gap can be caused by gastrointestinal loss of bicarbonate, renal loss of bicarbonate, rapid normal saline infusion, urologic procedures, ingestions, hypoaldosteronism, hyperkalemia, and toluene.[14]

Medical Screening

A. *Chief complaint:* Nonspecific, protracted diarrhea, panic attack
B. *Signs and symptoms*
  1. Confusion, somnolence
  2. Nausea, vomiting, diarrhea
  3. Hyperventilation
C. *Focused assessment*
  1. *Cardiac:* Tachycardia
  2. *Pulmonary:* Tachypnea, Kussmaul respirations
  3. *Neurological:* Altered mental status

Differential Diagnoses

A. See Table 21.3 for differential diagnoses of metabolic acidosis.

Diagnostic Testing

A. *Labs*
  1. Arterial blood gas (ABG)
    a. pH low
    b. $PaCO_2$ normal to low
    c. HCO_3 low (hallmark of metabolic acidosis)
  2. Basic metabolic panel (BMP) commonly shows concurrent electrolyte abnormalities.
  3. EKG to evaluate for conduction disturbances
  4. CO level for suspected carbon monoxide toxicity
  5. Calculate the anion gap to help with the differential diagnosis.

Management

A. *Pharmacologic therapies*
  1. Treat the underlying cause
  2. 0.9% normal saline for volume replacement
B. *Nonpharmacologic therapies*
  1. Maintain airway, breathing, circulation

TABLE 21.3 DIFFERENTIAL DIAGNOSES OF METABOLIC ACIDOSIS: MNEMONICS

HIGH ANION GAP METABOLIC ACIDOSIS: MUDPILES MNEMONIC	NORMAL ANION GAP METABOLIC ACIDOSIS: HARDUPS MNEMONIC
Methanol	**H**yperventilation
Uremia	**A**cetazolamide, **a**cids, **A**ddison disease
Diabetic ketoacidosis or alcoholic ketoacidosis	**R**enal tubular acidosis
Propylene glycol, **p**aracetamol	**D**iarrhea
Isoniazid (INH) and **i**ron	**U**reterosigmoidostomy
Lactic acidosis	**P**ancreatic fistulas
Ethylene glycol	**S**aline in large volumes
Salicylates and **s**olvents	

2. Establish intravenous (IV) or intraosseous (IO) access
3. Rapid sequence intubation (RSI) or bilevel positive airway pressure (BiPAP) for ventilatory support
4. Continuous cardiac monitor

C. *Consultation/collaboration*
1. Nephrology consult for toxin-induced metabolic acidosis that requires hemodialysis
2. Consult poison control for overdose and toxic ingestion.

Patient Disposition

A. *Consider admission for any of the following:* Altered mental status, cardiac dysrhythmias, concurrent electrolyte abnormalities, hemodynamic instability.

Metabolic Alkalosis

Metabolic alkalosis occurs when there is an increase in bicarbonate and a loss of hydrogen ions. This change is caused by an intracellular shift of hydrogen ions. The respiratory system will begin to compensate by decreasing ventilation and retaining carbon dioxide. The kidneys will try to excrete excess bicarbonate through the urine. Possible causes of metabolic alkalosis are prolonged vomiting, nasogastric suction, diuretics, severe potassium or sodium depletion, alcohol abuse, Bartter's syndrome, and massive transfusion, especially in renal insufficiency.[15]

Medical Screening

A. *Chief complaint:* Nonspecific, protracted vomiting

B. *Signs and symptoms*
1. Confusion, somnolence
2. Vomiting

C. *Focused assessment*
1. *Pulmonary:* Hypoventilation
2. *Neurological:* Altered mental status

Differential Diagnoses

A. Volume contraction alkalosis from diuretic use
B. Severe hypokalemia
C. Hypercalcemia
D. Massive transfusion

Diagnostic Testing

A. *Labs*
1. Arterial blood gas (ABG)
   a. pH high
   b. $PaCO_2$ normal to high
   c. HCO3 high (hallmark of metabolic alkalosis)
2. Basic metabolic panel (BMP) commonly shows concurrent electrolyte abnormalities.

B. *EKG:* To evaluate for conduction disturbances

Management

A. *Pharmacologic therapies*
1. Treat the underlying cause.
2. 0.9% normal saline for volume replacement

B. *Nonpharmacologic therapies*
1. Maintain airway, breathing, circulation.
2. Establish intravenous (IV) or intraosseous (IO) access.
3. Rapid sequence intubation (RSI) or bilevel positive airway pressure (BiPAP) for ventilatory support
4. Continuous cardiac monitor

C. *Consultation/collaboration:* Intensivist consult of ICU admission

Patient Disposition

A. *Consider admission for any of the following:* Altered mental status, cardiac dysrhythmias, concurrent electrolyte abnormalities, hemodynamic instability.

Respiratory Acidosis

Respiratory acidosis is caused by any condition that decreases ventilation. It is an increase in carbon dioxide partial pressure (PCO_2), while bicarbonate level can be decreased or normal. Respiratory acidosis is typically caused by a decrease in central nervous system (CNS) respiratory drive, muscular weakness, obstructive pulmonary disorders, and hypoxia. Respiratory acidosis can an acute or chronic condition.[16]

Medical Screening

A. *Chief complaint:* Nonspecific, respiratory arrest, unresponsive

B. *Signs and symptoms*
1. Confusion, somnolence, headache, anxiety
2. Nausea, vomiting, diarrhea
3. Ischemic chest pain

C. *Focused assessment*
1. *Cardiac:* Bradycardia, circulatory collapse
2. *Pulmonary:* Decreased minute volume
3. *Neurological:* Altered mental status, seizures, papilledema

Differential Diagnoses

A. Sedative overdose
B. Stroke
C. Pulmonary embolism
D. End-stage interstitial lung disease
E. Obstructive pulmonary disease
F. Toxins
G. Electrolyte disturbances
H. Congestive heart failure
I. Pneumothorax

Diagnostic Testing

A. *Labs*
1. Arterial blood gas (ABG)
   a. pH low
   b. $PaCO_2$ increased (hallmark of respiratory acidosis)
   c. HCO3 normal or high
2. Basic metabolic panel (BMP) commonly shows concurrent electrolyte abnormalities.

a. Hypochloremia is common.

B. *EKG:* To evaluate for conduction disturbances

C. *Toxicology screen*: For opiates, benzodiazepines, tricyclic antidepressants, and barbiturates

Management

A. *Pharmacologic therapies*

1. Treat the underlying cause.

B. *Nonpharmacologic therapies*

1. Maintain airway, breathing, circulation.
2. Establish intravenous (IV) or intraosseous (IO) access.
3. Rapid sequence intubation (RSI) or bilevel positive airway pressure (BiPAP) for ventilatory support
4. Continuous cardiac monitor

C. *Consultation/collaboration*

1. Intensivist consult of ICU admission
2. Consult poison control for overdose and toxic ingestion.

Patient Disposition

A. *Consider admission for any of the following:* Altered mental status, cardiac dysrhythmias, concurrent electrolyte abnormalities, hemodynamic instability

Respiratory Alkalosis

Respiratory alkalosis is noticed when there is an increase in ventilation. It is a decrease in carbon dioxide partial pressure (PCO_2) and an increase in the serum pH. The kidney helps in this maintenance by decreasing hydrogen secretion and increasing bicarbonate secretion. Causes of respiratory alkalosis can be from fever, acute onset of dyspnea, anxiety, trauma, recent surgery, thromboembolic disease, hypocalcemia, asthma, stroke (cerebrovascular accident [CVA]), and chronic obstructive pulmonary disease (COPD). Another cause is from toxic ingestions. A common cause is from salicylate toxicity.[15]

Medical Screening

A. *Chief complaint:* Nonspecific, anxiety-related hyperventilation

B. *Signs and symptoms*

1. Anxiety
2. Lip and hand paresthesias, carpopedal spasm, syncope
3. Hyperventilation

C. *Focused assessment*

1. *Cardiac:* Tachycardia
2. *Pulmonary:* Tachypnea, Kussmaul respirations
3. *Neurological:* Altered mental status

Differential Diagnoses

A. Salicylate toxicity
B. Anxiety
C. Caffeine overdose
D. Nicotine overdose
E. Anemia
F. Pulmonary embolism
G. Pulmonary edema
H. Pregnancy
I. Sepsis
J. Hyponatremia

Diagnostic Testing

A. *Labs*

1. Arterial blood gas (ABG)
   a. pH high
   b. $PaCO_2$ low (hallmark of respiratory alkalosis)
   c. HCO_3 normal or low
2. Basic metabolic panel (BMP) commonly shows concurrent electrolyte abnormalities.
   a. Hypocalcemia is common.
3. EKG to evaluate for conduction disturbances

Management

A. *Pharmacologic therapies*

1. Treat the underlying cause.

B. *Nonpharmacologic therapies*

1. Maintain airway, breathing, circulation
2. Establish intravenous (IV) or intraosseous (IO) access
3. Rapid sequence intubation (RSI) or bilevel positive airway pressure (BiPAP) for ventilatory support
4. Continuous cardiac monitor

C. *Consultation/collaboration*

1. Intensivist consult of ICU admission
2. Consult poison control for overdose and toxic ingestion.

Patient Disposition

A. *Consider admission for any of the following:* Altered mental status, cardiac dysrhythmias, concurrent electrolyte abnormalities, or hemodynamic instability.

Age and Developmental Considerations

A. *Pregnancy considerations*

1. A normal $PaCO_2$ and normal serum pH indicates hypoventilation in pregnant patients.

ONCOLOGIC EMERGENCIES

Cancer is one of the leading causes of death throughout the world. By 2040, it is estimated that there will be 29.5 million new cancer cases, with a death rate of 16.4 million patients (https://www.cancer.gov/about-cancer/understanding/statistics#). Because of the variability of where patients with cancer are cared for and the variety of reasons patients with cancer may come to the ED, it is difficult to estimate how many patients with oncologic emergencies present to the ED.[17] However, patients do come to the ED for care related to their cancer diagnoses. These patients are complex and require resources not always available in many EDs. Patients being treated for cancer will present for treatment-related effects. These include neurologic changes; fever; dyspnea; nausea, vomiting, diarrhea; electrolyte abnormalities; and tachyarrhythmias.[18]

The most common oncologic emergencies that may be encountered in the ED include febrile neutropenia, spinal cord compression, superior vena cava syndrome, and tumor lysis syndrome.

Febrile Neutropenia

Pathophysiology

Febrile neutropenia or neutropenic fever is a significant complication related to cancer therapy. It is estimated that 50% of patients with a solid tumor and 80% of patients with a hematologic cancer receiving therapies may suffer with febrile neutropenia.[19] Treatment of cancer with chemotherapy causes immunosuppression, which places the patient at risk for infection. The bone marrow is damaged and unable to produce immune cells (neutrophils). The most common chemotherapies that may cause neutropenia include anthracyclines, antimetabolites, alkylating agents, camptothecin, hydroxyurea, mitomycin C, vinblastine, and taxane class.[19] Other causes of neutropenia include hereditary disease such as Cohen syndrome; autoimmune diseases such as rheumatoid arthritis and Crohn's disease; infections from bacteria, viruses, and fungal sources; medications as noted; metals, such as gold and mercury, exposure; and nutritional problems such as B12 deficiency.[19]

Medical Screening

A. *Chief complaint:* Fever, patient who has received chemotherapy in the last 6 weeks

B. *Signs and symptoms*

1. Oral temperature ≥38.3°C or a temperature ≥38.0°C for 1 hour in a neutropenic patient
2. Mucositis
3. Cough
4. Skin infection(s)
5. Sinusitis
6. Diarrhea
7. Presence of an infected catheter used for chemotherapy
8. *Clostridium difficile*
9. Headache
10. Altered mental status

C. *Past medical history*

1. Cancer
2. Chemotherapy within the last 6 weeks
3. Adverse reactions to previous cancer treatments

Physical Examination

A. *General:* Distress and discomfort related to the level of fever, altered mental status

B. *Skin:* Presence of a wound, rash, central catheter for chemotherapy

C. *Ears, nose, and throat (ENT):* Sores in the mouth, mucositis, nasal congestion, nasal erosions

D. *Cardiac:* Signs of septic shock, hypotension, tachycardia, presence of a new murmur

E. *Pulmonary:* Congestion, sore throat, cough, decreased breath sound, wheezes, rales

F. *Neurological:* Altered mental status

G. *Gastrointestinal:* Abdominal pain, nausea, vomiting, diarrhea, decreased or absent bowel sounds indicating obstruction

Differential Diagnoses

A. Chemotherapy-induced toxicity

B. Infection from another source such as pneumonia not related to neutropenia

C. Reaction to other medications used to manage the patient's cancer

Diagnostic Testing

A. *Labs*

1. Complete blood count (CBC) with differential
2. Two sets of blood cultures (aerobic and anaerobic)
3. If a catheter is present for chemotherapy administration, one set of cultures should be taken from the lumen of the catheter.
4. Liver function tests
5. Renal function
6. Lactate level
7. Urinalysis
8. Wound culture
9. Fungal blood cultures may be requested by the oncologist.
10. Polymerase chain reaction (PCR) for influenza and respiratory syncytial virus (RSV)

B. *Imaging*

1. Chest radiograph
2. Other imaging may be indicated based on the patient's symptoms, for example, a CT or MRI of the brain of patient with an altered mental status.

Management

A. *Pharmacological management*[19]

1. Recommend consultation with patient's oncologist.
2. If patient does not require admission, patient may be treated with ciprofloxacin plus amoxicillin/clavulanate, or clindamycin.
3. Some centers are using single-agent moxifloxacin.

B. *Nonpharmacological therapies*

1. Patients should be placed in an isolated area to prevent any further of exposure.
2. Visitors should be limited to decrease risk of exposure.

Patient Disposition

A. All patients with febrile neutropenia should be emergent patients.

B. Determine how high risk the patient is, using the National Comprehensive Cancer Network Risk Criteria for Neutropenic Fever.[20]

C. High-risk patients will require admission.

D. Patient may need to be transferred to a higher level care for treatment.

Age and Developmental Considerations

A. Most patients with febrile neutropenia may not always have a source easily identified in the ED.
B. Older and younger patients are at higher risk for complications and need to be evaluated quickly.

Spinal Cord Compression

Pathophysiology

Malignant spinal cord compression (MSCC) can occur in 5% of patients who have cancer and can present as the initial symptom of malignant cancer. The most common cancers that cause this are lung, breast, prostate, and multiple myeloma (both Hodgkin and non-Hodgkin).[21] MSCC can occur from the spread of cancer to the vertebral column. It can also occur when a pathological vertebral fracture compresses the spinal column.

Medical Screening

A. *Chief complaint:* Back pain, neurologic changes, ataxic gait
B. Signs and symptoms
  1. Back pain
  2. Motor weakness and deficits
  3. Cauda equina syndrome
  4. Bowel and bladder incontinence
  5. Paralysis
  6. Tingling in lower extremities
C. *Past medical history*
  1. Multiple myeloma
  2. Lymphoma
  3. Lung, breast, or prostate cancer

Physical Examination

A. *General:* Generalized weakness, more pronounced depending on which area of the spinal cord is affected
B. *Neurological:* Muscle weakness in extremities, hypo- or hyperreflexia
C. *Musculoskeletal:* Pain with palpation over spinal column
D. *Gastrointestinal:* Decreased rectal tone, bowel incontinence
E. *Urological:* Urinary incontinence
F. *Gait:* Ataxic

Differential Diagnoses

A. Spinal column fracture
B. Spinal cord infection

Diagnostic Testing

A. *Labs*
  a. Complete blood count (CBC) with differential
  b. Two sets of blood cultures (aerobic and anaerobic)
  c. Liver function tests
  d. Renal function
  e. Lactate level
  f. Urinalysis
  g. Fungal blood cultures may be requested by the oncologist.
  h. Polymerase chain reaction (PCR) for influenza and respiratory syncytial virus (RSV)
B. *Imaging*[21]
  1. CT scan of the spine
  2. Gadolinium-enhanced MRI of the spine
  3. Myelography

Management[21]

A. *Pharmacological therapies*
  1. Corticosteroids to reduce vasogenic edema
B. *Nonpharmacological therapies*
  1. Radiation therapy for radiosensitive tumors
  2. Anterior corpectomy and then radiation therapy in some situations
  3. Stereotactic beam radiation therapy is more frequently used to prevent radiation toxicity.
  4. Surgical management may be indicated.

Patient Disposition

A. Patient should be considered emergent.
B. Patient will need to be admitted.
C. May require transfer to a higher level of care

Age and Developmental Considerations

A. Ambulatory status at the time of presentation to the ED will help determine the outcome of the patient.
B. Rapid assessment, diagnoses, and treatment will contribute to a positive outcome related to this emergency.

Superior Vena Cava Syndrome

Pathophysiology[21]

Superior vena cava syndrome (SVCS) is caused by a mechanical obstruction of the superior vena cava. This syndrome can result from malignancy or thrombosis. The primary malignancies that cause SVCS are lung cancer and non-Hodgkin lymphoma. SVCS results from direct compression of the vein before it enters the right atrium. Enlarged mediastinal lymph nodes and mediastinal and thoracic tumors can obstruct blood return to the heart.

Medical Screening

A. *Chief complaint:* Shortness of breath
B. *Signs and symptoms*
  1. Dyspnea
  2. Cough
  3. Facial edema
  4. Distended neck veins
  5. Distended chest veins
C. *Past medical history*
  1. Malignancies from lung cancer and non-Hodgkin lymphoma
  2. Intravascular devices that may cause thrombosis
  3. Syphilis

Physical Examination

A. *General:* Moderate to severe respiratory distress, facial edema, swelling in neck and upper extremities
B. *Skin:* Cyanosis
C. *Cardiac:* Jugular vein distention
D. *Pulmonary:* Congestion, cough, decreased breath sound, wheezes, rales
E. *Neurological:* Altered mental status

Differential Diagnoses

A. Congestive heart failure
B. Pulmonary embolus

Diagnostic Testing

A. *Labs*
1. Complete blood count (CBC) with differential
2. Liver function tests
3. Renal function
4. Lactate level
5. Urinalysis

B. *Imaging*[21]
1. CT of the chest with intravenous contrast
2. Chest radiograph
3. Magnetic resonance venography

Management

A. *Pharmacological Interventions*
1. Corticosteroids
2. Chemotherapy, depending on the type of malignancy

B. *Nonpharmacological Interventions*
1. Radiation therapy
2. Placement of intravascular stents

Patient Disposition

A. Patient should be considered emergent.
B. Patient will need to be admitted.
C. May require transfer to a higher level of care

Age and Developmental Considerations

A. Rapid assessment, diagnoses, and treatment will contribute to a positive outcome related to this emergency.

Tumor Lysis Syndrome[12]

Pathophysiology

Tumor lysis syndrome (TLS) results from massive cytolysis that causes the release of tumor cellular contents into the patient's systemic circulation. It is a grave oncologic metabolic emergency. The metabolic abnormalities that are the consequences of this syndrome include hyperkalemia, hyperuricemia, hyperphosphatemia, and hypocalcemia. These abnormalities can result in acute renal failure, cardiac dysrhythmias, seizure, acidosis, azotemia, and sudden death. TLS occurs following the initiation of cytotoxic chemotherapy. However, it can also occur with the administration of radiotherapy, immunotherapy, surgery, or from highly proliferative tumors.[12]

Medical Screening

A. *Chief complaint:* Cardiac arrhythmias, nausea, vomiting, diabetes insipidus, muscle cramps, extremity spasms
B. *Signs and symptoms:* Dependent upon the abnormalities in the electrolytes and end-organ damage (brain, heart, and kidney)
1. Cardiac arrhythmia
2. Seizures
3. Nausea and vomiting
4. Diarrhea
5. Low urinary output
6. Muscle cramps
7. Carpopedal spasms
8. Tetany
9. Altered mental status
10. Hallucinations

Physical Examination

A. *General:* Distress and discomfort related to the source of the electrolyte abnormalities
B. *Cardiac:* Irregular heartbeat, tachyarrhythmias, bradycardia
C. *Pulmonary:* Congestion, sore throat, cough, decreased breath sound, wheezes, rales
D. *Neurological:* Altered mental status, seizure activity, hallucinations
E. *Gastrointestinal:* Abdominal pain, nausea, vomiting, diarrhea, decreased or absent bowel sounds indicating obstruction
F. *Musculoskeletal:* Muscle cramps, paresthesia, tetany, carpopedal spasms

Differential Diagnoses

A. Congestive heart failure
B. Pulmonary embolus
C. Acute renal failure

Diagnostic Testing

A. *Labs*
1. Serum potassium
2. Phosphate
3. Calcium
4. Creatinine
5. Uric acid

B. *Imaging*
1. EKG
2. Chest radiograph

Management

A. *Pharmacological interventions*
1. Rasburicase
2. Allopurinol
3. IV rehydration

B. *Nonpharmacological therapies*
1. Continuous cardiac monitoring
2. Lab monitoring based on the severity of the TLS and the patient's symptoms
3. Emergent oncology consult
4. Renal consult if indicated

Patient Disposition

A. Patient should be considered emergent.
B. Patient will need to be admitted.
C. May require transfer to a higher level of care.

Age and Developmental Considerations

A. Rapid assessment, diagnoses, and treatment will contribute to a positive outcome related to this emergency.
B. May be first indication that the patient has a malignancyBraun, Barstow and Pyzocha (2015).

References and Additional Reading

References and Additional Reading for this chapter are online only and can be found at https://connect.springerpub.com/content/reference-book/978-0-8261-6091-5/part/part02/toc-part/ch21.

22. Infectious Diseases

NICOLE MARTINEZ

Learning Objectives

- Identify common infectious diseases that may be encountered in the emergency care environment.
- Use evidence-based guidelines to provide a comprehensive evaluation, treatment, and management of a patient with an infectious disease.
- Formulate a plan of care for patients with an infectious disease, including a plan for treatment and management, notification of appropriate authorities, decreasing risks for transmission, and follow-up care.

Infectious diseases remain one of the leading causes of death in developed and developing countries throughout the world. Infections can cause significant morbidity and mortality to our most vulnerable populations, including the very young, the elderly, those susceptible to health disparities, and the immunocompromised. The main types of pathologic organisms causing infectious diseases are viruses, bacteria, fungi, protozoa, and worms. The presentation and symptoms can range from mild to life-threatening.[1]

Disease transmission reflects the host–agent–environment interaction model[2] (Figure 22.1). The infectious agent is introduced to the host via an exogenous route from the environment or when an endogenous agent overcomes the host immunity. Common ways for these infectious agents to enter the body are through the skin, ingestion of contaminated food or water, bites from insect vectors, including ticks and mosquitos, inhalation of airborne microbes, sexual contact, or transmission from mothers to their unborn children.

Once the infectious agent has penetrated the body's defense barriers, an immune response is initiated. The host's immune system utilizes both innate and adaptive mechanisms to monitor, detect, and eliminate pathogenic microbes that may result in disease. An immunocompetent response includes contribution from many subsets of leukocytes: B cells, T cells, natural killer (NK) cells, NK-T cells, neutrophils, eosinophils, basophils, mast cells, monocytes, megakaryocyte, and erythrocytes.[3,4] Each cell has a specific role in the full complement of the immune system.

As clinicians in the ED, strict adherence to personal protective equipment (PPE) protocols is essential to prevent the spread of some infectious diseases with which patients may present. Protocols may range from the simple application of gloves to the application of an N95 mask, gown, gloves, and eye protection. The mode of transmission of each pathogen and disease determines the level and degree of PPE.

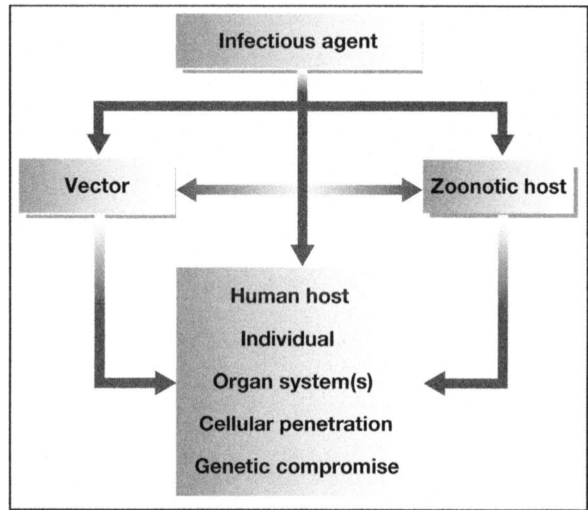

FIGURE 22.1 Host–agent–environment interaction model.
Source: Adapted from Fiske, C. & Bloch, F. (2019). Infectious diseases. In G.D. Hammer & S. J. McPhee (Eds.), *Pathophysiology of disease: an introduction to clinical medicine*, 8th ed. McGraw-Hill Education.[2]

Diphtheria

Once considered a major cause of death and illness among children, diphtheria is now rare in developed countries due to vaccination that is initiated early in childhood. The disease, however, continues to cause illness globally. The gram-negative bacillus *Corynebacterium diphtheriae* is the causative agent for this highly contagious disease.[5] Toxic strains of the bacterium produce an endotoxin that causes membranous nasopharyngitis, which can result in airway obstruction. The subsequent localized necrosis of the pulmonary mucosa can lead to cardiac or even neurologic complications, including myocarditis, central and peripheral neuropathies.[6] In fact, myocarditis is present in two-thirds of patients, and there is clinical evidence of cardiac dysfunction in 10% to 25% of patients. Neuropathies are noted in 5% of patients with severe disease, and cutaneous diphtheria may also produce lesions.[7,8] Incubation period for diphtheria is 2 to 5 days. Treatment of pharyngeal diphtheria, with penicillin or erythromycin, is intended to eradicate the bacteria while neutralizing the exotoxin.[6]

Predisposing Factors

A. Though it is rare in the United States, it should be considered in patients who are immunocompromised and nonimmunized.[7]

Physical Examination

A. *Chief complaint:* Sore throat, fever

B. *Signs and symptoms*

1. Sore throat, low- or high-grade fever, headache, nausea, fatigue, malaise lasting for 1 to 2 days. Patient may report history of travel to endemic areas in the previous weeks and/or a crowded living environment.

C. *Focused assessment*

1. Patients may have a low- or high-grade fever, but most will appear toxic in appearance. Tachycardia is common.
2. Head, eyes, ears, nose, and throat (HEENT)
   a. Thick gray-white pharyngeal membrane that covers the tonsils, oropharynx, nasopharynx, and uvula (Figure 22.2)

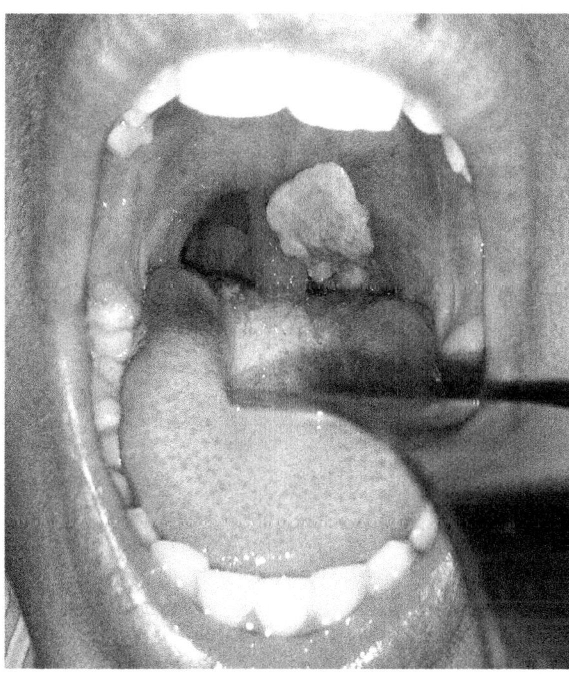

FIGURE 22.2 Dirty white pseudomembrane classically seen in diphtheria.

   b. Inflammation, erythema, and edema of pharynx
3. Respiratory
   a. Stridor
   b. Wheeze
   c. Cyanosis
   d. Accessory muscle use/retractions
4. Lymphatic
   a. Extensive anterior and submandibular cervical lymphadenopathy
5. Cardiac
   a. Cardiac dysrhythmias, atrioventricular blocks, ST-T wave changes
   b. Congestive heart failure
   c. Endocarditis
6. Neurological
   a. Assess for cranial nerve neuropathies.
   b. Cranial nerve deficits including ciliary paralysis, pharyngeal, facial, or laryngeal nervous dysfunction, and oculomotor deficits
   c. Peripheral neuropathy develops 10 days to 3 months post-onset of the pharyngeal disease.
7. Integumentary
   a. Painful erythematous pustule that breaks down to form an ulcer engulfed by a gray membrane[8,9]

Differential Diagnoses

A. Pharyngitis
B. Peritonsillar abscess
C. Mononucleosis
D. Epiglottitis
E. Retropharyngeal abscess
F. Rheumatic fever
G. Oropharyngeal/esophageal candidiasis
H. Myocarditis
I. Angioedema
J. Infective endocarditis
K. Septic shock

Diagnostic Testing[10]

A. *Labs*

1. Throat and pharyngeal cultures
2. Polymerase chain reaction (PCR) assay for the presence of the A and B subunits of the diphtheria toxin gene. The Centers for Disease Control and Prevention (CDC) does not perform this test to rule out diphtheria unless the antitoxin is requested.
3. Complete blood count (CBC) with differential
4. Urinalysis (UA) for serum pregnancy and to assess for transient proteinuria
5. Troponin I levels to assess severity of myocarditis

B. Chest x-ray (CXR) and soft tissue neck x-ray/CT or ultrasound (US) to assess for soft tissue swelling, enlarged epiglottis, or narrowing of the glottic region

C. EKG may exhibit ST-T wave changes, dysrhythmia, or heart blocks.[9]

Management

A. *Procedures*

1. *Airway management:* Endotracheal (ET) intubation, surgical airway
2. Laryngoscopy, bronchoscopy as indicated
3. Electrical pacing as needed for conduction abnormalities[9]

B. *Pharmacologic therapies*

1. *Adult:* Erythromycin
2. *Adult:* Penicillin V K or penicillin G

3. *Pediatric:* Penicillin or erythromycin (for patients 6 months of age and older)
4. Horse serum antitoxin can be obtained from the CDC on request. PCR must be ordered.[5]

C. *Consultation/collaboration*
1. Contact the CDC to report the case, to request antitoxin, and to test the specimens.
2. Infectious disease
3. Neurology as needed for complications
4. Cardiology as needed for complications
5. Ears, nose, and throat (ENT)/anesthesia as needed for airway maintenance
6. Pulmonary for bronchoscopy[9]

Patient Disposition

A. Hospitalization with standard and respiratory droplet precautions
B. Transition of care information
1. Respiratory isolation
2. Supportive care, including antipyretics
3. Continuation of antibiotic treatment
4. Serial EKGs to detect cardiac abnormalities
5. Physical therapy as needed for neurologic dysfunction[9]

Age and Developmental Considerations

A. Increased awareness and promotion for immunization is the key.
B. *Prevention and education:* Diphtheria is transmitted via airborne respiratory droplets or by contact with secretions and/or exudate from the skin lesions. Patients and family members should be provided with adequate education and preventative measures regarding its transmission, and infected individuals should be cautioned about being around immunocompromised, pregnant, elderly, and pediatric individuals.[5]
C. *Patient and family education and counseling:* Because of the high risk for transmission to close contacts, especially those in the household, a diphtheria toxoid booster should be administered and contacts should be provided with a 7- to 10-day course of antibiotics. Obtain throat and pharyngeal swabs from all close contacts. Household contacts should be closely monitored for disease progression, and antitoxin should be administered at the first signs of illness.[5]

Herpes Zoster—Shingles

Herpes zoster (HZ), commonly known as shingles, is caused by the virus that stems from a previous infection from or by vaccination with the varicella zoster virus (VZV).[11] VZV is a DNA virus in the *Herpesviridae* family.[12] After a VZV infection,[11] the virus will remain dormant within the basal root ganglia in the spinal cord, where it will reactivate, causing the HZ rash.[13] The reactivation is prompted by a compromised immune state with natural aging and can be exacerbated by stressful triggers, including comorbid diseases and stressful diseases that cause strain on the body.[14] Eruption typically occurs in individuals who previously had a varicella infection and very rarely in vaccinated individuals.[12, 15]

Physical Examination

A. *Chief complaint:* Painful rash
B. *Signs and symptoms*
1. HZ infection is defined by three stages
a. *Prodromal stage:* Flu-like symptoms, including fever, muscle and joint aches, lethargy, and headaches, may also accompany the prodromal phase. An acute HZ infection typically is preceded by a prodromal stage with sharp, dull, tingling, or burning pain in addition to paresthesia along the affected dermatome.
b. *Active stage:* Patients may complain of intense pruritus, and the pain may precede the active eruption of the classic vesicular rash by 1 to 10 days. Active or eruptive stage starts with the rash, which presents as linear, maculopapular lesions of erythema and then progresses to vesicles that scab and crust over within 10 to 12 days. Because of the dermatomal distribution, the rash never crosses the midline; however, some presentations may include adjacent dermatomes.
c. *Chronic stage*

C. *Focused assessment:* Full head-to-toe assessment
1. *General:* Fatigue, malaise
2. *Skin:* Assess for involvement of ophthalmic division of trigeminal nerve, Hutchinson sign to assess for HZ ophthalmicus. All chest, abdominal, pelvic, and back pain should have thorough skin assessment for lesions.
3. *Pulmonological:* Disseminated disease may cause pneumonitis.
4. *Abdominal:* Disseminated disease may cause hepatosplenomegaly (hepatitis)
5. *Neurological:* Disseminated disease may cause meningoencephalitis, peripheral neuropathy. Assess for postherpetic neuralgia (PHN).

Differential Diagnoses

A. Primary varicella
B. Herpes simplex virus (HSV)
C. Insect bites
D. Bullous impetigo
E. Trigeminal neuralgia
F. Cellulitis
G. Molluscum contagiosum

Diagnostic Tests

A. Clinical presentation is sufficient for diagnosis with most patients.
B. Labs may aid in patients with disseminated disease or if the diagnosis is not certain.
1. *Polymerase chain reaction (PCR):* Preferred method to detect the virus and distinguish VZV from herpes simplex virus. The sample should ideally be from an unroofed vesicular lesion and/or scab from a crusted lesion.
2. Other less sensitive and less specific tests include the Tzanck smear, viral culture, and serology testing.

C. If HZ ophthalmicus is suspected, evaluation of the eye with fluorescein stain and slit lamp examination is necessary.

Management

A. *Pharmacologic therapies*
1. Follow evidence-based guidelines when prescribing.
2. Generally, VZV is a self-limited disease; therefore, the goal of treatment is to decrease pain, treat the acute infection, and prevent complications, including PHN.
3. Immunocompetent patient
a. Antiviral agent should be initiated within 72 hours of rash onset
b. Antiviral agent
c. *Analgesics:* Ibuprofen, acetaminophen
d. Corticosteroids (controversial)
4. Immunocompromised patient
a. IV acyclovir
b. *Analgesics:* Ibuprofen, acetaminophen
c. Corticosteroids: Consider in patients with severe disease or central nervous system (CNS) involvement. Administer prednisone taper over 7 days.
5. HZ ophthalmicus
a. Ophthalmologist evaluation is essential.
b. Antiviral agent
c. IV acyclovir if immunocompromised
d. Erythromycin ointment for secondary infection
e. Topical cycloplegic if complicated with iritis
6. PHN
a. Antivirals are not indicated.
b. May need long-acting opioids.
c. Gabapentin and tricyclic antidepressants may be beneficial.

B. *Nonpharmacologic therapies*
1. Application of topical nonsteroidal anesthetic substances, such as calamine and oatmeal baths, helps with pain and itching and further aids in drying the lesions.

C. *Consultation/collaboration:* For suspicion of disseminated disease or in those who are immunocompromised

Patient Disposition

A. *Transition of care information*
1. Hospital admission for HZ is reserved for severe cases and is rarely necessary. If disseminated disease to the central nervous, pulmonary, or gastrointestinal systems is suspected, hospitalization and/or airway support may be indicated.
2. *Isolation:* Airborne precautions for all patients

B. *Discharge instruction*
1. Take all medications as directed.
2. Wound care instructions and return precautions for secondary infection risk
3. Return immediately for concern of worsening infections, signs of disseminated disease, PHN, or ophthalmic involvement.

Age and Developmental Considerations

A. *Pregnancy:* Zoster in pregnancy is not associated with increased risk on congenital varicella syndrome. Vaccine is contraindicated during pregnancy.

B. *Pediatric:* Occurrence in childhood is common when varicella occurred in utero or within the first 6 months of life. Neonatal zoster requires IV acyclovir.

C. *Prevention and education*
1. Postexposure prophylaxis
a. VariZIG is recommended within 72 hours of exposure for immunocompromised patients, pregnancy patients, exposed premature neonates born <28 weeks gestation, exposed premature neonates born >28 weeks gestation to a seronegative mothers, neonates born to mother with varicella between 5 days predelivery and up to 2 days postdelivery.

D. *Patient and family education and counseling*
1. Patients should be provided with anticipatory information of the progression of the disease and healing process of the lesions.
2. Recommend isolation from pregnant, immunocompromised, and nonvaccinated persons.
3. PHN may require a referral for a pain specialist.

HIV/AIDS

Symptoms of an acute HIV infection occurs in 50% to 90% of individuals, and diagnosis is overlooked in roughly 75% of cases, as the patients typically have nonspecific presentations and complaints.[16] Symptoms of an acute infection usually develop within 2 to 4 weeks of exposure and can last for several weeks there afterward. Early symptomatic identification is essential to prevent further complications and disease progression.[16,17]

Pathophysiology

A. AIDS is defined with evidence of a HIV infection with CD4 <400 or with an AIDS defining illness, including infection, malignancy, or other.

B. Primary infection (2–6 weeks after exposure): Fever, malaise, rash, flu-like illness, diarrhea. Up to 90% of patients are asymptomatic.

C. Advanced HIV disease (CD4 <200): Fever, night sweats, fatigue, cough, opportunistic infections

Predisposing Factors

A. IV drug use
B. Blood transfusions prior to 1985
C. Sexual promiscuity
D. Men who have sex with men
E. Unprotected intercourse with at-risk partners

Physical Examination

A. A full head-to-toe assessment should be completed on all patients suspected to have an HIV infection.

B. Generalized
1. Fever
2. Malaise
3. Flu-like illness with lymphadenopathy and hepatosplenomegaly
4. Weight loss
5. Night sweats

C. Respiratory
1. Dyspnea
2. Cough
3. Pharyngitis
4. Hemoptysis

D. Cardiac
1. Dyspnea

E. Neurologic
  1. Chronic low-grade headache
  2. Altered mental status
  3. Neuropathy
  4. Dementia
  5. Seizures
  6. Painless vision loss

F. Gastrointestinal
  1. Diarrhea (chronic/acute)
  2. Nausea

G. Integumentary
  1. Rash on face and trunk
  2. Alopecia

Differential Diagnoses

A. *Respiratory symptoms*
  1. TB
  2. Pulmonary emboli
  3. Pulmonary hypertension
  4. *Pneumonia:* Bacterial, viral, or fungal
  5. Malignancy
  6. Lymphocytic interstitial pneumonitis

B. *Cardiac*
  1. Endocarditis
  2. Pericarditis
  3. Myocarditis
  4. Pericardial effusion
  5. Acute coronary syndrome

C. *Neurologic*
  1. Neurosyphilis
  2. Meningitis
  3. Toxoplasmosis
  4. HIV or metabolic encephalopathy
  5. Cytomegalovirus (CMV) or herpes simplex virus (HSV) encephalitis
  6. Lymphoma
  7. Subarachnoid hemorrhage
  8. Cerebral infarct

D. *Gastrointestinal/genitourinary (GI/GU)*
  1. Infectious esophagitis (candida, CMV, HSV)
  2. Reflux esophagitis
  3. Hepatomegaly
     a. Hepatitis
     b. *Opportunistic infection:* CMV, mycobacterium avium complex (MAC), TB
  4. Diarrhea
     a. Parasites
     b. Bacteria
     c. Viral (CMV, HSV, HIV)
     d. Fungal
     e. HIV-associated enteropathy
  5. Renal disease
     a. Vasculitis
     b. Obstruction
     c. HIV nephropathy
     d. Drug nephrotoxicity

E. *Oral*
  1. Fungal infection (candida)
  2. Viral lesions (CMV, hairy leukoplakia, HSV)
  3. Bacterial lesions (periodontal disease, TB)
  4. Neoplasm
  5. Autoimmune (aphthous ulcers)

Diagnostic Testing

A. There is a 24-week window between primary infection and seroconversion. At this time, tests may be negative.

B. *Enzyme-linked immunosorbent assay (ELISA):* Detects IgG antibody.
  1. *Sensitivity and specificity:* 99%

C. Western blot
  1. Detects IgG antibody against HIV proteins.
  2. Utilized to confirm a positive ELISA.
  3. Can detect an infection during the 6-month seroconversion window period.
  4. Nearly 100% sensitive and specific

D. Rapid HIV testing
  1. Results available within 20 minutes
  2. Multiple types of tests are available: Oral swab and blood
  3. Positive tests require confirmation with ELISA or Western blot.
  4. *Specificity and sensitivity:* 99%

E. Absolute lymphocyte count
  1. General systemic symptoms
  2. Aerobic/anaerobic, fungal, AFB, and MAC blood cultures

F. Respiratory symptoms
  1. Chest x-ray (CXR)
  2. Sputum cultures, acid-fast bacteria (AFB), and Gram stain
  3. Blood cultures

G. *Serum lactate dehydrogenase (LDH):* Level will be elevated in *Pneumocystis* pneumonia (PCP).

H. Arterial blood gas (ABG)

I. Cardiac symptoms
  1. EKG
  2. Serum cardiac markers
  3. CXR
  4. Blood cultures if suspected endocarditis
  5. Toxicology screen to evaluate for amphetamine and cocaine abuse

J. Neurologic symptoms
  1. Lumbar puncture with opening pressure
  2. Evaluate cerebrospinal fluid (CSF) for glucose, protein, Gram stain and culture, cell count with differential, India ink stain, herpes simplex and *Cryptococcus* antigen, AFB smear, and Venereal Disease Research Laboratory (VDRL).
  3. Head CT with and without contrast

K. GI/GU symptoms
  1. Hepatic serology
  2. Ultrasound (US) if biliary symptoms present
  3. CT of abdomen and pelvis
  4. Stool for ova and parasites: Gram stain, culture, and *Clostridium difficile* assay
  5. *Female patient:* Urinalysis for pregnancy, pelvic examination with wet mount
  6. Gonorrhea and chlamydia culture if symptoms present

L. Ocular symptoms
  1. Slit lamp exam with fluorescein stain

Management

A. *Pharmacologic therapies:* Patients who are suspected to have bacterial infections should receive their first dose of antibiotics in the ED. HIV treatment should be initiated if there is a low CD4 or high viral load, if an AIDS-defining illness is noted, and if the patient is pregnant.

1. *Postexposure prophylaxis:* Start therapy within 72 hours if possible and continue for 4 weeks.
    a. Zidovudine + lamivudine
    b. Lamivudine + stavudine
    c. Stavudine + didanosine
    d. Three-drug regime indicated for very high-risk exposure

B. *Triple therapy* (highly active antiviral therapy [HAART])

C. *Oral candidiasis*
1. Clotrimazole

D. *Pneumocystis jiroveci pneumonia (PJP)*
1. Trimethoprim/sulfamethoxazole (TMP/SMZ)
2. *Sulfa allergy:* Pentamidine or dapsone

E. *Toxoplasmosis:* 6-week treatment
1. Sulfadiazine
2. Leucovorin
3. Pyrimethamine
4. Steroid for cerebral edema
5. *Cryptococcal meningitis:* Treat with medications below for 2 weeks, then with fluconazole for 8 weeks
6. Amphotericin B
7. Flucytosine

F. *Esophageal candidiasis:* 14- to 21-day treatment
1. Fluconazole

G. *MAC*
1. Clarithromycin
2. Ethambutol

H. *CMV retinitis*
1. Ganciclovir

I. *Consultation/collaboration*
1. All patients should be referred to primary HIV care for initiation and ongoing management.

Patient Disposition

A. *Disposition*
1. Discharge criteria include the patient's ability to maintain hydration, self-care, and mobility.
2. Admission criteria include hypoxemia, pericardial effusion, neutropenic fever, unexplained fever with central nervous system (CNS) involvement, seizures, pneumonia, TB, hemodynamic instability, intractable nausea, vomiting, and/ or diarrhea, inability to tolerate oral intake.

Age and Developmental Considerations

A. *Prevention and education*
1. Promote safe sexual practices.
2. Take medications as directed.
3. Report any cough or fever immediately to clinician.
4. Avoid contact with others who are ill.
5. Encourage cessation of drug, alcohol, and tobacco use.
6. Avoid pregnancy to prevent fetal transmission.

B. *Patient and family education and counseling*
1. Minimize exposure to blood and bodily secretions.
2. Do not share toothbrushes, razors, or drug paraphernalia.

Infectious Mononucleosis

Infectious mononucleosis, often called "mono," is a contagious disease that is most common among teenagers and young adults. The Epstein–Barr virus (EBV), a member of the herpes virus family, is the most common causal agent of infectious mononucleosis, but other viruses, including cytomegalovirus, adenovirus, and HIV, have also been found to cause the disease. Transmission of the disease is via oropharyngeal route through the saliva. Greater than 90% of adults on serologic testing have had a prior infection with EBV.

Pathophysiology

A. The initial immunologic response from the T-cells is responsible for an elevated absolute lymphocyte count as well as the associated symptoms. The EBV then infects and replicates in B cells that are then transformed into plasmacytoid cells.

B. Complications include airway edema, meningitis, glomerulonephritis, hepatitis, pericarditis, encephalitis, splenic rupture, pneumonia, and Guillain–Barré syndrome. These complications typically occur in the pediatric or geriatric populations.[18-20]

Physical Examination

A. *Chief complaint:* Sore throat and fever

B. ***Signs and symptoms:*** Incubation period is 4 to 6 weeks.
1. Prodromal fatigue, malaise, arthralgias, and myalgias
2. History of sore throat and fever
3. Lymphadenopathy
4. Headache
5. Abdominal pain is uncommon; however, it may be present in severe cases with splenic enlargement and/ or rupture.
6. Prior history of administration of amoxicillin or ampicillin

C. *Focused assessment*
1. *General:* Febrile (80%–90%), malaise, fatigue (90%–100%)
2. *Head, eyes, ears, nose, and throat (HEENT):* Exudative pharyngitis, tonsillar enlargement, symmetric tender lymphadenopathy (100%), may have eyelid edema, petechia can appear at the junction of the hard and soft palate.
3. *Abdominal:* Hepatomegaly (15%–25%), splenomegaly (50%–60%), jaundice
4. *Neurological:* May have findings consistent with encephalitis, aseptic meningitis, optic neuritis, or Guillain–Barré syndrome.
5. *Skin:* Morbilliform rash can be seen in patients who were given amoxicillin; petechiae.

Differential Diagnoses

A. Adenovirus
B. Streptococcal pharyngitis
C. HIV
D. Rubella
E. Hepatitis
F. Cytomegalovirus (CMV)
G. Mumps
H. Diphtheria

I. Leukemia
J. Lymphoma

Diagnostic Testing

A. Complete blood count (CBC) with differential
1. Typically, an elevated white blood cell count that peaks during week 2 of the illness
2. Lymphocyte count with >50% lymphocytes on differential
3. Absolute lymphocyte count >4,500
4. Elevated lymphocyte count with >10% atypical lymphocytes
5. Decreased neutrophils and/or platelets

B. Liver function tests (LFT)
1. Elevated with transaminases within three times that of normal is found in 85% of patients during the first 2 weeks of the disease.

C. *Monospot test:* Detects presence of heterophil antibodies which peak at 2 to 5 weeks and may persist for several months.
1. Moderately sensitive (85%) and highly specific (100%)

D. CT scan or ultrasound of abdomen for significant abdominal pain to identify splenic rupture and to rule out other pathology

Management

A. Avoid placing patient in the same general area of those who are high risk, including immunocompromised patients and post-transplant patients.

B. *Pharmacologic therapies*
1. Antipyretics for fever control
2. Analgesics for pain relief from sore throat
3. Steroids for significant pharyngeal edema (controversial)
a. Methylprednisone
b. Prednisone
c. Dexamethasone
4. Antibiotics if there is suspicion of bacterial infection

C. *Nonpharmacologic therapies:* Supportive therapy and rest

D. *Consultation/collaboration*
1. Infectious disease may be consulted if serology is not conclusive or if significant complications are present.
2. Ears, Nose, and Throat (ENT) may also be consulted for complications.

Patient Disposition

A. *Transition of care information*
1. Admission is warranted for significant airway edema that represents a potential for compromise, neurologic complications, severe hepatic or hematologic complications, and inability to take PO.

B. *Discharge instruction:* Most patients are managed outpatient.
1. Increased hydration, rest
2. Avoid transmitting the infection via saliva to others by avoiding kissing and sharing utensils and drinks with others.
3. Avoid contact sports or other strenuous exercise for the first 1 to 3 weeks of the illness regardless of spleen size.
4. Patient should follow up with primary care after the first 3 weeks of illness in order to reassess persistent symptoms and whether she or he is able to return to full activity. Patient may need further studies if splenomegaly is persistent.

Age and Developmental Considerations

A. *Pediatric considerations:* Children <4 years old are often asymptomatic. Children who are symptomatic typically present with atypical signs and symptoms, including neutropenia, pneumonia, and rash.

B. Prevention and education

C. Patient and family education and counseling

Measles, Mumps, and Rubella

Measles, mumps, and rubella (MMR) have infected millions of lives over the last century.[21,22] Despite the high incidence of vaccinated individuals, these highly communicable diseases continue to flourish within clusters of outbreaks throughout the United States. Emergency medicine clinicians play a key role in early recognition and diagnosis of the diseases, with an emphasis on prevention of widespread outbreaks.[23,24]

Physical Examination

A. *Chief complaint:* Fever, rash, cough, myalgia, swelling to face

B. Full comprehensive exam is necessary to rule out complications.

C. Signs and symptoms (Table 22.1)

Differential Diagnoses

A. Scarlet fever
B. Infectious mononucleosis
C. Enterovirus
D. Roseola
E. Secondary syphilis
F. Kawasaki disease
G. Erythema infectiosum
H. Toxic shock syndrome (TSS)
I. Drug reactions
J. Measles and rubella should also be on the differential list for each other.

Diagnostic Testing

A. Diagnosis is typically based upon clinical findings for all three diseases, however, confirmation of these infections may be achieved.

B. *Measles*
1. Immunoglobulin (Ig) M antibody
2. Polymerase chain reaction (PCR) performed on urine or a throat or nasopharyngeal swab
3. Chest x-ray (CXR) for suspected pneumonia

C. *Mumps*
1. Serum IgM antibody can be utilized to confirm active infection; however, vaccinated individuals may not mount a significant IgM response.
2. Reverse transcriptase-PCR (RT-PCR) performed on serum, buccal, or oral swab. Extremely sensitive and should be conducted within 3 to 8 days of onset of

TABLE 22.1 SUMMARY OF INFECTIOUS DISEASES, ROUTE OF TRANSMISSION, INCUBATION PERIOD, AND SIGNS AND SYMPTOMS

INFECTIOUS DISEASE	ROUTE OF TRANMISSION	INCUBATION PERIOD	SIGNS AND SYMPTOMS	RASH	CONTAGIOUS PERIOD
Measles virus (rubeola)	Airborne or droplet	7–21 days	Coryza, cough, conjunctivitis, fever greater than 101°F/38.3°C, Koplik spots on buccal mucosa, malaise Koplik spots appear 1–2 days before rash and disappear 48 hours after onset of rash.	3–5 days after initial symptoms. Red, maculopapular blanching rash that spreads from the head centrifugally downward and may become confluent. Palms and soles of the feet are rarely involved. Rash clears in 3–4 days.	4 days preceding rash and 4 days after rash resolves
Mumps	Airborne or droplet	12–25 days	Myalgia, mild to moderate fever, parotitis (unilateral or bilateral), jaw pain, otalgia, anorexia, headache, malaise, orchitis, oophoritis, pancreatitis Classic swelling of parotid glands occurs 48 hours after onset of prodromal period. It can last for 10 days. Parotitis is not present in all cases. Vaccinated individuals are less likely to present with severe symptoms.	None	2 days before and 5 days after parotid swelling (unilateral or bilateral)
Rubella (German measles)	Droplet	14–23 days	Low grade fever, lymphadenopathy, injected conjunctiva, cough, coryza, headache	Red macular rash that evolves to a pink-red maculopapular rash that begins on the face and spreads to the rest of the body, and coalesces on the trunk. Characteristically disappears in three days and may be pruritic.	7 days before and 7 days after rash resolves

Note: Disease description of route of transmission, incubation period, signs and symptoms, and contagious period was derived from the CDC (2017) Measles; Mumps; Rubella. Information on rashes was derived from Chamberlain, N. (2013). Skin rashes diseases: 1-6. Retrieved from https://www.atsu.edu/faculty/chamberlain/exanthems.htm#measles[25]

parotid swelling. Negative PCR in a vaccinated individual does not rule out mumps.

D. *Rubella*
   1. RT-PCR
   2. Enzyme-linked immunosorbent assay (ELISA) to detect rubella IgM antibodies[26]

Management

A. *Procedures*
   1. Lumbar puncture to assess for complications of measles, including encephalitis

B. *Pharmacologic therapies*
   1. Follow evidence-based guidelines when prescribing.
   2. Antipyretics
   3. IV hydration as needed
   4. WHO recommends vitamin A once a day for 2 days for children with measles when vitamin A deficiency is prevalent as it may decrease the risk of mortality.
   5. May treat with postexposure prophylaxis for the nonimmune.

C. *Consultation/collaboration*
   1. If major complications, including encephalitis, pneumonia, pericarditis, or myocarditis, are suspected, consultation with admission may be necessary.

Patient Disposition

A. *Admission criteria*
   1. Severe complications, including pneumonia, encephalitis, and dehydration
   2. Immunocompromised patients
   3. Older adult patients with comorbid conditions
   4. Isolate suspected cases

B. *Discharge criteria*
   1. No complications
   2. Educate regarding contagious period.

C. *Discharge instruction*
   1. Isolation precautions
   2. Increase hydration and rest

Age and Developmental Considerations

A. *Geriatric:* Those born before 1957 are generally considered to be immune.
B. *Pregnant:* Increased risk of spontaneous abortion. Women should not receive MMR vaccine during pregnancy. Disease is not reported to have any known birth defects.
C. *Pediatric:* MMR vaccine to be administered on or after 12 months of age. Second dose is to be administered before the start of school.
D. Prevention and education
 1. Primary prevention via immunization is key to preventing these highly communicable diseases.
 2. Patient and family education and counseling
  a. Emphasize the importance of isolation measures to prevent widespread outbreak.
  b. Provide supportive care with antipyretics, analgesics, and antiemetics for vomiting and dehydration.[27-29]

Tuberculosis

Tuberculosis (TB) remains a common disease throughout the world. It is most common in middle- or low-income countries. It is not as common in the United States, but patients present to EDs from many countries for care. The ED serves as a public health safety net, especially in poorer communities in the United States. TB in the United States is more frequently found in populations where access to healthcare is limited. It is more often found among racial and ethnic minorities, including Black or African American, Hispanic, and Asian populations. In 2019, the Centers for Disease Control and Prevention (CDC) reported 2.7/100,000 cases (www.cdc.gov/tb/statistics/default.htm). The CDC also has identified about 13 million people living in the United States with latent TB.[30, 31]

Pathophysiology

A. TB is a communicable disease. The cause is *Mycobacterium tuberculosis,* an aerobic acid-fast bacterium (AFB). It is spread through aerosolization of the bacteria from an infected person. Coughing is the most common cause of transmission. Aerosol droplets can remain the air for 30 minutes. Only people with active disease can spread TB.
B. Exposed patients may develop TB within weeks of exposure, where others may not develop it until years later or not at all. The exposed person's immune system plays the primary role as to whether the patient will develop TB.
C. Signs and symptoms of TB include a cough lasting longer than 3 weeks; no appetite; weight loss, hemoptysis, night sweats, chills, and fatigue.

Predisposing Factors

A. HIV
B. Transplant patients on immunosuppression
C. Renal failure and chronic dialysis
D. Malignancy
E. *Substance abuse:* Alcohol, smoking, drug use

Physical Examination

A. A full head-to-toe assessment should be completed on all patients with suspected TB. Because the disease could infect the clinician, it is important to use the appropriate personal protective equipment (PPE) to perform the examination.
B. *Generalized*
 1. Productive cough
 2. Fever
 3. Fatigue
 4. Weight loss
 5. Night sweats
C. *Respiratory*
 1. Dyspnea (more common in older patients)
 2. Productive cough
 3. Hemoptysis
D. *Cardiac*
 1. Dyspnea (more common in older patients)
 2. Chest pain
E. *Other symptoms*
 1. Will be seen based on the patient's medical problem (e.g., HIV infection)

Differential Diagnoses

A. *Respiratory symptoms*
 1. HIV infection
 2. Pulmonary emboli
 3. Pulmonary hypertension
 4. *Pneumonia:* Bacterial, viral, or fungal
 5. Malignancy
 6. Latent TB
B. *Cardiac*
 1. Endocarditis
 2. Pericarditis
 3. Myocarditis
 4. Pericardial effusion
 5. Acute coronary syndrome (ACS)
C. *Neurologic*
 1. **Neuro**syphilis
 2. Meningitis
 3. Toxoplasmosis
 4. HIV or metabolic encephalopathy
 5. Cytomegalovirus (CMV) or herpes simplex virus (HSV) encephalitis
 6. Lymphoma
 7. Subarachnoid hemorrhage
 8. Cerebral infarct
D. *Gastrointestinal/genitourinary (GI/GU)*
 1. Infectious esophagitis (candida, CMV, HSV)
 2. Reflux esophagitis
 3. Renal disease
  a. Vasculitis
  b. Obstruction
  c. Drug nephrotoxicity
E. *Extrapulmonary TB*
 1. Extension of TB into other organ systems
 2. Common in patients infected with HIV or other immunocompromised diseases
 3. TB within the central nervous system can cause meningitis, tuberculomas, or spinal arachnoiditis. TB meningitis is the most serious.

4. Pott disease is the most common form of musculoskeletal disease.
5. TB can affect the heart by causing pericarditis.
6. TB can affect the GU system, causing problems with the kidneys, bladders, and ureters.
7. TB can affect the terminal ileum, causing enteritis, ulceration, and strictures.
8. Cutaneous TB can manifest itself as *verrucose cutis* (purple-brown wart-like growths), *lupus vulgaris* (small, sharply defined red/brown lesions), *scrofuloderma* (firm, painless lesions that ulcerate with a granular base), or a *tuberculid* (a generalized exanthem or recurring nodule).

Diagnostic Testing

A. *Mycobacterium culture:* Limited use in the ED because it can take several weeks to a month for results.
B. Sputum microscopy with stains for AFB, followed by mycobacterial culture with drug susceptibility testing, again can take up to 2 to 3 weeks.
C. *Complete blood count (CBC):* Elevated white count, low Hb
D. Nucleic acid amplification tests (NAATs)
E. *Tuberculin skin testing (TST):* Used for latent TB
F. Gastric aspirate positive for AFB
G. Bronchoscopy and bronchoalveolar lavage (BAL)
H. Interferon-gamma release assays (IGRAs) QuantiFERON ®-TB Gold for active TB is 75% sensitivity; also used for latent TB.
I. Rapid HIV testing
  1. Results available within 20 minutes
  2. *Multiple types of tests available:* Oral swab and blood
  3. Positive tests require confirmation with enzyme-linked immunosorbent assay (ELISA) or Western blot.
  4. Specificity and sensitivity: 99%
J. Respiratory symptoms
  1. Chest x-ray (CXR)
  2. CT is more sensitive for pulmonary TB because it can reveal more lesions.
  3. Sputum cultures, AFB, and Gram stain
  4. Blood cultures
K. Arterial blood gas (ABG)
L. Cardiac symptoms
  1. EKG
  2. Serum cardiac markers
  3. CXR
  4. Blood cultures in suspected endocarditis
  5. Toxicology screen to evaluate for amphetamine and cocaine abuse

Management

A. *Pharmacologic therapies:* Patients who are suspected to have bacterial infections, such a pneumonia, should receive their first dose of antibiotics in the ED.
B. TB treatment medications
  1. *Isoniazid:* Adverse reactions include hepatitis/increased liver function tests (LFTs), seizures, and peripheral neuropathy.
  2. *Pyrazinamide:* Hepatitis/elevated LFTs, gout, and increased serum glucose can be a problem in patients with diabetes, arthralgias, and flushing.
  3. *Ethambutol:* Vision changes, neuropathy, and neuritis
  4. *Rifampin:* Hepatitis/elevated LFTs, GI symptoms, thrombocytopenia, anemia, orange discoloration of body fluids, drug-induced lupus
  5. *Rifapentine:* Hepatitis, thrombocytopenia
  6. *Rifabutin:* Used in patients who cannot tolerate rifampin
C. Consultation/collaboration
  1. All patients should be referred to primary HIV care for initiation and ongoing management.

Patient Disposition

A. Disposition
  1. Discharge criteria include the patient's ability to maintain hydration, self-care, and mobility. Patients should be instructed to isolate themselves and contact local public health departments for follow-up.
  2. Patients who are severely ill, hemodynamically unstable, or have other comorbidities should be admitted. The patients will need to be admitted to an isolation room.
  3. Patients who are not likely to follow recommended treatment for TB should also be admitted.

Age and Developmental Considerations

A. *Prevention and education*
  1. Promote appropriate isolation.
  2. Take medications as directed.
  3. Report any cough or fever immediately to clinician.
  4. Avoid contact with others who are ill.
  5. Encourage cessation of drug, alcohol, and tobacco use.
  6. Avoid pregnancy to prevent fetal transmission.
B. *Patient and family education and counseling*
  1. Minimize exposure to infected patient.
  2. Encourage patient's family members to be tested for TB.
  3. Provide continuous follow-up as recommended by current CDC guidelines.

Varicella

Varicella, or chickenpox, results from an infection from varicella zoster virus (VZV). It is a highly contagious disease that has a prodromal and vesicular stage. Cases typically occur in late winter and early spring. The rash starts on the trunk, where most lesions are clustered. The rates of varicella have dramatically decreased with significant vaccine coverage; however, cases do occur within unvaccinated populations and vaccinated populations, which seem to have a more mild and limited response.[32] Varicella causes a spectrum of diseases.

Pathophysiology

A. DNA virus that lies latent in the cranial nerve ganglia, dorsal root ganglia, and autonomic ganglia
B. Periodically activated
C. Virus is transmitted by the respiratory route and by coming into contact with lesion.

Predisposing Factors

A. Unvaccinated individuals
B. Immunocompromised patients

Physical Examination

A. Low-grade fever, headache, malaise, precedes rash by 1 to 2 days
B. Pruritic rash
C. Anorexia listlessness
D. Classic exanthem
  1. Lesions typically begin on the face and spread to the trunk and extremities.
  2. Lesions are papular, vesicular, or pustular on an erythematous base that measures approximately 2-3 mm.
  3. May involve the oropharyngeal, conjunctival, or vaginal mucosa.
  4. Duration of vesicle formation is 3 to 5 days and crust formation is by 7 to 10 days. Vesicles may continue to form, which results in lesions of various stages.
E. Adolescents and adults
  1. Presentation is similar to that as in children, but adolescents and adults are at a higher risk for severe disease and extracutaneous infections, including pneumonia.
F. Immunocompromised patients
  1. Prolonged healing with potential for severe complications, including pneumonia
  2. More numerous lesions with a hemorrhagic base
G. Pregnant patients
  1. Risk to fetus is greatest in first half of pregnancy.
  2. Risk to mother is greatest if infection is in second half of pregnancy.
H. Extracutaneous manifestations
  1. *Pneumonitis:* Occurs 3 to 5 days after onset of rash. Twenty-five times more common in adults, with highest risk in adult smokers and immunocompromised children
  2. *Cerebritis:* Develops 3 to 8 days after onset of rash. Symptoms include headache, meningismus, vomiting, fever, delirium, and malaise.
  3. *Cerebellar ataxia:* Develops 5 days after onset of rash. Symptoms include ataxia, vomiting, fever, slurred speech, and vertigo.
I. Reye's syndrome

Differential Diagnoses

A. Disseminated herpes
B. Measles
C. Scabies
D. Erythema multiforme
E. Disseminated coxsackie
F. Impetigo
G. Drug eruption

Diagnostic Tests

A. History and physical exam are typically sufficient.
B. Viral culture
C. Polymerase chain reaction (PCR): Diagnostic test of choice
D. Direct fluorescent antibody skin scrapings
E. Serologic test for varicella antibody
F. Extracutaneous manifestations
  1. *Pneumonitis:* Chest x-ray (CXR)
  2. *Cerebritis:* Lumbar puncture (LP) demonstrates elevated protein and lymphocytic pleocytosis.
  3. *Reye's syndrome:* Elevated LFTs, prothrombin time (PT), partial thromboplastin time (PTT), elevated ammonia

Management

A. Symptom treatment with antipyretics and antihistamines for all patients
  1. Infants/children
    a. *Acyclovir:* Not recommended in uncomplicated varicella in healthy children
    b. Reduces lesions by 25% and duration of fever by 1 day.
    c. Prophylaxis with varicella zoster immunoglobulin (VZIG) in susceptible patients and those who are immunocompromised. Susceptible children are at risk if they live in the same household as a patient with active varicella or HZ.
  2. Adolescents/adults
    a. Acyclovir recommended in adults with uncomplicated varicella. It should be initiated within the first 24 hours to prevent progression to disease dissemination.
  3. Pregnant women
    a. Need VZIG if patient reports no known history of childhood disease and if no antibodies to VZV is noted.
    b. Need antibody testing prior to administration of VZIG.
    c. May administer acyclovir or valacyclovir prophylaxis during second and third trimester.
  4. Immunocompromised patients
    a. IV acyclovir
    b. Should be started within 24 hours of onset of rash for maximum efficacy.
    c. VZIG prophylaxis for susceptible immunocompromised patients
  5. Extracutaneous
    a. IV acyclovir
B. *Pharmacologic therapies*
  1. Follow the evidence-based guidelines when prescribing.
  2. Acyclovir
  3. Valacyclovir
  4. Famciclovir
  5. Diphenhydramine
  6. Hydroxyzine
  7. VZIG
C. *Consultation/collaboration*
  1. Patients who are discharged need follow-up with primary care provider (PCP) to ensure resolution of the disease.

Patient Disposition

A. *Discharge instructions*
  1. Uncomplicated courses in immunocompetent children and adults without evidence of secondary bacterial infection or extracutaneous disease can be managed with antipyretics as an outpatient. Patients with pneumonia and those who are immunocompromised require admission. All admitted patients should be placed in isolation.

Age and Developmental Considerations

A. *Geriatric:* Increased risk for extracutaneous complications. Lower immunity results in potential for reactivation as HZ.
B. *Pediatric:* Increased risk for secondary bacterial infection with group A *Streptococcus* or *Staphylococcus* in 1% to 4% of health children, with possible progression to sepsis
C. *Pregnant*: Pregnant patients with no known history of childhood illness of varicella and a negative titer require VZIG. Varicella pneumonia during pregnancy is a medical emergency as it is associated with life-threatening respiratory compromise of the mother and ultimate fetal demise.
D. *Prevention and education*
   1. Vaccination has decreased incidence by 85%.
   2. Most common in early spring and late winter
   3. Virus is transmitted via respiratory route and direct contact with lesions.
   4. 10- to 21-day incubation period
   5. Infectious 48 hours before vesicle formation until vesicles have crusted. This cycle typically takes 3 to 7 days.
   6. Crop nails and practice good hygiene to help prevent secondary infection.
E. *Patient and family education and counseling*

Zoonotic Infections

Zoonotic diseases are very common throughout the world and the United States. According to the Centers for Disease Control and Prevention (CDC), three out of four new and emerging infectious diseases are spread from animals to humans, and the World Health Organization (WHO) reports that nearly 61% of all human diseases are zoonotic in origin. The transmission includes direct contact, indirect contact, foodborne, and vector borne. Animals can carry bacteria, fungi, viruses, and parasites, and all can be transmitted to humans. Humans are usually an accidental host that acquires disease through close contact, and for that reason, clinicians should ask about pets, travel, bites, and exposure history when taking a thorough history and while formulating a differential diagnosis.

(See Chapter 36, Soft Tissue Injuries, sections on mammalian bites and venomous animal injuries for further details.)

Physical Examination

A. *Chief complaint:* Fevers, rash, arthralgias, myalgias
B. Signs and symptoms, diagnostics, and complications (see Tables 22.2, 22.3, 22.4)

Differential Diagnoses

A. See Table 22.5 for summary of differential diagnoses for vector-borne zoonotic infections.

Management

A. *Procedures*
   1. Tourniquet test for dengue fever
   2. Lumbar puncture for suspected neurologic complications, including meningitis
   3. Head CT for encephalopathy
B. *Pharmacologic therapies*
   1. NSAIDs and/or acetaminophen to reduce pain and alleviate fever
   2. IV fluids to correct fluid and electrolyte deficits
   3. Platelet transfusion for severe thrombocytopenia
   4. Disseminated intravascular coagulation (DIC) therapy, if necessary
   5. Symptomatic treatment for all viral illnesses
   6. Malaria
      a. Follow evidence-based guidelines when prescribing.
      b. Artemether + lumefantrine
      c. Artesunate + amodiaquine
      d. Artesunate + mefloquine
      e. Artesunate + sulfadoxine/pyrimethamine
      f. Pyrimethamine

TABLE 22.2 TICK VECTOR ZOONOTIC DISEASES

DISEASE	INCUBATION PERIOD	SIGNS AND SYMPTOMS	DIAGNOSTICS	COMPLICATIONS
Lyme	Few days to a month after tick bite	Stage 1: 30%–50% recall tick bite. ECM (bull's eye rash), regional adenopathy, headache, low-grade fever, myalgia, fatigue, malaise. Stage 2 (secondary disseminated): Days to weeks after onset, triad of aseptic meningitis, cranial neuritis (Bell's palsy), and radiculoneuritis. Tachycardia, bradycardia, myopericarditis Stage 3: Onset >1 year after disease onset. Acrodermatitis chronica atrophicans, arthritis, hepatitis. Persistent disease: Articular and neurologic symptoms Disease has varying presentations dependent upon route of entry.	CBC: Leukocytosis, anemia, thrombocytopenia. ESR: >30 mm/hr CMP: Transaminitis CSF: Pleocytosis, elevated protein, obtain CSF spirochete antibodies. Obtain ELISA, IFA, and Western blot when ECM lesion is not present. PCR: Highly specific and sensitive	Neurologic and cardiac complications, including meningitis, encephalitis, and heart block

(continued)

TABLE 22.2 TICK VECTOR ZOONOTIC DISEASES (*CONTINUED*)

DISEASE	INCUBATION PERIOD	SIGNS AND SYMPTOMS	DIAGNOSTICS	COMPLICATIONS
Tularemia Natural vectors include ticks, mosquitos, biting flies, and wild rabbits. Natural hosts include rodents, domestic animals, and water and soil contaminated by infected animals.	3–5 days	Lesion typically begins as a papule accompanied by fever. Ulceroglandular: Most common presentation with lesion, adenopathy, fever, chills, myalgias, and headaches Glandular: Rare form, within lymphatic system through scratch or abrasion Oculoglandular: Rare form, organism enters via splash to eye. Edema, conjunctivitis, chemosis Pharyngeal: Rare form, from ingestion of contaminated food or water, severe throat pain with lymphadenitis Pneumonic: Secondary to inhalation, seen in farmers and landscapers. Fever, dry cough, pleuritic chest pain Typhoidal: May present with severe sepsis, meningitis, endocarditis, hepatitis, or renal failure	PCR and ELISA Serum antibody titers do not reach diagnostic level until >10 days after onset of illness.	Typhoidal tularemia
Rocky Mountain spotted fever	2–14 days	Reported tick bite within 14 days of rash. Rash: Begins in flexor surfaces of wrist and ankles and rapidly spreads to palms and soles, spreads centripetally, may involve face and trunk. Rash is macular, flat, and erythematous and becomes darker, papular, and dusky in 1–2 days, with eventual evolution to petechial or purpuric lesions that may coalesce. Nonproductive cough, chest pain, dyspnea, abdominal pain, meningismus, encephalitis, generalized edema, dehydration, myalgia, malaise	Clinical diagnosis supplemented by confirmatory lab findings. PCR and immunofluorescent antibody CBC: Thrombocytopenia, anemia CMP: Hyponatremia, elevated aspartate aminotransferase, lactate dehydrogenase Arterial blood gas for hypoxia and respiratory alkalosis. Coagulation profile for suspected DIC.	DIC, noncardiogenic edema, acute renal failure; may be fatal to those who are greater than 50 years of age, male gender, African American or G6PD deficiency.
Babesiosis		Gradual onset of malaise and fatigue with high fever 1–4 weeks after tick bite or 1–9 week after contaminated blood product transfusion Chills, sweats, headache, anorexia, arthralgia, nausea, and nonproductive cough Pharyngeal edema, hepatosplenomegaly, retinopathy, petechia, ecchymosis, ECM	Thin blood smear with Giemsa or Wright staining PCR can be utilized if stains are negative. Indirect immunofluorescent antibody testing can be used if other tests are negative. CBC: Anemia, thrombocytopenia Elevated LFTs Proteinuria, hemoglobinuria	Parasitemia, respiratory distress, shock, severe hemolysis, hepatic or renal failure

(*continued*)

TABLE 22.2 TICK VECTOR ZOONOTIC DISEASES (*CONTINUED*)

DISEASE	INCUBATION PERIOD	SIGNS AND SYMPTOMS	DIAGNOSTICS	COMPLICATIONS
Ehrlichiosis	Symptom onset 1–2 week following tick bite	Abrupt onset of fever, chills, malaise, headache, myalgias Rash may be macular, maculopapular, or petechial. Usually involves the trunk and spares the hands and feet. Lymphadenopathy, hepatosplenomegaly, abnormal neurologic and pulmonary findings dependent upon if complications are present	Culture, PCR, and antibody titer test are not routinely available. Wright stain of peripheral blood has low sensitivity depending on the technician. Potentially fatal tick-borne illness that is usually diagnosed clinically CDC defines illness as fever with one or more of the following: myalgia, anemia, leukopenia, thrombocytopenia, transaminitis, and headache + serologic evidence of IgG antibody or detection by PCR assay, or isolation of organism in cell culture.	ARDS, renal failure, shock, rhabdomyolysis, encephalopathy, DIC, meningitis

Note: Information regarding incubation period, signs and symptoms, and diagnostics is adapted from the CDC. Contact state health department and CDC for diagnostic testing and reporting. Samples will likely need to be sent to the CDC for confirmatory diagnosis.

The information herein regarding zoonotic infections is not all iclusive as there is a myriad of zoonotic infections. The information represents the most common infections which may present to the ED.

ARDS, acute respiratory distress syndrome; CBC, complete blood count; CDC, Centers for Disease Control and Prevention; CMP, comprehensive metabolic panel; CSF, cerebrospinal fluid; DIC, disseminated intravascular coagulation; ECM, erythema chronicum migrans; ELISA, enzyme-linked immunosorbent assay; ESR, erythrocyte sedimentation rate; G6PD, glucose-6-phosphate dehydrogenase; IFA, immunofluorescence assay; LFTs, liver function tests; PCR, polymerase chain reaction.[33–39]

Source: Anderson P. Babesiosis. In: Schaider JJ, Barkin RM, Hayden SR, Wolfe RE, Barkin RE, Rosen P, eds. *Rosen & Barkin's 5-Minute Emergency Medicine Consult.* Wolters Kluwer Health; 2015:120–121; Barkin R. Rocky mountain spotted fever. In: Schaider JJ, Barkin RM, Hayden SR, et al, eds. *Rosen & Barkin's 5- Minute Emergency Medicine Consult.* Wolters Kluwer Health; 2015:990–991; Barkin R, Edlow J. Ehrlichiosis. In: Schaider JJ, Barkin RM, Hayden SR, Wolfe RE, Barkin RE, Rosen P, eds. *Rosen & Barkin's 5-Minute Emergency Medicine Consult.* Wolters Kluwer Health; 2016:1170–1171; Biggs H, Behravesh C, Bradley K, et al. Diagnosis and management of tickborne tickettsial diseases: Rocky Mountain spotted fever and other spotted fever group rickettsioses, ehrlichiosis, and anaplasmosis- United States. https://www.cdc.gov/mmwr/volumes/65/rr/rr6502a1.htm?s_cid=rr6502a1_w; Kitch BB, Meredith JT. Zoonotic infections. In: Tintinalli JE, Stapczynski JS, Ma OJ, Yealy DM, Meckler GD, Cline DM, eds. *Tintinalli's Emergency Medicine: A Comprehensive Study Guide.* vol 1. 8th ed. McGraw-Hill Education; 2016; Lee M. Lyme disease. In: Schaider JJ, Barkin RM, Hayden SR, et al, eds. *Rosen and Barkin's 5-Minute Emergency Medicine Consult.* 5th ed. Wolter Kluwer Health; 2015:664–665; World Health Organization. Vector- borne disease. http://www.who.int/news-room/fact-sheets/detail/vector-borne-diseases [32–38]

TABLE 22.3 MOSQUITO VECTOR ZOONOTIC DISEASES

DISEASE	INCUBATION PERIOD	SIGNS AND SYMPTOMS	DIAGNOSTICS	COMPLICATIONS
Dengue	3–14 days	Fever, joint pain, headache, retro-orbital pain, myalgias, rash, arthralgias, extreme fatigue, and weakness. Rapid and weak pulse, cold, clammy skin, restlessness. At times, hemorrhagic symptoms, including positive tourniquet test, petechiae, ecchymosis, purpura, hematuria, hematemesis, or bloody stool may be present. Consistent with Dengue shock syndrome	RT-PCR: During first 5 days of symptoms and/or early convalescent phase MAC-ELISA: IgM antibodies will remain elevated for 2–3 months after illness. Both acute and convalescent phase specimens are needed to make a diagnosis. Neutropenia, elevated hematocrit, BUN, and creatinine, hyponatremia, thrombocytopenia (<100,000/mm3), transaminitis	Dengue shock syndrome and Dengue hemorrhagic fever
Zika	12 days	Many people are asymptomatic. Other clinical findings include acute onset of fever with maculopapular rash, arthralgias, myalgias, headache, or conjunctivitis.	RT-PCR MAC-ELISA: Qualitative detection of IgM antibodies in serum or CSF. Results may be difficult to interpret related to cross-reaction with other flaviviruses and possible nonspecific reactivity. Inconclusive tests should be sent to the CDC.	Birth defects, preterm birth and miscarriage. Neurologic complications including neuropathy, Guillain Barre syndrome, and myelitis

(*continued*)

TABLE 22.3 MOSQUITO VECTOR ZOONOTIC DISEASES (*CONTINUED*)

DISEASE	INCUBATION PERIOD	SIGNS AND SYMPTOMS	DIAGNOSTICS	COMPLICATIONS
Chikungunya	3–7 days	Majority of patients are asymptomatic. Fever and polyarthralgia (most common) Headache, joint swelling, conjunctivitis, nausea/ vomiting, maculopapular rash, myalgias	Laboratory diagnosis is achieved by testing serum or plasma to detect virus, viral nucleic acid, or virus-specific IgM and neutralizing bodies. Lymphopenia, thrombocytopenia, elevated creatinine, and elevated transaminases	Uveitis, retinitis, myocarditis, hepatitis, nephritis, meningoencephalitis, myelitis, Guillain–Barre syndrome, and cranial nerve palsies
Malaria	8–16 days	Malaise, chills, fever with classic malaria paroxysm (15–60 minutes of chills, followed by 2–6 hours of nondiaphoretic fever, followed by defervescence and profuse diaphoresis) Myalgias, nausea, vomiting, diarrhea, shortness of breath, rales, pulmonary edema, headache, seizures, mental status change Periodicity of the disease is reflective of the life cycle of the protozoan.	Oil emersion light microscopy of a thick-smear Giemsa stain CBC (anemia, thrombocytopenia, leukopenia), CMP (hyponatremia, renal failure, lactic acidosis), UA, LFTs (increased bilirubin and LDH).	Respiratory distress, pulmonary edema, seizure, circulatory collapse, jaundice, severe anemia, death
WNV	2–14 days	70%–80% are subclinical or asymptomatic. Acute febrile illness with headache, weakness, myalgia, or arthralgia, maculopapular rash, nausea, and vomiting	Routine laboratory studies are non- specific. In patients with neuroinvasive disease, CSF evaluation exhibits lymphocytic pleocytosis. WNV-specific IgM antibodies are usually detected after onset of illness and persist from 30–90 days. RT-PCR confirms infection.	Meningitis, encephalitis, and acute flaccid paralysis Cardiac dysrhythmias, myocarditis, rhabdomyolysis, optic neuritis, orchitis, pancreatitis, and hepatitis are rare.

Note: Information regarding incubation period, signs and symptoms, and diagnostics is adapted from the Centers for Disease Control and Prevention. Contact state health department and CDC for diagnostic testing and reporting. Samples will likely need to be sent to the CDC for confirmatory diagnosis. The above information regarding zoonotic infections is not limited to the information provided as there is a myriad of zoonotic infections. The information represents the most common infections which may present to the ED.

BUN, blood urea nitrogen; CBC, complete blood count; CDC, Centers for Disease Control and Prevention; CMP, comprehensive metabolic panel; CSF, cerebrospinal fluid; IgM, immunoglobulin M; LFT, liver function test; LDH, lactate dehydrogenase; MAC-ELISA, IgM antibody capture enzyme-linked immunosorbent assay; RT-PCR, reverse transcriptase-PCR; UA, urinalysis; WNV, West Nile virus.[37,40,41,42,43,44,45,46,47]

Source: Centers for Disease Control and Prevention. Chikungunya: clinical evaluation and disease. https://www.cdc.gov/chikungunya/hc/clinicalevaluation.html; Centers for Disease Control and Prevention. Chikungunya: diagnostic testing. https://www.cdc.gov/chikungunya/hc/diagnostic.html; Centers for Disease Control and Prevention. Dengue: laboratory guidance and diagnostic testing. https://www.cdc.gov/dengue/clinicalLab/laboratory.html; Centers for Disease Control and Prevention. West nile virus: clinical evaluation and disease. https://www.cdc.gov/westnile/healthcareproviders/healthCareProviders-ClinLabEval.html; Centers for Disease Control and Prevention. Traveler's health: world map of areas with risk of Zika. https://wwwnc.cdc.gov/travel/page/world-map-areas-with-zika; Centers for Disease Control and Prevention. Zika virus: types of Zika Virus tests. https://www.cdc.gov/zika/laboratories/types-of-tests.html; Freedman J. Dengue fever. In: Schaider JJ, Barkin RM, Hayden SR, et al, eds. *Rosen & Barkin's 5-Minute Emergency Medicine Consult.* Wolters Kluwer Health; 2015:298–299; Kitch BB, Meredith JT. Zoonotic infections. In: Tintinalli JE, Stapczynski JS, Ma OJ, Yealy DM, Meckler GD, Cline DM, eds. *Tintinalli's Emergency Medicine: A Comprehensive Study Guide*. vol 1. 8th ed. McGraw-Hill Education; 2016; Moskoff J. Malaria. In: Schaider JJ, Barkin RM, Hayden SR, Wolfe RE, Barkin RE, Rosen P, eds. *Rosen & Barkin's 5- Minute Emergency Medicine Consult.* Wolters Kluwer Health; 2015:672–673.[36,39–46]

TABLE 22.4 FLEA VECTOR ZOONOTIC DISEASE

DISEASE	INCUBATION PERIOD	SIGNS AND SYMPTOMS	DIAGNOSTICS
Murine typhus	7–14 days following exposure	Fever, chills, myalgias, anorexia, nausea, vomiting, cough, abdominal pain Rash typically occurs on day 5 of illness. Starts as maculopapular eruption on the trunk and spreads peripherally, sparing the palms and soles.	Clinical presentation and epidemiologic setting typically determine treatment and diagnosis. Confirmation can be determined by PCR, IFA to detect IgG or IgM antibodies.

Note: Information regarding incubation period, signs and symptoms, and diagnostics is adapted from the Centers for Disease Control and Prevention. Contact state health department and CDC for diagnostic testing and reporting. Samples will likely need to be sent to the CDC for confirmatory diagnosis. The above information regarding zoonotic infections is not limited to the information provided as there is a myriad of zoonotic infections. The information represents the most common infections which may present to the ED.

IFA, immunofluorescence assay; IgM, immunoglobulin M; PCR, polymerase chain reaction.[48]

Source: Centers for Disease Control and Prevention. Zoonotic diseases. https://www.cdc.gov/onehealth/basics/zoonotic-diseases.html.[48]

TABLE 22.5 DIFFERENTIAL DIAGNOSES FOR VECTOR-BORNE ZOONOTIC INFECTIONS

VECTOR FOR ZOONOTIC DISEASE	DIFFERENTIAL DIAGNOSES FOR SAME VECTOR ILLNESSES	DIFFERENTIAL DIAGNOSES FOR OTHER INFLAMMATORY OR INFECTIOUS DISEASES
Tick	Rocky Mountain spotted fever Lyme disease Ehrlichiosis Relapsing fever Tularemia Babesiosis Tick bite paralysis Colorado tick fever	Meningococcemia Measles Rubella Varicella Viral exanthem Kawasaki disease Typhus Scarlett fever Tuberculosis Toxoplasmosis Anthrax Diphtheria Legionnaires' disease Q fever Brucellosis Toxic shock syndrome Staphylococcal sepsis Infectious mononucleosis Disseminated gonococcal infection Secondary syphilis Allergic vasculitis Thrombotic thrombocytopenic purpura Juvenile rheumatoid arthritis
Mosquito	Malaria Zika Chikungunya virus Dengue virus West Nile virus Yellow fever virus Rift Valley virus St. Louis encephalitis virus Eastern equine encephalitis virus California serogroup viruses	Meningitis Encephalitis Stroke Acute renal failure Acute hemolytic anemia Typhoid fever Influenza Measles Rubella Scarlett fever HIV Mononucleosis Hepatitis Erythema infectiosum Roseola infantum Leptospirosis Sepsis Hepatitis Hypoglycemic coma Viral diarrheal illness
Flea	Murine typhus Rickettsiosis Plague Scrub typhus Epidemic typhus *Mycoplasma haemofelis* Tapeworm	Influenza Gastroenteritis Encephalitis Myocarditis Arthritis Sepsis pneumonia

(*continued*)

TABLE 22.5 DIFFERENTIAL DIAGNOSES FOR VECTOR-BORNE ZOONOTIC INFECTIONS (*CONTINUED*)

VECTOR FOR ZOONOTIC DISEASE	DIFFERENTIAL DIAGNOSES FOR SAME VECTOR ILLNESSES	DIFFERENTIAL DIAGNOSES FOR OTHER INFLAMMATORY OR INFECTIOUS DISEASES
Direct or indirect contact with an animal or bodily fluid, or handling of contaminated food	Rabies *Salmonella* *Escherichia coli* Psittacosis Avian influenza Hantavirus—deer mice	Influenza Gastroenteritis Encephalitis Myocarditis Arthritis Sepsis Pneumonia

Note: The differential list for these zoonotic infections is extensive and is not limited to the above mentioned list.[33, 34, 35, 36, 37, 40, 41, 42, 43, 49]

Source: Anderson P. Babesiosis. In: Schaider JJ, Barkin RM, Hayden SR, Wolfe RE, Barkin RE, Rosen P, eds. *Rosen & Barkin's 5-Minute Emergency Medicine Consult.* Wolters Kluwer Health; 2015:120–121; Barkin R. Rocky mountain spotted fever. In: Schaider JJ, Barkin RM, Hayden SR, et al, eds. *Rosen & Barkin's 5- Minute Emergency Medicine Consult.* Wolters Kluwer Health; 2015:990–991; Barkin R, Edlow J. Ehrlichiosis. In: Schaider JJ, Barkin RM, Hayden SR, Wolfe RE, Barkin RE, Rosen P, eds. *Rosen & Barkin's 5-Minute Emergency Medicine Consult.* Wolters Kluwer Health; 2016:1170–1171; Bentz S. Tularemia. In: Schaider JJ, Barkin RM, Hayden SR, Wolfe RE, Barkin RE, Rosen P, eds. *Rosen & Barkin's 5-Minute Emergency Medicine Consult.* Wolters Kluwer Health; 2015:1170–1171; Biggs H, Behravesh C, Bradley K, et al. Diagnosis and management of tickborne tickettsial diseases: Rocky Mountain spotted fever and other spotted fever group rickettsioses, ehrlichiosis, and anaplasmosis- United States. https://www.cdc.gov/mmwr/volumes/65/rr/rr6502a1.htm?s_cid=rr6502a1_w; Centers for Disease Control and Prevention. Chikungunya: clinical evaluation and disease. https://www.cdc.gov/chikungunya/hc/clinicalevaluation.html; Centers for Disease Control and Prevention. Chikungunya: diagnostic testing. https://www.cdc.gov/chikungunya/hc/diagnostic.html; Centers for Disease Control and Prevention. Dengue: laboratory guidance and diagnostic testing. https://www.cdc.gov/dengue/clinicalLab/laboratory.html; Centers for Disease Control and Prevention. West nile virus: clinical evaluation and disease. https://www.cdc.gov/westnile/healthcareproviders/healthCareProviders-ClinLabEval.html; Kitch BB, Meredith JT. Zoonotic infections. In: Tintinalli JE, Stapczynski JS, Ma OJ, Yealy DM, Meckler GD, Cline DM, eds. *Tintinalli's Emergency Medicine: A Comprehensive Study Guide.* vol 1. 8th ed. McGraw-Hill Education; 2016.[32–36,39–42,48]

7. Lyme disease
   a. First line
      i. *Stage 1:* Doxycycline (except pregnant women). Clinicians should never delay treatment while awaiting laboratory diagnosis.
      ii. Amoxicillin
      iii. Aspirin
      iv. Ceftriaxone
   b. Second line
      i. Cefuroxime
      ii. Azithromycin
      iii. Cefotaxime
      iv. Penicillin G
8. Tularemia
   a. Streptomycin
   b. Ciprofloxacin
   c. Doxycycline
9. Rocky Mountain spotted fever
   a. Doxycycline
   b. Chloramphenicol
10. Babesiosis
   a. Atovaquone
   b. Azithromycin
   c. Clindamycin
11. Ehrlichiosis
   a. Doxycycline
   b. Rifampin for pregnant patients, those allergic to doxycycline, and mildly affected children <9 years old.
12. Murine typhus
   a. Doxycycline

C. *Consultation/collaboration:* For immunocompromised patients and those with complications.

Patient Disposition

A. Admission for high-risk patients and those with severe disease with complications, including meningoencephalitis, cardiac arrhythmias

B. Discharge instructions

C. Increase hydration and rest.

D. Transition of care information

Age and Developmental Considerations

A. Neonatal dengue can occur by vertical transmission if mother is infected 0 to 8 days prior to delivery. Dengue hemorrhagic fever and Dengue shock syndrome are most common in children.

1. Sickle cell trait is protective of malarial infection.
2. Cerebral malaria is more common in children. Pregnant patients are at higher risk of malarial infections.
3. Facial paralysis is accompanied by aseptic meningitis in one-third of patients with Lyme disease.
4. Untreated children may have keratitis, but appropriately treated children have excellent prognosis for unimpaired cognitive functioning.
5. Transmission of babesiosis can occur in utero and during delivery.

B. Prevention and education

1. Clean hands after being around animals.
2. Prevent bites from mosquitos, fleas, and ticks.
3. Food safety
4. Avoid bites and scratches from animals.
5. Be vigilant and aware of zoonotic infections at all times, including at petting zoos, fairs, schools, stores, and parks. Research diseases before travel.
6. Choose a pet wisely.
7. Chemoprophylaxis for malaria with Malarone, chloroquine, doxycycline, primaquine, or mefloquine

References and Additional Reading

References and Additional Reading for this chapter are online only and can be found at https://connect.springerpub.com/content/reference-book/978-0-8261-6091-5/part/part02/toc-part/ch22.

23. Psychiatric and Mental Health Emergencies

DAVID T. HOUSE

Learning Objectives

- Identify signs and symptoms of patients presenting with psychiatric and/or mental health disorders.
- Ensure safety for the psychiatric/mental health patient and ED staff.
- Utilize various mental health screening tools to properly assess the patient who presents with psychiatric symptoms.
- Implement pharmacological interventions for acute psychosis and schizophrenia.
- Initiate the appropriate disposition for the psychiatric/mental health patient.

Mental illness is generally characterized by changes in mood, thought, or behavior. Mental illness consists of two broad categories that define these various conditions. Any mental illness (AMI) is defined as a mental, behavioral, or emotional disorder, which can vary in impact ranging from no impairment to mild, moderate, or even severe impairment. Serious mental illness (SMI) is defined as a mental, behavioral, or emotional disorder resulting in serious functional impairment, which substantially interferes with or limits one or more major life activities.

Prevalence

In 2016, nearly one in five adults aged 18 or older in the United States had any mental illness (AMI). This amounts to an estimated 44.7 million adults, representing 18.3% of the U.S. adult population. An estimated 10.4 million adults in the nation had a serious mental illness (SMI) in 2016, representing 4.2% of the U.S. adult population. In 2016, 3.1 million (12.8%) of adolescents aged 12 to 17 experienced a major depressive episode. Over the past decade, the percentage of adolescents and younger adults with AMI has risen. Prevalence is higher among women (21.7%) than men (14.5%) and young adults aged 18 to 25 (22.1%) have the highest prevalence of any mental illness.

General Approach

ED care for psychiatric and mental health patients is particularly challenging due to a lack of resources. Patients may have vague, nonspecific symptoms, and the assessment, diagnosis, and disposition is often time-consuming and difficult. Emergency psychiatric assessment should focus on:

A. Safety and stabilization
B. Identification of suicidal, homicidal, or dangerous behavior
C. Medical evaluation
D. Psychiatric consultation
E. Psychiatric diagnosis and severity assessment

Anxiety and Posttraumatic Stress Disorders

Anxiety disorders include disorders that share features of excessive fear, anxiety, and other related behavioral disturbances. This group of disorders consists of generalized anxiety disorder, panic disorder, and posttraumatic stress disorder (PTSD). Anxiety is anticipation of future threats, whereas fear is an emotional response to real or perceived imminent threat. Panic attacks are a part of anxiety disorders and are a type of fear response. PTSD is a type of stress-related disorder acquired when the patient is exposed to a stressful or traumatic event.

Pathophysiology

The cause of these disorders is multifactorial, but the underlying mechanism is not fully established. Both biological and neuropsychological factors predispose individuals to anxiety disorders. Genetic factors play a role along with neurotransmitters such as norepinephrine, serotonin, and gamma-aminobutyric acid (GABA). Psychological and environmental risk factors such as exposure to stressful events also contribute to anxiety disorders. In the event of a pandemic such as COVID-19, both the physiological risk of infection and psychological stress associated create fear and uncertainty, contributing to increased levels of anxiety and stress.

Prevalence

Generalized anxiety disorder affects approximately 6.8 million adults or 3.1% of the U.S. population. The prevalence for females is twice that of males. Anxiety disorders affect 25.1% of children between the age of 13 and 18 years old. Panic disorder affects 6 million adults (2.7%) of the U.S. population. Women are affected twice that of males. PTSD affects 7.7 million adults or 3.5% of the U.S. population and is higher for females than males across all age groups.

Physical Examination

A. *Chief complaint:* Chest pain, palpitations, shortness of breath, sense of impending doom

B. *Signs and symptoms*
   1. Shaking, trembling, or sweating
   2. Chest pain or discomfort, palpitations, tachycardia
   3. Shortness of breath, tachypnea
   4. Abdominal pain, nausea, or vomiting
   5. Numbness, tingling, lightheadedness, or dizziness

C. *Medication history for anxiety*
   1. *Selective serotonergic reuptake inhibitors (SSRIs):* Paroxetine, sertraline, citalopram
   2. *Serotonin-norepinephrine reuptake inhibitors (SNRIs):* Venlafaxine, duloxetine
   3. Buspirone
   4. *Benzodiazepines:* Alprazolam, clonazepam, diazepam, lorazepam

D. *Past medical history:* Pertinent to condition
   1. Previous medical history or diagnosis of psychiatric/mental health disorder
   2. Substance abuse history that includes alcohol, prescription drugs, caffeine, and nicotine
   3. Family psychiatric/mental health history
   4. Social history that screens for stressful life events (witnessed or experienced) and past sexual, physical, and emotional abuse, trauma, or emotional neglect

E. *Focused assessment*
   1. Screening instruments such as the Generalized Anxiety Disorder Seven-Item (GAD-7) Scale or the Hospital Anxiety and Depression Scale (HADS)
   2. *General:* Anxious, shaking, trembling
   3. *Cardiac:* Chest pain or discomfort, palpitations, tachycardia
   4. *Pulmonary:* Shortness of breath
   5. *Gastrointestinal (GI):* Abdominal pain or nausea
   6. *Neurological:* Numbness, tingling, lightheadedness or dizziness
   7. *Psychological:* Fear of losing control or dying, inability to concentrate

Differential Diagnoses

A. Anxiety
B. Panic reaction
C. PTSD
D. Acute myocardial infarction
E. Pulmonary embolus
F. Cerebrovascular accident (CVA)
G. Thyroid storm
H. Hypoglycemia
I. Substance abuse, intoxication, or withdrawal

Diagnostic Testing

A. Complete blood count (CBC) with differential
B. Serum chemistries
C. Thyroid function tests
D. Serum and urine toxicology screen
E. EKG

Management

A. *Procedures/management*
   1. Directed at stabilization, keeping patient and staff safety in mind

B. *Pharmacologic therapies*
   1. Follow evidence-based guidelines for prescribing.
   2. Pharmacologic treatment should be aimed at decreasing anxiety in the ED and not meant for outpatient treatment. Initiate a short-term benzodiazepine for acute episodes.
      a. Lorazepam, orally every 8 hours
      b. Clonazepam, orally every 12 hours
      c. Alprazolam, orally every 6 to 8 hours
      d. Diazepam, orally every 6 to 12 hours
      e. Initiating long-term antidepressant therapy for anxiety is not typical in the ED and is done outpatient by a psychiatric/mental health professional or primary care clinician with close follow-up.

C. *Consultation/collaboration*
   1. Psychiatric/mental health clinician
   2. Social work, care managers
   3. Primary care clinician

Patient Disposition

A. *Transition of care information*
   1. Admit for any suicidal, homicidal ideation, or with severe depression.
   2. Admit to rule out any life-threatening medical condition.
   3. Discharge and close follow-up with psychiatric/mental health services or primary care physician

B. *Age and developmental considerations*
   1. Patient and family education and counseling
      a. Education and reassurance about anxiety disorders
      b. Refer to community resources such as social services, counseling services, mental health professionals, or substance abuse organizations such as Alcoholics Anonymous.

C. *Documentation*
   1. Patient safety, education, and close follow-up

Eating Disorders, Bulimia, Anorexia

Eating disorders are a group of disorders causing serious and sometimes fatal alterations to a person's eating behavior. The patient may experience alterations in consumption or absorption of food that impact physical health or psychosocial functioning. Obsessions with body weight, food, and shape may signal an eating disorder. Common eating disorders include binge eating disorder, bulimia nervosa, and anorexia nervosa.

Pathophysiology

Eating disorders consist of both biological and psychosocial factors. Evidence exists that there is a familial connection composed of both genetic and behavior influences. Neurotransmitter systems have been found to be disrupted in anorexia nervosa. Deficits have been found in dopaminergic function (dopamine is thought to be involved with eating behavior, motivation, and reward) and serotonergic function (serotonin may be

BOX 23.1 SCOFF QUESTIONNAIRE

The SCOFF Questionnaire is a valid and reliable tool for detecting an eating disorder

Do you make yourself **S**ick because you feel uncomfortably full?
Do you worry you have lost **C**ontrol over how much you eat?
Have you recently lost more than **O**ne stone (14 pounds) in a 3-month period?
Do you believe yourself to be **F**at when others say you are too thin?
Would you say that **F**ood dominates your life?

*One point for every "yes"; a score of ≥2 indicates a likely case of anorexia nervosa or bulimia (sensitivity and specificity of 100% and 87.5%)

involved with mood, impulse control, and obsessional behavior). However, the exact pathogenesis is not well understood.

Incidence and Prevalence

For anorexia nervosa, there is an overall incidence rate of 8 per 100,000 person-years, with a prevalence of 0.9% in women and 0.3% in men. Bulimia nervosa has an overall incidence rate of 12 per 100,000 person-years, with an estimated lifetime prevalence of 1.5% in women and 0.5% in men. The prevalence of bulimia is higher in Latinos (2.03%) and African Americans (1.31%) than Whites (0.51%).

Physical Examination

A. *Chief complaint:* Weakness, fatigue, dizziness, syncope, bloating, nausea

B. *Signs and symptoms*
   1. Weakness, fatigue
   2. Dizziness, syncope, confusion
   3. Bloating, persistent nausea, pain with eating, hematemesis
   4. Anxious, depressed

C. *Focused assessment*
   1. Use screening instrument such as the SCOFF Questionnaire for eating disorders (Box 23.1), SIG-E-CAPS for depression screening, or SAD PERSONS for suicide risk (see Table 23.1 and Box 23.2).
   2. Psychiatric and general medical history
   3. Recent weight changes, efforts to control weight, meal patterns, binge eating, dietary restrictions, attitudes about eating, purging
   4. Mental status exam
   5. Physical examination to include height, weight, and body mass index (BMI)
   6. Ridged or brittle nails, dry skin, Russell's sign (callous or trauma to dorsum of the hand)
   7. Hypotension, bradycardia, tachydysrhythmia, murmur
   8. Menstrual status (females)
   9. Prescription or over-the-counter (OTC) medications such as weight loss medications or laxatives
   10. Family history of eating disorders
   11. Thoughts of suicide

Differential Diagnoses

A. Anorexia nervosa
B. Bulimia nervosa
C. Major depressive disorder
D. Mallory-Weiss tear
E. Hyperthyroidism
F. Human immunodeficiency virus
G. Intra-abdominal malignancy
H. Hyperemesis gravidarum

Diagnostic Testing

A. Complete blood count (CBC) with differential, blood glucose

TABLE 23.1 SAD PERSONS

Modified Suicide Risk Assessment Tool		
RISK FACTOR	**CRITERIA**	**SCORE**
S Sex	Male	1
A Age	<20 years; >45 years	1
D Depression	Major (depressed mood)	2
P Psychiatric History	Previous attempts	1
E Excessive Drug Use	Ethanol or other drug abuse	1
R Rationality Loss	Psychosis, severe depression	2
S Separated	Loss of spouse or other	1
O Organized plan	Developed suicide plan	2
N No Supports	No social support	1
S Sickness	Chronic illness	1

Note: Score less than 2: discharge with outpatient psychiatric evaluation;
Score of 3–6: consider hospitalization or close follow-up;
Score of 7 or greater: hospitalization.
Source: With permission from Patterson WM, Dohn HH, Bird J, Patterson GA. Evaluation of suicidal patients: The SAD PERSONS scale. *Psychosomatics.* 1983;24:343–345. 348–349.1

BOX 23.2 SIG E CAPS

Depressive Disorder Assessment Tool

S sleep amount increased or decreased
I interest (anhedonia)
G guilt
E energy level decreased
C concentration decreased
A appetite increased or decreased
P psychomotor activity increased or decreased
S suicidal ideation

B. Serum chemistries, electrolytes, thyroid function, hepatic function
C. Urinalysis, urine pregnancy test (females)
D. Serum and urine toxicology screen
E. Psychiatric medication drug levels such as lithium, valproic acid
F. EKG

Management

A. *Procedures/management*
  1. Management is directed at identifying any urgent or emergent conditions, electrolyte imbalances, or cardiac arrhythmias based on diagnostic results.
  2. Identify any risk of suicidal ideation.
B. *Pharmacologic therapies*
  1. Follow evidence-based guidelines when prescribing.
  2. If long-term pharmacotherapy is indicated, it should be initiated by a psychiatric/mental health clinician or primary care clinician.
  3. Avoid NSAIDs.
C. *Consultation/collaboration*
  1. Multidisciplinary approach, consultation with psychiatric/mental health clinician or primary care clinician

Patient Disposition

A. *Transition of care information*
  1. Treatment is based on stabilization of medical complications followed by hospital admission, transfer to inpatient psychiatric facility, or outpatient referral to a mental health specialist or primary care clinician.
  2. Society of Adolescent Medicine Criteria for hospitalization (Table 23.2)
B. *Age and developmental considerations*
  1. Patient and family education and counseling
    a. Establish healthy eating habits, recommended list of foods.
    b. Limit physical activity.
    c. Support groups, National Association of Anorexia Nervosa and Associated Disorders helpline 630-577-1330 or https://anad.org/
C. *Documentation*
  1. Documentation of baseline laboratory results, screening scales, and referral information to mental/behavioral health or primary care clinician

Physical Examination

A. *Chief complaint:* Changes in mood, thought, or behavior
B. *Signs and symptoms*
  1. Abdominal pain, nausea, vomiting, diarrhea
  2. Accidental injuries
  3. Altered mental status
  4. Decreased activity
  5. Chest pain or discomfort
  6. Combative, uncooperative
  7. Fatigue, weakness
  8. Hallucinations, delusions
  9. Shortness of breath
  10. Substance abuse
C. *Focused assessment*
  1. Simultaneous medical and psychiatric evaluation
  2. Document behavioral changes through history.
  3. Identify medical symptoms.
  4. Determine medical comorbidities.
  5. Obtain medication and drug history.
  6. Perform physical examination.
  7. Perform mental status and neurologic assessment.
  8. Determine medical clearance.

TABLE 23.2 SOCIETY OF ADOLESCENT MEDICINE CRITERIA FOR HOSPITALIZATION

ANOREXIA NERVOSA	BULIMIA NERVOSA
<75% of ideal body weight for age, sex, and height	Serum potassium <3.2 mmol/L
Heart rate <50 beats/min daytime, <45 beats/min nighttime	Serum chloride <88 mmol/L
Body fat <10% of body weight	Esophageal trauma and hematemesis
Dehydration	Vomiting unresponsive to antiemetics
Cardiac arrhythmia including QT prolongation	Dehydration
Temperature <96°F	Cardiac arrhythmia including QT prolongation
Orthostasis and syncope	Temperature <96°F
Acute psychiatric emergencies such as hallucinations or suicidality	Orthostasis and syncope
Systolic blood pressure <90 mmHg	Acute psychiatric emergencies such as hallucinations or suicidality
Ongoing weight loss despite outpatient treatment	Ongoing purging despite outpatient treatment

Differential Diagnoses

A. Anxiety, posttraumatic stress disorder
B. Mood disorder, depression, bipolar, dysthymia
C. Factitious disorders
D. Eating disorders, anorexia, bulimia
E. Suicidal ideation
F. Psychosis, schizophrenia
G. Substance use disorder

Diagnostic Testing

A. Vital signs
B. Point-of-care blood glucose
C. Lab diagnostics based on need for identification of underlying medical condition
- **1.** CBC with differential
- **2.** Serum chemistries
- **3.** Hepatic function tests
- **4.** Thyroid function tests
- **5.** Serum and urine toxicology screen
- **6.** Urinalysis and urine pregnancy (females)

D. EKG
E. CT scan of the head (altered mental state [AMS] or focal neurologic deficits)

Management

A. *Procedures/management*
- **1.** Directed at stabilization, keeping patient and staff safety in mind
- **2.** Patient-centered approach
- **3.** Ensure safety for patient and prevent self-harm by having patient change into a gown and remove possible weapons, clothing (belts, shoelaces), or medications that can inflict harm.
- **4.** Clear room of any potentially harmful objects.
- **5.** Close observation by trained patient specialists, sitter, or facility security

B. *Pharmacologic therapies*
- **1.** ED pharmacologic therapy is directed toward patient stabilization and reduction of patient anxiety or violence
- **2.** If long-term pharmacotherapy is indicated, it should be initiated by a psychiatric/mental health professional or primary care clinician.

C. *Consultation/collaboration*
- **1.** Psychiatric/mental health clinician
- **2.** Social work, care managers
- **3.** Primary care clinician

Patient Disposition

A. *Transition of care information*
- **1.** Admit unstable patients, advanced age, medical comorbidities, or no response to ED treatment.
- **2.** Transfer to psychiatric/mental health facility after medical clearance.
- **3.** Discharge home with family or support system, close follow-up with psychiatric/mental health clinician or primary care clinician

B. *Age and developmental considerations*
- **1.** Patient and family education and counseling
  - **a.** Education for psychiatric/mental health condition including verbal and written information
  - **b.** List of warning signs, risk factors, and follow-up instructions
  - **c.** List of coping strategies
  - **d.** Family or friends need to be educated with patient and be able to provide a support system.
  - **e.** Refer to community resources such as social services, counseling services, mental health professionals, or substance abuse organizations such as Alcoholics Anonymous.
  - **f.** Give the National Suicide Prevention Hotline number (1-800-273-TALK [8255])

C. *Documentation*
- **1.** Should reflect decision-making process, risk level, risk of imminent self-harm, patient safety, education, social support, and close follow-up plan

Mental Health Disorders of the Elderly

Delirium and dementia are common mental health disorders in the elderly and are often interrelated. Distinguishing between the two is important. Delirium is an acute change in cognition that fluctuates rapidly over time and is often reversible. Dementia is a gradual loss of cognitive functioning in two or more aspects of a person's life. Dementia is memory impairment and at least one of the following: aphasia, apraxia, agnosia, disturbance in executive functioning that impacts social, functional, or occupational activities. The most common form is Alzheimer's dementia.

Pathophysiology

Delirium occurs when there is impairment of normal sending and receiving of signals within the brain. One or a combination of factors, such as drug toxicity and/or medical conditions, can cause delirium. This onset of symptoms for delirium is usually a sudden process. Dementia is more of an insidious process. It may be caused by vascular changes (ischemia) within the brain or an abnormal build of proteins (Lewy bodies).

Prevalence

An estimated 7 million adults suffer from delirium in the United States. Delirium is a common, serious, and often fatal disorder that affects as many as 50% of elderly in the hospital setting. Typically, there is evidence of a medical and/or multifactorial etiology. There are an estimated 5.7 million adults in the United States who have Alzheimer's dementia. In 2015, Alzheimer's was the fifth leading cause of death in adults ≥ 65 years old.

Physical Examination

A. *Chief complaint:* Confusion, behavioral changes
B. *Signs and symptoms*:
- **1.** Changes in thinking and reasoning
- **2.** Confusion
- **3.** Parkinson's symptoms, including movement disorders
- **4.** Visual hallucinations
- **5.** Delusions
- **6.** Memory loss
- **7.** Sleep difficulties

C. *Focused assessment*
1. Mental Status Examination screening test such as the Confusion Assessment Method and the Mini-Cog
2. Screening for depression use SIG-E-CAPS.
3. Thorough history and physical—baseline mental status and level of functioning
4. Past medical history and recent illnesses
5. Medication lists, over-the-counter (OTC), anticholinergic medications
6. Substance abuse
7. Timing—acute and/or fluctuating

Differential Diagnoses

A. Alzheimer's disease
B. Vascular dementia
C. Dementia with Lewy bodies
D. Mixed dementia
E. Delirium
F. Parkinson's disease
G. Cerebrovascular accident (CVA)
H. Adverse medication reaction

Diagnostic Testing

A. Point of care glucose
B. Complete blood count (CBC) with differential
C. Basic metabolic panel, calcium, phosphorus, liver function tests, thyroid function studies
D. Urinalysis
E. Serum and urine toxicology studies
F. Lumbar puncture
G. Cardiac markers
H. Arterial blood gas (ABG)
I. EKG
J. Head CT if trauma, altered mental status (AMS), or focal neurologic deficits

Management

A. *Procedures/management*
1. Current strategies focus on identifying underlying disease and treating symptoms

B. *Pharmacologic therapies*
1. Cholinesterase inhibitors
2. Antipsychotic drugs
3. Antidepressants
4. Clonazepam
5. If long-term pharmacotherapy is indicated, it should be initiated by a psychiatric/mental health practitioner or primary care provider

C. *Consultation/collaboration*
1. Psychiatric/mental health services, neurology

Patient Disposition

A. *Transition of care information*
1. Hospitalization for further evaluation (delirium)
2. Discharge if patient returns to baseline or can be discharged to the care of a capable individual
3. Transfer to an appropriate facility

B. *Age and developmental considerations*
1. Patient and family education and counseling
   a. Safety and care of the patient
   b. Medication interactions
   c. Nonpharmacologic therapies and supportive care
   d. Community resources such as social services, counseling services, mental health professionals, national organizations such as Alzheimer's Association

C. *Documentation*
1. Documentation should reflect decision-making process, patient safety, education, social support, and follow-up plan with mental health specialist or neurologist.

BOX 23.3 SYMPTOMS OF MOOD DISORDERS

Five or more of the following symptoms must be present for a duration of 2 weeks; cannot be due to substance abuse or medical condition, and cause significant impairment in normal functioning. *At least one of the symptoms is either depressed mood or loss of pleasure.*

1. Depressed mood
2. Anhedonia (loss of pleasure)
3. Significant weight loss or gain
4. Insomnia or hypersomnia
5. Psychomotor agitation or retardation nearly every day
6. Fatigue or loss of energy
7. Feelings of worthlessness or inappropriate guilt
8. Diminished ability to think or concentrate
9. Recurrent thoughts of death, suicidal ideation without a specific plan, suicide plan, or attempt

Mood Disorders, Depression, Bipolar Disorder, Dysthymia

Mood disorders are classified into depressive and bipolar disorders. Depressive disorders are characterized by discrete episodes of at least 2 weeks' duration (see Box 23.3). A more chronic form of depression, persistent depressive disorder (dysthymia), can be diagnosed when the mood disturbance continues for at least 2 years in adults or 1 year in children. The bipolar I disorder criteria represents the classic manic-depressive disorder or affective psychosis. Bipolar II disorder, requiring the lifetime experience of at least one episode of major depression and at least one hypomanic episode. Major depression, bipolar, and mania may be accompanied by delusions and hallucinations.

Pathophysiology

The pathophysiology of mood disorders is not well established. Neurotransmitters such as serotonin and norepinephrine play a role in neurophysiology. Monoamine deficiency is hypothesized as a cause. Decreased levels of glutamate and gamma-aminobutyric acid (GABA) are seen. Another possibility is the hypothalamic-pituitary-adrenal (HPA) axis. Depression is a familial disorder but less heritable than bipolar disorder. Psychosocial factors such as stressful life events, lack of family support, and substance abuse are risk factors.

BOX 23.4 DIG FAST MNEMONIC

Primary symptoms of a manic attack
D Distractibility
I Impulsivity/Indiscretion (excessive involvement in pleasurable activities
G Grandiosity (inflated self-esteem)
F Flight of ideas
A Activity increase/psychomotor agitation
S Sleep deficit (decreased need for sleep)
T Talkativeness (pressured speech)

Prevalence

In 2016, the prevalence of major depressive episode among U.S. adults aged 18 and older was 6.7%. The prevalence was higher among females (8.5%) compared to males (4.8%) and highest among individuals aged 18 to 25 (10.9%). Among adolescents aged 12 to 17, the prevalence of major depressive episode was 12.8% of the U.S. population. Bipolar disorder affects about 2.6% of the U.S. population age 18 and older every year. More than two-thirds of those diagnosed with bipolar have at least one close relative with depression or bipolar disease.

Physical Examination

A. *Chief complaint:* Decreased attention, depression, elevated mood, flight of ideas, mania

B. *Signs and symptoms*

1. Depressed mood
2. Loss of interest or pleasure
3. Change in appetite or weight
4. Sleep disturbance
5. Fatigue or loss of energy
6. Suicidal ideation and/or behavior
7. Mania, irritability, delusional ideas (bipolar)

C. *Focused assessment*

1. General medical history, psychiatric history, physical examination
2. Screening for suicide risk use SAD PERSONS, depression use SIG-E-CAPS, and for bipolar, mania use DIG FAST (Table 23.1 and Boxes 23.2 and 23.4)
3. History and physical focused on mood disorder or other conditions such as drug abuse, medications, or underlying medication condition
4. Medication history to include lithium, valproic acid, carbamazepine, haloperidol, or a benzodiazepine
5. *General:* Poor eye contact, poor hygiene
6. *Psychological:* Mania, irritability, hypomania, delusions, hallucinations

Differential Diagnoses

A. Unipolar major depression (major depressive disorder)

B. Persistent depressive disorder (dysthymia)

C. Substance/medication-induced depressive disorder

D. Bipolar I disorder (manic episode)

E. Bipolar II disorder (hypomania)

F. Suicidal ideation/homicidal Ideation (SI/HI)

Diagnostic Testing

A. Complete blood count (CBC) with differential

B. Serum chemistries, thyroid function, hepatic panel

C. Urinalysis, urine pregnancy test (females)

D. Serum and urine toxicology screen

E. Psychiatric medication drug levels such as lithium, valproic acid

F. EKG

Management

A. *Procedures/management*

1. Directed at stabilization, keeping patient and staff safety in mind
2. Straightforward, non-threatening questions regarding SI/HI thoughts or intent
3. Ensure safety for patient and prevent self-harm by having them change into a gown and remove possible weapons, clothing (belts, shoelaces), or medications that can inflict harm.
4. Clear room of any potentially harmful objects.
5. Close observation by trained patient specialists, sitter, or facility security

B. *Pharmacologic therapies*

1. Follow the evidence-based guidelines when prescribing.
2. If long-term antidepressant pharmacotherapy is indicated, a psychiatric/mental health clinician or primary care clinician should initiate with close follow-up due to delayed onset and potential adverse side effects.
3. Bipolar pharmacotherapy should not be initiated by the ED provider except for treatment of acute agitation or to restart previously prescribed lithium or anticonvulsant medication.
   a. *Severe mania:* Lithium, valproic acid, or carbamazepine with or without an antipsychotic such as haloperidol or benzodiazepine
      i. Lithium, initial orally two or three times daily (may cause central nervous system [CNS] depression, serotonin syndrome)
      ii. Valproic acid, orally two or three times daily (nausea/vomiting [N/V], thrombocytopenia, hepatic failure)
      iii. Carbamazepine, orally one or two times daily (agranulocytosis, N/V, leukopenia, hyponatremia)
      iv. Aripiprazole in combination with lithium, orally once daily. (headache, N/V, extrapyramidal symptoms)
      v. Aripiprazole monotherapy, initial orally once daily (headache, N/V, extrapyramidal symptoms)
      vi. Risperidone monotherapy, initial orally once daily (extrapyramidal side effects, sedation, nausea)

C. Consultation and collaboration

D. Psychiatric/mental health clinician
E. Primary care clinician

Patient Disposition

A. *Transition of care information*
   1. Both depression and bipolar disorder patients who are at risk for harm to self or others need psychiatric evaluation for admission.
   2. Discharge home if supportive environment, close follow-up with mental health services, primary care provider or counselor, and no SI/HI
B. *Age and developmental considerations*
   1. Criteria for depression in children and adolescents are the same as for adults. However, they may present differently. Children and adolescents may experience interruptions in attention, poor concentration, increased irritability, oppositional behavior, withdrawal from daily activities, and substance abuse.
C. *Patient and family education and counseling:*
   1. Educate patient on signs and symptoms of depression, bipolar, mania, thoughts of suicide.
      a. Thoughts of suicide
         i. Call your provider and tell them it is urgent.
         ii. Call 911.
         iii. Go to the nearest ED.
         iv. Call the National Suicide Prevention Lifeline 1-800-273-8255.
      b. Create a support environment for patient.
      c. Substance Abuse and Mental Health Services Administration www.samhsa.gov
D. *Documentation*
   1. Thorough understanding of discharge instructions to include risk factors, close follow-up, and signs/symptoms to return immediately to the ED

Psychosis and Schizophrenia

Psychosis is defined as a fundamental derangement of the mind characterized by defective or lost contact with reality. Psychotic disorders include abnormalities in one or more of the five domains: Delusions; hallucinations; disorganized thinking; disorganized or abnormal motor behavior; and negative symptoms.

Schizophrenia is the most common type of psychosis. Schizophrenia patients have high rates of concomitant substance abuse and other medical comorbidities. Psychotic symptoms can increase patients' risk of harming themselves or others or being unable to meet their basic needs. Diagnostic criteria consist of two or more of the following symptoms and at least one must be disorganized speech or delusions:

A. Delusions (bipolar disorder, depression, and schizoaffective disorder ruled out)
B. Disorganized speech (significant impact to work, interpersonal relations, self-care)
C. Grossly disorganized or catatonic behavior
D. Hallucinations (at least 6 months)
E. Negative symptoms (not attributed to substance use or another medical condition)

Pathophysiology

Onset of schizophrenia is usually between the late teens and mid-30s and is preceded by a prodromal phase. Genetic and environmental predisposing factors contribute to schizophrenia. The dominate cause of schizophrenia is thought to be an excessive amount of dopamine along with environmental and genetic disorders leading to schizophrenia. Other neurotransmitters, such as adenosine and glutamate, may also contribute to schizophrenia.

Prevalence

Schizophrenia affects approximately 2.4 million adults in the United States and is considered the leading cause of chronic incapacity. The male-to-female ratio is 4:1. The incidence of schizophrenia is higher in certain minority ethnic groups and urban areas. The prevalence of schizophrenia is 0.5% to 1% worldwide. It is estimated that 13% to 23% of people experience psychotic symptoms at some point in their lifetime, and 1% to 4% percent will meet criteria for a psychotic disorder.

Physical Examination

A. *Chief complaint:* Hallucinations, delusions, agitation, aggression, disorganized thinking
B. *Signs and symptoms*
   1. Positive symptoms
      a. Hallucinations
      b. Delusions
      c. Thought disorders
      d. Movement disorders
   2. Negative symptoms
      a. Flat affect
      b. Reduced feelings of pleasure
      c. Difficulty beginning and sustaining activities
      d. Reduced speaking
   3. Cognitive symptoms
      a. Poor functioning
      b. Trouble focusing or paying attention
      c. Problems with working memory
   4. Agitation
   5. Combinative
   6. Thought disorganization
   7. Uncooperative
   8. Violent
C. *Focused assessment*
   1. Timeline of symptoms
   2. Psychiatric history, prior diagnosis, prior treatment
   3. Substance use history
   4. Family history for psychiatric history
   5. Medical history
   6. Medication history
   7. *Mental status examination:* Grooming, hygiene, general behaviors, mood, affect, thought processes, attention, memory function
   8. Screening with FIND ME (functional [psychiatric], infectious, neurologic, drugs, metabolic, endocrine)

Differential Diagnoses

A. Schizophrenia
B. Schizoaffective disorder
C. Substance-induced psychoses
D. Meningitis
E. Alzheimer's disease
F. Hypoglycemia
G. Hepatic encephalopathy

Diagnostic Testing

A. Complete blood count (CBC) with differential
B. Serum chemistries, Hepatic function panel
C. Thyroid function tests
D. Serum screen for syphilis
E. Serum and urine toxicology screen
F. Serum levels for measurable psychiatric medications (lithium, phenytoin, valproic acid)
G. Urinalysis and urine pregnancy
H. Vitamin B12 levels
I. EKG

Management

A. *Procedures/management*

1. The safety of the patient and ED staff is the principal concerns.

a. Ensure safety for patient and prevent self-harm by having them change into a gown and remove possible weapons, clothing (belts, shoelaces), or medications that can inflict harm.

b. Clear room of any potentially harmful objects.

c. Close monitoring and observation by trained patient specialists, sitter, or facility security

2. Evaluate for risk factors for violence.

3. Employ de-escalation techniques.

4. Medication to control agitation or sedation, monitor with continuous pulse oximetry, end title CO_2, cardiac monitoring

5. Physical restraints, protocol for monitoring, provider orders, reassessment

B. Pharmacologic therapies should be based on evidence-based recommendations from recognized sources, for example, the Centers for Disease Control and Prevention(CDC), or guidelines specific to the environment where the clinician practices."

1. Management for acute agitation or violent patient

a. Combination 5-2-1 pharmacologic treatment

i. Haloperidol intramuscularly (IM) once (atypical antipsychotic adverse effects such as acute dystonic reactions, anticholinergic effects, cardiovascular effects, and neuroleptic malignant syndrome)

ii. Lorazepam IM once

iii. Benztropine IM once

2. Single pharmacologic treatment

i. Ziprasidone IM once, consider lower dose in elderly patients. Typical antipsychotic medications tend to be sedative or are associated with extrapyramidal effects. Federal Drug Administration (FDA) black box warnings due to cardiac dysrhythmias such as QTc prolongation and/or torsade's de pointes.

ii. Lorazepam IV or IM. May give doses as frequently as every 10 minutes for severely agitated patients, standard suggested dose interval 30 minutes

iii. Midazolam IV or IM. In severely agitated patients, doses may be given every 3 to 5 minutes.

iv. Haloperidol IM. The onset of action is within 30 to 60 minutes. The dose should be decreased by one half in the elderly. May give repeat doses as frequently as every 15 to 20 minutes in patients with severe agitation until the desired level of sedation is achieved, but suggested doses may be repeated every 30 minutes

v. Droperidol IM onset of action ranges from 15 to 30 minutes, with a duration of 6 to 8 hours

vi. Ketamine IM onset of action 3 minutes, single dose for initial control of severe agitation

3. If long-term pharmacotherapy is indicated, it should be initiated by a psychiatric/mental health clinician or primary care clinician

C. Consultation/collaboration

a. Emergent psychiatric evaluation if patient is at risk of self-harm, violent, or unable to care for themselves

b. Psychiatric/mental health consultation in the ED for new-onset psychosis or worsening of existing psychotic symptoms

c. Consult probate judge concerning involuntary hospitalization.

Patient Disposition

A. *Transition of care*

1. Admit to inpatient psychiatric care if patient is medically stable and at risk for self-harm, violent behaviors, or unable to care for themselves

2. If medically stable, transfer to a psychiatric facility.

3. Outpatient management and follow-up with psychiatric services based on patient's functional level, safety, and recommendations from psychiatric services

B. *Age and developmental considerations*

1. Patient and family education and counseling

a. Safety education, signs and symptoms to seek emergent care

b. Treatment options, medications, mental health services

c. Family support and social support groups

C. *Documentation*

1. Supporting documentation

a. Use of restraint charting according to facility guidelines, timed provider orders, nursing flow sheet, patient reevaluation

b. Involuntary hospitalization requires certification and legal justification

c. Documentation should reflect decision making process, risk level, risk of imminent self-harm, social support, follow-up plan if patient is to be discharged.

Somatoform Disorder, Factitious Disorder, Malingering

Somatic symptom disorder (SSD) patients present with a variety of physical (somatic) symptoms in the absence of any detectable physical disease. Factitious disorders consist of intentionally produced or feigned signs or symptoms in the absence of any apparent external incentives. There are two types of factitious disorders: factitious disorders imposed on self (FDIS) and factitious disorder imposed on another (FDIA). Munchausen syndrome is the most common FDIS. Malingering is often associated with antisocial personality disorder. Characteristics of malingering may consist of antisocial behavior, poor cooperation during evaluation, vagueness about previous hospitalizations or treatments, or discrepancies between claimed disability and objective findings.

Pathophysiology

The pathophysiology is not well understood for SSD, factitious disorder, and malingering. Several genetic and biologic factors contribute to symptoms as well as previous traumatic experiences and cultural/social norms.

Prevalence

The prevalence of SSD, factitious disorders, and malingering is unclear. Risk factors based on previous studies include females, lower socioeconomic status, history of childhood chronic illness or sexual abuse, family history of chronic illnesses, fewer years of education, or concurrent psychiatric disorders.

Physical Examination

A. *Chief complaint:* Pain, fatigue, syncope, chest pain, shortness of breath
B. *Signs and symptoms*
  1. Abdominal pain
  2. Arthralgia
  3. Chest pain
  4. Hematuria
  5. Seizures
  6. Weakness
C. *Focused assessment*
  1. Thorough general medical and psychiatric history
  2. History of past and present illnesses
  3. Family and social history
  4. Physical and mental status exam
  5. Analysis of medical records
  6. Information from family and friends

Differential Diagnoses

A. Major depressive disorder
B. Anxiety disorder
C. Personality disorder
D. Malingering
E. Substance abuse disorder
F. Thyroid disease
G. Systemic lupus erythematosus
H. Multiple sclerosis

Diagnostic Testing

A. CBC with differential
B. Serum chemistries, thyroid function
C. Serum and urine toxicology screen
D. Urine and urine pregnancy
E. EKG

Management

A. *Procedures/management*
  1. Establish rapport; maintain a nonjudgmental, caring attitude.
  2. Review of previous medical records
  3. Review of previous diagnostic tests
  4. Interview family members
B. *Pharmacologic therapies*
  1. None unless an underlying medical condition
C. *Consultation and collaboration*
  1. Psychiatric/mental health clinician
  2. Primary care clinician

Patient Disposition

A. *Transition of care information*
  1. Outpatient referral to psychiatric/mental health clinician, primary care clinician
  2. Avoid hospitalization or referral to medical specialist if possible.
B. *Age and developmental considerations*
  1. Patient and family education and counseling
    a. Educate patient and reassure patient no acute life-threatening diagnosis exists, and further testing and additional medications are not needed at this time.
    b. Follow up with mental health specialist, primary care clinician, or counselor.
C. *Documentation*
  1. Careful, objective documentation of results, conversations with patient, and referral information

Substance Use Disorders

Substance use disorders (SUD) include the unhealthy use of alcohol, illicit drugs, and nonmedical use of prescription drugs. The *Diagnostic and Statistical Manual of Mental Disorders, Fifth Edition,* classifies SUD into categories from mild to severe. The severity is based on the number of criteria present: two to three is considered mild, four to five is moderate, and six or more is severe. The diagnosis requires two or more of the following criteria:

A. Taking substances in larger amounts or longer than originally intended
B. Expressed desire to reduce or failure to reduce despite previous attempts
C. Increased time to obtain, use, or recover from the substance
D. Craving alcohol or other drugs
E. Failure to fulfill major role obligations at home, work, or school
F. Continued use despite social or interpersonal problems

G. Social, occupational, or recreational activities reduced or stopped due to substance use
H. Recurrent use in situations where it is physically hazardous
I. Continued use despite knowledge of having persistent or recurrent physical or psychological problems caused by the substance
J. Tolerance
K. Withdrawal

Pathophysiology

Excessive substance use activates the brain reward system, which is involved in the reinforcement of behaviors and the production of memories. The pharmacological mechanisms by which each class of drugs produces reward are different. The drug typically activates the brain reward system and produces feelings of pleasure, often referred to as a "high." Individuals with lower levels of self-control, which may indicate brain inhibitory mechanism impairments, may be predisposed to develop SUD.

Prevalence

Opioid overdose deaths in the United States have doubled within the last decade. In 2018, there were 67,367 drug overdose deaths with a 10% increase from 2017 to 2018 involving opioids such as fentanyl and other synthetic narcotics, excluding methadone. However, opioid overdose-related events continue to be problematic in the ED setting.

Physical Examination

A. *Chief complaint:* Altered mental status (AMS)
B. *Signs and symptoms*
  1. AMS
  2. Hypertension, tachycardia
  3. Mydriasis
  4. Diaphoresis, track marks from injection drug use, skin abscess
  5. Urinary retention
  6. Seizures, coma
C. *Focused assessment*
  1. Thorough general medical and psychiatric history
  2. History of substance use, previous treatments
    a. Timeline of symptoms
    b. Type, frequency, and amount of substance use
  3. Family and social history
  4. Analysis of medical records
  5. Psychiatric history, prior diagnosis, prior treatment
  6. Medication history, include psychiatric medications
  7. Mental status examination
    a. General behaviors, mood, affect, thought processes, attention, memory function
  8. *Screening tools/questionnaires to identify substance use:* Screening, Brief Intervention, and Referral to Treatment (SBIRT), Single Screening Questions, or alcohol screening CAGE questionnaire (see https://www.mdcalc.com/cage-questions-alcohol-use)
    a. Single screening questions for alcohol and drug use
      i. Do you drink beer, wine, liquor, or distilled spirits? How many times in the past year have you had five or more (for men)/four or more (for women) drinks in a day?
      ii. How many times in the past year have you used an illegal drug or used a prescription medication for nonmedical reasons?

Differential Diagnoses

A. SUD
B. Anxiety disorder
C. Bipolar disorder
D. Depression
E. Posttraumatic stress disorder (PTSD)
F. Hypoglycemia
G. Drug intoxication
H. Intracranial hemorrhage
I. Meningitis

Diagnostic Testing

A. Complete blood count (CBC) with differential
B. Serum chemistries
C. Thyroid function tests
D. Serum and urine toxicology screen
E. Urinalysis and urine pregnancy
F. EKG

Management

A. *Procedures/management*
  1. Medical stabilization
  2. Patient-centered approach
  3. Ensure safety for patient and prevent self-harm by having them change into a gown and remove possible weapons, clothing (belts, shoelaces), or medications that can inflict harm.
  4. Clear room of any potentially harmful objects.
  5. Close monitoring and observation by trained patient specialists, sitter, or facility security
  6. Establish medical clearance.
B. *Pharmacologic therapies*
  1. Follow evidence-based guidelines when prescribing.
  2. Overdose acute treatment
    a. Naloxone, 0.4 to 2 mg every 2 to 3 minutes subcutaneously, intramuscularly, or intravenously; 1 mg each nostril intranasally, 0.8 to 5 mg every 2 to 3 minutes via endotracheal tube (ETT)
  3. Alcohol (ETOH) withdrawal
    a. Uncomplicated—no seizures, no hallucinations, no delirium
      i. Lorazepam, orally or IV every 1 to 2 hours
      ii. Diazepam, orally or IV every 2 to 4 hours
      iii. Chlordiazepoxide, orally
      iv. Ondansetron, IV q8h (vomiting)
    b. Seizures
      i. Lorazepam, IV
    c. Delirium tremens
      i. Lorazepam, IV every 15 minutes PRN
    d. Midazolam, IV hydration with NS 1 L, thiamine IV, and folate IV

4. Opioid withdrawal
   a. Buprenorphine/naloxone, 4 to 8 mg buprenorphine and 2 mg naloxone sublingual (may repeat 1–2 hours later for a maximum 8 mg buprenorphine)
5. If long-term pharmacotherapy is indicated, it should be initiated by a psychiatric/mental health practitioner or primary care provider as an outpatient.

C. *Consultation/collaboration*
   1. ED collaborative team consisting of psychologists, social workers, care managers, nurse specialists, peer alcohol and drug counselors

Patient Disposition

A. *Transition of care information*
   1. Admission if advanced age, medical comorbidities, or no response to ED treatment
   2. Discharge/transfer to detoxification unit.
   3. Discharge to supportive family environment and outpatient program if no suicidal ideation/homicidal ideation (SI/HI), no trauma, or no major medical comorbidities.

B. *Age and developmental considerations*
   1. Patient and family education and counseling
      a. Refer to community resources such as social services, counseling services, mental health professionals with close follow-up.
      b. Provide list of detoxification or treatment resources in the community and substance abuse organizations such as Alcoholics and Narcotics Anonymous.

C. *Documentation*
   1. Documentation should reflect decision-making process, risk level, risk of imminent self-harm, patient safety, education, social support, and follow-up plan.

Suicide

Suicide is defined as death caused by self-directed injurious behavior with intent to die as a result of the behavior. A suicide attempt is a nonfatal, self-directed, potentially injurious behavior with intent to die as a result of the behavior. Suicidal ideation refers to thinking about, considering, or planning suicide. Many suicide attempts occur during an acute crisis, such as the exacerbation of an underlying psychiatric disorder or personal loss.

Pathophysiology

Suicide is a complex mix of genetic, psychological, and social factors. While the mechanism is not clearly understood, research suggests suicide and depression involve serotonergic systems in the form of low serotonin levels or altered serotonin receptor function. Other potential mechanisms include low serum and cerebrospinal fluid levels of brain-derived neurotrophic factor, excessive noradrenergic neurotransmission, and hyperactivity of the hypothalamic pituitary.

Prevalence

Suicide is the tenth leading cause of death in the United States. In 2017, 47,173 Americans died by suicide, and there were an estimated 1.4 million suicide attempts. In 2017, men died by suicide 3.5 times more than women. In 2017, White males accounted for 78% of suicide deaths. The rate of suicide is highest in middle-aged white males. Adults between 45 and 54 years of age had a suicide rate of 20.2%. The second highest rate was in those 85 years or older (20.1%), followed by adolescents and young adults aged 15 to 24 (14.5%). In 2017, 50.6% of all suicide deaths were caused by firearms. The highest rates by ethnicity in 2017 were 15.9% Whites, 13.4% American Indians and Alaska Natives, and 6.6% among Black or African Americans. Risk factors include males, adolescence, older adults, sexual orientation (LGBT), alcohol or substance abuse, prior suicide attempts, family history, mental disorders, chronic illnesses, recent job or financial loss, and lack of social support.

Physical Examination

A. *Chief complaint:* Suicidal thoughts or behaviors

B. *Signs and symptoms*
   1. Unintentional overdose
   2. Accidental injuries
      a. Gunshot wounds
      b. Automobile crashes
      c. Lacerated wrists
      d. Falls from heights
   3. Thoughts of harming oneself with or without a plan

C. *Focused assessment*
   1. Screening for "red flag" risk factors for suicide, risk assessment using the Columbia-Suicide Severity Rating Scale or the Decision Support Tool
   2. Comprehensive suicide risk assessment using Suicide Assessment Five-step Evaluation and Triage (SAFE-T) tool card available at http://www.sprc.ord (see Table 23.3)
   3. Past history
      a. Any suicidal thoughts, plans, or behaviors
      b. Any prior medical and psychiatric conditions
      c. Any inpatient or outpatient treatment
      d. Current medications, drug, or alcohol use
      e. Concomitant medical illnesses
   4. Thorough physical exam to examine evidence for drug ingestion, trauma, medical illness, or evidence of self-harm behavior

Differential Diagnoses

A. Suicidal ideation
B. Suicidal behavior
C. Suicide attempt
D. Self-directed violence
E. Major depressive disorder
F. SUD

Diagnostic Testing

A. CBC and differential, blood glucose

TABLE 23.3 SAFE-T SUICIDE ASSESSMENT FIVE-STEP EVALUATION AND TRIAGE

1 Identify risk factors	Previous history or attempts Current/past psychiatric disorders Key symptoms: anhedonia, impulsivity, anxiety/panic Family history Precipitants/stressors/interpersonal: loss in the form of relationships, job, financial, chronic illness, intoxication, history of abuse Change in treatment Access to firearms
2 Identify protective factors	Internal: ability to cope with stress, religious beliefs External: responsibility to family, children, pets, social support
3 Conduct suicide inquiry	Ideation: frequency, duration (last 48 hours), intensity Plan: timing, location, availability Behaviors: past attempts, non-suicidal self-injurious actions Intent: extent to carry out plan
4 Determine risk level/intervention	Determine risk based on clinical judgment, after completing steps 1–3 Risk level: high, moderate, low
5 Document	Document: risk level, rationale, treatment plan to address/reduce risk, firearm instructions, interventions, and follow-up

B. Serum chemistries with liver function tests, ammonia, thyroid-stimulating hormone (TSH)
C. Coagulation studies
D. Urinalysis and pregnancy test in females of childbearing age
E. Serum and urine toxicology screening
F. Serum testing for potential toxic ingestion and ethanol level
G. Serum levels for measurable psychiatric medications (lithium, phenytoin, valproic acid)
H. EKG
I. Chest x-ray (CXR)
J. CT scan of the head (patients with altered mental state [AMS])

Management

A. *Procedures/management*
  1. Medical stabilization
  2. Patient-centered approach
  3. Ensure safety for patient and prevent self-harm by having them change into a gown and remove possible weapons, clothing (belts, shoelaces), or medications that can inflict harm.
  4. Clear room of any potentially harmful objects.
  5. Close monitoring and observation by trained patient specialists, sitter, or facility security
B. *Pharmacologic therapies*
  1. Follow evidence-based guidelines when prescribing.
  2. Therapy is directed at reducing agitation as needed with benzodiazepine or short-acting antipsychotic such as haloperidol or olanzapine.
  3. Intoxicated with CNS depressant (e.g., alcohol [ETOH])
    a. Haloperidol, intramuscularly/intravenously (IM/IV) once
    b. Droperidol, IM/IV once
    c. Haloperidol, IM/IV with Lorazepam IM/IV once
    d. Ziprasidone, IM once
    e. Olanzapine, IM once
  4. Cooperative by agitated patient
    a. Lorazepam, orally once
    b. Risperidone, orally once
    c. Olanzapine, orally once
  5. If long-term pharmacotherapy is indicated, it should be initiated by a psychiatric/mental health clinician or primary care clinician.
C. *Consultation/collaboration*
  1. Emergent evaluation by a psychiatric/mental health clinician
  2. Legal consultation, local probate judge for involuntary commitment

Patient Disposition

A. *Transition of care information*
  1. Inpatient hospitalization to stabilize medical condition
  2. Voluntary/involuntary hospitalization (voluntary preferred)
  3. Transfer to psychiatric facility.
  4. Outpatient management if risk of subsequent suicide is determined to be low, and support system is available with close follow-up with mental health specialist
B. *Age and developmental considerations*
  1. Screening for children and adolescents use HEADS-ED (home, education, activities, drugs and alcohol, suicidality, emotions and behaviors, discharge resources), ASQ (Ask Suicide-Screening Questionnaire), *Diagnostic and Statistical Manual of Mental Disorders*, Fourth Edition (*DSM-IV*) two-item screener for alcohol use disorder is adolescents
C. *Patient and family education and counseling*
  1. Education for suicide prevention including verbal and written information
  2. List of warning signs, risk factors, and follow-up instructions
  3. List of coping strategies

4. National Suicide Prevention Hotline number (1800-273-TALK [8255])
5. Secure or remove guns at home.

D. *Documentation*

1. Supporting documentation
   a. Use of restraint charting according to facility guidelines, timed provider orders, nursing flow sheet, reevaluations
   b. Involuntary hospitalization requires certification and legal justification.
   c. Documentation should reflect decision-making process, risk level, risk of imminent self-harm, social support, follow-up plan if patient is to be discharged.

Additional Reading

Additional Reading for this chapter are online only and can be found at https://connect.springerpub.com/content/reference-book/978-0-8261-6091-5/part/part02/toc-part/ch23.

III. Shock and Trauma

24. Shock: Cardiogenic, Hypovolemic, Neurogenic, Septic, Toxic

EDYTA PEDLOWSKA

Learning Objectives

- Define shock and general concepts associated with shock states, including physiologic response to shock and shock progression.
- Perform an assessment for a patient who might be experiencing signs of shock.
- Discuss initial diagnostic testing and management of the patient experiencing shock.
- Describe the septic type of distributive shock, including pathophysiology, clinical manifestations, diagnosis, and management.
- Discuss cardiogenic shock, including pathophysiology, clinical manifestations, diagnosis, and management.
- Explain nonseptic type of distributive shock such as toxic and neurogenic shock, including pathophysiology, clinical manifestations, diagnosis, and management.
- Describe hypovolemic shock, including pathophysiology, clinical manifestations, diagnosis, and management.
- Discuss the use of pharmacotherapy in the management of shock states.

General Approach to the Patient With Shock

It has been estimated that in the United States, each year more than 1 million cases of shock are seen in the ED.[1] The mortality from shock can range from 10% to 87% and is based on the type of shock, patient age, and comorbidities.[2] Prevention, awareness, early recognition, and compliance with evidence-based protocols lead to optimizing treatments, which then improve patient's outcomes.[3]

Shock is defined as circulatory system failure that is caused by insufficient cellular oxygen delivery, consumption, and utilization.[4] It is important to understand the physiology of tissue oxygenation in order to properly identify and treat shock.[1]

Most commonly, patients in shock will have decreased cardiac output and/or systemic vascular resistance; however, it is important to know that in early stage of shock and different forms of shock those values may be normal. Shock's initially reversible cellular oxygen imbalance can lead to irreversible multiorgan dysfunction or failure when not recognized and treated appropriately.[4]

Pathophysiology

A. Changes in systemic blood pressure (BP), cardiac output, and systemic vascular resistance can affect tissue perfusion, and thus can result in shock.[1]
B. BP is determined by cardiac output and systemic vascular resistance, where cardiac output is a product of heart rate and stroke volume.
C. Stroke volume is affected by preload, afterload, and myocardial contractility.[1] The mean arterial pressure is measured with cardiac output and systemic vascular resistance, and it is an important factor because when mean arterial pressure (MAP) decreases, so does the oxygen delivery to the tissues.[1]

Physical Examination

A. Temperature may be decreased or elevated.
B. Heart rate
  1. Commonly elevated, due to cardiac disease, beta-blocker use, or hypoglycemia
  2. Paradoxical bradycardia may be observed

C. Systolic blood pressure (SBP)
  1. Increased in early shock
  2. Decreases as the shock progresses

D. Diastolic blood pressure (DBP)
  1. Increased in early shock
  2. Decreases as the shock progresses

E. Pulse pressure
  1. Increased in early shock stage
  2. Decreases as the shock advances

F. MAP is commonly low (<65 mmHg).
G. *Central nervous system:* Altered mental status, delirium, restless, coma due to low cerebral perfusion
H. *Skin:* Pale, dusky, mottled, cyanosis, increased capillary refill >3 seconds
I. *Cardiovascular:* Jugular vein distention or flattening, tachycardias, arrhythmias, and pulmonary congestion
J. *Respiratory:* Tachypnea, increased minute ventilation, hypo- or hypercapnia
K. *Splanchnic organs:* Ileus, gastrointestinal bleed, pancreatitis, acalculous cholecystitis, mesenteric ischemia
L. *Renal:* Decreased glomerular filtration rate, oliguria
M. *Metabolic:* Hypoglycemia, hyperglycemia, hyperkalemia, metabolic acidosis[1]

Differential Diagnoses

A. Diagnosing a state of shock can be made by analyzing clinical, biochemical, and hemodynamic features.[4]
B. Obtaining patient's medical history can expedite the process of determining the cause of shock.

Diagnostic Testing

A. *Labs, including:* complete blood count (CBC) with differential, comprehensive metabolic panel (CMP), glucose, calcium, magnesium, phosphorus, blood urea nitrogen (BUN), creatinine, serum lactate, partial thromboplastin time (PTT), international normalized ratio (INR), arterial blood gases (ABG), liver function test (LFT), blood cultures, urinalysis, urine cultures, wound cultures, pregnancy test, and cortisol level.[1]
B. EKG, chest radiograph, CT of chest, abdomen, pelvis, and bedside ultrasound[1]

Management

A. Establishing airway (intubation, positive pressure ventilation)
B. Controlling the work of breathing (mechanical ventilation and sedation)
C. Optimizing circulation (fluid resuscitation with isotonic crystalloids, vasopressors)
D. Assuring adequate oxygen delivery (controlling oxygen consumption by providing analgesia, muscle relaxation, warm covering, anxiolytics)
E. Achieving end point resuscitations (stable blood pressure, heart rate, urine output, MAP >65 mmHg)[1]

Types of Shock

Shock can be differentiated into four categories: distributive, cardiogenic, hypovolemic, and obstructive.[5]

Distributive

A. Septic
 1. Gram-positive, Gram-negative, fungal, viral, parasitic, mycobacterium
B. Nonseptic
 2. Inflammatory shock, neurogenic shock, anaphylactic shock, toxic shock

Cardiogenic

A. Cardiomyopathic
 1. Myocardial infarction (involving >40% of the left ventricle or with extensive ischemia), severe right ventricle infarction, acute exacerbation of severe heart failure from dilated cardiomyopathy, stunned myocardium from prolonged ischemia (e.g., cardiac arrest, hypotension, cardiopulmonary bypass), advanced septic shock, myocarditis, myocardial contusion, drug-induced (e.g., beta-blockers).
B. Arrhythmogenic
 1. Tachyarrhythmia, bradyarrhythmia
C. Mechanical
 1. Valvular insufficiency, acute valvular rupture (papillary or chordae tendineae rupture, valvular abscess), critical valvular stenosis, acute or severe ventricular septal wall defect, ruptured ventricular wall aneurysm, atrial myxoma.[5]

Hypovolemic[6]

A. Hemorrhagic
 1. Trauma, gastrointestinal bleeding (e.g., varices, peptic ulcer), intraoperative and postoperative bleeding, retroperitoneal bleeding (e.g., ruptured aortic aneurysm), aortic-enteric fistula, hemorrhagic pancreatitis, iatrogenic (e.g., inadvertent biopsy of arteriovenous malformation, or left ventricle), tumor or abscess erosion into major vessels, ruptured ectopic pregnancy, postpartum hemorrhage, uterine or vaginal hemorrhage (e.g., infection, tumors, lacerations), spontaneous peritoneal hemorrhage from bleeding diathesis.[5]
A. Nonhemorrhagic
 1. Gastrointestinal losses (e.g., diarrhea, vomiting, external drainage)
 2. Skin losses (e.g., heat stroke, burns, dermatologic conditions)
 3. Renal losses (e.g., excessive drug-induced or osmotic diuresis, salt-wasting nephropathies, hypoaldosteronism)
 4. Third space losses into the extravascular space or body cavities (e.g., postoperative and trauma, intestinal obstruction, crush injury, pancreatitis, cirrhosis).[5]

Obstructive

A. Pulmonary vascular
 1. Hemodynamically significant pulmonary embolus, severe pulmonary hypertension, severe or acute obstruction of the pulmonic or tricuspid valve, venous air embolus
B. Mechanical
 1. Tension pneumothorax or hemothorax (e.g., trauma, iatrogenic), pericardial tamponade, constrictive pericarditis, restrictive cardiomyopathy, severe dynamic hyperinflation (e.g., elevated intrinsic positive end-expiratory pressure [PEEP]), left or right ventricular outflow tract obstruction, abdominal compartment syndrome, aortocaval compression (e.g., positioning, surgical retraction).[5]

This chapter focuses on septic shock, nonseptic such as neurogenic and toxic shock, cardiogenic, and hypovolemic shock.

Septic Shock

Sepsis

Before discussing septic shock, it is important to understand sepsis. According to the Centers for Disease Control and Prevention (CDC) in the United States more than 1.5 million of people get sepsis each year, and approximately 250,000 die from sepsis each year.[7]

The Third International Consensus Definitions for Sepsis and Septic Shock defines sepsis as a life-threatening organ dysfunction caused by a dysregulated host response to infection.[8] In sepsis, there is a simultaneous activation of inflammation and coagulation in response to a pathogen, with mortality rates of 20%.[9] Patients with sepsis who are more likely to have poor outcomes, and can be rapidly identified by using quick Sequential Organ Failure Assessment (qSOFA).[8] The qSOFA criteria include altered mental status, respiratory rate ≥22, and systolic blood pressure (SBP) ≤100 mmHg, with a score ≥2 indicating a poor outcome.[8]

"Septic shock is defined as a subset of sepsis in which underlying circulatory, cellular, and metabolic abnormalities are associated with a greater risk of mortality than sepsis alone."[10]

Septic shock mortality ranges between 60% and 80%.[9]

Due to quality measures, the Centers for Medicare & Medicaid Services (CMS) continue to define sepsis as:

- *Sepsis:* Two systemic inflammatory response syndrome (SIRS) criteria plus suspected infection
- *Severe sepsis:* Above plus lactate >2 or organ dysfunction
- *Septic shock:* Severe sepsis with hypoperfusion despite adequate fluid resuscitation or lactate >4[11]

SIRS criteria are defined as: tachycardia (heart rate >90 beats/min), tachypnea (respiratory rate >20 breaths/min), fever or hypothermia (temperature >38 or <36°C), and leukocytosis, leukopenia, (white blood cells >12 x 10^9/L or <4 x 10^9/L).[8]

Since 2015, the CMS has been enforcing the Surviving Sepsis Campaign sepsis bundle measure, which requires that within 3 hours of recognition of sepsis lactate measurement, blood cultures, antibiotic therapy, and fluid therapy 30 mL/kg is started, with reassessment at 3 to 6 hours at that time repeating a lactate and reassessing the need for additional fluid therapy.[11,12]

In 2018, the Surviving Sepsis Campaign bundle was revised, and the 3-hour and 6-hour bundles were merged into a single "hour-1 bundle" in order to begin the resuscitation and management of sepsis immediately.[3] This new bundle requires obtaining blood for serum lactate levels and blood cultures, administration of antibiotics and fluids and initiation of vasopressors if hypotension continues within the first hour of identifying sepsis.[3]

Although serum lactate does not specifically measure tissue perfusion, increase in levels has been associated with tissue hypoxia and poor outcomes; therefore, resuscitation should be guided by normalizing lactate levels and remeasuring the levels in 2 to 4 hours if initial level was >2 mmol/L.[3]

Obtaining blood cultures preferably two sets aerobic and anaerobic to identify the pathogen prior to initiation of antimicrobial therapy should be performed; however, it should not delay the administration of antibiotics.[3] Empiric, broad-spectrum antibiotics should be started and narrowed once the pathogen of the infection is identified.[3]

IV fluid resuscitation with at least 30 mL/kg crystalloid fluid should be administered immediately upon recognition of sepsis, and/or hypotension and elevated lactate levels.[3,12] Administration of fluids beyond the initial resuscitation should be carefully assessed because fluid overload has been associated with poor outcomes.[3]

When initial fluid resuscitation fails to increase blood pressure, vasopressors should be initiated within the first hour to achieve mean arterial pressure (MAP) ≥65 mmHg and adequately perfuse vital.[3]

Sepsis source can be from bacteria, viruses, fungi, or parasites.[9] The causative pathogen varies based on the anatomical site of infection; however, according to CDC,[7] the most common sources include lungs, kidneys, skin, gut, and the most common pathogens are *Staphylococcus aureus*, *Escherichia coli*, and some types of *Streptococcus*.

Predisposing Factors

A. Risk factors for sepsis include advanced age, ICU admission, bacteremia, immunosuppression, diabetes, cancer, community-acquired pneumonia, and previous hospitalizations.[11]

Medical Screening

A. Signs and symptoms
  1. Specific to the infectious source
  2. Most common clinical features of sepsis include fever, hypotension, tachycardia.[11]
  3. As sepsis progresses and end-organ dysfunction develops, cool skin and cyanosis may be seen with decreased capillary refill, skin mottling, oliguria, anuria, acute kidney injury, altered mental status, and restlessness.[13]

Diagnostic Testing

A. Laboratory findings[11]
  1. Complete blood count (CBC)
  2. Serum electrolytes
  3. Renal function panel
  4. Lactic acid panel
  5. Liver function panel
  6. Urinalysis, urine culture, blood cultures
  7. Arterial blood gas
  8. Type and screen
  9. Prothrombin time
  10. Activated partial thromboplastin
  11. Fibrinogen
  12. D-dimer

B. Imaging
  1. During early investigation of the source of sepsis, obtaining chest radiograph, abdominal radiograph, CT scan, and ultrasound must be considered.[11]

C. Septic shock should be recognized when:
  1. Septic patient continues to be hypotensive.
  2. Requires vasopressors to maintain MAP ≥65 mmHg
  3. Persists having a serum lactate level >2 mmol/L despite volume resuscitation[8]

Management

A. The treatment of sepsis and septic shock starts with recognizing its presence, early reversal of hemodynamic abnormalities, and controlling the infection.[11]

B. Improving tissue perfusion, preload, and cellular oxygenation are the goals of the resuscitation.[11]

C. Start with volume resuscitation and administer 30 mL/kg crystalloid fluid bolus within the first hour and reassess patient's responsiveness by observing increase in SBP ≥90 mmHg, MAP ≥65 mmHg, peripheral pulses, decrease in heart rate and increase in urinary output ≥0.5 mL/kg/hour.
  1. If blood pressure does not respond to the initial fluid bolus do not delay starting vasoactive agents in order to provide adequate perfusion pressure.[11]

2. The vasopressor of choice in septic shock is norepinephrine due to its vasoconstrictive effects with minimal change in heart rate.[12]

a. Vasopressin (up to 0.03 units per minute) may be used when additional agent is needed to raise MAP or to decrease norepinephrine dosage.[12]

b. Epinephrine can be also used in addition to norepinephrine or when norepinephrine is contraindicated

i. Increases aerobic lactate production and increases heart rate.[12]

c. Phenylephrine has been associated with possible splanchnic vasoconstriction; therefore, the use should be limited until more research is available.[12]

d. Dopamine should not be routinely used in management of septic shock due to potential arrhythmogenic effects, the surviving sepsis campaign suggests the use of dopamine only in selected patients such as patients with low risk of tachyarrhythmias and absolute or relative bradycardia.[12]

e. All vasoactive agents should be infused though central line to prevent local tissue necrosis.

i. If central access is unavailable, vasopressors can be administered slowly and at low concentrations through a large-bore intravenous catheter with continuous monitoring.[14]

ii. If extravasation occurs, infusion should be stooped, and proper extravasation protocol should be followed, including infiltration with an antidote such as phentolamine.[14]

D. Treating the sources of infection with broad-spectrum antibiotics should be initiated ideally within the first hour of identifying sepsis.

1. The coverage should be directed against Gram-positive, Gram-negative, and (if suspected) against fungi.[14]

Patient Disposition

A. Transition of care

1. Patients in sepsis and septic shock should be transferred to the ICU as soon and stabilized for further care.[1]

2. Documentation

3. Resuscitative efforts in the ED should be documented and clearly communicated to the critical care team for best continuity of care.[1] Although morbidity and mortality of patients in septic shock remain high, adherence to evidence-based protocols may improve the prognosis.[15]

Cardiogenic Shock

Cardiogenic shock is defined as systemic hypotension and hypoperfusion due to decreased cardiac output, resulting in inadequate tissue perfusion despite sufficient volume status.[15] Cardiogenic shock is the leading cause of death in patients with acute myocardial infarction (AMI), and it is more prevalent in patients with ST-segment elevation myocardial infarction (STEMI) than non-ST-segment elevation myocardial infarction (NSTEMI).[15] It has been estimated that approximately 10% of patients with AMI who will suffer from cardiogenic shock will have it upon arrival to ED, with time of onset after presentation of approximately 6 hours.[15] Mortality rates exceed 50%, and half of those deaths happen within the first 48 hours upon arrival.[15]

Most commonly, cardiogenic shock is caused by mechanical complications (e.g., left ventricular free wall rupture, ventricular septal defect, acute mitral regurgitation due to chordal rupture or papillary muscle dysfunction, right ventricular infarction, aortic dissection), depression of cardiac contractility (MI, sepsis, myocarditis, cardiomyopathy, medication toxicity, dysrhythmia), or mechanical blood flow obstruction (aortic stenosis, hypertrophic cardiomyopathy, mitral stenosis, left atrial myxoma, pericardial tamponade).[15]

Pathophysiology

When significant myocardial insult occurs, cardiac output will decrease, blood pressure (BP) will drop, organ hypoperfusion takes place, and catecholamine release, thus resulting in increased myocardial oxygen demand and decreased myocardial blood supply that can lead to rapid deterioration.[16] Cardiogenic shock is a serious syndrome that requires urgent diagnosis and adequate treatment. It is important to obtain patient's medical history upon presentation to the ED.

Predisposing Factors

A. Risk factors include:[15]

1. Advanced age
2. Female
3. History of diabetes
4. History of congestive heart failure
5. Previous MIs, coronary artery disease (CAD), or prior ischemic events in a setting of impaired ejection fraction, severe and extensive infarcts.[15]

Medical Screening

A. Patient may complain of chest pain, shortness of breath, and/or weakness.[15]

B. Clinical features of cardiogenic shock include[17]:

1. Hypotension
2. Tachycardia
3. Tachypnea
4. Jugular venous pressure (JVP)
5. Rales
6. Heart murmur and gallops
7. Cool extremities
8. Peripheral edema
9. Abdominal ascites
10. Hepatomegaly
11. Pulsatile liver
12. Pulsus alternans
13. Orthopnea
14. Restlessness
15. Dullness to percussion in lung bases
16. Parasternal lift

Diagnostic Testing

A. There are no cardiogenic shock-specific laboratory markers.

B. Helpful to obtain the following[15]:

1. Serial troponins
2. Serum lactate

3. Brain natriuretic peptide (BNP)
4. C-reactive protein (CRP)
5. Complete blood count (CBC)
6. Drug levels such as digoxin or illicit drugs
7. Basic metabolic panel (BMP)
8. Arterial blood gases (ABGs)
9. Serum electrolytes
10. Renal and liver panel.[15]

C. Tools that can aid in diagnosis include
1. *EKG:* (ST-segment elevations, elevation of RV leads
2. *Chest radiography:* Pulmonary edema, widened mediastinum indicative of aortic dissection, cardiomegaly, pulmonary congestion
3. *Echocardiography:* Papillary muscle rupture, acute ventricular septal defect, free wall rupture, mitral regurgitation, RV infarction
4. *Right heart catheterization:* Cardiac index <2.2 L/min/m^2 in setting of pulmonary capillary wedge pressure (PCWP) >18 mmHg.[18]

Management

A. Revascularization
1. Percutaneous coronary intervention or coronary artery bypass grafting to restore coronary blood flow to perfuse myocardial tissue.
2. Most important treatment for cardiogenic shock from ischemic insult and should not be delayed.[15]

B. Patients with AMI should receive aspirin if not contraindicated.

C. If hemodynamically permissible, they may receive morphine and nitroglycerin intravenously to relieve chest pain.[15]

D. Patients suffering from cardiogenic shock in ED should be stabilized by obtaining venous access, supplemental oxygen, cardiac monitoring, urine output monitoring, and correcting hypovolemia, hypoxemia, arrhythmias or electrolyte or acid–base abnormalities.[15]

E. Mechanical ventilation may be necessary for a respiratory failure setting, however, it may worsen hypotension.[15]

F. Crystalloid fluid boluses should be given based on clinical findings, and when pulmonary congestion develop vasopressors inotropes should be administered.[15]

G. Routine use of inotropes is not recommended, however, their use in cardiogenic shock has a role in maintaining systemic perfusion and reestablishing end-organ function.[17]

H. Most common inotropic medications used in cardiogenic shock include[15].
1. *Dobutamine:* May give if systolic blood pressure (SBP) ≥90 mmHg
2. *Dopamine:* Causes tachycardia
3. *Norepinephrine:* May use if SBP <70 mmHg also in combination with Dobutamine
4. *Epinephrine:* May cause acidosis and dysrhythmias
5. *Milrinone:* Lowers blood pressure (BP)

I. Fibrinolytic therapy
1. Proven to reduce mortality rates in patients who are in cardiogenic shock secondary to STEMI and are unable to undergo immediate revascularization
2. Least effective treatment modality compared to coronary intervention and intra-aortic balloon pump use.[15]

J. An intra-aortic balloon pump use has been associated with improved outcomes in patient in cardiogenic shock.
1. Increases myocardial oxygen perfusion and increases cardiac output.[17]

K. Percutaneous left ventricular assist devices (LVAD) have been successfully used as a temporary measure while patient is recovering from cardiogenic shock or waiting for a transplant.[15]

L. When all maximum medical treatments fail, extracorporeal membrane oxygenation (ECMO) may be used short term to provide full circulatory support while the patient is recovering from cardiogenic shock interventions or waiting for coronary intervention, LVAD, or transplant.[15]

Patient Disposition

A. Transition of care
1. Patients in cardiogenic shock should be treated in the ICU at a facility that can perform invasive revascularization.
2. Transfer should not be delayed.[15]

Neurogenic Shock

In the United States, there are approximately 17,700 new cases of spinal cord injury each year.[19] Neurogenic shock occurs in less than 20% of patients with spinal cord injury.[20] "Neurogenic shock occurs when the spinal cord is injured and sympathetic innervation to the heart along with vasomotor tone is lost, with prevailing parasympathetic innervation by the intact vagus nerve."[21]

Medical Screening

A. Presents most commonly with the injury to spinal cord above T6

B. Main causes of neurogenic shock are spinal cord trauma, spinal cord neoplasm, or (although rare) spinal/epidural anesthetic.[22]
1. Can occur within minutes to several weeks after the injury[23]

C. Two main clinical features are hypotension and bradycardia.[20]
1. Patients may also have warm, dry skin, and may be tolerating hypotension well due to "presumably normal" peripheral oxygen delivery.[20]
2. Cardiac dysrhythmias; motor and sensory deficits can also be present.[22]

Differential Diagnosis

A. Diagnosis of neurogenic shock starts by excluding other causes for hypotension and bradycardia.[20]

Diagnostic Testing

A. Diagnostic imaging to confirm the injury to the spine is done with plain radiographs, CT scan, and MRI scan.[20]

Management

A. After securing the airway, and ensuring ventilation is adequate, main treatment of neurogenic shock should focus on maintaining adequate perfusion and preventing secondary spinal cord damage.[22] Patients with traumatic causes of neurogenic shock should be immobilized to prevent further damage.[22]

B. Adequate management of neurogenic shock includes crystalloid fluid resuscitation (commonly patients in neurogenic shock are resistant to fluids, carefully administered fluids to prevent overhydration that can cause pulmonary and spinal cord edema).[21]

C. To avoid fluid overload, early use of vasopressors (no specific agent has been shown to be superior to others in this condition) is recommended with target of systolic blood pressure (SBP) ≥90 mmHg and mean arterial pressure (MAP) 85 to 90 mmHg.[20]

D. Atropine may be used when bradycardia persists.[20]

Patient Disposition

A. Transition of care information

1. Upon stabilization in the ED, patients should be treated in the ICU.
2. Follow-up from neurosurgeon

Toxic Shock Syndrome

Toxic shock syndrome (TSS) is a serious condition which, if not recognized and treated adequately, can be fatal, with mortality rates ranging from 30% to 80% in adults and 3% to 10% in children.[24] It has been estimated that every year 1.5 to 11 per 100,000 people were diagnosed with TSS.[24] TSS was found to occur more in the winter and spring months, and in adults aged >45 years, children <5 years.[24] The two most common organisms that are attributed to TSS are *Staphylococcus aureus* and *Streptococcus pyogenes*; other infections include *Streptococcus agalactiae, Streptococcus viridans*, Group C and Group G *Streptococcus*, and *Clostridium*.[24]

TSS occurs when these organisms begin to produce toxins that lead to systemic hemodynamic crisis and multiorgan dysfunction.[25] The immune response to the protein that is released by these organisms causes massive T and B-cell activation, and immense cytokine release that create the severe clinical features of this condition.[24] Staphylococcal TSS was linked to tampon use in 1980, however, after changing the production of tampons and their usage, the rates of menstrual-related Staphylococcus TSS significantly improved.[24] However, the rates of nonmenstrual-related staphylococcal TSS has increased and has been seen in patients postabortion, postsurgical postpartum, postintrauterine device, after burns, and soft tissue injuries.[24] Streptococcal TSS has been associated with higher morbidity and mortality rates than staphylococcal TSS and is seen in postviral infection, pharyngitis, and soft tissue trauma, deep infection sites (necrotizing fasciitis).[24]

Medical Screening

A. Clinical features of TSS are often based on the source of infection.

B. Most commonly, patients will present with fever, hypotension, and rash (initially erythrodermic rash, with skin and mucosal involvement, ulceration may be seen in severe cases) followed by chills, weakness, sore throat, abdominal pain, vomiting, diarrhea, headache, oliguria, peripheral edema, headache, confusion, agitation, pulmonary edema, and pleural effusions.[24]

C. Staphylococcal TSS in young patients presents more with flu-like symptoms, fever, diarrhea, vomiting, headache, sore throat, as well as change in mental status.[24]

D. Streptococcal TSS, 55% of the time will have more focal infection characteristics such as pneumonia, cellulitis, pharyngitis, necrotizing, fasciitis (50% of necrotizing fasciitis cases are by streptococcal organism).[24]

E. Acute respiratory distress syndrome has been seen in up to 45% of patients with invasive streptococcal TSS and hypotension.[24]

Differential Diagnoses

A. The Centers for Disease Control and Prevention (CDC) provides criteria to help differentiate between staphylococcal and streptococcal TSS:

1. Many of these criteria overlap with other illnesses such as septic shock, meningococcemia and develop in end stages of the TSS, making the diagnosis difficult.[24]

B. When four clinical and laboratory criteria are present the diagnosis of staphylococcal TSS is probable; when more than five are present, the diagnosis is confirmed. The criteria include:

1. Fever of >38.9°C or 102.0°F
2. Diffuse macular erythrodermic rash
3. Desquamation 1 to 2 weeks after rash onset
4. Systolic blood pressure (SBP) ≤90 mmHg (adults) or ≤5th percentile by age (<16 years old)
5. Multiorgan involvement (three or more systems):
   a. Gastrointestinal (vomiting/diarrhea)
   b. Muscular (severe myalgias or creatine kinase ≥2 times upper limit of normal)
   c. Mucous membrane involvement, renal (blood urea nitrogen [BUN] or Cr ≥2 times upper limit of normal or urinary sediment with pyuria with no urinary tract infection)
   d. Hepatic (total bilirubin, aspartate aminotransferase (AST) or alanine aminotransferase (ALT) ≥2 times upper limit of normal)
   e. Hematologic (platelets ≤ 100,000/mm^3)
   f. Neurologic (alteration in consciousness without focal neurologic signs when fever and hypotension are absent).
6. Laboratory criteria must be negative for blood or cerebrospinal fluid cultures (blood cultures may be positive for *S. aureus*) and negative for Rocky Mountain spotted fever, leptospirosis, or measles.[24]

C. To make the diagnosis of streptococcal TSS probable according to the CDC,[26] all criteria must be met with no other etiology for the illness and with isolation of group A *Streptococcus* from nonsterile site and to confirm the diagnosis all clinical criteria must be met and isolation of group A *Streptococcus* from sterile field obtained. The criteria include:

1. SBP ≤90 mmHg (adults) or ≤5th percentile by age (<16 years old)
2. Multiorgan involvement (two or more systems)[26]
   a. Gastrointestinal (vomiting/diarrhea)
   b. Muscular (severe myalgias or creatine kinase ≥2 times upper limit of normal)
   c. Mucous membrane involvement, renal (Cr ≥2 mL/dL or Cr >2 times upper limit of normal, >2-fold elevation from patient baseline)
   d. Hepatic (total bilirubin, ALT, AST ≥2 times upper limit of normal)
   e. Hematologic (platelets ≤100,000/mm^3, disseminated intravascular coagulation, or >2-fold elevation from patient baseline)
   f. Acute respiratory distress syndrome
   g. Skin (generalized erythematous macular rash that can desquamate)

h. Soft tissue necrosis (gangrene, myositis, necrotizing fasciitis)

Diagnostic Testing

A. TSS is a clinical diagnosis.
B. Helpful to obtain tests such as complete blood count (CBC), complete metabolic panel (CMP), liver function test (LFT), coagulation studies, creatinine phosphokinase level, blood culture, urinalysis, chest radiographs, EKG.[25]
1. Most common abnormalities seen are anemia, thrombocytopenia, elevated coagulation tests, leukocytosis, electrolyte imbalances (hyponatremia, hypophosphatemia, hypocalcemia, hypoalbuminemia), elevated blood urea nitrogen and creatinine (due to kidney injury), elevated creatinine kinase (rhabdomyolysis), and positive blood cultures (positive in approximately 60% of patients with streptococcal TSS, and 5% in staphylococcal TSS).[24]

Management

A. The initial management of patients in TSS in the ED should be based on treating the shock and source of infection using sepsis protocols.[24]
1. Aggressive fluid resuscitation should be initiated, along with broad-spectrum antibiotics with coverage for *S. aureus* and *S. pyogenes as well as* methicillin-resistant *S. aureus* (MRSA).
a. Vancomycin or Linezolid (should be used as first-line agents), with addition of Clindamycin (superior to other agents when given >2 hours after onset of illness), erythromycin, rifampin, or fluoroquinolones.[24]
B. The source of infection should be identified as soon as possible and treated appropriately (wound should be debrided, tampons, nasal packing removed).[24]
C. IV immune globulin should be given only when all other treatments failed to show improvement within the first 6 hours of treatment.[25]

Patient Disposition

A. Transition of care information:
1. Patients with TSS should be transferred and treated in the ICU
2. Follow-up from the infectious disease clinician

Hypovolemic Shock

Hypovolemic shock occurs when there is insufficient end-organ perfusion secondary to inadequate circulatory blood volume.[27]

Pathophysiology

A. Hypovolemic shock can develop from:
1. *Hemorrhagic conditions:* Trauma, gastrointestinal bleeding (e.g., varices, peptic ulcer)
a. Intraoperative and postoperative bleeding
b. Retroperitoneal bleeding (e.g., ruptured aortic aneurysm)
c. Aortic-enteric fistula
d. Hemorrhagic pancreatitis, iatrogenic (e.g., inadvertent biopsy of arteriovenous malformation, or left ventricle)
e. Tumor or abscess erosion into major vessels
f. Ruptured ectopic pregnancy
g. Postpartum hemorrhage
h. Uterine or vaginal hemorrhage (e.g., infection, tumors, lacerations)
i. Spontaneous peritoneal hemorrhage from bleeding diathesis[5]
2. *Nonhemorrhagic conditions*
a. Gastrointestinal losses (e.g., diarrhea, vomiting, external drainage)
b. Skin losses (e.g., heat stroke, burns, dermatologic conditions)
c. Renal losses (e.g., excessive drug-induced or osmotic diuresis, salt-wasting nephropathies, hypoaldosteronism)
d. Third space losses into the extravascular space or body cavities (e.g., postoperative and trauma, intestinal obstruction, crush injury, pancreatitis, cirrhosis).[5]
B. The mortality of hypovolemic shock is high, with hemorrhagic shock being the highest and ranging from 30% to 40%, with half of deaths occurring during the first 24 hours.[28]
C. When acute blood loss occurs and hypovolemic shock develops, physiologic compensatory mechanisms are activated in attempt to maintain perfusion.[28]
D. Hypovolemic shock triggers coagulation and massive inflammatory response that can lead to organ damage if not corrected.[28]

Medical Screening

A. Clinical features of hypovolemic shock include:[27]
1. Tachycardia
2. Hypotension
3. Narrowed pulse pressure
4. Decreased capillary refill with weak peripheral pulses
5. Cool and pale skin
6. Decreased urine output
7. Dry mucous membranes
8. Altered mental status corrected

Diagnostic Testing

A. In order to properly treat hypovolemic shock, it is important to estimate how much blood volume the patient lost.
B. Based on clinical signs, acute blood loss can be estimated by using hemorrhage classification system (Table 24.1).[6]
C. Imaging
1. Management of hemorrhagic shock focuses on rapid identification of the source of the bleed and replacement of intravascular volume.[29]
2. Diagnostic evaluation may include plain chest and pelvic radiography, echocardiography, ultrasonography, and focused assessment with sonography for trauma (FAST).[29]
3. If the source of the bleed is still uncertain, CT scan may be used once patient has been stabilized.[29]
D. Laboratory tests that are helpful in establishing severity of the shock:
1. Serum lactate
2. Blood gas analysis
3. Complete blood count
4. Complete metabolic panel

TABLE 24.1 ADVANCED TRAUMA LIFE SUPPORT (ATLS) HEMORRHAGE CLASSIFICATION SYSTEM

	CLASS I	CLASS II	CLASS III	CLASS IV
Blood loss in %	<15	15–30	30–40	>40
Pulse rate	<100	100–120	120–140	>140
Blood pressure	Normal	Normal	Decreased	Greatly decreased
Pulse pressure	Normal or increased	Decreased	Decreased	Decreased
Respiratory rate	14–20	20–30	30–40	>35
Mental status	Slightly anxious	Mildly anxious	Anxious, confused	Confused, lethargic
Urine output (mL/hour)	>30	20–30	5–15	Minimal

Source: The ATLS ® classification of hypovolemic shock. Committee on Trauma, American College of Surgeons. Advanced trauma life support for doctors–student course manual. 8th ed. American College of Surgeons, Chicago; 2008, Table 1.[29]

5. Coagulation panels prothrombin time/international normalized ratio (PT/INR), partial thromboplastin time (PTT), and electrolytes.[29]

Management

A. Massive Blood Transfusion Protocol should be activated.[29] In hemorrhagic shock, intravascular volume repletion is best achieved by administration of blood products in a 1:1:1 plasma-to-platelets-to-red cells ratio.
   1. Studies have shown that this ratio reduced short-term mortality in trauma patients with hemorrhagic shock.[29]
   2. Patients who are receiving large amounts of blood products should also receive IV calcium chloride due to blood products containing anticoagulant citrate that can become toxic, cause hypocalcemia, and life-threatening coagulopathy.[29]
   3. Isotonic crystalloids should be used for temporary intravascular volume expansion.[29]
      a. The recommended amount of crystalloids is limited to 3 L within first 6 hours of patient arrival to the ED, due to increased risk of complications such as respiratory failure, compartment syndrome, increased coagulopathy state from fluid overload.[29]

B. Procoagulant agent such as tranexamic acid has been widely used with massive blood transfusion to reduce need for more transfusions and reduce mortality.[29]
   1. Additional agents such as activated recombinant factor VII, prothrombin complex concentrate, and fibrinogen concentrate with patients on anticoagulants or with hemophilia may be considered in select patients.[29]

C. Another agent that has been shown to reduce the blood products transfusion and fluid requirement is vasopressin.[29]

D. Consultation and collaboration
   1. Surgical clinicians should be included in patient's management early in the care.

Patient Disposition

A. Transition of care information
   1. Once stabilized, patients should be transferred to ICU for further care and management.

References

References for this chapter are online only and can be found at https://connect.springerpub.com/content/reference-book/978-0-8261-6091-5/part/part03/toc-part/ch24.

25. Multisystem Trauma

MELINDA K. JOHNSON

Learning Objectives

- List and describe the components and order of the advanced trauma life support (ATLS) primary and secondary survey in the trauma patient.
- Consider how anatomic and physiologic differences in the pediatric, geriatric, and pregnant trauma patient inform injury patterns, response to injury, and outcomes.
- Recognize how the mechanism of injury can lead to specific patterns of injury.
- List differential diagnoses for exam findings in the trauma patient.
- Appropriately disposition the trauma patient, recognizing situations and presentations that require transfer to a higher level of care.

Blast/Concussive/Explosive Injuries—Special Considerations[1, 2, 4, 13, 14]

A. *Primary blast injury*: Supersonic overpressure wave that primarily affects air-filled structures, may have delayed presentation

1. Hollow viscus injuries
   a. *Signs:* Abdominal tenderness, rebound, guarding, sepsis/shock, absence of bowel sounds, bruising of abdominal wall
   b. *Symptoms:* Abdominal pain, nausea and vomiting, hematemesis (rarely), rectal pain, testicular pain
2. Tympanic membrane (TM) rupture
   a. *Signs:* Hemorrhage, effusion, hearing loss, TM rupture, nystagmus
   b. *Symptoms:* Pain, deafness, tinnitus, vertigo
3. Ocular injuries
   a. *Signs:* Lacerations, hyphema, eyelid injury, ecchymosis, open globe, pupillary changes, decreased visual acuity, decreased extraocular movements, embedded objects
   b. *Symptoms:* Blurry or decreased vision, photophobia, eye pain, foreign body sensation, floaters
4. Concussion
   a. *Signs:* Contusions, ecchymosis, open wounds to head
   b. *Symptoms:* Headache, altered mental status, repetitive questioning, neurologic changes
5. Chest/lung injuries
   a. *Signs:* Tachypnea, cyanosis, decreased breath sounds, dullness to percussion, diffuse coarse crackles, subcutaneous emphysema
      i. May be delayed by up to 48 hours
   b. *Symptoms:* Dyspnea, cough, hemoptysis, chest pain

B. *Secondary blast injury:* Flying objects and shrapnel

1. Penetrating injuries

C. *Tertiary blast injury:* Blunt or penetrating impact with surroundings as victim is propelled through the air

1. Fractures
2. Amputations
3. Crush injuries
   a. Compression of extremities or other body parts that causes muscle swelling and/or neurological disturbances of affected areas
   b. Concern for traumatic rhabdomyolysis, reperfusion syndrome, and compartment syndrome
   c. *Signs:* Hypotension, renal failure, metabolic abnormalities, compartment syndrome
4. Hemothorax or pneumothorax

D. *Quaternary blast injury:* —All injuries not classified as primary, secondary, or tertiary

1. Burns
2. Smoke inhalation
3. Chemical agent release
4. Radiation
5. Asphyxia
6. Exacerbations of chronic medical conditions due to the blast or blast effects

E. *Focused assessment* (advanced trauma life support [ATLS] guidelines)

1. Primary survey (ABCDE)
2. Secondary survey—AFTER primary survey completed
   a. *AMPLE history:* **A**llergies, **M**edication, **P**ast medical history, **L**ast oral intake, **E**vents leading to presentation
   b. Mechanism of injury
      i. Distance victim was from explosion
      ii. Enclosed versus open space
      iii. Surrounding environment
      iv. Quantity and type of explosive
      v. Any embedded shrapnel
      vi. Consider primary, secondary, tertiary, and quaternary blast effects
   c. Head-to-toe assessment
      i. Head and maxillofacial

(1) Traumatic brain injury (TBI)
(a) Shrapnel can create easily missed small entry wounds.
(b) Neuroimaging important early diagnostic tool
(2) Ocular injuries
(a) Eye examination needed for all moderately to severely injured blast victims.
(3) Ear
(a) TM rupture
- Check for bleeding or drainage.
- Assess if they are hearing clearly.
- Isolated TM rupture should have chest x-ray (CXR).

(b) Damage to ossicles leading to conductive hearing loss

ii. Cervical spine and neck
(1) Maintain immobilization.
(2) Assess entire spine by log rolling, palpating.

iii. Chest—pulmonary barotrauma
(1) Most common fatal primary blast injury
(2) Pulmonary contusion (hemoptysis)
(3) Pneumothorax
(4) Pulmonary edema
(5) Pneumomediastinum
(6) Air embolism (rare)

iv. Abdomen
(1) Gastrointestinal (GI) injuries less common, but rate increases with proximity to explosive device
(2) Usually from primary blast
(3) Intestinal injury or rupture
(4) Bleeding from liver, spleen, or kidneys
(5) Maybe occult—most common cause of delayed morbidity and mortality

v. Perineum and vagina
(1) Assess for bleeding.
(2) Rectal pain
(3) Testicular pain

vi. Musculoskeletal
(1) Fractures
(2) Amputations
(3) Crush injuries
(4) Compartment syndrome
(5) Do not let distracting injuries lead to missing other injuries.

vii. Neurologic
(1) Mental status (ongoing reassessment)
(2) Assess for pain, paralysis, and paresthesia.
(3) Sensation
(4) Motor function
(5) Deep tendon reflexes

F. *Patient management*

1. Lung injury
a. High flow O_2 to prevent hypoxemia (nonrebreather [NRB] mask, continuous positive airway pressure [CPAP], endotracheal [ET] tube)
b. Fluid management to ensure perfusion but avoid volume overload
c. ET intubation
i. Indicated for massive hemoptysis, impending airway compromise, respiratory failure
d. Decompression (chest tube)
i. Indicated for pneumothorax or hemothorax
e. If required, air transport or general anesthesia
i. Consider prophylactic chest tube.
f. Air emboli—May present as stroke, myocardial infarction (MI), acute abdomen, blindness, deafness, spinal cord injury, claudication
i. High flow O_2: Prone, semileft lateral, or left lateral position
ii. Consider hyperbaric O_2 therapy (transfer)

2. Abdominal injury
a. Work up similar to blunt and penetrating abdominal trauma
b. Injuries will be more severe with underwater blasts.
c. Laboratory studies
d. Radiologic studies
i. Plain abdominal films
ii. CT scan
iii. Focused Assessment with Sonography in Trauma (FAST)
e. Initial management
i. Airway, breathing, circulation (ABC)
ii. Nothing by mouth (NPO)
iii. Avoid removal of penetrating objects in ED.
iv. Antibiotics and tetanus prophylaxis
f. Serial abdominal examinations (presentation may be delayed) with high degree of suspicion for missed or delayed injuries

3. Ear injury
a. Standard trauma protocols and lifesaving measures should be prioritized first.
b. Tympanic membrane injury should raise suspicion and evaluation for additional primary blast injury.
c. External ear injury
i. Foreign body removal with cleaning and irrigation of wounds
ii. Do not leave exposed cartilage.
d. TM rupture
i. Suction any obscuring fluids so TM can be visualized
ii. Keep ear clean and dry.
iii. Referral to otolaryngologist
iv. Antibiotic ear drops
v. Excellent prognosis with spontaneous resolution in majority of cases
e. Middle ear injuries
f. Can be deferred until an otolaryngologist is available

4. Eye injury
a. Assume all eye injuries may be a ruptured globe.
i. IV antibiotics if ruptured globe is suspected
b. Do not force lids open to examine eye.

i. Defer eye exam if there is massive swelling or lid hematoma.

c. Use convex plastic or metal shield, or bottom of a clean paper or Styrofoam cup to protect the globe.

i. Do not patch or bandage eye.

d. Do not remove impaled objects.

e. Obtain visual acuity of each eye.

i. Light perception

ii. Hand motion

iii. Count fingers

f. CT orbits to identify foreign bodies

g. MRI contraindicated until it is proven no metallic foreign bodies are present

h. Tetanus as indicated

i. Antiemetics to reduce nausea and vomiting

5. Crush injury

a. Administer IV fluids prior to releasing the crushed body part (especially if prolonged crush >4 hours).

b. *Hypotension:* IV hydration (up to 1.5 L/hour)

c. *Renal Failure:* Maintain urine output of at least 300 mL/hour with intravenous fluids (IVFs)

d. *Acidosis:* IV sodium bicarbonate until urine pH reaches 6.5 to prevent myoglobin and uric acid deposition in kidneys

e. *Hyperkalemia/hypocalcemia:* Calcium gluconate or calcium chloride; sodium bicarbonate; regular insulin with dextrose; Kayexalate

f. Monitor for cardiac arrhythmias.

g. Monitor for compartment syndrome.

h. Treat open wounds with antibiotics and tetanus prophylaxis.

i. Observe all crush injuries, regardless of how well they look.

6. Extremity injury

a. Document a systematic musculoskeletal, neurological, and vascular exam.

b. Radiographs

c. Antibiotics and tetanus for all open fractures

d. Irrigation of contaminated wounds

e. Splinting for mechanical stability and pain relief

f. Surgery consultation for ongoing management as indicated

G. *Patient disposition*

1. Stabilize.

2. Determine the need for transport to definitive care.

3. Patient outcome is directly related to the time elapsed between injury and properly delivered definitive care.

Diagnostic Testing

A. *Labs*

1. Orders should be based upon clinical assessment and patient needs.

a. Type and screen if transfusion expected

b. Pregnancy test on all women of childbearing age

c. Complete blood count (CBC)

d. Electrolyte levels

e. Liver function studies

f. International normalized ratio (INR)

g. Lactate

h. Others as indicated

B. *Radiology*

1. X-ray

a. Use judiciously and do not delay care to obtain.

b. Can be taken portably in resuscitation area

c. CXR

i. Can identify life-threatening injuries

d. Pelvis x-ray

i. Can identify fractures that may require transfusion

2. Extended Focused Assessment with Sonography for Trauma (eFAST)

a. Quick detection of intraabdominal blood, pneumothorax, and hemothorax

3. CT

a. Abdominal pain or tenderness

b. Significant mechanism of injury

c. Head injury

Differential Diagnoses

A. *Altered mental status (AMS)*

1. Hypovolemia

2. Acute neurologic injury

3. Intoxication

4. Preexisting medical conditions

5. Adverse drug reactions

6. Hypoglycemia

7. Electrolyte abnormalities

8. Behavioral and mental health conditions

9. Seizures

10. Infection

11. Poisonings

B. *Shock*

1. Significant finding in a trauma patient

2. Hemorrhagic—most common cause of shock

3. Nonhemorrhagic

a. Tension pneumothorax

b. Neurogenic

c. Cardiogenic

d. Cardiac tamponade

e. Septic

C. *Pharmacologic*

1. Medications can cause medical issues that lead to trauma.

2. Drug overdose

3. Polypharmacy

4. Medication side effects

D. *Hypotension*

1. Concerning finding

2. Tension pneumothorax

3. Hemorrhage

4. Cardiac tamponade

5. Acute myocardial infarction (MI)

6. Cardiac contusion

7. Exsanguination

8. Neurogenic shock

E. *Hypo- and hyperglycemia*

1. Medications

2. Illness
3. New or chronic medical conditions

F. *Distracting injuries (amputations, open fractures)*
1. Avoid distraction.
2. Continue following a systematic approach so as to not miss anything.
3. Completely expose the patient and examine head to toe.

Disposition

A. *Stabilize.*

B. *Determine need for transfer to definitive care.*
1. Patients with injuries beyond the management capacity of a hospital with limited resources should be transferred to the nearest trauma center.
   a. Decision when to transfer an unstable patient should be made in collaboration between transferring and receiving clinicians.
   b. Decompensation in transit should be anticipated.
   c. Qualified personnel and necessary resuscitative equipment should accompany the patient.
2. Patient outcome is directly related to the time elapsed between injury and properly delivered definitive care.
   a. Do not delay transfer to perform diagnostic procedures that do not change the immediate plan of care.
   b. Transfer delays are associated with increased mortality.
3. Provide receiving facility with:
   a. Past medical history and mechanism of injury
   b. Physical examination findings
   c. Treatments received
   d. Patient response
   e. Diagnostic tests and results
   f. Rationale/need for transfer
   g. Mode of transportation
   h. Anticipated arrival time
4. Use of a transfer checklist can help ensure important information is not missed.

C. *Admission*
1. Decision to admit depends on the facility's capabilities to care for the patient.
   a. Patient condition
   b. Nature of injury
   c. Availability of needed resources
2. Transfer to operating room
3. Admission to surgical services

Epidemiology of Trauma[1,3,6,7,9,10,11,13,14]

A. *Trauma overview*
1. Leading cause of death among those under 46 years of age globally
2. Incidence of death from injury increases more than threefold with increasing poverty.
3. Economic cost of traumatic injuries and death is estimated in the hundreds of trillions of dollars.
4. Most common causes of mortality from trauma
   a. Hemorrhage
   b. Multiple organ dysfunction syndrome
   c. Cardiopulmonary arrest
5. Preventable causes of morbidity
   a. Unintended extubation
      i. Most common cause of preventable morbidity in trauma patients
   b. Technical surgical failures
   c. Missed injuries
   d. Intravascular catheter-related complications
6. Majority of deaths occur at the scene or within the first 4 hours after a patient reaches a trauma center.
   a. The "golden hour" concept
      i. Emphasizes the importance of intervention during the first hour after injury to reduce the risk of death
7. Few countries or regions globally have comprehensive systems of trauma care

B. *Motor vehicle collision statistics*
1. Globally
   a. Leading cause of death between ages 18 and 29
   b. Accounted for 1.25 million deaths in 2014 per the World Health Organization (WHO)
2. United States
   a. More than 32,000 people are killed and 2 million injured each year from motor vehicle crashes.
   b. In 2013, the U.S. crash death rate was more than twice the average of other high-income countries.
   c. Major risk factors for crash deaths in the United States
      i. Not using seat belts, car seats, booster seats
         (1) Front seat belt use is lower in the United States than in most other comparison countries.
      ii. Drunk driving
         (1) One in three crash deaths involved drunk driving.
      iii. Speeding
         (1) Almost one in three crash deaths involved speeding.

C. *Firearm statistics*[10]
1. Significant concern unique to the United States
2. 39,740 firearm-related deaths in the United States in 2018
3. Among the five leading causes of death for people ages 1 to 64 in the United States
4. The two major component causes of firearm injury deaths in 2017 were:
   a. Suicide (60%)
      i. Highest among adults 75 years of age and older
   b. Homicide (36.6%)
      i. Highest among teens and young adults 15 to 34 years of age
5. Nonfatal firearm injuries:
   a. Assaults
      i. Account for seven out of every 10 medically treated firearm injury
   b. Unintentional
      i. Account for two out of every 10 medically treated firearm injury

6. Males account for 85% of all victims of firearm death and 88% of nonfatal firearm injuries.
7. The rate of firearm-related mortality increased 2.0% for males from 2016 to 2017.
8. At age 12, firearm injuries double and steadily increase until age 22, then decrease afterward

D. *Sources of blunt trauma:*
   1. Motor vehicle collisions
   2. Pedestrian versus automobile
   3. Bicycle
   4. Falls

E. *Sources of pediatric trauma:*
   1. Blunt trauma accounts for 90% of all pediatric trauma.
      a. Pedestrian struck by motor vehicle
      b. Occupant in motor vehicle collision
      c. Fall from height
      d. Fall from a bicycle
   2. Injuries associated with motor vehicles are the most common cause of death in children of all ages regardless of if they are:
      a. Occupants
      b. Pedestrians
      c. Cyclists
   3. Drowning
   4. House fires
   5. Homicides
      a. Child maltreatment
         i. Majority of infant homicides
      b. Firearm injuries
         i. Most of the homicides for those over the age of 1 and adolescents
   6. Falls

Primary Survey (Advanced Trauma Life Support [ATLS] Guidelines)[1,9,12–14]

A. *Overview of primary survey (ABCDE)*
   1. Identifies life-threatening injuries
   2. Treatment in a prioritized sequence, addressing greatest threat to life first
      a. Secure the airway.
      b. Maintain ventilation.
      c. Control hemorrhage.
      d. Treat shock.
   3. 10-second assessment
      a. ABCD can quickly be assessed by:
         i. The clinician identifying themselves
         ii. Asking the patient for their name
         iii. Then asking what happened
      b. Appropriate response suggests:
         i. Ability to speak clearly indicates no major airway compromise
         ii. Can generate air movement to permit speech indicates breathing not severely compromised
         iii. Alert enough to describe what happened indicates level of consciousness (LOC) not markedly decreased

B. *Airway maintenance with restriction of cervical spine motion*
   1. Assess and maintain patency.
      a. Identify and remove any foreign bodies.
      b. Identify facial injuries that may cause airway obstruction.
      c. Suction to clear secretions and accumulated blood.
   2. Maintain cervical spine immobilization.
   3. Establish a definitive airway if there is any doubt on airway integrity.
      a. Surgical airway if intubation contraindicated or cannot be accomplished

C. *Breathing and ventilation*
   1. Airway patency adequate ventilation
   2. Provide supplemental oxygen; monitor oxygen saturation.
   3. Expose the patient's neck and chest and inspect for:
      a. Injuries
      b. Jugular venous distention
      c. Trachea position
      d. Chest wall excursion
   4. Auscultate for bilateral breath sounds.

D. *Circulation with hemorrhage control*
   1. Hemorrhage is the primary cause of preventable deaths after injury.
   2. Assess central pulse quality, rate, regularity.
   3. Evaluate skin color and temperature.
   4. Measure blood pressure.
      a. Assume hypotension is from blood loss due to injury once tension pneumothorax is ruled out.
   5. Definitive bleeding control
      a. Identify and control any external source of hemorrhage.
         i. Manual pressure, compression bandage, hemostatic dressing
         ii. Tourniquets for exsanguinating extremities
      b. Internal sources of bleeding most often chest, abdomen, retroperitoneum, pelvis, and long bones
         i. Source identified by exam and imaging
            (1) Chest or pelvic x-ray
            (2) Extended Focused Assessment with Sonography for Trauma (eFAST)
         ii. Management of internal bleeding
            (1) Immediate interventions
               (a) Chest decompression
               (b) Pelvic stabilizing device
               (c) Extremity splints
               (d) Resuscitative endovascular balloon occlusion of the aorta (REBOA)
                  – Emerging tool in the management of noncompressible torso hemorrhage
                  – Can manage life-threatening hemorrhage below the diaphragm in patients unresponsive to resuscitation
            (2) Definitive
               (a) Surgery
               (b) Interventional radiology
               (c) Pelvic and long bone stabilization
      c. Replace intravascular volume.

i. Place two large bore (18 gauge or larger) intravenous catheters.

(1) Intraosseous (IO) catheter is a second line option.

ii. Initial fluid resuscitation with 20 mL/kg of a crystalloid

iii. If no improvement after initial crystalloid therapy, transfuse with type O blood (O-negative for females of childbearing age).

iv. All intravenous solutions should be warmed.

d. Volume resuscitation is not a substitute for definitive control of hemorrhage.

i. Aggressive resuscitation before control of bleeding increases mortality and morbidity

6. Reverse anticoagulation

7. Emergency thoracotomy may be needed in patients without palpable central pulses.

E. *Disability (assessment of neurologic status)*

1. Neurological status

a. Consult neurosurgery once brain injury recognized.

2. Glasgow Coma Scale (GCS; see Table 26.1)

a. Score of 8 or less is concerning for a poorer prognosis

b. Decrease in LOC may indicate

i. Decreased cerebral oxygenation and perfusion

ii. Direct cerebral injury

c. Altered LOC

i. Immediately reevaluate oxygenation, ventilation, and perfusion.

(1) Assume central nervous system injury until proven otherwise.

(2) Other etiologies Hypoglycemia alcohol narcotics other substances:

3. Assess pupillary size and reaction.

4. Assess motor function—lateralizing signs or spinal cord injury.

F. *Exposure/environmental control*

1. Completely undress and carefully examine patient.

2. Prevent hypothermia, a life-threatening complication in trauma patients.

a. Cover with warm blankets.

b. Warm intravenous fluids.

c. Maintain a warm environment.

G. *Resuscitation* Prioritize interventions based on findings of primary survey.

1. Airway obstruction

2. Tension or open pneumothorax

3. Flail chest or pulmonary contusion

4. Massive hemothorax

5. Cardiac tamponade

H. *Adjuncts to the primary survey*

1. EKG monitoring

a. Dysrhythmias can indicate blunt cardiac injury.

b. Pulseless electrical activity (PEA) can indicate:

i. Cardiac tamponade

ii. Tension pneumothorax

iii. Significant hypovolemia

2. Pulse oximetry

a. Findings can be inaccurate.

b. Confirm findings with arterial blood gas (ABG).

3. Ventilatory rate, ABG, end-tidal CO_2 monitoring

4. Urinary and gastric catheter unless contraindicated

5. X-rays (chest and pelvis if indicated)

a. Mark potential points of entry with a radiopaque object for better radiographic evaluation.

6. eFAST

a. Negative eFAST does not exclude injury.

I. *Reassess airway, breathing, circulation (ABCs) and consider need for transfer.*

1. Do not delay transfer for a thorough diagnostic evaluation.

2. Only undergo testing that enhances resuscitation and stabilization efforts.

Role of the APRN in Trauma Resuscitation

A. Important trauma team member

B. Communicates effectively

C. Should practice to full scope of ability

Secondary Survey (ATLS Guidelines)

A. *Overview of secondary survey*

1. Rapid but thorough head-to-toe examination

a. Complete history

b. Physical examination

i. Each body region is completely examined.

ii. Consider likely injuries related to mechanism of injury.

c. Reassessment of vital signs

2. Begins after:

a. The primary survey (ABCDE) is completed

b. Resuscitative efforts are underway

c. Improvement of patient's vital functions

B. *AMPLE history*

1. Allergies

2. Medications carriage return

3. Past medical history

4. Last meal (time)

5. Events/environment surrounding injury

a. Time since injury

b. Post-injury symptoms

C. *Mechanism of injury*

1. Can provide clues to anticipated injuries

a. Blunt trauma

i. Automobile collisions

(1) Seat belt use

(2) Steering wheel deformation

(3) Airbag deployment

(4) Direction of impact

(5) Patient position in vehicle

(6) Ejection from vehicle

(a) Greatly increases likelihood of major injury

b. Penetrating trauma

i. Body region injured

ii. Organs in path of penetrating object

iii. Velocity of missile

iv. Firearm injuries

(1) Velocity

(2) Caliber

(3) Presumed path of bullet
(4) Distance from weapon to wound
c. Thermal injury
i. Thermal burns
(1) Eschar
(2) Occult trauma
ii. Electrical burns
(1) Cardiac arrhythmias
(2) Compartment syndrome
iii. Inhalation burns
(1) Carbon monoxide poisoning
(2) Airway swelling
(3) Pulmonary edema

Special Considerations—Penetrating Trauma[1,9,12–15]

A. Wide range of presentations depending on affected body area
B. Mechanisms of penetrating trauma
1. Gunshot wounds
2. Stabbings
3. Impaled objects
4. Propelled shrapnel
C. May present stable and decline precipitously
D. Vital sign abnormalities, especially hypotension, persistent tachycardia, or hypoxia should raise a red flag for underlying injury
E. Identification of entry and exit wounds can aid in the determination of potential patterns of injury.
1. Mark with radiopaque object for visibility on imaging.
F. Signs and symptoms
1. Head and neck
a. Altered mental status (AMS), loss of consciousness (LOC), headache, nausea and vomiting (N/V), foreign body sensation in throat, voice changes, jugular venous distention, focal neurologic deficits, bony step offs of skull or cervical spine
2. Chest/thorax
a. Dyspnea, air hunger, pleuritic chest pain, hypoxia, tachypnea, tachycardia, hypotension, hemoptysis, hypoperfusion, absent breath sounds on the affected side, hyperresonance or dullness to percussion, paradoxical chest wall movement, subcutaneous emphysema, pneumomediastinum, muffled heart tones
3. Great vessels
a. Exsanguination, hemothorax, tamponade, widening of the mediastinum on CXR
4. Abdomen and pelvis
a. Symptoms may be subtle or absent at initial presentation
b. Abdominal pain and tenderness, nausea, vomiting, rigidity, guarding, ecchymosis, auscultation of bowel sounds in the thoracic cavity, tachycardia, hypotension, peritoneal signs, fever
G. Focused Assessment (ATLS guidelines)
1. Primary Survey (ABCDE)
2. Secondary Survey—Diagnostic testing and management

a. Head and neck
i. Early endotracheal (ET) intubation in comatose patients
(1) Be cautious of the difficult airway with facial and/or neck trauma.
ii. Avoid nasal gastric tube with a midface injury; use oral route.
iii. Focused, serial neurological examination
iv. Hyperventilation in moderation
v. Elevated intracranial pressure (ICP)
(1) Mannitol—*not* if hypotensive
(2) Hypertonic saline
(3) Barbiturates
vi. Posttraumatic epilepsy
(1) *Anticonvulsants:* Only when necessary as they may inhibit brain recovery
vii. CT scan in all patients with penetrating head trauma
(1) Do not allow this to delay transfer to definitive care.
viii. Neurosurgery consultation
b. Chest
i. Tension pneumothorax
(1) Clinical diagnosis (do NOT wait for imaging)
(2) Immediate decompression
(a) Large caliber needle (temporizing measure)
(b) Chest tube (definitive treatment)
ii. Open pneumothorax
(1) Sterile, occlusive dressing that is taped on three sides
iii. Massive hemothorax
(1) Replenish lost blood volume.
(a) Crystalloids
(b) Blood product
(2) Decompression with chest tube
(a) Autotransfusion collection
iv. Cardiac tamponade
(1) Echocardiogram or eFAST
(2) Surgical intervention
(a) Pericardiocentesis if surgical intervention not possible (not definitive)
v. Cardiac arrest or pulseless electrical activity
(1) ED thoracotomy if indicated, performed by a qualified surgeon
vi. Simple pneumothorax
(1) Chest tube—fourth or fifth intercostal space, just anterior to the midaxillary line
(2) Avoid general anesthesia or positive pressure ventilation until chest tube placed.
vii. Tracheobronchial tree injury
(1) Immediate surgical consultation
c. Abdomen and pelvis
i. Serial physical examinations by the same clinician in alert patients
ii. Trending of vital signs and laboratory studies
iii. Early surgical consultation

iv. Pelvic stability should only be assessed once to prevent further hemorrhage
v. No urinary catheters in patients with a perineal hematoma or high riding prostate
vi. X-rays
(1) Upright CXR if penetrating trauma above the umbilicus
(2) Markers to all enter and wound sites
(3) Anteroposterior pelvic x-ray may help establish source of blood loss in patients with pelvic pain or tenderness and hemodynamic instability
vii. Focused Assessment Sonography in Trauma (FAST)
(1) Detect presence of hemoperitoneum
(2) Rapid, noninvasive, accurate, inexpensive
(3) Scans of pericardial sac, hepatorenal fossa, splenorenal fossa, pelvis (pouch of Douglas)
viii. Diagnostic peritoneal lavage (DPL)
(1) Rapid study to identify hemorrhage
(2) Less commonly used today
ix. CT
(1) Only in hemodynamically stable patients without indication for emergency laparotomy
(2) Should not delay treatment and transfer
(a) If there is obvious evidence the patient will need to be transferred, CT should NOT be done.
x. Exploratory laparotomy
(1) Any hemodynamically unstable patient with penetrating abdominal trauma
(2) Gunshot with transperitoneal trajectory
d. Impaled objects
i. Leave in place objects deeply impaled in the chest and abdomen.
ii. May cut or shorten external portion of impaled object outside of skin to facilitate transport
e. Shock
i. Recognize its presence.
(1) Any patient with an injury who is cool and tachycardic should be considered to be in shock until proven otherwise.
ii. Identify probable cause and treat accordingly.

Special Populations

A. *Pediatric trauma*
1. Assessment and management priorities same as for adults
2. Prearrival preparedness
a. Estimate weight beforehand.
i. Availability of a length-based resuscitation tape (e.g., Broselow Tape)
b. Precalculate and draw up commonly needed drugs.
c. Appropriate size equipment ready
3. Anatomic considerations
a. Higher body surface area to body mass
i. Greater risk of multisystem injuries
ii. Higher risk for hypothermia
b. Airway
i. Larynx visualization may be difficult due to larger tongue and tonsils.
ii. Secretions can pool in the retropharyngeal space due to the larynx being funnel-shaped
iii. Positioning for airway patency
(1) Position the plane of face parallel to the spine board by placing a one-inch layer of padding under the torso.
c. Head/brain
i. More serious head injury due to greater head to body ratio
ii. Predisposed to skull fractures due to thinner cranium
iii. Open sutures accommodate elevated intracranial pressure (ICP) which can delay recognition of important injury
iv. More prone to acceleration-deceleration injuries
v. Significant susceptibility to cerebral hypoxia and hypercarbia due to increased cerebral blood flow
vi. Traumatic brain injury (TBI) can occur without loss of consciousness (LOC).
d. Spine
i. More flexible interspinous ligaments and joint capsules
ii. Injury uncommon
iii. Larger heads in comparison to necks leads to higher angular momentum, causing higher level injuries (occiput to C3)
(1) <8 years susceptible to spinal cord injury without evidence of radiographic abnormality (SCIWORA)
(a) When in doubt, assume an unstable injury exists and limit spinal motion and obtain appropriate consultation.
e. Chest
i. Pliable chest wall can lead to pulmonary contusions and other injuries without skeletal injuries.
ii. More prone to tension pneumothorax due to mobility of mediastinal structures
iii. Most chest injuries in children can be identified with chest radiographs.
f. Abdomen
i. Internal organs more susceptible to injury due to anterior placement of liver and spleen and less protective overlying musculature
ii. Kidneys susceptible to deceleration injury as they are less protected and more mobile
g. Musculoskeletal system
i. Immature, more pliable bones with growth plates

(1) Less prone to fractures even with internal organ damage
(2) Fractures that do occur may be greenstick, buckle, or involve growth plates.

- **h.** Vascular access more difficult to secure

4. Developmental considerations
   - **a.** More susceptible to heat loss
     - **i.** Ensure appropriate temperature regulation
     - **ii.** Mild/moderate hypothermia has direct negative effects on cardiac function
   - **b.** Remarkable cardiovascular reserve
     - **i.** Consider compensated shock with tachycardia.
     - **ii.** Minimal signs of shock not present until 25% of blood volume is lost
   - **c.** Higher oxygen extraction and glucose utilization
   - **d.** Minimize separation of pediatric patients from parents/guardians.
   - **e.** Mental health issues are common in children following traumatic events.
     - **i.** Provide resources.

B. *Geriatric trauma*

1. Worse outcomes
2. Falls are the most common cause of fatal and nonfatal injury in those 65 years of age.
3. Motor vehicle crashes are the second most common cause of injury in the elderly.
4. More susceptible to serious injury from low-energy mechanisms
   - **a.** Have a higher suspicion for injury
   - **b.** Lower threshold for diagnostic testing
   - **c.** Lower threshold for admission
5. Decreased physiologic reserve
   - **a.** Less able to compensate
6. Vital signs are unreliable to detect hemodynamic instability in the elderly.
   - **a.** Underlying hypertension makes blood pressures misleading.
   - **b.** Include altered mental status (AMS), urine output, and skin perfusion in evaluation.
7. Polypharmacy
   - **a.** Increased risk of bleeding
   - **b.** Medications may alter vital signs.
8. Anatomic changes can complicate airway management.
   - **a.** Dentures
   - **b.** Cervical arthritis
   - **c.** Temporomandibular arthritis
9. Maintain a high suspicion for intentional injuries and injuries caused by neglect.
10. Consider concomitant medical issues.
11. Institute measures to prevent and evaluate skin breakdown.
12. Inquire about existing advanced directives.

C. Trauma in pregnancy

1. Care for mother = care for fetus
2. Trauma occurs in up to 8% of pregnancies.
3. Motor vehicle accidents (MVAs) and domestic partner violence account for most cases of major maternal trauma.
4. Consult obstetrics early.
5. Gravid uterus alters injury patterns.
6. Poor fetal outcome predicted by maternal hypotension and acidosis
7. Cardiovascular changes
   - **a.** Cardiac output increases by 20% at eight weeks gestation, continuing to rise until 30 to 32 weeks.
   - **b.** Increased intravascular volume allows for significant blood loss before tachycardia, hypotension and other signs of hypovolemia occur.
     - **i.** Fetus may be in distress despite normal maternal vital signs.
   - **c.** Increased preload, decreased afterload
   - **d.** Blood pressure falls 5 to 15 mmHg during the second trimester and returns to normal by term.
   - **e.** Supine position can lower cardiac output by 25% to 30%.
     - **i.** Place in left lateral decubitus position.
   - **f.** Heart rate increases 10 to 15 beats per minute over baseline by third trimester.
   - **g.** Flow murmurs common
   - **h.** Hypertension and proteinuria should raise concern for preeclampsia.
8. Pulmonary changes
   - **a.** Increased tidal volume causes increased minute ventilation.
     - **i.** Hypocapnia is common.
     - **ii.** $PaCO_2$ of 35 to 40 mmHg may indicate an impending respiratory failure during pregnancy.
   - **b.** Oxygen consumption increases
     - **i.** Reduced oxygen reserve at term
     - **ii.** Administer supplemental oxygen for goal of 95% saturation.
     - **iii.** Maternal hypoxia leads to fetal hypoxia, distress, and possible demise.
   - **c.** Upward displacement of diaphragm at 20 weeks
     - **i.** Twenty percent decrease in functional residual capacity
     - **ii.** Chest tubes should be placed higher to avoid intraabdominal placement.
9. Gastrointestinal
   - **a.** Delayed gastric emptying
     - **i.** Early decompression with gastric tube to reduce aspiration risk
10. Urinary/renal
    - **a.** Increased glomerular filtration rate (GFR) and renal blood flow
    - **b.** Decreased serum creatinine
    - **c.** Glycosuria common
11. Musculoskeletal
    - **a.** Symphysis pubis widens 4 to 8 mm.
    - **b.** Sacroiliac joint space increases by month 7.
    - **c.** Large engorged pelvic vessels
      - **i.** Can contribute to massive retroperitoneal bleeding and exsanguination
12. Neurologic
    - **a.** Eclampsia
      - **i.** Can mimic head injury

ii. May present as seizures with associated hypertension, hyperreflexia, proteinuria, and peripheral edema
iii. Maintain high level of suspicion.

13. Uterus
   a. Pelvic organ first 12 weeks of pregnancy
   b. Enlarged uterus increases risk of visceral injury.
   c. Uterine blood flow not autoregulated
      i. Decrease in maternal systolic blood pressure can negatively impact fetus.

Trauma Systems[1, 12, 14]

A. Systematic team approach such as advanced trauma life support (ATLS) required
   1. Rapid assessment
   2. Triage
   3. Resuscitation
   4. Diagnosis
   5. Therapeutic intervention

B. Prehospital care
   1. Care generally begins by emergency medical services (EMS).
   2. Prehospital goals
      a. Lifesaving interventions
         i. Airway maintenance
         ii. Control of external bleeding and shock
      b. Prevention of additional injuries
         i. Immobilization
      c. Rapid transport to the closest appropriate facility
         i. Preferably a verified trauma center
         ii. Minimize scene time.
   3. EMS should notify receiving ED of:
      a. Patient age, history, and sex
      b. Mechanism and time of injury
      c. Vital signs
      d. Apparent injuries

C. Hospital phase
   1. Advanced planning and teamwork essential
   2. Critical aspects
      a. Resuscitation area available
      b. Smooth handover between EMS and those at receiving hospital
      c. Properly functioning and strategically organized airway equipment
      d. Warmed intravenous crystalloid solutions
      e. Appropriate monitoring devices
      f. Protocols to quickly mobilize additional resources and personnel
      g. Transfer agreements with verified trauma centers

D. Trauma centers
   1. Verification process by the American College of Surgeons (ACS)
   2. Institutions are certified based on a commitment of personnel and resources to maintain level of readiness for critically injured patients.
   3. Care involves
      a. Multidisciplinary evaluation
      b. Diagnostic and therapeutic interventions
      c. Smooth transitions between departments
   4. Principles of ATLS followed
      a. Treat greatest threat to life first.
      b. Lack of definitive diagnosis should not impede treatment.
      c. Evaluation of the acutely injured can begin without a detailed history.

References and Additional Reading

References and Additional Reading for this chapter are online only and can be found at https://connect.springerpub.com/content/reference-book/978-0-8261-6091-5/part/part03/toc-part/ch25.

26. Head Trauma and Brain Injuries

MARISA LOSAVIO

Learning Objectives

- Explain the pathophysiology of brain injuries that occur from trauma.
- Identify predisposing risk factors of head trauma.
- Identify signs and symptoms of patients with brain injury.
- Use evidence-based guidelines to perform a comprehensive physical assessment on a trauma patient.
- Identify potential differential diagnoses for a patient who presents to the emergency department (ED) posttrauma.
- Develop plan of care regarding diagnostic testing, pharmacologic therapies, and overall management of a head injury patient including age and developmental considerations.
- Establish safe disposition plans for patients with mild, moderate, or severe head injuries.

Each year, approximately 1.7 million people in the United States sustain a head injury. Brain trauma is defined as an impairment to brain functioning as a result of an external direct or indirect force to the head. Clinical manifestations of brain trauma can range from scalp lacerations to brief loss of consciousness, coma, disability, or death. Injuries that can cause brain trauma include loss of consciousness from cardiac/neurological cause, fall, and accidental trauma from bike, motorcycle, car accident, gunshot wounds, and more. The leading causes of head injury are falls and motor vehicle collisions. Traumatic brain injury (TBI) is classified as mild, moderate, or severe based on the Glasgow Coma Scale (GCS). See Table 26.1 for the GCS.

TABLE 26.1 GLASGOW COMA SCALE FOR ALL AGE GROUPS

	4 YEARS TO ADULT	CHILD <4 YEARS	INFANT
EYE OPENING			
4	Spontaneous	Spontaneous	Spontaneous
3	To speech	To speech	To speech
2	To pain	To pain	To pain
1	No response	No response	No response
VERBAL RESPONSE			
5	Alert and oriented	Oriented, social, speaks, interacts	Coos, babbles
4	Disoriented conversation	Confused speech, disoriented, consolable, aware	Irritable cry
3	Speaking but nonsensical	Inappropriate words, inconsolable, unaware	Cries to pain
2	Moans or unintelligible sounds	Incomprehensible, agitated, restless, unaware	Moans to pain
1	No response	No response	No response
MOTOR RESPONSE			
6	Follows commands	Normal, spontaneous movements	Normal, spontaneous movements
5	Localizes pain	Localizes pain	Withdraws to touch
4	Moves or withdraws to pain	Withdraws to pain	Withdraws to pain
3	Decorticate flexion	Decorticate flexion	Decorticate flexion
2	Decerebrate extension	Decerebrate extension	Decerebrate extension
1	No response	No response	No response
Possible Score: 3–15			

Note: In intubated patients, the Glasgow Coma Scale verbal component is scored as a 1, and total score is marked with a "T" (or tube) denoting intubation (e.g., "8T").
Source: Cydulka RK, Cline DM, Ma O, Fitch MT, Joing S, Wang VJ. *Tintinalli's Emergency Medicine Manual.* 8th ed. McGraw-Hill Education; 2017.[1]

Pathophysiology

Primary brain injuries are the result of an insult associated with a moderate and severe TBI, which results from mechanical force that produces high levels of direct damage and strain to the brain parenchyma. Brain edema resulting from TBI can be especially dangerous as intracellular and extracellular water content rises. The brain swells, and the intracranial pressure increases, causing direct compressive tissue damage, vascular compression ischemia, and brain parenchyma herniation, and eventually brain death. The ultimate neurological outcome of a patient with head trauma is dependent on the extent of primary TBI occurring alone or along with secondary insults such as hypotension and hypoxia, which worsen the neurochemical and neuroanatomic pathophysiology. Primary injury causes permanent mechanical cellular disruption and microvascular injury, while secondary injury is a result of intracellular and extracellular derangement that is caused by the initial trauma. Ultimately, the amount of secondary brain injury can also be influenced by certain medical comorbidities, age of the patient, and other traumatic injuries.

General Approach

Predisposing Factors

A. Age (toddlers, teenagers, and the elderly)
B. Gender (males more commonly)
C. Mechanism of injury and severity of TBI (e.g., height of fall, impact surface condition, damage sustained to vehicle, airbag deployment, seat belt use, history of ejection from vehicle)
D. High association with motor vehicle collisions in children and young adults
E. High association with falls in the elderly
F. Use of anticoagulants and antiplatelet medications
G. Existing medical comorbidities such as preexisting coagulopathy
H. Abuse or assault like injury
I. Acute ethanol intoxication or other intoxicants
J. Seizure disorders
K. Syncope or dizziness as prodrome

Medical Screening

A. *Chief complaint:* Traumatic brain/head injury
B. *Signs and symptoms*
- **1.** Altered mental status ranging from mild lethargy, semiconscious, unconscious to coma with fixed and dilated pupils
- **2.** Confusion or amnesia
- **3.** Combativeness
- **4.** Hypoxia, respiratory distress
- **5.** Hypotension, shock, cardiac arrest
- **6.** Headache
- **7.** Nausea and vomiting
- **8.** Seizure
- **9.** Elevated intracranial pressure (ICP; >15 mmHg)
- **10.** Cushing's reflex that includes bradycardia, hypertension, and diminished respiratory effort in response to lethal increases in ICP, resulting in progressive neurological deterioration.
- **11.** Scalp or facial lacerations or hematoma
- **12.** Decerebrate or decorticate posturing in comatose patients.
- **13.** Blood in ear canal, hemotympanum, rhinorrhea, otorrhea, Battle's sign, raccoon sign, or cranial nerve deficits can be associated with basilar skull fracture.
- **14.** Postconcussive syndrome presents with headache, sensory sensitivity, memory or concentration difficulties, irritability, sleep disturbance, dizziness, depression, and amnesia.

Physical Examination

A. Follow Advanced Trauma Life Support (ATLS) algorithm (including primary and secondary surveys) to perform the trauma-focused examination while performing any lifesaving procedures as necessary.
- **1.** Protect the cervical spine during evaluation, treatment, and imaging.

B. *Assess and secure airway.*
- **1.** Provide oxygenation, endotracheal intubation, and ventilatory support as necessary

C. *Obtain details surrounding the event rapidly.*
D. *General and neurological*
- **1.** Assess mental status, including GCS score (Table 26.1), and assess pupils, including size and reactivity, motor strength and symmetry, and cranial nerve assessment as tolerated.
- **2.** If possible, obtain brief neurological examination prior to rapid sequence intubation (RSI)/intubation and administration of sedative or neuromuscular blocking agents

E. *Cardiac:* assess for hypotension, arrhythmia, brady-/tachycardia, hemodynamic stability
F. *Respiratory:* assess for tachypnea, abnormal lung sounds
G. *Head and neck examination* for external signs of trauma such as scalp laceration, contusion, abrasion, or avulsion, which can also give insight into risk of skull fracture

Differential Diagnoses

A. Cerebrovascular accident (CVA); thrombus versus hemorrhagic
B. Drug or alcohol intoxication
C. Cardiac or respiratory arrest
D. Hypoglycemia
E. Seizure
F. Attempted suicide or homicide
G. Child abuse/neglect

Diagnostic Testing

A. Cardiac monitoring, EKG
B. Pulse oximetry and capnography
C. Blood glucose
D. Determine if CT imaging of the head and cervical spine is dependent on patient's mechanism of injury, medical history, comorbidities, and signs and symptoms (see Box 26.1, Table 26.2).
- **1.** Several decision rules are in place for help in determining whether imaging is necessary including scales based on GCS, New Orleans, or Canadian Head CT rule. All decision-making rules exclude patients who are taking anticoagulation or antiplatelet therapy.

TABLE 26.2 NEW ORLEANS CRITERIA AND CANADIAN CT HEAD RULE CLINICAL DECISION RULES

NEW ORLEANS CRITERIA—GCS 15*	CANADIAN CT HEAD RULE—GCS 13–15*
Headache	GCS <15 at 2 hr
Vomiting	Suspected open or depressed skull fracture
Age >60 years	Age ≥65 years
Intoxication	More than one episode of vomiting
Persistent anterograde amnesia	Dangerous mechanism (fall >3 feet or struck as pedestrian)
Seizure	Any sign of basal skull fracture
IDENTIFICATION OF PATIENTS WHO HAVE AN INTRACRANIAL LESION ON CT	
100% sensitive, 5% specific	83% sensitive, 38% specific
IDENTIFICATION OF PATIENTS WHO WILL NEED NEUROLOGICAL INTERVENTION	
100% sensitive, 5% specific	100% sensitive, 37% specific

*Presence of any one finding indicates need for CT scan.
GCS, Glasgow Coma Scale.
Source: Cydulka RK, Cline DM, Ma O, Fitch MT, Joing S, Wang VJ. *Tintinalli's Emergency Medicine Manual.* 8th ed. McGraw-Hill Education; 2017.[1]

BOX 26.1 CT SCANNING FOR ADULTS WITH BRAIN INJURY: AMERICAN COLLEGE OF EMERGENCY PHYSICIANS GUIDELINES

- Adults with a Glasgow Coma Scale score of <15 at the time of evaluation should undergo CT imaging.
- Mild traumatic brain injury with or without loss of consciousness: If one or more of the following is present:
  - Glasgow Coma Scale score <15
  - Focal neurologic findings
  - Vomiting more than two times
  - Moderate to severe headache
  - Age >65 years
  - Physical signs of basilar skull fracture
  - Coagulopathy
  - Dangerous mechanism of injury (e.g., fall >4 feet)
- Mild traumatic brain injury with loss of consciousness or amnesia: If one or more of the following is present:
  - Drug or alcohol intoxication
  - Physical evidence above the clavicles
  - Persistent amnesia
  - Posttraumatic seizures

Source: Cydulka RK, Cline DM, Ma O, Fitch MT, Joing S, Wang VJ. *Tintinalli's Emergency Medicine Manual.* 8th ed. McGraw-Hill Education; 2017.[1]

E. Toxicologic screen
F. If there was prodrome to head injury or other medical complaints on arrival, this would require further testing such as labs.
  1. Complete blood count (CBC)
  2. Comprehensive metabolic panel (CMP)
  3. Coagulation studies
G. Further imaging as necessary including cervical spine, CT cervical spine, maxillofacial, thoracic, or lumbar spine
H. X-ray imaging as necessary for additional injuries
I. MRI may be necessary for some posttraumatic injuries

Management

A. *Procedures*
  1. Resuscitation of pulselessness and apneic patients and perform any lifesaving procedures as needed per the ATLS algorithm.
  2. Continuous cardiac monitoring and pulse oximetry to maintain cerebral perfusion and oxygenation
  3. Determination of oxygenation and ventilation to determine necessity of tracheal intubation (intubate for GCS <8) or oxygen via face or nasal mask in awake patients as tolerated.
  4. Prevent secondary injury by correcting hypoxia, hypercapnia, hyperglycemia, hyperthermia, anemia, or hypoperfusion.
  5. Implement spinal precautions.
  6. Recognize and treat elevated ICP.
  7. Arrange for neurosurgical intervention as indicated.
  8. Sedation and analgesia can decrease baseline ICP and prevent transient rises from agitation, coughing, and gagging.
  9. Prevent and control seizure activity.
  10. Control temperature.
  11. Treat elevated ICP by keeping the head of the bed at 30 degrees, ensuring good blood pressure, temperature control, and ventilation.
  12. Acute hyperventilation may be used to prevent or delay herniation while definitive resources are mobilized by reducing the carbon dioxide partial pressure (PCO_2) to the range of 30 to 35 mmHg as it will cause cerebral vasoconstriction. Prolonged hyperventilation is not recommended.
  13. Neurosurgery consultation for ICP monitoring and ventriculostomy for ICP management or other acute neurosurgical intervention.

Pharmacologic Therapies

A. Largely supportive care
B. Treat both hypoglycemia and hyperglycemia with dextrose or insulin as indicated.

C. Give antiepileptic drug if GCS <8, acute seizure with injury, or abnormal head CT scan including acute subdural or epidural hematoma, acute intracranial hemorrhage, depressed skull fracture or if with penetrating head injury.
D. Administer acetaminophen as needed for fever.
E. Consider osmotherapy with the use of osmotic diuretics to reduce acute cerebral edema.
F. Consider hypertonic saline (3% NaCl 250 mL/30 min) for refractory elevations in ICP.
G. Sedation and analgesia as necessary as keeping patients appropriately sedated can decrease ICP.
H. Consider use of general anesthetic that has minimal effects on blood pressure, respiratory rate, and cardiac output.
I. Normal saline or lactated Ringer's solution is typically used for resuscitation for trauma patients with hypovolemic hypotension.
J. Barbiturate therapy can reduce cerebral metabolic demands of injured brain tissue to help in reducing ICP. Pentobarbital is most often used.
K. Steroid use is NOT indicated, provides no benefit, and is associated with increased mortality in moderate to severe TBI.
L. Antibiotic prophylaxis may be used for penetrating head injury, open skull fractures, and complicated scalp lacerations.

Consultation and Collaboration

A. Immediate neurosurgery referral or transfer as necessary for advanced care for severe head trauma.
B. Brain injury related to trauma may require consultation from trauma/acute care surgery as indicated for additional injuries.
C. Transfer may be necessary to an institution that is capable of neurosurgical care and acute neurosurgical intervention if it is not available at the receiving hospital.

Patient Disposition

A. Patients with severe head injury will have consultation by neurosurgery team, and will likely require admission to either a neuro-ICU or a medical ICU.
B. Patients with moderate head injury should be admitted for observation, even if initial CT scan is normal. Patients will require frequent neurological exam and may require a repeat CT scan if symptoms do not improve, or if patients are on certain anticoagulants.
C. Patients with low risk or minor TBI can be discharged from the ED with normal examination findings and after an ED observation period of about 4 to 6 hours.
D. If any doubt exists regarding safety of discharge in a patient with minor head injury, a brief inpatient observation period (12–24 hours) is warranted.
  1. Discharge instructions should include instructions describing the signs and symptoms of delayed complications of head injury, and patient must have access to a telephone.
  2. Patients should only be discharged with someone to monitor in the posttrauma period by a sober and responsible adult.
  3. Patients who have sustained a concussion are at risk for prolonged morbidity, and athletes should not be allowed to return immediately to sports activities due to the risk of second impact syndrome. A graduated return to play protocol is typically used, which includes stages such as no activity, light aerobic exercise, sport-specific exercise, noncontact training, full-contact practice, and finally, then return to play.
  4. Include prevention and education tips including the use of helmets or headgear for all high impact sports, supervising children during activities, safe diving into bodies of water, and seat belt use.
E. Transition of care information
  1. Summary of care including any information or details from the mechanism of injury care given prehospital and in the ED.
  2. Findings from all diagnostic studies completed, and these should be transferred with patient if they require transfer for neurosurgical care.
  3. Current status including hemodynamic stability, vital signs, and any medications administered.
F. Prevention and education
  1. Emphasis on public education of preventing head injuries with safe practices.
  2. Education on risks of danger of ethanol use in conjunction with head injury.
  3. Parent education on adequate supervision of children when playing contact sports.
  4. Importance of wearing helmets/headgear in all contact sports.
  5. Importance of use of seat belt and child car seats.
  6. Education on postconcussive syndromes and safe reintroduction to activity.

Age and Developmental Considerations

A. Children may only be discharged to a competent adult.
B. Head injury is the leading cause of traumatic death in patients younger than 25 years.
C. GCS will be more difficult to assess in children and patients with difficulty communicating.
D. Must assess for intentional abuse in children or the elderly, as head injury from child abuse is common.
E. Severe head trauma in children has lower mortality.
F. Adult survivors of severe head trauma are usually severely disabled, whereas children older than 2 years who survive a severe head injury have a better outcome than adults as children's skulls are more distensible than adults.
G. Children with minor head trauma often have more pronounced symptoms such as lethargy, paleness, with frequent emesis and complaints of headaches and dizziness.
H. Children with concussions tend to be more symptomatic than adults.
I. The presence of a skull fracture in children is a predictor of TBI.

References

References for this chapter are online only and can be found at https://connect.springerpub.com/content/reference-book/978-0-8261-6091-5/part/part03/toc-part/ch26.

27. Spinal Injuries

JANE HOLSTON

Learning Objectives

- Identify, evaluate, and treat traumatic spinal injuries in ED or urgent care settings.
- Provide emergent treatment for patients with unstable spinal fractures.
- Provide treatment for respiratory compromise, spinal shock, neurogenic shock, or other life-threatening complications.
- Recognize spinal injuries that require immediate consult and make the appropriate consult.
- Order and interpret appropriate diagnostic tests and imaging for spinal injuries.
- Develop appropriate plans of treatment for spinal injuries.
- Choose the appropriate disposition for patients with spinal injuries.
- Provide appropriate patient education and follow-up care for optimal patient outcomes.

Injuries to the spine can be life-threatening; therefore, the importance of rapid and proper evaluation is crucial. Spinal cord injury (SCI) is the second leading cause of paralysis in the United States, with stroke being the leading cause at 33.7%, followed closely by SCI at 27.3%.[1] According to the National Spinal Cord Injury Statistical Center (NSCISC), there are an estimated 17,700 SCIs in the United States each year, excluding those who die at the scene.

Males with an average age of 43 years are predominately affected.

The most common cause is motor vehicle crashes (MVCs), followed by falls. Gunshot wounds and sports injuries are other common causes.[2] The majority of these patients will present to the Emergency Department (ED) for evaluation and treatment.

Prompt attention must be paid to assess for airway compromise, bleeding, and neurological impairment in any type of spinal injury.

Anatomy

A. The vertebral column consists of 33 vertebrae: 7 cervical, 12 thoracic, 5 lumbar, 5 fused sacral, and 4 fused coccygeal (Figure 27.1).

B. Intervertebral discs lie between each vertebra, with the exception of the fused sacral and coccygeal vertebrae.

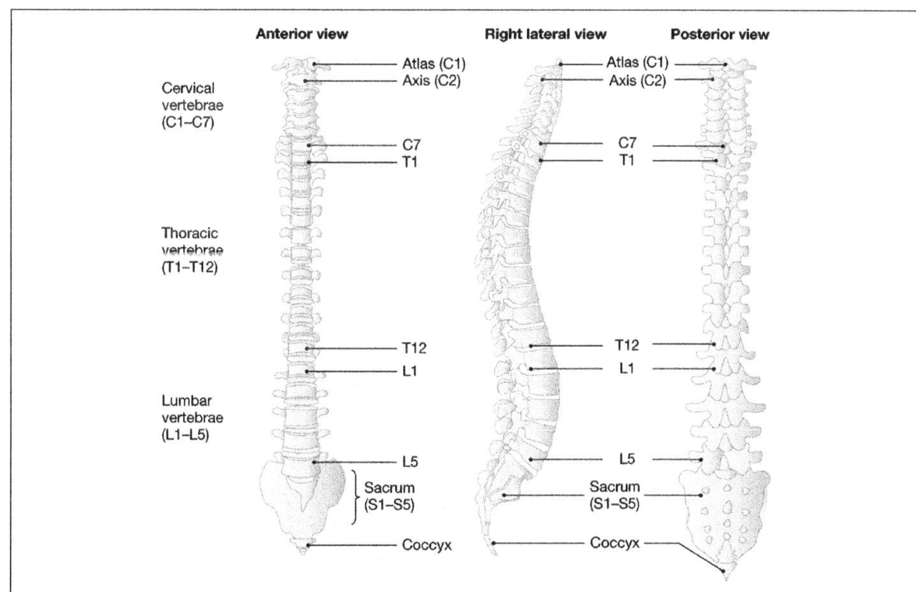

FIGURE 27.1 Spinal column.
Source: From Stutzman Z, Gawlik K. Evidence-based assessment of the musculoskeletal system. In Gawlik KS, Melnyk BM, Teall AM, eds. *Evidence-Based Physical Examination.* 1st ed. Springer Publishing Company, 2021: p. 311, Figure 15.5.[3]

1. Act as shock absorbers for the vertebral bodies
2. Consist of a tough outer layer known as the annulus fibrosis with a fibrous gel-like material known as the nucleus pulposus, contained within the discs, allowing them to absorb pressure exerted by activity

C. The vertebral canal is a cavity that runs through the center of each vertebra in the vertebral column that serves to surround and protect the spinal cord.[2]

1. Within the vertebral canal, other structures protecting the spinal cord include the meninges (dura, arachnoid, and pia mater) and the cerebrospinal fluid (CSF).
   a. CSF constantly flows and bathes the spinal cord in nutrients, helps to eliminate waste products, and serves as a cushion against impact, with approximately 600 mL being produced daily.[2]

D. The central nervous system (CNS) consists of the brain and the spinal cord.

1. The spinal cord begins at the base of the brain stem at the first cervical vertebra (C1) and ends approximately at the first lumbar vertebra (L1), in a cone-shaped structure, known as the "conus medullaris."
2. The bundle of nerves that make up the conus medullaris separate into the cauda equina, which gets its name from its resemblance to a horse's tail.[4]
3. The spinal cord has numerous vital functions, including motor, sensory, and autonomic function. Injury to the spinal cord can result in loss of sensation, loss of function, complete paralysis, and even death.
4. Much like the vertebral column, the spinal cord is divided into sections which include 8 cervical, 12 thoracic, 5 lumbar, 5 sacral, and 1 coccygeal, with nerve roots exiting out from foramina in the vertebra from each level (Figure 27.2). C8 is the eighth nerve root that exits between C7 and T1.[2,4]

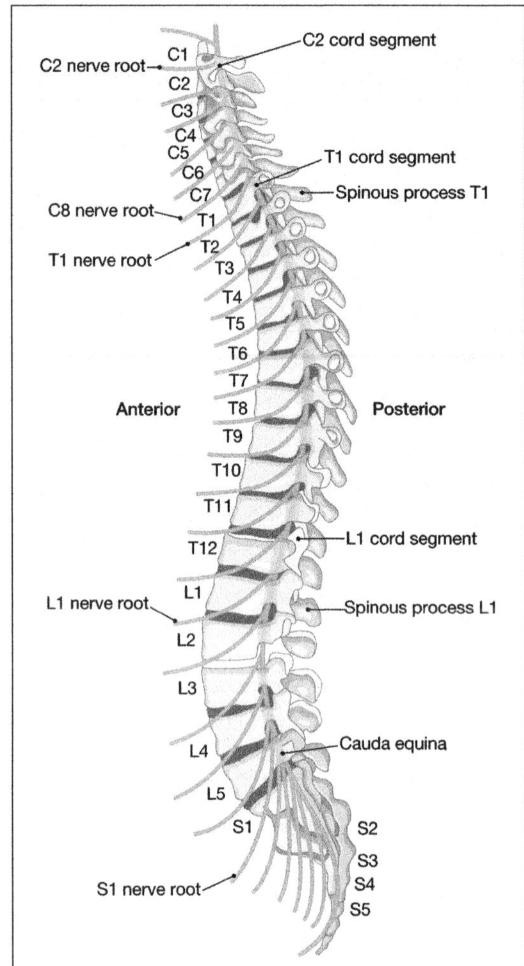

FIGURE 27.2 Lateral view of the spinal cord.
Source: From Simons L. Evidence-based assessment of the nervous system. In Gawlik KS, Melnyk BM, Teall AM, eds. *Evidence-Based Physical Examination*. 1st ed. Springer Publishing Company, 2021: p. 311, Figure 14.1.[5]

Pathophysiology

A. Injuries to the spine can occur in a variety of ways due to the multiple structures and functions of the spinal cord and spinal column.

B. Trauma to the cervical spine can occur through pronounced hyperflexion, hyperextension, lateral bending, rotation, and axial compression.[6]

1. Multiple forces may be exerted in one traumatic event such as a high-velocity rollover motor vehicle accident (MVA).
2. The neck is very vulnerable to life-threatening injury due to its high degree of flexion and mobility and the extent of the injury may not be apparent immediately, as a cascade of physiologic reactions may occur following the injury such as edema that can cause compression, alter blood flow, and cause neurogenic damage.[7]

C. Trauma to the thoracic and lumbar spine often occurs due to forceful mechanisms of injury such as MVAs, falls, sports/recreation activities, and acts of violence such as gunshot wounds.[2,8]

D. Primary injury is the degree of injury sustained at the time of the impact. Vertebrae can be fractured or displaced, causing injury to the spinal cord. Damage can range from minor bruising of the spinal cord to complete dissection.

1. A complete spinal cord injury (CSI) occurs when all motor and sensory function is lost from the level of the injury downward and occurs in approximately 50% of all spinal cord injuries (SCIs).
   a. Compromised blood flow from contusion and edema that compromises blood flow is seen in most CSIs, and the effects are bilateral.
2. An incomplete SCI occurs when the patient retains some function below the affected level, and deficits may occur unilaterally.[8]

E. Secondary injury results from the cascade of physiologic reactions that occur once an injury to the spinal cord has taken place, including edema that can lead to compromised blood flow, tissue ischemia, and cell and tissue death.[9]

F. Per the American Association of Neurological Surgeons (AANS, 2020), SCIs can be graded using the American Spinal Injury Association (ASIA) SCI scoring system:

1. *ASIA A:* Injury is CSI with no sensory or motor function preserved.
2. *ASIA B:* A sensory incomplete injury with complete motor function loss
3. *ASIA C:* A motor incomplete injury, where there is some movement, but less than half the muscle groups are antigravity (can lift up against the force of gravity with a full range of motion).
4. *ASIA D:* A motor incomplete injury where more than half of the muscle groups are antigravity.
5. *ASIA E:* Normal

Predisposing Factors

A. Sex and age[4,10]
  1. The average age for CSI to occur is currently 43 years of age and gender is predominately male (78%).
  2. Persons between the ages of 16 and 30 are predisposed to SCI from traumatic events with MVAs leading the way.
  3. Falls are the predominant cause in people >65 years of age.

B. Those who engage in risky behavior, including use of illicit drugs and alcohol, high-impact sporting events, reckless or high-speed driving, or those at increased risk for being involved in a violent crime have a higher incidence of sustaining an injury to the spinal cord.[4,10]

C. Persons with cancer resulting in weakening of bone and those with chronic conditions, such as osteoarthritis, osteoporosis, or ankylosing spondylitis, can also be predisposed to SCI due to decreased flexibility and resilience when an injury occurs.[4,10]

Medical Screening

A. When a patient presents with an injury, it is essential to obtain as much history as possible. This is especially true in patients with known or suspected spinal injuries.
  1. If the patient is able to speak, obtain as much information about the mechanism of injury and any symptoms that the patient may be experiencing.
  2. If the patient appears to have altered mental status (AMS), both traumatic brain injury (TBI) and SCI should be suspected.
  3. Family members, emergency medical services (EMS) personnel, and any other bystanders or witnesses to the incident may provide valuable information as well.[11]

B. A thorough history of present illness (HPI), past medical history, current medications, allergies, family history, surgical history, social history, and review of systems should be obtained as soon as possible but should not delay initial evaluation or treatment.

Physical Examination

Any patient who has suffered trauma, especially those showing signs of head or neck injury with a severe mechanism of injury and signs of neurologic compromise should be treated as though they have an SCI until proven otherwise. Assessing for and maintaining airway, breathing, and circulation, and excluding any obvious immediate life-threatening injuries in combination with immobilization are priorities during the primary survey. As with any traumatic injury, the primary survey can be performed using the acronym ABCDE and follows ATLS recommendations.

A. *Airway and cervical spine (per ATLS)*
  1. Assess for airway compromise. If the patient is unable to speak, perform the chin lift or **jaw thrust maneuver (especially if SCI is suspected)**. During assessment of the airway, observe for injuries to the face and neck such as lacerations, bruising, or obvious fractures or other deformities. When moving or rolling the patient over, ensure that at least two medical personnel are at the bedside in order to properly utilize the two-person spinal immobilization technique, to protect both the spine and the airway.[12]

B. *Breathing and ventilation*
  1. Inspect for obvious causes of ventilatory problems such as tracheal deviation, chest wounds, or signs of pneumothorax. Auscultate breath sounds, being prepared to perform a needle decompression if a tension pneumothorax is suspected. Provide supplemental oxygen initially to all trauma patients.[12]

C. *Circulation*
  1. Assess for signs of obvious blood loss by noting patient responsiveness using the AVPU mnemonic:
    a. A: Are they **A**lert?
    b. V: Do they respond to **V**erbal stimuli?
    c. P: Do they respond to **P**ainful stimuli?
    d. U: Are they **U**nresponsive to any stimuli?
  2. Assess the color and temperature of their skin, capillary refill, and pulses to determine whether hemorrhage could be occurring.[12]

D. *Disability*
  1. Neurologic status can be quickly assessed by performing the Glasgow Coma Scale (GCS), which assesses eye-opening, verbal, and motor response.[12]

E. *Exposure and environment*
  1. The patient should be undressed to assess for any injury hidden by clothing or objects causing pressure such as wallets or car keys, then quickly recovered with a blanket to prevent hypothermia.[11,12]
  2. The primary survey listed earlier should be performed rapidly, followed by a focused neurologic exam, keeping in mind that head injuries often occur with SCIs. The examiner should develop a systematic approach and should use it routinely. The neck and back should be inspected for signs of laceration, bruising, deformity, or other obvious injuries. Paraspinal muscles and spinous processes should be palpated for tenderness, paying special attention to the level where any tenderness is noted.[9] The level of potential injury can be determined by assessing motor function as noted in the image below:
  3. Dermatomes should be tested for any sensory deficit using pain and light touch (Figure 27.3). Deep tendon reflexes of the bilateral upper and lower extremities should be tested for presence and symmetry on a 0 to 4+ scale, with 0 being no response and 4+ being hyperactive with clonus. Strength of the upper and lower extremities should be tested if possible, on a 0 to 5 scale with 0 being no contraction or movement and 5 being full strength. Saddle anesthesia, sensory loss to the perineal area, buttocks, and inner thighs (think parts of the body that would touch a saddle when horseback riding), could indicate injury to the cauda equina, also

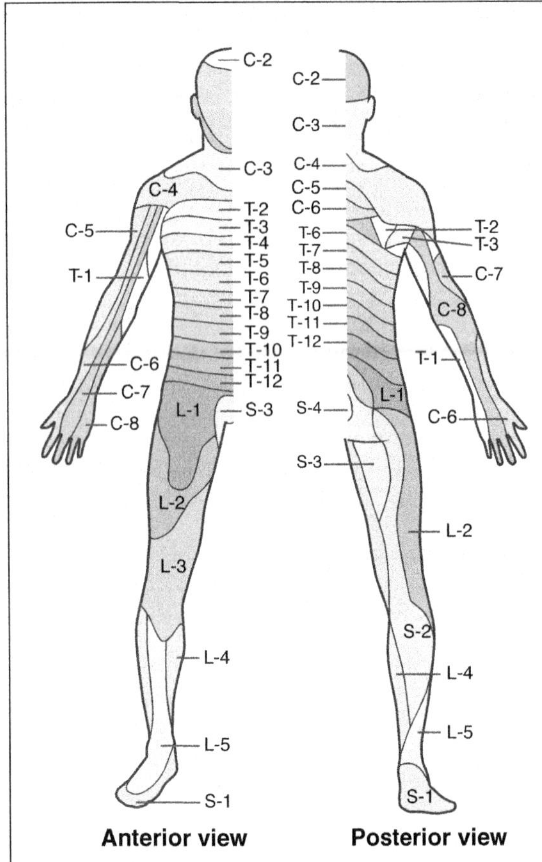

FIGURE 27.3 Dermatomes, anterior and posterior view.
Source: From Chiocca EM. *Advanced Pediatric Assessment.* 3rd ed. Springer Publishing Company; 2019: Figure 22.6[31]

known as cauda equina syndrome and is always considered a medical emergency. Bowel or bladder dysfunction may also occur with spinal injury, so assess for incontinence or retention of urine and/or stool. Anogenital reflexes such as the bulbocavernosus reflex, anal wink reflex, cremasteric reflex, and abdominal reflexes should all be tested if indicated. Note that priapism in males can be a sign of a complete spinal cord lesion.[9,11,14]

Differential Diagnoses

A. Formulating differential diagnoses in the trauma patient with the potential for acute spinal injury can be complicated by chronic conditions. The presence of preexisting pathology of the spine, such as ankylosing spondylitis, osteoporosis, or degenerative disc disease, may put the patient at risk for more serious injury and complications following the injury.

B. Some differential diagnoses include:

1. Muscle strain (whiplash if cervical injury)
2. Herniated nucleus pulposus (HNP)
3. Vertebral fracture
4. Vertebral dislocation
5. Vertebral dislocation fracture
6. Contusion
7. Pelvic fracture
8. Spinal hematoma
9. Epidural abscess

Diagnostic Testing

A. Clinical decision-making tools that have undergone extensive clinical testing for validity and reliability such as the Nexus Criteria for C-Spine Imaging and the Canadian C-Spine Rule can be quickly used to determine whether imaging should be performed in suspected cervical spine injures. These tools should only be used in adult patients who are awake and stable.[15]

1. These criteria were created largely due to overuse of radiography in patients with suspected cervical spine injuries and have been widely tested across the United States using large numbers of participants.
2. Consideration of these guidelines can greatly reduce radiation exposure to patients, in addition to time and healthcare costs by eliminating unnecessary testing.[16,17]
3. The entire spine should be imaged in any patient with a confirmed or strongly suspected SCI.[18]

B. The NEXUS Criteria use the acronym NSAID:

1. *N:* Neurologic deficit
2. *S:* Spinous process tenderness
3. *A:*Altered mental status (AMS) or level of consciousness
4. *I:* Intoxication
5. *D:* Distracting injury
6. This tool should only be used in patients > 1 and <55 years of age.
7. The Canadian C-Spine Rule takes into account factors such as the age of the patient, mechanism of injury, paresthesias of extremities, ability to sit up, ability to ambulate, and mobility of the neck.

C. Using electronic tools to calculate these scores such as MDCalc can quickly give the clinician an objective score and both can be performed in a matter of minutes at the bedside.[19]

D. Although helpful in reducing unnecessary imaging, no set of criteria is 100% reliable, and these tools should always be used in combination with history, physical examination, and the skills and knowledge of the clinician. Regardless of what tool is used, the mechanism of injury, symptoms or physical findings and age, and condition of the patient should all be taken into account and imaging should be done for any suspicion of spinal injury.

E. Determining imaging type if indicated

1. Older patients, multitrauma patients, and patients with a high suspicion for fracture should be sent directly for a CT scan.
2. Cervical x-rays may be sufficient for patients with lower risk factors and lower suspicion of fracture.[19] Plain films can be performed quickly at the patient's bedside with minimal radiation exposure as compared with CT; however, CT is more reliable.
3. If the clinician feels as though plain films only are indicated, ordering the correct views is very important.

4. Five views are often necessary to adequately rule out a cervical fracture, and all seven vertebrae must be included. These views include:.

a. Anteroposterior (AP) gives views of the vertebral bodies and intervertebral spaces.

b. Lateral evaluates spinous processes, soft tissue, the position of the vertebrae, and the facet joints.

c. Odontoid evaluates for injury to C1 and C2.

d. AP oblique images provide views of the intervertebral foramina, joints of the spine, and the pedicles from the side further from the image receptor.

e. PA oblique images provide the same view, but from the side closest to the image receptor.[20]

5. Advancements in technology have placed CT as the gold standard above plain films for evaluating spinal injuries. CT has become the chosen method of imaging in the ED, due to its high reliability, availability, and the fact that it can be performed quickly to evaluate for fractures and other bony abnormalities. CT of the cervical, thoracic, and lumbar spine are typically ordered without contrast. In the event that the CT is negative, but an acute neurologic deficit is present, an MRI should be ordered to evaluate for edema, hemorrhage, and other injuries to the spinal cord, the nerve roots that exit from the spinal cord, and the surrounding soft tissues.[11,21]

F. Spinal cord injuries can occur without evidence of radiographic abnormality (SCIWORA), which may occur in 6% to 19% of spinal injuries in children and 9% to 14% in adults. It is seen most commonly with sudden and extreme hyperextension of the neck, such as in a rear-end collision or a blow to the face.[22] Although abnormal findings on x-ray and CT may be absent, neurologic findings such as signs of spinal shock (apnea, bradycardia, and hypotension), and neurologic deficits such as numbness, tingling, weakness, and paralysis to the extremities can often be seen, however, may be delayed.[23] This underscores the importance of performing and documenting a comprehensive neurologic exam in any patient suspected of having an SCI. Therefore, if the clinician has any clinical suspicion of SCI, an MRI should be ordered.[23]

G. Lab tests such as a complete blood count (CBC) and arterial blood gas (ABG) may be necessary to assess for bleeding or respiratory compromise, a lactate level can assist in monitoring perfusion if shock is present, and additional tests such as a comprehensive metabolic profile (CMP) and a urinalysis may be ordered to evaluate for any preexisting or underlying disorders.[18,11]

Management

A. Initial management of the trauma patient with a suspected spinal injury includes immobilization and assessing and maintaining airway, breathing, and circulation.

B. If spinal instability is suspected, the cervical spine should be immobilized using a rigid cervical collar with the head stabilized with supportive blocks and straps, and a long backboard to prevent further or secondary injury to the spinal cord.

1. Recent studies have shown that spinal cord immobilization is not only unnecessary for most trauma patients but can potentially cause harm.[11,24,25]

2. Regardless of recent evidence, patients who have sustained almost any type of traumatic injury putting them at risk for a spinal injury and brought in by EMS will still be immobilized.

3. Tools such as the NEXUS Criteria or the Canadian C-Spine Rule can help to determine whether patients are at risk and can be used to guide the extent of immobilization necessary in the field. Using this logic, patients with altered level of consciousness, intoxication, spinous process tenderness, focal neurologic symptoms, distracting injury, or obvious spinal deformity should be immobilized.[11,24,25]

4. A report issued by the American College of Emergency Physicians (ACEP) in 2015 also supported the idea that the use of strict immobilization using backboards and rigid cervical collars lacked evidence to support benefit and were unnecessary in most instances, and added that the increased pain produced by immobilization devices can lead to an increase in unnecessary diagnostic imaging.

a. Prolonged immobilization can lead to increased pain, anxiety, agitation, pressure ulcers, respiratory compromise, tissue breakdown, and aspiration, and can not only make the physical exam more difficult but can increase the difficulty of necessary procedures such as intubation.

b. Cervical collars can compress the jugular veins leading to increased intracranial pressure, which could further compound a head injury.[24,25]

C. Every effort should be taken to prioritize the immobilized patient and to remove the backboard as soon as possible.

1. The log roll technique or the use of an assistive device such as a slider board should be used to main tain in-line spinal stabilization and depending on the type of injury and condition of the patient, an adequate amount of staff should be at the bedside to ensure that spinal motion restriction (SMR) of the entire spine and is maintained until the patient can be properly evaluated.[11,26]

2. A minimum of three medical personnel is required to properly maintain in-line stabilization.

a. The person at the head of the bed maintains cervical spine immobilization and directs the rest of the team.

b. The remaining two team members should stand on one side of the bed to ensure SMR of the lumbar and thoracic spine.

c. Until evaluation takes place, a rigid cervical collar can be replaced by a semirigid one.

d. The patient should be kept supine if possible, but if unable to lie supine, such as with a patient who is vomiting, the lateral position is acceptable, but SMR must still be maintained.[11]

D. Airway, breathing, and circulation are always priorities, but if a spinal injury is suspected, careful attention to ensuring SMR should be maintained while any resuscitative procedures are being performed. A designated member of the medical team should focus on maintaining spinal immobilization during resuscitation. If intubation is required, rapid sequence orotracheal intubation is preferred.[11]

E. Shock is commonly seen in trauma patients. Shock can occur due to the SCI causing neurogenic shock or more commonly, due to hypovolemia as a result of blood loss, either internally or externally.

1. The majority of shock seen in patients with SCI is due to blood loss, so assume that this is the cause until proven otherwise.

2. Patients with hypovolemic shock will typically be tachycardic and have decreased capillary refill, whereas patient with neurogenic shock are typically bradycardic with normal capillary refill. IV fluid resuscitation should begin immediately and volume replacement using blood products should be begun if hemorrhage is suspected.[11]

a. Evaluation and treatment for the source of the bleeding should be begun immediately as well.

b. Depending on the condition of the patient, diagnostic testing for the source of hemorrhage can include CT, peritoneal lavage, and the Focused Assessment with Sonography for Trauma (FAST) exam, which can be performed quickly at the bedside.[27]

3. Neurogenic shock, also known as vasogenic shock, is a life-threatening condition that can result in multiorgan dysfunction and death.

a. It should be considered a diagnosis of exclusion until other causes of hypotension, such as blood loss, are ruled out.[9]

b. It is seen in patients who have sustained spinal cord injuries, and more commonly with complete spinal cord injury.

c. The classic symptoms are hypotension and bradycardia (systolic blood pressure [SBP] <100 mmHg and heart rate [HR] <80 bpm) and usually presents within the first 2 hours following the injury.[28,29]

d. It mainly occurs in SCIs at or above the level of T6 and is caused by the loss of sympathetic tone below the level of the injury, resulting in autonomic dysregulation and hemodynamic instability. Initial treatment is IV fluid resuscitation with an isotonic crystalloid solution to treat the hypotension while the cause(s) of the symptoms are being further evaluated.

e. The initial amount of IV fluid should be limited to 2 L due to the risk of pulmonary edema and the potential for the development of acute respiratory distress syndrome (ARDS).

f. The goal of treatment includes SBP of 90 to 100 mmHg, HR of 60 to 100 bpm in normal sinus rhythm (NSR), and urine output of >30 mL/hr.

g. Supplemental oxygen should be provided to maintain optimal perfusion, and care should be taken to prevent hypothermia. If the patient remains hypotensive despite aggressive fluid resuscitation, vasopressors to promote vasoconstriction, and inotropes to increase cardiac contractility are considered the second line.[27,28,30]

h. Norepinephrine treats both hypotension and bradycardia; therefore, it is a preferred initial treatment.[27]

i. Phenylephrine should be avoided in these patients, as it can worsen bradycardia.[21,29]

j. A urinary catheter should be placed to monitor urine output, which should be at least 0.5 mL/kg/hr and can be used to measure the patient's response to treatment.[11]

4. Spinal shock should not be confused with neurogenic shock. It is similar in presentation to neurogenic shock and is characterized by hypotension, bradycardia, and hypothermia.

a. Initially, neurologic changes may occur above the level of the injury in patients with spinal shock but subside after a few days.

b. Other key features include a loss of muscle tone, voluntary muscle movement, and reflexes due to pathophysiologic changes that take place following high-impact trauma to the spinal cord.

c. Spinal shock typically resolves within 24 hours but can last days to months following a spinal injury.[9,11,27,31,32]

d. Although difficult to treat, initial ED management of spinal shock is the same as treatment for neurogenic shock but is an ongoing process that will be continued in the ICU and will require a multidisciplinary healthcare team for the optimum outcome of the patient.[32]

F. Of note, although still commonly used, there is no clinical evidence to support the routine use of steroids in the treatment of acute spinal cord injuries. Risks of steroid use can include increased rate of sepsis, hyperglycemia, pulmonary embolism, and delayed wound healing.[9,18]

G. Head injuries are commonly seen in patients who have sustained an SCI. It is important to perform an neurologic exam to determine whether imaging of the brain is needed. If changes in mental status, focal neurologic deficits, or seizure activity is noted, a head CT without contrast should be performed to assess for an intracranial abnormality.[11]

H. Other complications that can occur following a spinal cord injury include bladder dysfunction, gastric ileus, and aspiration. Unless contraindicated, a urinary catheter should be placed to address any urinary incontinence or retention and to accurately measure urine output. Paralytic ileus following an SCI is common, so the patient should be placed nothing by mouth (NPO) initially, and once SCI is confirmed, a nasogastric tube to intermittent low wall suction should be considered. Due to the high potential for aspiration, antiemetics should be given to any patient with an SCI and suctioning should be available at the bedside for all patients and used frequently for patients with altered level of consciousness and for those who cannot control their secretions.[11]

Patient Disposition

A. Patients with spinal cord injuries will require an emergent consult with an orthopedic surgeon or a neurosurgeon.

B. The majority of patients with spinal fractures will require admission for surgical stabilization, pain management, and ongoing evaluation and treatment to prevent or reduce secondary injury.

C. While in the ED, spinal immobilization should be maintained, and the patient should be monitored closely for any changes in neurologic status and for respiratory compromise. During this time, careful assessment for any other injuries should take place and treated as indicated.

D. Cervical spine injuries

1. Most fractures and dislocations to the cervical spine will require admission to the hospital, but admission to the ICU is required for any fracture that is unstable or if a neurologic deficit is present.

2. Patients who have no radiographic abnormalities and no neurologic deficits may be discharged in most cases.

3. Acute muscle strain (whiplash) and other musculoskeletal injuries with mild to moderate pain may be treated with muscle relaxants and NSAIDs and an orthopedic or neurosurgery referral.

4. Patients who report higher levels of pain in the absence of neurologic deficits and abnormalities on imaging should be discharged home with a rigid cervical collar and referred to an orthopedist or neurosurgeon for further evaluation.[33]

E. Thoracic and lumbar spine injuries

1. The majority of traumatic fractures to the lumbar spine will require admission to the hospital, but patients with unstable fractures or neurologic deficits require admission to the ICU.

2. In some cases, patients with stable fractures and no neurologic deficits may be discharged after evaluation by a spine surgeon or neurosurgeon.

3. An example of a stable fracture that can be considered for discharge home after careful evaluation and in the absence of neurologic deficits is a compression fracture, which is also known as a wedge fracture.

F. Prior to considering any patient with a spinal fracture for discharge, ensure that the patient has been properly evaluated with a CT scan and flexion–extension x-rays to evaluate for stability and that no neurologic deficits are present. The social history of the patient should also be evaluated to ensure that the patient has someone at home to assist them and to monitor for any changes in their neurologic status. Admission should be strongly considered if the patient does not have a stable support system.[34]

G. Any patient with any type of spinal injury that is discharged home should be given strict return precautions. These patients should be advised to return to the ED immediately if they experience any new or worsening symptoms, including neurologic deficits, loss of function, or increased pain. The importance of follow-up with the appropriate orthopedic or neurology specialist should be emphasized.

References

References for this chapter are online only and can be found at https://connect.springerpub.com/content/reference-book/978-0-8261-6091-5/part/part03/toc-part/ch27.

28. Neck Injuries

ALLIE T. GILBERT | CHRIS GISNESS

Learning Objectives

- Identify common traumatic neck injuries.
- Discuss the initial management of neck trauma.
- Identify the zones of the neck.
- List the soft and hard signs of neck trauma.
- Identify specific diagnostic testing for neck trauma.
- Discuss the treatment of specific neck injuries.

Neck trauma is most often due to blunt or penetrating trauma, and accounts for about 1% of traumatic injuries. Vascular injuries, which are the most common cervical neck injury, occur in up to 40% of patients with penetrating neck trauma.[1] The emergency clinician must be able to recognize and treat the complications of neck trauma because they may be life-threatening due to airway compromise and hemorrhage.

Motor vehicle crashes are the major cause of blunt trauma. Other causes are secondary to assaults, falls, and strangulation, including from hanging. Blunt vascular neck injury occurs in about 1% of this type of injury and is considered rare. Loss of airway, rather than hemorrhage, is the major cause of death.[2]

Penetrating trauma is usually secondary to ballistic injuries and stab wounds. High-velocity missiles can penetrate soft tissue and bones, and most often, their pathway is predictable. Flying debris and sharp penetrating objects can impale into the neck and cause significant injury. Gunshot wounds are more likely to cause vascular injury and injury to the digestive esophageal system. The leading cause of death in penetrating neck injuries is vascular injury.[3,4]

Anatomy

A. The neck is composed of many vital structures, and trauma to the neck can result in damage to various organs and systems including

1. Respiratory
2. Vascular
3. Skeletal
4. Gastrointestinal
5. Nervous
6. Endocrine
7. Lymphatic

B. The neck is divided into three zones to guide management of injuries (see Table 28.1). Dividing the neck into zones also makes for easier communication when describing the injury and other possible injuries.[5]

1. Zone I
   a. Includes the base of the neck and extends from the cricoid cartilage to the sternal notch and clavicles

TABLE 28.1 ANATOMIC ZONES AND STRUCTURE OF THE NECK

	ZONE I	ZONE II	ZONE III
Anatomic landmarks	Clavicles to the cricoid cartilage	Cricoid cartilage to the angle of the mandible	Angle of the mandible and the base of the skull
Structures contained	Proximal common carotid artery	Carotid artery	Distal carotid artery
	Vertebral artery	Vertebral artery	Vertebral artery
	Subclavian artery	Larynx	Distant jugular vein
	Major vessels of upper extremity	Trachea	Salivary and parotid glands
	Apices of the lungs	Esophagus	Cranial nerves IX–XII
	Esophagus	Pharynx	Spinal cord
	Trachea	Jugular vein	
	Thyroid	Vagus nerve	
	Thoracic duct	Recurrent laryngeal nerve	
	Spinal cord	Spinal cord	

Source: Adapted from Bean, AS. Trauma to the neck. In: Tintinalli JE, Stapczynski JS, Ma OJ, Yealy DM, Meckler GD, Cline DM, eds. *Emergency Medicine: A Comprehensive Guide*. 9th ed. McGraw-Hill; 2020: 1722.[1]

b. Injury to this area can affect the mediastinal structures.
c. The proximal carotid and vertebral arteries, major thoracic vessels, superior mediastinum, lungs, esophagus, trachea, thoracic duct, and spinal cord are major structures in this area.
2. Zone II
a. Area of the midneck between the cricoid cartilage and the angle of the mandible
b. It is the most exposed area and is of high concern for injuries that penetrate the platysma muscle.
c. Major structures include the carotid and vertebral arteries, jugular veins, esophagus, trachea, larynx, and spinal cord.
d. Common areas that are injured include the common carotid artery, internal jugular vein, esophagus, and trachea.[4,6]
e. These injuries typically require surgical exploration.
f. Zone II injuries are the most common type of neck injuries, but Zone I has the highest mortality.[6]
3. Zone III
a. This zone is the area of the upper neck and extends from the angle of the mandible to the base of the skull.
b. The major structures in this area include the distal carotid and vertebral arteries, pharynx, and spinal cord.[1]

C. The neck is additionally divided into triangles and fascial planes.
1. The anterior and posterior triangles are separated by the sternocleidomastoid muscle.
a. The anterior triangle
i. Composed of many vital structures
ii. The anterior triangle is composed of the area bordered
(1) Anteriorly by the midline of the neck
(2) Posteriorly by the sternocleidomastoid muscle
(3) Superiorly by the lower mandibular edge
b. The posterior triangle
i. The posterior triangle is composed of the area bordered
(1) Posteriorly by the anterior border of the trapezius muscle
(2) Anteriorly by the sternocleidomastoid muscle
(3) Inferiorly to the clavicle
c. The anterior neck structures are particularly vulnerable to injury compared to posterior neck injuries, which have a better outcome with the exception of spinal trauma.[6]
2. The fascial layers are composed of the superficial cervical fascial layer and the deep cervical fascial layer.
a. Superficial cervical fascia
i. Composed of platysma muscle, a thin layer of muscle overlying the sternocleidomastoid muscle spanning from the facial muscles to the thorax[5]
ii. Wounds penetrating through the platysma muscle are considered deep wounds and warrant further evaluation.
iii. Wounds that do not penetrate through the platysma are considered superficial and are less concerning for serious injury because they do not affect deeper neck structures.
b. Deep cervical fascia
i. Composed of the investing, pretracheal, and prevertebral fascia.
ii. Carotid sheath is also located within the deep cervical fascia.
iii. The continuity of the pretracheal fascia with the anterior mediastinum makes patients with aerodigestive injuries specifically at risk for developing mediastinitis.
iv. Hemorrhage may be confined to any single compartment, but pressure from large hematomas can cause airway compromise.

D. Neck circulation
1. With any vascular injury to the neck, a multitude of injuries can occur and must be considered in the differential diagnosis.[7]
2. Vascular structures in the neck are considered high risk for injury and include the
a. Carotid arteries
b. Subclavian arteries
c. Vertebral arteries
d. Internal and external and jugular veins
3. Anterior brain circulation
a. Composed of anterior and middle cerebral arteries
i. Arise from internal carotid arteries and supply the forebrain.
(1) Originate from the circle of Willis
(2) Give rise to branches that supply the cortex and that penetrate the
(a) Basal ganglia
(b) Thalamus
(c) Internal capsule
(3) Middle cerebral artery branch goes into the lenticulostriate arteries that supply the
(a) Basal ganglia
(b) Thalamus
4. Posterior brain circulation
a. Composed of arterial branches arising from the posterior cerebral, basilar, and vertebral arteries.
b. Supply blood to the midbrain, cerebellum, occipital lobe, and medial temporal lobes.
c. The circle of Willis, which communicates between the anterior and posterior circulation, is intact in approximately 20% of people.[6]

Pathophysiology

A. The pathophysiology of neck injuries varies with the location and mechanism of injury. Structures of the neck are discussed in the Anatomy section of this chapter.

B. This chapter divides the pathophysiology of neck trauma into

1. Penetrating or blunt
   a. Tracheobronchial
   b. Pharyngoesophageal
   c. Laryngotracheal (LT)
   d. Vascular
2. Blunt
   a. Strangulation

C. Penetrating neck injuries

1. Penetrating neck injuries involve only a small percentage of traumatic injuries; however, the mortality rate can be as high as 10%.[1]
   a. These wounds are caused by bullets, glass, shrapnel, and knives.
   b. Bullets from guns cause aerodigestive and vascular injuries.
   c. Injuries due to a higher velocity are more likely to cause death.
2. Gunshot wounds are divided into low and high velocity.
   a. Shots from low-velocity weapons follow irregular trajectories along a pathway of least resistance and can result in a pellet embolus to the heart or other organs.[1,6]
   b. A high-velocity weapon produces more extensive damage than a low-velocity weapon.
   c. Gunshot wounds usually cause greater injury because they can penetrate deeper into the body and cause cavitation.
   d. A gunshot wound to the neck usually requires surgical exploration.[5,6]
3. A stab wound is unpredictable, and the depth and path of penetration may violate the platysma muscle and be misleading.
4. Wounds that enter the platysma muscle require a surgical consult,[5,6] and wounds with hard signs of injury usually require immediate operative exploration.[4]

D. Tracheobronchial injuries (TBIs)

1. TBIs are rare but potentially life-threatening, and occur between the cricoid cartilage and right and left main-stem tracheal bifurcation.[8]
   a. Injuries that occur within 1 inch of the carina have a high mortality rate and are most commonly caused by penetrating mechanisms.
   b. A clothesline injury, which is a direct blow to the neck, may cause this injury.
2. TBIs can occur
   a. In the trauma setting and be caused by instrumentation during intubation and tracheostomy placement.
   b. In blunt trauma in a patient with multiple severe injuries that involve the intrathoracic trachea.
   c. Following hyperextension injuries or direct force such as weightlifting injuries, strangulation, or seat belt injuries.
   d. Immediately following a direct impact of the neck against the steering wheel.
3. Penetrating injuries are most likely secondary to gunshot wounds or stab wounds and account for about 5% to 10% of traumatic neck injuries.[3,4]
4. In children, the larynx may be injured but typically does not fracture because of the flexibility of the cartilage.

E. Pharyngoesophageal injuries (PEIs)

1. PEIs, which are rare and often occult, are associated with a high morbidity and mortality.[3]
2. PEI often occurs during a sudden acceleration or deceleration mechanism in which the neck was fully extended.[1]
3. Signs and symptoms upon presentation may be subtle, and their onset is often delayed.
4. Patients who present with a suspected aerodigestive injury should undergo an endoscopy to define their injury.

F. LT injuries

1. LT injuries can occur in 2% to 5% of patients with penetrating trauma.[1]
2. Patients with hard signs of LT injury need early airway control and operative intervention (Table 28.2).

TABLE 28.2 SOFT AND HARD SIGNS OF NECK INJURY

SOFT SIGNS	HARD SIGNS
Minor hemoptysis	Rapidly expanding or pulsatile hematoma
Nonpulsatile, nonexpanding hematoma	Massive hemoptysis
Oropharyngeal bleeding	Air bubbling from wound
History of arterial bleeding	Severe hemorrhage
Hypotension in the field	Shock unresponsive to intravenous fluids
Dysphonia	Decreased or absent radial pulses
Dysphagia	Vascular bruit or thrill
Neurologic findings	Stridor, hoarseness, or airway compromise
Proximity wound	Cerebral ischemia
	+/- Massive subcutaneous hematoma
	Hematemesis

Source: Adapted from Bean, AS. Trauma to the neck. In: Tintinalli JE, Stapczynski JS, Ma OJ, Yealy DM, Meckler GD, Cline DM, eds. *Emergency Medicine: A Comprehensive Guide*. 9th ed. McGraw-Hill; 2020:1724, Table 260-5.[1]

3. Blunt LT injury occurs in less than 1% of patients. The mechanism of injury is usually secondary to a motor vehicle crash from a direct force from a shoulder restraint or the neck striking the dash or steering wheel.[6]

a. Clothesline injuries, hangings, assaults, and attempted strangulation are examples of the mechanism of injury.

4. The larynx is protected by the mandible, making these injuries rare, although the cricoid cartilage can be fractured and cause death.

G. Vascular neck injuries

1. Complications of vascular neck trauma include the following:

a. Exsanguination, secondary to penetrating injuries

b. Distortion of the airway

c. Hematoma formation that can lead to vascular occlusion or embolization from a penetrating wound, such as from a gunshot

2. Blunt vascular injuries are rare and have been termed blunt cerebrovascular injury.

a. The mortality rate for blunt vascular injuries is around 60%.[6]

b. The internal carotid artery is most often injured, followed by the vertebral artery.[6]

c. If a vascular neck injury is found, a complication such as carotid dissection should be considered.

d. Although not discussed in this chapter, blunt neck trauma can cause injury to the spinal column.

3. Penetrating vascular injuries occur in about 25% of all neck injuries; 37% of deep penetrating injuries have some vascular injury involvement.[6]

a. Trauma to the neck that penetrates a large vessel can lead to hemorrhage or shock and may produce a hematoma that occludes the airway.

b. Deep large lacerations in the jugular veins can produce an air embolism, causing hypotension and respiratory distress.

c. If the injury involves the platysma muscle and hard signs of injury are present, the patient may require interventional angiography.

d. If there is no involvement within the platysma muscle, the patient may be observed.

e. If there are soft signs of injury and any suspicion for LT injury, an endoscopy is done.

f. In most of these cases, a CT angiogram (CTA) should be done.[6,7]

4. Ongoing evaluation should continue because vascular injuries may not be readily apparent and occur later in the physical examination.

H. Strangulation injuries

1. Strangulation injuries are considered blunt neck trauma. The mechanism of injury may be

a. Hanging

b. Postural strangulation

c. Ligature strangulation

d. Manual strangulation

e. Accidental

i. An individual may become entangled in machinery.

ii. An individual may experience autoerotic asphyxia, that is, choking oneself during sexual stimulation, or self-strangulation by another person, with a ligature to produce a euphoric state caused by cerebral hypoxia[9]

2. Hanging is the second most common means of suicide in the United States.

3. Death in strangulation is due to cerebral anoxia and ischemia from obstruction of cerebral venous return, rather than from acute airway compromise.

a. When both external and internal jugular veins are simultaneously compressed and occluded, cerebral vascular congestion and edema and unconsciousness result. Once limp, the force on the neck can tighten further and lead to complete arterial occlusion, brain injury, and death.

b. A LT fracture, cervical spine injuries, and carotid artery injury may also occur.

c. Vagal reflexes can cause fatal dysrhythmias and increased sympathetic tone from pericarotid pressure.

d. Survivors of hangings may have hypoxic-ischemic brain injury. Pulmonary injury may occur from neurogenic sequelae, such as hemiplegia, paraplegia or quadriplegia, postobstructive, and cardiogenic pulmonary edema.[10]

Predisposing Factors

A. The neck is susceptible to injury secondary to the location and mechanism of trauma. There are many critical structures in the neck that if injured can cause significant and life-threatening complications, such as airway compromise, hemorrhage, and neurological injuries.

B. Flying debris and/or sharp penetrating objects can impale into the neck and cause significant injury.

C. Gunshot wounds and penetrating objects are more likely to cause injury to the aerodigestive system, as well as vascular injury than other mechanisms.

D. Blunt trauma to the neck is most likely due to motor vehicle crashes, assaults, falls, and strangulation.

E. Loss of airway rather than hemorrhage is the major cause of death in neck trauma, except for penetrating trauma in which death is usually from hemorrhage.[1]

Physical Examination

A. The initial physical examination in trauma is best accomplished by following the Advanced Trauma Life Support (ATLS) guidelines.[2] An initial rapid but thorough examination is essential to determine the type and severity of all injuries.

1. Airway

a. Physical examination begins with the airway, looking for signs of airway obstruction or compromise.

b. Signs of airway obstruction include

i. Stridor; must have a low threshold for intubation if this occurs

ii. Agitation

iii. Confusion, suggesting hypoxia

iv. Intercostal retractions

v. Supraclavicular retractions
vi. Low oxygen saturation

c. Cyanosis, indicating hypoxemia, which may be difficult to see in a pigmented skin, and can be a late sign

d. A patient with neck trauma should be assumed to have a difficulty with airway. The clinician should consider the following elements for neck trauma:

i. Several mnemonics can be used, but SOAP-ME from Sulton, Middlebrooks, and Taylor is appropriate for neck trauma.[11] This mnemonic includes the following:

(1) *Suction:* Appropriately sized suction catheter and tonsillar suction catheter

(a) Airway obstruction can result from bleeding or vomitus, which require suctioning.

(2) *Oxygen:* Adequate oxygen supply, flow meters, and appropriate delivery devices

(3) Airway: Appropriately sized airway equipment, nasopharyngeal airway, oral airway, laryngoscope blades in working condition, and bag-valve mask

(4) *Pharmacy:* All resuscitation medications, all reversal drugs, and sedatives and sedative antagonists

(5) *Monitors:* Pulse oximeter, blood pressure cuffs, electrocardiogram (EKG), stethoscopes, and end-tidal carbon dioxide monitoring

(6) *Extra equipment:* Surgical supplies for a difficult airway, videoscopes, and fiber optics

e. Equipment required for securing an airway may include

i. Basic oxygen nasal cannula
ii. Bag-valve mask
iii. Laryngeal mask airway (LMA)
iv. Endotracheal (ET) tubes for intubation
v. Needle cricothyrotomy supplies; surgical cricothyrotomy may be necessary.
vi. Tracheostomy supplies; tracheostomy may be required but would be deferred to a trauma surgeon.

f. A patient with significant vascular injury can develop a hematoma, which can cause displacement and obstruction of the airway.

2. Breathing

a. Breathing is assessed by auscultating for breath sounds.

b. Snoring, gurgling, stridor, or hoarseness may be a sign of airway obstruction.

c. Hemothorax and tension pneumothorax can occur in patients with penetrating neck trauma.[2]

i. Hemothorax may occur in patients with neck trauma, depending on the site of injury.[2]

(1) Signs include flat neck veins, decreased breath sounds, dullness on percussion, and trachea at the midline.

(2) If hemothorax is suspected, a 28- to 32-French chest tube is inserted at the fifth intercostal space, anterior to the midaxillary line.

(a) If 1500 mL of blood or more is returned, blood transfusion is indicated.

(b) The patient may require a thoracotomy, at which time a trauma surgeon who is experienced and trained should perform this procedure.

ii. Tension pneumothorax occurs when air leaks from the lung through the chest wall and is forced into the pleural space without escaping.[12]

(a) Signs include a mediastinal shift to the opposite side, which decreases venous return and compresses the lung, unilateral breath sounds, hyperresonant sounds upon percussion, hypotension, and respiratory distress.

(b) Late signs include distended neck veins and tracheal deviation.

(c) Tension pneumothorax and pericardial tamponade may be confused because the signs are similar. However, a tension pneumothorax would percuss hyperresonant and unilateral or decreased breath sounds are usually heard on the side of the injury. In cardiac tamponade, the key finding is muffled heart sounds.[2]

(d) Treatment involves emergent needle decompression; if the intervention is needed, it should be performed according to the latest version of the American College of Surgeons Advanced Trauma Life Support Course (ATLS).[2]

(e) The patient requires supplemental oxygen, end-tidal carbon dioxide monitoring, and continuous pulse oximetry.

3. Circulation

a. Bleeding to the point of exsanguination is a common cause of death in penetrating neck injury.

i. Direct pressure to the wound is essential in controlling bleeding; avoid the application of pressure to both carotid arteries at the same time.
ii. Blindly clamping neck vessels is not recommended.
iii. Open wounds should be covered and compressed to control bleeding and prevent an air embolus.
iv. Neck wounds are not probed to avoid the chance of massive hemorrhage or blood clots being dislodged.
v. If bleeding is heavy and continues, a trauma surgeon should be consulted.
vi. Shock is treated with intravenous fluids and blood, as indicated per ATLS protocols[2]:

(1) O-positive blood for males and O-negative blood for females of child-bearing age[13]

(2) Two large-bore intravenous catheters should be inserted but placed in the extremity on the opposite side of the injured neck.
(3) A 16- or 18-French gauge urinary catheter may be inserted into the wound to stop bleeding, but a trauma surgeon should be consulted.

b. A venous or arterial air embolism is a complication that can cause shock or cardiac arrest and is usually unresponsive to intravenous fluids and/or a thoracotomy.

i. If an air embolism is suspected, the patient should be placed in a head-down, left-lateral decubitus position. This position will cause intracardiac air to accumulate in the apex of the right ventricle.[3]

ii. Aspiration of the air from the right apex of the ventricle can be done using ultrasound-guided pericardiocentesis.

(1) Placing the patient in the left-lateral decubitus position may buy time until the trauma surgeon is available. The procedure is controversial; some believe the patient should be put in a more neutral position.[3]

c. An extended focused physical examination with sonography in trauma (eFAST) should be part of the circulation evaluation.[2] This exam is aimed at identifying the free fluid in the abdomen and the pericardium, along with a possible pneumothorax, and free fluid in the pleural space.

4. Exposure

a. The patient should be completely undressed, including the removal of all jewelry, and thoroughly exposed to assess for all injuries, particularly in the neck.

b. The axilla, perineum, scalp, and skin folds should be examined.

c. The patient should be kept warm by warming lights, a heated room, and blankets.

5. Additional adjuncts

a. A nasogastric (NG) tube is a relative contraindication in a patient with penetrating neck injury and should be avoided in case there is neck distortion. Exceptions may include if positive pressure ventilation is used.

b. A patient with a known vascular or suspected vascular or aerodigestive injury should undergo invasive interventions under the care of a trauma surgeon.

c. Frequent and thorough examination is required, and the patient should be reassessed frequently to avoid overlooking any injuries.

d. The patient with a penetrating neck trauma is at risk for injury if the platysma muscle is violated and should be assessed for vascular, upper, and esophageal injuries.

e. The severity of neck trauma and management of neck trauma can be evaluated by the use of hard and soft signs, which are included in Table 28.2.[1]

f. Never probe a wound. Assume that a deeper structure is involved.[14]

g. Any impaled objects should be stabilized to prevent displacement and should never be removed.

6. Disability

a. Spinal cord injury can occur in patients with penetrating neck injuries and is most often evident at the time the patient presents to the ED.

b. In an awake, alert, neurologically intact patient with no distracting injuries, a cervical collar is unnecessary in most cases because the collar can obscure the neck and eliminate proper evaluation and physical examination of the neck.[3]

c. A patient with an altered mental status (AMS) before the exam needs a cervical collar placed.

Differential Diagnoses

A. It is important to distinguish a seat belt sign from a neck hematoma.

1. A neck hematoma is a more concerning finding because this injury could lead to airway compromise.

B. Although rare, esophageal injuries are easy to miss and are critical to the early identification of complications from leakage of orogastric contents, which can lead to infection or mediastinitis.[6]

C. Differential diagnoses

1. Massive hemorrhage of the neck secondary to penetrating trauma
2. Tension pneumothorax secondary to penetrating neck trauma
3. Pharyngeal perforation secondary to penetrating neck trauma
4. Mediastinitis secondary to penetrating PEI
5. Blunt cerebral vascular injury secondary to hyperextension of the neck resulting in dissection
6. Pseudoaneurysm secondary to blunt carotid or vertebral artery injury to the neck
7. Airway occlusion secondary to expanding neck hematoma
8. Occult esophageal injury secondary to penetrating neck trauma
9. Aspiration pneumonia secondary to near-hanging, strangulation

Diagnostic Testing

A. Diagnostic testing in the ED for neck trauma is most often reserved for the stable patient.

1. Hemodynamically unstable patients typically go straight to surgery, bypassing diagnostic testing.
2. CT angiography (CTA) is recommended.
3. Patients with soft signs of trauma who have stable vital signs will have diagnostic imaging done to further assess injures.

B. Diagnostic tests include the following:

1. Radiographs of the head, neck, and chest can be done to assess for fragments, pneumothorax, or hemothorax. The transfer of a patient to another facility or to surgery should never be delayed to obtain any radiographs of the head and neck.
2. Bedside eFAST ultrasound

3. Diagnostic imaging, such as CT scan and CTA, in stable patients with penetrating trauma can reduce unnecessary surgical explorations, and in turn, can reduce cost, length of stay, and morbidity and mortality.[15] New generation scanners produce high-quality pictures. Some literature recommends CTA as the diagnostic study of choice for a patient who is hemodynamically stable and does not have hard signs of trauma to assess for aerodigestive track and vascular injuries.[15]
   a. CTA is the preferred imaging in patients with penetrating neck injury that do not require immediate surgery.
   b. Angiography remains the gold standard.[5,10]
   c. If a significant injury is suspected, there should be no delay in obtaining advanced images.
4. Color flow Doppler ultrasound is highly sensitive for detecting important vascular injuries, is portable and noninvasive, has no ionizing radiation, and is less costly than other medical imaging modalities. Disadvantages include the inability to scan through subcutaneous tissues, hematoma formations, and bone, and it cannot be used to evaluate the aerodigestive structures of the neck. And it is not the recommended test of choice.[1,3]

Emergency Care for Specific Neck Injuries

A. Penetrating neck injuries
   1. Physical examination
      a. Patients with penetrating neck injuries may present with many signs and symptoms, but they may be subtle, nonspecific, and minimal. During the initial physical examination, external wounds can be easily missed; therefore, the clinician must know what injuries and structures could be involved. Signs and symptoms such as stridor, dyspnea, drooling, external bleeding, or hematoma formation should be monitored frequently. Signs and symptoms may also include decreasing mental status, respiratory distress, dysphagia, hematemesis, stridor, crepitus, and focal neurologic deficit.[3] The clinician should look for soft and hard signs of injury. Refer to Table 28.2.
   2. Management
      a. Anticipate that airway management may be difficult. All equipment should be available at the bedside. The SOAP-ME mnemonic (**S**uction, **O**xygen, **A**irway, **P**harmacy, **M**onitors, **E**xtra equipment) helps with management of neck injuries, since anatomical airways may be distorted and will likely call for advanced airway procedures. Table 28.1 identifies the significant structures involved.
      b. For the patient who arrives in a cervical collar is stable, and has no neurologic deficits, the collar may be removed to better evaluate for injuries.
      c. A cervical collar is often used for patients who have hard signs of injury, such as air bubbling from the wound, pulsatile bleeding, expanding hematoma, a thrill, or bruit, and in a patient younger than 50 years old or with any signs of cerebrovascular injury or hematemesis. Once the cervical spine is cleared, the collar would most likely be removed, but the patient would need to go to surgery for exploration.
      d. After the airway is established, breath sounds and vital signs should be frequently assessed.
      e. If there are signs of tension pneumothorax, this condition should be treated with a needle thoracostomy followed by a chest tube.
      f. Impaled objects should be stabilized.
      g. Two large-bore intravenous catheters should be placed in the contralateral extremity to the penetrating neck wound, if possible.
      h. The bleeding should be stopped initially by direct pressure and shock treated.
      i. If there are signs of vascular injury that would cause neurological deficits, such as hemiplegia, absent pulses, bruits, thrills, or expanding hematoma, consult a trauma surgeon and/or neurosurgeon, depending on the type of injury, and add to the trauma team.[3]
      j. Penetrating wounds that do not violate the platysma may be managed in the ED, and the patient may be discharged according to recommendations of a trauma surgeon. Patients with significant injury are likely to be admitted and their care transferred to a surgeon.[6]
      k. If there are no hard signs and a low suspicion of injury, the patient is observed. If there is a suspicious wound on CT or signs of aerodigestive injury, the patient requires direct laryngoscopy, bronchoscopy, esophagogastroduodenoscopy, or upper GI (gastrografin then barium).

B. Tracheobronchial injuries
   1. Physical examination
      a. The patient with traumatic brain injury (TBI) is likely to present with
         i. Hemoptysis
         ii. Subcutaneous emphysema
         iii. Pneumothorax
         iv. Respiratory distress, such as dyspnea, decreased or absent breath sounds, tachypnea, stridor, or hoarseness
         v. Associated spinal injury
      b. The patient with penetrating injuries is likely to present with
         i. An air leak or bubbling from the neck wound
         ii. Mediastinal emphysema
         iii. Hemoptysis
         iv. Possible spinal injury[8]
   2. Diagnosis
      a. Specific findings on imaging, such as CT scan or bronchoscopy, that would confirm or be considered for TBI include the following:
         i. Air in soft tissue
         ii. Hyoid bone elevated above the third cervical vertebrate
         iii. Pneumothorax
         iv. Air in the wall of the trachea or mainstem bronchus

b. A patient with TBI may have an abnormal endotracheal intubation or distended endotracheal tube cuff from protrusion from the trachea.[8]
c. The definitive diagnosis is made upon seeing the injury during the clinical examination or doing surgical exploration or bronchoscopy.

3. Management
a. If TBI is suspected, a trauma surgeon and/or anesthesiologist should be called for immediate intervention. The patient is admitted under the care of a trauma surgeon.
b. The preferred management of TBI is endobronchial intubation over a flexible bronchoscope that can aid in the identification, location, and severity of the injury.[2,8,12,16] A smaller endotracheal tube or emergency cricothyrotomy may be indicated.[12]

C. PEIs
1. Physical examination
a. Patients may present with subtle signs that can result in delay of care and an increase in mortality.
b. There are no hard signs of injury, but soft signs to consider are listed in Table 28.2.
c. The patient may present with
i. Subcutaneous emphysema
ii. Dysphagia
iii. Odynophagia
iv. Blood in the salvia
v. Hematemesis
d. Other signs and symptoms to consider include
i. Neck pain
ii. Hoarseness
iii. Cough
iv. Stridor
v. Decreased neck range of motion
e. PEI with air leaking from the wound is the most common sign of an esophageal or airway injury.
f. Contamination can occur secondary to orogastric contents with bacteria and can lead to abscess formation, mediastinitis, and sepsis.[6] Death can occur from sepsis and mediastinitis.[12]

2. Diagnosis
a. Radiographs of the neck and chest may reveal esophageal perforation if pneumomediastinum, hydrothorax, or retropharyngeal air is present.
b. Contrast esophagography may be done.
c. CTA is the image of choice to evaluate the vasculature and soft tissues.
d. CTA without contrast is not supported, although a CT scan may see the trajectory if a bullet was the mechanism of injury and is secondary to a penetrating injury.
e. Symptomatic patients who do not meet criteria for neck exploration can be evaluated by direct esophagoscopy or swallowing studies. Esophagoscopy is more sensitive.
f. Patients who are asymptomatic can be evaluated for injuries with a multidetector computed tomographic angiography (MDCTA).

3. Management
a. Patients with PEIs are likely surgical candidates and may receive intravenous antibiotics.
b. Small pharyngeal perforations may be managed nonsurgically.
c. Perforations greater than 2 cm require surgical repair. The patient is admitted and care transferred to the consulting team.

D. LT injuries
1. Physical examination
a. Signs of blunt LT injuries may not appear initially, but progress because of airway edema and/or hematoma that can result in an airway obstruction.
b. The individual may have mucosal disruption, exposed cartilage, or a displaced fracture.
c. Bubbling air from the wound is considered a hard sign and indicates injury if subcutaneous air is palpated over the larynx, indicating a fracture until proven otherwise.
d. Presenting signs and symptoms include[1,3,6]
i. Tenderness over the larynx
ii. Hemoptysis
iii. Loss of anatomic landmarks
iv. Dysphonia
v. Aphonia
vi. Dyspnea
vii. Stridor
e. Patients with LT may not tolerate lying flat and need the head of the bed elevated.[6]
f. LT may be overlooked secondary to other multisystem trauma.

2. Diagnosis
a. Flexible fiberoptic laryngoscopy may be used to determine the extent of the injury and can define airway patency.
b. CT is the imaging of choice for the patient without airway compromise.
c. Plain radiographs may be done to evaluate for edema, foreign body, and fracture.

3. Management
a. Secure the airway.
b. Airway disruption can occur immediately but is often delayed; therefore, the patient requires close monitoring. Patients who have no identified injury with neck pain may be monitored in the ED for 12 hours and discharged with the recommendation of a trauma surgeon.[6]
c. If an LT injury is suspected, early laryngoscopy should be done.
i. Fiberoptic-guided oral intubation is the best choice. A video laryngoscope may be used with consideration to perform a surgical airway, which may be done in the ED. A tracheostomy is done in the operating room if time permits.
d. Care of the patient with an LT injury is typically transferred to a consulting trauma surgeon.
e. Small mucosal injuries can be managed with humidified air, analgesia antireflux medications, vocal rest, and clear diet.[6]

E. Strangulation
1. Physical examination
a. Presenting signs
i. Visual disturbances, subconjunctival petechiae
ii. Swollen tongue or oropharynx, mild cough, hoarseness
iii. Blood in the oropharynx
iv. Facial edema or edema to the neck
v. Altered mental status (AMS)
vi. Seizures
vii. Symptoms of stroke[10]
b. The patient should be evaluated for hard signs of neck trauma (Box 28.1).

BOX 28.1 HARD SIGNS OF STRANGULATION

- Visual disturbances
- Conjunctival or facial petechial hemorrhages
- Swelling of the tongue or oropharynx
- Blood or vomit in the oropharynx
- Facial swelling, lacerations abrasion bruising
- Neck abrasions, ligature marks, tenderness over the larynx
- Hoarseness or stridor
- Crepitus palpated
- Cyanosis or hypoxia
- Respiratory distress, rales wheezes, cough
- Dysrhythmias
- Altered mental status, seizures, stroke-like symptoms
- Incontinence

Source: From Dunn RJ, Smock W. Strangulation injuries. 2017. StatPearls. https://www.ncbi.nlm.nih.gov/books/NBK459192/.[16]

c. The external neck should be checked for visible signs of petechiae, contusions, and ligature marks.[10]
d. The patient may be asymptomatic upon presentation.
e. Tardieu's spots, which are highly correlated with asphyxial deaths, are petechial hemorrhages seen in the conjunctiva, mucous membranes, and skin cephalad to the ligature marks.
f. Thyroid cartilage or hyoid bone fractures may be seen along with tenderness to palpation over the larynx or hoarseness.
2. Diagnostic testing
a. Patients who present with a strangulation injury should have a brain CT and neck CTA.
b. Endoscopy may be required if there are symptoms of a laryngeal injury. If so, a laryngobronchoscopy may be needed.
3. Management
a. Initial management should follow the Advanced Trauma Life Support (ATLS) guidelines of airway, breathing, circulation, and disability, including cervical spine immobilization. Endotracheal intubation may be required.
b. Monitor for cardiac dysrhythmias.
c. Patients with platysma muscle injury should be admitted to surgical services.
d. A patient with altered mental status should be considered to have cerebral edema and increased intracranial pressure and treated as such.
e. In strangulation injuries, the signs and symptoms may be delayed. Therefore, the patient should be frequently monitored to allow for early identification and treatment of visceral or vascular injury.
f. Patients with abnormal findings on CT scan or CTA should be admitted; patients with normal findings should be closely observed.
g. The patient should be evaluated thoroughly by psychiatry and checked frequently for signs of self-harm.
h. Patients who are asymptomatic with normal mental status may be discharged home to a family or friend who can provide monitoring.
i. Strict return to the ED instructions should be explained, including delayed respiratory or neurological signs and symptoms.
i. Strangled patients or victims of domestic violence need social service and possible safe shelter placement.

F. Vascular neck trauma
1. Physical examination
a. Most signs and symptoms develop between 10 and 72 hours of onset; up to one-third of patients may not develop any symptoms for more than 24 hours.[6]
b. If the injury involves the platysma muscle and there are hard signs of vascular injury, the patient may require interventional angiography or go directly to surgery.
c. The major concern for vascular neck trauma includes dissection of carotid or vertebral vasculature and subsequent stroke.
d. Presenting signs and symptoms
i. Any real or potential arterial hemorrhage from the neck, mouth, nose, or ear
ii. Expanding cervical hematoma
iii. Cervical bruit in patients under the age of fifty
iv. Ataxia, emesis, dizziness, or visual field deficits may be signs of vertebral injuries.[6]
v. The majority of patients with blunt cerebrovascular injury have no acute neurologic indicators at the onset of presentation, and signs tend to occur several hours later.[7]
e. Risk factors for vascular neck trauma include patients with
i. Injury from high-velocity mechanisms
ii. Significant facial trauma
iii. Complex skull fractures
iv. Basal skull fractures
v. Occipital condyle fracture
vi. Petrous bone fracture
vii. Diffuse axonal injury with Glasgow Coma Scale (GCS) score less than 8
viii. Cervical vertebral fractures, subluxation, or ligamentous injury with thoracic injury

ix. Blunt cardiac rupture
x. Upper rib fractures
xi. Expanding hematoma
(1) A seat belt injury with swelling and altered mental status must be evaluated to rule out an expanding hematoma.

f. In children, the incidence of blunt vascular injury is lower but must be evaluated; management is the same as for adults.

2. Diagnosis
a. Rapid diagnosis and treatment are essential when a blunt vascular injury of the neck is suspected.
b. CTA is the gold standard for the diagnosis of blunt cerebral vascular injury.
c. Ultrasound is not recommended and should not be used.
d. Magnetic resonance angiogram (MRA) has a variable sensitivity and should not be used unless the patient has absolute contraindications to iodinated contrast (bean tint).

3. Management
a. An airway should be established and maintained.
b. Life-threatening injuries are treated according to the ATLS protocols submitted by the college of surgeons.
i. Shock should be treated per ATLS protocols.[2]
c. Blunt vascular injury management depends on the type of injury and may include anticoagulation, but care is likely to be transferred to a consulting team.
d. Stroke should be considered and antithrombotic agents, such as aspirin, clopidogrel, or heparin, given.
e. The trauma team should be consulted early.
f. Preparing for the patient for surgery is necessary for an acute injury.

Patient Disposition

A. Most patients with penetrating or blunt injuries to the neck are admitted to a trauma center.
B. Patients with significant injuries may be taken to surgery for resuscitation and stabilization.
C. Hospital admission is usually required for any patient with penetrating trauma that violates the platysma and for those patients with significant blunt trauma.
1. If the platysma is intact and has been evaluated thoroughly, after a period of observation the patient may be discharged, with follow-up with a surgeon.
D. Patients who present with initially nonthreatening injuries, but have injury to the airway or aerodigestive tract, and those with a possible visceral or vascular injury should be admitted for close observation for potential worsening of injuries.
E. Patients who present with strangulation or hanging, especially those with clinical findings, should be admitted for close observation to assess for deterioration and to have further evaluation with psychiatry.
1. These patients are at risk for posttraumatic stress disorder.
2. Social services follow-up is recommended.
F. If interpersonal violence was involved, those patients should be referred to social service for a safe place to return.[10]
G. Patients who present with strangulation should be observed for delayed noncardiogenic pulmonary edema.[6]
H. Superficial neck wounds can be managed according to practice standards. Repair clean wounds, but high-risk wounds or wounds greater than 12 hours should be left open to heal by secondary intention.
I. Wound care instructions should be provided.
J. Tetanus toxoid should be administered, as indicated.
K. Pain medication and antibiotics may be prescribed for penetrating neck wounds.
L. Antibiotics may be prescribed for PEIs.
M. Blunt cerebral vascular trauma patients may be prescribed antithrombotic agents.[1]

References

References for this chapter are online only and can be found at https://connect.springerpub.com/content/reference-book/978-0-8261-6091-5/part/part03/toc-part/ch28.

29. Abdominal Trauma

TIFFANY ANDREWS

Learning Objectives

- Discuss the incidence and epidemiology of abdominal trauma.
- Identify the anatomic regions of the abdomen that are critical in assessing and managing trauma patients.
- Recognize a patient who is at risk for abdominal and pelvic injuries based on mechanism of injury.
- Explain an abdominal assessment as part of a trauma exam.
- Discuss prehospital and ED management of abdominal and pelvic injuries.
- Use the appropriate diagnostic procedures to determine whether a patient has ongoing hemorrhage and/or other injuries that cause delayed morbidity and mortality.
- Identify ED care transfer and ED assessment tools.
- Identify patients who require surgical consultation and possible surgical and/or catheter-based intervention.

Principles of Trauma

A. Blunt abdominal trauma
   1. Injury results from a sudden increase of pressure to the abdomen, typically by compressive, sheering, or stretching forces.
   2. Solid organs are injured more frequently than hollow viscous organs.
   3. Solid organ injury usually manifests as hemorrhage.
   4. Hollow viscus injuries result in bleeding and peritonitis from contamination with bowel contents.
   5. Liver and spleen are the most frequently injured organs, followed by the intestines and retroperitoneal structures.
   6. Less frequently injured are the mesentery, pancreas, diaphragm, urinary bladder, urethra, and vascular structures.

B. Penetrating abdominal trauma
   1. Solid organ injury usually results in hemorrhage.
   2. Injury to both thoracic and abdominal structures occurs in 25% of cases.
   3. Most injured structures include the small bowel, liver, colon, abdominal vascular structures.

Overview of the Emergency Medicine Issue

A. Abdominal trauma is a major cause of morbidity and mortality in the United States, especially because it can be very difficult to recognize clear symptoms early.

B. In blunt force abdominal trauma, the spleen and liver are the most injured organs, with a mortality rate of roughly 8.5%.

C. Many forms of blunt abdominal trauma injuries involve vehicles. The injury pattern of blunt abdominal trauma is often diffuse and involves a compression or crushing mechanism by direct energy transmission, which can exceed the tolerance limits of the organ tissue, causing damage.

D. Injury can also be caused by movement of the abdominal organs within the body.

E. Penetrating abdominal trauma has a slightly higher mortality and morbidity rate, depending on the mechanism of injury, ranging up to about 12%.

F. Gunshot and stab wounds combine to cause 95% of penetrating abdominal injuries, with the most serious morbidities arising from wound site infections and development of intra-abdominal abscesses.

Assessment

A. It is important to do a thorough assessment of all trauma patients utilizing a systematic and comprehensive approach that includes Advanced Trauma Life Support (ATLS®) guidelines, in the order outlined, to identify injuries early and reassessing often.
   1. Primary survey
   2. Adjuncts to primary survey (including diagnostics)
   3. AMPLE history (allergies, medications, past medical history, last meal or other intake, and events leading to presentation)
   4. Secondary survey

Signs and Symptoms

A. Vital sign abnormalities, particularly tachycardia, hypotension, mild alterations in mental status, tachypnea, and/or hypoxia must prompt a thorough search for the underlying injury.

B. Blunt injuries
   1. Patients may present with a spectrum of symptoms from abdominal pain, signs of peritoneal irritation to hypovolemic shock.
   2. Delayed presentation possible with small bowel injury or splenic injuries

C. Penetrating injuries
  1. High-velocity projectile can cause extensive direct tissue damage.
  2. Exit wound may be larger than entrance wound, but small entrance wounds can conceal massive internal damage.

Signs

A. Rigidity, distention, guarding, ecchymosis (e.g., seat-belt sign, flank, periumbilical), abrasions, absence of bowel sounds (late finding), auscultation of bowel sounds in the thoracic cavity, tachycardia, hypotension, peritoneal signs, fever, open wounds on abdomen, back, or chest, Cullen's sign
B. Hypotension, narrow pulse pressure, tachycardia may reflect blood loss and significant injury.

Symptoms

A. Abdominal pain and tenderness, nausea, vomiting, labored respirations from diaphragmatic irritation or upper abdominal injury, left shoulder pain with inspiration (Kehr sign) from diaphragmatic irritation.

Associated Injury Mimics

A. Fractures, thoracic injuries, and abdominal wall injuries may mimic intra-abdominal injuries.

Focused Assessment (Advanced Trauma Life Support Guidelines)

A. General
  1. Evaluate and stabilize airway, breathing, and circulation first.
  2. Primary objective is to determine need for operative intervention.
  3. Primary and secondary surveys in trauma are repeated frequently to identify any change in patient's status and determine additional interventions.
B. Primary survey (ABCDE)
  1. Airway
    a. Assess and maintain patency.
    b. Cervical spine control
    c. Establish definitive airway with a cuffed, secured tube in the trachea if any doubt patient can maintain airway integrity.
  2. Breathing and ventilation
    a. Expose chest and neck, observing for any entry wounds.
    b. Respiratory rate and depth
    c. Tracheal deviation (late finding of tension pneumothorax)
    d. Symmetry of chest wall movement
    e. Accessory muscle use
    f. Bilateral breath sounds
  3. Circulation assessment with hemorrhage control
    a. Level of consciousness can be diminished when blood volume or perfusion is diminished.
    b. *Assess pulse quality, rate, regularity:* Tachycardia (rapid and thready) is indicative of hypovolemia.
    c. *Evaluate skin color and temperature:* Grey, ashen facial skin is indicative of hypovolemia.
    d. Measure blood pressure (BP).
    e. Determine external and potential internal sources of bleeding.
  4. Disability assessment
    a. Neurological status
      i. Glasgow Coma Scale (GCS)
      ii. Pupillary size and reaction
      iii. Lateralizing signs or spinal cord injury
  5. Exposure and environment
    a. Completely undress patient
    b. Prevent hypothermia, that can occur quickly and can be potentially lethal.
C. Resuscitation: Prioritize interventions based on findings of primary survey.
  1. Aggressive and continued volume resuscitation is not a substitute for definitive control of hemorrhage.

AMPLE History

A. Ask emergency medical services (EMS), family, bystanders, and so on, if patient unable to answer
B. Allergies
C. Medications: Inquire about anticoagulation use.
D. Past medical history
E. Last meal (time)
F. Events surrounding injury
  1. Time since injury
  2. Postinjury symptoms
  3. Blood loss at the scene/en route
G. Mechanism of injury
  1. Type and specifics of injury, history surrounding injury
  2. Penetrating abdominal trauma
    a. In left thoracoabdominal area can injure the left diaphragm, spleen
    b. In right thoracoabdominal area can injure the liver
    c. Abdominal visceral injury possible peritoneal penetration
    d. Type and specifics of weapon (e.g., knife, gun, type of ammunition, type of gun)
    e. Location of injury
    f. Number of shots fired
  3. Blast trauma: Can penetrate organs from fragments or blunt injuries
  4. Blunt abdominal trauma
    a. Direct blow, shearing injuries, deceleration injuries
    b. Most injured organs are spleen, liver, and small bowel.
    c. Motor vehicle crash (MVC)
      i. Greatest cause of blunt abdominal trauma
      ii. Type of crash (e.g., head-on, rear-ended, t-boned, sideswiped) and direction of impact
      iii. Frontal impact injuries with bent steering wheel, knee imprint on dashboard, or bull's eye fracture of windshield

(1) Fractured spleen, liver
(2) Posterior fracture/dislocation of hip and/or knee
(3) Traumatic aortic disruption

iv. Side impact injuries
(1) Traumatic aortic disruption
(2) Diaphragmatic rupture
(3) Fractures spleen/liver/kidney depending on side of impact
(4) Fractured pelvis

v. Use of seatbelt and type of seatbelt (i.e., lap belt or shoulder harness)
(1) Lap belt injuries
(a) Tear or avulsion of bowel mesentery
(b) Thrombosis of iliac artery or abdominal aorta
(c) Rupture of small bowel or colon
(d) Pancreatic or duodenal injury
(2) Shoulder harness injuries
(a) Rupture of abdominal viscera
(b) Rib fractures

vi. Sitting location in the car

vii. Deployment of airbags (consider airbag contact injury)

viii. Degree of damage to the vehicle the victim was in; whether the vehicle rolled over

ix. High-risk MVC includes intrusion, including roof of >12 inches (30 cm) on occupant side of vehicle or >18 inches on any side, ejection (partial or complete), death in same passenger compartment, vehicle telemetry data with high risk of injury

x. Pedestrian or bicyclist versus auto thrown, run over, or with >20 mph impact can cause significant injury, including traumatic aortic dissection and abdominal visceral injuries.

xi. If crush injuries, ascertain weight and force of the object.

d. Assault
i. Type of assault (e.g., fists, kick, belt, bat, or blunt object) and location of impact on body

e. Fall
i. Height of fall, number of stairs (if relevant)
(1) Fall from >20 feet or 6 meters (2 stories) in adults and >10 feet or 3 meters (2–3 x height of child) indicates high-energy injury.
(a) Falls from height can injure both solid organs as well as the hollow viscous.
(b) Retroperitoneal injuries are associated with significant blood loss because force is transmitted up the axial skeleton.
(c) Can sustain abdominal visceral injuries or fractured pelvis

ii. What the patient landed on can help determine where injury may have occurred.

iii. Cause of fall (e.g., seizure, syncope, chest pain, dyspnea versus mechanical)

H. Reassess airway, breathing, circulation (ABC) and consider need for transfer.

I. Secondary survey AFTER primary survey completed. Head-to-toe assessment

1. Head and maxillofacial area
a. Traumatic brain injury
b. Facial fractures

2. Cervical spine and neck
a. Maintain spinal immobilization.
b. Assess entire spine by log rolling, inspection, and palpation.

3. Chest
a. Flail chest
b. Simple pneumothorax
c. Hemothorax
d. Tracheobronchial tree injury
e. Diaphragmatic Injury

4. Abdomen assessment
a. In hypotensive patients, goal is to rapidly identify an abdominal or pelvic injury as a potential cause.
b. In hemodynamically stable patients without signs of peritonitis may give a more detailed evaluation to determine presence of injuries.
c. A normal initial examination does not exclude significant injury.
d. Significant blood loss can be present in the abdominal cavity without a dramatic change in the external appearance or dimensions of the abdomen and without obvious signs of peritoneal irritation.
e. The boundaries of the abdomen include the diaphragm superiorly (nipples anteriorly, inferior scapular tip posteriorly) and the intragluteal fold inferiorly and encompass the entire circumference.
f. Inspection/auscultation/percussion/palpation
i. Thoroughly assess front and back of patient for ecchymosis or wounds.
ii. Assess abdomen/pelvis for tenderness or guarding, distention, rigidity, bruising over the iliac wings, pubic, labia, scrotum.
iii. Skin folds can mask penetrating injuries and make assessment more difficult.
iv. Look for signs of intra-abdominal bleeding or peritoneal irritation; exam is limited in detecting intraperitoneal blood.
v. Percussion causes slight movement of the abdomen and can elicit signs of peritoneal irritation.
vi. Absence of bowel sounds does not necessarily correlate with injury.
vii. Injury in the retroperitoneal space or intrathoracic abdomen is difficult to assess by palpation.
viii. Rectal examination should be done to assess for bony trauma or blood as well as anal wink and good tone.
ix. Penetrating abdominal wound with evidence of intrathoracic injury should raise suspicion for diaphragmatic rupture.

x. Examine penis, perineum, external meatus.
(1) Look for blood at the meatus, perineal hematoma, vaginal laceration, vaginal or rectal foreign body (FB); do prostate examination (should be normal).

5. Musculoskeletal
   a. Fractures
   b. Compartment syndrome
   c. Do not let distracting injuries lead to missing other injuries.
6. Neurologic
   a. Mental status including Glasgow Coma Scale (GCS; ongoing reassessment)
   b. Assess for pain, paralysis, and paresthesia.
   c. Sensation
   d. Motor function
   e. Deep tendon reflexes (DTR)

Diagnostic Reasoning

A. General considerations
   1. Lower thoracic injury may cause abdominal pain.
   2. Fractures (rib, pelvis) may cause abdominal pain.
   3. If penetrating upper abdominal wounds, consider the possibility of intrathoracic injury.
   4. If penetrating wounds to the lower thoracic area, consider the possibility of intra-abdominal injury.
   5. Diagnoses of intra-abdominal injuries from gunshot wounds to the abdomen are typically made by laparotomy.
   6. Diagnostic laparoscopy is useful in diagnosing diaphragmatic injury, spleen or liver lacerations.

Prehospital Treatment

A. Titrate fluid resuscitation to clinical response. Target SBP of 90 to 100 mmHg.

B. Normal vital signs do not preclude significant intra-abdominal pathology.

C. Apply sterile dressings to open wounds and moistened sterile dressings to eviscerated bowel.

D. Secure impaled foreign objects in place; do not remove them.

Initial Stabilization/Therapy

A. Ensure adequate airway.
   1. Intubate if needed.
   2. O_2 100% by nonrebreather (NRB) face mask

B. Two large-bore IV lines with warmed crystalloid infusion

C. Begin infusion of packed red blood cells if no hemodynamic response to 1 L of crystalloid.

D. If patient is in profound shock, consider immediate transfusion of O-negative blood.

E. Consider tranexamic acid (TXA) for hemorrhage.

F. Consider anticoagulation reversal as needed.

G. Surgical intervention with laparotomy by a qualified surgeon is indicated for uncontrolled shock, findings of hemoperitoneum, clinical signs of peritonitis, or clinical deterioration during observation.

Adjuncts to Primary Survey and Resuscitation

A. EKG

B. Pulse oximetry

C. Ventilatory rate, capnography

D. Labs
   1. Check hemoglobin/hematocrit, which initially may be normal secondary to isovolumic blood loss.
   2. Check coagulation markers (e.g., platelets, prothrombin [PT], and partial thromboplastin time [PTT]).
      a. Effects of some anticoagulants may not be accurately reflected in lab values.
   3. Metabolic panel
   4. Type and screen are essential.
      a. Crossmatch packed red blood cells (PRBCs) for unstable patients.
   5. Urinalysis for blood
      a. Microscopic hematuria in the presence of shock should prompt genitourinary (GU) evaluation.
   6. Pregnancy test for females of child-bearing age
   7. Ethanol concentration
   8. Toxicology screen
   9. Arterial blood gas (ABG)
      a. Base deficit may suggest hypovolemic shock and help guide the resuscitation.
      b. Low pH and base excess levels indicate shock.

Imaging

A. Do obtain essential x-ray/CT scan after the initial resuscitation process, even in pregnant patients.

B. Extended focused abdominal sonography for trauma (eFAST)
   1. To detect free intraperitoneal fluid
   2. Ultrasound (US) is rapid, requires no contrast agents, and is noninvasive.
   3. Operator dependent
   4. Does not exclude intra-abdominal injury.

C. CT
   1. Use in patients in whom the initial exam does not indicate need for emergency laparotomy.
   2. Most useful in assessing the need for operative intervention and for evaluating the retroperitoneal space and solid organs
   3. Not reliable for detection of hollow viscus or diaphragmatic injuries

D. Peritoneal lavage
   1. Few indications for diagnostic peritoneal lavage in a hemodynamically stable patient when CT is readily available. POCUS has reduced the DPL rates as well especially eFAST.
   2. Locally explore stab wounds to anterior abdomen
      a. If the wound penetrates the anterior fascial layer, the patient should undergo diagnostic peritoneal lavage or bedside US.

E. Chest x-ray (CXR)
   1. Can aid in detection of pneumoperitoneum or ruptured diaphragm.

F. Abdominal x-ray
  1. Localization of foreign body (FB), missiles, associated fractures, free air
G. Pelvic x-ray
  1. Fracture of the pelvis and gross hematuria may indicate GU injury.
  2. Further evaluation of these structures with retrograde urethrogram or cystogram

Emergency Department Management

A. Pharmacologic therapies
  1. Follow evidence-based guidelines when prescribing.
  2. Tetanus toxoid booster for patients with open wounds
  3. Tetanus immunoglobulin for patients who have not had complete series
  4. Intravenous broad-spectrum antibiotics should be administered with laparotomy as indicated
  5. Correct coagulopathy when clinically indicated.
  6. Administer analgesia when needed. Avoid NSAIDs due to risk of bleeding.
B. Nasogastric (NG) tube
  1. If a fracture of the cribriform plate is known or suspected, insert a gastric tube orally to prevent intracranial passage.
  2. Evacuate stomach, decrease distention, and decrease risk of aspiration.
  3. May relieve respiratory distress if caused by a herniated abdominal content through the diaphragm.
  4. Blood in NG tube may indicate gastric injury.
C. Urinary catheter
  1. Insert after ruling out urethral injuries.
  2. Facilitates rapid assessment of genitourinary (GU) injury.
  3. Assists in monitoring urinary output.
D. Pelvic binder
  1. Reduces the fracture and lessens the bleeding by increased pressure between fractured ends of the bones.
  2. Can use a sheet, pelvic binder, or other devices applied at the level of the greater trochanters of the femur.

Consultation and Collaboration

A. Indications for emergent surgical/trauma consultation and/or laparotomy
  1. Blunt abdominal trauma with hypotension with a positive focused assessment with sonography for trauma (FAST) or clinical evidence of intraperitoneal bleeding or without another source for bleeding
  2. Hypotension with an abdominal wound that penetrates the anterior fascia
  3. Gunshot wounds that traverse the peritoneal cavity
  4. Evisceration
  5. Bleeding from the stomach, rectum, or genitourinary (GU) tract following penetrating trauma
  6. Peritonitis
  7. Free air, retroperitoneal air, or rupture of the hemidiaphragm
  8. CT that demonstrates ruptured gastrointestinal (GI) tract, intraperitoneal bladder injury, renal pedicle injury, or severe visceral parenchymal injury after blunt or penetrating trauma
  9. Blunt or penetrating abdominal trauma with aspiration of GI contents, vegetable fibers, or bile from diagnostic peritoneal lavage (DPL), or aspiration of 10 mL or more of blood in hemodynamically abnormal patients

Specific Issues

Diaphragm Injuries

A. Overall incidence from blunt trauma is 5%.
B. Blunt tears can occur anywhere, but most often are in the left hemidiaphragm.
C. Penetrating injuries usually produce 1 to 2 cm perforations, but can also cause larger lacerations because of the curved nature of the diaphragm.
D. Blunt injuries usually result in a larger laceration, tearing in a radial fashion involving the posterior lateral diaphragm. Commonly 5 to 10 cm in length
E. On CXR may see elevation or blurring of the hemidiaphragm, hemothorax, or gastric tube positioned in the chest.

Abdominal Compartment Syndrome

A. Consequence of elevated pressure in a confined space or limited space
B. Pressures increase secondary to increased interstitial fluid or cell swelling.
C. Circulation, function, and viability of the tissues or structures within are compromised.
D. Abdominal wall becomes stiffer, compliance falls.
E. Venous return is diminished typically from decreased inferior vena cava (IVC) flow and elevation of the diaphragm.
  1. Caused by retroperitoneal pooling of blood, obstruction by diaphragmatic cura, decreased venous outflow from legs.
F. Visceral blood flow declines with increased intra-abdominal pressure, resulting in visceral ischemia.
G. Renal blood flow, glomerular filtration rate, and urine output are diminished.
  1. Oliguria seen at intra-abdominal pressure (IAP) of 15 to 20 mmHg; anuria >20 mmHg
H. Thoracic cavity is compressed by abdominal distention and lung compliance falls.
  1. Increased ventilatory pressures, pulmonary artery (PA) pressures, pulmonary vascular resistance
  2. Arterial blood gas (ABG) may show hypoxemia, hypercarbia, and acidosis (combined respiratory and metabolic components).
I. Cardiac output is depressed secondary to decreased stroke volumes, despite compensatory tachycardia.
  1. Preload is decreased secondary to decreased venous return and increased pressure.
  2. Afterload is increased secondary to elevated systemic vascular resistance (increased heart rate [HR],

systemic vascular resistance [SVR], pulmonary artery pressure [PAP], pulmonary capillary wedge pressure [PCWP], central venous pressure [CVP], peak airway pressure).

J. Traumatic causes
  1. Intra-abdominal bleeding, ruptured abdominal aortic aneurysm, pneumoperitoneum
  2. Hypoperfusion of the viscera with hemorrhagic shock, large volume resuscitation, tight abdominal closures s/p laparotomy, use of positive pressure ventilation, swelling of intestines

K. Compounding factors
  1. Premorbid illness (e.g., cardiac, pulmonary, renal)
  2. Massive fluid volumes
  3. Trendelenburg positioning (increases diaphragmatic compression by abdominal contents)
  4. Positive end-expiratory pressure (PEEP)
  5. Other associated injuries

L. Five features of abdominal compartment syndrome
  1. Elevated ventilatory pressures
  2. Elevated central venous pressures
  3. Decreased urinary output
  4. Massive abdominal distention
  5. Reversal of these derangements with abdominal decompression

M. Normal intraperitoneal pressure = 0 mmHg
  1. Intra-abdominal pressures measured directly (needle connected to manometer placed directly into peritoneal cavity) or indirectly (measured across the wall of the abdomen using an indwelling structure such as a Foley)
  2. Bladder pressures most used and correlate with pressures of 5 to 70 mmHg
  3. Grading system
    a. *I:* Bladder pressure 7 to 11 mmHg (can be normal postoperatively)
    b. *II:* 11 to 18 mmHg (close monitoring indicated)
    c. *III:*18 to 26 mmHg (most require decompression)
    d. *IV:* >26 (all require decompression, surgical emergency, and can progress to fatal organ dysfunction and cardiac arrest)

Liver Injuries

A. Most injured organ

B. Common injury mechanisms are penetrating trauma, with about 20% from blunt trauma.

C. Patients with right-sided rib fractures have a higher incidence of liver injury.

D. Rapid deceleration may be responsible for avulsion of the hepatic veins or retro-hepatic inferior vena cava injuries.

E. Penetrating injuries usually discovered intraoperatively. Blunt injuries usually diagnosed with peritoneal lavage, CT, or ultrasound (US).

F. CT has high sensitivity and specificity. US has specificity of 80% and sensitivity of 99%. Diagnostic peritoneal lavage (DPL) has poor specific ranging from 25% to 67%, although 98% sensitive.

G. Biliary duct disruption with formation of bile collection may occur, but rarely clinically significant.

H. Mortality from liver injuries is less than 10%.

I. Liver injury scale
  1. *I:* <10 % subscapular. Laceration <1 cm (15%)
  2. *II:* 10% to 50% subscapular. Laceration 1 to 3 cm (55%)
  3. *III:* >50% subscapular or ruptured or expanding, large intraparenchymal hematoma (25%)
  4. *IV:* Parenchymal disruption 25% to 75% liver (3%)
  5. *V:* >75% parenchymal disruption. Major vascular injury (2%)
  6. *VI:* Hepatic avulsion (<1%)

J. Management
  1. 20% to 50% of blunt liver injuries require operative management.

K. Nonoperative
  1. Hemodynamically stable without peritoneal signs
  2. Liver-related transfusion requirement minimal
  3. No associated hallow visceral injuries
  4. Occasionally embolization via angiography may provide vascular control and arrest bleeding in the stable patient.

L. Operative exploratory laparotomy

Biliary Injuries

A. Penetrating injury is the most common cause.
  1. Stab wounds cause transection or laceration of biliary tree or gallbladder.
  2. Gunshot wound–caused laceration or crushing injuries are commonly associated with vascular injuries.
  3. Typically injured by direct injury with compression over the spine or during rapid deceleration events at the points of fixation
  4. May be contused, lacerated, avulsed
  5. Prognosis is predicted by associated injuries; gallbladder injury alone has excellent prognosis (rare).
  6. Patients typically present with a retroperitoneal or intraperitoneal leak of bile.
  7. Diagnosed by exploratory laparotomy, CT (shows fluid collection in retroperitoneum, around duodenum or ascites), or US
  8. Delayed presentations
    a. Obstructive jaundice, biliary ascites, sepsis
    b. Diagnosed by hepatobiliary iminodiacetic acid (HIDA) scan or endoscopic retrograde cholangiopancreatography (MRCP).

Splenic Injuries

A. Splenic rupture is most common cause of major abdominal injuries.

B. Motor vehicle crash (MVC) is the most common cause.

C. History of trauma involving left upper abdomen or lower chest

D. Signs and symptoms
  1. Abdominal pain and tenderness
  2. Rib fractures of the left lower chest
  3. Pain referred to the left shoulder tip
  4. Progressive anemia by serial hematocrit
  5. Rising leukocyte count (>15,000 u/L)
  6. Signs of shock (e.g., tachycardia, hypotension)
  7. Positive signs

a. Enlargement of spleen, fractured ribs in left lower chest, displacement of gas in transverse colon

8. Can have a delayed rupture in 5% of blunt trauma (usually within 2–3 weeks of injury).
   a. Usually from intraparenchymal hemorrhage or bleeding contained within peritoneal folds or omentum
   b. With breakdown of hematoma and liquefaction of cells, there is an increased osmotic pressure leading to increased water within hematoma, expanding size and increasing pressure leading to rupture.
9. Diagnosis
   a. Exploratory laparotomy, CT, US
10. Organ injury scaling
   a. Subscapular, nonexpanding hematoma, <10% depth, nonbleeding; capsular tear <1 cm parenchymal surface area
   b. Subscapular nonexpanding hematoma, 10% to 50% surface area, intraparenchymal nonexpanding hematoma, <2 cm in diameter; capsular tear with active bleeding, 1 to 3 cm parenchymal depth, not involving trabecular vessel
   c. Subscapular hematoma with >50% surface area or expanding, ruptured subscapular hematoma with bleeding; intraparenchymal hematoma with > 2cm or expanding. Tear >3 cm parenchymal depth or involving trabecular vessels
   d. Ruptured intraparenchymal hematoma with bleeding. Laceration involving the segmental or hilar vessels, producing major devascularization (>25% of the spleen)
   e. Completely shattered spleen. Hilar vascular injury that devascularizes the spleen
11. Management
   a. Nonoperative
      i. Fifty percent of ruptured spleens in adults. Immunocompromised adults should have spleens preserved if possible.
      ii. Ninety percent of children
      iii. Non-life-threatening hemorrhage, blunt trauma with subscapular bleeding, or very small amounts of intraparenchymal bleeding
      iv. Spleen is only injured organ.
      v. Serial CT scans
   b. Operative
      i. Minor lacerations and capsular tears can be managed by electrocautery, argon beam coagulation or hemostatic gel, absorbent mesh.
      ii. Debridement or surgical repair
      iii. Partial splenectomy
         (1) If there is preservation of part of the spleen
      iv. Indications for total splenectomy
         (1) Irreparable injury to the spleen (grade 4–5)
         (2) Severe blood loss leading to hemodynamic instability
         (3) Multiple injuries with extensive repairs
         (4) Coagulopathy, hypothermia, and associated medical/surgical conditions that preclude lengthy surgery

Gastric Injuries

A. Blunt trauma is not common (<1%), usually occurs when stomach is full and direct force is applied to it (MVC, fall from height).
B. Penetrating injury occurs in about 20%, typically involves other organs as well.
C. Gastric necrosis
   1. Ingested corrosives
D. Signs and symptoms
   1. Mechanism of injury (stab, gunshot wound, blunt trauma, ingestion)
   2. Tenderness, guarding, rebound tenderness (leaking gastric juice causes peritoneal irritation)
   3. Liver dullness may disappear as free gas overlies the liver.
   4. Peritonitis
   5. Diagnosis
      a. Chest/abdominal x-ray (XR) shows free gas in abdomen or under diaphragm; can be unreliable.
      b. Peritoneal lavage (DPL) may reveal blood and gastric contents.
      c. CT with contrast indicates gastric perforation, extraluminal air and fluid.
      d. Management is operative repair.

Duodenal Injury

A. Relatively uncommon (3%–5%); mortality rate about 17% to 35%
B. Penetrating injuries account for three-fourths of all injuries; combined duodenal/pancreatic injuries are usually secondary to penetrating trauma.
C. Blunt injury usually caused by abrupt deceleration, crushing the retroperitoneal duodenum against the spine or by causing a blowout of an air-filled, closed duodenal loop.
D. Sharp blows to the epigastric region, such as steering wheel or handlebars, are the most common causes of blunt injuries.
E. Unrestrained drivers in frontal impact collisions
F. Fifty percent of duodenal hematomas in children are attributed to child abuse,
G. Volume of fluid traversing the duodenum ranges from 5 to 10 L daily. This large volume of fluid, with its activated digestive enzymes and bile, is responsible for the profound inflammatory response associated with duodenal injuries.
H. Diagnosis
   1. Intraoperatively
   2. DPL has limited role.
   3. XR
      a. Useful in suggesting duodenal perforation when gas bubbles are present in the retroperitoneum adjacent to the right psoas muscle, around the right kidney, or anterior to the upper lumbar spine.
      b. Fractures of the transverse processes of the lumbar vertebrae are indicative of forceful retroperitoneal trauma and can serve as a predictor of duodenal or pancreatic injury.

4. CT shows retroperitoneal air or extravasated oral contrast medium and constitutes proof of injury.
5. US is understudied in this area.

I. Injury severity classification
1. *I:* Hematoma involving a single portion of the duodenum or a partial thickness laceration without perforation
2. *II:* Hematoma involving more than one portion of the duodenum or laceration with disruption of <50% circumference
3. *III:* Laceration with 50% to 75% disruption of circumference of D2 or 50% to 100% circumference of D1, D3, D4
4. *IV:* Laceration with disruption of >75% of circumference of D2 and involving ampulla or distal common bile duct
5. *V:* Laceration with massive disruption of the duodenopancreatic complex or devascularization of the duodenum

J. Management
1. Nonoperative
a. Nasogastric (NG) decompression and parenteral nutrition
b. Hematoma resolution in about 10 to 14 days
2. Operative laparotomy

Pancreatic Injury

A. Uncommon (7%); mortality 18%
B. Majority from penetrating trauma followed by sharp blows to the epigastrium
C. Mostly associated with liver injuries, stomach injuries, and major vascular structures, followed by injuries of the small bowel and colon, spleen, kidney, duodenum, or biliary tract
D. Over 90% of patients have at least one other intra-abdominal injury.
E. Diagnosis
1. Amylase is not a reliable indicator of pancreatic injury; however, if normal, there is a 95% likelihood of no injury to the gland.
2. Intraoperatively (most common)
3. X-ray and DPL unreliable, ERCP plays no role
4. CT can reveal abnormality or adjacent structures, but they can take days to appear.
F. Injury severity grading
1. *I:* Minor contusion without duct injury, superficial laceration without ductal injury
2. *II:* Major contusion without ductal injury or tissue loss, major laceration without ductal injury or tissue loss
3. *III:* Distal transection or parenchymal injury with a duct injury
4. *IV:* Proximal transection or parenchymal injury involving ampulla of Vater
5. *V:* Massive disruption of the pancreatic head

Small Bowel Injuries

A. Incidence in penetrating trauma is highest (>80%) for gunshot wound, lower for stab wounds (30%–50%).
B. Not common in blunt abdominal trauma (5%–15%)
C. Most commonly from shearing, crushing, or bursting
D. Seatbelt injuries
E. Proximal jejunum and terminal ileum are the most injured because the small bowel is sheared away from its anchoring points.
F. Can be injured by being crushed against the spine or pelvis.
G. A compressed loop of small bowel may also be ruptured due to high intraluminal pressure.
H. Assessment
1. Retroperitoneal injury is often difficult to assess because intact perineum may prevent blood and intestinal content spillage into the abdominal cavity.
2. Abdominal tenderness, pain, guarding, rebound tenderness, absence of bowel sounds, increasing leukocytosis, elevated amylase, fever
I. Diagnostics
1. Labs including amylase, white blood cell (WBC) count
2. XR not helpful
3. CT scan with triple contrast (IV, oral, enema)
4. DPL
5. Exploratory laparotomy
J. Management
1. Nonoperative
a. Not all hematomas/lacerations need to be explored.
2. Operative
a. Hemodynamic instability
b. Peritoneal signs and symptoms penetrating torso wounds below the nipple
c. Intraperitoneal free air
d. Bullet or pellet
e. Positive DPL
f. High index of suspicion

Colon Injuries

A. Incidence of penetrating trauma from gunshot wound 25%–30%, from stab wounds 5%–10%
B. Blunt trauma injuries (3%–10%)
1. Most commonly from shearing, crushing, or bursting
2. Seatbelt injuries
C. Assessment
1. Retroperitoneal injury is often difficult to assess because intact perineum may prevent blood and intestinal content spillage into the abdominal cavity.
2. Abdominal tenderness, pain, guarding, rebound tenderness, absence of bowel sounds, increasing leukocytosis, elevated amylase, fever
D. Diagnostics
1. Labs including amylase, WBC
2. XR not helpful
3. CT scan with triple contrast (IV, oral, enema)
4. DPL
5. Exploratory laparotomy
E. Management
1. Operative
a. In general, blunt colon injuries usually require resection secondary to the larger colon destruction.

Rectal Injuries

A. Rare (3% to 5% of all colon injuries)
B. Typically, from penetrating injuries or foreign objects inserted into rectum
C. Pelvic fractures can lacerate rectum.
D. Blunt trauma from high pressure blowing out the pelvic floor may cause a rectal injury.
E. Assessment
  1. Rectal examination
    a. Evaluate for blood.
    b. Perianal laceration in association with weak anal tone suggests anal or sacral injury.
F. Diagnosis
  1. Rigid sigmoidoscopy
  2. Gastrografin enema
G. Management
  1. Primary closure
    a. Stable, minimal contamination, no other associated injuries
  2. Operative management

Genitourinary Trauma

A. Contusions, hematomas, and ecchymosis of the back or flank are markers of potential underlying renal injury.
B. Gross hematuria is an indication for imaging.
C. Penile injuries
  1. Zipper firmly attached to foreskin
    a. Cut zipper from garment, ring block the penis; if fails, patient needs operative management.
  2. Dog bite
    a. Broad-spectrum antibiotics and DO NOT suture primarily (can be sutured 1– 2 weeks later)
  3. Fracture
    a. There is not a bone in the penis (unlike in a walrus).
    b. Refers to a tear of the fibrous wall of the corpus cavernosum caused by forceful bending of the erect penis and usually results from a thrust executed with more enthusiasm than accuracy.
    c. Sudden pain followed by rapid swelling, deviates away from site of injury
    d. The tear can extend to the urethra, in which case there is blood in the external meatus.
    e. Treatment is surgical repair.
  4. Degloving injury
    a. Usually an industrial or agricultural injury in which the patient's trousers and penile skin get caught in a moving belt or chain
    b. Penile skin is often devitalized.
    c. Treatment is surgical repair.
D. Testicular injuries
  1. Penetrating injuries need surgical exploration and/or removal.
  2. Traumatic hematocele (blood within the tunica vaginalis) may indicate rupture.
    a. US can confirm this condition; management is surgical repair.

Urethral Injuries

A. Hematuria indicates urinary injury.
B. Urethrogram can diagnose rupture of the bulbar urethra. Typically presents as tender swelling of perineum and inability to pass urine.
C. Penetrating injuries require surgical repair.
D. Patient with fractured pelvis and blood at external meatus is diagnostic of rupture of the urethra.
  1. High-riding prostate identified on rectal exam suggests a complete rupture of the urethra.
  2. Suprapubic cystoscopy or surgical repair

Bladder Injuries

A. Can be caused by blunt trauma in a patient with a full bladder.
B. Labs can show a disproportionate increase in blood urea nitrogen (BUN) versus creatinine because urea is more readily absorbed by the peritoneum than creatinine.
C. Anuria suggests possible ruptured bladder with extravasation of urine into the abdomen and can be accompanied by penile and scrotal edema.
D. Cystography is used to diagnose bladder rupture.
  1. Full bladder and drainage films can demonstrate extraperitoneal and intraperitoneal rupture.
  2. Can yield a false negative result if there is a plug in the omentum or a knuckle of the bowel temporarily sealing the bladder rupture.
E. Extraperitoneal bladder rupture can be treated by urethral catheterization in the absence of other injuries.
F. Penetrating injuries require surgical repair.

Ureteral Injuries

A. Most causes are iatrogenic.
  1. Hysterectomy, removal of ovarian mass, colectomy, aortic aneurysm surgery, extraction of a calculus from the ureter, ureteroscopic procedures
B. Penetrating trauma requires surgical repair.
C. Patient with fever, drainage of pus, followed by watery fluid from the vagina after surgery is indicative of a urinary fistula.
  1. If it is urine, creatinine concentration is many times higher than serum creatinine.

Renal Injuries

A. Diagnosis by CT with contrast can define the extent of the injury and can differentiate viable from devascularized renal tissue.
B. Positive microscopic blood in the urine without shock, rib fractures, loin contusion, or abrasions do not need to be investigated further; frank hematuria should be investigated.
C. Operative management in patients with persistent hemorrhage, shattered kidney or one with multiple lacerations, or a vascular injury

Pelvic Injuries

A. Blunt trauma, especially MVC followed by falls, crushing injuries, and explosions
B. Elderly, osteoporotic patients can sustain injury from a minor fall.
C. Carry high mortality rate
  1. Typically associated with other injuries, hemorrhage, and shock
D. If a crushing injury is severe enough to cause pelvic fracture, it can also cause diaphragmatic rupture.
E. Assessment

1. Patient may be unable to bear weight without pain, even with a less severe fracture.
2. Severe deformity in extreme cases with bruising and hematoma formation also points to fracture.
3. Stability of the pelvis
   a. Anteriorly, pressure should be placed over symphysis pubis.
   b. Laterally, pressure should be placed over iliac wings and the hip joint should go through a full range of motion.
   c. If pain is felt or if difficulty is experienced with the movements, fracture should be suspected.
4. Bleeding from pelvic fractures
   a. Torn or lacerated pelvic arteries and veins
   b. In a closed, nondisplaced fracture, pelvic and retroperitoneal bleeding may amount to as much as 4 L and can be fatal if fluid replacement does not take place.
   c. Open fracture requires surgical repair.
5. Soft tissue injuries associated with pelvic fractures
   a. *Muscle:* Most common injury, leading to hematomas, pain, and inability to ambulate
   b. *Urinary system:* Urethra and bladder can be ruptured, particularly with displaced fractures.
   c. Genitals/vaginal injuries
   d. *Intestinal tract:* Rectal, large and small bowel injuries
6. Diagnostics
   a. XR (include ap, lateral, and oblique)
   b. CT
7. Management
   a. *Priorities:* Respiratory/circulatory injuries first, then abdominal sources of bleeding, then pelvis
   b. Crystalloid infusion, blood if fast bleeding or hematocrit very low
   c. Pelvic bleeding can be controlled by external fixators, angiography with embolization, surgical packing at laparotomy.
   d. *External fixators:* Reduces the fracture and lessens the bleeding by increased pressure between fractured ends of the bones.
      i. Can use a sheet, pelvic binder, or other devices applied at the level of the greater trochanters of the femur.
   e. If bleeding persists after external fixation, angiography with embolization is required, and if that does not work, then requires surgical repair.
   f. Military antishock trousers (MAST) are useful in treatment to allow more time to perform angiography or embolization, but can lead to respiratory compromise due to pressure on the abdomen leading to an elevated diaphragm and possible increase in blood pressure causing increased bleeding above the level of MAST suit.
   g. Definitive fixation of the fracture is not urgent and can wait until patient stabilizes.
   h. Uncomplicated, nondisplaced, closed fracture
      i. Anterior portion of pelvis does not contribute to weight bearing; bedrest until pain subsides, then mobilized as tolerated.
      ii. Posterior fractures should have injuries to the lumbosacral region ruled out and mobilization is more gradual because this is a no weight bearing area.

Patient Disposition and Transition of Care Information

A. Admission criteria
   1. Patients who require surgical intervention
   2. Equivocal findings of Focused Assessment with Sonography for Trauma (FAST) exam or CT
   3. Unstable patients

B. Discharge criteria
   1. Patients with isolated blunt abdominal trauma who are clinically stable and have a negative abdominal CT (w/IV contrast) can be considered for safe discharge.
   2. No patient with suspected high-risk intra-abdominal injury should be discharged.
   3. Patients with stab wounds without fascial penetration may be discharged after thorough evaluation in the ED and evidence of clinical stability.

C. Transfer criteria
   1. Do not delay transfer to perform diagnostic procedures that does not change the immediate plan of care.
   2. Patients should be resuscitated and attempts made for stabilization as possible prior to transfer.
   3. Whenever the patient's treatment needs exceed the capability of the receiving institution, transfer should be considered.
   4. Treatment before transfer (as able)
      a. Airway
         i. Establish definitive airway with cuffed tube in the trachea as indicated.
         ii. Suction
         iii. Gastric tube
      b. Breathing
         i. Oxygen supplementation
         ii. Mechanical ventilation as needed
         iii. Insert chest tube with known or suspected pneumothorax.
      c. Circulation
         i. Control external bleeding (note time of tourniquet placement).
         ii. Two large-bore IVs, crystalloid infusion
         iii. Indwelling urinary catheter
         iv. Cardiac monitoring
         v. Tilt pregnant patients on left side to improve venous return.
      d. Central nervous system (CNS)
         i. Mannitol or hypertonic saline if needed and when advised by receiving trauma specialist
         ii. Restrict spinal motion
      e. Diagnostic studies
         i. Perform diagnostic studies as indicated but DO NOT delay transfer for this.
      f. Wounds
         i. Clean and dress wounds after controlling external hemorrhage.

ii. Tetanus
iii. Antibiotics as indicated
g. Fractures
i. Splinting and traction as able
5. Provide receiving facility with
a. Past medical history and mechanism of injury
b. Physical examination findings
c. Treatments received and patient response
d. Diagnostic tests and results
e. Rationale/need for transfer
f. Mode of transportation
g. Anticipated arrival time

Age and Developmental Considerations

A. Pregnancy
1. When you care for the mother, you are also caring for the fetus.
2. Fetal and maternal injury after the first trimester is associated with increased rate of fetal loss, but not necessarily maternal mortality.
3. Likelihood of fetal injury increases with severity of maternal insult.
a. Minor trauma can also lead to fetal injuries (50% of fetal losses).
4. Physiologic hypervolemia of pregnancy may lead to an underestimation of blood loss.
a. Clinical shock may be apparent only after a 30% maternal loss.
5. Gravid uterus alters injury patterns and are typically less evident.
6. Injury severity score (ISS) >9 associated with worse outcome
7. Increased probability of injury to bowel, liver, or spleen if entrance of penetrating object is in upper abdomen
8. Poor fetal outcome predicted by maternal hypotension and acidosis
9. One in three pregnant women admitted to the hospital for trauma deliver during hospitalization.
10. Less frequent bowel injury, more frequent retroperitoneal hemorrhage due to the engorgement of pelvic organs and veins
11. Increased morbidity and mortality with pelvic fractures due to pelvic and uterine engorgement
12. Fetal or uterine trauma includes
a. Placental abruption, fetal-maternal hemorrhage (FMH), premature labor, uterine contusion or rupture, fetal demise, premature membrane rupture, hypoxemic or anatomic fetal injury (skull fracture)
13. Abruption occurs in up to 60% of severe trauma cases and 1% to 5% of minor injuries.
a. Most common cause of isolated fetal death
b. Accounts for up to 50% of fetal loss
c. May occur with no external bleeding (20%)
d. Occurs after 16 weeks gestation
e. Can present with abdominal pain, cramping, and/or vaginal bleeding.
f. Hallmark is uterine contractions.
14. Uterine rupture
a. Usually in patients with prior C-section
b. Nearly universal mortality
c. Ten percent maternal mortality
15. Pelvic fracture
a. May be an independent predictor of fetal death
b. Fatal insults to fetus can occur in all trimesters.
c. Ten percent fetal mortality in patients with minor fractures
16. FMH occurs in >30% of severe trauma.
a. Isoimmunization of Rh-negative mothers can occur with as little as 0.03 mL of FMH.
17. Penetrating trauma results in direct injury to fetus, maternal shock, and premature delivery.
18. Fetal mortality is 73%, and maternal mortality is 66% following penetrating trauma.
19. Falls and slips in one out of four pregnant women cause
a. 4.4-fold increase in preterm birth
b. 8-fold increase in placental abruption
c. 2.1-fold increase in fetal demise
d. 2.9-fold increase in fetal hypoxia
20. Burns
a. If body surface area (BSA) involved is >40%, the maternal and fetal mortality approaches 100%.
21. Intentional trauma and domestic violence increase the risk for preterm birth 2.7-fold and low birth weight 5.3-fold.
22. Risk factors for domestic violence include substance abuse, low socioeconomic status, unintended pregnancy, history of domestic violence prior to pregnancy, history of witnessed violence, unmarried status.
23. Electrocution is a significant cause of fetal mortality.

B. Pediatrics
1. Children have less body fat and, therefore, more intense energy transmission.
2. Children can lose large amounts of intra-abdominal blood quickly due to lower blood volumes.
3. Given the smaller size of the intrathoracic abdomen, the spleen and liver are more exposed to injury because they lie partially outside the boney rib cage.
4. Unrecognized pediatric abdominal trauma is a significant contributor to mortality among traumatic injuries to children.
5. Fewer than 10% of pediatric injuries are considered abdominal trauma in nature; however, more than 80% of pediatric abdominal injuries are caused by blunt force trauma.
6. Be suspicious of pediatric abdominal injuries, as many are caused by abuse.
7. In more than 90% of cases, bleeding from an injured spleen, liver, or kidney is self-limited, and less than 15% of cases require surgery.
8. Duodenal hematomas and blunt pancreatic injuries are commonly caused by blunt trauma from handlebars of a bicycle, kicks, or impact during contact sports.
9. Initial volume resuscitation consists of a 20 mL/kg crystalloid bolus (can be repeated).
10. If abnormal hemodynamics persist, administer 10 mL/kg PRBC.

C. Geriatrics
   1. Risk of injury/death increases after age 55.
   2. Systolic blood pressure (SBP) <110 mmHg may represent shock after age 65.
   3. Comorbid disease such as coronary artery disease (CAD), renal disease, arthritis, and pulmonary disease can decrease physiologic reserve, which can make recovery more difficult.
   4. Falls are the most common cause of injury after age 65, followed by motor vehicle crashes (MVCs).
   5. Hip fractures are the single most common diagnosis and can frequently be the cause of hypovolemia and blood loss in the elderly.
   6. Vital signs are unreliable to detect hemodynamic instability in the elderly.
      a. Include altered mental status (AMS), urine output, and skin perfusion in evaluation.
   7. Polypharmacy
      a. Increased risk of bleeding
      b. May alter vital signs
   8. Consider advanced directives.

Patient and Family Education and Counseling

A. Establish family contact and engagement.
B. Provide and ensure safety and security.
C. Avoid discussion of event as this may intensify symptoms.
D. Provide appropriate resources related to coping and signs/symptoms of distress.
E. Connect with appropriate follow-up resources.

Additional Reading

Additional Reading for this chapter are online only and can be found at https://connect.springerpub.com/content/reference-book/978-0-8261-6091-5/part/part03/toc-part/ch29.

30. Genitourinary Trauma

TRACY BROWN | TRACIE GADLER

Learning Objectives

- Evaluate and treat genitourinary trauma involving the upper internal structures of the system.
- Evaluate and treat genitourinary trauma involving the lower internal structures of the system.
- Evaluate and treat genitourinary trauma involving external genitourinary structures, male or female.
- Identify injuries requiring specialist consultation.
- Identify and order appropriate laboratory studies and radiographic imaging needed as it relates to the location of the injury.

Trauma to the genitourinary (GU) tract is usually found with other injuries to adjacent structures. The system consists of upper and lower tract internal structures and external structures. The treatment of patients with injuries to this organ system should always begin with treatment associated with any other trauma patient. This chapter discusses specific variables associated with the GU system itself.

Pathophysiology and Assessment of the Genitourinary Tract[1–4]

A. *Kidney:* Located in the retroperitoneal region. Back muscles and the lower rib cage protect the kidneys. Clinical signs include pain in the flank region, flank ecchymosis, and symptoms of adjacent injuries to include abdominal pain, gross hematuria, rib pain, spine pain, and shock. Injuries are graded on a I to V scale, beginning with contusions progressing to complete vascular disruption.[5,6] Hematuria is absent in over 50% of penetrating injury.

B. *Ureter:* Back muscles and the pelvis protect the structures. Clinical signs are nonspecific. Late signs include flank pain, development of palpable flank mass known as a urinoma, and fever. Seventy-five percent of injuries to the ureters occur from surgical causes. Initial assessment of the ureteral introitus is essential to determine whether blood is present.

C. *Bladder:* Usually protected by the pelvis in blunt trauma unless fracture is involved, especially when the bladder is empty. Clinical signs include microhematuria greater than 25 red blood cells/high power field in 99% of all blunt bladder trauma cases. Gross hematuria is seen in over two-thirds of injury cases. Other symptoms include the inability to void and lower abdominal pain. Symptoms of peritonitis with intraperitoneal urine leakage. The bladder wall is thinnest at the top of the structure nearest to the peritoneum. Bladder injuries are classified into three categories: contusion, extraperitoneal, and intraperitoneal ruptures. Extraperitoneal rupture can only occur with penetrating trauma.

D. *Urethra:* The structure is divided into two sections: anterior and posterior urethra. Clinical signs include gross hematuria, voiding problems, scrotal or perineal ecchymosis, and blood at the urethral introitus. Anterior urethra is relegated to male patients and associated with the penis. Female patients have only the posterior urethra, which is mostly mobile given minimal attachment sites to the pubic region, is very short, and thus rarely injured. The bulbomembranous junction is the posterior urethral weak point. Specifics noted in external genital injury section below.

E. Male- and female-specific reproduction organ assessment should not be left out. Urology or gynecology consultations for specific evaluation should be included in care. Lack of assessment of both vaginal and rectal vaults can often result in undiagnosed injuries. Gender specifics noted in the individual external trauma sections below.

Diagnostic Testing[1–4,7]

A. *Urinalysis:* Capturing initial urine output is important to identify any hematuria that may not be seen after fluid resuscitation begins. In blunt trauma, gross hematuria is highly sensitive for GU injury. In penetrating trauma, the absence of gross hematuria does not exclude some form of injury. The severity of hematuria in either type of injury does not correlate with injury severity. Microscopic hematuria is not always a result of injury. Patient treatment is based on the severity of the microscopic hematuria results.

B. *Radiograph imaging:* Useful in identification of bone trauma (lower rib fractures, pelvic fractures, and vertebral fractures), retained penetrating projectiles. External marking of penetrating injuries is helpful in determining trajectory of projectile. Typically, anteroposterior and lateral imaging is done.

C. *Ultrasound:* This form of imaging identifies free fluid, suggestive of internal organ injury. The limits of ultrasound include a lack of differentiation between blood, urine, or other types of fluid. Ultrasound cannot rule out injury of kidneys, ureters, or bladder. Ultrasound is also used for testicular evaluation including blood flow.

D. *CT scanning:* The imaging of choice for renal trauma. The initial images performed do not have sufficient contrast to definitively identify injury; delayed imaging with appropriate amounts of contrast is needed.

E. *Retrograde urethrogram:* Used in evaluation of urethral injury. Progression to CT scan and pelvic angiography should be performed to identify life-threatening injuries. Contrast from the urethrogram can affect interpretation of the other imaging. The study is performed by injecting sterile saline diluted contrast into the urethral meatus, either by using a 60-mL syringe with a Christmas tree adapter or by placing a urinary catheter tip 2 to 3 cm into the urethra and blowing up the balloon. Avoid spillage or leakage by ensuring tight fittings.

F. *Retrograde cystogram:* Cannot be performed until urethral trauma has been ruled out. The study can be done with plain imaging or via CT. Baseline imaging should be obtained prior to insertion of 400 mL of diluted contrast solution through a urinary catheter by gravity. The catheter tip syringe should be held above the level of the bladder without the plunger to allow for natural filling. Only forceful injection should be done if the bladder is contracted, and then 50 mL of full concentration contrast should be used. The goal is to have the bladder expanded enough to allow for leakage from rupture site. The urinary catheter will need to be clamped after filled, second set of images obtained. A third set of images are obtained once the bladder is allowed to drain after unclamping the urinary catheter. Intraperitoneal and extraperitoneal ruptures will appear differently, either leakage around the bladder or as a flame-like area.

G. *Retrograde pyelography:* Only done by the urologist during cystoscopy.

H. *Intravenous pyelography (IVP):* This form of imaging has been overtaken by CT imaging. Previously a one-image AP supine view (single-shot IVP) was done to identify blunt renal trauma. The test is now used to evaluate the function of the noninjured kidney and ureteral trauma when the patient is unstable to go to CT, when the urologists deem it indicated. To perform imaging 2 mL/kg contrast dose is given IV, and the image is shot 10 minutes later.

General Management

A. Treatment of shock and massive injuries should be initiated to stabilize patients. Follow recommendations as noted in Chapter 24. Treatment of GU-specific injuries varies in surgical and nonsurgical care, dependent on the severity of the injury.

Consultation Considerations

A. Recommendations should come from the urologist assuming responsibility for follow-up care. Transfer to a consulting facility should occur for specialist care after initial stabilization of the patient. Identification of any injury to the GU structures should prompt urology consultation.

Upper Genitourinary Tract Injury Specifics[3,4,8]

A. Kidney trauma
  1. Nonsurgical management is recommended for Grades I to II. Grade V results in complete nephrectomy.[5] See Resources for the grading of kidney injuries.
  2. Penetrating trauma increases the severity of damage, placing the injury into Grade III to V categories, thus increases likelihood of nephrectomy.[6]

B. Ureteral trauma
  1. In cases of hematuria without other urethral injury signs, one attempt of urinary catheter placement can be made. The urinary catheter placement should be aborted if resistance is met.
  2. Blunt trauma accounts for one-third of nonoperative injuries. The structure is torn at the ureteropelvic junction from deceleration forces.

Lower Genitourinary Tract Injury Specifics[3,4,9]

A. Bladder trauma
  1. Bladder decompression is often needed via suprapubic cystostomy tube. Prior to removal, repeat cystography is preferred to verify healing.
  2. Extraperitoneal injuries are, for the most part, handled nonoperatively, while intraperitoneal requires surgical intervention.
  3. Penetrating trauma will most often require surgical repair.

B. Urethral trauma
  1. Ureteral care posttrauma can be as simple as urinary catheter placement so the urethra can heal via secondary intention. If urine must be diverted to aid in repair or healing of the urethra, a suprapubic cystostomy tube may need placement.
  2. Operative management will encompass stent placement and, in some cases, repair over the stent intraoperatively.
  3. Specific male injuries discussed in the Penile Trauma section.

External Genital Trauma: Female[3,4,10,11]

A. Vulvar hematoma
  1. Hematoma resulting from trauma is frequently seen with falls associated with straddling objects. It is common to see nonrepairable tears associated with the hematoma.
  2. Urinary retention can be seen from either swelling that obstructs the urethra to avoiding urination because of the pain associated with the tears. Encourage urination in the bathtub with warm water or after viscous lidocaine application to tears.
  3. A urinary catheter may be required in extreme cases involving obstruction of the urethra from swelling.
  4. Conservative care centers around ice pack usage.

5. This injury can also be seen with human bites during oral–genital sex.

B. Human bite wounds
   1. Treatment for these wounds needs to follow information in human bite section; see Chapter 35.

C. Vaginal lacerations
   1. These injuries may be seen with coitus; however, water sports contribute to more severe trauma deep into the vaginal vault to include the cervix. The "water douche" from water skiing falls and Jet Ski falls are usually the culprits. Initial care involves controlling bleeding and hemodynamic stabilization. Consultation of a gynecologic specialist for repair is needed. Recommendations for preventive treatment for infection with antibiotics from bacteria in both the water and the vagina are not specifically addressed.

D. Foreign body retention
   1. Early-onset retrieval of tampons and contraceptive sponges is usually all that is required. Late stage, patients complain of foul odor, vaginal discharge, and tenderness. Emergent concerns include toxic shock syndrome. Treatment of this problem is noted in Chapter 24. Pessary complications are discussed in Chapter 18.

E. Injuries associated with sexual assault are addressed in Chapter 55.

Penile Trauma

Penile injuries can occur from a myriad of causes, including automotive accidents, self-inflicted, occupational accident, fracture from forceful sexual encounters, burns, bites, or mechanical injury such as a zipper injury.[12]

Medical screening

A. *Chief complaint:* Penile pain

B. Signs and symptoms
   1. Depends on the cause
   2. Pain, penile soft tissue injury, bleeding, penile edema, penile ecchymosis

C. Focused assessment
   1. GU, and possibly psychiatric evaluation depending on cause

Diagnostic Testing

A. Diagnosis typically made from clinical presentation

B. *Ultrasound:* Useful for penetrating trauma; not beneficial in penile fractures

C. *MRI:* Useful in evaluation of lesions to the corpus cavernosum

D. *Urinalysis:* Assists in identifying urethral involvement

E. Surgical preparation depending on the extent of injury

Medical Decision-Making/Differential Diagnoses

A. Injuries noted to the urethra require immediate referral and surgical intervention. Early surgical intervention for fractures of the penis results in better patient outcomes.[12]

Management

A. *Pharmacologic therapies:* Pain management

B. *Consultation and collaboration:* Urology referral

Age and Developmental Considerations

A. Many patients underreport penile injuries due to moral and psychological reasons.[13]

Prevention and Education

A. Depending on cause. Avoid injury. Circumcision can decrease the risk of penile zipper entrapment. Secondary complications may include pain with an erection or sexual encounter, erectile dysfunction, and curvature of the penis.[12]

Additional Resources

Grading of Kidney Injury: https://faculty.washington.edu/jeff8rob/trauma-radiology-reference-resource/6-abdomen/aast-kidney-injury-scale/

References

References for this chapter are online only and can be found at https://connect.springerpub.com/content/reference-book/978-0-8261-6091-5/part/part03/toc-part/ch30.

31. Peripheral Vascular Injuries

KELLY TOFFOLI

Learning Objectives

- Define peripheral vascular injury.
- Identify signs of peripheral vascular injury.
- Use and interpret common diagnostic modalities in the evaluation of peripheral vascular injuries.
- Evaluate criteria and scoring tools available.
- Determine management goals with regard to peripheral vascular injury.
- Summarize special considerations associated with peripheral vascular injury presentation.

Peripheral vascular injuries can be devastating and threatening to life, limb, or both. These injuries may be the result of an accident, from a motor vehicle, a fall, an athletic injury, or an assault. Individuals with blunt and penetrating trauma are at risk for peripheral vascular injury. Peripheral vascular injuries present a challenge for clinicians. An injury to a vital blood vessel may be subtle and difficult to identify. Delay of diagnosis can lead to complicating hemorrhage, aneurysm formation, arteriovenous fistulization, and gangrene. Irreversible tissue damage due to ischemia can occur in as few as 4 to 6 hours.[1] Delay of diagnosis can complicate repair and present an increased risk for amputation and permanent physical disability.[2] To limit associated morbidity and mortality, it is vital for clinicians to quickly identify peripheral vascular injuries and intervene accordingly. A detailed history, including the mechanism of injury and physical examination, is necessary to identify the potential for vascular compromise. This chapter covers definitions of peripheral vascular injury, assessment findings or common presentations, diagnostic evaluation options, criteria for scoring, treatment goals, and management of peripheral vascular injuries.

General Approach to Peripheral Vascular Injury

Anatomy and Pathophysiology

A. *Vasculature*
   1. Functionally, arteries and veins are responsible for transporting blood throughout the body, maintaining the viability of extremities and organs.
   2. A vascular injury refers to an injury of a blood vessel, usually referring to an artery or a vein.
   3. Vascular injuries are divided into five different types[3]:
      a. Intimal injuries that include subintimal hematomas, flaps, and disruptions
      b. Total wall defects with bleeding hematomas, or pseudoaneurysm
      c. Total disruption with bleeding and/or occlusions
      d. Arteriovenous fistulas
      e. Spasm

B. *Vascular trauma*
   1. Categorization of trauma is dependent upon mechanism of the injury.
      a. Blunt trauma injury usually occurs as a result of a crush or stretch mechanism.
         i. May occur secondarily as a result of a fracture or dislocation of a bone
      b. Penetrating injury can occur with a tear or puncture.
         i. Examples of penetrating trauma are a gunshot wound, propelled object, or stab-type wounds.
      c. Combination injuries with both blunt and penetrating components are possible as well.
         i. Blunt and penetrating injuries can lead to clot formation or thrombosis causing interruption of blood flow or result in life-threatening hemorrhage.[4]

C. *Central versus peripheral vascular injuries*
   1. Vascular injuries can be central or peripheral. The focus in this chapter is primarily on peripheral injuries.
   2. Greatest morbidity and mortality related to peripheral vascular injury was associated with supracondylar fracture of the humerus, posterior knee dislocation, or tibial plateau fracture.[5]
      a. Penetrating extremity trauma is the leading cause of peripheral vascular injuries, accounting for 75% to 80% of injuries.[6]
      b. Projectiles from handguns account for 50% of injuries, followed by stab wounds (30%), and shotguns (5%).
         i. Femoral and popliteal arteries were most commonly affected, which occurred in 50% to 60% of injuries followed by brachial artery injury, estimated to account for 30% of traumatic arterial injuries.
         ii. Blunt trauma injuries accounted for 5% to 25% of peripheral vascular injuries.

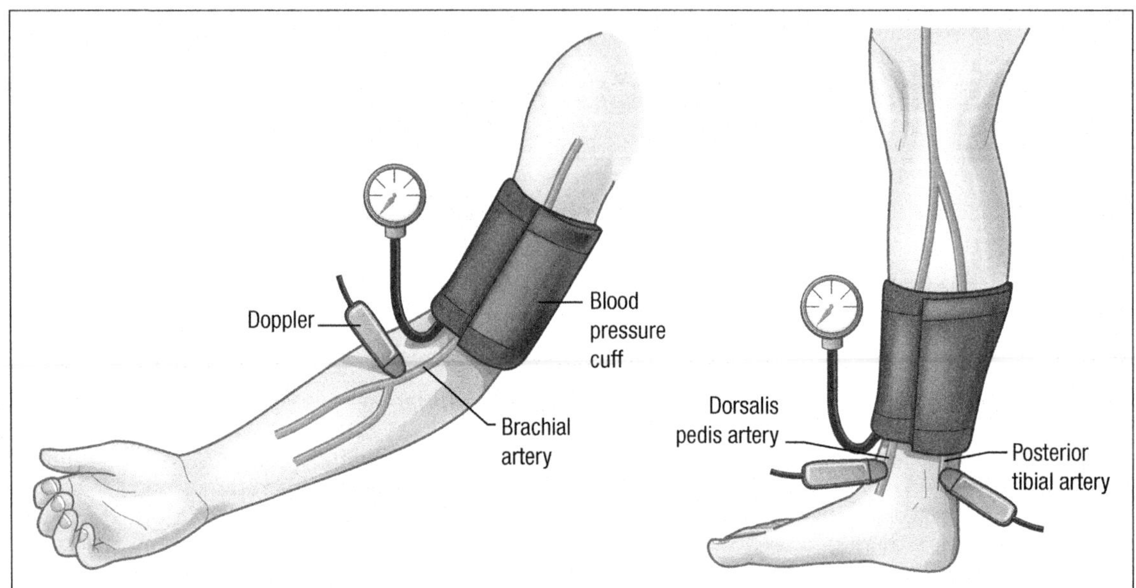

FIGURE 31.1 Arterial pressure indices (API) measurement.

Medical Screening

A. *Signs and symptoms*

1. Active hemorrhage
2. Expanding hematoma with or without pulsation
3. Absent or diminished distal pulses
4. Palpable thrill or audible bruit
5. Signs of ischemia or occlusion
   a. Dark or blue discoloration of the extremity
   b. Extremity that is cold or cool to touch
   c. "Six P's" of acute arterial occlusion are "hard signs" of high probability of vascular injury[7]:
      i. Pulselessness
      ii. Pallor
      iii. Paresthesias
      iv. Pain
      v. Paralysis
      vi. Poikilothermia or loss of thermoregulation
   d. "Hard signs" may also be considered "absolute" signs, indicating the need for immediate vascular intervention, necessary to salvage the extremity.[2]
6. "Soft signs" of vascular trauma[7]
   a. Trauma with significant hemorrhage (on scene or in transit)
   b. Unexplained hypotension or shock
   c. Small, stable, nonexpanding, and nonpulsatile hematoma
   d. Diminished distal pulses
   e. Neurologic deficit
   f. Close proximity of injury to major vascular structures
   g. Associated significant bony injury
   h. Also referred to as "relative" signs as they warrant further investigation and meticulous monitoring[2]

B. *Physical examination*

1. Physical examination was found to be sensitive with regard to evaluation of lower extremity trauma.
2. Physical examination was found to be especially sensitive for vascular injuries requiring reperfusion intervention.[8]

Diagnostic Evaluation

A. *Ankle-brachial index (ABI) or arterial pressure indices (API)*

1. Utilized to assess vascular integrity
   a. ABI are indicated to evaluate for peripheral vascular disease by measuring and comparing systolic blood pressure (SBP) readings of the extremities, specifically between the ankle and forearm.
   b. API compares SBP of injured extremity compared to an uninjured extremity using the following steps:
      i. Measure injured extremity blood pressure (BP), then measure contralateral uninjured extremity SBP (Figure 31.1).
      ii. If the arm is injured, utilize standard brachial systolic pressure; if the leg is injured, utilize ankle systolic pressure in which the BP cuff is applied to the calf.
      iii. Dorsalis pedis pressure and posterior tibial pressure is measured in the lower extremities.
      iv. A Doppler should be utilized to obtain the first sound as the cuff is deflated.
      v. API may not be feasible if the injury is sustained too distal for application of a sphygmomanometer cuff. The following calculation is utilized:
         (1) API = (SBP of injured extremity)/(SBP uninjured extremity)
      vi. API measuring >0.9 mmHg suggests the artery is intact (no injury)
      vii. An API cutoff of <0.9 mmHg is >95% sensitive and specific for arterial injury. A finding of <0.9 mmHg should be followed by immediate surgical consultation and/or consideration of an emergent CT angiography (CTA).[7]

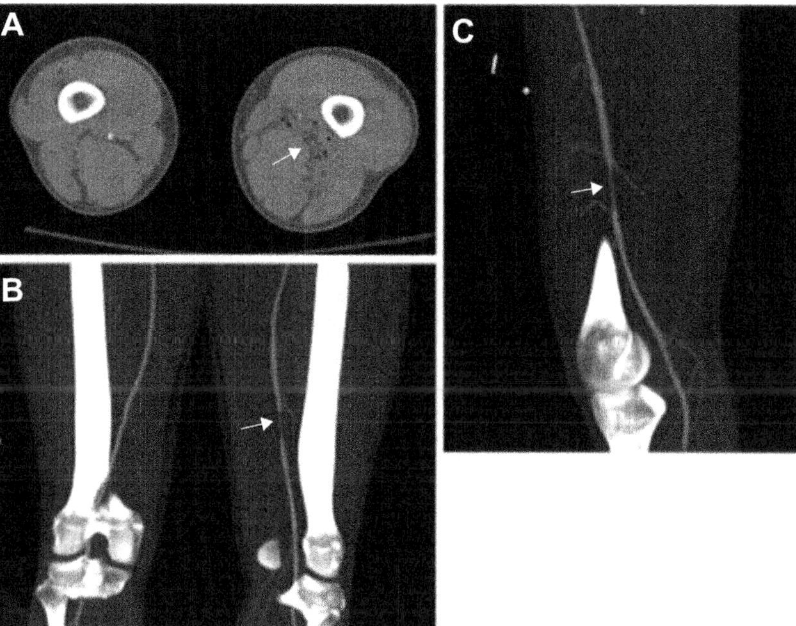

FIGURE 31.2 An 18-year-old man who sustained a gunshot wound to the left thigh. (A) CT angiogram reveals gas and focal narrowing/spasm of the left superficial femoral artery (arrow). (B) Projection in the coronal (arrow) and (C) sagittal planes (arrow) show the same injury. In this case, the patient was treated nonoperatively.
Source: Adibi A, Krishnam MS, Dissanayake S, et al. Computed tomography angiography of lower extremities in the emergency room for evaluation of patients with gunshot wounds. *Eur Radiol.* 2014;24(7):1586–1593. https://doi.org/10.1007/s00330-014-3174-1.[9]

B. *CTA*

1. CTA is considered the gold standard of imaging for the evaluation of vascular injury.[10]

2. CTA has been identified as almost 100% sensitive and specific in the diagnosis of vascular injury, specifically in the lower extremity after penetrating trauma.[8]

3. CTA has been found to be an effective tool in the evaluation of the upper extremities as well.

a. Used to investigate "soft signs" of vascular trauma

i. CTA imaging is an excellent noninvasive diagnostic tool given its accessibility, speed of acquisition, sensitivity, and specificity.

4. CTA runoff is optimal for evaluation of the lower extremities (Figure 31.2).

5. Run-off CTA images extend from the costo-diaphragmatic recess to the forefoot of the lower extremity.

6. To obtain a CTA, contrast material is injected into a large-bore venous access prior to obtaining images.

7. *Drawback:* Contrast material injected for the examination has the potential to cause contrast nephropathy in 1.0% to 4.8% of patients.[8]

8. Baseline renal function, such as a serum blood urea and nitrogen (BUN) and serum creatinine are indicated, if time warrants.

9. Drawback: multiple CT scans have been associated with an increased cancer risk.[8]

C. *Magnetic resonance angiography (MRA)*

1. MRA utilizes a magnetic field to evaluate the integrity of vasculature with favorable contrast resolution providing a luminal map of the arterial tree.

2. Provides stack three-dimensional (3D) images generating a volumetric representation that highlights vascular pathology.

3. Utilizes nonionizing radiation in a noninvasive manner. Gadolinium is delivered through a venous catheter, prior to obtaining images.

4. The contrast material used for MRA is believed to have fewer adverse effects as compared with injected contrast agents used for CTA. [11]

5. The greatest disadvantages are related to cost and time.

a. Cost of MRA is significantly higher than a CTA.

b. An MRA can take up to an hour or more to obtain depending on the study, whereas most CTA evaluations are completed in <10 minutes.

6. Another disadvantage is related to the use of a magnetic field, patients who have an implanted devices such as pacemakers, metal in the eyes, implanted orthopedic devices, and those individuals with certain surgical clips would not be candidates for this type of diagnostic examination.

D. *Duplex ultrasonography*

1. Point-of-care ultrasound (POCUS) is widely accessible in the ED and can aid in the identification and diagnosis of peripheral vascular injury.

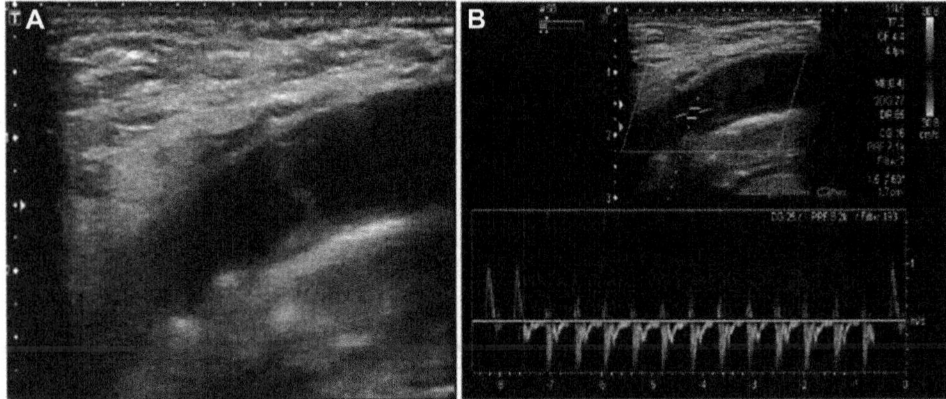

FIGURE 31.3 (A) Posttraumatic femoral artery intimal flap B-mode small echogenic flap into the lumen. (B) Turbulent flow with change of direction of the flow was seen moving the sample volume near the moving flap. *Source:* Montorfano MA, Pla F, Vera L, Cardillo O, Nigra SG, Montorfano LM. Point-of-care ultrasound and Doppler ultrasound evaluation of vascular injuries in penetrating and blunt trauma. *Crit Ultrasound J*. 2017;9(1):5. https://doi.org/10.1186/s13089-017-0060-5.

a. Color flow duplex Doppler translates returning ultrasound waves into a color-coding, based on velocity and direction of blood flow.
b. POCUS is a reliable tool found to have a sensitivity of 95% to 97% and specificity of 95% to 98% with regard to the evaluation of vascular trauma.[10]
c. POCUS has been effectively utilized specifically for patients presenting with soft signs of vascular trauma or for those individuals suspicious of vascular injury.
d. POCUS is useful in the identification of an acute arterial injury through the presence or absence of flow, the presence of pseudoaneurysms, waveform and flow velocity abnormalities, and changes in the quality of the Doppler signal.[12]
e. When utilizing POCUS, it is important to consider directionality of blood flow that is generated by adjacent collateral vessels, which can cause retrograde flow that may mimic a normal examination.

2. High-frequency linear ultrasound transducers are utilized for higher resolution and a lower penetration (Figure 31.3).
a. Patients with large hematomas may require a convex probe for higher penetration.[10]
b. When evaluating the affected area, explore vessels in a transverse and longitudinal manner with B-mode.
c. Proximal and distal flows with color flow duplex Doppler ultrasound is recommended.
d. Explore the contralateral extremity for comparison as needed. Normal veins appear oval and are completely compressible with the ultrasound probe. Waveform Doppler will display a continuous wave flow pattern. Arteries are round in shape with an echogenic wall. Arteries are noncompressible with the ultrasound probe. Arteries of the extremities show a triphasic waveform pattern. The triphasic pattern has a first positive phase corresponding with systole of the left ventricle, a second negative phase corresponding with the closure of the aortic valve, and a third positive phase is produced by the elasticity of the arterial walls.
i. Loss of the triphasic pattern is always pathologic, the absence of triphasic pattern can be acute (traumatic injury or obstruction) or chronic (atherosclerotic process, diabetes, and with aging).[10]

Criteria for Scoring Peripheral Vascular Injuries

Several scoring tools are available for utilization in the presence of a peripheral vascular injury. For the purposes of our discussion, the predictive salvage index (PSI) and the mangled extremity severity score (MESS) will be

BOX 31.1 CATEGORIES AND SCORING OF PREDICTIVE SALVAGE INDEX

SITE	SCORE
ARTERY	
Supra popliteal level	1
Popliteal level	2
Infra popliteal level	3
BONE	
Mild	1
Moderate	2
Severe	3
MUSCLE	
Mild	1
Moderate	2
Severe	3
INTERVAL TO OPERATING ROOM	
<6	1
6-12	2
>12	3

reviewed. Both tools attempt to predict limb salvage in the presence of a peripheral vascular injury. Both have been criticized with regard to usefulness and validity.

A. PSI

1. The PSI by Howe et al. in 1987 was proposed in an attempt to avoid unnecessary salvage of a limb and was based on a retrospective analysis of a small group of patients. The study analyzed factors that determined amputation or salvage of a lower limb. Variables of importance (Box 31.1) include:

a. Extent of vascular injury
b. Degree of bone damage
c. Degree of injury to muscle
d. Warm ischemia time

2. Sensitivity of 78% and a specificity of 100% was reported. The cutoff value of 8 or greater was a determinant for amputation.[14]

3. The PSI was found to be especially useful in those individuals who had a combination of lower limb injury with associated vascular injury.

B. MESS (Table 31.1)

1. The MESS was created to be utilized as an objective tool to assist with stratification and the prediction for potential salvage of a severe limb injury.

2. The MESS stratifies the injured limb based on:

a. Severity of skeletal/soft tissue injury
b. Degree and time of limb ischemia
c. Severity of shock
d. Patient age

3. A score can range from 2 to 14.

a. A score of 7 or higher correlates with a greater risk for amputation.

4. MESS is controversial with regard to its utilization and its application due to the emergence of more contemporary operative techniques.[7]

Management

A. As with all trauma management, initial resuscitation, diagnostic evaluation, and management are guided through the utilization of a systematic and concise approach according to the protocols from the Advanced Trauma Life Support (ATLS) program, established by the American College of Surgeons Committee on Trauma.[15]

B. ATLS emphasizes rapid and accurate assessment, resuscitation, and stabilization according to priority, determination of needs, and proper transfer if necessary to ensure optimization of care in order to prevent the deterioration of a patient's condition during the evaluation, resuscitation, and the transfer process.

C. Hemorrhage

1. Hemostasis or control of extremity hemorrhage is a primary goal with regard to management.

2. Hemorrhage is one of the leading causes of death in trauma patients.[16]

3. Hemorrhage is best managed with a multidisciplinary approach.

a. Damage control resuscitation is an approach that includes arrest of active hemorrhage, limiting intravenous crystalloid administration, early initiation of blood product administration, allowing for permissive hypotension, requesting early surgical consultation, and restoration of baseline physiologic function while averting the lethal triad of hypothermia, coagulopathy, and acidosis or excessively stimulating the immune-inflammatory system.[17]

b. Permissive hypotension allows for a mean arterial pressure (MAP) of >50 mmHg or an SBP of 70 to 90 mmHg.

TABLE 31.1 MANGLED EXTREMITY SEVERITY SCORE (MESS)

	FACTORS	SCORE
Skeletal/soft tissue injury	Low energy (stab; simple fracture; pistol gunshot wound)	1
	Medium energy (open or multiple fractures, dislocation)	2
	Medium energy (open or multiple fractures, dislocation)	3
	Very high energy (high-speed trauma + gross contamination	4
Limb ischemia	Pulse reduced or absent but perfusion normal	1*
	Pulseless; paresthesias, diminished capillary refill	2*
	Cool, paralyzed, insensate, numb	3*
Shock	Systolic BP always > 90 mmHg	0
	Hypotensive transiently	1
	Persistent hypotension	2
Age (years)	30	0
	30–50	1
	>50	2

*Doubled score for ischemia > 6 hours. A MESS score of 7 means a 100% prognosis value in favor of amputation.

BP, blood pressure.

Source: With permission from Johansen K, Daines M, Howey T, et al. Objective criteria accurately predict amputation following lower extremity trauma. *J Trauma.* 1990;*30(5)*:568–573. doi:10.1097/00005373-199005000-00007[13]

c. This approach may avoid the adverse effects of early, high-dose fluid resuscitation, such as dilutional coagulopathy and acceleration of hemorrhage.[18]

4. Active hemorrhage: swift intervention is key
   a. Obvious hemorrhage in a compressible area should be initially treated with direct digital pressure.[19]
      i. Direct pressure should be attempted for approximately 10 to 15 minutes if the patients remains hemodynamically stable.
      ii. Should direct pressure fail, a tourniquet can be applied.
         (1) Pneumatic tourniquets (PTs) have effectively been utilized to control extremity hemorrhage.
         (2) This technique was found to improve survival in patients without shock.[20]
         (3) Suggested placement of the PT cuff is at least 5 cm proximal to the bleeding wound, pressure should be <250 mmHg, for not more than 2 hours continuously to avoid ischemic complications.[21]
         (4) Consideration with regard to tourniquet removal should include the possibility of significant blood loss, acidosis, hyperkalemia, and hypotension.
         (5) Careful timing, rewarming, resuscitation, coagulopathy correction, and collaborative surgical consultation should take place prior to the withdrawal of the tourniquet.[7]
5. Pharmacologic intervention
   a. Off-label tranexamic acid (TXA)
      i. The utility of TXA in acute trauma is well established; knowledge gaps and limitations still exist.[22]
      ii. TXA is administered as an intravenous infusion for severe hemorrhage. TXA is administered within 3 hours of injury as an immediate intravenous dose of 1 g and may be followed by a 1 g continuous infusion over 8 hours.[23]
      iii. TXA has been associated with a reduction in all-cause mortality associated with hemorrhage.[16] TXA effectively blocks the lysine-binding sites on plasminogen, hence inhibiting fibrinolysis, resulting in inhibition of clot degradation.[23]
      iv. TXA was found to have a limited incidence of adverse events[16] but should be avoided in those individuals with known thromboembolic disease.[23]
6. The cessation of life-threatening hemorrhage supersedes that of limb salvage. In severe cases of bleeding, temporary aortic balloon catheter tapenade can be used as a temporizing measure in patients with devastating abdominal, pelvic, and lower limb hemorrhage.[17]

D. Osseous injury
1. The presence of vascular injury may be accompanied by fracture of regional osseous structures or occur with associated joint injury.
2. Approximately 33% of vascular injuries are combined with fractures, and approximately 17% are associated with nerve injuries.
3. Fracture is an independent risk factor for amputation.[2]
4. Management strategies are focused on pain management, preservation of function, and prevention of infection.
   a. Preservation of functionality may require reduction, relocation, and stabilization with splinting, and sometimes traction fixation of the extremity is necessary to prevent further injury.[7]
   b. Infection of osseous structures can occur when integument is compromised or with open wounds.
      i. Penetrating injuries are considered open.
      ii. Multiple classification systems are available to categorize open fractures, such as the Gustilo-Anderson classification.
      iii. This system stratifies injuries within three types and subtypes; higher scores correspond with worsening severity and prognosis, particularly with regard to infection.[24]
      iv. Early antibiotic administration usually within 3 hours of injury has been shown to have a significant positive impact on the prevention of infection in patients with open fracture.[25]
      v. Type I and Type II injuries have been associated with gram-positive organism infection such as those caused by *Staphylococcus aureus* and *Streptococcus* species infection, therefore a first-generation cephalosporin, such as cefazolin 2 g intravenous is recommended.
      vi. Type III injuries receive the same antibiotic coverage, a first-generation cephalosporin, such as cefazolin 2 g, in addition to coverage against gram-negative organisms, which would include the addition of an aminoglycoside such as gentamycin dosed at 6 mg/kg as an intravenous infusion.[7]
      vii. Additionally, consider high-risk contaminated wounds such as those associated with farmyard injuries, dirty water, fecal contamination, marine injuries, and human or animal bites. These injuries have a particularly high risk for infection, often with unusual organisms like *Clostridia*, *Pseudomonas*, *Vibrio*, or *Aeromonas*, they require organism-specific coverage.[24]
      viii. For patients who are allergic to penicillin and/or cephalosporin, vancomycin and ciprofloxacin may be given.[26]

E. *Wound management*
1. Wound management principles focus on hemostasis, identification of the extent of injury, pain management, and prevention of infection.
2. Wounds should be irrigated until foreign material has been sufficiently removed. Exact amount of irrigation varies; one study suggested 250 mL of irrigation fluid per 5 cm of wound length or approximately 50 mL per centimeter of wound length.[27]
3. In the ED setting, an isotonic saline solution is often utilized.

a. Studies have shown that tap water and distilled water irrigation may be just as effective for wound irrigation.[28,29]

4. Each wound should be evaluated in a bloodless field to fully evaluate depth and for the possibility of retained foreign body.

5. Consider radiographic or ultrasound imaging if there is concern for retained foreign body.

6. Ultrasound can effectively determine the presence of foreign body with regard to depth, size, and proximity of foreign body to adjoining nerves, vessels, or tendons.[30]

7. If there is concern for deep or complicated foreign body, surgical consultation should be obtained before removal.

F. *Infection prevention*

1. Vascular injury with associated osseous structure injury will require prompt antibiotic therapy.

2. Early administration of antibiotics can reduce infection in these patients.[31]

3. The administration of prophylactic antibiotics has been proven necessary in multiple previous studies and is incorporated in current guidelines proposed by ATLS.[32]

4. Additionally, consider that individuals who have underlying conditions such as those with vascular disease, those who smoke, are those who are immunocompromised including diabetic patients, or those who have significantly contaminated wounds may have a greater risk for infection.

5. If infection with methicillin-resistant *S. aureus* is a possibility broader coverage can be obtained by using trimethoprim/sulfamethoxazole, clindamycin, doxycycline, or vancomycin.[26]

6. As with all open wounds, tetanus status must be evaluated and updated according to Centers for Disease Control and Prevention (CDC) guidelines.[33]

G. *Consultation*

1. The care team will identify those individuals with potential for vascular injury based on history and physical examination findings.

2. Hard signs or absolute signs of vascular injury require immediate vascular evaluation and often intervention by a vascular surgeon.

a. In some cases, an interventional radiologist can be consulted to perform image-guided procedures such as stenting and embolization in an interventional suite.

3. An orthopedic surgeon should be consulted for associated bone and joint injuries.

4. Peripheral vascular injuries are often complicated and often require a multidisciplinary approach for treatment.

Special Considerations

A. *Nerve-related injury*

1. Nerve injury may accompany peripheral vascular injury due to the proximity of vascular structures in relation to nerve bundles. Suspect primary nerve injury if nerve deficit symptoms occur immediately following the injury. If the symptoms are delayed, vascular causes of neuropathy such as nerve compression and compartment syndrome are more likely.

B. *Specific trauma*

1. The subclavian and axillary structures are technically intrathoracic but are closely associated with the periphery, therefore, were included in this brief discussion. Gupta[34] identified specific vascular injuries and the suggested associated imaging and considerations for each:

a. Subclavian artery and vein injury are uncommon, often a result of penetrating trauma, manifesting as hemorrhagic shock. Associated pneumothorax or hemothorax, and injury to mediastinal structures is common. Severe nerve injury can occur and should be considered in these individuals. A chest x-ray, and even CTA may be warranted. Ultrasound is not the best diagnostic for evaluating subclavian artery and vein injuries due to overlying pulmonary structures. Subclavian vein injury is more dangerous than subclavian artery injury due to a high risk of air embolus. Patients should be placed in Trendelenburg if vein injury is suspected.

b. Axillary artery and vein trauma often result from a shoulder dislocation and denervation due to plexus injury. Axillary vascular injury and plexus injury are associated with a high risk for amputation.

c. Forearm artery injury involves injury to the radial or ulnar arteries. These injuries are associated with intermittent claudication and often require repair.

2. Lower leg injuries are associated with a high risk for compartment syndrome and require close monitoring. Acute compartment syndrome can occur after a long bone fracture. Tibial fractures are the most common cause of compartmentalization, followed by distal radius fractures that account for 75% of cases of acute compartment syndrome.

References

References for this chapter are online only and can be found at https://connect.springerpub.com/content/reference-book/978-0-8261-6091-5/part/part03/toc-part/ch31.

32. Orthopedic Injuries

MARY JO CEREPANI | MICHAEL SWEENEY

Learning Objectives

- Differentiate simple fractures from complex fractures.
- Compare and contrast a variety of musculoskeletal complaints.
- Demonstrate the ability to identify red flags of common and complex musculoskeletal complaints.
- Differentiate diagnosis based on pathophysiology, clinical assessment, and diagnostic testing.

Bursitis

Bursitis is an inflammation of any of the many bursae located in the human body. The synovial lining becomes thickened and produces an excessive amount of lubricating fluid, which results in swelling and pain.

Anatomy

There are approximately 160 bursa located in various parts of the body. A bursa is a saclike structure between skin or between bones, ligaments, and tendons. The bursae are lined with synovial tissue that produces fluid that serves as a lubricant between the structures that reduces friction.

Pathophysiology

A. Causes
 1. Overuse injuries
 2. Traumatic events
 3. Gout/pseudogout
 4. Infectious disease
 5. Hemorrhagic disorders
 6. Improper injection of vaccinations into the subdeltoid and subacromial bursa
 7. Autoimmune disorders
  a. Reactive arthritis. Psoriatic arthritis, rheumatoid arthritis (RA)
  b. Ankylosing spondylitis
  c. Scleroderma
  d. Systemic lupus erythematosus (SLE)
  e. Pancreatitis
  f. Oxalosis
  g. Uremia
B. Septic bursitis
 1. Most common at the superficial bursae
 2. 50% to 70% of cases are the result of microorganisms directly introduced to the bursae via traumatic injury or cellulitis.
 3. 10% of cases are infection of deep bursae, which is due to contiguous septic arthritis or bacteremia.
 4. *Staphylococcus aureus,* most common pathogen in 80% of cases
 5. Additional organisms have been identified in infectious bursitis.

Medical Screening

A. *Chief complaint:* Localized pain and swelling at a bursae
B. Signs and symptoms
 1. Localized tenderness
 2. Pain worse with joint manipulation, tendon manipulation, or both
 3. Edema
 4. Erythema
 5. Reduced movement
 6. Warm to hot at the location of the bursae
C. Focused assessment
 1. Most common locations (Figure 32.1)
  a. Subacromial
   i. Tenderness noted over the greater tuberosity
   ii. Difficulty with abduction
   iii. Frequently associated with supraspinatus tendonitis
   iv. Elevation of the arm with repetitive activity such as pitching a baseball or repetitive lifting activity
  b. Olecranon
   i. Most common location for septic bursitis due to common location for trauma of the skin and surrounding tissues
   ii. Often needle aspiration is recommended because of the frequency of septic bursitis.
   iii. Chronic stress from repetitive leaning forward positions with pressure on the elbows
   iv. Common nontraumatic causes of olecranon bursitis are gout, pseudogout, and RA, and uremia.
  c. Trochanteric (greater trochanteric bursitis)
   i. More common in women in their fourth to sixth decade of life
   ii. More common in runners, athletes, or ballet dancers
   iii. Patients report chronic, intermittent aching pain that radiates down the lateral hip.
   iv. Walking or laying on the affected side exacerbates pain.
   v. Pain can be reproduced with hip abduction (superficial bursitis) or resisted active abduction (deep bursitis).

d. Prepatellar
   i. Often well-circumscribed warm edema over the lower pole of the patella. Knee flexion causes increased tension over the bursa and increased pain.
   ii. The knee joint does not have evident pain with flexion and extension.
   iii. Common in professions or repetitive activities causing trauma or constant friction between the skin and the patella
   iv. Delayed traumatic bursitis may be the result of an injury that occurred a week or more prior to the onset of symptoms.
   v. *Caution:* Recognize that the superficial nature of the bursa makes it vulnerable to the introduction of microorganisms and predisposes to septic arthritis. Therefore, it is strongly recommended that needle aspiration of fluid be performed if there is a higher index of suspicion for septic bursitis.
e. Infrapatellar
   i. Located more distally than prepatellar bursitis
   ii. Result of frequent kneeling, gout, or syphilis
   iii. Can be mistaken for Osgood–Schlatter disease (OSD)
   iv. Key pain with flexion and extension at the extremes of the range of motion and edema on both sides of the patellar tendon.

Differential Diagnoses

A. Infectious bursitis
B. Noninfectious bursitis
C. Gout and pseudogout
D. Occult trauma
E. Septic arthritis
F. Cellulitis

Diagnostic Testing

A. *Labs:* Routine laboratory blood work is generally not useful in making the diagnosis of infectious versus noninfectious bursitis. However, lab work is warranted when

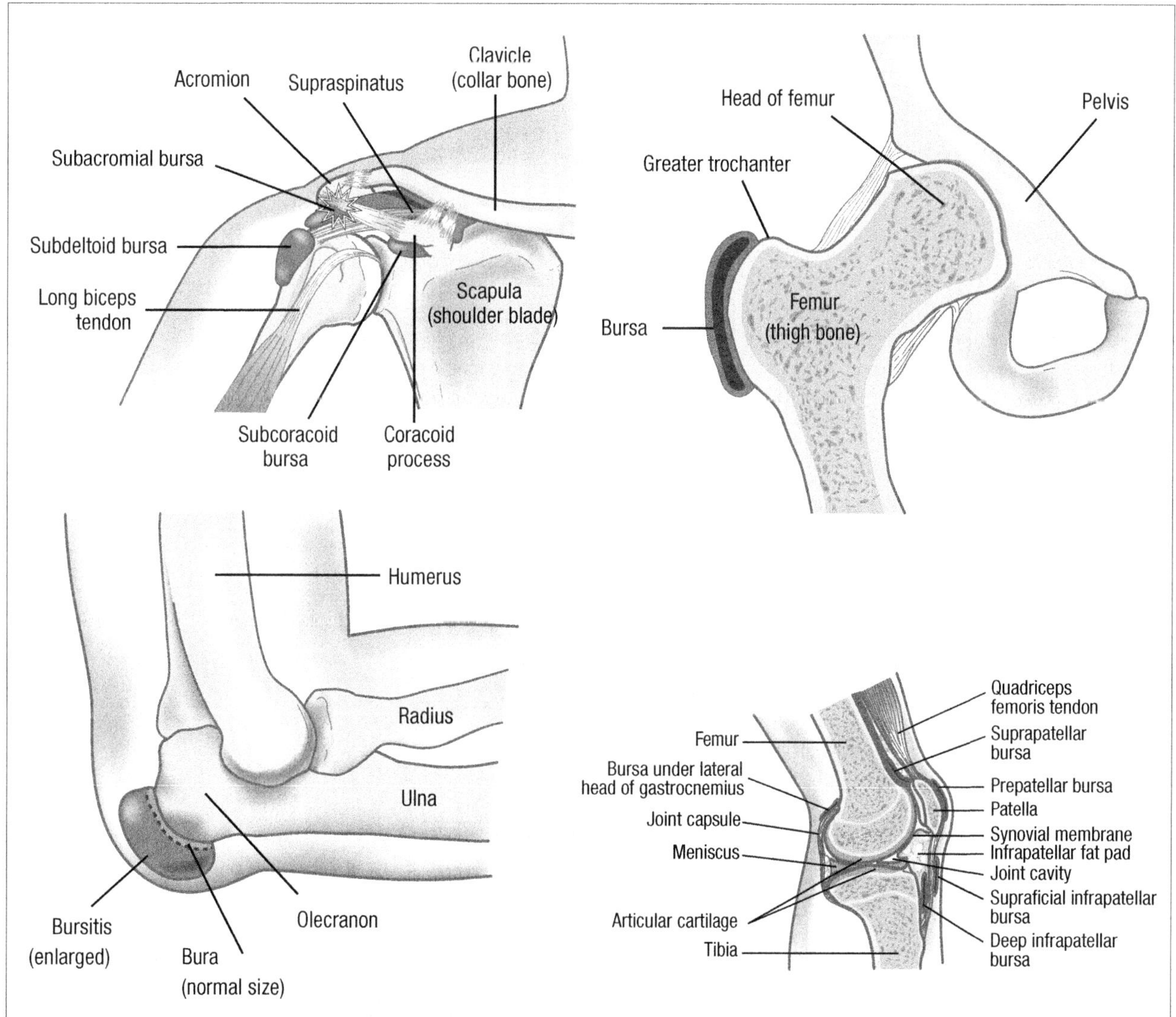

FIGURE 32.1 Locations of bursitis in subacromial (A), greater trochanteric (B), olecranon (C), and prepatellar or infrapatellar (D) spaces.

suspected septic bursitis and/or autoimmune-related disease is suspected.

B. Imaging

1. *X-ray:* Limited utility in the presence of bursitis. However, maybe warranted in the joint if the diagnosis is unclear.

2. *Ultrasound:* Significant utility when the diagnosis is unclear to identify bursae fluid. Additionally, prudent to aid in needle aspiration of the bursae fluid.

3. *MRI:* Although MRI is sensitive for the identification of bursitis, it is unnecessary and has limited utility from the ED.

C. *Needle aspiration of the bursae:* Refer to the procedure section listed below.

Management

A. Procedures

1. Needle aspiration of bursa

a. Basic techniques are like arthrocentesis technique

b. Utilization of ultrasound

i. Can improve the success of the procedure

ii. Can identify the location of the fluid

iii. This can be landmarked for entry (or) use ultrasound linear probe in the longitudinal or use aseptic technique.

c. Use sterile gloves.

d. Appropriate identification of the location of the bursa, avoiding tendons, major vessels, and major nerve branches

e. Do not perform if overlying cellulitis is suspected.

f. Aspirated fluid

i. Cell count

(1) Nonseptic bursitis has cell counts <2,000 mcL

(2) PMNs versus mononuclear cells

(3) White cell count usually lower than in septic arthritis

ii. Gram stain

(1) Limited utility due to variable sensitivity. Negative Gram stain does not exclude septic arthritis.

iii. Protein/glucose

(1) Infected bursa fluid can have an elevated protein and a low glucose level. However, this does not have accurate sensitivity in identifying septic arthritis

iv. Culture

(1) Is the conclusive test for diagnosis of septic bursitis

v. Crystals:

(1) Monosodium urate crystals are seen in gout.

(2) Calcium pyrophosphate crystals are seen in pseudogout.

(3) Cholesterol crystals are seen in rheumatoid-related bursitis and chronic effusions.

B. Pharmacologic therapies

1. Follow evidence-based guidelines for prescribing.

2. NSAIDs

3. Narcotic pain management

4. Topical lidocaine patches

5. May consider intrabursal steroid injection based on the patient's history and current condition

C. Nonpharmacologic treatments

1. Rest

2. Cold treatments

3. Heat treatments

4. Elevation

5. Compression with elastic wrap dressing

6. Immobilization

D. Consultation and collaboration

1. *Orthopedic surgeon:* If it is unclear if the joint or the bursae is infected, then seek the assistance of an orthopedic consultant.

2. *Emergency medicine physician:* Consider collaboration with the ED physician where the diagnosis is unclear.

Patient Disposition

A. Discharge

1. Most patients without findings of infection can be discharged to follow up with the primary doctor or appropriate specialist.

B. *Admission:* Identification of infectious septic arthritis or in cases where the diagnosis is unclear admission is suggested.

C. Age and developmental considerations

1. Prevention and education

2. Patient and family education and counseling

D. *Documentation:* It is important to clinically document in the medical decision-making why infectious bursitis is or is not suspected as well as septic joint. It is imperative that the documentation for these patient's assessment, treatment, reassessment, and timeline of disposition, is clearly documented. It is vital to document all findings, procedures, timely consultations with specialists, and medical decision-making.

Compartment Syndrome

Compartment syndrome occurs when the pressure within a closed muscle compartment exceeds the perfusion pressure and impairs blood outflow. This results in a lack of oxygenated blood flow and accumulation of waste products. It frequently is the result of direct trauma to the muscle group. This results in muscle and nerve ischemia. Prolonged muscle hypoxia leads to necrosis and permanent posttraumatic muscle contracture: Volkmann's ischemia.

Anatomy

A. Upper extremity compartments

1. The forearm (three compartments) most prone to compartment syndrome (Figure 32.2)

a. Volar

b. Dorsal

c. Mobile wad

2. *The hand:* Complicated multiple compartments within this confined space

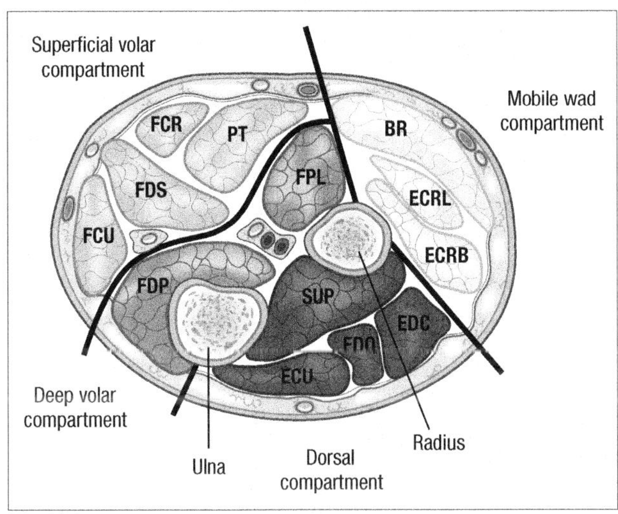

FIGURE 32.2 Four compartments of the forearm.

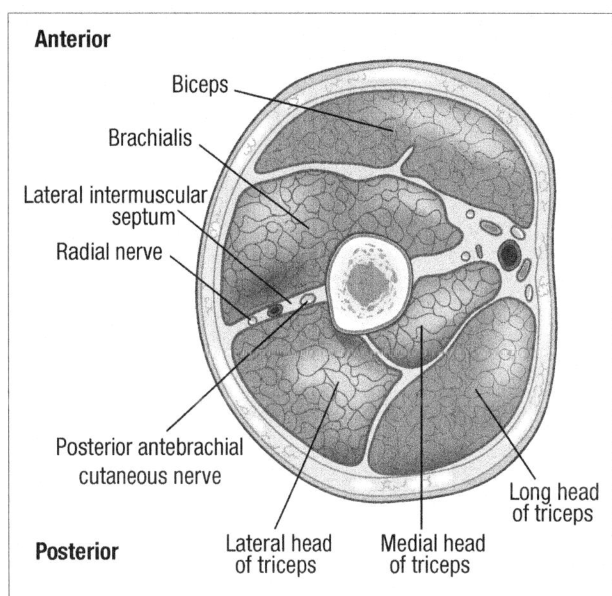

FIGURE 32.3 Two compartments of the arm.

3. *The upper arm* (Figure 32.3): Compartment syndrome is uncommon in this area.

B. Lower extremity compartments
   1. The lower leg (four compartments; Figure 32.4)
      a. Anterior
      b. Deep posterior
      c. Lateral
      d. Superficial
   2. The thigh (three compartments)
      a. *Anterior:* Femoral artery and nerve transverse located here
      b. Medial
      c. Posterior
   3. The buttocks (three compartments)
      a. Tensor
      b. Medius/minimus
      c. Maximus
   4. *The foot:* Complicated with nine compartments within this confined space

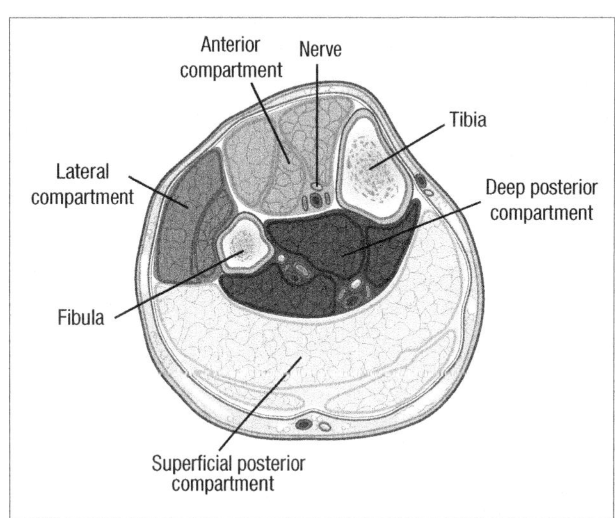

FIGURE 32.4 Compartments in the lower leg.

Pathophysiology

A. Common causes
   1. *Orthopedic:* Tibial fractures, forearm fractures
   2. *Vascular:* Ischemic reperfusion injury, hemorrhage
   3. *Iatrogenic:* Vascular puncture in anticoagulated patients, IV/intra-arterial drug injection, constrictive cast
   4. *Soft tissue injury:* Prolonged limb compression, crush injury, burns

Medical Screening

A. *Chief complaint:* Pain resulting from one of the following events:
   1. Crush injury
   2. High-pressure injuries
   3. Prolonged immobilization
   4. Blunt trauma

B. Signs and symptoms
   1. Pain out of proportion is the earliest finding and classic symptom.
      a. Ischemic muscle pain
         i. Pain exacerbated by active muscle contraction.
         ii. Pain exacerbated by stretching the muscle.
         iii. Poorly localized
         iv. Difficult controlling pain with normal dosing of appropriate analgesia
      b. Paresthesia a classic symptom
         i. Decreased sensation to pinprick
         ii. Decreased sensation to light touch
         iii. Decreased sensation to two-point discrimination
      c. Pallor
      d. Paresis
      e. Pulse deficit
   2. More negative predictive value than positive predictive value
   3. Signs and symptoms do not generally develop until tissue pressure has reached a critical level.

C. Focused assessment
1. Forearm is the most common location for compartment syndrome.
a. Educating the risk of compartment syndromes is important for fractures of the forearm with swelling and splinting.
2. Anterior tibial compartments most common site of compartment syndrome in the lower extremity.
3. Even with diligent clinical care, it is often difficult to identify cases of compartment syndrome before injury to muscle occurs. This becomes very evident in the uncooperative, unconscious, or critically injured patient who is unable to report symptoms.

Differential Diagnoses

A. Necrotizing soft tissue infections
B. Gas gangrene
C. Cellulitis
D. Peripheral vascular injuries
E. Rhabdomyolysis
F. Cnidaria envenomation
G. Deep venous thrombosis (DVT)

Diagnostic Testing

A. Imaging
1. X-rays
a. X-rays are often normal but can show signs of soft tissue swelling.
b. X-ray region localized to swelling for fracture or foreign body.
2. Ultrasound
a. Utilized to rule out DVT or Doppler ultrasonography to evaluate blood flow to the extremity
B. Laboratory testing
1. Complete blood count (CBC)
2. Comprehensive metabolic panel (CMP)
3. Serum and urine myoglobin
4. Creatine kinase
5. Urinalysis (UA)
6. Coagulation Studies

Management

A. The goal of the clinician is rapid assessment and diagnosis and early intervention with an orthopedic specialist.
B. There are several groups of patients whose clinical findings are difficult to obtain or interpret and who would benefit from measurement of compartment pressures.
C. Procedures
1. Measuring compartment pressure devices
a. Stryker (reusable)
b. Centurion (single-use disposable)
c. Self-calibrating disposable pressure transducer with integrated digital display
2. Single-use pressure monitoring
a. Indication
i. When clinical evaluation cannot make the diagnosis of compartment syndrome because the assessment is equivocal or unclear
b. Contraindication
i. Absolute: none
ii. Relative: coagulation disorder, overlying infection, cellulitis, burns
3. General procedure
a. Needle insertion is typically 18G.
b. Perpendicular insertion to the compartment
c. Insert cautiously to avoid nerve and blood vessels.
i. Stryker method
(1) Place the 18-gauge needle with a side port on the tapered stem of the diaphragm chamber.
(2) Screw a 3 mL prefilled saline syringe onto the back of the diaphragm chamber, which has a black disk.
(3) Place the diaphragm chamber assembly into the pressure monitor, black disc side down. Ensure that the chamber is well seated in the device.
(4) Snap the cover closed into place. Do not force.
(5) Hold the needle at a 45-degree angle up from level horizontal and press the plunger slowly to advance the saline through the system and purge the air.
(6) Turn the pressure monitor on. It should read between 0 and 9 mmHg.
(7) Hold the pressure monitor at the intended angle of insertion and press the "ZERO" button to calibrate. At this time, the device display should read "00."
(8) Clean the skin
(9) Administration of topical or injectable anesthetic is necessary (but not required).
(10) Insert the device into the compartment being measured.
(11) Slowly inject a maximum of 0.3 mL of saline into the compartment and wait for the device to record and display the pressure.
ii. Centurion Compass UniversalHG
(1) Remove Compass Universal from its sterile packing.
(2) Remove the proximal Luer Cap and connect Compass UniversalHG to 18G needle and saline-filled syringe.
(3) Prime Compass UniversalHG and needle with saline.
(4) With the Compass UniversalHG and needle positioned at the insertion angle, activate and calibrate Compass UniversalHG by depressing the power button for approximately one second until the display reads "00 mm."
(5) Insert needle tip and inject 0.3 mL of saline.
(6) Pressure is displayed on Compass UniversalHG LCD.
(7) See Centurion Medical Products Corp., www.centurionmp.com.
d. Focused extremity
i. Forearm
ii. Upper arm
iii. Lower leg
iv. Thigh
e. Pressure reading interpretation (Table 32.1)
D. Pharmacologic therapies
1. Follow evidence-based guidelines for prescribing.

TABLE 32.1 LABORATORY STUDIES TO DIAGNOSIS ORTHOPEDIC CONDITIONS

BLOOD TEST	EXAMPLES
Alkaline phosphate level	Increased with healing fractures, metabolic bone disease, osteoporosis, and metastatic tumors of bone
Calcium level	Increased with metastatic bone cancer, dehydration, Paget's disease Decreased with hypoparathyroidism, renal failure, and rhabdomyolysis
Creatine kinase level	Increased in dehydration, hyperthyroidism, renal failure, and rhabdomyolysis
Phosphorus level	Increased in bone metastases and hypoparathyroidism
ALT, AST	Increased in myositis
Uric acid level	Increased in gout, multiple myeloma, and acute tissue destruction because of starvation or excessive exercise
C-reactive protein	Increased in acute inflammatory changes and rheumatoid arthritis
Antinuclear antibodies	Positive in rheumatoid arthritis, systemic lupus erythematosus, and polymyositis
Serum rheumatoid factor	Positive in rheumatoid arthritis and some chronic inflammatory diseases

ALT, alanine aminotransferase; AST, aspartate aminotransferase.

2. Appropriate analgesia
3. NSAIDs
4. IV fluids

E. Consultation and collaboration
1. Orthopedic surgeon
a. Early consultation is strongly advised. Due to the concerning nature of this pathology and that it can be limb altering, contact the specialist early. These cases are time-sensitive and a 6-hour to fasciotomy time frame.
2. ED physician
a. It is strongly suggested that you collaborate with an attending physician to aid in decision-making process and facilitate rapid diagnosis and intervention.

Patient Disposition

A. Admission versus operative management
1. Most patients will require disposition to an operative suite. Most of these cases will require an operative setting to perform a fasciotomy. However, in the cases where the compartment pressure measurement is equivocal or nondiagnostic of the pathology, the patient will be admitted for serial neurovascular checks and serial compartment pressure analysis.

B. Transfer
1. Depending on the clinical setting, it may be required to transfer this patient to a tertiary center for evaluation and surgical intervention by an orthopedic specialist.

C. Age and developmental considerations
1. *Elderly:* Due to complications with dementia, decreased pain sensorium, and immobility; it will be difficult for the patient to assess an extremity fracture or musculoskeletal injury for developing compartment syndrome. Therefore, clear discharge instructions must be written for family, friends, or nursing facility so that they may reassess the injury.
2. *Children:* In cases with the risk for developing compartment syndrome exists, age of the patient will determine the ability to reassess their injury. Parents often need to be educated on musculoskeletal injury risk for compartment syndrome.
3. *Disabilities:* Patients with mental retardation (MR), autism, or similar conditions will require a third party to be educated on the risks of compartment syndrome related to musculoskeletal injuries.

D. Prevention and education
1. *Risk:* Educating patients with musculoskeletal trauma, fractures, minor crush injuries, or swelling to a specific extremity on the risk of compartment syndrome.
2. *Delayed process:* Patients should be aware that there may be a delay in the development of compartment syndrome and should be taught about reassessing their injury and signs/symptoms that should alert the patient return to the ED for reassessment.

E. Patient and family education and counseling
1. The diagnosis of compartment syndrome can result in lifelong musculoskeletal damage. Family and patient need counseling on the seriousness of this pathology and the possible disfigurement with a fasciotomy or extremity deformity related to the extremity ischemia.
2. Based on the location of the injury, instruct the patient and family to the correct position of the injured limb to prevent further injury.

F. Documentation
1. Documentation should focus on:
a. Medical decision-making that describes the thought process of the clinician's suspicion for compartment syndrome
b. Rapid diagnosis of compartment pressure
c. Documentation with the orthopedic specialist
i. Times of communication and evaluation
ii. Plan identified with specialist
d. Documentation of peripheral pulses, capillary refill, and sensory function
i. Document multiple assessments of neurovascular status

Hip Injuries (Fractures/Dislocations)

The hip is generally a stable ball-and-socket joint. The head of the femur is deeply situated in the acetabulum and ligamentous with strong support from surrounding musculature. Therefore, hip fractures and dislocations are often the results of significant force. The hip anatomy includes the acetabulum and the proximal femur 2 to 3 inches below the lesser trochanter. The hip structure is weakest posteriorly.

Anatomy

A. Landmarks

1. *Greater trochanter:* Muscle attachment for abductors and short rotator muscle

2. *Lesser trochanter:* Muscle attachment for iliopsoas muscle

3. The result is rich blood supply, collateral blood supply, and conductive to healing.

4. *Femoral head:* Very delicate blood supply making the risk for avascular necrosis and poor bone healing

Medical Screening

A. *Chief complaint:* Often a combination of hip pain and immobility

B. Signs and symptoms

1. Pain

a. Directly over the hip

b. Pain with motion

c. Anterior groin pain or thigh pain

d. Acute versus gradual pain

i. Acute pain: Usually more the result of acute traumatic event

ii. Gradual pain: Anterior groin pain increased with activity is suggestive of the stress fracture.

2. Shortened extremity

a. Affected leg shortens because the muscles acting on the joint are dependent on the continuity of the joint to perform.

b. May be an indication of a fracture or dislocation

3. Visualization should prompt the clinician to assess arterial vascular supply to the extremity by assessing the peripheral pulses, check Doppler pulses, assess capillary refill.

4. Lateral rotated extremity

5. Limited painful range of motion

6. Pain on passive range

7. Ecchymosis may or may not be present.

8. Limp or antalgic gait

9. Palpation of the inguinal area produces discomfort.

10. Inability to bear weight

C. Focused assessment

1. Hip fracture

a. Intracapsular

i. Location

(1) Capital (uncommon)

(2) Subcapital (common)

(3) Trans- or midcervical (rare)

(4) Basicervical (uncommon)

ii. Fracture and dislocation

(1) Specific focused concern on patients with intracapsular fractures because these fractures/dislocations often cause femoral neck blood vessels to be compromised or kinked because of tear or compression secondary to hemarthrosis.

b. Extracapsular

i. Location

(1) *Intertrochanteric:* Most common

(2) Subtrochanteric

2. Dislocation

a. Posterior dislocation

i. Occurs in 90% of hip dislocations

ii. Shortened, internally rotated, adducted

iii. High-energy impacts such as motor vehicle accidents (MVAs) and falls from height

iv. Very painful

b. Anterior dislocation

i. Occurs in 10% of hip dislocations

ii. Mechanism

c. Prosthetic hip dislocations

i. Dislocates with simple movements

ii. Most commonly within 1 month of hip replacement

iii. Often reoccurs

iv. If reoccurring then likely will need orthopedic revision

3. Older adults

a. High index of suspicion because the incidence doubles each decade over the age of 50. Also two to three times higher in women than men; 9 out of 10 fractures occur in patients over the age of 65. Bleeding from closed pelvic and long-bone fractures can be aggressive in the older adult population.

4. High-energy trauma

a. Fractures and dislocations of the hips are often high-energy impacts alerting the clinician that the assessment should not be isolated to the hip in question. It is pertinent that a complete head-to-toe assessment be completed to ensure no other coexisting injuries are present.

D. Neurovascular assessment

1. It is imperative that the clinician perform a thorough neurovascular assessment of the affected extremity.

2. The sciatic nerve sits just inferoposterior to the hip joint and is injured in 20% of all hip dislocations. The nerve may be contused or lacerated.

3. Assessment should include assessment for peripheral sensory deficit along sciatic nerve root, L5/S1 dorsiflexion/plantar flexion weakness, or vascular compromise. This should alert the clinician that emergent reduction is necessary.

Medical Decision-Making and Differential Diagnoses

A. It is important to stress that fractures of the hip and dislocations of the hip have similar presentations. Objectively, it is important to identify if there was a traumatic event or hip pain without trauma. The nontraumatic assessment is focused on excluding a septic joint.

B. Differential diagnosis includes the following:
1. Hip fracture
2. Hip dislocation
3. Femur injuries and/or fracture
4. Pelvic injuries and/or fracture
5. Femoral head avascular necrosis
6. Femoral neck fracture
7. Hip pointer
8. Hip tendonitis/bursitis
9. Iliopsoas tendonitis
10. Slipped capital femoral epiphysis

Diagnostic Testing

A. Imaging studies
1. X-rays
a. X-rays are the mainstay of evaluation for hip fracture versus dislocation.
b. Anteroposterior (AP) views of the pelvis and hip and cross-table lateral
c. X-rays are sufficient to evaluate potential fractures. If the extremity can be rotated internally or externally, this can increase the sensitivity of successful identification of fractures.
2. CT scan
a. If there is high index of suspicion for a fracture or the patient is unable to bear weight and the x-rays do not identify a fracture, CT imaging may be helpful in identifying an occult fracture.
3. MRI/bone scan
a. Although these are perfectly accurate in identifying occult fractures, they have limited utility in the ED due to lack of access by the clinician.

B. Laboratory testing
1. If the diagnosis of the hip pain is unclear, laboratory testing may help direct the differential diagnosis.
2. Complete blood count (CBC)
3. Basic metabolic panel (BMP; electrolytes and renal function)
4. Urinalysis (UA)
5. Prothrombin time/international normalized ratio (PT/INR), partial thromboplastin time (PTT)

C. Admission requirement
1. Patients that require admission for hip fracture repair or hip reduction often have preoperative testing completed.
a. EKG
b. Chest x-ray (CXR)
c. CBC, BMP, PT/INR, PTT
d. Blood type and screening

Management

A. Primary management is focused on pain management and stabilization of extremity until diagnosis of fracture or dislocation can be identified. Ensuring there is no vascular compromise is vital. Once identified, determination for orthopedic consultation, stabilization versus reduction, or operative management is the goal.

B. Aggressive management in the elderly population. Morbidity and mortality associated with hip fractures are primarily the result of patient immobilization and the development of DVT or pulmonary embolism (PE). Even with modern surgical intervention, mortality following hip fractures ranges from 15% to 35% within 1 year.

C. Procedures
1. Conscious sedation
a. Sedation will likely be required for hip dislocation reduction.
b. IV, monitor, oxygen, resuscitation equipment
c. Ensure that the patient is medicated appropriately.
d. Ensure the patient remains nil per os (NPO) while in the ED for surgery or other procedures.
e. Ensure adequate assessment of medical history and physical examination to assess for risk complications related to the procedure.
2. Hip reduction techniques
a. Allis Technique
i. Patient is laying supine with unaffected leg flat. One clinician is stabilizing the pelvic with their palms, while the second clinician is grabbing the proximal end of the lower leg just below the knee. With the thumbs over the medial and lateral collateral ligaments, pull traction in a 45-degree angle. While continuing to pull traction, transition to pull vertically. While continued upward traction, external and internal rotation should be performed until completion of reduction can be identified.
b. Whistler Technique (Figure 32.5)
i. Position the patient supine with both knees flexed to 130 degrees. The clinician instructs an assistant to stabilize the pelvis, and the clinician places their arm under the affected knee and grabs the other knee. The clinician anchors the ankle to the bed with the other hand. Using the arm under the knee as a lever, the clinician raises the shoulder and elevates the affected knee.
c. Captain Morgan Technique (Figure 32.6)
i. The patient is placed supine with the knee flexed. The clinician places their flexed knee under the patient's knees. The clinician applies force with their leg in an upward direction, internally and externally rotating the hip as needed to facilitate reduction.
d. East Baltimore Lift Maneuver (Figure 32.7)
i. The East Baltimore lift is another method of reducing a posterior hip dislocation. For this method (after considering sedation or analgesia), the patient is placed supine. The affected leg is flexed at right angles at both the hip and the knee. The clinician and assistant stand on opposite sides of the patient (pelvis level), and each place an arm under the patient's calf, cradling the leg and resting their hand on the shoulder of the person opposite. Traction is applied by anterior lift while the leg is stabilized by the clinician maintaining the knee's right angle. A third person is required to stabilize the pelvis.
e. Rocket Launcher Maneuver (Figure 32.8)

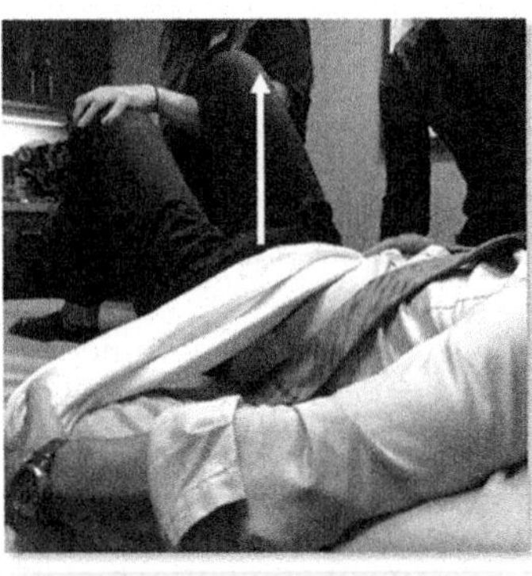

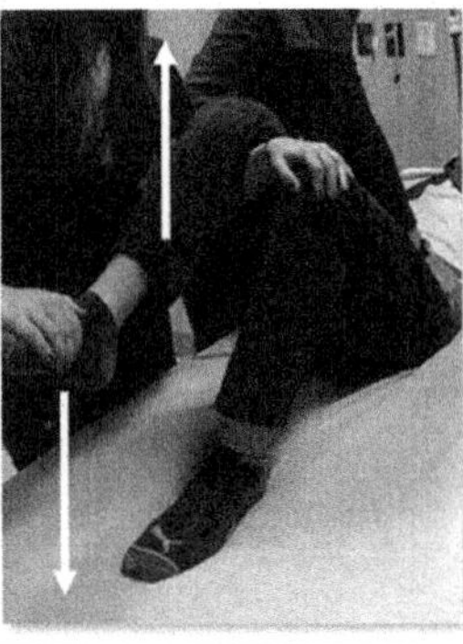

A B

FIGURE 32.5 Whistler technique. (A) Second clinician provides counter pressure to the pelvis using direct pressure or sheet to stabilize pelvis. (B) Using the arm under the knee as a lever, the clinician raises the shoulder and elevates the affected knee.

A B

FIGURE 32.6 Captain Morgan technique. (A) The clinician places the flexed knee under the patient's knee. The clinician applies force with the leg in an upward direction, internally and externally rotating the hip as needed to facilitate reduction. (B) The second clinician provides counter pressure to the pelvis.

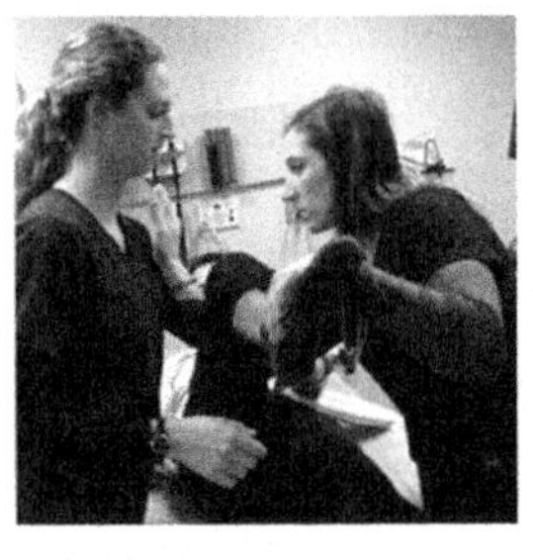

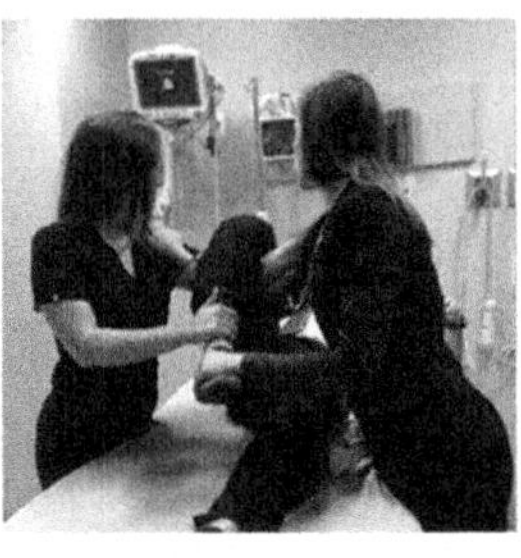

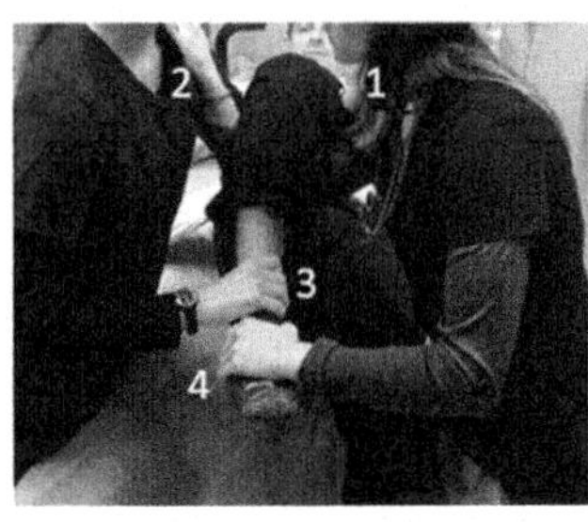

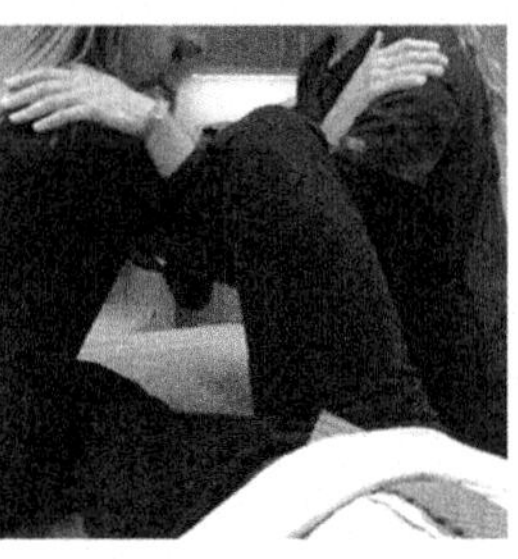

A B C D

FIGURE 32.7 East Baltimore Lift maneuver. (A) The affected leg is flexed at right angles at both the hip and the knee. (B) The clinician and assistant stand on opposite sides of the patient (pelvis level), and each place an arm under the patient's calf, cradling the leg and resting their hand on the shoulder of the person opposite in the order shown (C). (D) Traction is applied by anterior lift while the leg is stabilized by the clinician maintaining the knee's right angle. A third person is required to stabilize the pelvis.

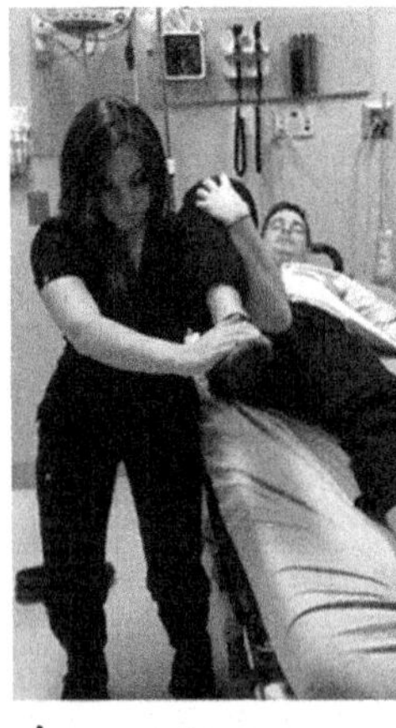

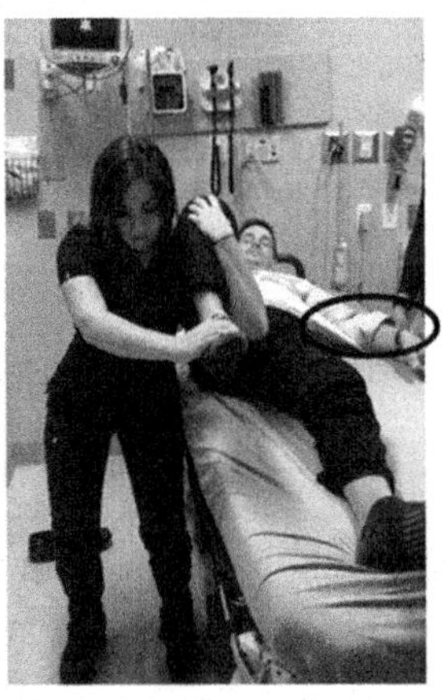

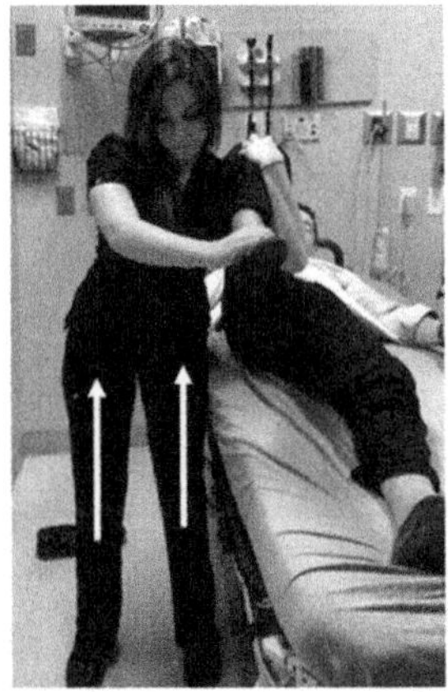

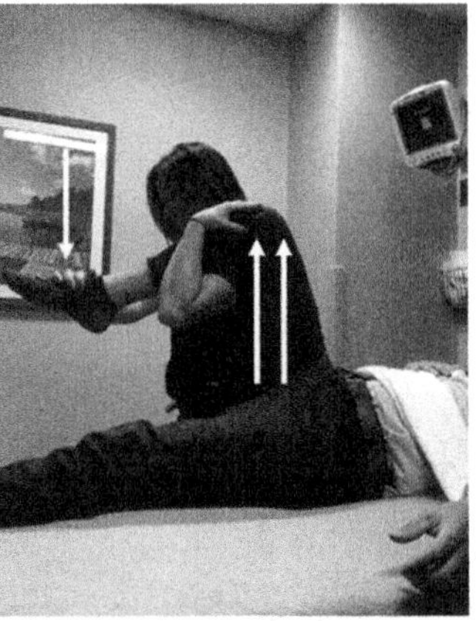

A B C D

FIGURE 32.8 Rocket launcher maneuver. (A) Start with knees flexed. (B) Second person to provide pelvic counter pressure directly or with sheet. (C) Use lower body strength to create vertical counter traction. (D) Note location of hands.

D. Pharmacologic therapies
1. Follow the evidence-based guidelines when prescribing.
2. *Narcotic analgesia:* Most hip fractures and dislocations require analgesia. Safe use of an opioid will be needed. Ensure that you assess the patient's pain pre- and postadministration.
3. *NSAIDs:* Toradol or ibuprofen are acceptable non-narcotic analgesia that may help with swelling and pain.

E. Consultation and collaboration
1. Management of hip fractures and dislocations is centered around early consultation with orthopedic specialist. Early consultation is suggested on cases where there is potential vascular compromise, open fractures, combination fracture/dislocations, prosthetic hip joint, or recent surgery with dislocation.
2. Collaboration is recommended for the clinician for any complicated dislocation or fracture with the ED attending. Collaboration will be required with the ED physician for conscious sedation reduction because the procedure requires one clinician to perform the reduction technique and one to monitor the patient during the procedure.

Patient Disposition

A. *Hip fractures:* After stabilization of the patient's pain and extremity, discussion with orthopedics, the patient will likely require admission for operative management. In a select few cases, disposition to discharge and non-weight bearing may be initiated but only after discussion with orthopedic specialist.

B. *Hip dislocation:* After stabilization of the patient's pain and extremity, identifying high-risk cases requiring prereduction orthopedic consultation, reduction can be performed. Successful reduction and successful postsedation recovery allow the patient to likely be discharged. Most dislocations without fracture can be discharged if they can be reduced and ambulated postreduction. Failure to successfully complete reduction, recent hip surgery with dislocation, and hardware dislocations, may all require operative management.

C. Documentation
1. Documentation should encapsulate the following data:
a. Neurovascular assessment pre- and postprocedure
b. Pain management and immobilization
c. Radiographic findings
d. Physical examination to exclude other injuries that may be the result of the identified trauma
e. Also, it is important to document the patient's ability to successfully ambulate postreduction of hip.

Age and Developmental Considerations

A. Prevention and education
1. Older adult patients:
a. Recommend ambulation assisting devices to reduce risk of fall.
b. Home risk assessment

B. Patient and family education and counseling
1. Fractures
a. Patient and family must be aware that the process for recovery will likely be a few months.
b. Patient and family education must encompass surgical intervention, recovery, and rehabilitation processes.
c. Discussion on stressed early intervention and treatment
d. Discussion on postsurgical complications
2. Dislocations
a. Patient discussion on reduction and technique
b. Patient discussion on risk and complications of conscious sedation should be identified.
c. Postmanagement with abductor pillow and high-risk body movements that could create a secondary dislocation.
d. Discussion on the importance of orthopedic specialists for follow-up

Lower Back Pain

Back pain is the second leading reason why patients visit their primary and the leading cause of work-related disability in persons <45 years. Although most of the back pain etiology does not cause life-threatening etiology or neurologically impairing, there are serious dangers exist in this chief complaint. Due to the sheer number of patients that visit the ED for this complaint, it is easy to develop an indifference to the complaint and overlook crucial history and physical clues that direct the clinician toward significant pathology.

Medical Screening

A. *Chief complaint:* Localizing back pain to the region of the pathology.

B. Signs and symptoms
1. Symptoms
a. A significant part of assessing the patient with back pain is recognizing that much of the examination is subjective information provided by the patient. A careful focused history to review the subjective data and symptoms that the patient reports. A clear understanding of medical history, surgical history, prior back dysfunction, duration of symptoms, and identification of associated symptoms to the back pain is key. The associated symptoms with the back pain will direct the clinician to exclude the concerning pathologies in the back pain differential.
b. See Table 32.2 for back pain red flags.

C. Physical examination (Tables 32.3 and 32.4)
1. *Vital signs:* Abnormal vital signs (fever, tachycardia, hypertension, hypotension) should raise concern for a more urgent pathologic cause of back pain.
2. *General appearance:* Most benign back pain patients are comfortable lying still. However, when the patient appears with excessive pain, consider acute spinal infections, abdominal aortic aneurysm, or nephrolithiasis.
3. *Abdominal assessment:* Auscultation for bruits and palpation for masses, tenderness, and an enlarged aorta. If the clinician has clinical ultrasound skills,

TABLE 32.2 ASSESSMENT OF PERIPHERAL NERVE INJURIES

NERVE	FREQUENTLY ASSOCIATED INJURIES	ASSESSMENT FINDINGS
Radial	Fracture of humerus, especially middle and distal thirds	Inability to extend thumb in "hitchhiker's sign"
Ulnar	Fracture of medial humeral epicondyle	Loss of pain perception in tip of little finger
Median	Elbow dislocation or wrist or forearm injury	Loss of pain perception in tip of index finger
Peroneal	Tibia or fibula fracture; dislocation of knee	Inability to extend great toe or foot; may also be associated with sciatic nerve injury
Sciatic and tibial	Infrequent with fractures or dislocations	Loss of pain perception in sole of foot

TABLE 32.3 COMMON FRACTURES

FRACTURE LOCATION	MECHANISM OF INJURY	CLINICAL FINDINGS	TREATMENT
Hand Phalanges Proximal to midphalanx fractures	Direct trauma or crush injury	Pain in digit, ligament laxity	Splint: finger splint Reduction may be required
Distal phalanx	Direct blow, crush injury	Subungual hematoma nail injury	Trephination or nail removal and repair of nail bed if macerated
Distal phalanx fracture	Sudden blow to tip of the extended finger	Flexion posture or "droop" of the distal interphalangeal joint (mallet finger)	Mallet splint or aluminum extension splint applied to the dorsal surface of the finger, which includes the distal and middle phalanges for 6–8 weeks; may require surgery
Metacarpal Second-fifth metacarpals	Crushing force or direct blow on the distal dorsal aspect of the closed fist	Swelling, rotational deformity of fingers or palm of the hand	Radial or ulnar gutter splint to the fingertips with the metacarpophalangeal joints flexed 70–90 degrees; may need surgery
Base of thumb (Bennet's fracture)	Axial load against a flexed thumb; fist fight, fall on hyperabducted or hyperflexed thumb	Pain and swelling dorsum of thumb, limited range of motion of metacarpophalangeal joint	Thumb spica splint with wrist in 30 degrees of extension, interphalangeal joint free and orthopedic referral
Humerus Neck	Fall on outstretched arm (may occur with dislocated shoulder)	Ecchymosis of shoulder, upper arm, and chest wall	Immobilize with sling, may splint or internally reduce if severe
Shaft	Direct trauma, twisting of arm	Radial nerve injury often occurs with fracture of lower third of bone	Immobilize with sling: use hanging arm cast if able to be mobile
Supracondylar	Fall on outstretched arm (usually occurs in children)	Swelling: pain on lateral side of elbow; decreased range of motion in elbow; may have associated wrist injury	Admit to hospital for close neurovascular observation and definitive care
Radius Head	Fall on outstretched arm	Swelling: pain on lateral side of elbow; decreased range of motion in elbow	Immobilize: treatment varies according to range of motion and possible dislocation
Radius Shaft	Usually occurs with falls, altercations, and motor vehicle crash	Pain along bone	Splint for comfort
Distal	Colles' fracture angulated dorsally, FOOSH	Distal fragment is deviated dorsally (dinner fork deformity)	Immobilize with splint; reduce if displaced, cast
Distal	Smith's fracture (angulated toward volar surface) fall onto dorsum of hand, FOOSH	Reverse Colle's fracture	Immobilize with splint reduce if displaced, cast
Galeazzi's fracture	Oblique fracture at junction of middle and distal thirds of radius with disruption of distal radioulnar joint: fall or blow on dorsal and lateral side of wrist and distal radius	Wrist and radial shaft tenderness and shortening	Usually unstable needs open reduction

(*continued*)

TABLE 32.3 COMMON FRACTURES (*CONTINUED*)

FRACTURE LOCATION	MECHANISM OF INJURY	CLINICAL FINDINGS	TREATMENT
Ulna Monteggia's fracture	Fracture of proximal third of ulna with anterior dislocation of radial head	Pain and swelling around elbow, pain worse with attempts at rotation; radial dislocation may be missed if elbow not included	Immobilize for comfort: closed reduction for children, open for adults Consult orthopedics
Nightstick fracture	Isolated, undisplaced fracture of midshaft of ulna as result of sharp blow	If ulna is angulated, injury to radius is also present	Immobilize fracture; requires ≥8 weeks to heal Consult orthopedic
Wrist Carpal fractures	Usually occurs with falls on outstretched hand or direct blow: common in young men whose strong muscles prevent injury to lower radius (navicular longest of carpal bones)	Pain in wrist, most severe in anatomic "snuff box" swelling (indicating scaphoid fracture): radiographs should include oblique view	Immobilize cast for at least ≥2 months to be sure fracture has reunited Consult orthopedics
Pelvis	Low velocity; elderly people; high velocity all age groups: MVC's, falls, and crushing forces	Hypovolemia; retroperitoneal space can hold 4 L of blood associated with multisystem trauma; especially genitourinary; tenderness with ilial wing compression or palpation of symphysis ecchymosis (late sign) in flank and peritoneal area	Splint to immobilize, begin fluid resuscitation, using caution as needed, Consult orthopedic immediately admit to hospital
Knee Head or neck (intracapsular)	Caused by fall or spontaneous break (osteoporosis)	Pain in hip or referred to knee; leg shortened and externally rotated	Splint; orthopedic referral surgical repair
Trochanter (extracapsular)	Caused by fall or spontaneous break (osteoporosis)	Pain in hip or referred to knee; leg shortened and externally rotated	Splint for comfort; Consult orthopedic surgical repair
Shaft	Associated with high force	Powerful muscle groups cause angulation and overriding to produce deformity; severe pain, blood loss into tissue and from intravascular volume	Traction splint; consult orthopedic admit patient
Tibia Plateau (extends into knee joint)	Fall on extended leg, direct blow, rotation stress on extended leg (pedestrian)	If radiographs are questionable or normal may aspirate joint; usually associated with soft tissue injuries	Splint for comfort, compressive dressing; refer to orthopedic specialist for definitive care
Shaft	Direct trauma—its position at distal end of leg exposes it to more trauma (e.g., car bumper); or rotation and leverage strain (as with stepping into deep hole while running) Open fractures more common because bone is subcutaneous on its anterior or medial surfaces	Associated with fractures in rest of body (ipsilateral extremity or elsewhere); must determine whether fibula is also fractured, because it acts as splint if intact Prone to complications: 1. Increased incidence of compartment syndrome. 2. Arterial injuries common with fractures of upper third.	Splint for comfort; refer to orthopedic specialist for evaluation and definitive care
Fibula Proximal	Direct blow to the side of leg	May have concomitant peroneal nerve injury associated with ankle injuries such as Monteggia fractures	Splint, orthopedic specialist, crutches
Ankle	Twisted, fall, or trauma of the ankle by inversion or eversion injury	Swelling, tenderness, and loss of alignment and function	Splint, orthopedic specialist may need an open reduction, due to joint instability and need for accurate alignment
Toes Second-fifth	Stubbing injury or heavy object being dropped on toes	Pain, swelling, ecchymosis, possible subungual hematoma	Buddy taping to adjacent toe with gauze padding between toes

FOOSH, fall on outstretched hand; MVC, motor vehicle crash.

TABLE 32.4 COMMON DISLOCATIONS

BODY AREA	MECHANISM OF INJURY	CLINICAL FINDINGS	TREATMENT
Phalanges Dorsal dislocations	Hyperextension of the joint (ball handling)	Deformity of phalanx at the proximal or distal interphalangeal joint (PIP dislocations)	Radiographs with a lateral view, reduction, and splint
Thumb dislocations	Radial stress on the ulnar collateral ligament	Painful swollen metacarpophalangeal joint of the thumb, tenderness over ulnar collateral ligament	Splint in a thumb spica and orthopedic referral
Shoulder Anterior	Fall on outstretched arm or direct impact on shoulder	Arm abducted, cannot bring elbow down to chest or touch opposite ear with hand	Splint in position of comfort, reduce as soon as possible
Posterior	Rare: strong blow in front of shoulder; with violent convulsions, seizures, or electrocution injuries	Arm held at side, unable to rotate externally	Splint in position of comfort, reduce as soon as possible
Elbow Radius and ulna	Fall on outstretched hand with elbow in extension	Loss of arm length, painful motion, and rapid swelling, nerve lesions may occur	As above surgical repair if dislocation is associated with fracture to radial head or olecranon
Radius Head (children)	Pulled or nursemaid's elbow caused by sudden pull, jerk, or lift on child's wrist or hand	Pain, refusal to use arm, limited supination, can flex and extend at elbow may have no deformity	Reduce, may place in sling advise parents that this may recur until age 5. Do not use sling at night
Hip Usually posterior	Blow to knee while hip is flexed and adducted (sitting with crossed knees); common in passengers seated in front seat	Hip flexed, adducted internally rotated and shortened; may have associated fracture of femur sciatic nerve injury (lies posterior)	Splint in position of comfort reduce as soon as possible
Patella	May be spontaneous	Knee flexed; can palpate patella lateral to femoral condyle	Reduce (may occur spontaneously) immobilize with cast or splint
Patella	Associated with other trauma	Excessive swelling tenderness, and palpable soft tissue defect	Surgical repair of soft tissue injury or fractures
Knee (rare)	Direct severe blow to upper leg or forced hyperextension of knee	Ligamentous instability (requires disruption of structures); inability to straighten leg; peroneal nerve and popliteal artery injury common, must assess distal neurovascular function	Immediate neurovascular assessment, reduce
Ankle	Ankle is complex, joint with multiple ligament providing stability; dislocation is usually associated with other injury such as fracture and soft tissue trauma	Swelling tenderness and loss of alignment and function	Splint, usually necessitates open reduction because this joint has complex motion and must have accurate alignment

PIP, proximal interphalangeal joint.

then a bedside visualization of the aorta should be performed.

4. Back examination
   a. Redness, warmth, drainage, wound
   b. Point tenderness
   c. Cerebrovascular accident (CVA) tenderness
   d. Straight leg raise
      i. Patient lying supine, passively lifting each leg separately to approximately 70 degrees in an attempt to reproduce the pain
      ii. A positive test results in reproduction of the patient's sciatic pain or radicular pain into the affected leg below knee.
         (1) Pain with dorsiflexion worse
      iii. Pain less with ankle plantar flexion
      iv. A positive test is highly specific but insensitive for nerve root compression by a herniated disc.

D. *Focused assessment:* History risk factors

Medical Decision-Making and Differential Diagnoses

A. See Table 32.5 for lower back pain differentials.

Diagnostic Testing

A. Imaging studies
   1. *X-rays:* Lumbar plain films when fracture, tumor, or infection is suspected. Anterior posterior and lateral views are usually adequate starting point.
      a. Routine x-rays are not indicated in all back pain patients.
   2. *MRI:* MRI is the definitive imaging modality in most emergent situations involving back pain. It offers the best resolution for assessment for lesions in vertebral bodies, spinal canal, spinal cord, and disk disease.
   3. *CT:* CT is most useful in evaluating the vertebral fractures, facet joints, and posterior elements of the spine.

TABLE 32.5 CHRONIC DISEASES RESPONSIBLE FOR PATHOLOGIC FRACTURE

	OSTEOARTHRITIS	RHEUMATOID ARTHRITIS
Pathology	Degenerative joint disease with degeneration of the articular cartilage	Systemic autoimmune disease causing inflammation of connective tissue
Age	Men before age 45 Women after age 55	Common in women more than men between ages of 35 and 50 years of age
Signs and symptoms	Pain and swelling in one, two, or more joints Limitation of joint motion in weight bearing and finger joint Heberden's nodes—DIP Bouchard's nodes—nodular bony enlargements occur in PIP Usually better in morning, worse as day progresses	Swelling, warmth, and tenderness of the joints, involves more than three joints Affects proximal joints of hands or wrist Fatigue Weakness Malaise Usually worse in the morning
Diagnostic procedures	Radiograph—bony hypertrophy, spur formation, and cartilage disruption Arthrocentesis—aspiration of joint fluid for analysis to exclude infection, gout, other diseases	Radiographs of joins, cysts, swelling, erosion CBC with differential ESR: elevated
Pharmacologic therapy	Non-narcotic analgesics NSAIDs	NSAIDs
Education	Weight reduction program	Physical therapy Exercise low impact Stress reduction
Referral	PCP or Orthopedic clinicial	Rheumatology specialist

CBC, complete blood count; DIP, distal interphalangeal joints; ESR, erythrocyte sedimentation rate; PIP, proximal interphalangeal joint.

a. CT is poor resolution for the spinal cord and spinal canal. It becomes useful in settings where MRI is not available or unsuitable for the patient. CT myelography is best suited when MRI not available.

B. Laboratory studies

1. Laboratory testing is indicated where there is clinical concern for infection, tumor, or rheumatological causes for back pain.
   a. Complete blood count (CBC)
   b. Basic metabolic panel (BMP): Assessing renal function specifically
   c. Erythrocyte sedimentation rate (ESR)
   d. *UA: Urinalysis: (UA)*Urinary tract infection (UTI), blood in urine, or renal cause for back pain
   e. *Pregnancy test:* All patients of childbearing age need a pregnancy test.

Management

A. *Procedures:* No indicated procedures in the ED are identified for this pathology.

B. Pharmacologic therapies

1. Follow evidence-based guidelines when prescribing.
2. NSAIDs
3. Appropriate analgesia
4. Muscle relaxers
5. Topical lidocaine patches
6. Steroid therapy
   1 Nonpharmacologic management of low back pain
7. Massage
8. Acupuncture
9. Yoga
10. General fitness program including weight loss when indicated
11. Lumbar stabilization exercises focusing on the core muscles of specific areas, specifically the abdominal, gluteal, and spinal extensor groups

C. Consultation and collaboration

1. *Spinal surgeon/neurosurgical specialist:* Early consultation in cases where there is a suspicion for spinal fractures, suspected spinal cord injuries, spinal infections, or noted neurologic deficits.
2. *Emergency medicine physician:* Consider collaboration with the ED physician where the diagnosis is unclear. Any case where neurologic deficits are identified consider collaborative discussion. Although rare, identification of red flag risk factors in combination with neurologic deficits poses significantly devastating consequences. Therefore, additional clinician help may be indicated to facilitate rapid intervention by the specialist.
3. *Tertiary subspecialties:* Identification of other pathologic causes of back pain not related to the spine or spinal cord may warrant other specialty consultation. Identification of abdominal aortic aneurysm will require consultation with vascular surgery, or identification of unknown pregnancy may require consultation with obstetrics specialist for preterm or term labor.

Patient Disposition

A. *Discharge:* Most patients without neurologic findings can be discharged to follow-up with the primary doctor or specialist.

B. *Admission:* Identification of neurologic pathology that is concerning for spinal cord compression or evidence of neurologic deficit requires admission for recurrent neurologic assessment for progression of disease, medical management, or surgical management.

C. *Transfer:* In certain medical facilities where there are limited resources or the necessary evaluation cannot be completed in time-sensitive cases, transfer to a tertiary facility may be required.

D. Documentation

1. It is imperative that the documentation for these patient's assessment, treatment, reassessment, and timeline of disposition, is clearly documented. Clearly, document history negatives that raise suspicion for more concerning pathology. It is vital to document all neurologic findings, timely consultations with specialists, and medical decision-making.

Age and Developmental Considerations

A. Prevention and education

1. For nonpathologic back pain prevention and education should be directed at proper lifting techniques, proper body mechanics, education or exercise and building core muscles, and weight control.

B. Patient and family education and counseling

1. Most patients with back pain will be discharged home, and the symptoms will likely improve with supportive treatment. However, if red flag risk factors are identified, or if history is concerning without any acute findings, the diagnosis should be nonspecific back pain. Patient should be clearly educated on signs and symptoms of neurologic concerns which necessitate immediate return to the ED.

Musculoskeletal Injuries

Musculoskeletal injury is one of the most common types of injuries seen in the ED and is a significant cause of disability. Primary mechanisms for these injuries include motor vehicle crashes (MVCs), assaults, falls, sports and recreation, and injuries sustained at work or home. Bone, soft tissue, and associated neurovascular injuries are rarely emergent unless accompanied by a life-threatening hemorrhage as in certain amputations and pelvic fractures. Fractures and soft tissue injuries are primarily designated as urgent because of potential neurovascular injury with resultant limb disability and pain. Early intervention enhances preservation of limb and function. It is imperative the emergency nurse practitioner provides a focused assessment to determine the level of care the patient needs at the initial evaluation and ongoing management of musculoskeletal injuries. The goal is to obtain a focused assessment by performing the primary and secondary survey to manage the musculoskeletal injuries in the ED by nurse practitioners.

Anatomy and Physiology

A. The musculoskeletal system and related neurovascular structures consist of bones, joints, tendons, ligaments, muscles, vessels, and nerves.

B. The skeletal system contains 206 bones, which provide support, strength, movement, and protection to the body and organs.

1. Bones store several minerals, including calcium and phosphorus, and are involved in blood cell production.

2. Bones are characterized by shapes as long, short, flat, or irregular, with the shape of a particular bone suited for a unique function or purpose.

3. The skeleton is composed of two types of bones: cancellous and cortical. Cancellous (spongy) bone is found in the skull, vertebrae, pelvis, and long-bone ends. Cortical (dense) bone is found in the long bones.

4. Bones are supplied by blood vessels, nerves, and lymphatic vessels that nourish bone tissue and allow the bone to repair injuries.

5. The periosteum covers the bones and provides a point for attachment of muscle, as well as the blood supply for underlying bone tissue.

C. Bone is connected to other bone by stabilizing bands of elastic, fibrous connective tissue called ligaments.

1. Nonelastic fibrous cords that connect muscle to bone are tendons.

2. Dense connective tissue is found between the ribs, in the nasal septum, ear, larynx, trachea, bronchi, between vertebrae, and on articulating surfaces is known as cartilage.

3. Cartilage has a limited vascular supply, whereas bone tissue has abundant vascular structures.

D. Joints are classified as nonsynovial (immovable and slightly immovable) and synovial (freely movable).

1. Synovial joints have two articulating surfaces covered with cartilage and are surrounded by a two-layered synovial membrane sac. The entire joint is encapsulated by dense, ligamentous material.

2. Joints provide mobility and stability, flexion and extension, medial and lateral rotation, and abduction and adduction. Joint movement is enhanced by muscles and ligaments that overlie the joint.

E. Nerves and arteries lie near bones and muscle groups, with arterioles distributed throughout the periosteum to provide nutrients. Nerves provide sensation and movement. The closeness of arteries and nerves to bone structures increases their risk for injury with trauma to soft tissue, muscles, bones, or joints.

Medical Screening

A. Chief complaint

1. Mechanism of injury

2. Primary and secondary assessment/resuscitation

B. Focused assessment

1. Assessment of musculoskeletal injuries begins with assessment of the airway, breathing, and circulation (ABC).

a. Rapid assessment identifies major injuries of the head, cervical spine, chest, and abdomen and prioritizes essential interventions.

b. After ensuring that no life-threatening injury has been left unattended, the nurse practitioner assesses and stabilizes any extremity injuries.

c. Assessment of musculoskeletal injuries includes inspecting for swelling, deformity, ecchymosis, abrasions, lacerations, or puncture wounds and palpating for crepitus and point tenderness.

2. A focused neurovascular evaluation is conducted for any injuries identified, noting the presence and/or

absence of pain, pulses, paralysis, paresthesia, pallor, temperature, and capillary refill.

3. Before immobilization, open fractures should be stabilized, and bleeding controlled. Open fractures with obvious bone protrusion or a deep laceration should be rinsed with sterile normal saline to remove gross contamination and covered with a dry sterile dressing.

4. Puncture wounds over a fracture site should not be irrigated because this can force bacteria deeper into the wound. Reduction of an open fracture should not be attempted in a prehospital setting because this may force contaminants into the wound, increasing the risk for infection.

5. To control bleeding apply pressure directly to the injury site, edges of the wound, or an adjacent pressure point. The use of a tourniquet for hemorrhage control should be considered only as a last resort (life over limb) because of potential neurovascular compromise.

Diagnostic Testing

A. Laboratory studies (Table 32.6)
   1. Complete blood count (CBC) with differential
   2. Erythrocyte sedimentation rate (ESR)
   3. Arterial blood gases (ABG)
   4. Blood cultures
   5. Urinalysis (UA); pregnancy test for female patients of childbearing age

B. Imaging studies
   1. Determine which radiologic films would be necessary after your primary and secondary survey was completed.
   2. Always include the bone above and below the joint.
   3. CT scan used for diagnosis
      a. Fractures involving articular surfaces such as tibial plateau, talus, calcaneus
      b. Fracture/dislocations that are difficult to visualized or manipulate
      c. Fracture of scapula, carpal bones, tarsal bones, dislocations of humeral and femoral heads, radio-ulnar or sternoclavicular joints
      d. Stress fractures
      e. Bony changes, metastatic processes
   4. Angiography; used to diagnose and treat vascular injuries, prevent hemorrhage

Management

A. Pharmacologic therapies
   1. Follow evidence-based guidelines when prescribing.
   2. Patients being discharged with musculoskeletal injuries may require NSAIDs, narcotic analgesics, and muscle relaxers. Open fractures will require antibiotics. Tetanus immunization should be up to date.
   3. Short-term use of an opioid may be indicated.

B. Procedural sedation for reductions and traumatic injuries may need to be used in the ED.

C. Soft tissue injuries
   1. The soft tissue of the extremities includes the skin, muscles, tendons, ligaments, nerves, and blood vessels. Injuries may occur with or without a bony injury, and in some cases it is difficult to make the diagnosis. A careful clinical examination along with radiologic studies to rule out skeletal trauma is necessary to identify the problem. Certain disorders may result from chronic overuse and may not have an acute history of injury.
   2. Classification of soft tissue injuries
      a. Sprains
      b. Strains
      c. Abrasions
      d. Contusions
      e. Hematomas
      f. Laceration
      g. Skin tears
   3. Strains and sprains
      a. Injuries to the structures around a joint are usually due to excessive stretch or sudden force. This results in pulling on the structures, which causes tears in muscle and/or tendon.
         i. A sprain is the stretching, separation, or tear of a supporting ligament, and a strain is the separation or tear of a musculotendinous unit from a bone.
         ii. Injury may result in pain, inability to weight bear fully, and swelling of the affected area.
         iii. Sprains and strains are rare in small children whose epiphyseal plates are still open and less vulnerable to forces. Athletes and obese patients resuming physical fitness are at risk for these types of injuries. Both are classified by the amount of damage.
      b. *First degree:* Minor tear in the fibers, minimal swelling, minor discomfort, absent or minor ecchymosis
      c. *Second degree:* Partial tear, joint intact, more severe swelling, visible ecchymosis

TABLE 32.6 EPIDURAL ABSCESS STAGING AND ASSOCIATED SYMPTOMATOLOGY

EPIDURAL ABSCESS STAGING	SYMPTOMATOLOGY
Stage 1	Back pain, tenderness, fever
Stage 2	Radicular pain, reflex abnormalities
Stage 3	Sensory abnormalities, motor weakness, bowel, or bladder dysfunction
Stage 4	Paralysis that rapidly becomes permanent without surgical intervention

Not all patients will progress sequentially through these stages

d. *Third degree:* Complete disruption of ligament; joint may be open; minimal to severe swelling; resultant separation of muscle from muscle, muscle from tendon, or tendon from bone

4. Contusions/hematoma

a. A contusion is a closed wound in which a ruptured blood vessel has hemorrhaged into the surrounding tissues. The blood may form a hematoma if bleeding is sufficient and has been contained. This may result from blunt external forces or exertional stresses. Symptoms may include swelling, discoloration, and tenderness. Populations at risk are those involved in physical activities, sports, or abusive relationships, and patients who are on anticoagulant therapy or who have a history of clotting disorders.

5. Treatment

a. *RICE:* Rest, ice, compression, and elevation

b. *Disposition:* If pain is severe, decreased sensation, increased swelling and cyanosis, patient may need to be admitted with an orthopedic consult.

D. Fractures (Tables 32.7–32.9)

1. A fracture is a disruption or break cortex of the bone. Patients may arrive in the ED with angulation, deformity, pain, and point tenderness, swelling, immobility, and/or crepitus. Other findings might include bony fragment protrusion, impaired neurovascular status, and occasionally shock.

2. Fractures are divided into two general categories: closed and open (Table 32.7).

a. With closed or simple fractures, the bone is broken, but the skin is intact.

b. Open or compound fractures are characterized by bone protrusion or puncture wounds in which the bone punctures the skin or a foreign object penetrates the skin and bone, causing a fracture.

E. Dislocations

1. A dislocation occurs when the articular surfaces of bones forming a joint are no longer in contact and lose their anatomic position. Bone ends may move because of congenital weakness, diseases that affect the articular and periarticular structures, and associated trauma.

2. Dislocations are considered an emergency because of the danger of injury to adjacent nerves and blood vessels in the form of compression, stretching, or ischemia.

a. Dislocations are described in terms of the distal segment in relation to the proximal segment (anterior, posterior, lateral, medial dislocations). Joint subluxations occur when part of the articular surface contact remains but is not complete.

3. A person with a suspected or known orthopedic injury should be carefully assessed for both fracture and dislocation. If either one is suspected, the limb should be splinted, a neurovascular examination performed, radiographic examination completed for confirmation of diagnosis and then the injury should be reduced as soon as possible. Table 32.10 provides specific findings and treatment of common dislocations.

F. Immobilization

1. Immobilization should be accomplished as soon as possible to minimize further damage or complications secondary to bone fragments or neurovascular injury and to reduce pain in the injured limb.

a. A splint should include the joints above and below the injury. Neurovascular status must be checked before and after immobilization.

b. If neurovascular status is initially compromised, gradual traction may be used to promote

TABLE 32.7 INTERPRETATION OF COMPARTMENT PRESSURE READING

PRESSURE	INDICATION
>30	Emergency
10–20	Threatens, repeat compartment pressures
10	No immediate concern
Calculating delta pressure = diastolic BP – compartment pressure	**Abnormal if the delta pressure is <30 mmHg.**

TABLE 32.8 PELVIC FRACTURE CLASSIFICATION AND ASSOCIATED KEY FINDINGS

PELVIC FRACTURE CLASSIFICATION	(TILE CLASSIFICATION SYSTEM)
Type	**Findings**
Type A: Stable pelvic ring fracture	**A1:** Avulsion of innominate bone (most common) **A2:** Iliac wing (Duverney) fracture **A3:** Transverse fracture of the sacrum/coccyx
Type B: Partially stable pelvic ring injuries (rotationally unstable/vertically stable)	**B1:** Unilateral open book (disruption symphysis pubis + SI hinge rotation) **B2:** Bucket handle (double rami) fractures (most common) **B3:** Bilateral open book fracture
Type C: Unstable pelvic ring fractures rotationally and vertically unstable) **** MOST LIFE THREATENING **** **70% WITH ASSOCIATED INJURIES**	**C1:** unilateral; (a) iliac fracture, (b) sacroiliac fracture/dislocation, (c) sacral fracture **C2:** Bilateral with one side Type B and one side Type C. **C3:** Bilateral with both sided type C

Note: Additional classification can be found by using Young–Burgess classification system for pelvic fractures.

TABLE 32.9 BACK PAIN RED FLAG RISK FACTORS

HISTORICAL RISK FACTORS	CONCERN
Pain > 6 weeks	Tumor, infection
Age <18, >50	Congenital anomaly, tumor
Major trauma	Fracture
Minor trauma in elderly	Fracture
History of cancer	Tumor
Fever and rigors	Infection
Weight loss	Tumor, infection
Injection drug use	Infection
Immunocompromised	Infection
Night pain	Tumor, Infection
Unremitting pain even when supine	Tumor, Infection
Incontinence	Epidural compression
Saddle anesthesia	Epidural compression
Severe/progressive neurologic deficits	Epidural compression

TABLE 32.10 DEFICITS WITH NERVE ROOT DYSFUNCTION

ROOT	PAIN	SENSORY LOSS	WEAKNESS
L4	Hip, anterior thigh	Anteromedial thigh to medial aspect of foot	Weak quadriceps; decreased knee jerk
L5	Lateral thigh/calf; dorsal foot, big toe	Lateral calf, dorsal foot, big toe	decreased extensor hallucis longus
S1	Posterolateral thigh, calf, heel	Back of thigh and calf, toes lateral heel	Gastrocnemius; decreased ankle jerk
S2–S4	Perineum	Perineum	Bowel/bladder; cremasteric

return of neurologic or vascular function before splinting.

c. If neurovascular status is compromised after splinting or traction, the splint should be removed and reapplied or the traction should be decreased.

d. Angulation should be corrected only if it prevents immobilization or if neurovascular compromise is present.

e. Splinting is best accomplished with an assistant to support the limb while a padded splint is placed and wrapped with a noncompressive bandage. Neurovascular status is rechecked after splinting.

2. Four basic types of splints exist, including soft splints such as pillows; hard splints such as padded board, cardboard, aluminum, plaster, fiberglass, or a ladder splint; inflatable air splints or vacuum splints; and traction splints, which reduce angulation and provide support.[1]

a. Common splints that are used to immobilize the thumb/finger, wrist/forearm, elbow, and lower extremities are thumb spica, volar splint, boxer splint, sugar tong, and posterior splints.

b. Air splints were used extensively when first developed because they conformed well and provided visualization of the injured extremity. However, an air splint that is not open on the distal end does not allow for neurovascular checks without deflating or unzipping the splint. An air splint should be inflated only to the point where a finger can be slipped between the splint and the skin. Excessive pressure in the splint can compromise circulation. Air splints also stick to the skin, cause irritation, and are difficult to remove in patients with excessive diaphoresis.

3. After immobilization, the limb should be elevated and an ice pack applied to minimize swelling. Caution is advised because overzealous elevation may compromise arterial circulation and excessive, prolonged cold may damage tissues.

4. The patient should be completely disrobed and examined for anterior injuries and then log rolled to identify posterior injuries while maintaining adequate cervical spine protection. Rings should be removed if the injury involves the hand, arm, foot, or toes. Elevation and cooling measures should be maintained, and neurovascular status should be checked periodically.

5. Careful history should include circumstances of the injury, time and mechanism of injury, and significant medical history, including acute and chronic alcohol use, medications, allergies, and tetanus immunization status. The time of last oral intake should be recorded, and the patient should be allowed nothing by mouth (NPO) if procedural sedation or surgical intervention is a possibility.

Patient Disposition

A. Documentation
  1. Chief complaint in patient's words
  2. Nature of incident
    a. History and mechanism of Injury
    b. Past medical history
    c. Past hospitalizations and surgeries
  3. Medications
  4. Immunizations (e.g., tetanus)
  5. Allergies
  6. Family history
  7. Social history
  8. Physical examination
    a. Level of distress
    b. Vital signs (VS) including pulse oximetry
    c. Inspection for deformity, swelling, discoloration, erythema, compare injured extremity to opposite extremity
    d. Range of motion, note decreased, active, passive
  9. Procedure note
  10. Medical decision-making
  11. Diagnosis
  12. Plan of care
  13. Disposition and discharge instructions

Age and Developmental Considerations

A. Pediatric
  1. Growth- and development-related
    a. Child's bone structure different from adult's; children considered skeletally immature
    b. Skeleton of infant and young child is largely cartilaginous
      i. Bones narrow and flexible
    c. Periosteum is thicker and resists disruption
      i. Provides circulation and nutrients to bone
      ii. Allows bone to be more elastic and resists fracture
    d. *Greenstick*: Shaft of bone (diaphysis) fractured on one side, but cortex intact on other side
    e. *Torus*: Compression fracture of the bone at the junction of the metaphysis and diaphysis causing "buckling"; patient often presents with pain but no deformity.
  2. Children have open epiphysis (growth plate) until after adolescence; this area is more susceptible to trauma; fractures to epiphysis constitute one third of all fractures and are described according to Salter–Harris classification system:
    a. *Type I:* Epiphysis separated from metaphysis
    b. *Type II:* Epiphyseal plate slipped with metaphyseal fracture, producing triangular fragment in metaphysis (most common type of fracture)
    c. *Type III:* Intra-articular fracture involving epiphysis, which is also slipped (surgery is required to maintain blood supply and prevent growth disturbance)
    d. *Type IV:* Fracture that includes intra-articular space, epiphysis, epiphyseal plate, metaphysis (surgical repair is required)
    e. *Type V:* Crush injury of epiphyseal plate, resulting in arrested growth; poor prognosis for normal growth
  3. Child's ligaments are more resistant than epiphysis to trauma.
    a. Dislocations rare
    b. Fractures often accompany dislocation.
    c. Sprains (ligaments tear) unusual in young children but do occur in adolescents
  4. General appearance
    a. Observe legs while child is walking.
    b. Infants have bowlegged (genu varum) appearance from birth to 2 or 3 years.
    c. Infants tend to evert feet and walk on inner aspects of feet.
    d. At 18 to 36 months, child may appear knock-kneed (genu valgum).
    e. Normal leg configuration should be present at approximately 6 to 7 years.
    f. Feet appear flatfooted
      i. Medial longitudinal arch normally obscured by fat pads until approximately 2 years
      ii. Arch better visualized when child not weight bearing, such as when seated or on tiptoe
    g. Child may normally walk with in-toeing (pigeon-toed).
      i. Rotational alignment of legs changes as skeleton matures, producing spontaneous correction.
      ii. Pathologic changes may be produced by disorders of feet, lower legs, hips.
  5. Pearls
    a. Fractures result from significant force: history should be appropriate for pattern of injury.
    b. Warning flags to consider child abuse in children: fracture in infant <1 year, spiral fracture, unwitnessed or unexplained injury, fracture in various healing stages, history of other fractures, fracture that does not fit mechanism of injury stated
    c. Approximately 25% of fractures in children < 3 years caused by nonaccidental trauma
    d. Torus/buckle fractures unique to children
    e. Pulling injury to arm can result in "nursemaid's elbow" (subluxation of the radial head) in child commonly seen in age 2 to 3 years of age.
    f. Limping in children uncommon; suspect hip disorder if found
    g. Unwillingness to bear weight requires further investigation

B. Geriatric
  1. Aging related
    a. Loss of bone minerals and mass
      i. Regeneration prolonged
      ii. Bones become more brittle.
      iii. Loss of vertebral body height results from compression that occurs with normal aging, which leads to kyphosis.
    b. Muscles lose ability to regenerate new fibers to replace ones lost because of age (atrophy).
      i. Decreased muscular strength and endurance, shuffling gait
      ii. Longer contraction time and tendency to fatigue more easily, which may cause muscle tremors, even at rest

TABLE 32.11 FUNCTIONAL MOTOR TESTING/DERMATOMAL SENSORY TESTING/REFLEX TESTING

NERVE ROOT	MOTOR EXAM	FUNCTIONAL TEST	PIN-PRICK	REFLEX
L3	Extend quadriceps	Squat down and rise	Lateral thigh and medial femoral condyle	Patellar tendon
L4	Dorsiflex ankle	Walk on heels	Medial leg and medial ankle	Patellar tendon
L5	Dorsiflex ankle	Walk on heels	Lateral leg and dorsum of foot	Medial hamstring
S1	Stand on toes	Walk on toes	Sole of foot and lateral ankle	Achilles tendon

2. Pearls
   a. Joint stiffness and degenerative changes contribute to decreased mobility.
   b. Posture is affected by age-related changes.
   c. Gait is affected by posture, balance, strength, flexibility.
   d. Changes in feet are common.
      i. Foot size decreases because of loss of subcutaneous fat.
      ii. Skin is drier; corns and calluses form at pressure points; epidermis thins and loses natural moisture.
      iii. Decreased circulation from peripheral vascular disease may delay healing; venous stasis or arterial occlusion produces ulceration.
      iv. Toenails thicken, affecting shoe fit.
      v. Bunion and toe overlapping or under-riding may occur.
   e. Osteoporosis promotes fractures, especially in vertebral bodies, ribs, proximal femur.
   f. Osteoarthritis (degeneration of movable joints) affects mostly weight-bearing joints of knees, vertebrae, small joints of hand and feet.
   g. Rheumatoid arthritis (systemic disease of connective tissue resulting in joint inflammation) produces swelling, stiffness, ankylosis, redness, warmth of joints.
   h. Pathologic fracture may be due to other chronic diseases (Table 32.11).
   i. Paget's disease
      i. Metabolic disease that causes excessive bone resorption and deposits
      ii. Middle-aged and older men primarily affected
      iii. Affected bones tend to fracture easily.

Pelvic Fractures

The pelvis acts as a body support structure, connecting the axial skeleton with the appendicular skeleton of the lower extremities. It is a conduit for the neurovascular structure and provides some housing and protection to the genitourinary/reproductive organ systems. Pelvic fractures alert the clinician for concern with associated organ system injuries because of the energy/force required to induce a fracture to the pelvic ring structures. Pelvic fractures can cause significant deformity, pain, and disability, especially if unstable/pelvic ring disruptions occur.

Anatomy

A. Bony structure
   1. The pelvic ring contains two innominate bones that connect anteriorly at the symphysis pubis and posteriorly at the sacrum via the sacroiliac (SI) joints.
      a. Ilium
      b. Ischium
      c. Pubis
      d. Sacrum
      e. Coccyx
B. Pelvic ring
   1. No inherent stability. Ligaments give stability.
   2. Anterior sacroiliac ligaments (SIL) resist external rotation
   3. Posterior SIL and iliolumbar ligaments (ILL) provide posterior stability by tension band.
   4. Strongest in the body
   5. *Sacrotuberous:* Resists shear, flexion of SI joint
C. Vascular structures
   1. The common iliac blood vessels enter the false pelvis into the external and internal iliac vessels. These vessels subdivide multiple times through the pelvis. Although a discussion about the extensive vascular supply within the pelvis is beyond the scope of this educational material, it is important for the clinician to acknowledge that a fractured pelvis should alert the clinician to assess and monitor for bleeding within the pelvic structures.
D. Neurologic structures
   1. Lumbar plexus and sacral plexus
      a. Key L2–S3 pass through the pelvis
      b. Therefore, neurovascular compromise may be present because of spinal nerve impingement, sciatic nerve, and other local nerve bundles.

Medical Screening

A. Chief complaint
   1. Primary complaint may be varied in these patients due to the high mechanisms required and the varying associated injuries. Primarily pain in the pelvic region or directly at the fracture site may be identified.
B. Signs and symptoms
   1. Focused signs
      a. *Pain:* Limit manual manipulation to gentle palpation. Manual compression may dislodge existing clot resulting in hemorrhage.
      b. Deformity
      c. Crepitus
      d. Visualization of soft tissue injuries
         i. Localized contusions

ii. Localized lacerations
iii. Localized abrasions
iv. Fractures and deformity of the proximal femur/hip
e. Identification of hemorrhagic shock
i. Tachycardia
ii. Hypotension
iii. Tachypnea
iv. Diaphoresis
v. Altered mental status
2. Neurovascular symptoms
a. Peripheral paresthesia
b. Peripheral weakness on assessment
c. L5–S1 decrease loss of dorsiflexion or plantar flexion
3. Urethral injuries
a. Male
i. *Blood at the meatus:* Indicates urethral disruption
ii. Hematuria
iii. Perineal and genital swelling
iv. Genital paresthesia
v. Genital bruising
vi. *Digital rectal examination:* High riding prostate on exam suggestive of urethral disruption
b. Female
i. Spontaneous hematuria
ii. Perineal and genital swelling
iii. Genital paresthesia
iv. Genital bruising

C. Focused assessment (Table 32.12)
1. High-energy-associated injuries
a. Due to the energy required to induce a fracture to the pelvic structures, it is imperative that the patient have a thorough full-body physical examination. The force required to fracture the pelvis should alert the clinician to observe for associated injuries that may require stabilization and management.
2. Inside the pelvic ring assess for
a. Hemorrhage
i. Most hemorrhage associated with a fracture is the result of vascular exposure at the fracture site, soft tissue injury, and localized venous bleeding.
ii. Arterial bleeding, although less common than venous, is alarming because of the large potential space that exists for blood loss.
iii. Hemorrhage within this space can also be the result of organ tissue structures within the pelvic girdle being injured.
iv. There is a large vascular supply to this region of the body, and therefore fracture should raise the clinician's index of suspicion for hemorrhage.
b. Neurovascular injury
c. Pelvic organ damage
3. Outside the pelvic ring assess for
a. Head injuries
b. Chest injuries
c. Spinal cord injuries (SCI)
d. Lower extremity Injuries
4. Anticoagulation therapy and antiplatelet therapy patients
a. Careful review of patient history to identify potential utilization of blood thinning agents (e.g., history of pulmonary embolism, deep vein thrombosis, atrial fibrillation, valvular transplant)
b. Medication list review for anticoagulation therapies

Medical Decision-Making and Differential Diagnoses

A. Decision-making
1. Pelvic fractures from the emergency clinician perspective is primarily an evaluation and stabilization of acute fracture, assessment for associated injuries within the pelvic ring (bleeding, neurovascular disruption, or injury to protected internal organs within the pelvis), identification of associated trauma of other body systems, and either immobilization for trauma surgical evaluation, orthopedic surgical evaluation, or transfer to a tertiary facility.

B. Differential diagnosis
1. Because the mechanism is traumatic in nature, the differential is delineating which injured body part is causing the symptoms.
a. Pelvic fracture
b. Hip fracture
c. Hip dislocation
d. Femur fracture

TABLE 32.12 TYPES OF FRACTURES

TYPE	ETIOLOGY
Transverse fracture	Sharp, direct blow
Oblique fracture	Twisting force
Spiral fracture	Twisting force while foot is firmly planted
Comminuted fracture	Severe direct trauma causes more than two fragments
Impacted fracture	Severe trauma, causes bone ends to jam together
Compression fracture	Severe force to top of head, sacrum, or os calcis (axial loading) forces vertebrae together
Greenstick fracture	Compression force; usually occurs in school-age children
Avulsion fracture	Forceful contraction of a muscle mass; causes a bone fragment to break away at the insertion point
Depressed fracture	Blunt trauma to a flat bone; usually associated with significant soft tissue damage

e. Soft tissue injuries
f. Coccyx fracture
g. Genitourinary (GU)-related injures
h. Gastrointestinal (GI) injuries
i. Hemorrhagic shock
j. Spinal trauma

Diagnostic Testing

A. Imaging
1. *X-ray:* Anteroposterior (AP) pelvis will often identify majority of pelvic fractures.
2. *Ultrasound:* A FAST (Focused Assessment with Sonography for Trauma) examination
3. *CT studies:* CT scan best for visualizing fracture for sacrum and SI joint
a. Easier to identify rotation and posterior displacement. Also, due to the high association with other injuries CT scan will help identify abdominal trauma.

B. Laboratory studies
1. Complete blood count (CBC), serial hemoglobin/hematocrit (H/H) if concern for hemorrhage
2. Type and screen
3. Comprehensive metabolic panel (CMP)
4. Urine drug screen (UDS)
5. Urinalysis (UA)

Management

A. Initial management centers on resuscitation
1. Following ABCDE as established in advanced trauma life support (ATLS) guidelines.
a. Airway
b. Breathing
c. Circulation
d. Disability
e. Exposure
2. Stabilization of pelvis
3. Pain management
4. Identifying and treating associated injuries
5. Observing for signs/symptoms of hypovolemic shock and treating as per the Advanced Trauma Support Guidelines.
6. Evaluation by trauma surgeon or orthopedic surgeon
a. Primarily has been nonoperative management in stable fractures
b. Operative management in unstable fractures
c. Increase in operative management due to operative medicine advances

B. Procedures
1. Placement of large-bore IVs ×2
2. Pelvic stabilization with binder
a. *Bedsheet:* Without moving the patient significantly, wrap a sheet around the patient back to front, around the greater trochanters and tighten the sheet and tie in a knot anteriorly.
3. Commercial pelvic binders
a. SAM sling (Sam Medical Products)
b. T-POD Pelvic Stabilizing Device (Pyng Medical Corp)

C. Pharmacologic therapies
1. Narcotic analgesia, likely will be required for most patients
2. Avoid NSAID analgesia.

D. Consultation and collaboration
1. Consultation
a. Early consultation is suggested with the following specialist:
b. Orthopedic surgeon
c. Trauma surgeon
i. If there are area-associated injuries, early subspecialty surgical evaluation may be required.
d. Vascular surgeon
e. Urologist
f. Gynecologist
2. Collaboration
a. Emergency physician collaboration is recommended in these cases. These cases can be labor intensive depending on the nature of the case. Additionally, for any patient that you are uncomfortable managing independently, it is suggested that you collaborate with an emergency physician.

Patient Disposition

A. Most patients with a pelvic fracture will require admission to the hospital. In community hospital settings, free-standing EDs, clinics, or remote locations, it may require transfer to a tertiary trauma center. This will likely be through aeromedical evacuation.

B. Documentation
1. Documentation should be focused on evaluating for life-threatening injuries and associated injuries.
2. Documenting assessment, injury identification, thought process in assessing for associated injuries because of the pelvic fracture identification, treatment
3. It is imperative that the clinician document early consultation with a trauma or orthopedic specialist.
4. If the patient requires transfer to tertiary center for evaluation, documentation of interaction between the receiving center, mode of transfer, and receiving attending collaboration should be documented.

Age and Developmental Considerations

A. Elderly patients are likely to have pelvic fractures with lower impact mechanisms due to the frailty of their bone density. Additionally, they will be more likely to have associated fractures such as hip and femur.

B. Prevention and education
1. Elderly
a. Fall risk and assessment
b. Ambulation aids (e.g., walker, cane, assistant)
2. Male patients between 15 and 28 years of age
a. These are the largest epidemiologic group with pelvic fractures.
b. *Seatbelt and automobile safety:* Many pelvic fractures in this age group occur via motor vehicle crashes.

C. Patient and family education and counseling
1. These injuries often have associated injuries and lengthy recovery times.

2. Discussion regarding the gravity of the injury, associated injuries, recovery times, and hospitalization should be initiated.

Rhabdomyolysis

Rhabdomyolysis is a syndrome caused by injury to the skeletal muscle. Myoglobin, a myocyte compound released into the plasma. Muscle injury can result in the release of massive plasma myoglobin levels, which then become involved in glomerular filtration. This creates a cascade effect that results in acute kidney injury and electrolyte disturbances. The terminal event is disruption of the NA+K+ATPase pump and calcium transport, resulting in increased intracellular calcium and subsequent muscle cell necrosis and production of free radicals.

Medical Screening

A. Signs and symptoms
- **1.** It is important to identify that ***musculoskeletal symptoms are present in only 50% of the cases identified*** and therefore a clear history, focused assessment, and high index of suspicion is necessary.
- **2.** Classic triad
  - **a.** Myalgias
  - **b.** Generalized weakness
  - **c.** Darkened urine
- **3.** Other signs/symptoms
  - **a.** Vague "flu-like" symptoms
  - **b.** Nausea/vomiting (N/V)
  - **c.** Fever
  - **d.** Abdominal pain
  - **e.** Muscle pain and tenderness
  - **f.** Decreased muscle strength
  - **g.** Soft tissue swelling

B. Focused assessment
- **1.** History
  - **a.** It is important to identify that there are many causes of rhabdomyolysis. The more common or likely "red flags" in the ED setting are listed below:
  - **b.** Drug and alcohol abuse
    - **i.** Involved in >80% of the cases of rhabdomyolysis. A thorough review of the patient's recreational drug use is essential.
    - **ii.** Alcohol abuse
      - **(1)** Nutritional compromise (these all increase risk of rhabdomyolysis)
        - **(a)** Hypokalemia
        - **(b)** Hypomagnesemia
        - **(c)** Hypophosphatemia
      - **(2)** Direct compression on the muscles due to stupor
      - **(3)** Coma related to intoxication (e.g., Saturday night palsy)
    - **iii.** Drug abuse
      - **(1)** Cocaine (common)
      - **(2)** Amphetamines (e.g., ecstasy)
      - **(3)** Lysergic acid diethylamide (LSD)
      - **(4)** Heroin
      - **(5)** Phencyclidine (PCP)
  - **c.** Medication induced:
    - **i.** It is vital that a focused history reviews the medications the patient is currently taking to assess for possible causes of rhabdomyolysis.
      - **(1)** *Statins:* Atorvastatin (Lipitor), fluvastatin (Lescol), lovastatin (Mevacor, Altoprev), pravastatin (Pravachol), rosuvastatin (Crestor), simvastatin (Zocor)
      - **(2)** Diuretics
      - **(3)** Benzodiazepines
      - **(4)** Corticosteroids
      - **(5)** *Phenothiazides:* Antipsychotics (e.g., chlorpromazine [Thorazine], fluphenazine [Prolixin])
      - **(6)** Tricyclics (e.g., amitriptyline, doxepin, nortriptyline)
      - **(7)** Narcotics
      - **(8)** Theophylline
  - **d.** Viral/bacterial illness:
    - **i.** Influenza A or B
    - **ii.** Legionella
    - **iii.** Other viral and bacterial causes have been cited.
  - **e.** Direct muscle injury:
    - **i.** Crush injury
    - **ii.** Compartment syndrome
    - **iii.** Electrical or lightning injury
  - **f.** Excessive muscular activity:
    - **i.** Sports and basic training
    - **ii.** Seizures
    - **iii.** Delirium tremens, dystonia, psychosis
  - **g.** Hyperthermia/hypothermia
- **2.** Physical examination
  - **a.** It is important to recognize that the patient more commonly has a normal physical exam and therefore it is vital in the diagnosis to elicit focused history cues to direct evaluation (e.g., cocaine or alcohol abuse).
  - **b.** In a small number of the cases, swelling and tenderness over the involved muscle groups and hemorrhagic discoloration of overlying skin may be observed. Muscle swelling may not be evident until after IV hydration.
  - **c.** Tachycardia
  - **d.** Altered mental status (AMS)

Differential Diagnoses

A. Medical decision-making revolves around obtaining a strong history. Since the patient's physical examination will likely be normal, it is important to identify the cause of the rhabdomyolysis.

B. The differential diagnosis is similar to the actual causes of rhabdomyolysis. A high index of suspicion for the disease process is required.

C. Traumatic injuries

D. Viral infections

E. Myalgias from other etiologies

F. Bacterial infections

G. Cold exposure

H. Malignant hyperthermia

I. Hyperosmotic conditions

J. Guillain–Barré (GB) syndrome
K. Inflammatory myositis
L. Medication side effect

Diagnostic Testing

A. Labs
1. *Creatine phosphokinase (CPK):* Most accurate indicator
a. 5X high end of normal
b. Range somewhere above 1,000 u/L
2. CBC
3. Metabolic panel to include potassium, sodium, chloride, magnesium, calcium, phosphorus
4. Lactic acid
5. An elevated CPK is suggestive of rhabdomyolysis, consider ordering the following if the cause is unknown:
a. Urine drug screen (UDS)
b. ETOH (alcohol level)
c. Troponin I
d. Urine myoglobin
i. Elevation occurs before creatine kinase (CK).
ii. Problem is clear 1 to 6 hours after injury.
iii. Limited utility but myoglobinuria is present when urine dip is positive for blood but no red blood cells (RBCs) on the microscopic examination.
e. Coagulation studies (e.g., prothrombin time/international normalized ratio [PT/INR], activated partial thromboplastin time [aPTT])
i. Rhabdomyolysis places patients at risk for developing disseminated intravascular coagulation (DIC).
ii. Admitted patients should consider having a DIC screening panel.
f. Aldolase, in-patient utility higher
B. Imaging
1. X-ray imaging if fractures suspected
2. MRI has utility on the in-patient evaluation but limited in the ED.
3. Ultrasound has a limited role in this diagnosis.

Management

A. Resuscitation measures as indicated by the patient's level of illness
B. Aggressive IV rehydration resuscitation
C. Careful monitoring of urinary output
D. General recommendations
1. Fluid resuscitation
2. Prevent end-organ damage
3. Correction of electrolyte imbalances
E. Obtain an EKG evaluating and treating hyperkalemia
F. Repeat assessments for the following:
1. Hyperkalemia
2. DIC
3. Compartment syndrome evaluation and assessment for orthopedic evaluation and emergent fasciotomy
G. End goal is stabilization and addressing life and limb threatening conditions
H. Procedures
1. IV access for IV hydration
2. Compartment pressures for suspected compartment syndrome
3. Urinary catheter placement if significantly noted renal failure, urinary retention, or obstructive uropathy noted
I. Pharmacologic therapies
1. Follow evidence-based guidelines for prescribing.
2. Fluid resuscitation
a. May require large doses of IV fluid
b. No clinical data to suggest the appropriate requirements
c. IV hydration adults
i. *Initial:* 2 L isotonic saline
ii. *Followed by:* 400 mL to 1,000 mL/hr
iii. *Maintain urine output:* 200 mL/hr
iv. Adolescence
(1) *Initial:* 20 mL/kg
(2) *Maintenance:* two to three times normal maintenance suggested
(3) Limited studies to make exact recommendations
v. Pediatrics
(1) *Initial:* 20 mL/kg
(2) *Maintenance:* two to three times normal maintenance suggested
(3) Limited studies to make exact recommendations
d. Repeating CPK and electrolytes every 6 to 12 hours
3. Correct electrolytes.
4. Consultation and collaboration
a. *Emergency attending:* ED attending should be consulted on cases when the diagnosis is not clear, complicated management, or where additional expertise will help in management of the patient.
b. *Nephrologist:* Consult nephrology for patients with significant rhabdomyolysis that show evidence of renal failure, severe electrolyte abnormalities, or needing hemodialysis. Discussion with nephrology should occur in cases of rhabdomyolysis with hyperkalemia, severe acid–base disturbances, refractory pulmonary edema, or progressive renal failure.
c. *Orthopedic surgeon:* Consult orthopedic surgeon for patients with rhabdomyolysis with limb fractures or suspected compartment syndrome.

Patient Disposition

A. Once the patient has been stabilized, disposition can be determined. Most cases of rhabdomyolysis, regardless of the cause, will likely benefit from admission, hydration, and renal filtration. Patient may need to be transferred to another institution for care.
B. Age and developmental considerations as previously noted
C. Prevention and education and patient and family counseling
1. If a preventable cause is identified, then the patient should be educated on the cause and identify efforts

to avoid this activity. Drugs and alcohol should be avoided if they are related to the cause of the patient's rhabdomyolysis.

2. Compliance with prescribed medications
   a. Avoiding illicit drugs
   b. Avoid allowing patients to lay in positions for a long period of time that may result in pressure necrosis.
   c. Encourage appropriate hydration when working out aggressively, for athletics, or in temperatures of extreme or significant humidity.

D. *Documentation:* Rhabdomyolysis and acute kidney injury

Medical Decision-Making and Differential Diagnoses

A. Differential diagnosis
   1. Bacterial sepsis
   2. Brain abscess
   3. Diskitis
   4. Endocarditis
   5. Fever of unknown origin
   6. Herniated nucleus pulposus
   7. Psoas abscess
   8. Vertebral osteomyelitis
   9. Epidural abscess

Diagnostic Testing

A. Laboratory studies
   1. CBC
   2. Erythrocyte sedimentation rate (ESR)
   3. Blood cultures
      a. + in 40% of patients with osteomyelitis
      b. + higher with epidural abscess

B. Imaging studies
   1. *X-ray:* Utility in osteomyelitis. No utility in epidural abscess.
      a. Common radiographic findings in suspected osteomyelitis are
         i. Bony destruction
         ii. Irregularity of vertebral end plates
         iii. Disc space narrowing
   2. *MRI:* Gold standard for making accurate diagnosis of osteomyelitis and epidural abscess.
   3. *CT:* Better at picking up osteomyelitis than in plain films

Management

A. The essential problem with spinal epidural abscess is that early diagnosis is vital. Permanent neurologic deficits and possible mortality can be avoided or reduced, but treatment must be in a rapid timely fashion. Treatment for both epidural abscess and osteomyelitis is likely surgical in nature.

B. Pharmacologic therapies
   1. Follow evidence-based guidelines when prescribing medication
   2. Antibiotic therapy
      a. When possible, hold empiric antibiotics until a microbiologic diagnosis is confirmed.
         i. Do not withhold antibiotics in septic patients.
         ii. Do not withhold antibiotics in patient with neurologic compromise.
      b. Broad spectrum coverage
         i. Cover gram-positive, gram-negative, aerobes, anaerobes (including methicillin-resistant *Staphylococcus aureus* [MRSA]).
      c. Most vertebral osteomyelitis is caused by *S. aureus*.
   3. Analgesia
      a. This can be a very painful pathology and adequate and regular opioid analgesia may be required.
      b. Administer with appropriate monitoring.
   4. IV resuscitation
      a. If the patient is septic, in shock, or has an elevated lactate level IV hydration with isotonic solution is recommended.

C. Consultation and collaboration
   1. *Spinal surgeon/neurosurgical specialist:* Early consultation in cases where there is suspicion for epidural abscess or osteomyelitis. Inquiry about whether they want to initiate antibiotic therapy prior to or after operative management should be queried.
   2. *Infectious disease specialist:* Consider consulting infectious disease specialist for clarification for optimal antibiotic choice based on the patient's comorbidities, medication allergies, and likely cause of the pathology.
   3. *Emergency medicine physician:* Consider collaboration with the ED physician where the diagnosis is unclear. Additionally, these cases are often time-sensitive operative management cases, with significantly devastating consequences. Therefore, additional clinician help may be indicated to facilitate rapid intervention by the specialist.

Patient Disposition

A. Admission
   1. If the services required to treat this patient are offered at your facility, the patient will likely be admitted to the hospital. If there is any neurologic deficit, the patient may require ICU level care for recurrent neurologic assessment and treatment for septic shock. The patient may require operative management immediately or this may be delayed based on the specialist clinical decision-making.

B. Transfer
   1. If the services required to manage the pathology are not offered at the clinician's facility or if operative management cannot be facilitated in a time=sensitive manner, the patient will likely require transfer. This will likely be in the form of aeromedical evacuation.

C. Documentation
   1. It is imperative that the documentation for these patient's assessment, treatment, reassessment, and timeline of disposition, is clearly documented. These

are high-risk cases that have the potential for poor outcomes, and therefore it is vital to document all neurologic findings, timely consultations with specialists, and medical-decision-making.

Age and Developmental Considerations

A. Pediatric
  1. Children with vertebral osteomyelitis and associated diskitis usually present with an abrupt onset of malaise, fever, and back pain. Often demonstrating back stiffness, restricted motion, guarded walking, and spine tenderness.
  2. Babinski reflex normal in up to 2 years old
B. Prevention and education
  1. Preventative education for these patients is mostly related to the patients that are utilizing IV drug use. Educating them on the dangers of reusing needles and suggesting rehabilitation therapy may be pertinent.
C. Patient and family education and counseling
  1. Patients and family need to be educated on the serious nature of this pathology. They need to be educated on the possibility for paralysis, gait dysfunction, or loss of motor/sensory function related to the pathology.

Spinal Infections

A. Vertebral osteomyelitis
  1. Spinal infections are infectious disease process that affects the vertebral body, intervertebral disc, or adjacent paraspinal tissue. Between 2% and 7% of all musculoskeletal infections. Vertebral osteomyelitis is the most encountered form of vertebral infection. It can result from direct open spinal trauma, from infections in adjacent structures, or from hematogenous spread of bacteria to the vertebra, or postoperatively. Left untreated may result in permanent neurologic deficits, significant spinal deformity, or death. Additionally, it can result in compression of the neural structures due to epidural abscess formation. This forms from pathologic fracture from the bone softening.
B. Epidural abscess
  1. In the same category of infections, epidural abscess is also a diagnosis that must be excluded with similar presentation. Epidural abscess is a rare but potentially life-threatening disease that requires prompt diagnosis and intervention. It involves a collection of pus between the dura of the skull or spine. Epidural abscesses form in two types: (a) spinal epidural abscess and (b) intracranial epidural abscess. They are delineated based on where they occur in the central nervous system (CNS) system.

Medical Screening

A. Chief complaint
  1. Back or neck pain is the most common symptom.
B. Signs and symptoms
  1. Classic triad for spinal abscess: (only present in 15% of patients)
    a. Fever
    b. Spinal pain
    c. Neurologic deficit
  2. Most symptoms are the result of enlargement of the abscess and surrounding inflammation (Table 32.13).
    a. Back pain
    b. Rigors/chills
    c. Radicular pain
    d. Motor weakness
    e. Sphincter dysfunction
    f. Sensory changes
    g. Paralysis
C. Focused assessment
  1. History
    a. Identify the following types of patients as high risk:
      i. IV drug abuse (IVDA)
      ii. Invasive spinal procedures
      iii. Open spinal trauma
      iv. Immunocompromised
      v. Diabetes
      vi. Dialysis
      vii. Tuberculosis (TB)
      viii. Cancer
      ix. Organ transplantation
    b. History of present illness
      i. Insidious presentation
      ii. Back pain is the most common symptom.
      iii. Usually patients report prolonged symptoms. In >50% of the patients, symptoms were present for >3 months.

TABLE 32.13 LOWER BACK PAIN DIFFERENTIAL

PATHOPHYSIOLOGY	DIFFERENTIAL
GI	Abdominal aneurysm/dissection, pancreatitis, cholecystitis, ulcer
Trauma	Acute lumbosacral strain, vertebral compression fracture, retroperitoneal bleeding
Infection IV drug use, HIV, immunocompromised	Spinal epidural abscess, discitis, osteomyelitis, pyelonephritis, perinephric abscess
Neurologic	Cauda equina syndrome, herniated disc, spinal stenosis
Rheumatologic	Fibromyalgia, rheumatoid arthritis, spondylitis, osteoarthritis
GYN/GU	Nephrolithiasis, ectopic pregnancy, labor
Neoplasm	Malignancy (multiple myeloma), bony metastasis

iv. Pain is initially localized and gradually worsens to a point where it does not respond to pain medication.
v. Eventually bed rest will not relieve symptoms.
vi. Unfortunately, neurologic symptoms are not present until late in the disease course.
vii. In severe cases, some patients may present with acute illness with fever, night sweats, elevated leukocyte counts, and signs and symptoms of shock.

c. Physical examination
i. Typical presentation will have mild symptoms and only mild tenderness over the spinous process of the involved vertebrae.
ii. Only half the patients will be febrile.
iii. Decreased overall range of motion
iv. Examination of the affected area for evidence of localized infection or scars that could aid in explaining the patient's pain. Additionally, look for track marks for potential IV injection points (e.g., between fingers, toes, arms, feet, neck)
v. Detailed motor examination should be performed that includes motor strength in all extremities.
vi. Sensory assessment
(1) *Rectal tone:* Normal, weak, or none
(2) *Perineum/perianal sensation:* Assess for saddle paresthesia or perianal paresthesia
(3) Presence or absence of Babinski sign:
(a) *Abnormal (+):* Big toe curls toward head and fanning of toes.
(4) Presence or absence of clonus
vii. Neurologic examination should be reassessed at regular intervals and documented for reference of improvement or deterioration.

Tendonitis

Tendonitis is inflammation of one of the many tendons in the body that causes pain at the tendon insertion site in the bone. Most pain related to tendons is not inflammatory in nature. The common term that we utilize as tendonitis is *tendinopathy*. This is defined as common clinical condition that affects the tendons and causes pain, swelling, or impaired performance. The exact cause of tendinopathy is unclear. This pathology is more common in the middle-aged population and is often described as the result of overuse of repetitive function of specific joints.

Medical Screening

A. *Chief complaint:* Painful range of motion of a specific joint

B. Signs and symptoms
1. Sign and symptoms vary at specific locations but can be generalized in the following manner:
a. Localized pain to the specific joint with range of motion of the tendon
b. Point specific tenderness over the tendon in question on flexion
c. Swelling

C. Focused assessment
1. Common sites of tendinopathy
a. Rotator cuff shoulder
i. Most common with repetitive activities overhead
ii. Describes as deep pain and significant pain with range of motion
iii. Physical testing:
(1) Palpation over greater tuberosity at supraspinatus tendon insertion
(2) *Jobe test (supraspinatus):* Both arms abducted at 90 degrees, held in front of the patient in full pronation. Test resistance and compare strength. Difficulty holding an arm up or presence of pain is a suggestive finding for rotator cuff pathology
(3) *Hawkins test (supraspinatus):* Forward flexion of affected arm to 90 degrees and then forcibly internally rotates the shoulder. This is accomplished by the clinician grabbing the elbow with one hand and the wrist with the other rotating in opposite directions to internally rotate the shoulder.

b. Bicipital tendonitis/tendinopathy
i. Pain in the anterior shoulder and over the bicipital groove
ii. Worse with flexing shoulder
iii. Worse with supination of the forearm
iv. Physical testing
(1) Pain with bicep resistance
(2) *Speed test:* Arm straight, makes a fist, with supination; clinician places their hand over the forearm and tests resistance to flexing the bicep

c. Epicondylitis of the elbow
i. Medial epicondylitis:
(1) Pain over the medial aspect of the elbow
(2) Common in golfers, bowlers, pitchers, and carpenters
ii. Lateral epicondylitis:
(1) Pain over the lateral aspect of the elbow
(2) Worse with grasping and twisting
(3) Common in tennis-type sports and manual labor workers

d. Knee: patellar and popliteal tendons, iliotibial band
i. Patellar:
(1) Localized pain to the anterior knee
(2) Often referred to as "Jumper's knee"
(3) Common in jumping sports like basketball, volleyball, high jump, and running

(4) Pain is common when ambulating uphill or when changing from the sitting to standing position.
(5) Tenderness over the lower pole of the patella where the tendon inserts

ii. Popliteus:
(1) Lateral knee pain
(2) Associated mechanism running downhill
(3) Tenderness just above joint and anterior to the lateral collateral ligament

e. Iliotibial band
i. Lateral knee pain
(1) Most common overuse syndrome of the knee
(2) Common in cyclist, runners, football players, dancers
(3) Aggravated by running downhill, long stride running, or sitting for lengthy periods of time with the knees flexed

f. Tibial tendon of the leg (shin splints)
i. Pain is noted over the anteromedial aspect of the lower leg.
ii. Mechanism has been from overpronation or repetitive running on hard surfaces.

g. Achilles tendon of the heel
i. Pain in the heel
ii. Pain in the heel with plantar flexion
iii. Common in runners with increased distances, change in running surface or poor footwear

Differential Diagnoses

A. Compartment syndrome
B. Bursitis
C. Deep vein thrombosis (DVT)
D. Gout/pseudogout
E. Reactive arthritis
F. Rheumatoid arthritis (RA)
G. Region-specific
1. Hand
a. Carpal tunnel syndrome
b. Soft tissue injuries
c. Hand infections
2. Foot/ankle
a. Soft tissue injuries
b. Plantar fasciitis
3. Knee
a. Soft tissue injuries
b. Infection superficial/septic arthritis
4. Rotator cuff
a. Soft tissue injuries
b. Dislocation

Diagnostic Testing

A. Laboratory studies
1. There is no utility for laboratory studies in many of these diagnoses unless there is concern that there is a joint infection, bursitis, or if it is unclear if tendinopathy is present.

B. Imaging
1. *X-rays:* Radiographic studies have limited utility but may provide clues. Occasionally, an avulsion fracture may be visualized, focusing on the potential tendon dysfunction. Additionally, calcium deposits may be present on imaging to suggest calcified tendinopathy.
2. *MRI/ultrasound (US):* These imaging studies are reserved for cases where the diagnosis is unclear. It should be noted that bedside US may provide useful examination if the clinician is skilled in tendon assessment. A discussion of bedside US is beyond the scope of this text, and the clinician can review findings in a variety of emergency medicine texts that focus on US diagnostics.

Management

A. General treatment goal is reduction of pain and return the patient to full activity.
1. Rest; however, continue to range joint at a decreased activity level.
2. Ice for the first 24 to 48 hours.
3. Splinting or immobilization
4. Sling if indicated
5. Strength and stretching exercises after the acute period and pain has subsided

Procedures

1. *Transcutaneous electrical nerve stimulation (TENS).* Useful but has not proven to be any more beneficial than other conservative treatment therapies.
2. Corticosteroid injections may be considered for failed conservative treatment; however, it should be noted that their effectiveness is controversial. No Achilles tendonitis should be injected with steroids due to the high risk for tendon rupture related to corticosteroid injection.

B. Pharmacologic therapies
1. Follow evidence-based guidelines for prescribing
2. NSAIDs are the mainstay of treatment for these complaints.
3. Oral or topical application are acceptable modes of administration.

C. Consultation and collaboration
1. Most cases do not require consultation by orthopedist specialist. Most cases do not require an emergency medicine physician consultation. However, cases where the diagnosis may not be clear, a collaborative opinion may be advised.

Patient Disposition

A. Most of these patients are dispositioned to discharge. Additionally, they should be referred for orthopedic follow-up.

B. Age and developmental considerations
1. Careful review of the patient's medications and medical history is advised before prescribing NSAID treatment.

C. Prevention and education

D. Patient and family education and counseling
1. Patients should be educated on their diagnosis, treatment, and need for follow-up.

2. It is important to identify concerning sign/symptoms or findings that should have the patient return to the ED.

E. Documentation

1. Clear documentation of evaluation, assessment, treatment, and follow-up are advised.

2. Documentation of medical decision-making that explains the clinician's suspicion for the pathology and explanation of elimination of high-risk diagnoses is advised.

Additional Reading

Additional Reading for this chapter are online only and can be found at https://connect.springerpub.com/content/reference-book/978-0-8261-6091-5/part/part03/toc-part/ch32.

33. Soft Tissue Injuries

KRISTINA DAVIS | SUSANNA RUDY | AUDREY SNYDER | RENEÉ SEMONIN HOLLERAN

Learning Objectives

- Identify the causes of specific soft tissue injuries that may be seen in the emergency or urgent care environments.
- Discuss the management of specific soft tissue injuries managed by the emergency nurse practitioner (ENP) in the emergency or urgent care environments.
- Identify high-risk soft tissue injuries seen in the emergency or urgent care environments.
- Discuss patient disposition and education related to the management of soft tissue injuries in the emergency or urgent care environments.
- Identify the causes of envenomation.
- Identify high-risk patients with envenomation injuries.
- Discuss the management of envenomation in the emergency or urgent care environments.
- Discuss patient disposition and education related to the management of patients who have suffered an envenomation injury.

Wound Management

KRISTINA DAVIS

A. Soft tissue injuries often result from traumatic injury. This section will discuss soft tissue injuries related to amputation, avulsion, degloving, laceration, and puncture wounds.

B. Amputation

1. Amputations can occur through a crush, tearing, or guillotine-type injury, causing the loss of a body part. An additional injury that could cause loss of a limb would be cold exposure (frostbite), which is covered in Chapter 36. The most common amputation injury involves the hands, specifically the fingers. Amputations may be replanted based on certain criteria and the type of injury. The treatment goal is to preserve use, control pain, minimize and create favorable healing, prevent neuromas, and, for fingertip amputations, preserve nails.

C. Avulsion and degloving

1. Avulsion occurs when skin and subcutaneous tissue is forcefully torn away from the muscle, fascia, or bone. An avulsion can occur from a high-energy or low-energy injury. Due to thin skin, geriatric patients are at greater risks of avulsions. The injury can be complete or partial. A degloving injury typically occurs from a shearing and/or high-energy injury. Avulsions can be repaired based on the vascularity of the flap, surrounding tissue, flap damage, and base ratio versus length. Degloving injuries are more difficult to repair and typically require extensive surgical reconstruction. Based on the time of injury determines the viability of the avulsed skin, <8 hours.

D. Laceration

1. A laceration is a disruption to the skin that may extend through several layers of tissue. The goal of laceration care is to avoid infection, provide the best cosmetic outcome, and control bleeding. Laceration repair is determined by the laceration location, age of laceration, and type of laceration.

E. Puncture wounds

1. Puncture wounds occur from a sharp object or the case of an animal bite, teeth, penetrating the skin and are described as the depth being greater than the width. Puncture wounds cause deep tissue injury and can involve tendons, joints, bones, or vascular injuries. Often puncture wounds are seen in the foot from a patient stepping on an object. Additionally, puncture wounds can also occur from animal bites of which there are many sources including domestic and wild animals.

Emergent Issues

A. Hemorrhage
B. Shock secondary to hypovolemia or infection
C. Loss of limb/body part
D. Disruption of skin
E. Infection
F. Pain

Assessment

A. Medical history

1. Tetanus status
2. Tobacco history
3. Extremity dominance
4. Occupation/hobbies
5. Allergies
6. Medications, especially those that may increase bleeding.
7. Medical history that will compromise healing and/or increase bleeding (e.g., hematologic disorders, diabetes, hypertension, peripheral vascular disease).
8. Details of injury
9. Time of injury

B. Focused assessment

1. *Concurrent injuries:* Care must be taken to avoid distraction from life–threatening injuries. A primary survey must be completed.

2. Type of injury

3. Skin color and temperature

4. *Vascular injury:* Assess amount of bleeding and blood loss, assess pulses that are distal and immediately proximal of the injury, hematoma, and ischemia.

5. *Sensation:* Two-point discrimination

6. Motor function to include strength

7. Level of injury including potential proximal and distal injuries

8. Contaminates (foreign bodies)

9. Exposure and/or injury to bone, tendon, and arteries

C. Injury-specific assessment

1. Amputation

a. Fingertip amputation classification "Allen and Fassler"

b. Ribbon sign, which is the twisting appearance of an artery

c. Amputated part accessibility

d. Viability of amputated part. Crush injuries are less likely to successfully be replanted than a guillotine injury.

2. Degloving

a. High potential of underlying fracture

b. *Extent of injury:* How many layers are involved epidermis, dermis, subcutaneous, fascia, muscle, and bone

3. Laceration

a. *Scalp:* Vascular, likely to bleed. Inspect for galea laceration. A galea laceration >0.5 cm requires suturing with absorbable suture prior to skin closure. Assess for skull involvement.

b. *Hand/finger:* Higher risk of nerve and/or tendon injury. Suspected tendon injury, major vascular injury, laceration penetrating the joint, requires a specialty. Active and passive range of motion (ROM) should be performed including against resistance. Assess for injury to the joint.

c. *Joints:* Lacerations that overly joints should be accessed for a joint injury. Joint injuries that accompany a laceration need a specialty consult.

d. *Face:* Since injuries to the face can occur over nerves and vessels that may impact wound healing, cosmetic effects, and neurologic damage, consider a plastic surgery consult for wounds that have a potential for poor cosmetic outcome. Staples should be avoided.

i. *Forehead:* Facial movement, symmetry, and sensation need evaluation prior to anesthesia and repair. For superficial lacerations that do not extend into the muscle, a single layer suturing technique can be done. For lacerations that extend into the muscle, layer must be repaired in multiple layers. The muscle should be repaired with absorbable suture material and then the outermost layer closed with sterile glue, skin closure strips, or nonabsorbable sutures. Suture cosmetically significant facial features first to facilitate proper alignment. Vertical lacerations have a poorer cosmetic outcome than horizontal lacerations. A flap laceration can cause a "trapdoor" effect. A mattress suture and subcutaneous tissue approximation may decrease the "trapdoor" effect.

ii. *Intraoral:* Evaluate for airway compromise, secure airway if a compromise is present. Access for dental trauma and mandible fracture. Most often heals well without wound closure; consider closure for large lacerations >1 cm, uncontrolled hemorrhage, gaping wound, or chance poor healing without repair. Tongue margin lacerations and through-and-through lacerations require suturing. Inspect all intraoral wounds for broken teeth fragments. May require multiple suturing layers. Suture loosely to allow for swelling and to avoid necrosis.

iii. *Lip:* For lips, the vermillion border is cosmetically significant. If the laceration crosses the vermillion border, the first suture should properly align the border vermillion.

iv. *Cheek:* Assess for injury to the parotid gland, parotid duct, and facial nerves. For suspected injury consult a specialist. For a through-and-through laceration, the intraoral layer should be repaired first with absorbable suture.

v. *Eyelid/eye:* Any injury suspected to the lacrimal duct, orbicularis oculi muscle, tarsal plate, injury to inner eyelid, and eyelid margins should have an immediate ophthalmology or plastic surgery consult. Lacerations that are at the lid edge and <1 mm will heal spontaneously and do not require suturing. An ophthalmic examination including extraocular movements (EOM), evaluation of ptosis, slit lamp, and fluorescein examination is necessary to access for concurrent injury.

vi. *Eyebrows:* Do not shave eyebrows. Extra care should be taken to anatomically align the edges; malalignment is obvious.

vii. *Ear:* Lacerations that occur from blunt trauma need an ophthalmoscope evaluation to access the tympanic membrane as well as evaluation for hemotympanum, impaired hearing, or otorrhea. Evaluate cranial nerve VII and the parotid gland for lacerations that extend anteriorly from the ear. Hemostasis should be accomplished to prevent a hematoma. Exposed cartilage should be covered. A specialty consult is necessary for ear avulsions, lacerations that are through-and-through, nerve involvement, or middle ear injury. During repair, care should be taken to cover expose cartilage with tissue. Anesthesia can be accomplished through a nerve block at the great auricular nerve.

viii. *Nose:* Anesthesia should be accomplished through a nerve block. Assess for a septal hematoma and underlying bony involvement in injuries related to blunt trauma. Septal hematoma must be drained if present to prevent septal necrosis. Ensure that exposed cartilage is covered. Care should be taken to align the alar margins.

4. Puncture wound
   a. Depth of the puncture wound
   b. *Infection:* Assess for signs/symptoms of infection including an abscess. Symptoms of infection include pain that has increased over several days, pain with movement, drainage, fever, tachycardia, pain out of proportion, or lymphangitis.

Differential Diagnoses

A. Hypovolemic shock
B. Vascular injury
C. Bony injury
D. Nailbed injury
E. Tendon injury
F. Nerve injury
G. Fracture
H. Foreign body
I. Diagnostic testing
   1. X-rays to injured area
      a. Assess bony involvement.
      b. Assess for foreign bodies (note wood and plastic can be radiolucent).
      c. Evaluate for osteomyelitis for infected puncture wounds.
   2. CT scan
      a. Head, for suspected closed head injury
      b. Face, for suspected facial fractures
      c. Cervical spine, for suspected injury
      d. With contrast for evaluation of suspected arterial damage

Management

A. Treatment
   1. General
      a. *Control hemorrhage:* Direct pressure or tourniquet
      b. Hypovolemic treatment: Fluids and blood products if necessary
      c. *Wound care:* Should be aimed at decreasing contaminants and bacteria. Irrigation with saline under pressure, which can be achieved with a 35- to 65-mL syringe and a 19-gauge needle to achieve a psi of 5 to 8. Avoid cleansers inside the wound due to tissue toxicity.
      d. *Wound closure:* Sterile technique is not required. Wound closure timing is based on the type of wound. Lacerations that occur from a clean object can be repaired up to 18 hours after injury without increased infection. Clean facial wounds can be closed up to 24 hours after injury.
         i. *Suture:* Lacerations that extend through the dermis, jagged wound edges, and require close approximation. Good for areas of high tension. Suturing material is based on the type and location of the injury.
         ii. *Staple:* Lacerations that extend through the dermis. Linear wounds. Areas without cosmetic perspective. Works well with scalp wounds, do not need to trim hair. Good for areas of high tension.
         iii. *Sterile glue:* Skin tear, flap laceration, or linear wounds that are under low tension should not be used on mucosa or eyes.
         iv. *Steri-Strip:* Skin tear, flap laceration, or linear wounds that are under low tension
         v. *Splint:* for areas of high tension
      e. *Tetanus prophylaxis:* Update if not received in the past 5 years
      f. Parenteral antibiotics with coverage directed toward gram-positive and gram-negative bacteria should be initiated within 6 hours for injuries with bony involvement.
      g. *Antibiotics:* Based on location of wound; wounds to lower extremities are at higher risk of infection while wounds that are in vascular areas such as the face and scalp are less likely to become infected. For underlying bony involvement, a dose of paternal antibiotics is recommended. Lacerations that occur due to an animal bite, animal scratch, human bite, or human scratch require prophylaxis antibiotics. A patient's medical history related to increased risk of infection should be considered when deciding on antibiotics. Overall healthy individuals do not need prophylaxis antibiotics. In older wounds, antibiotics may be considered depending on what caused the wound, presence of infection, and how the wound was initially managed.
         i. Plantar puncture wound through the sole of the shoe require antibiotics cover *Staphylococcus aureus* (cephalosporin) and *Pseudomonas aeruginosa* (fluoroquinolones).
      h. Local anesthesia or regional nerve block; for smaller amputations such as fingers or toes a digital block can be done
      i. Opioid pain control
      j. Consider need for rabies prophylaxis when wound was caused by a mammal including exposure to saliva.
      k. Consultation with a hand surgeon, orthopedic surgeon, trauma surgeon, or plastic surgeon depending on type and extent of injury
   2. Treatment specific to **amputation**
      a. Splint the injury in a functional position.
      b. *Amputated part:* Rinse with saline and then wrap in saline moistened gauze and cool indirectly. Do not place directly on ice. An amputated part's viability is increased from warm ischemia time of 6 to 8 hours to 12 to 24 hours. Keep the amputated part with the patient.
      c. *Fingertip amputations:* Treatment should include the goals of maintaining length, nail preservation, sensation, and function. Amputations that are distal and are <1 cm^2 without nailbed involvement or bone exposure can heal by secondary intention. Amputations that are distal to the distal interphalangeal (DIP) joint and do not involve bone can most likely be managed in the ED. A small amount of bony exposure can be managed through rongeur and closure or healing by secondary intention.

However, consultation and close follow-up with a hand surgeon is warranted.

d. Plastic surgery, orthopedic surgeon, or trauma surgeon consult should be strongly considered.

e. Replantation is less successful in adults over the age of 50 due to vascular regeneration.

f. Pediatric patients have a more successful replantation rate.

3. Treatment specific to avulsion and degloving

i. *Airway management:* For degloving or avulsion injuries that involve the face or neck and compromise the airway. Consider secondary edema.

ii. *Wound closure:* Determined by the extent of injury (small area), vascularity of flap, and vascularity of surrounding tissue.

iii. Plastic surgery consult should occur early for avulsion/degloving injuries.

B. Consultation and collaboration

1. Consult with hand or orthopedic surgeon for injuries with tendon or nerve injury.

2. Consult with a plastic surgeon for patients with complicated facial lacerations or concerns for poor cosmetic outcome.

3. Consult a vascular surgeon for arterial injury.

4. General surgery consult for surgical debridement.

5. For degloving and amputation injuries consider transfer to a trauma facility.

Patient Disposition

A. Transition of care information

1. Transfer to trauma facility versus transfer to operating room (OR) versus discharge.

a. Depending on the resources at the facility patients with major traumatic **amputations** will either be transferred or admitted.

b. Patients with minor **amputations**, such as the tip of a finger may be discharged directly from the ED. However, for any injury that extends beyond the fingernail, a consultation should be completed prior to discharge.

c. Based on the extent of injury, if the patient is transferred and avulsed skin is available, send with patient.

d. Consider transfer to trauma facility for extensive injuries.

e. **Puncture** wounds may need to be transferred to the OR. Other wounds that need surgical intervention include those that have a complex abscess, associated osteomyelitis, or require surgical debridement.

B. Discharge instructions

1. *Wound care:* Keep area clean and dry. After 24 hours patients may get area wet briefly but should not submerge the area such as baths or swimming. Antibiotic ointment should be applied to the wound.

2. Instruct patient to return for pain out of proportion

3. Educate patient on signs/symptoms of infection including redness and swelling at wound site, purulent drainage from site, and warm to touch.

4. Consider prophylactic antibiotics for patients who are at high risk (e.g., those with diabetes, immunocompromised patients, or plantar puncture wound through the sole of the shoe).

5. *Splint care:* Instruct patients on signs/symptoms of neurovascular compromise.

6. *Animal bite:* Lacerations from an animal bite or scratch need prophylaxis antibiotics such as Amoxicillin/clavulanate. Additionally, the animal's rabies status needs to be verified. If necessary, the patient should receive rabies prophylaxis.

7. Head injury precautions for scalp or facial injuries from blunt trauma

8. Suture/staple removal based on suture/staple location

9. Wound care location considerations is specific based on location and wound closure material. For Steri-Strips or sterile glue, avoid getting area wet until healed. Do not use antibiotic ointment on sterile glue or Steri-Strips. Wound closure areas may be bandaged, but patient should be encouraged to allow the area to be open to air regularly.

a. *Scalp:* Sutures/staples removed in 10 to 14 days.

b. *Hand/finger:* For wounds in a high-tension area patients may benefit from a splint placement.

c. *Face:* For wounds that may have a poor cosmetic outcome advise patient to follow-up with a plastic surgeon.

i. *Forehead:* Due to the "trapdoor" effect patients need to have a follow-up with a plastic surgeon for potential revision. A compression dressing may be needed to decrease hematoma or dead space within the wound.

ii. *Intraoral:* Consider oral antibiotics for through-and-through facial wounds.

iii. *Lip:* Suture removal in 5 to 7 days. Plastic surgery follow-up for cosmetic concerns.

iv. *Cheek:* Suture removal in 5 days. Plastic surgery follow-up for cosmetic concerns or identified nerve injury.

v. *Eyebrow:* Suture removal in 5 to 7 days

vi. *Eyelid/eye:* Ophthalmic antibiotic ointment should be used for any tissue near the eye. Close ophthalmology follow-up. Sutures should be removed in 3 to 5 days.

vii. *Ear:* Sutures should be removed in 5 to 7 days. A pressure dressing should be applied to prevent a perichondrial hematoma. Patient should return in 24 hours for dressing change and reevaluation or have a specialty follow-up in 24 hours. The dressing does not need to be reapplied in the absence of a hematoma. Antibiotic prophylaxis necessary for injuries that involve the cartilage.

viii. *Nose:* Sutures should be removed in 3 to 5 days. Otolaryngology follow-up in 5 to 7 days for displaced nasal fractures. Antibiotic prophylaxis necessary for injuries that involve the cartilage.

C. Prevention and education

1. Discuss the possibility of scarring.

2. Specialty follow-up for injuries that required a specialist consult or high-risk injuries.

3. Fingertip amputation and partial amputations are susceptible to fingernail deformity, poor cosmetic outcome, and usage disability.
4. Patients with amputation injuries are at risk for developing painful neuromas, have poor cosmetic outcomes, loss of sensation, loss of work, and increased need for rehabilitation services.

Burns

AUDREY SNYDER

Burns are an injury to the skin that may be caused by thermal (heat), electrical, chemicals, or radiation. The skin is the largest organ in the body and encompasses approximately 15% of total body weight. It maintains several very important bodily functions: protective barrier against infection, regulates fluid loss, temperature regulation, Vitamin D absorption, and sensation. The epidermis of the skin is the thicker outer layer of stratified, squamous epithelium. The dermis below contains blood vessels, hair follicles, nerve endings, and sebaceous (sweat) glands (Figure 33.1). When the skin is compromised, vital functions are also impacted. Cells are destroyed, fluids and electrolytes depleted, the risk of infection increases, and the ability to regulate temperature is impacted.

A first degree is a superficial partial-thickness burn involving only the epidermis, that is usually painful, dry, red, and may have mild swelling. Pain improves with cooling. First-degree burns usually heal spontaneously and have a low risk of infection. A sunburn is an example of a first-degree burn.

Second-degree burns can be classified as superficial partial-thickness or deep partial-thickness. Superficial partial-thickness burns extend beyond the epidermis and are very painful and sensitive to temperature changes and air exposure. Skin may appear red with moist blisters and weeping. These burns typically heal in 7 to 21 days but may develop pigmentation scarring. A deep partial-thickness may or may not be sensitive to touch, but is often sensitive to air exposure. Healing is prolonged over several weeks and scarring is likely. With deep partial-thickness burns, the infection barrier is destroyed increasing the risk for infection.

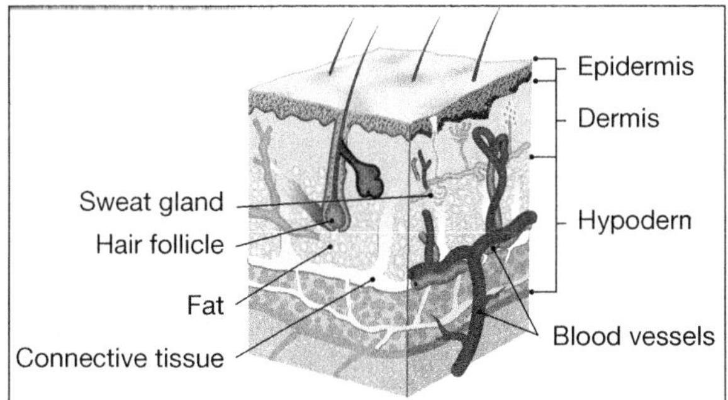

FIGURE 33.1 Anatomy of the skin.
Source: Ousley LE, Gentry RD. Evidence-based assessment of skin, hair, and nails. In: Gawlik KS, Melnyk BM, Teall AM, eds. *Evidence-Based Physical Examination: Best Practices for Health and Well-Being Assessment.* Springer Publishing Company, 2021. Fig. 9.1.[1]

Third-degree burns are full thickness extending through the epidermis and dermis and may have destruction of subcutaneous tissue, fascia, muscle, and bone. Third-degree burns often are not painful due to damage to the nerves. Surrounding second-degree areas will be painful. Third-degree burns can appear dry, charred, or translucent. Eschar or leathery devitalized tissue may develop. Treatment may require escharotomy, fasciotomy, and/or skin grafting. Healing is prolonged and severe scarring is anticipated.

Burns are classified as minor, major, or severe. *Minor* burns may be partial-thickness and encompass no more than 15% of total body surface area (TBSA), full thickness <2% TBSA, not involving eyes, ears, hands, feet, face, or perineum, excludes electrical or inhalation burns, age is <60 years with no preexisting medical conditions or additional injuries. *Major* burns are usually partial thickness, which are 15% to 25% TBSA, can be full thickness 2% to 10% TBSA in an adult <60 years of age with no chronic cardiac, endocrine, and/or pulmonary comorbidities at the time of the burn and does not involve eyes, ears, hands, face, or perineum, excludes electrical or inhalation injuries, and there are no complicated injuries in addition to the burn. *Severe* burns are >25% of the TBSA in the adult, full-thickness burns >10% TBSA, burns involving the eyes, ears, hands, face, feet, or perineum, includes electrical or inhalation injury, in an adult >60 years of age, or patient has chronic cardiac, pulmonary, or metabolic disorder at the time of burn injury, or burns are accompanied by other injuries.

Globally an estimated 180,000 deaths per year are the result of burns. Thermal burns are the most common type of burn and can be caused by flames, scalding, or contact with hot objects. Radiation burns can occur with exposure to ultraviolet light, x-ray, or prolonged radiation and should be managed as burn severity indicates.

Burns occur mainly in the home and workplace. Burns are cared for in all types of emergency settings. Effective burn care to restore form and function requires the collaboration of an interdisciplinary team of clinicians. Burns can result in profound hypovolemic shock due to fluid shifts from intravascular to interstitial. Burn care requires a methodical approach using a primary and secondary survey assessment and the development of a plan including consultation and transport to a burn or trauma center if appropriate.

Medical Screening

A. Chief complaint and history
   1. Key components of history from emergency medical services (EMS), patient, and family
   2. Mechanism of injury
   3. Past medical history
   4. Medications
   5. Allergies
   6. Tetanus immunization status
B. Signs and symptoms
   1. Direct injury

2. Impact on vital function

C. Focused assessment

1. Primary assessment is the same as for all trauma patients.

a. Assess mental status, verbalization.

b. Airway management (with C-spine stabilization if trauma mechanism in history)—assess for airway patency.

i. Assessment for smoke inhalation injury. Patients who have a history of being in a closed space with flames and smoke or where an accelerant or other chemicals were involved are at greatest risk of inhalation injury.

(1) Stages of smoke inhalation injury

(a) Acute hypoxia with asphyxia occurs at the time of injury.

(b) Upper airway and pulmonary edema in the first hours to days after injury

(c) Infectious complications occur later.

(2) Signs of laryngeal edema and potential for airways obstruction

(a) Burn to face

(b) Singed nasal hair or eyebrows

(c) Soot in nares or mouth

(d) Hoarse voice

(e) Drooling or inability to maintain secretions

(f) Difficulty swallowing or talking

(g) Increased work of breathing

ii. Toxic exposure from byproducts of combustion

iii. Direct thermal injury

iv. Airway placement and management for laryngeal edema to prevent airway obstruction. Follow a process of basic jaw-thrust or chin lift, oral airway placement, endotracheal (ET) intubation, or surgical airway to secure a definitive airway. Consider rapid sequence intubation (RSI).

v. *Oxygenation:* If exposure to carbon monoxide provide 100% oxygen for at least 6 hours to reduce the half-life of carbon monoxide in plasma.

c. Breathing assessment

i. Assess for breathing.

ii. Auscultate breath sounds.

iii. Ensure effective ventilation with mechanical airway.

iv. Ventilator management

v. Escharatomy if circumferential burns imped respirations

d. Circulation

i. Monitor pulse rate and peripheral pulses; anticipate tachycardia, rate of 100 to 120 bpm due to catecholamine release. Higher rates should be evaluated for hypovolemia, other trauma, or inadequate pain management

ii. Assess capillary refill in children.

iii. Monitor for burn shock.

iv. Place all patients with major burns on a cardiac monitor and continuous pulse oximetry. If definitive airway is placed monitor continuous end-tidal CO_2.

v. Obtain vascular access and initiate fluid resuscitation (IV line or intraosseous may be placed through burned skin if necessary).

e. Disability and exposure

i. Alert/Verbal/Painful/Unresponsive (AVPU) to establish baseline mentation. If deficits exist, consider carbon monoxide, chemical exposure, and traumatic injury.

ii. Burn patients should be fully undressed to assess for the full extent of injuries. All jewelry should be removed to prevent constriction. For all burn patients, it is imperative to stop the burning process. Patients may arrive at the ED with charred clothing still in place continuing the burning process. Flush with cool to warm water. Once cooled, discontinue the application of water or wet dressings.

iii. Assess for compartment syndrome.

iv. Calculate the percentage of the burn area.

v. Maintain environmental control as patients lose thermoregulatory ability.

(1) Warm IV fluids.

(2) Warm room temperature.

(3) Cover exposed skin.

(4) Use warming blanket or external warming device such as a Bair Hugger.

2. *Secondary assessment:* Head-to-toe examination to identify life-threatening injuries

a. Associated injuries

b. Shock

c. Infection prevention

3. Burn assessment using a standardized method

a. Burn depth and severity

b. Burn area

i. Rule of 9s (www.allhealthpost.com/rule-of-nines/)

(1) Each arm 9%

(2) Each leg 18%

(3) Thorax front 18%, back 18%

(4) Head 9%

(5) Perineum area/genitals 1%

ii. Lund and Browder Chart is used with infants and children as it is more specific to age and body part burned (aironline.info/lund-browder-chart-45/)[2]

iii. Palmar surface of the patient's hand equates to 1% body surface area (BSA)

c. Risk of increased mortality

i. Morbidity and mortality rise with increased burn surface area.

ii. Age

(1) Children <4 years

(2) Adults >60 years

iii. Comorbidities

(1) Cardiac disease

(2) Respiratory disease
(3) Impaired renal function
(4) Altered endocrine function (diabetes)

Medical Decision-Making and Differential Diagnoses

A. Assess for inhalation injury caused by smoke or hot air causing respiratory damage.
B. Consider potential for airway compromise as swelling occurs.
C. Evaluate for additional injuries if the burn was associated with a blast.

Diagnostic Testing

A. Radiology
  1. Chest x-ray (CXR)
  2. Bronchoscopy
B. Laboratory data
  1. Complete blood count (CBC)
  2. Electrolytes
  3. Serum lactate level to monitor for adequate resuscitation
  4. Blood alcohol level
  5. Toxicology screening
  6. Base deficit
  7. Arterial blood gas with focus on pH
  8. Type and screen
  9. Beta-human chorionic gonadotropin (hCG) test in female patients of childbearing age
  10. Carboxyhemoglobin level
  11. Urine for myoglobin
  12. Creatinine kinase (CK)

Management

A. Emergent phase begins at the time of injury and ends with restoration of vascular permeability. In small burns, maximum edema is seen in 12 to 24 hours, whereas in large burns, maximum edema is seen at 24 to 48 hours.
B. Rinse burn with water in large quantity until the burn is cooled.
  1. Resuscitation begins with initiation of fluid resuscitation and ends with reduction of fluid volume shifts. Fluid resuscitation is calculated based on the time of injury with a goal to not under-or over-hydrate. Patients with BSA <30% without airway compromise may be candidates for oral fluid resuscitation. When IV fluids resuscitation is indicated, between 2 to 4 mL/kg body weight per percentage burn surface area should be administered within the first 24 hours following injury. Calculated fluid volumes are only a guide to initial resuscitation. Subsequent fluids are titrated to urine output.
    a. Obtain height and weight or use weight-based resuscitation tape for measurement in children.
    b. Brooke Formula (modified) 2 mL × weight in kg × TBSA% burn and Parkland Formula 4 mL/ × weight in kg × TBSA% burn. Half of fluids are given in the first 8 hours following injury and the remaining fluid given over the next 16 hours.[3] Pediatric patients' maintenance fluids should include a source of glucose.
    c. Large-bore IV placement, intraosseous placement if emergent.
    d. Ideal fluid choice—crystalloids, balanced salt solutions (lactated Ringer's) warmed[4]
    e. Assessment of urinary output: Ideally 30 to 50 mL/hour (0.3–9.5 mL/kg/hour in adults) or 1 mL/kg/hour in children. Fluid resuscitation is adjusted based upon output.
  2. Maintain normothermia with warm fluids, warm blankets, head coverings, warming lights.
  3. Patients with upper airway burns should have the head of the bed elevated in a semi-upright position to facilitate venous and lymphatic drainage allowing gravity to reduce airway edema.
  4. Monitoring
    a. Vital signs with goal of normalization of blood pressure and heart rate
    b. Acid–base balance
      i. Metabolic acidosis is anticipated in the early resuscitation phase.
      ii. Hyperkalemia is anticipated during the first 24 to 48 hours post-burn.
      iii. Electrolyte replacement
    c. Urine output
    d. Oxygen saturation
    e. Temperature regulation
  5. Procedures
    a. Intubation and airway management for identified or potential inhalation injury. Intubation should be considered prior to transfer. Humidification of inhaled gases.
    b. Placement of urinary catheter to monitor output
    c. Gastric tube placement if patient requires intubation, vomits, or has burns >20% BSA
    d. Bronchoscopy
    e. *Escharotomy:* Circumferential burn to an extremity can result in significant edema and impaired perfusion. Significant burns to the chest and abdomen can result in compartment syndrome with cardiovascular and respiratory compromise. Both may require escharotomies. Abdominal compartment syndrome may require abdominal decompression.
  6. Burn wound management
    a. First-degree or superficial burn
      i. Cool compresses
      ii. Keep moist.
      iii. Bacitracin ointment
      iv. Vaseline petroleum gauze or Xeroform dressings[5]
    b. Second-degree or partial thickness
      i. Clean with antimicrobial cleanser such as Hibiclens and cover.
      ii. Gentle washing if contaminated and cover with clean linens.
    c. Third-degree or full thickness
      i. Echaratomy if needed
      ii. Debridement with collagenase (Santyl)
      iii. Surgical skin grafting later
      iv. Transfer to burn center if available and transfer criteria met.

BOX 33.1 AMERICAN BURN ASSOCIATION CRITERIA FOR TRANSFER TO BURN CENTER

A. Partial thickness burns >10% TBSA
B. Burns that injury to face, hands, feet, genitalia, perineum, or major joints
C. Third-degree burns in any age group
D. Electrical burns including lightning injury
E. Chemical burns
F. Inhalation injury
G. Children with burns in hospitals that do not have appropriate personnel or equipment for the care of children
H. Burn injury in any patients with preexisting medical conditions that could result in complications for management, prolong recovery, or affect mortality.
I. Any patient with burns with trauma in which the burn creates the greatest risk of morbidity/mortality. If trauma is at greatest risk, patient should be cared for at the trauma center and then transferred to the burn center when stable.
J. Patients with burns who require or will require special emotional, social, or rehabilitative intervention.

TBSA, total body surface area.
Source: Excerpted from Guidelines for the Operation of Burn Centers. Resources for Optimal Care of the Injured Patient. Committee on Trauma, American College of Surgeons; 2006:79–86. http://ameriburn.org/wp-content/uploads/2017/05/burncenterreferralcriteria.pdf.[7]

v. If delayed transport, apply silver sulfadiazine (Silvadene), aqueous 10% mafenide solution if surgical delay, or appropriate antibiotic ointment and occlusive dressing[6]

7. Pharmacologic therapies
   a. Pain management (ketamine, fentanyl, morphine, methadone, hydrocodone, gabapentin, hydromorphone)
   b. Anxiolytics (Versed, Ativan) in small doses
   c. Topical antibiotics
   d. Silver-impregnated barrier dressings
8. Consultation and collaboration
   a. Trauma team
   b. May require transfer to burn center (Box 33.1). Improved outcomes have been documented for burns >50% TBSA, children <12 years of age, and inhalation injuries at verified burn centers.
   c. ICU admission
   d. Pulmonary consult for bronchoscopy
   e. Surgery for debridement, escharotomies, or abdominal decompression
   f. Hyperbaric chamber for carbon monoxide exposure with carboxyhemoglobin levels >25%.

Chemical Burns

Chemical burns are caused by necrotizing agents that can be acid, alkali, or organic compounds, although acids are the most common insult.

A. Acid (cleaning products, industrial applications)
B. Alkali (sodium, potassium, and ammonia)
C. Organic compounds (petroleum)

Management

A. Initial care
   1. Remove from chemical source immediately, remove clothing, and brush off dry substances.
   2. For liquid and petroleum, rinse with copious amounts of water.
   3. Consult Material Safety Data Sheet (MSDS) and contact the poison control center and regional burn center for additional guidance.

Electrical Injury

Electrical injury is caused by heat from electrical current passing through the body and damaging tissues. Cardiac arrest may occur with electrical injury. Exposure to voltage <1,000 volts produces cutaneous injury and exposure to an electrical source that is >1,000 volts has a greater potential for deep injury to nerves, muscles, and vascular bed.[7]

A. Types of electrical injuries
   1. Entrance and exit wounds—circumscribed deep wounds at the point of contact with the electrical source or ground, usually hand or feet.
   2. Cutaneous burns can occur from arc injuries, flash injuries, or flames if clothing or material nearby catches fire.
   3. Deep soft tissue injuries to the muscles, nerves, or vascular bed.
   4. Lighting injury may be considered exposure to a large amount of direct current. Cutaneous injuries can occur. Initial management of airway, breathing, and circulation (ABC) is imperative.

Medical Decision-Making and Differential Diagnoses

A. Early referral to burn center
B. Early surgery team involvement for possible fasciotomy for limb burns
C. Abdominal surgery consult for abdominal compartment syndrome
D. Early neurosurgery consultation for head injury
E. Ophthalmology consult to exclude erosion or ulceration of cornea
F. Cardiology consult

Diagnostic Testing

A. EKG
B. Creatinine kinase (CK)
C. Urine myoglobin

Management

A. Cardiopulmonary resuscitation
B. Assess for associated injuries related to falls and violent muscle contractions.
C. Multiple system trauma care
D. Removal of necrotic tissue
E. Decompression of compartments

F. Complications
   1. Risk of cardiac injury
   2. Ileus formation
   3. Myoglobinuria from muscle destruction
   4. Rhabdomyolysis—if myoglobin in urine or elevated CK resuscitate to increased urine output to 3 to 4 mL/kg/hour until rhabdomyolysis resolves. Alkalinization of urine may decrease nephrotoxic potential with iron release. A higher urine output is desired.

G. Procedures
   1. Muscle compartment pressure monitoring
   2. Escharatomy
   3. Fasciotomy

Patient Disposition

A. Discharge instructions
   1. Hand hygiene education
   2. Maintain clean environment for burned areas and with dressing changes.
   3. Dressing change instructions.

B. Transition of care information
   1. Mechanism
   2. Time of injury
   3. Percentage total body surface area (TBSA)
   4. Amount of fluid resuscitation
   5. Identified injuries

C. Patient and family education and counseling
   1. Do not use ice on burn.
   2. Do not use lotions, toothpaste, lard, butter, or other products on burns.
   3. Stop the burning process with water.

D. Documentation
   1. Time of injury to guide resuscitation
   2. Percentage TBSA
   3. Serial vital signs including temperature
   4. Total fluid resuscitation

Age and Developmental Considerations

A. Consideration of abuse

B. Prevention and education
   1. Keep matches, lighters, firecrackers, gasoline, and explosives out of reach of children.
   2. Always test bathwater.
   3. Install smoke detectors.
   4. Check smoke alarms regularly.
   5. Use back burners on the stove when cooking and children are present.
   6. Do not leave children unattended in the bathtub.
   7. Do not leave children unattended near a fireplace.
   8. Never hold a child when working with or around hot objects.
   9. Set water heaters to <120°F (48.9°C).

Envenomations

SUSANNA RUDY AND RENEÉ SEMONIN HOLLERAN

Envenomation or envenoming is the process of injecting a poison or toxic mixture of venom into another animal or human by the bite, touch, spray, or sting of a venomous animal, insect, or marine mammal. There are numerous species that produce evolved chemical toxins, which are used as a targeted defense or to incapacitate through discomfort, paralysis, or death of their prey. Most envenomations in the United States are indigenous, caused by local fauna, animal life of a particular region or time period. Unfortunately, an estimated $10 billion annual exotic animal black market trade industry has complicated the problem by increasing risk of exposure to rare and nonnative species that can result in fatal medical consequences. Invertebrates, those without a backbone, constitute 95% of all animal species and make up the majority of envenomation's presenting to the emergency care setting. These include arachnids and arthropods (e.g., spiders), scorpions, insects (e.g., bees, wasps, ants, caterpillars, and centipedes), cnidarians (e.g., jellyfish, sea anemones, sea urchins, and coral), and cephalopods (e.g., blue-ringed octopus). Venomous vertebrates, animals with a backbone, include certain saltwater fish and stingrays and freshwater fish such as the catfish as well as reptiles (e.g., snakes, lizards), amphibians (e.g., newts and frogs) and unassuming mammals (e.g., mole, platypus, shrew, solenodon, and the slow loris).

Snakebites

Epidemiology

Certain venomous snakebites carry a high potential for morbidity and mortality. There are over 3,000 species of snakes in 160 countries worldwide, of them, 600 are venomous and of those, 250 are recognized by the World Health Organization (WHO) as being medically important due to potential lethality from local and systemic complications of hematologic, neurotoxic, and myotoxic sequelae. In June 2017, WHO added snakebite envenoming to a priority list of neglected tropical diseases due to incidence. The most recent WHO epidemiologic findings estimate an average prevalence of five million annual snakebites worldwide, and 2.7 million envenoming's resulting in clinical illness, 400,000 amputations and 138,000 deaths annually; there are many more unreported. Of those snakebites that are fatal, it is estimated that about 50% to 75% occur before victims can reach the hospital for antivenom treatment.

North America is home to 25 species of snakes from the two largest families of venomous snakes. The United States has four groups of venomous snakes: copperheads, cottonmouths, rattlesnakes (pit vipers), and coral snakes. Identifying physical characteristics of venomous snakes include nostril pits (heat-sensing organs), a triangular-shaped head, elliptical pupils, and subcaudal plates arranged in a single row. Coral snakes are the eastern and western species that inhabit the United States are smaller and brightly colored with red, yellow, and black rings.

A common mnemonic to differentiate snakes with similar rings is "red on yellow, kill a fellow; red on black, venom lack." Cobras, mambas, and kraits are members of the family Elapidae but are not indigenous to the Americas. Two-thirds of snakebites occur on the hands or upper extremities. Initial bites can be misleading, there may be no significant initial symptoms followed by rapid respiratory deterioration and shock. Severity and outcome depend on bite location, amount of venom injected, promptness, and effectiveness of initial treatment and management. Snakebite envenomation poses a complicated treatment management due to its complexity of composition as it contains a multitude of toxin components and complex biochemical interactions from 26 protein families.

Pathophysiology

Snakebite envenoming is a potentially life-threatening disease that results from the injection of a mixture of complex toxins ("venom") following the bite of a venomous snake, but not all venomous snakebites result in envenomation; only 50% to 55% of all bites result in exposure to a toxin; the remaining are considered "dry bites." Snake venoms are complex mixtures of protein and peptide toxins, varying from one species to another. Venom is formed in the modified glands through a duct in the snake's fangs and injected into prey.

Venom dosage per bite depends on multiple factors: the elapsed time since the last bite, the degree of threat perceived by the snake, and size of the prey. Venom is made of complex 26 proteins but predominantly water and four types of toxic proteins: cytotoxins that cause local tissue damage, hemotoxins cause internal bleeding neurotoxins affect the nervous system, and cardiotoxins that act directly on the heart. It is the action of these enzyme proteins, proteases, collagenase, arginine ester hydrolase, and neurotoxins that facilitates the destructive properties in venom. Envenomation causes inflammation and muscle damage can lead to metabolic acidosis, hyperkalemia, hypotension, increased creatine phosphokinase (CPK), and myoglobin ultimately leading to acute renal failure and/or cardiac arrest. The hyaluronidase allows rapid spread of venom through subcutaneous tissues by disrupting mucopolysaccharides; phospholipase A2 perpetuates hemolysis secondary to the esterolytic effect on red cell membranes leading to muscle necrosis. Thrombogenic enzymes promote the formation of a weak fibrin clot, which, in turn, activates plasmin and results in a consumptive coagulopathy, decreased platelet count <10,000/mm^3 within 1 hour leading to internal bleeding, and its hemorrhagic consequences leading to systemic multiorgan dysfunction.[8,9]

Medical Screening

A. *Chief complaint:* Witnessed snakebite or tooth scratch, localized pain

B. *Signs and symptoms:* Specific to the snake, general symptoms may include the following:

1. Fang marks
2. Swelling at the site of the envenomation
3. Drowsiness
4. Nausea and vomiting
5. Increased salivation
6. Fasciculations
7. Weakness
8. Hypotension
9. Cardiovascular collapse

C. Past medical history

1. Increased risk of severe reaction if patient has been exposed to venom

D. Focused assessment

1. *General:* Altered mental status
2. *HEENT (head, eyes, ears, nose, and throat):* Visual acuity, loss, diplopia, photophobia
   - **a.** *Eyes:* Venom ophthalmia (Pit Viper) often presents with pain, hyperemia, blepharitis, blepharospasm, and corneal erosions. Delay or lack of treatment may result in corneal opacity, hypopyon, and/or blindness.
3. *Cardiac:* Hypotension, hypovolemic distributive shock, cardiotoxicity, cardiac failure
4. Pulmonary:
   - **a.** Paralysis of the diaphragm and respiratory failure due to neuromuscular blockade
   - **b.** Capillary leak and interstitial fluid in the lungs
   - **c.** Increased minute ventilation
5. *Gastrointestinal:* Ischemic bowel from gut ischemia
6. *Renal:* Acute kidney injury, myoglobinuria, and rhabdomyolysis
7. *Neurologic:* Local extremity pain, neuromuscular paralysis, persistent nerve damage
   - **a.** *Venom opthalmia:* Cranial nerve VII may be affected by local spread of spat venom to the eye. No evidence of systemic dissemination in humans from spit venom.
8. *Musculoskeletal:* Myolysis (muscle degeneration) and myonecrosis, compartment syndrome
9. *Integumentary:* Localized soft tissue swelling, ecchymosis, bloody fang punctures, marks, local tissue and skin necrosis from demand vasoconstriction, ischemia, gangrene, tissue loss
10. *Hematologic/Lymph:* Regional lymphadenopathy, thrombosis, hemorrhage, coagulopathy, and prolonged disruption of hemostasis resulting in disseminated intravascular coagulation (DIC).
11. *Metabolic:* Lactic acidosis
12. *Psychologic:* Fear and psychologic damage

Medical Decision-Making and Differential Diagnoses

A. Diagnoses of snakebite is made with identification of the snake and presence of symptoms of envenomation

B. Differential Diagnoses

1. Anaphylaxis
2. Deep venous thrombosis (DVT)
3. Extremity vascular trauma
4. Scorpion envenomation
5. Septic shock
6. Serum sickness
7. Wasp stings
8. Wound care
9. Wound infection

Diagnostic Testing

A. Labs:

1. Complete blood count (CBC) count with manual differential and peripheral blood smear

2. Prothrombin time (PT) and activated partial thromboplastin time (APTT), international normalized ratio (INR)
3. Creatine kinase myocardial band (CK-MB)
4. Fibrinogen and split products
5. D-dimer
6. Blood type and cross-match
7. Blood chemistries, including electrolytes, blood urea nitrogen (BUN), creatinine
8. Urinalysis for myoglobinuria
9. Arterial blood gas (ABG) determinations and/or lactate level for patients with systemic symptoms

B. Imaging studies:
1. Baseline chest radiograph in patients to evaluate for and trend/ pulmonary edema
2. Plain radiograph to rule out retained fang(s) or foreign bodies

Management

A. The Antivenom Index is a database containing indications for antivenom administration and location of the antivenom. The information is updated and maintained by the Association of Zoos and Aquariums and the University of Arizona, funded by the Health Resources and Services Administration (HRSA) through the Poison Center Stabilization and Enhancement Program Grant and administered by the University of Arizona College of Pharmacy and the Venom Immunochemistry, Pharmacology, and Emergency Response (VIPER) Institute.

B. Snakebite severity score (SSS; Table 33.1), severity of envenomation (SOE; Table 33.2), and pain local effect index (PLEI) should be used to determine dosing amount of antivenom. Estimation of dose of antivenom depends on amount of venom delivered. Prediction of amount is based on severity of symptoms at presentation. Localized to evolution of systemic symptoms.

C. Pharmacologic therapy
1. *Antivenom therapy:* Cornerstone of management. Administer immediately.
2. May need additional doses of antivenom if progression of symptoms noted.
3. If administration is delayed, increase the initial dose.
4. Not necessary to do skin testing for allergy prior to administration

TABLE 33.1 SNAKEBITE SEVERITY SCORE

Date							
Time							
Pulmonary Symptoms							
0. No signs/symptoms	0	0	0	0		0	1
1. Dyspnea, minimal chest tightness, mild/ vague discomfort, respirations of 20–25 bpm	1	1	1	1		2	3
2. Moderate respiratory distress, 26–40 bpm	2	2	2	2			
3. Cyanosis, air hunger, extreme tachypnea, or respiratory insufficiency/failure	3	3	3	3			
3. Cyanosis, air hunger, extreme tachypnea, or respiratory insufficiency/failure	3	3	3	3			
Cardiovascular System							
0. No signs/symptoms	0	0	0	0	0	0	1
1. HR 100–125 bpm, palpitations, generalized weakness, benign dysrhythmia, or hypotension	1	1	1	1	1	2	3
2. HR 126–175 bpm, or hypotension with SBP > 100 mmHg	2	2	2	2	2		
3. HR > 175 bpm, or hypotension with SBP < 100 mmHg, malignant dysrhythmia, or cardiac arrest	3	3	3	3	3		
Local Wound			0	0	0	0	1
0. No signs/symptoms	0	0	1	1	1	2	3
1. Pain, swelling, or ecchymosis within 5–7.5 cm of bite site	1	1	2	2	2	0	0

(continued)

TABLE 33.1 SNAKEBITE SEVERITY SCORE (*CONTINUED*)

Date							
Time							
2. Pain, swelling, or ecchymosis involving less than half the extremity (7.5–50 cm from bite site)	2	2	3	3	3		
3. Pain, swelling, or ecchymosis involving half to all of extremity (50–100 cm from bite site)	3	3	4	4	4		
4. Pain, swelling, or ecchymosis extending beyond affected extremity (more than 100 cm of bite site)	4	4					
Gastrointestinal System							
0. No signs/symptoms	0	0	0	0	0	0	1
1. Pain, tenesmus, or nausea	1	1	1	1	1	2	3
2.Vomiting or diarrhea	2	2	2	2	2		
3. Repeated vomiting, diarrhea, hematemesis, or hematochezia	3	3	3	3	3		
Hematologic Symptoms							
0. No signs/symptoms	0	0	0	0	0	0	1
1. Coagulation parameters slightly abnormal: PT <20 sec, PTT <50 s, platelets 100–150 K/mL, or fibrinogen 100–150 mcg/mL	1	1	1	1	1	2	3
2. Coagulation parameters abnormal: PT <20–25 sec, PTT <50–75 s, platelets 50–100 K/mL, or fibrinogen 50–100 mcg/mL	2	2	2	2	2	2	4
3. Coagulation parameters abnormal: PT <50–100 sec, PTT <75–100 s, platelets 20–50 K/mL, or fibrinogen <50 mcg/mL	3	3	3	3	3		
4. Coagulation parameters markedly abnormal, with serious bleeding or the threat of spontaneous bleeding; unmeasurable PT or PTT, platelets <20 K/mL, undetectable fibrinogen, severe abnormalities of other laboratory values also fall into this category	4	4	4	4	4		
Central Nervous System							
0. No signs/symptoms	0	0	0	0	0	0	1
1. Minimal apprehension, headache, weakness, dizziness, chills, or paresthesia	1	1	1	1	1	2	3
2. Moderate apprehension, headache, weakness, dizziness, chills, paresthesia, confusion, or fasciculation in the area of bite site	2	2	2	2	2		
3. Severe confusion, lethargy, seizures, coma, psychosis, or generalized fasciculation	3	3	3	3	3		
TOTAL							

bpm, beats per minute; HR, heart rate; PT, prothrombin time; PTT, partial thromboplastin time; SBP, systolic blood pressure; SSS, snakebite severity score.

Source: Fowler AL, Hughes DW, Muir MT, et al. Resource utilization after snakebite severity score implementation into treatment algorithm of crotaline bite. *J Emerg Med.* 2017;53(6).[10]

TABLE 33.2 SEVERITY OF ENVENOMATION

Signs and Symptoms	Minimal	Moderate	Severe
Local	Swelling, erythema, or ecchymosis confined to bite site	Progression of swelling, erythema, or ecchymosis beyond bite site	Rapid swelling, erythema, or ecchymosis involving the body part
Systemic	No systemic signs or symptoms	Non-life-threatening signs or symptoms (nausea/vomiting, mild hypotension, perioral paresthesias, and myokymia)	Markedly severe signs and symptoms (hypotension [systolic < 80 mmHg], altered sensorium, tachycardia, tachypnea, and respiratory distress)
Coagulation	No coagulation abnormalities or other laboratory abnormalities	Mild abnormal coagulation profile without significant bleeding	Abnormal coagulation profile with bleeding (INR, aPTT, fibrinogen, platelet count < 20,000 μL)
Snakebite severity score	0–3	4–7	8–20

aPTT, activated partial thromboplastin time; INR, international normalized ratio.

Source: Adapted with permission from Moriarity RS, Dryer S, Repogle W, Summers RL. The role for coagulation markers in mild snakebite envenomations. *Western J Emerg Med.* 2012;12(1):68–74. Table 1. https://doi.org/10.5811/westjem.2011.6.6729.[11]

D. *CroFab:*

1. Patients are eligible for therapy with *CroFab* if they have moderate or severe envenomation as described or any degree of envenomation with progression of the envenomation syndrome.

2. *Note:* As the antivenom dose reflects venom size, not patient size, the U.S. Food and Drug Administration (FDA) recommends the same initial and subsequent doses for pediatric patients. Data show efficacy and safety for patients as young as 14 months.

3. *Adverse effects of antivenom:* Anaphylaxis, urticaria, rash, and delayed onset of serum sickness

4. *If CroFab indicated:* Loading dose: four to six vials: dose is same for adults/children

5. Assess SSS hourly.

6. If symptoms increased, repeat loading dose of four to six vials and ICU admission. Continue hourly assessment until symptoms improve.

7. *Symptoms decreased or improved:* Start maintenance dosing of two vials every 6 hours × three doses.

8. Reassess every hour for 6 hours and then every 6 hours for 24 hours and then every 12 to 24 hours until symptoms stabilized or decreased.

E. *Pain management:* Acetaminophen (Tylenol), NSAIDs (Motrin, Advil, Aleve), opioids

F. *Antihistamine:* Given after antivenom: do not prevent adverse reactions from antivenom administration

G. *Small Molecule Therapeutics (SMT):* Naturally occurring or synthetic molecules that target G-coupled proteins to delay venom toxicity. This can be used as an adjunct therapy to antivenom. Can be given in the field, in hospital, and on discharge (D/C) in oral and IV form. Increases efficacy of the antivenom. Low allergenicity, and superior tissue penetration due to small molecular size and compatible with antivenom. Expands the time to development of neurotoxicity that results in irreversible complications such as respiratory paralysis.

1. Not yet FDA approved for use.

H. Venom ophthalmia:

1. Vasoconstrictor with epinephrine (mydriatic analgesia)

2. Topical cycloplegics to prevent posterior synechiae, ciliary spasm, and pain

3. Local anesthetic with topical Tetracaine (limit use)

4. Prophylactic topical antibiotics

5. Antihistamines for allergic keratoconjunctivitis

6. Do not administer topical or IV antivenom for venom opthalmia (contraindicated).

I. *Procedures:* Fluorescein stain with slit-lamp examination to exclude corneal abrasions.

J. *Supportive therapy:* Immobilization of extremity and pressure to puncture or bite wound delays systemic absorption of venom from the bite site.

1. *Venom ophthalmia:* Urgent decontamination with copious irrigation (saline solution)

K. *Consultation/collaboration:* Medical toxicologist. Resource familiar with snakebite envenomations can create cost savings for a healthcare institution.

Patient Disposition

A. Transition of care information

1. May need to be transferred to a higher level of care for management.

B. Age and developmental considerations

1. Young children and older adults may be at greater risk of the effects of envenomation.

2. Prevention and education

a. Become familiar with poisonous snakes within the local environment where one lives.

b. If traveling, become familiar with poisonous snakes within the local environment.

c. Carry first aid for initial treatment of envenomation.

3. Patient and family education and counseling

a. Become familiar with poisonous snakes within the local environment where one lives.

b. If traveling, become familiar with poisonous snakes within the local environment.

c. Carry first aid for initial treatment of envenomation.

Poisonous and Venomous Arthropods

Arthropods (e.g., insects, arachnids, and crustaceans) are invertebrate animals with exoskeletons, segmented body, and paired appendages. They are known for molting (i.e., shedding exoskeleton and replacing it). There are over one million species, representing 80% of all animal species. Arthropods use toxins for defense or to kill prey. Spiders and scorpions are of the subphylum Chelicerata and Arachnida class. Collectively, they cause more venomous injuries to humans worldwide than any other species; their stings are notable in their ability to cause systemic infection and death.

Spiders

Spiders are arachnids, a branch of arthropods. The arachnid class has very diverse membership, more than 100,000 species of spider have been identified. There are 4,000 species of spiders in North America. All spiders, except for two small groups in the arachnid family, have poison glands and release venom from sacs near their chelicerae (fangs). Spider bites are common, but only a few can cause severe and life-threatening symptoms or death. Most of these venomous spiders are found in Latin America, one in Australia and a few in North America. There are only two species in North America that are venomous and cause illness: the black widow spider (*Latrodectus mactans*) and the brown recluse spider (*Loxosceles reclusa*).

Three important syndromes are caused by spider bites: latrodectism (black widow), loxoscelism (brown recluse), and funnel web spider syndrome (funnel web spider).

Venomous Spiders: Brown Spiders (Brown Recluse)

Epidemiology

Spiders live in dark, dusty environments. They are shy and only bite when pressed or handled. Envenomation from a recluse can occur when the spider is trapped against a person's skin. The spider will bite in self-defense. Most spider bites occur when people are putting on shoes or other clothes, particularly those left on the floor. Envenomation from a recluse is known as cutaneous loxoscelism.

Pathophysiology

A. The most important component of their venom is sphingomyelinase D, an enzyme that destabilizes vessel walls and red blood cell membranes and causes extensive skin necrosis and hemolysis with the risk of acute renal failure (the latter is seen in 5% of patients). In a few hours, an extremely painful ischemic area with pallor, cyanosis, and erythema develops, creating the characteristic *marble plaque*. The plaque may also have hemorrhagic blisters. Full necrosis manifests in approximately 7 days, resulting in a blackened and insensitive eschar adhered to the deep skin layers.[12] The deployment of the eschar occurs after approximately 1 month, leaving an extensive and deep ulcer with a granular base and raised edges.

B. *Treatment:* Depends on the stage of the envenomation and there is no established time frame for the use. Moderate cases (systemic changes without hemolysis) may need five ampoules and severe cases (with hemolysis) may require up to 10 ampoules. When there is necrosis without hemolysis, it is possible to use sulfone, which acts by blocking neutrophil diapedesis and inhibiting the extension of necrosis. The administration of oral corticosteroids is controversial but indicated in some protocols. In later stages, extensive and slow healing ulcers can be treated with skin grafts.

Medical Screening

A. *Chief complaint:* Pain or pinprick at the site of the bite; witnessed spider leaving the scene or falling out of one's clothes.

B. Signs and symptoms of bite:
1. May or may not feel pain at the bite site
2. *Within 2 to 6 hours:* Maybe mild to severe pain, pruritus, erythema
3. *12 hours:* Small blister may appear.
4. *12 to 24 hours:* May turn from erythematous will turn to violaceous, may or may not turn to necrosis
5. *48 hours:* If necrosis is to occur, wound may not blanch.
6. *3 to 4 days:* Necrosis will occur.
7. *5 to 7 days:* Eschar formation
8. *7 to 14 days:* The central area of the wound will have darkened, slightly depressed, necrotic area and hardened; eschar will slough.
9. 2 to 4 months before healing

C. Signs and symptoms of systemic loxoscelism:
1. Rare occurrence
2. Hemolytic anemia
3. Acute renal injury
4. Venom acts on metalloproteinases in red blood cells and cause lysis
5. Can be fatal within 12 to 0 hours if this happens

D. Past medical history
1. Increased risk with wound healing with diabetes
2. Increased risk with renal disease

E. Focused assessment:
1. *General:* Fever, chills, arthralgias
2. *Neurologic:* Altered mental status (AMS)
3. *HEENT (head, eyes, ears, nose, and throat):* Scleral icterus
4. *Skin:* Petechial, scarlatiniform, or morbilliform eruptions on the trunk, jaundice

Medical Decision-Making and Differential Diagnoses

A. Hemolytic anemia
B. Renal failure
C. Envenomation from another source

Diagnostic Testing

A. Complete blood count (CBC)
B. Chemistry
C. Bilirubin

D. Liver enzymes
E. Urinalysis
F. Chest radiograph

Management

A. Support respiratory system when indicated.
B. Support circulatory system when indicated.
C. Antivenin as indicated
D. Wound care for the bite

Venomous Spiders: Black Widow Spiders

Epidemiology

A. Found worldwide and the most important species in the Americas, for the severity of the envenomation.
B. There are three black widow spiders: southern *(Latrodectus mactans)* and western black widow *(Latrodectus hesperus);* the brown widow *(Latrodectus geometricus)* is a common spider that causes less serious injury. These spiders have a characteristic red or orange hourglass design on the ventral abdomen.

Pathophysiology

A. Envenomation by a black widow is known as latrodectism. The venom of the widow spider works on the neuromuscular junction, which causes the release of neurotransmitters causing muscles to contract. Because it blocks the reabsorption of the neurotransmitters back into the presynaptic, there is prolonged stimulation and painful contractions.
B. *Treatment:* Requires widow antivenom, dosage depends on the severity of the symptoms. Antivenom is made from horse serum. Benzodiazepines are also used to promote muscle relaxation.

Medical Screening

A. *Chief complaint:* Pain at the bite site, muscle contractions
B. *Signs and symptoms:* Drooling, nausea, vomiting, hypotension, circulatory shock, death
C. Past medical history pertinent to condition:
   1. Patient with respiratory problems such as asthma can be at increased risk of anaphylaxis
D. Focused assessment:
   1. *Respiratory:* Distress
   2. *Skin:* Diaphoresis in different regions of the body; bite wound erythema
   3. *Abdomen:* Rigid abdominal muscles
   4. *Musculoskeletal:* Fasciculations

Medical Decision-Making and Differential Diagnoses

A. Envenomation from another spider
B. Acute abdomen

Diagnostic Testing

A. Complete blood count (CBC)
B. Chemistry
C. Bilirubin
D. Liver enzymes
E. Urinalysis
F. Chest radiograph

Management

A. Support respiratory system when indicated.
B. Support circulatory system when indicated.
C. Antivenin as indicated.
D. Wound care for the bite
E. Monitor for anaphylaxis.

Patient Disposition

A. Transition of care information
   1. May require transfer for critical care management
   2. Consult experts such a poison control or management or local entomologist
B. Age and developmental considerations
   1. Prevention and education
      a. Shake clothing before getting dressed.
      b. Avoid areas where spiders may live.
   2. Patient and family education and counseling
      a. Shake clothing before getting dressed.
      b. Avoid areas where spiders may live.

Scorpions (Venomous Arthropod)

Epidemiology

A. Scorpions are venomous live in hot climates. The most lethal in North America is the bark scorpion *(Centruroides exilicauda)* found primarily in the southwestern desert.
B. The scorpion uses a stinger on the telson, the last segment of the tail.

Pathophysiology

A. The release of neurotoxins and neurologic transmitters leads to central and peripheral nervous system effects causing prolonged neurologic manifestations with tetany and twitching. The venom disrupts the autonomic nervous system by dissociating the parasympathetic and sympathetic nervous systems

Medical Screening

A. *Chief complaint:* Reported sting by patient, localized pain at the site of the sting.
B. Signs and symptoms:
   1. Localized tenderness at the site of the sting
   2. Hypertension
   3. Tachycardia
   4. Muscle fasciculations
   5. Disconjugate gaze—most common in children
   6. Weakness
   7. Agitation
   8. Opisthotonos
C. *Past medical history:* Increased risk of complications with asthma and diabetes.
D. Focused assessment:
   1. *General:* Altered mental status. The sting causes intense local pain.
   2. *HEENT (head, eyes, ears, nose, and throat):* Visual acuity, loss, diplopia, photophobia, mydriasis/myosis, disconjugate gaze
   3. *Cardiac:* Tachycardia/bradycardia, intense sweating, hypertension, hypotension, shock, arrhythmia, death
   4. *Pulmonary:* Pulmonary edema
   5. *Gastrointestinal:* Abdominal cramps

6. *Genitourinary (GU):* Priapism
7. *Neurological:* Salivation, hypothermia
8. *Integumentary:* Minor inflammation at site of sting

Medical Decision-Making and Differential Diagnoses

A. Neurological disease
B. Neurological infection
C. Envenomation from another source

Diagnostic Testing

A. Complete blood count (CBC)
B. Chemistry
C. Bilirubin
D. Liver enzymes
E. Urinalysis
F. Chest radiograph
G. Consider CT if neurologic source is suspected.

Management

A. Most patients do not need medical treatment. Recommend 24 hours of observation.
B. General treatment is supportive—cold compressed to affected area for comfort.
C. Pharmacologic therapy
   1. *Pain control:* Mild cases: nerve block with 2% lidocaine (3–4 mL)
   2. Can be repeated at 0–30–60 minutes.
   3. *Oral pain medications:* Nonsteroidal anti-inflammatory medications: Motrin, Advil
   4. *Severe cases:* Antivenom serum: Can use either antiarachnidic or antiscorpionic serum, dosage depends on the severity of the envenomation.
D. Procedures
E. Supportive therapy:
   1. Most patients only need home supportive therapy.
   2. Treatment within 2 hours of sting is most effective.
   3. Clean wound with soap and water and dry.
   4. Cool compresses × 10 minutes as needed.
   5. May repeat as needed every 20 minutes: slows spread of venom
F. Consultation and collaboration

Patient Disposition

A. Transition of care information
   1. May require transfer for critical care management
   2. Consult experts such as poison control or management or local entomologist or zoologist
B. *Age and developmental considerations:* Young children at greatest risk of developing complications from scorpion stings.
   1. Prevention and education
      a. Shake clothing before getting dressed.
      b. Avoid areas where scorpions may be.
   2. Patient and family education and counseling
      a. Shake clothing before getting dressed.
      b. Avoid areas where scorpions may be.

Marine Envenomation

The marine environment provides the habitat for dangerous marine fauna. Many marine animals have evolved sharp teeth and spines or venom glands for defense and predation.

Encounters with marine life may result in traumatic injury or envenomation, requiring emergency medical management.

Epidemiology

The most common reported U.S exposures are to jellyfish (31%), stingrays (16%), venomous fish (including lionfish, catfish, and others) (28%), and gastropods (6%). The world's most venomous marine animals include the pufferfish, porcupine fish, ocean sunfish, and the triggerfish.

Pathophysiology

The venomous fish releases neurotoxins, and it depends on the type of species what type of neurotoxins are injected. Tetrodotoxin (TTX) is a sodium channel blocker affecting the sodium channel pathway and prevents the nervous system from carrying messages and thus muscles from flexing in response to nervous stimulation. TTX is more poisonous than cyanide. Poisoning occurs through consumption. The most poisonous parts were the liver and eggs enters the body through ingestion, injection, inhalation, or through abraded skin. It can cause paralysis of the diaphragm, loss of intercostal muscles resulting in death from respiratory failure.

Medical Screening

A. *Chief complaint:* Respiratory distress
B. *Signs and symptoms:* Generally appear within 4 to 6 hours. If the patient survives 24 hours, recovery without any residual effects will usually occur over a few days.
C. Past medical history pertinent to condition
D. *Focused assessment:* Symptoms appear within 17 minutes of ingestion
   1. *General:* Altered mental status
   2. *HEENT* (head, eyes, ears, nose, and throat): Paresthesias of lips, tongue, hypersalivation, visual acuity, loss, diplopia, photophobia, mydriasis
   3. *Cardiac:* Hypotension, shock, cardiac arrhythmias
   4. *Pulmonary:* respiratory distress, diaphragm paralysis, respiratory failure
   5. *Neurologic:* Paresthesias of extremities, weakness, lethargy, headache, incoordination, tremor, paralysis
   6. *Gastrointestinal:* Nausea, vomiting, diarrhea, and abdominal pain
   7. *Integumentary:* Diaphoresis, cyanosis
   8. Hematologic

Medical Decision-Making and Differential Diagnoses

A. Neurologic disease
B. Neurologic infection
C. Envenomation from another source

Diagnostic Testing

A. CBC
B. Chemistry
C. Bilirubin
D. Liver enzymes

E. Urinalysis
F. Chest radiograph
G. Consider CT if neurologic source is suspected

Management

A. Pharmacologic therapy
  1. No specific antidotes or antivenins in many cases
  2. Pain management related to wounds and injuries needs to be initiated.
  3. Alpha-adrenergic agonists
  4. Anticholinesterase agents
  5. Monoclonal antibodies available through USAMRIID
B. Supportive therapy
  1. Aggressive and early with IV fluid and hemodynamic support
  2. Early airway management
  3. Removal of stingers when indicated
  4. Wound care
C. Consultation and collaboration
  1. Toxicology
  2. USAMRIID

Patient Disposition

A. Transition of care information
  1. Transfer to appropriate facility for management.
B. Age and developmental considerations
  1. Children tend to be at greater risk of complications from injuries of envenomation.
  2. Prevention and education
    a. Keep away from dangerous areas.
    b. Become familiar with possible sources of envenomation or injury.
    c. Know where to obtain resources for prevention and treatment.
  3. Patient and family education and counseling
    a. Keep away from dangerous areas.
    b. Become familiar with possible sources of envenomation or injury.
    c. Know where to obtain resources for prevention and treatment.

Human Bites

Epidemiology

A. Human bites are the third most common bite and account for up to 26% of all bite presentations to the ED.
B. The human bite can be more serious than an animal bite, in part due to the quantity and range of polymicrobial organisms found in the inoculum. Human mouths have more bacteria than most animals. The human bite contains over 100 million organisms originating from roughly 190 different species of bacteria, a broad but relatively equal mixture of gram-positive and gram-negative aerobes and anaerobes manifesting in the gingiva of the human dentition as tartar. Gram-positive *Staphylococcus aureus* and gram-negative *Eikenella corrodens* have been isolated in up to 30% of human bite wounds. Bacteria may also originate from the microbiome of ingested food or the victim's own skin during penetration. Any break in the skin has a potential for infection and requires evaluation and treatment by a healthcare provider. Most human bites involve the legs, arms, or hands (60%). Head and neck bites account for approximately 30%. Hands have a much higher rate and risk of infection with poor or limb-threatening outcome than any other location and require priority evaluation and management.

Pathophysiology

The mechanisms of injury and action for sustaining a human bite are primarily facilitated by two mechanisms: an occlusive bite and the clenched fist method. Of the two, punching someone in the teeth with a closed fist has a higher associated risk of skin laceration, infection, joint penetration, extensor tendon laceration, and bone fracture due to the location of injury. Most injuries occur in the dominant hand over dorsal aspect of the third and fourth metacarpophalangeal (MCP) or proximal interphalangeal joint (PIP). Once the skin is broken, bacteria can travel up the extensor tendons of the hand with a natural extension of the fingers after impact. Occlusive bites can occur anywhere on the body but are predominantly seen on the hands, fingers, head, and neck. Injuries to these areas can result in superficial abrasion type injuries to extensive avulsion; deep puncture bites can result in localized crushing tissue injury that will need to be closely evaluated. Infection can be local, superficial, form abscesses, cellulitis/or progress to systemic infection. Human bites also pose a risk of infectious disease transmission through saliva. HIV and hepatitis B are high-risk infectious disease with hepatitis B having the higher risk of transmission.

Medical Screening

A. *Chief complaint:* human bite, punch in the mouth
B. Signs and symptoms:
  1. *Injury:* Laceration, puncture wound, ecchymosis, abrasion, avulsion injury
  2. *Cellulitis:* Redness, warmth, localized or progressive, red streaking
  3. Abscess
  4. *Systemic:* Risk of sepsis
  5. Febrile, white blood count (WBC) >12,000, hyper-/hypothermia, tachycardia, hypotension, tachycardia, bradycardia
C. Past medical history pertinent to condition
  1. *History of presenting problem:* Circumstances leading up to injury, risk of assault or abuse, patient safety concerns, play or aggressive behavior associated with injury, time of injury, mechanism of injury, infectious disease, and immunosuppression status of both parties. Immediate medical treatment provided.
  2. *Pertinent medical history:* Diabetes, hypertension, peripheral vascular disease, renal disease, immunosuppression, infectious disease, lymphadenopathy
  3. I Tetanus status (within the last 5 years)
D. Focused assessment:
  1. *General:* Overall appearance on presentation
  2. *Cardiovascular:* Pulses, capillary refill

3. *Integumentary:* Document skin integrity and describe wounds.
4. *Musculoskeletal:* Area affected, range of motion, joint spaces, crepitus, edema, flexor and extensor tendon integrity; evaluation of tenosynovitis
5. *Neurologic:* Parasthesias, paralysis, any loss of motor function, two-point discrimination test.
6. *Diagnostics:* Imaging to rule out fracture of affected limb or presence of retained foreign body (teeth).

Medical Decision-Making and Differential Diagnoses

A. Animal bites
B. Cellulitis
C. Hand infections
D. Insect bites
E. Foreign body
F. Penetrating trauma
G. Puncture wound

Management

A. Pharmacologic therapy
1. *Pain management:* Oral or IV pain medication may be required to evaluate the extent of the wound.
2. *Tetanus:* Human bites can transmit *Clostridium tetani* in rare cases. Tetanus booster is indicated if patient received three previous tetanus doses and no follow-up booster within 5 years of injury; otherwise not indicated if current on immunization.
3. *Antibiotics:* The Infectious Diseases Society of America (IDSA) clinical guidelines recommend all human bite wounds of the hands, puncture wounds over joint spaces, bone, tendons, or if patient is high-risk receive prophylactic antibiotics. No antibiotics indicated if no epidermal layer penetration.

B. Document wound(s) measurement (L, W, Depth) in mm or cm. Tissue loss

C. In assault cases involving bite marks:
1. *Photodocument injuries:* Before and after cleansing (use ruler, pt identifier, anatomic identifier)
2. Wound diagram, arch pattern, canine width

D. *Procedures:* Wound care and management
1. *Control external bleeding:* Direct pressure, gauze dressing
a. *Wound cleaning:* Soak in basin with Hibiclens, sterile water, sterile saline solution, or warm soapy water to remove gross external contaminants
b. *Wound irrigation:* Copious amounts of sterile isotonic sodium chloride, dilute hydrogen peroxide, or dilute betadine (if no diagnostic evidence of fracture)
c. Debridement of devitalized tissue
d. *Closure of wound bed:* Do not close any wound >12 hours old, hand or puncture wounds. Head and neck wounds should consult plastic surgery if available. Close using simple, interrupted suture technique. Do not overlay or embed sutures in these injuries. Puncture wounds should be left open and not closed due to risk of infection from deeply penetrated bacteria.

E. Supportive therapy
1. Telfa nonstick overlay, gauze, loosely applied kling/ace wrap if on hands or extremities. Elevate and immobilize extremity in the position of comfort for no longer than 48 hours to avoid stiffness of joints.

F. Consultation and collaboration
1. *Surgical management:* May be required. Wound exploration, debridement, and extensive closure
2. Wounds to face and ears require plastic surgery evaluation. Head and neck injuries require evaluation by an ear, nose, and throat specialist (ENT).

Patient Disposition

A. Transition of care information
1. Patient may require transfer to a higher level of care.

B. *Age and developmental considerations:* Human bites may be a sign of potential abuse.
1. Prevention and education
2. Patient and family education and counseling

References and Additional Reading

References and Additional Reading for this chapter are online only and can be found at https://connect.springerpub.com/content/reference-book/978-0-8261-6091-5/part/part03/toc-part/ch33.

IV. Environmental Emergencies

34. Frostbite and Nonfreezing Cold Injuries

AMY BIGHAM | RENEÉ SEMONIN HOLLERAN

Learning Objectives

- Describe the pathophysiology of nonfreezing cold injuries and predisposing factors.
- Differentiate between superficial and deep frostbite on physical examination.
- Demonstrate correct management of the patient with nonfreezing cold injuries, including factors to consider in patient disposition.

Nonfreezing cold injury (NFCI) is an injury of the hands or feet resulting from exposure to wet conditions and temperatures just above freezing, typically found in soldiers. NFCI is due to microvascular endothelial damage, stasis, and vascular occlusion. At first, the tissue is cold and anesthetic, progressing to hyperemia in 24 to 48 hours. Hyperemia is accompanied by an intense painful burning sensation as well as blisters, redness, and, possibly, ulcerations. NFCI management raises frustration in both medical officers and commanders. Most authorities are not aware of or remain unimpressed with the severity of NFCI, nor do they realize that it produces lifelong symptomatology.[1,2]

Anatomy

A. Frostbite (also known as frostnip) occurs as a result of prolonged cold exposure (outdoors as well as indoors) constricting blood vessels in the extremities, which diverts warm blood flow and oxygen to central vital organs.
B. As the body temperature continues to drop, the brain permanently constricts vessels in extremities to maintain warmth in vital organs, and frostbite begins.
C. Cell death occurs due to exposure. Ice crystals form in the space outside cells and cells become dehydrated.
D. Injury can occur locally to the feet and toes of the lower extremities, the hands and fingers of the upper extremities, the nose and cheeks of the face, and the auricle of the ears.

Pathophysiology[1,2]

A. As the temperature body lowers, blood flow is shunted from the periphery to the central circulations.
- **1.** This results in lower temperatures of the skin in the extremities.
- **2.** As the temperature lowers, cells deteriorate from the lack of oxygen and water.
- **3.** The lining of the blood vessels becomes damaged.
  - **a.** This damage results in the leaking of blood into the soft tissue on rewarming and reperfusion.
  - **b.** Small clots form, causing blood flow difficulties and inflammation.
  - **c.** The inflammation causes further tissue damage.

Predisposing Factors[1,2]

A. Duration of exposure
B. Temperature
C. Wind
D. Precipitation
E. Lack of appropriate clothing
F. Level of outside activity (e.g., skiing, running)
G. Alcohol (ETOH)
H. History of tobacco use
I. Use of drugs that can impair level of consciousness or interferes with circulation
J. History of diseases such as cardiovascular disease or diabetes

Physical Examination[1,2]

A. *Superficial frostbite*
- **1.** *Look for color changes:* Light skin will become red and ruddy; dark skin will appear lighter than surrounding tissue. Both will blanche followed by color changes
- **2.** *Feel area for pliability:* Does the area feel frozen, or is it still soft and pliable?
- **3.** *Ask patient how it feels:* Early frostbite will retain sensation, and pain will increase as reperfusion occurs. The patient may also report numbness, tingling, and/or burning.

B. *Deep frostbite*
- **1.** Look at the skin appearance. Unlike superficial frostbite, the skin will appear to lack all underlying color from the lack of perfusion. Skin will appear white and waxy, and will turn mottled or blotchy, then to grayish yellow to grayish blue as injury progresses.
- **2.** Look for swelling and blistering.
- **3.** *Gently palpate:* Does surface feel frozen with no pliability in underlying tissue?

4. *Ask patient how it feels:* Deep frostbite may be painful as nerve endings are damaged, or there may be a complete loss of sensation.

Differential Diagnoses

A. Frostnip
B. Hypothermia
C. Alcohol intoxication

Diagnostic Testing

A. Depth of injury is difficult to estimate on initial exam.
B. Initial classification is superficial or deep.
C. Diagnosis is clinical; no labs or films needed.

Management[1,2]

A. Remove patient from cold environment.
  1. *Outside:* Place patient in heated ambulance, wrap in blankets, remove wet clothing.
  2. *Inside:* Turn up heat while working in patient's home, wrap in blankets, and move to heated ambulance.
B. Gently handle frostbitten areas.
  1. Do not rub affected areas.
  2. Ice crystals in tissues cause further damage.
C. Wrap affected area gently and loosely with gauze.
  1. Patient may complain of tingling/burning; these are normal sensations.
D. If patient does not respond to simple treatment, begin care for deep frostbite.
  1. Provide high-concentration oxygen to improve oxygenation to damaged tissue.
  2. Advise patient not to smoke or consume caffeine or alcohol (vasoconstrictors, raise blood pressure).
  3. Do not allow patient to use affected part or walk on affected feet.
  4. Place area in warm circulating water.
  5. Treat with parenteral opiates as indicated by level of pain.
E. Do not debride blisters.
F. Apply aloe vera cream every 6 hours and dry dressing.
G. Administer tetanus immunization as indicated.
H. Meticulous local care of the injured area to prevent wound infection
I. Optional antibiotic prophylaxis

Patient Disposition

A. Consider admission if social circumstances are questionable: for example, a homeless patient.
B. Local frostbite can be discharged home with sufficient guideline for self-care.

References

References for this chapter are online only and can be found at https://connect.springerpub.com/content/reference-book/978-0-8261-6091-5/part/part04/toc-part/ch34.

35. Heat-Related Emergencies

TRACY BROWN

Learning Objectives

- Identify specific heat-related illnesses and injuries likely to present to the ED.
- Determine treatments associated with heat illnesses and injuries.
- Apply current cooling techniques available for the treatment of heat illness and injuries.
- Describe prevention and specific strategies to prevent heat-related illnesses and injury.

Heat-related illnesses and injuries are seen year-round and throughout the world. Those who practice in elevated temperature environments are well versed in treatment of these illnesses and injuries. Clinicians in areas of the country not accustomed to heat-related illness and injury, however, may find themselves needing to care for these types of patients. Areas of the country that do not typically see high environmental temperatures less frequently, need to have in place necessary mechanisms for combating the problem (e.g., air-conditioned homes, cars, and workplaces). People in these parts of the country are not acclimatized to elevated temperatures. Even those who have acclimatized to the higher temperature environments can succumb to the illnesses and injuries discussed in this chapter. Since there is a growing use of emergency medicine clinicians in field environments for missionary and humanitarian work, sporting events, and expeditions, additional information on preventive care and planning has been included.

Pathophysiology[1–3]

A. Heat regulation

1. *Conduction:* The transfer of heat between two surfaces in contact with one other.
2. *Convection:* Air or water movement across a surface thereby transferring heat away from the surface.
3. *Evaporation:* Vaporization of water removing heat from the surface. Elevation in humidity will affect the body's ability to perform this function.
4. *Radiation:* The electromagnetic transfer of heat into the environment surrounding. Once the outside temperature rises over 95°F or 35°C, the body can no longer perform this function.

B. Thermoregulators

1. *Hypothalamus:* When central nervous system (CNS) receptors are activated due to an internal temperature change, the hypothalamus responds by sending signals to the body to prompt vasodilation and sweating, or vasoconstriction, shivering, and hormone thermogenesis.
2. *Thermosensors and the CNS actions:* Activation of peripheral vasodilation and sweating. Increases the blood flow to the skin.

C. *Acclimatization:* Refers to the body's adaptation to its surroundings to more efficiently regulate heat loss in higher temperature climates. The setpoint for thermoregulation is reset to begin triggering vascular changes and sweating (with less sodium) much sooner. A minimum of 1 week of constant exposure to the environment is needed to make the adjustment. The adjustment will again change with the exposure to a new environment. Specific protocols will be discussed further in this chapter.

D. Considerations

1. Risk factors[4,5–7]
   - a. Age (decreased cardiac reserve in older years), poor physical fitness and health, obesity
   - b. Hydrations status, use of alcohol
   - c. Inappropriate clothing and equipment
   - d. Lack of acclimatization, amount of exertion of activity
   - e. Lack of air conditioning, social isolation
   - f. Congenital and developed conditions affecting the sweat glands
   - g. Excessive scars, severe sunburn affecting sweating
2. Medication contributors[4,8]
   - a. There are two ways medications can predispose a person to heat injury:
     - i. The drug's action increases heat production.
     - ii. Thermoregulatory centers become compromised, diminishing their ability to function effectively.
   - b. Examples
     - i. Hypertension (HTN) medication (beta-blockers, calcium channel blockers)
     - ii. Antihistamines
     - iii. Decongestants
     - iv. Anticholinergics
     - v. Amphetamines
     - vi. Tricyclic antidepressants
     - vii. Diuretics
     - viii. Neuroleptics
     - ix. Antipsychotics
     - x. Selective serotonin reuptake inhibitors (SSRIs)

3. Occupational injuries relative to heat exposure should also be considered. While the field of medicine does not have specific research on the subject, the areas of occupational health and occupational safety are beginning to investigate the relationship between the two. A literature review done through the occupational health arena revealed research from around the world to include the United States, Canada, Australia, Italy, Spain, Thailand, and China.[9] Most research data regarding temperatures during the study window came from local weather stations around the world. Injury data, for the most part, came from some type of health and safety record or a worker's compensation claim. The type of job evaluated varied widely. Further research into the relationship is needed to determine whether the concept is noted across multiple industries. Injury prevention programs should address traumatic, heat-related injuries on the job.[10]

Special Conditions

A. Exercise-associated hyponatremia (EAH)[11] is identified with endurance activities as the leading cause of morbidity and mortality. The diagnosis is made solely on the serum sodium levels seen up to 24 hours after the activity.[12]

1. There are two mechanisms associated with the development of EAH: overhydration and excessive secretion of antidiuretic hormone (ADH), which impairs the excretion of water in the urine.[11,13]

2. Up to 50% of cases are asymptomatic.[14,15]

3. Symptoms can include

- **a.** Headache, dizziness, altered mentation, seizures, and coma
- **b.** Weakness, fatigue
- **c.** Respiratory distress
- **d.** Tachycardia, hypotension
- **e.** Nausea and vomiting
- **f.** Changes in urination from diuresis to oliguria

4. Diagnosis identification may easily be mistaken for simple dehydration, heat illness, and even high-altitude illnesses. On site serum, sodium analysis has been recommended by the International Exercise-Associated Hyponatremia Consensus Development Conference.[12] For the ED, good history taking of events in the patient's past 24 hours can clue a clinician into the possibility of the diagnosis. Identification of the problem before excessive hypotonic fluid hydration begins can prevent worsening of the diagnosis or delaying improvement of the patient's symptoms.[16,17]

5. Treatment in the field[12]

- **a.** Observation of athlete for the initial hour after completing activity or event
- **b.** Oral intake of salty snacks or small amounts of hypertonic fluids includes bouillon or soup until the athlete begins urinating.
- **c.** If the individual has neurological changes beyond having a headache a hypertonic solution should be used. Oral version is 3 to 4 bouillon cubes diluted in ½ cup water (125 mL).
- **d.** Individuals unable to tolerate oral intake should be given an IV 3% hypertonic saline infusion according to current evidence-based guidelines. This treatment has been shown to have no undo side effects in the field and reduces cerebral edema caused by hyponatremia.

6. Treatment in the ED

- **a.** Assessment
  - **i.** Blood sodium level
  - **ii.** Evaluation for cerebral edema
  - **iii.** Additional testing associated with ruling out any differential diagnosis suspected
- **b.** Management
  - **i.** O_2 as needed for respiratory concerns
  - **ii.** Minimal fluid intake until Na levels are confirmed unless critical hypotensive state exists
  - **iii.** *Na levels below 125:* Above hypertonic saline recommendations can be initiated. After such time standard sodium replenishment can be initiated or allow for natural correction with free water excretion in the urine

7. Prevention

- **a.** Avoiding overhydration by educating athletes to drink according to how thirsty they are.
- **b.** Avoid overuse of sodium supplements. If an athlete has appropriate fluid intake, the sodium supplements will not change blood serum sodium levels.[18] Those who do not drink enough, usually seen in exercisers, can end up with elevated sodium blood levels.[19]
- **c.** Monitoring body weight is commonly used with ultramarathon events to evaluate for overhydration. Weight loss alone should not be used to diagnose EAH because EAH has been seen in athletes, in some environments, with extreme weight loss during the event.[14]

B. Rhabdomyolysis is the damage of skeletal muscle. The problem can be seen in isolation or as a part of exertional heat illness.

Special Populations

A. Older adults

1. Long-term mobility issues increase susceptibility.

2. Preexisting conditions increase susceptibility.

3. Medication regimens may affect thermoregulation.

4. Heat edema is typically seen in the population as a result of not being acclimatized. New onset of the problem will require workup for new-onset congestive heart failure or deep vein thrombosis problems.

5. Living conditions involving the age of the home, availability of air-conditioning, and fixed income over budget utility costs

B. Pediatric

1. Young children do not have well-developed sweating and thermoregulatory systems.

2. Age will affect ability to escape emergent situations (i.e., being trapped in an enclosed space).

3. Preteen and teens may not exercise sufficient judgment to stop activities in humid and temperature elevated environments.

4. Acclimatization response for school sports requires 10 to 14 days. Heatstroke deaths during practice occur usually within the first 4 days before acclimatization occurs.

Prevention and Planning

A. Individual

1. *Personal risk reduction:* Minimize or abstain from alcohol use, smoking, and elicit substance use. Establish a healthy weight. Use sunscreen to prevent severe sunburn.[4] Some research has identified that severe sunburn can impede sweating capability.[4,20]

2. *Acclimatization planning:* Individuals need to plan their acclimatization based on the specific activity and location the activity is to take place. Different organizations have slightly different guidelines. Wilderness Medicine Society (WMS) recommends 1 to 2 hours of exertional activity in the heat each day for 8 days.[4] The National Athletic Trainer's Association guidelines, put out in 2016, noted a 7- to 14-day time window for acclimatization. The process focuses on gradual adding of equipment, duration of the training, and intensity.[21] The need for guidelines associated with high school football has been shown in many studies that have evaluated exertional heat illness and death with and without guideline implementation. Guideline implementation has diminished episodes of heat illness and incidence of death.[22-24]

3. Dietary changes to decrease endogenous production of heat include decreased protein intake with increased carbohydrate intake. Digestion of protein results in increased production of heat in the human body.[25,26]

4. Precooling techniques have been used in preparation for heat exposures. The concept is used by endurance athletes. Precooling has been found helpful in prolonged activity. The concept, however, is detrimental in sprint length activities.[27] Protocols for precooling include the use of cold packs, cold vests, cold water emersion or swimming, cold oral fluid intake, and air-conditioned rooms. The most effective form and most feasible is cooling packs or vests, and cold drinks.[28] Each individual may choose to adopt a protocol for their own benefit to reduce heat injury risks.

5. Become educated to recognize early problems associated with heat injuries.[21,24,29]

6. *Heat tolerance testing (HTT):* A test used after an episode of heatstroke to determine if an athlete can return to their sport to participate safely.[30] There are several forms of the test, the Israeli Defense Force (IDF). HTT is the most frequently used design. The IDF original design began in the 1970s and has adapted over the years. Currently, there is now a predictive value component, known as the probability of heat tolerance (PHT), which allows borderline tolerant cases to be evaluated objectively.[31] HTT testing is not something handled in the ED. Referral to the patient's primary care clinician should be a part of the discharge plan. Recommending this type of evaluation to patients having suffered a heat injury may prevent a repeat occurrence, the results of which could be more devastating.

Activity[4,25]

A. Reschedule or decrease strenuous activity until temperature is lower.

B. Use of a preactivity checklist to identify participants who may be at increased risk for heat injuries. The information to gather should include:

1. The individual's history of exertional heat stroke or exhaustion. Details of the event, from when the incident occurred to return to activity, and any complications

2. History of any previous incidents or problems in the heat while exercising

3. Information on the individual's recent training regimen should also be included. Training in the heat and humidity over the past 2 weeks in acclimatization prep

4. Type of training program the participant followed over the past 2 months and their current condition

5. Include questions regarding fluid drinking habits, sweating habits (e.g., salty), and any supplement usage.

C. Establishment of guidelines for sports practice in elevated temperature conditions. Provide cooling and rehydration breaks frequently. Equipment and clothing adjustments as needed. Guidelines should be based on wet-bulb globe temperature (WBGT). When involving sports activities, guidelines should include trainer authority to stop or change practice programs or drills for the safety of the athletes.[21,22,32]

Clothing and Equipment

A. Lightweight clothing, breathable fabrics

B. Clothes should fit loosely against the body.

C. Clothes should be well ventilated to aid in cooling.

D. Replacement of saturated clothing (evaporation becomes limited) with dry garments

E. Minimize equipment that occludes large areas of skin, compromising the body's natural cooling mechanisms.

F. Mandated equipment usage and reduction guidelines are based on WBGT thresholds. Examples include military occupational guidelines, sports medicine guidelines.[21,29]

G. Wet Bulb Globe Temperature (WBGT)[8,36] is a measurement in direct sunlight of heat stress on the human body. It takes into consideration not only the temperature but also humidity, sun angle, and cloud coverage, and wind speed. This type of reading differs from common weather warnings such as the heat index. The heat index accounts for humidity and temperature in the shade.

a. This form of temperature reading is used in safety policies associated with athletics and the military. It guides training recommendations, clothing, gear, and exercise or drills.[25,37,38] Having this information will be useful for those who practice emergency medicine outside the confines of the ED.

b. Clothing will affect the accuracy of WBGT usage.

c. There are now modern thermometers that measure and calculate the WBGT.

d. To calculate the WBGT using the three types of thermometer readings:

$$WBGT = 0.7T^{w} + 0.2T^{g} + 0.1T^{d}$$

T^{w} = Natural wet-bulb temperature
T^{g} = Globe thermometer temperature
T^{d} = Dry-bulb temperature

Cooling Techniques[1,4,32]

A. Topical cooling (field or hospital setting) with ice packs to regions of the groin, neck, and axilla have had questionable results; studies have been limited. Traditional ice packs have proven more effective than chemical cooling packs.[33] A recent study evaluated the placement of ice to palms and soles of the hands and feet along with the cheeks and actually found these locations provide twice the cooling rate from the traditional sites. Further research is required.[34] Either approach can be used in conjunction with other methods to accelerate cooling.
B. Evaporative cooling (field or hospital setting) should be implemented when immersion therapy is not available. The process involves removing or loosening clothing and pouring cold water all over the patient to maximize evaporation from the skin. Adding fanning of the patient brings into play convection of heat from the body, decreasing the cooling time. Cooling time is still twice as long as emersion therapy but is still effective when the alternative is not available.[35]
C. Immersion cooling (limited to location with available tank)[32]

1. Parameters involve cooling patients at a rate of 1°C per 5 minutes (1°F per 3 minutes). The goal is to reach core body temperature of 38.3°C to 38.9°C (101°F–102°F).[32]
2. Iced water should be used.
3. If space in the submersion tank is limited, ensure the trunk is under the water.
4. Continuous circulation of the water is important during immersion.
5. Pt is immersed in cold water for 15 to 20 minutes.
6. If rectal temperature monitoring is not available, the patient should be immersed in the cold-water bath till the patient begins shivering.[32]
7. Immersion therapy is the gold standard for heatstroke treatment and, in young healthy individuals, boasts a zero-fatality rate in the research.[35]

D. Cardiopulmonary bypass (limited to an available facility with the capability) is reserved for refractory cases of heatstroke. The setup is time-intensive for mainstream usage, even with capability.
E. Cooling blankets (hospital setting) are easy to use, but the use will prevent being able to use other methods. More effective measures, such as evaporation and conduction methods, should be used first.
F. Body cavity lavage (hospital setting) has limited research data to establish the effectiveness. The method is time-intensive to set up. There is concern over fluid absorption into the body, which hasn't been evaluated as to its effects.

Environmental Considerations[4,21-24]

A. *Acclimatization guidelines for the region and or activity/event:* Follow the most rigid program.
B. Emergency plans for the care of heat injuries established in the region or in association with the event or activity
C. Available equipment and equipment proximity, for treatment of heat injuries
D. Avoid direct sunlight, seek shade.
E. Precooling options available in the area, should an individual opt for the practice.

Prehospital Care[4]

A. Prevention via adjustment in activity should initially be implemented.
B. Fluid and electrolyte replacement for mild illness
C. With moderate illness, add movement to cool or shaded areas, and make modifications to enhance the body's own cooling mechanisms, that is, equipment removal and clothing adjustments.
D. Airway, breathing, circulation, disability, exposure (ABCDEs) should be addressed first in severe illness and then begin cooling measure immediately in the field, cold water emersion if possible. Rectal temperature monitoring, as noted previously, is the gold standard, but is not usually possible in the field, thus you should cool the patient until either they begin shivering or treat with emersion therapy for 15 to 20 minutes, specific parameters are below.

Diagnostic Studies Used in Heat Injury Evaluation[1,39]

A. *Blood work:* Complete blood count (CBC), chemistry, liver enzymes, arterial blood gas (ABG), coagulation studies, lactate, myoglobin level, creatinine phosphokinase level (CPK)
B. *Additional studies:* Urinalysis (UA), EKG, lumbar puncture (LP) studies
C. *Imaging:* Chest x-ray (CXR), CT scan of the brain

Hydration

A. Water intake recommendations vary based on the individual's activity. Urination is key to removing any excess water burden.

1. The National Athletic Trainers' Association (NATA) position statement recommends pushing oral fluids even when not thirsty.[25]
2. Wilderness Medicine Society (WMS) prevention recommendations prefer fluid intake to be guided by thirst to balance dehydration vs overhydration. The concept is much more important when looking at endurance events and training.[11,40,41]
3. Fluid preloading has not been shown to help in tolerating heat or aiding in body precooling.[42]

B. Water purification is a topic to discuss briefly here for those clinicians involved in providing care in a less than optimal environment. The clinician may be called upon to aid in making available drinkable water to missionary team members, general populations in a disaster area, or even a small group caught in an austere environment when supplies have been exhausted.

1. Purification method of choice should be based on[43]
   a. The number of people who will need to be supplied with drinkable water.

b. Amount of area available to accommodate holding treated water.
c. Quality and source of water to be treated.
d. Fuel available for treatment.
e. Individuals' taste associated with final treated water.

2. Water treatment is a two-step process[43]:
   a. Clarification is used to remove particles.
      i. *Absorption:* Usually granular activated charcoal, for the removal of organic chemicals, pesticides, and some heavy metals.
      ii. *Sedimentation:* Allow particles to settle at the bottom of a container and then siphon water off the top, or pore water through some type of filter.
      iii. *Coagulation and flocculation:* Add chemical that will bind with particles and then mix to promote binding. This method works well for heavy medals.
   b. Disinfection is used to kill any bacterial agents, viruses, protozoa, and other parasites.
      i. *Heat:* The World Health Organization (WHO) recommends bringing water to a rapid boil at a temperature over 140°F (60°C) and then allow to cool without any use of rapid cooling techniques.[44] The Centers for Disease Control and Prevention (CDC) recommends a rolling boil at a temperature over 140°F (60°C) for 1 minute. This allows for a margin of safety.[45]
      ii. *Ultraviolet light:* Range of 200 to 280 nm. This method is hindered by free-floating particles.
      iii. *Filtration:* Water pressurized through a filter. This is used at a municipal level. Today, however, personal-sized products are now available
      iv. *Chemical disinfection:* Iodine and chlorine are most widely used.
         (1) Iodine usage is frequently seen with a small group or individual treatment plans. The WMS warns of groups that should not be exposed to excessive iodine (e.g., those with thyroid disease, pregnant women, individuals who are iodine sensitive, or individuals from regions of the world that are chronically deficient in iodine).[46]
         (2) Chlorine is the preferred treatment for large-scale operations by both WHO and the CDC.[47,48]
      v. *Reverse osmosis:* A filtration desalinization seen used on ocean-faring vessels
3. Products for personal use will note their effectiveness rating or the particulate size that can be filtered.
   a. Decide your choice of product based on the region to be traveled and possible threats.
   b. Threats to consider
      i. *U.S. wilderness: Escherichia coli, Salmonella, Giardia*
      ii. *International:* Industrial toxins and chemicals, *E. coli, Vibrio, Giardia, Cryptosporidium, Shigella,* hepatitis A
4. *Considerations:* Whether taking a history of a patient who presents with illness after travel or preventing illness in advance of travel
   a. Brushing teeth with boiled water or bottled water
   b. Vegetable washing using boiled water
   c. Consider any recent disaster evacuation in the destination region.

C. *Salt usage*[1,4,21,25]: The use of sodium tablets specifically for the prevention of complications associated with sodium losses is controversial in the literature. The argument for salt loading in anticipation of expected losses (long-distance endurance activities and sporting events) is countered by the argument regarding the risk of developing hypertonic hypernatremia (the weekend outdoor enthusiast). The use may be considered with a good working knowledge of the individuals who have heavy salt losses noted by white stains with sweating. The use of fluids and foods with increased sodium is however universally recommended in treatment regimens. Average sports drinks contain 25 mg to 200 mg/240 mL of sodium.

Types of Heat Injuries[1]

A. *Classic injuries*: Do not require any physical activity and are seen in heat-stress-elevated environments. Heat stress involves the combination of elevated humidity with elevated temperatures. Classic injuries are slow in onset, up to days, resulting in both electrolyte and volume changes.

B. *Exertional*: The most common cause of death seen in young athletes.[49] These are seen with elevated heat stressors and heat production activity from muscle usage, either with exertional jobs or athletic events. Dehydration and hyperpyrexia are seen because of lack of cooling resulting in organ failures.

C. *Hyperpyrexia*: A body temperature that exceeds 106°F (41.1°C) from fever. Hyperpyrexia is seen frequently in other parts of the world such as the tropics. Fevers associated with excessive isolated muscle activity or deliriums can elevate to hyperpyrexia levels. The problem is seen in many infectious fevers as well. Examples of these include malaria that has invaded the brain and meningitis associated with tetanus. Neither are seen with any regularity in the United States. Other febrile infections that have been associated with the concept of hyperpyrexia include staphylococcal sepsis, thyrotoxic crises, and streptococcal erysipelas sepsis, along with any damage to the mid-brain.[50] Exposure to very high external temperatures when someone is not acclimatized can also result in hyperpyrexia.

D. *Confinement hyperpyrexia (CH)*: A type of hyperpyrexia associated with nonexertional elevation in body temperature. This type of hyperpyrexia is more commonly seen in the United States than those associated with the type discussed above. Examples of CH involve individuals being locked in confined spaces (e.g., cars, train cars, enclosed workspaces, or living spaces not air-conditioned). The spaces develop extremely high temperatures thus elevating the human body's temperature.[1]

Minor Heat Illnesses[1-4,8,32]

A. Prickly heat

1. *Signs and symptoms:* Classic sign is a rash with itching. Sweat ducts are blocked by inflammation and subsequently rupture under the skin.

2. *Treatment:* Includes antihistamines for itching. Topical steroids, calamine lotion, oral vitamin C, and salicylic acid can also be of benefit.[51]

B. Heat edema

1. *Signs and symptoms:* Swelling of the hands, feet, and ankles from pooling of interstitial fluid as a result of gravity. Antidiuretic and aldosterone hormones will be elevated.

2. *Treatment:* Support hose and extremity elevation

C. Heat cramps

1. *Signs and symptoms:* Involuntary, intermittent spasms of skeletal muscle. Usually seen once resting begins after extreme activity in unacclimated individuals. The pathophysiology of the problem involves a decrease in potassium and sodium intracellularly. Patients have usually rehydrated with large quantities of water. This is not to be confused with muscle spasms associated with exercise in athletes, which last much longer. Muscle spasms of this nature are relieved with massage and stretching.

2. *Treatment:* To replenish electrolytes. Over-the-counter electrolyte solutions may be used, flavored is more palatable and thus preferred. Avoid taking solid salt tablets because of the gastric irritability, dissolve the tablets first per the package instructions.

D. Heat syncope

1. *Signs and symptoms:* Collapse associated with activity in hot conditions. This can be the result of extended standing or sudden change from sitting to standing after being in elevated temperature conditions. Elderly patients exposed to heat can experience the incidence without movement or exertional activity. Blood volume is decreased as a result of peripheral vasodilation and loss in vasomotor tone.

2. *Treatment:* Simple cooling and rehydration efforts lead to treatment. Removing the patient from the elevated temperature environment should first be addressed.

Major Heat Illnesses[1-3,8,32]

A. *Heat exhaustion:* Can be identified with the body's thermoregulatory abilities intact along with keeping the body's temperature below 104°F (40°C). The problem can be caused by the lack of fluid intake since most people tend to only replace two-thirds of what they lose. It may also be from excessive water intake in unacclimated individuals resulting in hyponatremia.

1. Signs and symptoms
   a. Headache
   b. Dizziness
   c. Ataxia
   d. Malaise
   e. Judgment impaired
   f. Nausea
   g. Muscle cramping
2. Physical examination
   a. Hypotension
   b. Tachycardia
3. Diagnostic studies
   a. CBC
   b. Chemistry
   c. Liver enzymes
   d. Any additional testing that is required to rule out any differential diagnosis
4. Differential diagnoses
   a. Heatstroke
   b. Infectious processes
   c. Toxicological problems
   d. Neurologic problems
5. Treatment
   a. Continue any cooling techniques started in the field until return of normothermic conditions.
   b. Fluid replacement guided by laboratory studies
6. Ongoing care
   a. Young patients frequently require fluid replacement and can be discharged home.
   b. Older patients require admission for fluid and electrolyte replacement and monitoring.

B. *Heatstroke:* Defined by temperatures over 104°F/4°C AND altered mental status (AMS). There is a loss in the body's ability to control temperature with the normal thermoregulatory functions.

1. Signs and symptoms
   a. Those noted in heat exhaustion but on a more profound level
   b. Progressive disorientation to unresponsiveness
2. Physical examination
   a. Hypotension
   b. Tachycardia
   c. Tachy arrhythmias
   d. Tachypnea
   e. Widened pulse pressure
3. Diagnostic and imaging studies[1,39]
   a. Complete blood count (CBC)
   b. Blood chemistry
   c. Liver enzymes
   d. *Coagulation studies:* prothrombin time (PT), partial thromboplastin time (PTT), fibrinogen
   e. CPK
   f. Lactate
   g. Arterial blood gases (ABG)
   h. Urinalysis (UA)
   i. EKG
   j. Chest x-ray (CXR)
   k. Lumbar puncture (LP) to evaluate for other causes associated with altered mental status (AMS). Cerebrospinal fluid (CSF) studies cell count, glucose, protein, culture if there is clinical suspicion, fungal studies, mycobacterial infection studies, and atypical infection studies.
   l. CT brain, again to rule out other causes of altered mental status.
4. Differential diagnosis
   a. *Neurological:* Status epilepticus, stroke, hypothalamic injury
   b. *Toxicological:* Overdose, substance withdrawals, malignant hyperthermia, neuroleptic malignant syndrome, serotonin syndrome

c. *Infections:* Encephalitis, meningitis, malaria, tetanus, typhoid
d. *Endocrine:* Thyroid storm, diabetic ketoacidosis (DKA), pheochromocytoma

5. Treatment ED resuscitation[32]
   a. Traditional evaluation of the ABCDEs (airway, breathing, circulation, disability, exposure) needs to be the start of evaluation.
   b. Continued rapid cooling if expected goal has not yet been met. Immersion is the most effective, but equipment needed for this type of cooling is not frequently seen in the ED. Additional cooling options for the ED are listed in the following.
   c. Frequent vital sign (VS) monitoring to include heart rate (HR), blood pressure (BP), respiratory rate (RR), pulse oximetry, and core temperature via rectal method. Central venous pressure (CVP) monitoring may be indicated for fluid resuscitation if renal function is affecting the output reliability. Cardiac rhythm monitoring.
   d. Resuscitation complications[3]
      i. *Aspiration and hypoxia:* Given seizure activity and cold-induced muscle rigidity, accompanied by frequently unconsciousness of the patient, intubation is necessary. Supplemental oxygen is needed because of the significant increase in demand from the thermal stressors. Anticipate acute respiratory distress syndrome (ARDS), pneumonitis, pulmonary infarction, and bleeding.
      ii. Fluid intake expectations higher than predicted. Patients with heat stroke often present with the appearance of right-sided heart failure that has been heat induced, putting them in a hyperdynamic state initially. As the presentation begins correcting itself, the patient will require additional fluids for resuscitation.[3]
      iii. Issues with hypotension and the type of vasoconstrictor medications are dependent on normal body temperatures. Dopamine and dobutamine are recommended. Alpha-adrenergic stimulating drugs, that is, norepinephrine can cause significant vasoconstriction resulting in slowing of cooling attempts.
      iv. Treatment of tachyarrhythmias resulting in need for defibrillation requires a cooled myocardium before being attempted.
      v. Coagulopathies are usually not seen until the day after injury. Monitoring for disseminated intervascular coagulation (DIC) and then implementing treatment (fresh frozen plasma and platelets) should be implemented.

6. Ongoing care[1-3]
   a. Mental status reevaluation
   b. Rectal temperature readings are the only form of temperature measurement that should be used in heat-related emergencies, other forms of registering body temperature are not accurate enough to base adjustments to emergent cooling measures.[52,53] Rectal temperature readings should be taken every 10 minutes to guide cooling and resuscitative efforts. While the use of urinary catheter temperature probes are widely used within the field of medicine, the use is not discussed in the arena of hyperthermic emergencies for temperature monitoring. This may be because the availability of urinary catheter placement allows for an internal cooling option.
   c. *Muscle tone monitoring:* Rigid muscles are an indicator of malignant hyperthermia versus flaccid musculature in exertional heatstroke, or intermittent muscle activity such as seizures or cold tonic–clonic muscle movement.[25,54]
   d. Ongoing cooling measures based on core temperature should continue until the goal temperature has been achieved.
   e. *Ongoing fluid resuscitation:* In nonexertional heatstroke, cardiac output can be severely affected. IV fluid (IVF) administration may be required despite exam findings suggestive of pulmonary edema.
   f. *Monitoring and early intervention of complications:* Acute renal failure, acute liver failure, rhabdomyolysis, and DIC. In exertional heat stroke, patients can develop systemic inflammatory syndrome (SIRS).[26,55] Treatment should follow SIRS guidelines.
   g. Therapeutic hypothermia has been found effective in severe heatstroke patients and thus might be considered in care. The study identified the use of noninvasive forms of cooling only.[56]

7. Types of heatstroke and their unique differences[1]
   a. Classic
      i. Type of patient
         (1) Older aged patients usually with predisposing factors such as
         (2) Sedentary lifestyle
         (3) Prior medical histories
         (4) Medication usage
      ii. Presentation
         (1) Decreased or absent urine production
         (2) Lack of sweating
         (3) CNS problems
      iii. Laboratory changes:
         (1) Mild lactic acidosis
         (2) Mild coagulation study changes
         (3) Mild CPK elevation
         (4) Normal calcium level
         (5) Normal potassium level
         (6) Normal sodium level
         (7) Normal glucose level
   b. Exertional
      i. Type of patient
         (1) Young patients
         (2) Healthy without a predisposing medical diagnosis
         (3) Those involved in exercise
      ii. Presentation
         (1) Diaphoresis
         (2) Organ injury to include cardiac, renal, and liver injuries or failures
      iii. Laboratory changes:
         (1) Severe lactic acidosis
         (2) Rhabdomyolysis

(3) DIC
(4) Hypocalcemia
(5) Hyperkalemia
(6) Hyponatremia
(7) Hypoglycemia

8. Complications of heatstroke[1]
   a. *Cardiac:* Heart failure progressing to injury and infarction of the myocardium.
   b. *Gastrointestinal:* No overt early symptoms, but development of liver injury progressing to failure. Injury progressing to infarction of the intestines.
   c. *Hematological:* No overt early symptoms but development of thrombocytopenia and DIC.
   d. *Metabolic:* Decreased potassium with progression to elevated potassium. If there is a decreased sodium, this can cause an increase in uric acid in the bloodstream, and if the sodium is elevated, the calcium blood levels can decrease.
   e. *Neurological:* Symptoms begin with an altered mental status, progressing delirium to coma and seizures, and then the development of cerebral edema and encephalopathy.
   f. *Pulmonary:* Pulmonary edema develops early and will progress to ARDS.
   g. *Renal:* Significant decrease to absence of urinary output progressing to rhabdomyolysis and acute renal failure.

Specialty Consultation

A. *Nephrology:* Monitoring and treatment of acute kidney injury.
B. *Surgery:* Monitoring or intervention in compartment syndrome.
C. *Gastroenterology:* Liver specialist or transplant; monitoring or intervention in acute potential liver failure and possible need for transplantation.
D. Admission requirements
   1. Heat stroke diagnosis will need ICU monitoring capability. If invasive monitoring is not available, transfer to a facility of higher care is needed. Any complex interventions will require hospital capabilities.

E. New treatments being evaluated for heatstroke complications
   1. Acute liver failure resolution with N-acetylcysteine (NAC). There was an isolated case involving a military recruit who developed heatstroke with a rectal temp of 107.9°F. The patient had initial aggressive external cooling measures before being transferred to a definitive care facility. The patient was admitted to the ICU, he improved cognitively, but laboratory studies identified both renal and liver failure progression. By day 3 of admission, a liver transplant team was consulted. The recommendation from the service was to start NAC. The dosing began with loading dose of 150 mg/kg over 1 hour, then 12.5 mg/kg/hr for the next 4 hours, and then 6.25 mg/kg/hr for the remainder of a 72- hour administration plan. The patient recovered with resolution of organ failure.[57]
   2. Renal failure and the use of allopurinol alone or in conjunction with sodium bicarbonate. It is thought that chronic kidney disease from a heat injury may be a result of hyperuricemia. Allopurinol inhibits xanthine oxide, thereby reducing serum urate. Low doses of allopurinol can decrease inflammatory markers in the kidney as in the liver. High doses of allopurinol can cause renal toxicity. The research thus far has involved mice with the use of either allopurinol alone or in combination with sodium bicarbonate.[58,59]
   3. Liver failure and the use of allopurinol alone or with sodium bicarbonate. There is significant inflammatory marker elevation with liver injury from heat injury. The inflammatory markers are significantly lowered with the use of allopurinol.[58,59]

References

References for this chapter are online only and can be found at https://connect.springerpub.com/content/reference-book/978-0-8261-6091-5/part/part04/toc-part/ch35.

36. Lightning and Electrical Injuries

DAVID T. HOUSE | ALEXANDER F. WRYNN

Learning Objectives

- Discuss current statistics surrounding electrical and lightning injuries.
- List common mechanisms of electrical injury.
- Discuss basic electrical physics and how they relate to patients who have experienced an acute electrocution.
- Discuss mechanisms of injury associated with lightning injuries.
- Discuss occupational exposures and how they are related to electrical injuries.
- Identify pertinent exam findings associated with electrical injuries.
- List what should be obtained in a routine work-up on patients who have experienced acute electrocution.
- Discuss fluid resuscitation of patients with electrical burns.
- Describe the patient who should be transferred to a burn center.
- Discuss which electrical burns require admission versus which can be safely discharged.
- Discuss awareness of long-term consequences of electrical injuries.

Electrical injuries are rare but often devastating events. Electrical burns account for an estimated 5% of burn admissions in developed countries.[1] In the United States, there are around 30,000 nonfatal shock incidents and 1,000 electricity-related deaths reported annually.[2] Lightning strikes are an extreme form of electrical injury, and they are the leading cause of weather-related deaths.[3] The estimated odds of being struck by lightning are only one in 500,000, and in 2018 there were 20 lightning strike fatalities in the United States.[3,4] Proper ED management of acutely electrocuted patients is of utmost importance. Missteps in management could lead to a lifetime of disability or even death.

Pathophysiology

Electricity is the flow of electrons through a conductor. These electrons flow from an area of high concentration to low concentration. There are four properties of electricity that can help determine or predict patient outcomes; they are voltage, current, resistance, and conductance.[5-8] Voltage is a measure of electromotive force. Current is the flow of electricity. Resistance is a material opposition to the passage of electrical force, while conductance is its ability to transmit a current.[8] Electricity can cause injury through three primary mechanisms, which are as follows[5]:

A. Electricity causing direct tissue damage. Electricity alters cell membrane potentials and leads to tetany.

B. Conversion of electrical energy to thermal energy leading to tissue damage and coagulation necrosis

C. Mechanical injury with direct trauma from falls or violent muscle contractions

Injury severity is determined by the magnitude of electrical energy, resistance encountered, current pathway, and duration of contact. Degree of injury is directly related to the magnitude of force. Electrical current is measured in amperes (A). Amperage is directly related to voltage and indirectly related to resistance. This relationship is defined using Ohm's Law, which is determined using the following equation[5-7]:

$$\text{Ohm's Law: } I = V/R$$

where I = current, V = voltage, R = resistance.

As stated previously, current is the flow of electricity. Current exists in two forms: direct and alternating current (AC). Direct current (DC) flows in one direction. When a person is injured by DC current, they experience one single muscle spasm from the shock. DC is typically seen in batteries and train rail lines. AC electricity, which is commonly seen in household wall sockets, changes direction periodically, leading to continuous muscle contraction in a person in contact with it. This continuous muscle contraction makes it difficult to let go of the source of electricity. The "let-go threshold" is the current level that prevents release of an electrical source. If the current is above this threshold, it can lead to a "locked-on" or "no let-go" phenomenon. Electrical injuries from AC can be significantly more devastating. Prolonged grip to the electrical source increases exposure time, which can lead to complications from respiratory arrest to cardiac arrhythmias. Lightning can exist as either form of current but typically closely resembles DC.[8]

When assessing voltage, electrical injuries are classically defined as being either low voltage (<1,000 volts) or high voltage (>1,000 volts). Most household injuries are considered low-voltage injuries. They commonly cause local damage at the site of electrical contact. High-voltage injuries classically happen in the workplace or an industrial setting. Higher voltage currents cause more severe damage and travel distally from the origin of the shock.

These types of injuries can lead to breakdown of deep muscles, placing patients at risk for developing rhabdomyolysis.[5] Lightning is always considered a high-voltage injury and can reach voltage levels as high as 110,000. Table 36.1 offers a summary of the voltage of commonly encountered electrical sources.[8]

Resistance is the ability to impede the flow of electricity, while conductivity is the amount of electrical current a material can carry.[5] Electricity can generate more heat in a more resistant conductor. If a tissue is highly resistant, it gives off increased thermal injury, leading to burns and damage to surrounding tissues. This property is the cause of the majority of thermal burns associated with electrical injuries, and what makes burn care of electrical injuries so difficult, as burns are often far worse than they appear externally.

When applying the above principles, one could understand how degree of electrical injury can vary significantly from one injury to the next. The same person could be exposed to the same level of voltage at different sites of their body and have drastically different burns and injury secondary to the resistance of tissues in that area.[5,6] High-resistance body tissues include bones, fat, and tendons, while nerves, blood vessels, muscles, and mucous membranes are some of the least resistant tissues. Skin has intermediate resistance, and there are a few factors that determine its resistance. Thicker skin has higher resistance, and things like wet skin or breaks in the skin can decrease its resistance (Box 36.1).[5]

The same basic principles can be applied to lightning injuries. Lightning strikes are always considered a high-voltage injury. Additionally, lightning strikes should always be viewed as a traumatic injury. Many clinicians are aware of burn injuries that can occur from lightning strikes but should be more astute to the multisystem trauma that can occur. It is important for the emergency nurse practitioner (ENP) to be aware of the various mechanisms from which lightning can cause injury. They are as follows[9]:

A. *Direct strike:* When the person has direct contact with lightning. It is hypothesized that this is the most fatal mechanism of lightning strikes; however, there is no direct research or evidence to support this.
B. *Contact voltage:* When lightning hits an outside source and travels through a pathway until it makes contact with someone holding onto an energy transmitter. The classic example of this strike is someone showering or turning on a faucet during a thunderstorm.
C. *Sideflash or splash:* This mechanism is created when lightning strikes an object, for example, a tree; it travels down that object and makes contact with a person before it hits the ground.
D. *Ground voltage*: Lightning travels through the ground and makes contact with a person.
E. *Upward streamer:* Thunderstorms have the potential to create an electrical field. They can charge surrounding objects, and these objects can possess enough energy to injure a person.[10]

An ENP can use these properties of electricity to assist them in the evaluation of patients who have sustained electrical injuries. When working with someone who has suffered an electrocution, ask oneself the following questions:

A. Was this high or low voltage?
B. AC or DC?
C. What was the area of contact?
D. What was the pathway of the current?
E. Was there anything that altered resistance (e.g., wet skin)?

TABLE 36.1 VOLTAGE LEVEL OF COMMON SOURCES OF ELECTRICAL INJURY

SOURCE	VOLTAGE (VOLTS)
High Voltage	
Lightning	110,000+
Rail network	25,000
Power lines	1,500
Low Voltage	
Mine	960
Subway third rail	750
Domestic (United States)	110

BOX 36.1 BODY TISSUE ELECTRICAL RESISTANCE

Listed in order of least-to-greatest resistance

A. Nerves
B. Blood vessels
C. Mucous membranes
D. Muscle
E. Skin
F. Tendon
G. Fat
H. Bone

Physical Examination

It is best to approach every electrical injury like a traumatic injury.[11] Following the Advanced Trauma Life Support (ATLS) algorithm will result in quicker identification and treatment of emergent complications. This is especially true with lightning strikes. With a significant number of electrocutions being occupationally related, it is important to conduct a thorough physical examination of these patients. All physical examination findings should be well documented, as several of these events have high likelihood of future litigation. It is more likely that high-voltage sources will cause more injury; however, one should always be aware that low-voltage burns could still cause serious complications, including arrhythmias and seizures.

Medical Screening

A. Presentation varies based on severity of injury.
B. *Chief complaint:* Initial findings, responsiveness, witnessed, prehospital treatments, include type of electrical injury, type of current, voltage, and duration of contact, and environmental conditions
C. Signs and symptoms
  1. Cardiac arrest
  2. Altered mental status (AMS)

3. Focal neurologic complaints
4. Seizures
5. Hearing loss
6. Blindness
7. Burns

D. History
1. Medical
2. Surgical
3. Social
4. Family history
5. Allergies
6. Medications
7. Immunizations

E. Focused assessment
1. System-to-system physical examination
a. *Skin*[6,12]: Electricity always has the capacity to cause burns. Skin burns can vary from mild first-degree burns to significant third-degree burns. The classic electrical burn is a depressed and charred central area with surrounding edema. Cutaneous skin burns from electricity are often called contact points. Every patient should be examined for different areas of contact, as they can assist the ENP with estimating potential areas of internal injury. There are select categories of burns to be aware of.
i. *High-voltage burns*: The classic electrical burn with central necrosis. Do not use the size of the surface burn to estimate internal injury, which one could significantly underestimate the extent of.
ii. *Arc burns*: The arc of electricity travels from an area of high to low resistance, creating a high temperature pathway that causes lesions at the contact point and ground point. Classically, these burns have dry centers and surrounding swelling. They will not occur with low-voltage injuries.
iii. *Flash burns*: Caused by the heat of the electrical arc. Often appear as small "splash-like" areas of superficial burn.
iv. *Flame burns*: Caused by ignition of clothing or surrounding objects. Thermal burns are commonly seen with flame injuries.
v. *Lichtenberg figures*[8]: A fine rash that resembles bare tree branches. Commonly seen after a lightning injury. This superficial rash requires no treatment; advise patients that it will dissipate within a few weeks.
b. *Ear, nose, throat (ENT)*[6,8,12]
i. The ENP should check the mouth of any young child suspected of having an electrical injury. These burns can be misleading and may not appear significant for 2 to 3 days, when they commonly start to form an eschar. Oral eschars have been noted to cause life-threatening bleeding from the labial artery. Any oral burn warrants involvement of both burn and oral surgery.
ii. Assess tympanic membranes (TMs) on every patient. TMs are a low-resistance electrical pathway, making them particularly vulnerable to injury. Electrical injuries place patients at risk of having ruptured TMs. Up to 50% of patients who have experienced electrical shocks have either ruptured TMs or some degree of hearing loss. Lightning strike victims are particularly vulnerable to TM rupture.
c. *Eyes*[8]
i. Ocular damage is common following a lightning strike. Once stable, these patients benefit from a detailed eye exam. Retinal damage can occur, so these patients should always follow up with ophthalmology.
d. *Cardiovascular*[13-16]
i. Electricity can damage the heart in two ways: direct myocardial injury and disruption of the heart's electrical system leading to arrhythmias. The heart is most sensitive to both high-voltage and AC injuries. It only takes a fraction of a second for 30 mA of AC or 300 to 500 mA of DC to cause severe myocardial damage and ventricular fibrillation.
ii. First and foremost, examine the chest wall for burn marks that could suggest passage through the thorax. Both horizontal (hand-to-hand) and vertical (head-to-foot) current pathways can pass through the thorax.
iii. Arrhythmias are the most common cardiac complication after electrical injuries. These are further discussed in the diagnostic work-up section of this chapter. During the initial physical examination, auscultate the patient's chest to identify irregular rhythms. In rare cases, electrical injuries have been noted to cause new-onset atrial fibrillation. Point-of-care ultrasound views of the heart could reveal wall motion abnormalities suggestive of myocardial injury.
e. *Pulmonary*[6,17,18]
i. Pulmonary complications of electrical injuries are rare. High-voltage injures are often associated with respiratory arrest secondary to spasm of the diaphragm or direct injury to the respiratory control center.
ii. As one would do with any burn injury, inspect the patient's airway for any signs of edema or burns. Routine auscultation of the chest should always be performed. Several case studies have revealed rare electricity-related pulmonary complications include pulmonary edema and pneumothorax. Utilize point-of-care ultrasound to evaluate for B-lines and proper lung sliding.
f. *Neurologic*[6,8]
i. Direct electrical injury to the central nervous system (CNS) is rare. One of the common CNS injuries associated with electricity is damage to the respiratory control center. Rare instances of cranial nerve damage and seizures have been reported. Spinal cord injuries have been documented with violent tetany and contractions associated with "locked on" electrical injuries.

ii. Any patient who has experienced a significant electrical shock should have a full neurologic examination. Many patients who suffer high-voltage injuries are often flung by the electrical source. This event places them at risk for several neurologic complications, from head injuries to spinal cord injuries.

iii. Keraunoparalysis is a transient paralysis that has been associated with lightning injuries. It is hypothesized that this condition occurs because of overstimulation of the autonomic nervous system, which results in vascular spasms. Lower extremities are more frequently affected. Common exam findings are loss of motor, sensation, pulse, and pallor of the affected extremity. Any sensory or motor deficit should be considered a spinal cord injury (SCI) until proven otherwise, and these patients should remain in spinal precautions and have advanced imaging of their cervical spine.

g. *Musculoskeletal*[6,17,19]

i. The violent muscle contractions and tetany often associated with electrical shocks place patients at high risk for fractures and muscular damage.

ii. Clinicians should be aware that patients who have been acutely electrocuted, especially ones who have experienced a high-voltage injury, are at risk for developing compartment syndrome. These symptoms may not develop within the first 48 hours. If the emergency nurse practitioner (ENP) has any suspicion of compartment syndrome, compartment pressures must be checked and early fasciotomy should be considered.

iii. Electrical injuries can predispose patients to having postburn contractures. Poor acute burn care management often leads to increased contractures.[20] Contractures can lead to permanent disability for patients. It is important to get a burn surgeon involved early in any patient who experienced a significant electrical injury. Early surgical intervention has been shown to reduce permanent contractures.

h. *Peripheral vascular*[6]

i. Thermal energy produced by electrical resistance causes burns and damages surrounding tissue. As stated previously, blood vessels are low-resistance tissues and are particularly vulnerable to injury. Coagulation necrosis is a common complication associated with electrical injuries. If a patient is having any degree of pain in an injured extremity, perform and document a full vascular assessment. If there is any decrease in peripheral pules or pallor to the extremity, consider getting an ultrasound or CT angiography to assess for clots.

Differential Diagnoses

A. It is often evident that a patient has experienced an electrical injury based on traumatic mechanism or presentation.

B. If the patient is unable to provide a clear history, look for clues of electrical injury, like characteristic cutaneous burns that are often associated with electricity.

C. Electrical injury should be the top differential for any patient with unexplained cardiac arrest that was near a high-energy power source or outside during a thunderstorm.

D. Additionally, the ENP should always be cognizant of the broad differential of complications that can be associated with electrical injuries. These include the following:

1. Thermal burns
2. Rhabdomyolysis
3. Ocular burns
4. Seizures and status epilepticus
5. Syncope
6. Cardiopulmonary arrest

Diagnostic Testing

A. There is currently no evidence-based work-up for a patient who has sustained an electrical injury. However, based on common complications associated with electrical injury, the ENP should consider ordering the following diagnostics tests:

1. EKG[13-16,21]

a. Damage to the heart muscle can occur as a result of several different mechanisms. There can be direct damage from the electrical current, infarction from coronary spasm, coronary thrombosis secondary to thermal energy, myocardial contusions from CPR, and injury from extensive catecholamine release. Changes to the patient's EKG may not be clear. Patients may have clear ischemic changes to their EKG (T wave changes, ST segment changes); they may also have a transient Brugada pattern. The sinoatrial (SA) node and atrioventricular (AV) node seem to be particularly vulnerable to injury, and sinus tachycardia, sinus bradycardia, and varying degrees of heart block have all been commonly associated with electrical injuries. In some rare cases, there have been reports of new-onset atrial fibrillation.

2. Labs[6,22]

a. There is currently no set of recommended labs for patients following an electrical injury.

b. Obtain routine labs such as a comprehensive blood count (CBC) and basic metabolic panel (BMP). Pay close attention to the patient's creatinine, as these patients are high risk to develop rhabdomyolysis.

c. Send a urinalysis (UA) to assess for myoglobinuria. Check a serum myoglobin if urine is myoglobin positive. Serial UAs should be sent to assess for clearing of myoglobinuria, and urine color should clear as myoglobin clears.

d. Creatinine kinase (CK) should be tested on every patient who has experienced a high-voltage injury. These patients are very high risk for rhabdomyolysis.
e. If the pathway of the shock is through the thorax or if cardiac injury is suspected, serum troponin levels should be evaluated. Take caution with troponin in patients who have experienced electrocutions. While troponin is considered the gold standard for evaluating myocardial damage, it is not as reliable in the setting of an electrical injury.[6,23]
f. Obtain a urine pregnancy test in all female patients of childbearing age.

Diagnostic Imaging[6]

A. *X-rays:* Obtain plain films on any painful or deformed bony areas. Pay close attention to shoulder pain; posterior dislocations are common with electrocutions and often missed on plain films. Obtain shoulder CT scans on patients with persistent pain and limited range of motion despite negative plain films.[24] Chest x-rays should be obtained in any patient in cardiopulmonary arrest, or with a complaint of chest pain or shortness of breath.
B. *CT scans:* Any patient with extensive injury, altered level of consciousness, or focal neurologic deficits should get a head CT scan. Obtaining a cervical spine CT should be considered in any patient with the above findings. The need for further CT imaging, including the chest, abdomen, and pelvis, should be based on the patient's presentation and exam findings.
C. *Ultrasound:* Perform a Focused Assessment with Sonography for Trauma (FAST) exam on all patients to assess for abdominal pathology. Add on cardiac views to assess wall motion abnormalities, which could suggest myocardial damage.

Management

A. Emergent management[25-29]
1. Follow basic ATLS and Advanced Cardiovascular Life Support (ACLS) protocols. Initiate immediate CPR and other resuscitative efforts in any patient in cardiac arrest. Be aggressive with CPR and other resuscitative efforts; electrical injuries often have better resuscitative outcomes than other cardiac arrest pathologies, even in the setting of asystole. Assess the patient for any signs and symptoms of respiratory distress. If there are signs of airway compromise, establish a definitive airway. Do not delay establishing a definitive airway; literature has suggested delays in airway management lead to more difficult intubations and worse patient outcomes. Fully undress and remove all jewelry from the patient to assess the extent of burns; look for multiple contact points that could suggest the electrical current's path. Once the patient is stable, obtain a STAT EKG.

General Management

A. Cardiac monitoring[13]
1. A mainstay of treatment. Any patient who experienced a high-voltage injury, loss of consciousness, or any cardiac arrhythmia on their EKG is a candidate for long-term monitoring.

B. Fluid resuscitation[6,30]
1. Proper fluid resuscitation is essential, especially in patients who have experienced a high-voltage injury. The common equation used for fluid resuscitation in electrical injuries is 4 mL × total body surface area (TBSA; %) × body weight (kg). 50% of this fluid is administered in the first 8 hours and the remainder over the next 16 hours. Fluid resuscitation is from the time of burn injury and should start within 2 hours of injury. TBSA is a problem area in electrical injury management. Cutaneous burns from electricity are often small; however, patients may have deeper injuries as a result of the passage of electrical current. Over-resuscitation also causes patient complications, most notably compartment syndrome from swelling secondary to fluid overload. To avoid under- and over-resuscitation, it is best to follow urine output. Current American Burn Association (ABA) guidelines suggest urine output goals of 1 mL/kg/hour. Place a urinary catheter for close fluid monitoring.
C. Wound care
1. Clean burned areas of skin and dress in an antibiotic wound dressing. Update tetanus immunization as needed. Burned patients are at high risk for infection. However, antibiotic prophylaxis is controversial, and there is no clear literature to support its utility.[31]
D. Consult services[6]
1. Care of the patient with an electrical injury can be complicated. It often requires a team of specialists to assist with the patient's management. The following are common consults one may obtain for these patients:
a. *Burn surgery:* Burn surgeons are probably the most important service to reach out to for patients who have sustained significant electrocutions. They can assist with early surgical interventions that have been proven to reduce mortality and disability following an electrocution.
b. *Trauma surgery:* Electrical injuries often result in multisystem trauma. Getting the trauma surgery team involved early can help streamline the management of these patients.
c. *Orthopedic surgery:* Fractures and other musculoskeletal injuries are common. Orthopedics should also be consulted on any patient with suspected compartment syndrome.
d. *Cardiology:* For patients with any concerning EKG changes or arrhythmias
e. *Ear, nose, throat (ENT):* Early ENT consult on any patient with concerns about oral mucosal injury
f. *Ophthalmology:* Any patient following a lightning strike, once stabilized, should have a detailed eye exam, as lightning injuries can cause retinal damage.[8]

Special Considerations

A. Pregnant patient[32]
1. Research on maternal–fetal outcomes following electrical injuries is limited. In previous studies, fetal mortality rate following electrical shock has been as high as 76%. High-voltage injuries result in fewer

fetal deaths. It is hypothesized that this is because of shorter exposure times associated with high-voltage injury. Fetal demise can occur instantly after the event, but can occur up to 3 to 7 days after. Common fetal complications include oligohydramnios and growth restrictions. Manage the pregnant mother as any other electrical injury. Follow ATLS and ACLS protocols for resuscitation; perform the same wound care and proper fluid resuscitation. Obtain an ultrasound to assess the fetus. Admission for fetal monitoring is necessary. Advise all pregnant patients that they should follow up with their OB/GYN clinician and have a repeat ultrasound within 2 weeks.

B. Pediatrics[6,33]

1. Children more frequently experience low-voltage injuries, but are still at high risk for complications. They have thinner skin, less body surface area, and decreased resistance to electricity. As stated previously, be very cautious with any pediatric patient with an oral burn; they are at high risk for labial artery bleeding. Arterial bleeds can be either acute or delayed by up to 2 weeks. Early ENT consult is essential. Adolescents, especially teenaged boys, are at risk for high-voltage injuries in the community given their affinity for high-risk behaviors.

C. Patients with pacemakers and defibrillators[13]

1. External electrical sources can cause damage and malfunction of both implanted pacemakers and defibrillators. Malfunction can lead to asynchronous pacing or unnecessary shocks from an implanted defibrillator. Device interrogation should always be performed on these patients.

D. Taser injuries[6]

1. Taser devices fire a metal projectile that implants in a person and delivers multiple shocks to subdue a person. The initial voltage is around 50,000 V. There have been reported cases of Taser-induced ventricular fibrillation. Patients may present with accompanying minor traumatic injuries. These are often from falls or altercations with law enforcement. Injuries rarely occur from the Taser darts themselves. Taser injuries should be approached the same way as any traumatic injury. Always remember to obtain an EKG and take complaints of chest pain and shortness of breath seriously.

Patient Disposition

A. Transfer to burn center[34]

B. ABA guidelines recommend prompt transfer to a burn center for any patient who has experienced a high-voltage injury, lightning injury, or low-voltage injury with serious cutaneous burns or diagnostic work-up abnormalities. Do not delay transfer for further diagnostic work-up.

C. Admission criteria[6,8,13,22]

1. There is no set time frame for cardiac monitoring, and there are no clear admission criteria for electrical injuries. As stated earlier, any patient with extensive burn injuries should be evaluated and treated at a burn center. Patients with significant traumatic injury should be evaluated and admitted to a trauma center for further trauma care. The following patients should be admitted to the hospital for 24 hours of ICU monitoring:

a. High-voltage and lightning injuries
b. Arrhythmias
c. Loss of consciousness
d. EKG abnormalities
e. Elevated or rising troponin

2. If anomalies continue during the hospitalization, patients may need further work-up with echocardiograms and/or coronary angiography. Pregnant patients should be admitted for fetal cardiac monitoring.

D. Discharge

1. Patients who experienced a low-voltage injury, and who are asymptomatic in the ED with a normal EKG, are safe to be discharged home with close follow-up. Advise patient to follow up with their primary care doctor within a week; follow-up EKGs may be needed. Patients with minor cutaneous burns may need to follow up in a burn clinic.

2. Discharge education

a. Advise the patient to follow up with proper clinicians. Offer education on any wound care that may be necessary. Recommend use of acetaminophen or ibuprofen for pain as needed. Make patient aware of any long-term symptoms that may develop as a result of the injury. Advise the patient to seek emergency care if they develop chest pain, shortness of breath, palpitations, lightheadedness, have a syncopal episode, or have worsening pain. If the patient has a burn wound, provide education of signs and symptoms of wound infections.

E. Long-term sequelae

1. No matter how minor they may seem, electrical injuries should be discharged with close follow-up and some degree of caution. Proper patient education could increase patient awareness of late complications often associated with lightning and electrical injuries. Some common long-term issues are listed below.

a. *Pain*[35]: Pain is a common long-term issue following electrical injuries. This pain is often difficult to classify and does not fit the pattern of any common neuropathic pain. Patients can benefit greatly from psychosomatic treatment.

b. *Ocular manifestations*[6,8,36]: The head is a common contact point of electricity, leading to various ocular manifestations, most notably, cataracts. About 6% of patients will develop cataracts. Patients should be advised to follow up with their ophthalmologist for continued eye exams following any type of electrical injury to the head, especially lightning injuries. Some other common manifestations that may occur are retinal damage, macular cysts, and macular holes.

c. *Peripheral neuropathies*[1,35,37]: Symptoms of numbness, tingling, and neuropathic pain can present days to months following injury, even from low-voltage injuries. Possible causes of these neuropathies include hemorrhage, cerebral edema, or chromatolysis of pyramidal cells. The exact pattern and timeline of symptoms are not fully understood.

d. *Return to work*[38]: Patients with minor injury should be able to return to work without difficulty. However, for some, return to work may be a slow process. In one study of patients who had sustained significant electrical injury, 61% of patients were able to return to their pre-injury occupation. Over half of those who returned to work required modified duties and scheduling. Median return time to work was 166 days from the date of injury. Again, the data highlights the importance of documentation with any electrical injury. These factors will often have some degree of impact on the patient's function.

e. *Psychological*[35,38-43]: Victims of electrical accidents commonly report psychiatric complications. Posttraumatic stress disorder (PTSD), depression, generalized anxiety, nightmares, and flashbacks are all commonly reported in the months following an accident. It is important to make patients aware that they may experience some degree of psychiatric disturbance from these accidents. Patients should be encouraged to seek proper care for these complications as an outpatient.

Predisposing Factors

Electrical injury can occur at any age. Males are more frequently affected than females. Children experience more low-voltage injuries since they are mostly victims of household electrocutions.[41] Younger children are commonly injured after inserting things in sockets or chewing on electrical cords, while older children experience injury from engaging in high-risk activities outdoors, making them more susceptible to high-voltage injury.[6,33] Adults are frequently injured in the workplace. Studies have found up to a third of electrical injuries occur in the workplace. One study that examined workplace electrical injuries from 2007 to 2016 reported that 1,651 workers died from electrical injury, with construction and extraction workers being at the highest risk.[42] This study did show a drop in electricity-related deaths throughout the 10-year period. Another study conducted by the National Institute for Occupational Safety and Health (NIOSH) listed the following as high-risk scenarios that can lead to fatal electrocutions[43]:

A. Direct contact with an energized line (28%)
B. Direct contact with energized equipment (21%)
C. Boomed vehicle contact with an energized power line (18%)
D. Improperly installed or damaged equipment (17%)
E. Conductive equipment, typically metal ladders, making contact with energized power lines (16%)

In the United States, lightning injuries occur most frequently in the summer months of May to September. Again, males are more frequently affected than females. Texas and Florida account for the most U.S. lightning strike deaths.[8] There is no clear "safe space" from lightning, but there are ways to prevent lightning strikes. Being indoors during a thunderstorm is the safest place to be, but avoid running water from household faucets and stay away from doorways and windows. Avoiding high mountain peaks during afternoons in summer months is advised. If a person wishes to mountain climb during the summer, they are advised to be "up by noon, and down by two."[8]

References

References for this chapter are online only and can be found at https://connect.springerpub.com/content/reference-book/978-0-8261-6091-5/part/part04/toc-part/ch36.

37. Scuba Diving and Dysbarism

JASMINE JOHNSON

Learning Objectives

- Describe the physics behind barotrauma and mechanism of diving injuries.
- Evaluate patients for common diving-related ailments occurring during descent, at depth, and during ascent.
- Determine life-threatening injuries based on history and physical examination.
- Perform initial treatment, including resuscitation and stabilization, and escalate level of care, including transfer as needed.
- Explain diving safety and injury prevention methods to patients.

Humans have been diving for thousands of years. Technology has developed that allows us to descend deeper and remain underwater longer. The underwater environment is very different than what we experience on land, and physiologic effects and injuries related to submersion can occur. Collectively, these injuries are commonly referred to as dysbarism.

An important step in assessing a patient with injuries related to diving and dysbarism, as with any patient presentation, is to collect information about the mechanism of injury and symptoms experienced. Information especially useful for patients with diving emergencies includes the depth at which symptoms began, length of dive, and timing of ascent. Depending on patient condition on arrival, information-gathering may need to be done simultaneously with resuscitation. It is also important to remember that patients sustaining injury at depth may present with complaints related directly to their injury, or a secondary event related to the injury (i.e., a symptom of nitrogen narcosis is vertigo, which may cause the patient to become confused and have a drowning event).

Divers may also experience environmental injuries such as hypothermia, sunburn, trauma, drowning event, marine animal attack, or envenomation. The presentation, diagnosis, and management of these environmental injuries are discussed elsewhere within Section IV: Environmental Emergencies.

To understand the mechanisms by which diving injuries occur, one must have a basic understanding of the laws of physics that determine behavior of gasses. The pressure of gasses can be measured in many different units. In this chapter, pressure is referred to using atmospheres (atm), millimeters of mercury (mmHg), and feet of seawater (fsw) 1 atm = 760 mmHg; thus, for every 33 feet of depth gained in seawater, the pressure is increased by 1 atm (or 1 atm for every 34 feet of freshwater). If a diver at sea level (1 atm) descends to 66 feet of depth, the pressure exerted on the diver will now be 3 atm.

Injuries Occurring at Depth

Anatomy and Pathophysiology

A. Dalton's law states that the total pressure exerted by a mixture of gasses is equal to the sum of the partial pressures of each gas in the mixture.

B. Henry's law states that at equilibrium the amount of a gas that will dissolve in a liquid is proportional to the partial pressure of that gas.

C. Together, Dalton's and Henry's laws explain why divers breathing compressed air at depth have uptake of inert gasses into their tissues.

  1. At deeper depths/higher pressures, more gasses dissolve into solution in the blood and tissues.

  2. There are many factors that can affect the uptake of gas into the body, such as the mixture of compressed air the diver is breathing in and the length of time the diver is submerged at depths >100 fsw.

D. Nitrogen narcosis

  1. "Rapture of the deep" occurs when tissue nitrogen concentrations are increased enough to cause intoxicating effects similar to those seen in alcohol intoxication. Poor judgment can cause divers to put themselves in dangerous situations.

E. Cerebral oxygen toxicity

  1. Oxygen becomes toxic to the central nervous system (CNS) and lungs at elevated partial pressures; generally occurs at deep depths with short exposure.

F. Pulmonary oxygen toxicity

  1. Secondary to diving, condition is very uncommon, as it occurs with prolonged exposure at lower partial pressures.

G. Hypercarbia and carbon monoxide poisoning

  1. Another potential complication of diving includes contaminated air in the diver's tank, generally from carbon monoxide or carbon dioxide. See Chapters 45 to 47.

H. The exact mechanism by which immersion pulmonary edema occurs is not known but is noted to be more common in cold water, likely related to vasoconstriction and a subsequent increase in afterload. Hypertension is a risk factor for these patients.

Medical Screening

A. Nitrogen narcosis

1. *Chief complaint:* May vary, including motor or cognitive complaint

2. *Signs and symptoms:* Disorientation, impaired motor skills or mental process

3. *Physical examination:* Normal examination—symptoms resolve with ascent.

B. Oxygen toxicity (cerebral)

1. *Chief complaint:* Neurologic problem

2. *Signs and symptoms:* Paresthesia, vertigo, nausea, seizures

3. *Physical examination:* Vomiting, focal neurological abnormalities

C. Immersion pulmonary edema

1. *Chief complaint:* Difficulty breathing

2. *Signs and symptoms:* Dyspnea, cough

3. *Physical examination:* Frothy sputum, crackles, cyanosis, hypoxia

Differential Diagnoses

A. Symptoms of nitrogen narcosis worsen with increasing depth and should resolve with ascent. If a patient has persistent symptoms of nitrogen narcosis, alternative causes (e.g., decompression sickness [DCS], cerebral arterial gas embolism [CAGE], and contaminated air) should be explored.

B. It is important to obtain in history what type of air mixture the diver was breathing as this information will help narrow the differential. Some mixtures with a high fraction of oxygen can cause cerebral oxygen toxicity at relatively shallow depths.

Diagnostic Testing

A. Suspicion of pulmonary edema should be confirmed by chest x-ray (CXR).

Management

A. There is nothing to do for nitrogen narcosis, as it resolves with ascent. These patients should be educated about safe diving practices, as nitrogen narcosis can lead to a dive emergency.

B. Oxygen toxicity secondary to diving is managed no differently than oxygen toxicity occurring on land. Reduce exposure to high fractions of inhaled oxygen. If the patient seizes or loses consciousness underwater, priority is ascent and resuscitation.

C. Immersion pulmonary edema is treated like any other cause of pulmonary edema: diuresis and positive pressure ventilation.

Patient Disposition

A. *Discharge:* Patients being discharged must be clinically stable.

B. Transition of care information

1. Any patient with oxygen toxicity or pulmonary edema should be admitted for monitoring and treatment.

2. Handoff should include pertinent diving history, including any respiratory distress or neurological symptoms (seizures) reported in the field and treatments initiated.

C. Prevention and education

1. Due to the increased danger of nitrogen narcosis during deeper dives, compressed air should not be used for diving below 120 feet.

2. Do not dive alone; if your partner displays abnormal behavior, assist them with controlled ascent.

Injuries Occurring During Ascent

Anatomy and Pathophysiology

A. As a diver ascends to shallower depths, gasses in the bloodstream will come out of solution and expand.

1. With appropriate rate of ascent, gasses circulate back to the lungs and are exhaled before there is enough expansion or accumulation to cause damage.

2. If a diver ascends more rapidly than the body can accommodate, gas expansion can cause trauma to tissues and bubble formation can cause obstructive and inflammatory effects on body systems.

3. The U.S. Navy dive tables provide recommendations for ascent based on depth and length of dive, but even experienced divers can become disoriented at depth or experience other emergencies that force them to rise too quickly to the surface.

B. Alternobaric vertigo

1. Air in the middle ear expands during ascent and exits passively through the eustachian tube. If an obstruction such as mucosal edema or thickened eustachian tubes prevents equilibration, the increased pressure will cause alternobaric vertigo.

C. Large volume air expansion within body cavities can become problematic. In the gastrointestinal (GI) system, air expansion is usually benign but rarely can cause surgical emergencies such as hernia incarceration/strangulation or gastric rupture. Ascension with a closed glottis may cause pulmonary barotrauma. Expanding air may rupture a lung, causing pneumothorax, especially in shallow water. Overinflation and increased pressure in the chest cavity can also force air bubbles across the alveolar-capillary membrane. This air can dissect into the pulmonary tissues causing pneumomediastinum and subcutaneous emphysema. Ruptured alveoli may result in alveolar hemorrhage or lead to an arterial gas embolism (AGE).

D. AGE

1. Occurs secondary to diving when gas bubbles cross the alveolar-capillary membrane and enter the arterial bloodstream, causing a physical barrier to circulation.

2. Complications of AGE are related to where the occlusion occurs. Cerebral arterial gas embolism (CAGE) leads to stroke-like symptoms. AGE can also occur in other vessels, including the coronary arteries, causing arrhythmia or cardiac arrest.

E. Decompression sickness

1. Nitrogen gas that dissolves into blood and body tissues during a dive will come out of solution and form bubbles during ascent. An ascent that occurs too quickly for the body to accommodate these bubbles leads to a phenomenon called decompression sickness (DCS), in which these small bubbles cause inflammation that leads to thrombosis, obstruction, and ischemia. Like AGE, manifestations of DCS are related

to where the injury occurs and can be very nonspecific, so history is important in making this diagnosis. There are two types of DCS.

a. Type 1 is generally not life-threatening and involves only the joints, skin, and lymphatic system.

b. Type 2 can include the inner ear, spine, central nervous system (CNS), respiratory system, and circulatory system.

Predisposing Factors

A. Injuries related to ascent are generally secondary to an ascent that is too rapid. Inexperience, disorientation, panic, difficulty regulating buoyancy, or running out of air are frequently associated.

B. Asthma doubles the risk of pulmonary barotrauma.

C. AGE is one of the most common causes of death in divers.

D. Patent foramen ovale (PFO) is a risk factor for DCS.

Medical Screening (AGE, DCS)

A. Alternobaric vertigo

1. *Chief complaint:* Ear problem
2. *Signs and symptoms:* Vertigo nausea
3. *Physical examination:* Nystagmus vomiting

B. GI barotrauma

1. *Chief complaint:* Abdominal pain
2. *Signs and symptoms:* Bloating, cramping, flatulence
3. *Physical examination:* Abdominal distension, tenderness to palpation, +/- rebound, and guarding

C. Pulmonary barotrauma

1. *Chief complaint:* Chest pain breathing problem
2. *Signs and symptoms:* Dyspnea, chest pain, cough, neck or chest fullness, voice change, dysphagia
3. *Physical examination:* Hypoxia, hemoptysis, crepitus, abnormal or unilateral breath sounds

D. CAGE

1. *Chief complaint:* Neurologic problem
2. *Signs and symptoms:* Confusion, disorientation, dizziness, visual disturbances, headache
3. *Physical examination:* Altered mental status (AMS), focal neuro deficits, seizures, loss of consciousness, apnea

E. DCS Type 1

1. *Chief complaint:* Skin or joint complaint
2. *Signs and symptoms:* Joint or muscle pain, skin discoloration or rash, pruritis
3. *Physical examination:* Cutis marmorata (skin mottling), erythematous rash, lymphadenopathy, extremity edema

F. DCSs Type 2

1. *Chief complaint:* Varies
2. *Signs and symptoms:* Nausea, vertigo, paresthesias (generally progress distal to proximal), weakness or paralysis, incontinence, headache, visual disturbance, dyspnea, cough, chest pain
3. *Physical examination:* Vomiting, nystagmus, focal neuro deficit, loss of rectal tone, AMS, cyanosis, hypotension

Differential Diagnoses

A. Interstitial pulmonary emphysema is indicative of more severe pulmonary barotrauma.

B. AGE should also be considered in all patients who show signs of pulmonary barotrauma.

C. Any diver arriving unconscious should be assumed to have AGE and treated as such.

D. AGE symptoms have a sudden onset and occur during ascent or within 10 minutes of surfacing.

E. DCS manifestations generally occur within several hours of surfacing, but occasionally can take up to 24 hours. If the patient flies or continues to higher altitude, symptoms can occur days after a dive.

F. Inner ear DCS has very similar presentation to inner ear barotrauma but occurs on ascent rather than descent—history is key in distinguishing these disorders.

G. Types 1 and 2 DCS and AGE can all coexist, and presentation may be a mixed picture.

Diagnostic Testing

A. Patients with peritoneal signs (rebound tenderness, guarding) after diving should receive abdominal imaging, including chest/abdominal x-ray to look for free air, and possibly CT if rupture or incarcerated/strangulated hernia is suspected.

B. Chest x-ray (CXR) can indicate pneumothorax or pneumomediastinum. If CXR is negative but there is high clinical suspicion, consider CT.

C. Familiarity with bedside ultrasound (US) can be helpful in diagnosing GI rupture (eFAST [expanded Focused Assessment with Sonography in Trauma]) or pneumothorax (absent lung sliding).

D. AGE can sometimes be visualized on imaging including CT, but the air bubble may be reabsorbed so frequently only secondary signs may be seen. Because of this, diagnosis is primarily clinical and cannot be excluded based on negative test results.

E. Microbubbles in DCS can sometimes be visualized on imaging including CT and MRI, but these tests are not sensitive enough to exclude the diagnosis based on negative imaging alone.

F. Inflation of a blood pressure cuff over a painful joint in Type 1 DCS should relieve the pain but is not always a reliable test.

G. Patient with pulmonary DCS may show right ventricular (RV) strain on US and EKG.

Management

A. The symptoms of alternobaric vertigo are usually self-limited. Decongestants may help symptoms resolve sooner. Consider treatment for vertigo and nausea.

B. Patients with mild GI discomfort can be treated symptomatically for excess gas and cramping.

C. GI rupture patients should be monitored for hemodynamic instability and given broad-spectrum antibiotics. Surgery should be consulted for management.

D. Pulmonary barotrauma patients should receive high-flow 100% oxygen. High-flow oxygen can resolve pneumomediastinum or a small pneumothorax over time, but a larger pneumothorax (especially if associated with instable vital signs) should be managed with needle decompression and/or tube thoracostomy. All patients with pneumothorax should have the pneumothorax drained prior to recompression therapy.

E. Pneumomediastinum symptoms generally resolve within a few days. Rarely, pneumomediastinum may require intubation and a cardiothoracic surgery consult.
F. Patient with AGE or DCS should be treated as critical (airway, breathing, circulation [ABC]). Apply high-flow 100% oxygen and initiate recompression therapy as soon as possible.
G. Keep AGE patients in a horizontal position.
H. Lidocaine may have neuroprotective effects in CAGE patients, although dosing has not been standardized.

Patient Disposition

A. Discharge: Alternobaric vertigo patients should follow up with ear, nose, and throat (ENT).
B. Transition of care information
  1. Handoff should include pertinent diving history, condition on arrival, procedures, and treatments initiated.
  2. When transporting a patient with AGE or DCS via aircraft to a facility with hyperbaric capabilities, guidelines for altitude and cabin pressurization should be followed.
C. Prevention and education
  1. Asthmatics should be cleared for diving by a pulmonologist after having pulmonary function testing.
  2. Pregnant women should not scuba dive due to the increased risk of fetal DCS.

Injuries Occurring During Descent

Anatomy and Pathophysiology

A. During descent, gas contained in body cavities is compressed and the volume decreases.
B. The ears are often affected by this pressure change, which causes the tympanic membrane to bend inward.
  1. Valsalva maneuver: Performed by divers to equalize pressure in the inner ear.
    a. Involves forcing air through the eustachian tubes, but when this fails, injury to the tympanic membrane can occur (middle ear barotrauma).
  2. A similar phenomenon occurs when the external auditory canal is occluded by cerumen, causing the tympanic membrane to bend outward (external ear barotrauma).
C. Inner ear barotrauma
  1. Serious condition that is the result of an inward-bending tympanic membrane that causes damage to cochleovestibular structures.
  2. A history of injury that occurred during descent is an important part of differentiating inner ear barotrauma from other conditions with similar presentations, such as decompression sickness (DCS), cerebral arterial gas embolism (CAGE), and alternobaric vertigo (discussed later in this chapter).
  3. If the tympanic membrane bends to the point of rupture, cold water may flow in and induce panic. A diver who becomes disoriented and cannot surface may drown.
D. Air-filled spaces of the body (lungs, sinuses, middle ears, and bowel) are affected by changes in pressure as a diver changes depth.
E. Boyle's Law
  1. At constant temperature, the pressure (P) and volume (V) of gas are inversely proportional ($P_1 \times V_1 = P_2 \times V_2$).
  2. Boyle's Law also applies to gasses in breathing supplies, such as tanks, tubing, and masks. The amount of gas volume changes with descent and ascent and is greatest near the surface, so the risk of barotrauma is higher at shallow depths.
F. The same mechanism causing ear injury can also result in damage to other areas of the body. Barosinusitis occurs when the sinus ostia are occluded by mucosal thickening, pus, or structural abnormality (deviated septum, polyps and the sinus cavities cannot equalize during descent. Mucosal edema develops and, in some cases, sinus mucosa may be stripped from the bone. The opposite can happen during ascent (sometimes referred to as "reverse squeeze") as pressure increases in the sinuses, but this painful condition is generally self-limited. Facial barotrauma is the result of negative pressure within the mask that covers the diver's face and nose. This condition can be avoided by exhaling through the nose to equalize pressure within the mask. Dental barotrauma can occur during ascent or descent as air spaces at the roots of infected teeth or under a filling can contract or expand, causing pain. In rare cases, the change in air volume can cause a tooth to crack or damage a filling.

Predisposing Factors

A. Middle ear barotrauma is the most common injury associated with scuba diving.
B. Barosinusitis is the second most common injury associated with scuba diving.
C. Inner ear barotrauma is much less common than middle ear barotrauma but is associated with greater morbidity.

Medical Screening

A. External ear barotrauma
  1. *Chief complaint:* Ear problem
  2. *Signs and symptoms:* Otalgia
  3. *Physical examination:* External auditory canal hemorrhage, tympanic membrane hemorrhage
B. Middle ear barotrauma
  1. *Chief complaint:* Ear problem
  2. *Signs and symptoms:* Otalgia, reduced hearing, sensation of ear fullness
  3. *Physical examination:* Conductive hearing loss, tympanic membrane hemorrhage, hemotympanum
    a. Note: If the patient has a ruptured tympanic membrane, signs and symptoms may also include nausea, vertigo, visual difficulty, disorientation, facial heaviness, and inability to move facial muscles. Physical examination may also include transient nystagmus, vomiting, and facial nerve palsy.
C. Inner ear barotrauma
  1. *Chief complaint:* Ear problem
  2. *Signs and symptoms:* Sudden onset symptoms—unilateral tinnitus, sensation of ear fullness, nausea, vertigo

3. *Physical examination:* Sensorineural hearing loss, vomiting, nystagmus, ataxia

D. Barosinusitis
1. *Chief complaint:* Facial, sinus, or nose problem
2. *Signs and symptoms:* Facial or sinus pain, bleeding from nose
3. *Physical examination:* Mucosal edema, submucosal hemorrhage, epistaxis

E. Facial barotrauma
1. *Chief complaint:* Facial, nose, or eye problem
2. *Signs and symptoms:* Facial pain, sinus pressure, ophthalmalgia, visual changes
3. *Physical examination:* Facial petechiae, ecchymosis, and edema, sinus tenderness, conjunctival injection or hemorrhage, impaired extraocular movements, exophthalmos

F. Dental barotrauma
1. *Chief complaint:* Tooth problem
2. *Signs and symptoms:* Dentalgia, broken tooth
3. *Physical examination:* Structural damage to tooth or dental work, tooth or gingival tenderness, evidence of infection (e.g., fluctuance, induration, inflammation)

Differential Diagnoses

A. Onset of symptoms is during descent. History may include difficulty equilibrating.

B. Inner ear barotrauma can be difficult to distinguish from DCS (discussed in the following). If there is any concern for DCS, recompression therapy should be initiated immediately. Other differentials include CAGE and alternobaric vertigo.

Diagnostic Testing

A. Ear complaints should have audiometry performed.

B. Eye complaints should have visual acuity and intraocular pressure measured.

C. CT if sinus rupture is suspected

D. *Perilymph fistula test:* Pressure applied to the tympanic membrane via insufflation will cause contralateral nystagmus in some patients with inner ear barotrauma.

Management

A. Most treatment is symptomatic, including analgesia.

B. Damage or rupture to the tympanic membrane should be treated with prophylactic antibiotics with coverage of *Vibrio* bacteria; fluoroquinolones, Bactrim, or doxycycline are preferred. If symptoms are severe, decongestants and a steroid taper may be prescribed.

C. Patients with inner ear barotrauma should have urgent otolaryngology evaluation and recommendations for management, which may range from conservative bed rest to exploration of the inner ear. Meclizine can be given to control vertigo, and measures should be taken to reduce spikes in intracranial pressure (e.g., stool softeners, decongestants).

D. Patients with barosinusitis should receive decongestants and prophylactic antibiotics (e.g., Augmentin or azithromycin), as they are at high risk for developing bacterial sinusitis secondary to bleeding in the sinuses. Those with severe symptoms may also benefit from a course of prednisone, but ensure that the patient does not show symptoms of a bacterial infection prior to prescribing steroids.

E. Depending on the location of epistaxis, nasal packing may be useful. An otolaryngology consult is necessary if bleeding cannot be controlled. Observe the patient for airway compromise (see Chapter 3 for epistaxis management).

F. Dental barotrauma should be referred to a dentist. Patients with dental barotrauma secondary to infection should be started on antibiotics.

Patient Disposition

A. Discharge
1. Patients with inner ear barotrauma or ruptured tympanic membrane should be referred to as otolaryngology for formal audiometry, vestibular function testing, and follow-up.
2. Patients with dental pain, infection, or structural damage to the teeth should be referred to a dentist for management and follow-up.

B. Prevention and education
1. Any person who cannot equalize the pressure in their ears should avoid diving. The same applies to those who have had a recent upper respiratory infection (URI).
2. If a diver experiences symptoms of a ruptured tympanic membrane, he or she should avoid panic and slowly ascend to the surface of the water. The person should not dive again until cleared by a specialist.
3. Do not dive within 24 hours after a dental treatment.
4. Ear plugs, tight-fitting wetsuit hoods, and eye goggles should not be worn while diving to prevent injury to the ears or eyes.
5. Prophylaxis with pseudoephedrine 12 to 24 hours prior to a dive may reduce the instance of barotrauma. Antihistamines should not be taken prior to a dive.

Additional Reading

Additional Reading for this chapter are online only and can be found at https://connect.springerpub.com/content/reference-book/978-0-8261-6091-5/part/part04/toc-part/ch37.

38. Altitude Injuries and Conditions

JASMINE JOHNSON

Learning Objectives

- Describe the normal adaptation process that occurs after travel to high altitudes.
- Evaluate patients for high-altitude illness based on history and physical exam.
- Perform initial treatment, including resuscitation and stabilization, and escalate level of care including transfer as needed.
- Outline prevention of high-altitude illness for patients.

High-altitude travel and recreation are increasingly common in today's society. Travelers who do not live at high altitude and who ascend quickly without proper acclimatization are at risk for high-altitude illness. High-altitude illness includes a set of syndromes that can be directly attributed to the hypoxia that can result from exposure to lower barometric pressures found in high-altitude environments.

The concentration of oxygen in the environment is constant at 20.9% of the barometric pressure. As altitude increases, barometric pressure decreases, and the partial pressure of oxygen (PaO_2) decreases proportionally. For this reason, though the fraction is constant, air at higher altitudes contains fewer oxygen molecules than air at sea level.

Because oxygen supplementation has been shown to prevent symptoms of altitude illness and hypoxia at sea level does not cause symptoms of altitude illness, we can deduce that altitude illness is caused by the combination of hypoxia and hypobaria rather than each alone.

Some similar pathological entities exist at sea level such as hypoxic ischemic encephalopathy or negative pressure pulmonary edema, but it is the unique combination of low oxygen levels and very low pressures couple by an austere environment with few treatment options in a patient population under physical stress that can make the following problems difficult to address.

The body adapts to decreased PaO_2 at altitude initially by increasing ventilation, a process known as the hypoxic ventilatory response. Hyperventilation causes a respiratory alkalosis, in turn compensated for by decreased renal bicarbonate reabsorption, which improves this pH imbalance. The process of ventilatory acclimatization and renal compensation takes about 4 to 7 days to equilibrate. If a person continues to ascend into lower barometric pressures (and therefore lower PaO_2), the process continues. Additionally, decreased CO_2 levels with ascent to higher altitudes causes peripheral venous constriction and relative increases in central blood volume. Cardiac output and renal blood flow both increase, inducing diuresis, an effect balanced by the secretion of antidiuretic hormone (ADH) and aldosterone. This is considered a normal response to ascent.

Within hours of arrival at high altitude, erythropoietin secretion increases and stimulates increased production of new red blood cells. Long-term exposure leads to a decrease in total blood volume, plasma volume, and an increase in hemoglobin concentration and relative red blood cell mass (hematocrit).

An individual's response to changes in altitude depends on multiple factors, including preexisting medical conditions, altitude of origin, rate of ascent, and sleeping altitude. Cardiovascular and pulmonary diseases—such as congestive heart failure (CHF), coronary artery disease (CAD), and chronic obstructive pulmonary disease (COPD)—can be exacerbated by hypoxia. Individuals who have a poor respiratory drive, low vital capacity, inherently low hypoxic ventilatory response, or who suffer from sleep apnea or morbid obesity do not compensate as well for the lower oxygen levels at altitude and are at greater risk for developing altitude illness. While maintaining physical fitness can reduce comorbidities associated with altitude illness, physical fitness itself does not decrease the risk of developing altitude illness. High-altitude travel is contraindicated in those who have sickle cell anemia with history of crises, symptomatic pulmonary hypertension, severe COPD, or poorly controlled heart failure.

Gradual ascent is essential to preventing high-altitude illness, as this allows time for necessary physiologic changes to occur. Hypoxemia is greatest during sleep; therefore, an important factor to consider is sleeping altitude. It is recommended that the first night should not be spent at an altitude >9,200 feet (2800 m), and sleeping altitude should not increase by >1,600 feet (500 m) per day. Individuals who are residents of high-altitude environments are already partially acclimatized compared to those coming from lower altitude or sea level.

Other injuries common to high-altitude and mountainous environments include cold injuries (e.g., frostbite and hypothermia, see Chapter 34), trauma (Chapter 25), dehydration, sunburn (Chapter 35), and lightning injury (Chapter 36).

Acute Mountain Sickness

Pathophysiology

Acute mountain sickness (AMS) is the mildest form of altitude illness, typically characterized by headache plus one or more additional systemic symptoms. The exact pathophysiology is not fully understood but is likely related to increased cerebral blood flow and volume from hypoxemia, which can cause blood–brain barrier leakage, vasogenic edema, and increased intracranial pressure. Hypobaria also plays a role in the development of AMS but the mechanism is unclear. Additionally, individuals with altitude illness usually do not experience the typical diuresis that occurs with a gain in elevation. In these persons, hypoxemia leads to altered fluid homeostasis and antidiuresis, and generalized fluid retention may be noted.

Medical Screening

A. *Chief complaint:* May vary, can involve multiple body systems

B. *Signs and symptoms*

1. Headache
2. Fatigue
3. Anorexia/nausea/vomiting
4. Lightheadedness
5. Sleep disturbance

C. *Physical examination*

1. Typically normal examination without abnormal pulmonary or neurologic findings; infants may display increased fussiness and decreased appetite.

Prevalence

A. Approximately 20% of people who ascend to 2,500 meters and 40% who ascend to 3,000 meters will develop symptoms.

Medical Decision-Making and Differential Diagnoses

A. A diagnosis of AMS requires history of a recent rapid gain in altitude to 2,000 meters or higher.

B. Symptoms may develop within hours to days of arrival at altitude.

C. Headache alone does not indicate AMS.

D. Viral syndrome and excessive alcohol intake (hangover) can present with similar symptoms.

E. If serious illness with similar symptoms is suspected, descent is warranted to eliminate confounding factors.

Diagnostic Testing

A. There are no confirmatory diagnostic tests; however, the Lake Louise AMS self-report questionnaire can help classify severity of illness.

B. MRI may show vasogenic edema, but this has also been seen in patients without AMS, and the clinical significance of this finding is unclear.

Management

A. Symptoms generally resolve within 1 to 4 days.

B. Halting ascent allows the body to acclimatize and can prevent progression of illness.

C. Reduce exertion and provide supportive care with fluids, analgesics, and antiemetics as indicated. (Narcotic medications can reduce respiratory drive and should be avoided.)

D. Supplemental oxygen (1–2 L/min) may improve symptoms.

E. Follow evidence-based guidelines when prescribing.

1. Acetazolamide may improve symptoms by inducing renal bicarbonate diuresis, which causes metabolic acidosis; the body responds by increasing ventilation. The overall effect is decreased hypoxemia and decreased fluid retention. It also lowers cerebrospinal fluid (CSF) volume, which may help prevent and relieve symptoms.
2. Dexamethasone may improve symptoms by reducing inflammation, cerebral blood flow, and nausea.

F. Descent typically relieves symptoms rapidly.

G. Findings of ataxia or altered mental status indicate progression to high-altitude cerebral edema, addressed below in this chapter.

H. Dyspnea on exertion is typical at high altitude; dyspnea at rest is an early indication of high-altitude pulmonary edema (HAPE), addressed later in this chapter.

Patient Disposition

A. *Discharge*

1. Most patients with AMS are stable for discharge home.
2. Patients can resume ascent once AMS symptoms have resolved.
3. Discharged patients should understand that if symptoms worsen or do not resolve within the typical time frame, they should descend because they are at risk for developing more serious altitude illness.

B. *Prevention and education*

1. Patients who develop AMS are more likely to have symptoms again during repeated exposures to altitude.
2. As discussed earlier, gradual ascent and lower sleeping elevation are key to prevention.
3. Avoid opioids and heavy alcohol consumption, especially before sleep, as this can increase sleep hypoxemia.
4. Acetazolamide can be taken as prophylaxis for high-altitude illness but should always be avoided in patients with severe allergy to sulfa as there is a small risk of cross reactivity.
5. Use of dexamethasone for prophylaxis is controversial and should generally be used only by those who must make a rapid ascent (such as rescue personnel) and who are allergic to acetazolamide.
6. Supplemental oxygen can be cumbersome or expensive, but may be used to prevent development of AMS.

High-Altitude Cerebral Edema

Pathophysiology

High-altitude cerebral edema (HACE) is a progression from acute mountain sickness (AMS) to global encephalopathy. It is the least common but most severe form of altitude illness. Because it is on the same spectrum as AMS, the pathophysiology is the same. It is more common with longer duration at altitude and higher sleeping altitude.

Medical Screening

A. *Chief complaint*: Neurologic problem(s)
B. *Signs and symptoms*
  1. Headache
  2. Altered mental status
  3. Nausea and vomiting
C. *Physical examination*
  1. Lethargy, altered mentation, ataxia, coma; cranial nerve palsy, papilledema, and retinal hemorrhage may also be present.

Medical Decision-Making and Differential Diagnoses

A. Symptoms typically develop 1 to 4 days after arrival at altitude; however, delayed onset may occur as late as 9 days after ascent.
B. Concurrent high-altitude pulmonary edema (HAPE) may also be present.
C. Early signs include altered consciousness and cerebellar ataxia; the cerebellum is particularly sensitive to hypoxia.
D. Presence of seizures, focal neurologic deficits, fever, and meningismus are atypical for HACE and alternative diagnoses should be considered (such as stroke, encephalitis, meningitis, or intracranial bleeding).
E. Persistence of symptoms despite adequate treatment should prompt further evaluation.

Diagnostic Testing

A. CT or MRI imaging of the head may help evaluate for other causes.
B. MRI shows vasogenic edema correlating with symptoms.

Management

A. Follow evidence-based guidelines when prescribing.
  1. Steroids aid recovery and reduce residual neurologic deficits; patients should receive dexamethasone.
  2. Acetazolamide can also be added.
B. Illness can progress to coma or death within hours; prompt diagnosis and treatment is essential and ABCs (airway, breathing, circulation) should be prioritized, including intubation for airway protection as indicated.
C. Immediate descent is key to treatment; if descent is not immediately possible, patients should be given supplemental oxygen while waiting and placed in a portable hyperbaric bag if available.
D. Severe cases may require hyperbaric therapy, which simulates lower altitude by increasing barometric pressure within the chamber.
E. If moving the patient is not possible due to terrain or weather conditions, rescue personnel may be able to drop supplies such as oxygen or portable hyperbaric bag to help temporize the patient's condition.
F. All patients should receive high-flow oxygen, which reduces intracranial blood flow at high altitude.
G. Additional methods of lowering ICP such as hyperventilation, diuretics, and hypertonic solutions such as mannitol can be considered in severely ill patients with caution.
H. Duration of HACE can vary from hours to weeks or longer depending on severity.

Patient Disposition

A. *Admission*
  1. Patients with suspected or diagnosed HACE have high risk of deterioration and should be admitted for observation and treatment.
B. *Transition of care information*
  1. Depending on location, clinicians may be giving handoff to emergency medical services (EMS) for transport to lower altitude or receiving a patient from mountain rescue personnel.
C. *Prevention and education*
  1. Prevention methods are the same as for AMS, including gradual ascent and low sleeping elevation.
  2. Long-term neurologic deficits can occur after an episode of HACE.

High-Altitude Pulmonary Edema

Pathophysiology

High-altitude pulmonary edema (HAPE) is a noncardiogenic form of pulmonary edema that is responsible for the most deaths due to altitude illness. Lower partial pressure of oxygen at elevation causes increased pulmonary artery resistance and pulmonary hypertension. Severely high microvascular pressure can result in capillary wall damage and fluid leakage, causing interstitial and alveolar pulmonary edema. Uneven pulmonary vasoconstriction contributes to development of HAPE due to over perfusion of some areas of lung vasculature.

Strenuous exercise, cold stress, rapid ascent, and longer duration of visit are associated with HAPE. Most cases occur above 10,000 feet of elevation but can also occur at lower altitudes. Respiratory infection present during ascent increases susceptibility to HAPE, especially in children. Preexisting pulmonary hypertension from any cause significantly increases risk, and high-altitude travel should be avoided in these individuals or undertaken only with physician approval and preventative measures such as supplemental oxygen and prophylactic medications.

Medical Screening

A. *Chief complaint:* Respiratory problem
B. *Signs and symptoms*
  1. Shortness of breath
  2. Cough (initially dry, progresses to clear or bloody sputum)
  3. Fatigue

C. *Physical examination*

1. Low-grade fever, tachycardia, severe hypoxia (pulse oximetry frequently as low as 40%–70%), crackles/rales on lung exam, dyspnea at rest, increased work of breathing/respiratory distress, cyanosis

Medical Decision-Making and Differential Diagnoses

A. Symptoms typically develop 1 to 4 days after arrival at altitude.
B. Individuals can develop HAPE with or without preceding acute mountain sickness (AMS).
C. Chest x-ray (CXR) findings typical in cardiogenic pulmonary edema (batwing infiltrates, Kerley B lines, cardiomegaly) are absent in HAPE.
D. It can be difficult to differentiate between HAPE and pneumonia at high altitude; if there is any question about diagnosis, empiric antibiotics should be started in addition to HAPE treatment.
E. Pulmonary embolism (PE) should also be considered, as high altitude effects can cause hyperviscosity and hypercoagulability—risk is further increased by prolonged immobility during traveling and sometimes by sleeping in a restrictive sleeping bag.

Diagnostic Testing

A. CXR can show patchy infiltrates, usually bilateral with pleural effusion present in severe cases.
B. EKG may show evidence of right heart strain.
C. Ultrasound may provide additional evidence of pulmonary edema (B lines) and elevated pulmonary artery pressures.
D. Brain natriuretic peptide level and echocardiogram can evaluate for possible cardiac component of edema in patients with history or exam findings concerning for heart failure.

Management

A. As with high-altitude cerebral edema (HACE), illness can progress to coma or death within hours; prompt diagnosis and treatment are essential and ABCs (airway, breathing, circulation) should be prioritized, including intubation and positive pressure ventilation as indicated for severe hypoxemia or respiratory distress.
B. Immediate descent is key to treatment of severe HAPE; if descent is not immediately available, patients should be given supplemental oxygen (6–8 L/min) while waiting, if possible.
C. Severe cases may require hyperbaric therapy, which simulates lower altitude by increasing barometric pressure within the chamber.
D. If moving the patient is not possible due to terrain or weather conditions, rescue personnel may be able to drop supplies such as oxygen or portable hyperbaric bag to help temporize the patient's condition.
E. Supplemental oxygen administration increases rate of recovery by lowering pulmonary artery pressure and improving oxygenation; delivery by continuous positive airway pressure (CPAP) is more effective at clearing alveolar fluid than nasal cannula or nonrebreather.
F. Keep the patient warm and reduce activity; mild cases may resolve with bed rest alone.
G. Nifedipine at recommended dose every 12 hours can lower pulmonary artery pressure.
H. Phosphodiesterase inhibitors (such as sildenafil or tadalafil) can be used as an alternative agent to nifedipine, and have less risk of inducing systemic hypotension.
I. Inhaled beta agonists (such as salmeterol) can help clear alveolar fluid.
J. Diuretics should not be used in HAPE as they are not effective and can worsen systemic volume depletion
K. Digoxin and ACE inhibitors should not be used as the pathophysiology differs from typical pulmonary edema and these drugs provide no benefit in HAPE.
L. If treated promptly, symptoms generally resolve within 24 to 48 hours.

Patient Disposition

A. *Discharge*

1. Patients with mild to moderate cases treated without descent should have a period of observation for serial examinations to evaluate for progression of disease or alternative pathology, then if improving can be discharged with supplemental oxygen.

B. *Transition of care information*

1. Depending on location, clinicians may be giving handoff to EMS for transport to lower altitude or receiving a patient from mountain rescue personnel.
2. Patients who cannot maintain pulse oximetry levels acceptable for the current altitude should be admitted to the hospital.
3. Patients with a heart murmur on physical exam should undergo evaluation for cardiac structural anomalies that may have predisposed them to developing HAPE.

C. *Prevention and education*

1. Patients who develop HAPE will generally have symptoms again during repeated exposures to altitude.
2. Nifedipine, sildenafil, or tadalafil should be taken prophylactically during ascent by patients who have had prior HAPE.
3. Dexamethasone, inhaled salmeterol, and acetazolamide also have some evidence of utility in prevention of HAPE.
4. Discharged patients should be educated that if they are planning air travel, additional recovery time or supplemental oxygen is advised (standard cabin pressure is equivalent to approximately 8,000 feet of elevation).

Additional Reading

Additional Reading for this chapter are online only and can be found at https://connect.springerpub.com/content/reference-book/978-0-8261-6091-5/part/part04/toc-part/ch38.

39. Drowning Injuries

MARISA LOSAVIO

Learning Objectives

- Explain the pathophysiology of drowning or submersion injury on the body.
- Identify signs and symptoms of a patient following a drowning event.
- Identify potential differential diagnoses for a patient who presents to the emergency department (ED) incapacitated.
- Use evidence-based guidelines to provide a comprehensive evaluation of a drowning trauma, including the patient's physical and cognitive state.
- Use an evidence-based algorithm do determine treatment of drowning patients, including diagnostic therapy, pharmacologic therapy, and procedures.
- Provide a safe disposition plan for a well, asymptomatic patient and transition of care of ill patients to inpatient setting.
- Develop preventative educational resources for at-risk groups.

Drowning is submersion into a liquid medium resulting in respiratory difficulty or respiratory arrest. Drowning occurs in people of all ages and backgrounds.

According to the Centers for Disease Control and Prevention (CDC), about 10 people die each day from unintentional drowning.

It ranks fifth among the leading causes of unintentional deaths in the United States.

Pathophysiology

A. During a drowning event, after submersion, the degree of hypoxic insult to the central nervous system (CNS) will determine the severity of injury and outcome to a patient.

B. When unexpected submersion occurs, it triggers breath holding, panic, and a struggle to get to the surface resulting in air hunger and hypoxia.

1. Breath holding eventually becomes overcome by laryngospasm, resulting in involuntary gasps causing aspiration of large quantities of water.
2. The amount of fluid that is aspirated, not composition, will determine the eventual pulmonary derangement.

C. Multiple factors influence the pathophysiology sequence after submersion events and affect the chance of survival including the following:

1. Age
2. Water temperature
3. Duration
4. Degree of hypothermia
5. Resuscitative efforts

D. Brain resuscitation after significant warm water drowning has been dismal, whereas recovery after asystole in cold water, though rare, is more likely.

E. Drowning in cold water (below 5°C or 41°F) leads to rapid hypothermia, which slows cerebral metabolism.

1. This postpones the effects of anoxia, which is associated with better prognosis.

F. Most importantly, asystole, either on location of drowning or in the ED, is a universal sign of poor prognosis.

Predisposing Factors

A. *Age:* Toddlers and older teenagers

B. *Sex:* Males more commonly

C. Race

1. Drowning rate for American Indians/Alaska Natives was twice the rate for Whites and the rate for African Americans was 1.4 times the rate for Whites. Black children ages 11 to 12 drown in a swimming pool at 10 times the rate of White children, and the greatest disparities were in swimming pools with swimming pool drowning rates were 5.5 times higher among Blacks aged 5 to 19 than that of the rate of Whites.[1]

D. Lack of swimming ability

E. Lack of barriers such as pool fencing

F. Lack of close supervision

G. Abuse (intentional drowning)

H. Failure to wear life jackets

I. Acute ethanol intoxication or other intoxicants

J. Seizure disorders

K. Syncope

L. Autism, behavioral issues, dementia

M. Prolonged QT syndrome as cold water extends QT interval

N. Cold versus warm water drowning

Medical Screening

A. *Chief complaint:* Respiratory distress after submersion event

1. Obtain details surrounding the event rapidly.

B. *Signs and symptoms*

1. Pulmonary injury noted by hypoxia, cyanosis, respiratory distress/arrest
2. Hypotension, shock, cardiac arrest
3. Tachypnea, audible rhonchi, rales, or wheezes

4. Pink froth from the mouth and nose, which would indicate pulmonary edema
5. Gastric distention secondary to aspiration and positive pressure ventilation
6. Vomiting
7. Hypothermia
8. Altered mental status (AMS) ranging from mild lethargy, semiconscious, unconscious to coma with fixed and dilated pupils
9. Decerebrate or decorticate posturing in comatose patients
10. Cardiac dysrhythmias, bradycardia, and tachycardia
11. Acute renal impairment as result of lactic acidosis/prolonger hypoperfusion
12. Coagulopathy (including disseminated intravascular coagulation) as result of hypothermia
13. Significant aspiration would predispose to development of acute respiratory distress syndrome (ARDS).

Physical Examination

A. Assess and secure airway
   1. Provide oxygenation, endotracheal intubation, and ventilatory support as necessary.
B. General and neurological
   1. Assess mental status, including Glasgow Coma Scale (GCS) score; assess pupils including reactivity.
C. Cardiac
   1. Assess for hypotension, arrhythmia, brady/tachycardia, hemodynamic stability.
D. Respiratory
   1. Assess for tachypnea, abnormal lung sounds.
E. Trauma survey should always be considered.

Differential Diagnoses

A. Drug (possible overdose) or alcohol intoxication
B. Cardiac arrest
C. Hypoglycemia
D. Seizure
E. Attempted suicide or homicide
F. Child abuse/neglect

Diagnostic Testing

A. Cardiac monitoring/electrocardiogram
B. Pulse oximetry, capnography
C. Core temperature with rectal temperature monitoring
D. Arterial blood gas (ABG)
E. Blood glucose
F. Serum creatinine
G. Electrolyte values (sodium, potassium, calcium, and magnesium)
H. Toxicologic screen
I. Liver function panel
J. Chest radiograph: may show aspiration of fluid initially, whereas late findings may include pulmonary edema or (ARDS)
K. Head/spine CT scan if indicated for trauma

Management

A. *Procedures*
   1. See Figure 39.1.
   2. Remove wet clothing, dry off, apply warming adjuncts to hypothermic patients.
      i. Blankets, warming devices, warm IV fluids
   3. Resuscitation of pulselessness and apneic patients
   4. Continuous cardiac monitoring and pulse oximetry
   5. Monitor core temperature
   6. Determination of oxygenation and ventilation to determine necessity of tracheal intubation
   7. Oxygen via face or nasal mask in awake patients as tolerated
   8. Patients with significant submersion injury typically benefit from mechanical ventilation, as super normal levels of positive end-expiratory pressure (PEEP) may be used to recruit fluid filled lungs and aid oxygenation.
   9. Hypothermia with cardiac arrest is an indication for extracorporeal rewarming and ECMO (extracorporeal membrane oxygenation).

Pharmacologic Therapies

A. Largely supportive care
B. Administration of corticosteroids does not improve outcome.
C. Induced coma and neuromuscular blockade do not improve neurological outcome.
D. Empirical antibiotics only to patients who were submerged in grossly contaminated water or who show signs of infection/sepsis
E. Efforts to control cerebral edema including use of mannitol, loop diuretics, hypertonic saline, and fluid restriction have not shown benefit.
F. May consider administration of naloxone if overdose is suspected

Consultation and Collaboration

A. May require immediate critical care consultation for management and admission for respiratory complications related to submersion injury
B. Submersion injury related to trauma may require consultation from trauma/acute care surgery or neurosurgery as indicated.

Patient Disposition

A. Asymptomatic patients on arrival to ED, who have no chest x-ray (CXR) or arterial blood gas abnormality, can be observed for 6 hours then discharged.
B. Asymptomatic to mildly symptomatic drowning victims should be observed for 4 to 6 hours.
C. If patients are asymptomatic, they should be monitored closely and observed for an 8-hour period and admitted if there is any deterioration or change in physical exam. If vital signs, pulse oximetry, pulmonary examination, CXR all remain normal, they can be discharged with appropriate follow-up. Verbal and written discharge instructions should be given regarding any respiratory or other problems, and if it is a pediatric patient they must be accompanied by a responsible adult.[3]
D. Admit symptomatic patients or those with history of apnea, unconsciousness, hypoxia, dysrhythmia, or abnormal CXR.

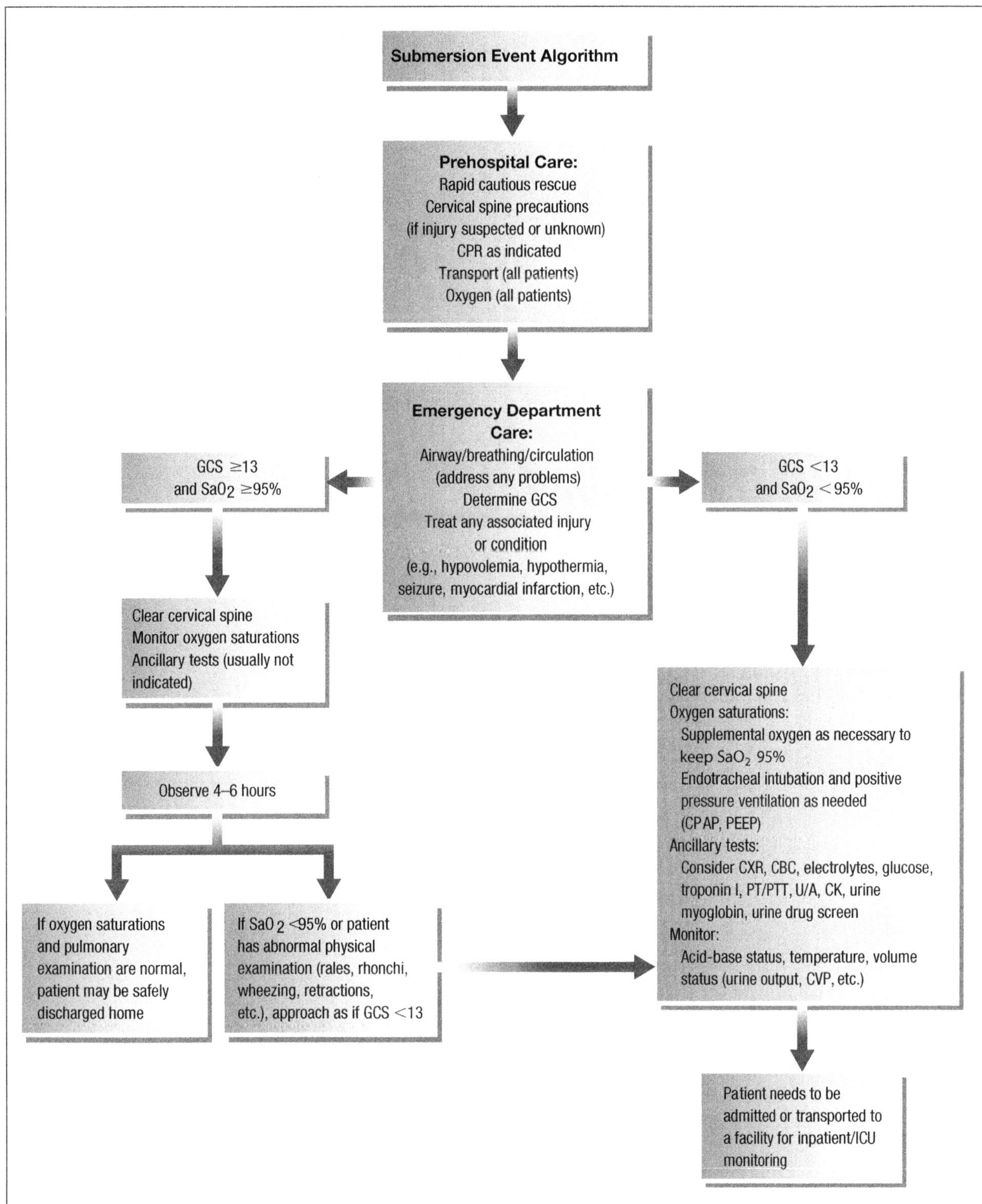

FIGURE 39.1 Algorithm for the treatment of a submersion event.
GCS, Glasgow Coma Scale.
Source: From Cydulka RK, Cline DM, John Ma O, et al. *Tintinalli's Emergency Medicine Manual.* 8th ed. McGraw-Hill Education; 2017.[2]

E. Patients who require ED resuscitation should be admitted to ICU for continuous cardiopulmonary and neurological monitoring.
F. Cerebral death cannot be diagnosed until core temperature reaches 32°C to 35°C.
G. If patient is normothermic upon arrival to ED and in cardiopulmonary arrest/asystole, considering discontinuing resuscitation efforts as recovery without profound neurologic complication is rare.
H. Discharge instructions
   1. Careful instructions about signs and symptoms of delayed pulmonary complications and strict return precautions including respiratory distress
   2. Careful instructions about signs and symptoms of delayed head injury complications and strict return precautions including headache, nausea, vomiting, and altered mental status (AMS)
   3. Include prevention and education tips
I. Transition of care information
   1. Summary of care including any information or details from the submersion injury, care given prehospital and in the ED
   2. Findings from all diagnostic studies completed
   3. Current status, including hemodynamic stability and vital signs.

Age and Developmental Considerations

A. Children may only be discharged to a competent adult.
B. Older adults have increased risk of bathtub drowning, related to comorbidities and medication use.
C. Toddlers primarily drown after falling into swimming pools or open water, but also in bathtubs or buckets at home.
D. Must assess for intentional drowning in young children as an act of child abuse.
E. Must assess for intentional drowning in teenagers as suicide/homicide/domestic abuse.
F. Prevention and education
   1. Emphasis on public education of CPR.
   2. Education on risks of danger of ethanol use in conjunction with water-related activities.
   3. Parent education on adequate supervision of children playing in or near water.
   4. Adequate and fully circumferential fencing around residential pools.
   5. Life jackets can be used to reduce risk in drowning's associated with boat activities.
   6. Educate on importance of never swimming alone, and swimming in places that have a lifeguard on duty.
   7. Include extra safety precautions for those swimming with medical comorbidities (e.g., seizures).

References and Additional Reading

References and Additional Reading for this chapter are online only and can be found at https://connect.springerpub.com/content/reference-book/978-0-8261-6091-5/part/part04/toc-part/ch39.

40. Radiation Injuries

M. ALLEN MCCULLOUGH

Learning Objectives

- Identify and describe the four types of ionizing radiation particles and characteristics of penetration.
- Discuss how ionizing radiation interferes with cellular function.
- Identify common complaints resulting from ionizing radiation exposure.
- Identify diagnostic test to consider in the presentation of ionizing radiation exposure.
- Explain nonpharmaceutical therapies for ionizing radiation illness.
- Summarize pharmaceutical therapies for ionizing radiation illness.
- Determine admission criteria for ionizing radiation illness.

Historically, devastating consequences have resulted from both incidental releases of nuclear materials and intentional releases such as those that may occur in acts of war. However, radiation exposures may occur in the absence of major releases of nuclear materials. Radiation is the emission or propagation of energy in the form of waves or particles through a material medium, such as the body. Radiation may be natural or manmade and may cause local or systemic damage to body tissues based on such factors as radiation type, dose, nature, and time of exposure countered by the nature of shielding. Exposures may occur accidentally or intentionally.

Pathophysiology

Types of Ionizing Radiation

A. Alpha particles are helium nuclei that are not capable of penetrating the skin beyond a shallow depth.
B. Beta particles are high-energy electrons that penetrate the skin causing damage into the dermal and subcutaneous tissues.
C. Neutrons are neutral particles with variable penetration and are capable of emitting alpha and beta particles as well as gamma rays.
D. Gamma rays are short-wavelength electromagnetic rays capable of penetrating deep into internal tissues and organs.[1]

Measurements of Radiation

A. The roentgen (R) measures the ionizing ability of rays in air.
B. The radiation absorbed dose (RAD) is the energy absorbed per unit of mass.
C. The roentgen equivalent in man (REM) is the RAD dose mathematically corrected by a quality factor.[1]

Types of Exposure

A. Irradiation is exposure to radiation but not to radioactive materials.
B. Contamination is retention of a radioactive material, usually in the form of liquid or dust on or inside the body that poses continued risk to the patient and may present risk to others in the patient's immediate surroundings.[1]

Pathology

A. Ionizing radiation interferes with cellular proliferation, denatures proteins, and may result in cellular death.
  1. Effects are variable to the radiosensitivity of the involved tissue and influenced by the nature of the irradiation as well as the dose, duration, and time of exposure and the effectiveness of shielding.
  2. Undifferentiated cells and tissues with high metabolic rate are most vulnerable to radiation insult.[1]

B. Children and unborn infants are particularly susceptible to radiation insult.[2]
C. Localized exposure causes radiation burn injury, whereas generalized whole-body exposure may cause systemic dysfunction known as acute radiation syndrome (ARS).
  1. While severe exposures may result in rapid death, ARS generally occurs in stages that may include a prodromal phase, a latent phase, and illness phase, and an outcome that may be death or recovery.
  2. The prodromal phase is characterized by acute inflammation and lasts for up to 48 hours.
  3. The latent phase is characterized by resolution of the inflammatory response and may last for up to 2 weeks.
  4. The illness phase is characterized by variable systemic dysfunction that may result in single or multisystem organ failure.
  5. Infection is the most common etiology of delayed death, but recovery with variable chronic effects is possible.[2]

Medical Screening

A. *Chief complaints:* Burn insult, nausea and vomiting, weakness, altered mental status, fever, diarrhea, bleeding, hair loss

B. *Signs and symptoms*

1. *Local exposure:* Erythema, blisters, tissue necrosis

2. *Systemic exposure:* Nausea, vomiting, fever, diarrhea, altered mentation, generalized weakness, bleeding, hair loss

C. *Medical history:* History of exposure

Focused Assessment

A. *General:* Evaluate for radiation using a Geiger counter (available from radiology or nuclear medicine department).

B. *Skin:* Hair loss, poor wound healing

C. Eyes

D. Ears, nose, throat

E. Neck

F. *Cardiac:* Weakness, low blood pressure

G. Pulmonary

H. *Neurological:* Dizziness, disorientation, fever, headache, fatigue

I. *Gastrointestinal/genitourinary:* Nausea and vomiting, diarrhea, loss of appetite

Differential Diagnoses

A. *Skin injury:* Chemical burn, ischemic ulcer, brown recluse spider bite, pyoderma gangrenosum

B. Leukopenia, hematologic malignancy, immunosuppression, HIV

C. Exposure to chemical warfare agents or other toxins

Diagnostic Testing

A. Complete blood count (CBC) with differential q4–6h until stable

B. Absolute lymphocyte count

C. Nasal swabs to detect contaminants

D. Type and crossmatch

E. 24-hour stool and/or urine for radioassay if internal contamination is suspected

F. Diagnostic imaging

G. Whole-body gamma camera

H. Cytogenetics (draw 24 hours postexposure into lithium-heparin tube or EDTA tube)

Management

A. *Nonpharmacologic therapies*

1. Utilize appropriate personal protection.

2. Remove clothing and decontaminate with soap and water (priority areas: wounds, mucous membranes, intact skin).

3. Minimize staff exposure.

4. Assess patient contamination, external and internal.

5. Treat life threats.

B. *Pharmacologic therapies*

1. Antiemetic therapy for nausea and vomiting; consult most current evidence-based guidelines and recommendations for ondansetron.

2. Isotonic IV fluids for rehydration

3. Decorporation agents appropriate to the specific radionucleotide

4. Cytokines and transfusion for exposures exceeding 200 RAD

5. Potassium iodide (if within 4 hours of contamination)

C. *Consultation/collaboration*

Patient Disposition

A. *Admission criteria*

1. Lymphocyte count $<1,000$ or decreased by 50% at 24 to 48 hours postexposure

2. Suspected acute exposure >200 RAD

3. Significant trauma or other illness

4. Uncontrolled vomiting

B. *Discharge criteria*

1. No residual contamination

2. No evidence of acute exposure >100 RAD

3. Tolerates oral fluids

Age and Developmental Considerations

A. Pregnant caregivers should be excused from caring for potentially contaminated patients.

Resources

National Library of Medicine's Radiation Emergency Medical Management (REMM) website Online, downloadable, and mobile apps. http://www.remm.nim.gov/

Centers for Disease Control and Prevention. Emergency preparedness and response: radiation emergencies. http://www.bt.cdc.gov/radiation/

Oak Ridge Institute for Science and Education. Radiation emergency assistance center/training site (REAC/TS). http://orise.orau.gov/reacts/

References

References for this chapter are online only and can be found at https://connect.springerpub.com/content/reference-book/978-0-8261-6091-5/part/part04/toc-part/ch40.

V. Toxicology, Overdose Management, Substance Use Disorder

41. Approach to the Poisoned Patient

VICKI BACIDORE | MICHAEL D. GOOCH

Learning Objectives

- Recall the essential aspects of the history and physical examination when evaluating the suspected poisoned patient.
- Identify essential diagnostic studies that should be considered when evaluating the suspected poisoned patient.
- Recall the importance and types of decontamination that can be used when managing the suspected poisoned patient.
- Utilize practice guidelines to develop a management and patient education plan.
- Utilize evidence-based practices to develop a plan for referral, consultation, or transition of care.

Poisoning is the leading cause of injury death in the United States with both illicit and pharmaceutical drugs causing the majority of poisoning deaths. According to the Centers for Disease Control and Prevention's National Center for Health Statistics (NCHS) Provisional Overdose Death Count, 70,237 persons died from drug overdoses in 2017, with opioids as the main driver of drug overdose deaths.[1]

Most adult presentations to the ED acutely for poisoning are due to drug overdoses. Over 5 million ED visits annually are associated with drug abuse or misuse.[2] Other toxicological presentations include accidental poisonings in children, exposures from chemicals or the environment, adverse medication reactions, and envenomation.[3]

The clinical effects of poisoned patients depend on a number of different factors, including the dosage, the length of time exposed to an agent, and the comorbidities of a patient. If poisoning can be recognized early, and appropriate treatment is rendered, the patient can have a positive outcome.

In caring for the poisoned patient, it is recommended that the regional poison control center be consulted. The poison control center can be contacted through the centralized phone number of the American Association of Poison Control Centers (AAPCC), 800-222-1222. The poison center is staffed 24/7 by a medical toxicologist who can provide emergent consultation, including real-time recommendations for diagnostic testing, emergency treatment, and monitoring.[4] The initial approach to managing the poisoned patient in the ED is based on patient assessment, toxidromes, diagnostics, resuscitation, stabilization, and supportive care.

General Approach to Overdose and Poisonings

Assessment

A. History
  1. Acute poisoning should be considered in patients who have an altered mental status, are unresponsive, or if they have unexplained respiratory, cardiovascular, or metabolic problems.
  2. Focus on key elements of the history from the patient, family members, friends, witnesses, or emergency medical services clinicians, including:
    a. The pharmaceutical agent(s) or toxin(s) ingested and any co-ingestions or alcohol
    b. The quantity of the agent ingested
    c. The time since ingestion
    d. Route of exposure
      i. Oral ingestion
      ii. Inhaled, snorted, or smoked
      iii. Dermal contact
      iv. Injected or parenteral
      v. Ocular exposure
      vi. Rectal or vaginal
    e. A history of any toxic effects or symptoms from the poisoning
    f. Events prior to ED presentation
    g. Any suicidal ideation
  3. Corroborate the history in an alert and cooperative patient but understand that information may be inaccurate or incomplete.[5]
  4. Consider other useful sources of information:
    a. Prior medical records
    b. Online prescription drug monitoring programs
    c. The pharmacy the patient uses
    d. The prescribing clinician's name listed on medication bottles
    e. Counting the number of pills in bottles
    f. Using resources to identify unknown tablets[3]
  5. Inquire about other mechanisms of possible exposure, including occupational (chemicals, pesticides, acids, heavy metals, and carbon monoxide) or a bioterrorism or other environmental event.[6]

TABLE 41.1 VITAL SIGNS AND CORRESPONDING TOXINS TO CONSIDER

VITAL SIGNS	TOXINS TO CONSIDER
Hyperthermia	Aspirin, cocaine, anticholinergics
Hypothermia	Opioids, sedatives
Hypertension	Stimulants, tricyclics, antihistamines
Hypotension	Antihypertensives, opioids
Tachycardia	Stimulants, vasodilators, anticholinergics
Bradycardia	Beta-blockers, calcium channel blockers, clonidine, digoxin
Tachypnea	Aspirin, amphetamines, carbon monoxide
Bradypnea	Narcotics, clonidine, alcohol

B. Physical examination

1. A detailed physical exam is secondary to immediate resuscitation and stabilization. A brief, focused exam can provide diagnostic clues that may suggest specific toxic agents.

2. Assessment of vital signs, neurological status, pupils, and respiratory/cardiac and gastrointestinal systems may point to toxicity from a category of poisons. See Table 41.1.[7]

3. When examining an unresponsive patient, it is important to consider possible concomitant conditions, such as central nervous system (CNS) infections, trauma, and intracranial pathology.[3]

4. General appearance

a. Examine patient and clothing for any pill bottles, needles, alcohol, patches, and drug paraphernalia.

b. Observe the general state of health of the patient, dress, hygiene, and affect.

c. Note any unusual odors that may suggest a diagnosis.

i. Fruity odors may be caused by ethanol, isopropyl alcohol, chlorinated hydrocarbons, or acetone.

5. Skin

a. Remove all clothing.

b. Assess skin for:

i. Color, temperature, and moisture

ii. The presence of bites (envenomation), rashes, and bullous lesions

iii. Check for medication patches.

iv. Observe for track marks in the antecubital fossa of the upper extremities.

(1) Less common areas such as sublingual and the dorsum of the feet

6. Neurologic

a. A systematic neurologic exam is essential if altered mental status:

i. Pupils, cranial nerve assessment sensation, strength, reflexes, and cerebellar function

ii. The Alert/Verbal/Painful/Unresponsive (AVPU) scale and Glasgow Coma Scale (GCS) can be obtained for baseline and trending neurological status.

7. Respiratory

a. Depending on the poisoning, patients can present to the ED unresponsive and at risk for airway obstruction and aspiration.

b. Control airway and provide high flow 100% oxygen if necessary.

c. Consider intubation early.

i. Many agents affect the patient's respiratory status, which can result in bronchospasm, pulmonary edema, hypoxia, and respiratory failure.

ii. Assessment of the patient's work of breathing and lung sounds is essential.

8. Cardiovascular

a. Various agents can affect hemodynamics as well as cardiac rhythm and intervals.

b. Many agents cause tachycardia.

c. Bradycardia can be caused by beta-blockers and calcium channel blockers.

d. Tricyclic antidepressants can cause QRS widening, and QT prolongation.

9. Gastrointestinal

a. Bowel sounds may be altered if the patient has ingested an agent that affects the cholinergic nervous system.

b. Melena or hematochezia could indicate anticoagulant toxicity.

c. Inspect the rectum and vagina for packets of illicit substances such as cocaine, heroin, or amphetamines which can rupture.

i. "Body packers" swallow or insert drug-filled packets into a body cavity for smuggling or evading law enforcement.

ii. Can lead to life-threatening bowel obstruction, perforation or toxicity if these packets rupture in the gastrointestinal tract.

Toxidromes

A. Toxidromes are a grouping of agents according to the signs and symptoms that they produce in a patient.

B. They can be useful in the identification of unknown agents and can direct initial patient treatment, but often times there are multiple drug ingestions and patient comorbidities that may alter a patient's presentation and do not point to a clear toxidrome.[7,8] See Table 41.2.

Diagnostics

A. Serum glucose and electrolyte levels are the two most indicated lab tests in the management of poisoned patients.[9]

B. Complete blood count (CBC)

C. Comprehensive metabolic profile (CMP)

1. If the serum bicarbonate is low, make the calculation to determine whether there is an elevated anion gap.

2. Anion gap metabolic acidosis can be considered using the mnemonic: GOLD MARK. This acronym represents, Glycols (ethylene and propylene), Oxoproline, L-lactate, D-lactate, Methanol, Aspirin, Renal failure, and Ketoacidosis.[10]

D. Coagulation studies

E. Serum osmolality and osmolar gap

F. Salicylate level

TABLE 41.2 SUMMARY OF TOXIDROMES AND CORRESPONDING SIGNS/SYMPTOMS

TOXIDROME	SIGNS/SYMPTOMS	AGENTS
Anticholinergic	("Hot as a hare, dry as a bone, red as a beet, mad as a hatter, blind as a bat.") Agitation, dry mucous membranes, flushed/dry/hot skin, blurred vision, hallucinations, mydriasis, tachycardia, urinary retention, constipation, seizures, and decreased bowel sounds	Diphenhydramine, antihistamines, atropine, antipsychotics, baclofen, phenothiazines, Jimson weed, tricyclic antidepressants
Cholinergic	SLUGBAM (salivation, lacrimation, urination, GI distress (diarrhea/vomiting), bronchorrhea/bronchospasm/bradycardia, abdominal cramps, miosis), sweating, muscle weakness, and muscle fasciculations	Organophosphates, pilocarpine, carbamates, muscarinic mushrooms, bioterrorism
Ethanolic	*Early:* Mild CNS depression, abdominal pain *Late:* Visual blurring/blindness, hypotension, hypopnea, seizures, flank pain, hematuria, oliguria, coma	Methanol, ethylene glycol
Hallucinogenic	Anxiety, dysphoria, hallucinations, hyperthermia, mydriasis	LSD, PCP, ketamine
Hypoglycemic	Altered mental status, diaphoresis, tachycardia, hypertension, seizures, slurred speech	Insulin, sulfonylureas
Opioid	CNS and respiratory depression, confusion, somnolence, coma, shallow respirations, bradypnea, bradycardia, hypotension, hypothermia, decreased bowel sounds, hyporeflexia, and miosis	Clonidine, codeine, buprenorphine, heroin, methadone, morphine, meperidine, hydromorphone, hydrocodone, oxycodone, fentanyl, tramadol
Salicylate	Tinnitus, hearing loss, dizziness, nausea, vomiting, tachypnea, hyperpyrexia, diaphoresis, ataxia, anxiety, altered mental status, seizure, cardiac arrhythmias, renal failure, acute lung injury, shock	Aspirin, acetylsalicylic acid
Sedative/hypnotic	Sedation–with progressive CNS depression and minimal or no respiratory depression, ataxia, delirium, hallucinations, hypotension, bradycardia, nystagmus, hyporeflexia, decreased bowel sounds, miosis or mydriasis	Anticonvulsants, benzodiazepines, barbiturates, ethanol, methocarbamol, propoxyphene, trazodone, zolpidem, zaleplon, eszopiclone
Serotonin	Altered mental status, fever, tremor, shivering, agitation, hyperreflexia, diaphoresis, ataxia, diarrhea	SSRI (fluoxetine, sertraline, paroxetine, fluvoxamine, citalopram), SRI (venlafaxine, nefazodone, mirtazapine
Sympathomimetic	Excessive speech, restlessness, tremor, insomnia, anorexia, hyperreflexia, seizures, hallucinations, rhabdomyolysis, tachycardia, hypertension, hyperactive bowel sounds, diaphoresis	Amphetamines, methamphetamine, caffeine, cocaine, ephedrine, LSD, methylphenidate, nicotine, PCP

CNS, central nervous system; GI, gastrointestinal; LSD, lyseric acid diethylamide; PCP, phencyclidine, SRI, serotonin reuptake inhibitor; SSRI, selective serotonin reuptake inhibitor

G. Acetaminophen level
   1. Serum acetaminophen level should be ordered in all poisoned patients.
   2. Early acetaminophen poisoning can exhibit without symptoms.
   3. There is no identifiable toxidrome when antidotes are efficacious.
   4. Order in patients with altered mental status, suspicion for self-harm, or when unable to obtain a complete history.[7]

H. Other labs
   1. Arterial blood gas (ABG) analysis
   2. Troponin level
   3. Creatine kinase
   4. Serum ethanol levels
   5. Specific drug levels
   6. Urine pregnancy for all women of child-bearing age

I. Urine drug screen
   1. False-positive screens can result with amphetamines as they are present in many other drugs, such as ephedrine, pseudoephedrine, ranitidine, trazodone, and chlorpromazine.
   2. A positive initial result may not be able to pinpoint the drug causing the acute poisoning as some drug detection levels do not produce clinical effects.
      a. Certain "designer" drugs (benzodiazepine metabolites, amphetamines) made in labs and frequently sold over the internet may result in a false-negative result due to the inability to detect certain drugs.[11]
      b. General toxicology screening tests have limitations as they are nonspecific, using enzyme-immunoassays that only detect typical classes of drugs.
         i. Opioid screens do not detect meperidine.
         ii. Assays are cross-reactive.
            (1) Pseudoephedrine tests positive for amphetamines and carbamazepine tests positive for tricyclic antidepressants.[12]

J. Diagnostic imaging can be useful in diagnosis confirmation, monitoring gastrointestinal decontamination, and identifying complications of exposure.
   1. Conventional radiography is used most often in the ED, but CT, ultrasound, transesophageal echocardiography (TEE), MRI, angiography, and PET can be used.
   2. An abdominal CT may reveal the presence of elongated packets of body packers.[8]
   3. Agents that are most likely to be revealed on plain radiographs are chlorinated hydrocarbons, heavy

metals, salicylates, enteric-coated drugs, iodinated compounds, and packets of drugs.[13]

K. Electrocardiograms are diagnostic for patients with exposures to agents that induce cardiac arrhythmias.

1. Tricyclic antidepressant exposure can result in prolongation of the QRS.
2. Ventricular bradycardia can be seen with digoxin and cardiac glycoside toxicity.
3. Nonspecific ST changes in all leads can be indicative of lithium toxicity.[9]

General Management of the Poisoned Patient

A. Resuscitation and supportive care

1. Resuscitation should take priority in any poisoning patient and advanced life support procedures should be followed.
2. Supportive care is the mainstay of treatment for most poisoned patients and is required for stabilization and to prevent additional complications until detoxification is completed.
3. Ensuring airway/breathing control, initiating venous access, and cardiac and pulse oximetry monitoring are essential.
4. Patients with CNS depression or seizures are at risk for airway compromise and aspiration, especially during gastrointestinal decontamination.
   a. Prophylactic endotracheal intubation may be required to protect the airway of agitated patients that may require sedation, anticonvulsant, antipsychotic, or neuromuscular blocking agents.
5. Hemodynamic monitoring, along with transvenous cardiac pacing, intra-aortic balloon pump, or extracorporeal membrane oxygenation may be required in some patients. A bedside echocardiogram can assess cardiac output and norepinephrine is a first-line agent for patients unresponsive to fluid resuscitation.[13]

B. General antidotes

6. Table 41.3 outlines common poisoning agents and their antidotes.

TABLE 41.3 COMMON POISONING AGENTS AND THEIR ANTIDOTES

AGENT	ANTIDOTE
Anti-muscarinic	Atropine, pralidoxime
Antiarrhythmics	Benztropine
Benzodiazepines	Calcium
Beta-blockers	Cyproheptadine
Bupivacaine	Deferoxamine
Calcium channel blockers	Digoxin-specific antibody fragments (Fab)
Carbon monoxide	Ethanol
Clonidine	Methylene blue (1% solution)
Cyanide	Atropine, pralidoxime
Digoxin	Naloxone
Dystonic crisis from antipsychotics	Succimer (Chemet)
Heparin	L-Carnitine
Iron	Deferoxamine
Isoniazid	Protamine
Lead, mercury, arsenic	Vitamin K
Magnesium	Glucagon
Methanol, ethylene glycol	Naloxone
Methemoglobinemia	Calcium
Methotrexate	Folinic acid (Leucovorin)
Opiates	Physostigmine
Organophosphate	Sodium bicarbonate
Serotonin syndrome	Sodium bicarbonate
Tricyclic antidepressants	Benztropine
Valproate	Cyproheptadine
Warfarin	Oxygen, hyperbaric

C. General management

1. Hypoglycemia
   a. Symptomatic patients that are hypoglycemic should be immediately given intravenous dextrose.
   b. Occasionally, patients may need larger doses to achieve a positive response.
   c. Glucagon is not usually recommended due to a delay in the onset of action and should be reserved for patients where intravenous access cannot be obtained.
      i. Glucagon may also not be effective in patients with depleted glycogen stores, as in alcoholics, cancer patients, and the elderly.
      ii. Gastric lavage and catharsis are not likely to benefit patients with insulin overdoses.
   d. Patients should be monitored for recurrent hypoglycemia.
      i. Nondiabetics are prone to significant hypoglycemia as they lack insulin resistance and may need dextrose infusions.
      ii. In patients that overdose on sulfonylureas or meglitinides, initial control of hypoglycemia with glucose should be done, the patient should be fed, and octreotide should be used because of the risk of glucose-stimulated insulin release.[8]
2. Cardiac arrhythmias
   a. Various dysrhythmias are common.
   b. Antiarrhythmic medications are not the initial treatment for toxicity-related arrhythmias, which usually respond if hypoxia, electrolyte, and acid/base imbalances are corrected, and an appropriate antidote is given.[12]
   c. If digoxin toxicity is suspected and the patient is severely bradycardic, digoxin Fab can be given (see Table 41.2).
3. Seizures
   a. Many agents as well as withdrawal syndromes can result in seizure activity.
      i. Manage hypoglycemia, electrolyte imbalances, secure an airway, provide adequate

oxygenation, and give appropriate first-line medications such as benzodiazepines.

ii. Barbiturates can be used if the patient does not respond to benzodiazepines.

iii. Phenytoin should not be given for the treatment of seizures related to toxins as it could worsen toxicity.[13]

iv. Assessment of other potential causes of seizures (intracranial pathology) should be considered.

4. Agitation

a. Treat with benzodiazepines.

b. Monitor airway.

c. Antipsychotic medications are not recommended due to negative anticholinergic and extrapyramidal effects.[12]

5. Hyperthermia/hypothermia

a. Hyperthermic core temperature readings in poisoned patients require aggressive cooling measures to prevent complications such as disseminated intravascular coagulation (DIC), rhabdomyolysis, and multiorgan failure.

b. Salicylates, sympathomimetics, methamphetamines, and serotonin syndromes are examples of toxicities that may cause hyperthermia.

c. Toxicities from ethanol, phenothiazines, and opioids can cause hypothermia where active warming measures would need to be employed (see Table 41.1).

D. Decontamination

1. Ocular

a. Treatment should begin with instilling tetracaine 0.5% ophthalmic drops for anesthesia and providing copious irrigation with a crystalloid solution.

b. Alkali ocular exposures produce more damage as they penetrate the tissues more than acids. Irrigation should be prolonged.

c. Once irrigation is complete, the conjunctival sac pH can be tested. Irrigation should continue until the pH reading is less than 7.4.

d. Obtaining an ophthalmologic consult is required in all exposures.

2. Gastrointestinal

a. Orogastric lavage is rarely indicated due to serious risks and has been proven to be less effected than single-dose activated charcoal.[14]

b. Single-dose activated charcoal can be beneficial if a known substance that can be absorbed by activated charcoal is given orally as a slurry within 1 hour of ingestion time.

c. Activated charcoal will not absorb metals, alcohols, and corrosive substances.

d. The patient must be alert, cooperative, have an intact airway, and be willing to drink it themselves.

e. In adult patients, the dose is typically 25 to 100 g and in children, the dose is weight-based at 0.5 to 1 g per kg to a maximum dose of 50 g.[15]

3. Whole-bowel irrigation (WBI)

a. Various substances are not fully bound by utilizing activated charcoal.

b. To decrease gastrointestinal transit time, polyethylene glycol (PEG), an osmotically balanced electrolyte solution can mechanically force toxins through the gastrointestinal track if given in large quantities.

c. The goal of this treatment is to decrease gastrointestinal absorption of the toxin and enhance elimination.

d. Patients must be fully alert, cooperative, have good airway control, be in upright position with active bowel sounds.

e. WBI is controversial and remains a possible option for patients who have ingested sustained-release, enteric-coated medications, iron, lead, zinc, or packets of illicit drugs.[16,17]

4. Multi-dose activated charcoal

a. Repeated doses of activated charcoal (20–30 g or 0.5–1 g/kg every 2–3 hours) given orally or via gastric tube is simple and noninvasive way to shorten the half-life of many drugs.

b. Activated charcoal in the intestines can reduce blood concentrations of a drug or toxin.

c. Should not be used in patients with ileus, obstruction, or if there is concern about fluid/electrolyte disturbance from diarrhea. There currently are no clinical trials that show this method has altered patient outcomes.[18]

5. Urinary manipulation

a. Obligatory diuresis may increase the glomerular filtration rate of the kidneys and ion trapping by urinary pH manipulation can enhance the elimination of lipid soluble agents.

b. Urinary alkalization is typically utilized in salicylate overdoses, but fluid overload can occur if diuresis of up to 1 liter per hour occurs.[18]

6. Extracorporeal methods

a. Used to increase the clearance of many water-soluble exogenous chemicals

i. Typically done in the ICU and are limited to patients with significant poisoning, as they require extensive resources and are not without complications.

b. Hemodialysis can be performed with clearance rates that can reach 200 to 300 mL per minute. This method requires anticoagulation, but fluid and electrolyte abnormalities are corrected concurrently.

c. Peritoneal dialysis is easier to perform and is continuous, but is less effective due to poor extraction ratios and slower clearance rates (10–15 mL per minute).

i. Not frequently used in the treatment of acute poisoning

d. Continuous renal replacement therapy can be considered for patients needing rapid drug removal less urgently.

i. Minimally invasive and has slower clearance rates, similar to peritoneal dialysis

ii. Less complications, impact on hemodynamics and can be performed continuously.

iii. The role of continuous renal replacement therapy remains unclear in treating patients with acute poisonings.[18]

Safe Disposition/Prevention of Recurrence

A. Emergency patients should be observed for at least 6 to 8 hours prior to discharge or transfer and if deterioration occurs, admission is necessary.

B. Consideration should be taken for delayed complications resulting from certain medications with slowed absorption.

C. Any patient with suicidal ideation or intent should have a psychological evaluation and be monitored closely.

D. Children should be evaluated for the possibility of a nonaccidental ingestion.

E. Women of childbearing age should be checked for pregnancy.

F. It is recommended that a regional poison center toxicologist be consulted (1-800-222-1222) to assist in treatment, observation, and admission decisions.[18]

References

References for this chapter are online only and can be found at https://connect.springerpub.com/content/reference-book/978-0-8261-6091-5/part/part05/toc-part/ch41.

42. Toxicology

VICKI BACIDORE | MICHAEL D. GOOCH

Learning Objectives

- Recall common toxins and their specific management.
- Recall the role of high-dose insulin and intralipid therapy when managing a patient with a suspected cardiotoxic emergency.
- Identify toxic emergencies that may benefit from hemodialysis.
- Recognize the importance of collaboration with toxicologists and other specialists.
- Utilize practice guidelines to develop a management and patient education plan.
- Utilize evidence-based practices to develop a plan for referral, consultation, or transition of care.

Acetaminophen

Acetaminophen is commonly found in numerous over-the-counter (OTC) medications used for relief of pain, cough and colds, and fevers. Acetaminophen is also found in several prescription oral analgesics, and may be administered by mouth, rectally, or by intravenous infusion in some settings. Unlike other commonly used OTC analgesics and antipyretics, acetaminophen only inhibits prostaglandins centrally, and has not been shown to increase the risk of gastric ulcers or renal complications. Acetaminophen is rapidly absorbed from the small intestines, with a plasma half-life of 2 hours. Acetaminophen is commonly noted in accidental and intentional ingestions. Current recommendations are to limit daily doses to no more than 4 g in adults, which is well below the toxic dose. Ingestions over 150 mg/kg in any patient are considered toxic.

Pathophysiology

Acetaminophen undergoes hepatic biotransformation via two pathways. In the less common pathway, acetaminophen is oxidized to a toxic metabolite, however at therapeutic doses, very little of this toxic metabolite is formed. This metabolite is then rapidly converted to a nontoxic form by glutathione. However, in an overdose or with hepatic dysfunction, this process is altered, which may lead to increased formation of the toxic metabolite, rapid depletion of glutathione, and reduced detoxification of the metabolites. These toxic metabolites build up, damage hepatic cells, lead to hepatic failure, and eventually cause multiorgan failure. Acetaminophen toxicity is often described in four stages (Table 42.1).

Medical Screening

A. *Chief complaint:* Overdose/ingestion, suicidal ideations
B. *Signs and symptoms* (depend on time elapsed since ingestion)
  1. *Gastrointestinal distress:* Nausea, vomiting, and anorexia
  2. Malaise
  3. Right upper quadrant (RUQ) pain
  4. Jaundice
C. *Focused assessment*
  1. Airway, breathing, circulation (ABC)
  2. Mental status
  3. Cardiovascular and respiratory examination
  4. Abdominal examination
  5. Psychiatric examination

Medical Decision-Making/Differential Diagnoses

A. Always consider other toxins or poisons.
B. Determine the time of ingestion.
C. Monitor mental status.
D. Assess for coagulopathy.

Diagnostic Testing

A. Complete metabolic panel (CMP)
B. Prothrombin time/international normalized ratio (PT/INR), partial thromboplastin time (PTT)
C. Venous blood gas (VBG)
D. Lactate

TABLE 42.1 STAGES OF ACETAMINOPHEN TOXICITY

STAGE	TIME SINCE INGESTION	CLINICAL MANIFESTATIONS
1	≤24 hours	Anorexia, nausea, vomiting, and malaise
2	24–72 hours	Right upper quadrant pain, elevated liver function tests, prolonged PT/INR, and reduced urine output
3	72–96 hours	Gastrointestinal symptoms return, hepatic enzymes peak, jaundice; death may occur
4	4 days–2 weeks	If patient survives: Asymptomatic and labs return to baseline

E. *Acetaminophen level:* First level needs to be 4 hours from the time of ingestion if known
F. Aspirin level
G. Urinalysis (UA)
H. Urine drug screen—utility varies
I. Pregnancy test, if indicated

Management

A. *Procedures:* Manage airway and ventilation, if indicated.
B. *Pharmacologic therapies*
  1. Support perfusion with crystalloids, then vasopressors, if needed.
  2. Administer activated charcoal if the ingestion was <4 hours (1–2 hours preferred), and the airway is maintained or secured.
  3. NAC, if levels are toxic after 4 hours from the time of ingestion, and/or patients are symptomatic.
    a. Replaces glutathione
    b. Best within 8 hours, little benefit after 24 hours
C. *Consultation/collaboration*
  1. Consult poison control or toxicology.

Patient Disposition

A. *Transition of care information*
  1. Admit or transfer for inpatient intensive care.
  2. Monitor mental status, vital signs, urine output.

Age and Developmental Considerations

A. *Prevention and education*
  1. Keep all medications secure, out of reach of children.
  2. Read contents of all medications, including OTC products.
  3. Consult clinician or pharmacist with questions about medications.

Anticholinergics

Anticholinergics are substances that block the action of acetylcholine at nicotinic, muscarinic, and sympathetic or parasympathetic receptors, with muscarinic being one of the most concern. Muscarinic receptors are located throughout the CNS, in smooth muscles, and salivary and sweat glands. Antihistamines, antipsychotics, and tricyclic antidepressants are some of the medications that have this antagonistic effect. There are several plants including jimson weed, deadly nightshade, and some mushrooms, which have antimuscarinic effects when ingested.

Pathophysiology

During toxic exposures or ingestions, receptors are blocked throughout the CNS and throughout the body. Central effects can include confusion, hallucinations, tremors, and eventually comatose state. Peripheral manifestations include mydriasis, dry mouth, urinary retention, tachycardia, hypertension (HTN), and hyperthermia. Not all patients will experience both central and peripheral changes. Anticholinergic toxicity is summed up in the mnemonic: blind as a bat, red as a beet, dry as a bone, mad as a hatter, hotter than Hades, and sick like a seizure.

Medical Screening

A. *Chief complaint:* Overdose/ingestion, suicidal ideations, altered mental status (AMS), fever
B. *Signs and symptoms* (depend on time elapsed since ingestion/exposure)
  1. Confusion, agitation
  2. Hyperthermia
  3. Tachycardia
  4. HTN
  5. Mydriasis
C. *Focused assessment*
  1. ABC
  2. Mental status
  3. Cardiovascular and respiratory examination
  4. Psychiatric examination

Diagnostic Testing

A. CMP
B. VBG
C. Lactate
D. Creatinine kinase (CK)
E. Acetaminophen and aspirin levels
F. Urinalysis (UA)
G. Urine drug screen—utility varies
H. EKG
I. Pregnancy test, if indicated

Medical Decision-Making/Differential Diagnoses

A. Always consider other ingestants.
B. Determine the time of ingestion.
C. Monitor mental status.
D. Sympathomimetic exposure
E. Serotonin syndrome
F. Neuroleptic malignant syndrome
G. Hyperthyroidism

Management

A. *Procedures*
  1. Manage airway and ventilations, if indicated.
  2. Initiate external cooling measures if core temperature >104°F (40°C).
    a. Consider intubation, sedation, and paralysis if needed.
B. *Pharmacologic therapies*
  1. Consider activated charcoal if the ingestion was <2 hours if symptomatic and the airway is maintained or secured.
  2. Administer sodium bicarbonate 50 mEq IV for QRS widening >120 ms.
    a. Repeat if needed, goal is QRS <110 ms.
  3. Use benzodiazepines to control agitation and seizures.
  4. Consider use of physostigmine to manage severe delirium and hallucinations.
    a. 1–2 mg IV push over 5 minutes or intramuscularly (IM)

b. Avoid in patients with narrow-angle closure glaucoma, bradycardia, AV heart block, and seizures as a result of the toxicity.

C. *Consultation/collaboration:* Consult poison control or toxicology.

Patient Disposition

A. *Transition of care information*
  1. Admit or transfer for inpatient intensive care
  2. Monitor mental status, vital signs, EKG, urine output

Age and Developmental Considerations

A. *Prevention and education*
  1. Keep all medications secure, out of reach of children.
  2. Read the contents of all medications, including over-the-counter (OTC) products.
  3. Consult clinicians or pharmacists with questions about medications.

Aspirin

Aspirin has been used for hundreds of years and has many uses due to its analgesic, anti-inflammatory, antiplatelet, and antipyretic properties. Acetylsalicylic acid inhibits prostaglandins both centrally and peripherally. It is often taken orally but can be given rectally and applied topically. Numerous over-the-counter (OTC) products contain some form of acetylsalicylic acid. An ingestion of 150 mg/kg or more is considered toxic.

Pathophysiology

Aspirin is rapidly absorbed from the gastrointestinal tract and peaks in 2 to 4 hours after ingestion. Aspirin is metabolized to free salicylic acid and excreted through the kidneys. With therapeutic doses, it undergoes first order kinetics, but with large ingestions, zero kinetics is often noted, leading to reduced biotransformation and excretion. Elevated salicylate levels directly stimulate the medullary respiration center leading to hyperventilation initially, as a metabolic acidosis develops, this too triggers tachypnea. As salicylate levels rise, oxidative phosphorylation is inhibited, leading to anaerobic metabolism and eventually a metabolic gap acidosis.

Due to its prostaglandin inhibition, renal blood is reduced, reducing excretion and worsening acidosis, as well as causing an acute kidney injury. The toxic effects of aspirin impact several systems and may lead to noncardiogenic pulmonary as well as cerebral edema, hyperthermia, and eventually coagulopathy.

Medical Screening

A. *Chief complaint:* Overdose/ingestion, tinnitus

B. *Signs and symptoms* (depend on time elapsed since ingestion)
  1. *Gastrointestinal distress:* Nausea, vomiting, and anorexia
  2. Tachypnea
  3. Hyperthermia
  4. Hypoglycemia
  5. Hypokalemia

C. *Focused assessment*
  1. Airway, breathing, circulation (ABC)
  2. Mental status
  3. Cardiovascular and respiratory exam
  4. Abdominal exam
  5. Psychiatric exam

Medical Decision-Making/Differential Diagnoses

A. Always consider other ingestants.
B. Determine the time of ingestion.
C. Monitor mental status.
D. Sepsis
E. Diabetic ketoacidosis (DKA)

Diagnostic Testing

A. Complete metabolic panel (CMP)—calculate anion gap
B. Prothrombin time/ international normalized ratio (PT/INR), partial thromboplastin time (PTT)
C. Venous blood gas (VBG)
D. Lactate
E. Acetaminophen level
F. Aspirin level
G. Urinalysis (UA)
H. Urine drug screen—utility varies
I. Pregnancy test, if indicated

Management

A. *Procedures*
  1. Manage airway and ventilations, if indicated.
  2. If intubation is required, must match the patient's preintubation minute volume

B. *Pharmacologic therapies*
  1. Support perfusion with crystalloids, then vasopressors, if needed.
     a. Maintain urine output of 2 to 3 mL/kg/hour.
  2. Administer activated charcoal if the ingestion was <4 hours (1–2 hours preferred) and airway is maintained or secured.
  3. Administer sodium bicarbonate infusion to achieve urine alkalization.
     a. Three amps of sodium bicarbonate in 1 L of D5W infusing at 2 to 3 mL/kg/hour
  4. Correct hypokalemia.

C. *Consultation/collaboration*
  1. Consult poison control or toxicology.
  2. Consult nephrology for hemodialysis.

Patient Disposition

A. *Transition of care information*
  1. Admit or transfer for inpatient intensive care.
  2. Monitor mental status, vital signs, urine output.

Age and Developmental Considerations

A. *Prevention and education*
  1. Keep all medications secure, out of reach of children.
  2. Read contents of all medications, including OTC products.

3. Consult clinician or pharmacist with questions about medications.

Cardiotoxic Medications

Beta-blockers, calcium channel blockers, and digitalis are used to manage various cardiovascular problems. Beta-blockers and calcium channel blockers are often used to manage HTN, coronary artery disease, and some arrhythmias. Digitalis has been used for years to manage atrial fibrillation and heart failure. Its use has declined due to newer medicines. There are several plants that have digitalis effects, including oleander, lily of the valley, and foxglove. These are sometimes consumed and can lead to toxicity.

Pathophysiology

Beta-blockers competitively block catecholamines at the beta receptors exerting negative inotropic, dromotropic, and chronotropic effects. This blockade may be limited to beta-1 receptors or both beta-1 and beta-2 depending on the medication. At toxic levels, all beta receptors are affected. Blockade of beta-2 receptors can lead to smooth muscle relaxation leading to vasodilation, and glycogenolysis, and gluconeogenesis.

Calcium channel blockers block slow L-type calcium channels in the myocardium and vascular smooth muscles. This blockade also leads to a negative inotropic, dromotropic, and chronotropic effect. Dihydropyridines have more of a vascular effect, this vasodilation often triggers a reflex tachycardia due to the drop in the systemic vascular resistance. At toxic levels, other channels are blocked leading to an increased release of insulin, in addition to bradycardia, heart blocks, and hypotension.

Digitalis inhibits the Na^+–K^+ pump that leads to an increase in intracellular sodium, which in turn increases intracellular calcium. This causes a positive inotropic effect to improve contractility and decreases atrioventricular node conduction to slow the ventricular response to fast rhythms such as atrial fibrillation. At toxic concentrations, vagal activity is increased leading to bradycardia, heart blocks, and eventually hypotension. The patient may also experience tachyarrhythmias. Due to the inhibition of the Na^+–K^+ pump, hyperkalemia is common with digitalis toxicity.

Medical Screening

A. *Chief complaint:* Overdose/ingestion, weakness, dizziness

B. *Signs and symptoms* (depend on time elapsed since ingestion)

1. *Gastrointestinal distress:* Nausea, vomiting, and anorexia
2. Weakness, fatigue
3. Altered mental status (AMS)
4. Bradycardia
5. Hypotension
6. Hyperglycemia (beta-blockers)
7. Hypoglycemia (calcium channel blockers)
8. Visual changes, including chromatopsia (digoxin)

C. *Focused assessment*

1. Airway, breathing, circulation (ABC)
2. Mental status
3. Cardiovascular and respiratory exam
4. Abdominal exam
5. Psychiatric exam

Medical Decision-Making/Differential Diagnoses

A. Always consider other ingestants.

B. Determine the time of ingestion.

C. Monitor mental status and perfusion.

Diagnostic Testing

A. Complete metabolic panel (CMP)

B. Venous blood gas (VBG)

C. Lactate

D. Digoxin level

E. Urinalysis (UA)

F. EKG

G. Pregnancy test, if indicated

Management

A. *Procedures:* Manage airway and ventilation, if indicated.

B. *Pharmacologic therapies*

1. Support perfusion with crystalloids, then vasopressors, if needed.
2. Administer activated charcoal if the ingestion was <4 hours (1–2 hours preferred) and airway is maintained or secured.
3. Manage bradycardia
   - a. Atropine
   - b. Transcutaneous pacing
   - c. Chronotropic infusion (e.g., epinephrine, dopamine)
4. Beta-blockers and calcium channel blockers specific
   - a. Consider IV calcium.
   - b. Consider IV glucagon 5 to 10 mg slow IV.
     - i. Predose with antiemetic.
     - ii. Follow by infusion.
     - iii. *Pediatrics:* 0.05 to 0.1 mg/kg
   - c. Consider high-dose insulin therapy.
     - i. 1 unit/kg IV, titrate to effect.
     - ii. Monitor glucose and potassium
     - iii. Administer dextrose infusion to prevent hypoglycemia.
   - d. Consider intralipid therapy.
     - i. IV bolus 1.5 mL/kg bolus over 3 to 5 minutes
     - ii. Infusion of 0.25 mg/kg/min
   - e. Sodium bicarbonate 1 to 2 mEq/kg IV for QRS widening
5. Digoxin specific
   - a. Manage hyperkalemia.
     - i. The use of calcium is controversial; the latest evidence supports its use.
   - b. Administer Fab fragments (DigiFab)
     - i. Indications

(1) Severe ventricular arrhythmias
(2) Severe refractory bradycardia
(3) Hyperkalemia
(4) Coingestion with other cardiotoxic medications
(5) Acute ingestion of >10 mg with one of the above
(6) Steady serum >6 ng/mL with one of the above

c. Phenytoin to manage tachyarrhythmias, if needed

C. *Consultation/collaboration*
1. Consult poison control or toxicology.
2. Consult nephrology for hemodialysis.

Patient Disposition

A. *Transition of care information*
1. Admit or transfer for inpatient intensive care.
2. Monitor mental status, vital signs, urine output.

Age and Developmental Considerations

A. *Prevention and education*
1. Keep all medications secure, out of reach of children.
2. Read the contents of all medications and supplements.
3. Consult clinician or pharmacist with questions about medications.

Iron

Iron is essential for the proper function of hemoglobin and transportation of gases throughout the body. The incidence of iron poisoning has dramatically dropped over the last several decades due to changes in labeling of supplements. Iron poisoning is often encountered from an acute ingestion of iron replacement tablets, some oral contraceptives, and especially prenatal vitamins that contain larger amounts of iron than most preparations. Toxicity is most often encountered in children. Ingestion of 20 to 60 mg/kg of elemental iron may produce symptoms, greater than 60 mg/kg is considered toxic and patients will be symptomatic.

Pathophysiology

Iron supplements contain varying amounts of elemental iron, some are instant release, and others are time released, which can impact toxicity. As toxic amounts of iron are absorbed, the normal pathways and storage of iron are overwhelmed. This excess iron is absorbed by cells, especially cardiac, hepatic, and neurons, leading to mitochondrial dysfunction and eventually cellular death. Toxicity also impairs capillary permeability, inhibits oxidative phosphorylation, and inhibits thrombin. In addition to the cellular insult, large amounts have a caustic effect on the intestinal lining leading to erosion and sometimes perforation. Iron toxicity is described in five phases (Table 42.2).

Medical Screening

A. *Chief complaint:* Ingestion, gastrointestinal distress, suicidal ideations

B. *Signs and symptoms*
1. See Table 45.5.

C. *Focused assessment*
1. Airway, breathing, circulation (ABC)
2. Mental status
3. Cardiovascular and respiratory exam
4. Abdominal exam

Medical Decision-Making/Differential Diagnoses

A. Always consider other exposures.
B. Determine the type of tablets and time of ingestion, if possible.
C. Monitor mental status.
D. Consider other agents that cause vomiting and acidosis (e.g., aspirin).

Diagnostic Testing

A. Serum iron concentration
1. 3 to 5 hours after ingestion is most useful.
2. Repeat at 6 to 8 hours after ingestion.
3. Levels
a. 350 mcg/dL—minimal toxicity
b. 350 to 500 mcg/dL—moderate toxicity
c. 500 mcg/dL—severe toxicity

B. Complete blood count (CBC)
C. Complete metabolic panel (CMP)
D. Venous blood gas (VBG)
E. Prothrombin time/partial thromboplastin time (PT/PTT)
F. Type and crossmatch
G. *Abdominal x-ray:* May show iron tablet fragments in the lumen of the bowel
H. Pregnancy test, if indicated

Management

A. *Procedures*
1. Manage airway and ventilation, if needed.
2. Gastric tube placement may be needed to facilitate whole bowel irrigation.

TABLE 42.2 CLINICAL MANIFESTATIONS OF IRON TOXICITY

PHASE	TIME FRAME	CLINICAL MANIFESTATIONS
1 GI	Within 6 hours	Vomiting, diarrhea, hematemesis, hematochezia
2 Latent	6–24 hours	GI symptoms resolve, metabolic acidosis, altered mental status, tachycardia, tachypnea
3 Systemic	12–24 hours	Renal failure, coagulopathy, GI symptoms return, worsening altered mental status, cardiovascular collapse → shock, respiratory distress/failure
4 Hepatic	2–5 days	Fulminant hepatic failure, coagulopathy—death often occurs during this phase
5 Obstructive	3–6 weeks	Bowel scarring and obstruction, if patient survives

B. *Pharmacologic therapies*

1. Support perfusion with crystalloids, then blood products, if needed.
2. If iron tablet fragments are noted on the x-ray, administer a whole bowel irrigation.
    a. Polyethylene glycol electrolyte (PEG) solution
3. Administer deferoxamine 15 mg/kg/hour IV for elevated iron concentrations.
    a. Chelating agent
    b. May turn urine pink
    c. May lead to acute respiratory distress syndrome (ARDS) in some patients

C. *Consultation/collaboration:* Consult poison control or toxicology.

Patient Disposition

A. *Transition of care information*

1. Admit or transfer symptomatic patients for inpatient intensive care.
2. Patients who are asymptomatic and have an 8-hour postingestion level <300 mcg/dL may be discharged home, in accidental cases.
3. Monitor mental status, vital signs, urine output.

Age and Developmental Considerations

A. *Prevention and education*

1. Keep all medications secure, out of reach of children.
2. Read contents of all medications, including over-the-counter (OTC) products.
3. Consult clinician or pharmacist with questions about medications.

Opioids

Opioids are one of the more common agents seen in toxic or poisoned patients. Whether from accidental overdose or ingestion or from the abuse of substances, opioids are encountered often and in all patient populations. Examples include scheduled analgesics such as morphine, hydromorphone, fentanyl, methadone, loperamide, oxycodone, and hydrocodone. Common opioids of illicit use include those previously mentioned and heroin. Patients may accidentally consume an excess amount in an attempt to control pain, overdose purposefully, or succumb to the adverse effects during recreational use. Ingestion by inquisitive pediatric patients also occurs. Opioids are not only physically but psychologically addictive and lead to tolerance, which requires larger doses to achieve the desired effect the more frequently they are taken. The agents may be coingested with other depressants including ethanol and sedatives. Some patients may swallow and transport condoms or bags containing opioids, which have been known to rupture, leading to rapid absorption. Some oral agents are combined with acetaminophen and during an overdose, this can present two toxic problems.

Pathophysiology

Opioids are easily absorbed and distributed with a rapid onset of action. The agents stimulate opioid receptors, especially mu receptors, leading to euphoria and central nervous system (CNS) depression. The CNS depression can range from miosis, an altered mental status to a comatose state, respiratory depression to respiratory arrest, and eventually death. Many opioids have active metabolites that can prolong their effects. Loperamide and methadone are associated with prolongation of the QRS and/or QT; this can be exacerbated with overdoses.

Medical Screening

A. *Chief complaint:* Drowsiness, alerted mental status, ingestion/overdose, suicidal ideations

B. *Signs and symptoms*

1. Altered mental status
2. Bradypnea
3. Slurred speech
4. Miosis
5. Hypoactive bowel sounds

C. *Focused assessment*

1. Airway, breathing, circulation (ABC)
2. Mental status
3. Cardiovascular and respiratory exam
4. Integumentary

Medical Decision-Making/Differentials

A. Always consider other exposures.

B. Monitor mental status and respiratory drive.

C. Acute respiratory distress syndrome (ARDS) is associated with some opioid overdoses.

D. Cerebrovascular accident (CVA)

E. Hypoglycemia

Diagnostic Testing

A. Basic metabolic panel (BMP)

B. Venous blood gas (VBG)

C. Ethanol level

D. Acetaminophen and aspirin levels

E. Urine drug screen—utility varies

F. EKG

G. Pregnancy test, if indicated

Management

A. *Procedures*

1. Manage airway and ventilation, if indicated.
    a. Intubate to secure airway, if needed.
    b. Monitor $ETCO_2$.

B. *Pharmacologic therapies*

1. Support perfusion with crystalloids, then vasopressors, if needed.
    a. Administer naloxone (Narcan) IV/intramuscularly (IM) or intranasal.
        i. Dose varies with severity
        ii. May require larger dose with some substances
        iii. Goal is to restore respiratory drive but not fully reverse in most patients due to withdrawal symptoms.
        iv. The half-life of naloxone is 60 to 90 minutes, less than most opioids.
    b. Consider administering a whole bowel irrigation if there is concern for body packing.

i. Polyethylene glycol electrolyte (PEG) solution

c. Sodium bicarbonate 1 to 2 mEq/kg IV for QRS widening

C. *Consultation/collaboration:* Consult poison control or toxicology.

Patient Disposition

A. *Transition of care information*

1. Observe any patient who required reversal for at least 4 hours, if no other intervention needed, consider discharge.
2. Admit or transfer for inpatient intensive care if multiple doses of naloxone are required.
3. Monitor mental status, vital signs.

Age and Developmental Considerations

A. *Prevention and education*

1. Keep all medications secure, out of reach of children.
2. Read the contents of all medications, including over-the-counter (OTC) products.
3. Consult clinician or pharmacist with questions about medications.
4. Consider prescribing a naloxone autoinjector to those at risk.

Sedatives and Anxiolytic

Sedatives are substances used for their calming or sleep-inducing effect. Anxiolytics are agents that reduce anxiety. Benzodiazepines are the most commonly used class of sedatives, and the most common class of medications used during suicide attempts. Barbiturates are less frequently used now compared to benzodiazepines but are more potent. Benzodiazepine like sleep aids, including zolpidem, zaleplon, and eszopiclone, structurally are unlike other agents, but have a similar effect, but less potent. Gamma-hydroxybutyrate (GHB) is an illicit substance that mimics gamma-aminobutyric acid (GABA), the primary inhibitory neurotransmitter in the central nervous system (CNS). GHB is used for its rapid onset and euphoria. Sedative agents are usually ingested or injected. Alcohol ingestion is often seen as a coingestion. Sedative agents may be used during sexual assaults and should be considered when there is amnesia to the events after an assault. Most sedatives have addictive properties, and patients may experience withdrawal symptoms during abstinence.

Pathophysiology

Most sedatives are rapidly absorbed and distributed with a rapid onset. They rapidly enter the CNS and exert their calming effect by enhancing the effects of GABA. Depending on the amount of the substance, the person may experience drowsiness or could become comatose. Some agents, especially benzodiazepines and barbiturates, can lead to respiratory depression, hypotension, and arrest if a significant amount of the medication is ingested or injected.

Medical Screening

A. *Chief complaint:* Drowsiness, alerted mental status (AMS), ingestion/overdose, suicidal ideations

B. *Signs and symptoms*

1. Bradypnea
2. Dizziness
3. Slurred speech
4. Ataxia

C. *Focused assessment*

1. Airway, breathing, circulation (ABC)
2. Mental status
3. Cardiovascular and respiratory examination

Medical Decision-Making/Differential Diagnoses

A. Always consider other exposures.
B. Monitor mental status and respiratory drive.
C. Cerebrovascular accident (CVA)
D. Hypoglycemia
E. Hypothyroidism

Diagnostic Testing

A. Basic metabolic panel (BMP)
B. Venous blood gas (VBG)
C. Lactate
D. Ethanol level
E. Urine drug screen—utility varies
F. EKG
G. Pregnancy test, if indicated

Management

A. *Procedures*

1. Manage airway and ventilation, if indicated.
   a. Intubate to secure airway, if needed.
   b. Monitor $ETCO_2$.

B. *Pharmacologic therapies*

1. Support perfusion with crystalloids, then vasopressors, if needed.
2. Consider flumazenil for reversal of benzodiazepines and benzodiazepine like sleep aids in severe cases or those who are not chronic users.
   a. Risk of withdrawal seizures

C. *Consultation/collaboration:* Consult poison control or toxicology.

Patient Disposition

A. *Transition of care information*

1. Admit or transfer for inpatient intensive care.
2. Monitor mental status, vital signs.

Age and Developmental Considerations

A. *Prevention and education*

1. Keep all medications secure, out of reach of children.
2. Read the contents of all medications, including over-the-counter (OTC) products.
3. Consult clinician or pharmacist with questions about medications.

Sympathomimetics

Sympathomimetics are one of the most commonly abused class of drugs. This class includes cocaine, ecstasy, amphetamines, methamphetamines, and newer street drugs including synthetic cannabinoids (e.g., K2, Spice, bath salts, and Molly's plant food). These highly addictive substances are often inhaled, insufflated, injected, ingested, and now vaped. The newer illicit street drugs are very popular given their availability online and in retail stores. One of the most attractive attributes of these substances is that they are synthetic and not detectable by routine drug screens. One of the other concerns is that often these substances contain other substances, and users may receive the effects of multiple drugs. Some patients may swallow and transport condoms or bags containing stimulants, which have been known to rupture, leading to rapid absorption and sometimes death. Recently, there have been documented cases of patients developing severe coagulopathies after using synthetic marijuana, which was contaminated with brodifacoum, a vitamin K antagonist commonly found in rat poisons. These patients should be managed similarly to patients requiring reversal of warfarin.

Pathophysiology

These agents increase the release and/or inhibit the reuptake of epinephrine, norepinephrine, and serotonin. These increased levels can cause significant stimulation of the central nervous system (CNS) and cardiovascular system. Some of the CNS effects include euphoria, increased energy, paranoia, agitation, excited delirium, mydriasis, hyperthermia, and seizures. Cardiovascular effects may include hypertension, tachycardia, arrhythmias, and coronary vasospasms. Some drugs have been associated with suicidal and homicidal ideations. Hyperthermia may lead to volume depletion and rhabdomyolysis. Some amphetamines, such as ecstasy, increase the release of antidiuretic hormone, which reduces the thirst response and can worsen dehydration. Some users are aware of this effect and may increase their water intake, which can lead to volume overload and hyponatremia, and eventually seizures.

Medical Screening

A. *Chief complaint*: Anxiety, palpitations, chest pain

B. *Signs and symptoms* (depend on time elapsed since ingestion)

1. Tachycardia
2. Hypertension
3. Hyperthermia
4. Agitation
5. Seizures

C. *Focused assessment*

1. Airway, breathing, circulation (ABC)
2. Neurologic exam
3. Cardiovascular and respiratory exam
4. Abdominal exam
5. Psychiatric exam

Medical Decision-Making/Differential Diagnoses

A. Always consider other ingestants.
B. Determine the time of ingestion.
C. Monitor mental status and perfusion.
D. Thyrotoxicosis
E. Serotonin syndrome
F. Neuroleptic malignant syndrome

Diagnostic Testing

A. Complete metabolic panel (CMP)
B. Creatinine kinase
C. Troponin
D. Venous blood gas (VBG)
E. Lactate
F. Urinalysis (UA)
G. Urine drug screen—utility varies
H. Coagulation studies, if indicated based on findings or if concerned for vitamin K antagonist exposure
I. EKG
J. CT scan head, if altered
K. Pregnancy test, if indicated

Management

A. *Procedures*

1. Manage airway and ventilation, if indicated.
2. Initiate external cooling measures if core temperature >104°F (40°C).

B. *Pharmacologic therapies*

1. Support perfusion and urine output with crystalloids, if needed.
2. Administer activated charcoal if the ingestion was <4 hours (1–2 hours preferred) and the airway is maintained or secured
3. Administer benzodiazepines (e.g., midazolam, to manage HTN, hyperactivity, seizures, and chest pain).
   a. Continuous infusion may be needed.
4. Consider vasodilators and/or alpha/beta blockers (e.g., labetalol, phentolamine) if HTN is refractory to benzodiazepines.
   a. Avoid pure beta-blockers (e.g., metoprolol).
5. Sodium bicarbonate 1 to 2 mEq/kg IV for QRS widening
6. Consider administering a whole bowel irrigation if there is concern for body packing.
   a. Polyethylene glycol electrolyte (PEG) solution

C. *Consultation/collaboration*

1. Consult poison control or toxicology.

Patient Disposition

A. *Transition of care information*

1. Admit or transfer for inpatient intensive care.
2. Monitor mental status, vital signs, urine output.

Age and Developmental Considerations

A. *Prevention and education*

1. Keep all medications and substances secure, out of reach of children.
2. Consult clinician or pharmacist with questions about medications.

Additional Reading

Additional Reading for this chapter are online only and can be found at https://connect.springerpub.com/content/reference-book/978-0-8261-6091-5/part/part05/toc-part/ch42.

43. Poisoning by Other Toxins

VICKI BACIDORE | MICHAEL D. GOOCH

Learning Objectives

- Identify other toxins that can cause poisoning and their specific management.
- Identify the diagnostics that are helpful in evaluating these toxic emergencies.
- Recognize the importance of collaboration with toxicologists and other specialists for the management of these poisonings.
- Implement practice guidelines to develop a management and patient education plan.
- Use evidence-based practices to develop a plan for referral, consultation, or transition of care.

Alcohols

Ethanol is often associated with toxic ingestions. Ethanol is readily available and is rapidly absorbed once ingested. Depending on the amount, it can lead to slowing of reflexes, alteration in mental status, depressed protective reflexes, coma, and death. There are other alcohols besides ethanol that may be encountered and can be very dangerous.

Methanol, a wood alcohol, is colorless and sweet tasting. Methanol is most often used as a solvent, fuel additive, and fuel source. It can be found in some windshield wiping fluids, antifreeze, and embalming fluid. Ethylene glycol is found in many formulations of antifreeze and deicing solutions. It, too, is colorless and sweet tasting. Isopropyl alcohol, a common form of rubbing alcohol, is often used as a disinfectant but is found in some solvents. Ingestions of these three alcohols are often seen in children, and as an ethanol substitute in alcoholics. These three alcohols are rapidly absorbed and can lead to intoxication as with ethanol. Isopropyl is considered more potent than ethanol, leading to rapid intoxication but is less toxic.

Pathophysiology

Alcohols are rapidly absorbed and metabolized by alcohol dehydrogenase (ADH) in the liver. Unlike most substances, alcohols undergo zero-order kinetics; their metabolism is not affected by serum concentration and occurs at a steady state. Coingestions are common, and the presence of ethanol will slow the metabolism of other alcohols, given ADH's affinity to ethanol. Isopropyl alcohol, similar to ethanol, is not usually fatal and does not lead to a metabolic gap acidosis. Isopropyl is metabolized to acetone and eventually glucose or other substances.

Methanol and ethylene glycol are often called toxic alcohols as they have severe toxic effects. Both are usually ingested, but methanol can be absorbed through the skin as well. Methanol is metabolized to formaldehyde and eventually formic acid. Formic acid inhibits oxidative phosphorylation, which leads to a metabolic gap acidosis. Formic acid collects in the central nervous system and damages neurons, and especially the optic nerve that leads to blindness in many cases. Acidosis worsens and death will occur without rapid treatment.

Ethylene glycol undergoes several phases of metabolism resulting in the formation of glyoxylic acid and oxalic acid, leading to a metabolic gap acidosis. Oxalic acid binds with calcium to form calcium oxalate crystals, which deposit in the renal tubules, as well as other vital organs. Renal failure rapidly develops, leading to a worsening metabolic acidosis, and eventually death without intervention.

Medical Screening

A. *Chief complaint:* Overdose/ingestion; suicidal ideations; intoxication

B. Signs and symptoms
1. Altered mental status (AMS); intoxication
2. Nausea, vomiting
3. Visual changes (methanol)
4. Tachypnea
5. Fruity acetone breath (isopropyl)
6. Tachycardia

C. Focused assessment
1. Airway, breathing, circulation (ABC)
2. Mental status
3. Cardiovascular and respiratory exam
4. Abdominal exam
5. Psychiatric exam

Medical Decision-Making/Differential Diagnoses

A. Always consider other toxins

B. Electrolyte imbalances

C. Other causes of a gap acidosis

Diagnostic Testing

A. Comprehensive metabolic panel (CMP)—calculate the anion gap.

B. Venous blood gas (VBG)

C. Lactate

D. Acetaminophen and aspirin levels

E. Ethanol, methanol, and ethylene glycol levels

F. Serum osmolarity

G. Urinalysis (UA)
H. Examine urine with black light; may fluoresce if ethylene glycol was ingested.
   1. The absence does not rule out ingestion; the presence confirms ingestion.
I. Urine drug screen—utility varies
J. Pregnancy test, if indicated
K. CT or MRI of brain, once stabilized

Management

A. Procedures
   1. Manage airway and ventilation, if indicated.
B. Pharmacologic therapies
   1. For ethanol and isopropyl ingestions, management is supportive.
   2. For methanol and ethylene glycol ingestions; in the presence of toxic levels, osmolar and gap acidosis, renal failure, or evidence of organ dysfunction
      a. *Fomepizole:* blocks ADH, prevents metabolism to toxic metabolites
         i. 15 mg/kg IV loading dose
         ii. Then 10 mg/kg IV every 12 hours for the specified time frame
      b. Ethanol administration, if fomepizole is not available
         i. Goal is to maintain ethanol level of 100 to 150 mg/dL
      c. Sodium bicarbonate infusions to correct acidosis
C. Consultation and collaboration
   1. Consult poison control or toxicology
   2. Nephrology

Patient Disposition

A. Transition of care information
   1. Admit or transfer for inpatient intensive care and hemodialysis.
   2. Monitor mental status, vital signs, and urine output.

Age and Developmental Considerations

A. Prevention and education
   1. Keep all medications and chemicals secure, out of reach of children.

Carbon Monoxide

Carbon monoxide (CO) is a colorless, odorless, and tasteless gas produced during the incomplete combustion of carbon-containing substances. Exposure may occur during an enclosed-space fire, other sources include mechanical and automotive exhaust, flame-type furnaces, heaters, cooking appliances, and poorly ventilated fireplaces and grills. CO is considered the most common cause of death from poisoning or toxic exposure. Accidental exposures are often encountered during disasters and severe weather events, which may cause prolonged electrical power outages leading people to attempt to produce heat from nonconventional sources and obtain power from portable generators without adequate ventilation.

Pathophysiology

CO has a high affinity for hemoglobin and combines with hemoglobin at least 200 times stronger than oxygen, forming carboxyhemoglobin (COHb). In addition to impairing oxygen transport, the creation of COHb impacts the ability of oxygen to dissociate from hemoglobin and shifts the oxyhemoglobin dissociation curve to the left. CO also inhibits oxidative phosphorylation causing a shift to anaerobic metabolism. The end result is severe tissue hypoxia leading to organ dysfunction, acidosis, and eventually death. CO also binds to myoglobin and can lead to rhabdomyolysis with severe levels. In some cases, patients may develop severe neurologic sequelae due to the hypoxic insult and reperfusion injury.

Medical Screening

A. *Chief complaint:* Headache; altered mental status (AMS); unresponsive
B. Signs and symptoms
   1. Headache
   2. Dizziness
   3. Vision changes
   4. Seizures
C. Focused assessment
   1. ABC
   2. Mental status
   3. Cardiovascular and respiratory examination
   4. Neurologic examination

Medical Decision-Making/Differential Diagnoses

A. Always consider other exposures
B. Consider CO poisoning in patients with unusual or persistent headaches
C. Monitor mental status
D. Recall that standard pulse oximetry is not reliable

Diagnostic Testing

A. Complete blood count (CBC)
B. Comprehensive metabolic panel (CMP)
C. Arterial blood gas (ABG)
D. COHb level
E. Lactate
F. EKG
G. Pregnancy test, if indicated

Management

A. Procedures
   1. Manage airway and ventilation, if indicated.
   2. Consider indications for hyperbaric oxygen therapy.
      a. Cardiac ischemia
      b. Pregnancy
      c. Levels >25%
   3. Evaluate with CO-oximeter, if available
B. Pharmacologic therapies
   1. Administer high-flow oxygen, despite pulse oximetry readings.
      a. Reduces half-life of CO
   2. Support perfusion with crystalloids, then vasopressors, if needed.

C. Consultation and collaboration
   1. Consult poison control or toxicology.

Patient Disposition

A. Transition of care information
   1. Admit or transfer for inpatient intensive care.
   2. Monitor mental status, vital signs, and urine output.

Age and Developmental Considerations

A. Prevention and education
   1. Keep areas with open flames, running machines, or vehicles well ventilated.
   2. Before using a fireplace for the first time in a season, be sure the flue is clean and open.
   3. Need for CO detectors in structures with gas heat or appliances.

Caustics

"Caustic" is a term used to describe chemicals that are known to cause significant tissue damage upon contact, usually due to their extreme pH. These chemicals are grouped based on their pH: acidic (pH <7) and alkaline (pH >7). Exposures may occur as an accidental or intentional ingestion or exposure, or incidental as an occupational exposure. Many of these are found in various household products and others may only be found in industrial settings, usually in a more concentrated form. Some common acids are acetic acid or vinegar, sulfuric acid that is found in some batteries and drain cleaners, hydrofluoric acid that is used in glass etching and to remove rust and to clean certain metals including some jewelry, and hydrochloric acid that is used in some cleaning products, in metal cleaning, and is found in some swimming pool products. Common alkalis include sodium hypochlorite or bleach, calcium hydroxide that is a common ingredient in cement and some hair products, potassium hydroxide that is found in some drain cleaners, and sodium tripolyphosphate that is an active ingredient in many detergents.

Pathophysiology

The severity of the tissue damage is dependent upon the pH, the formulation, and the concentration of the chemical, the duration of contact, and the presence of any protective equipment. The more concentrated the chemical and the further the pH of the chemical is away from 7.0, the more significant the potential tissue injury. Depending on the route of exposure, a solution may cause more damage than a solid. Contact with an acid causes coagulation necrosis. The hydrogen ions in the acid cause immediate cell death and eschar-like formation, which limits the ability of the chemical to penetrate deeper and cause more tissue trauma. In the case of an ingestion, the acid may leave the gastrointestinal (GI) tract and cause systemic effects, including severe acidosis and renal failure. Hydrofluoric acid is unique in that it can penetrate deeper, causing more tissue damage and pain. As free fluoride ions are released, they bind to magnesium and calcium, which can cause significant imbalances and inhibit the sodium–potassium pumps. Unlike acids, alkalis cause a liquefaction necrosis and can penetrate deeper and cause more tissue damage. Like acids, ingestion can cause significant injuries to the GI tract, though an alkaline ingestion can also cause multiorgan injuries.

Medical Screening

A. *Chief complaint:* Burns, ingestion, pain, vomiting
B. Signs and symptoms
   1. Burns
   2. Respiratory distress
   3. Coughing
   4. Stridor
   5. Dysphagia
C. Focused assessment
   1. Airway, breathing, circulation (ABC)
   2. Mental status
   3. Cardiovascular and respiratory examination
   4. Abdominal examination

Medical Decision-Making/Differential Diagnoses

A. Always consider other exposures.
B. Attempt to identify the chemical, but do not delay treatment.
C. Monitor mental status, airway, breathing, and perfusion.

Diagnostic Testing

A. Venous blood gas (VBG)
B. Comprehensive metabolic panel (CMP)—evaluate for an anion gap
   1. Obtain an ionized calcium, if hydrofluoric acid
C. Complete blood count (CBC)
D. Urine analysis (UA)
E. Lactate
F. EKG, especially if hydrofluoric acid
G. Type and screen
H. If intentional, consider acetaminophen and salicylate levels.
I. Chest x-ray (CXR)
J. Scans and endoscopy once stabilized

Management

A. Procedures
   1. Don appropriate personal protective equipment (PPE), remove all clothing, and decontaminate the skin.
   2. Manage airway and ventilation, if needed, manage as if a difficult airway.
   3. Avoid gastric tube placement until after endoscopic evaluation.
B. Pharmacologic therapies
   1. Follow evidence-based guidelines when prescribing.
   2. Establish IV access and fluid resuscitate or administer blood products as needed.
   3. Do not give medications to attempt to decontaminate the GI tract.
   4. If hydrofluoric acid: Calcium administration
      a. *Topical application for superficial burns:* 3.5 g of calcium gluconate powder in 5 oz of water-soluble lubricant, or 25 mL of 10% calcium gluconate in 75 mL of water-soluble lubricant

b. *Intradermal injection:* 0.5 mL of 10% calcium gluconate per square centimeter of burned skin
c. *IV and/or intra-arterial infusions:* 10 mL of a 10% calcium gluconate solution and 40 mL of 5% dextrose in water and infused over 4 hours
d. Chloride may be used if gluconate is not available.
e. May also need magnesium replacement

C. Consultation and collaboration
1. Consult poison control or toxicology, endoscopic service, and/or burn surgery.

Patient Disposition

A. Transition of care information
1. Admit or transfer patient to an appropriate level of care.
2. Monitor mental status, airway, vital signs.

Age and Developmental Considerations

A. Prevention and education
1. Keep all chemicals, cleaning supplies, detergents, and toxins secure and out of the reach of children.
2. Always read instructions before using chemicals.

Cyanide

Cyanide has several commercial uses, including photography, the manufacturing of plastics and rubber, preparation of animal hides, and as a fumigant. Cyanide is also important during the refining process of precious metals. Cyanide is most often encountered in patients with smoke inhalation injuries from an enclosed-space fire, or the burning of wood, plastics, and rubbers. In addition to inhalation, exposure can result from exposure to cyanide in its liquid or solid form. Lastly, cyanide toxicity is a side effect of long-term infusions of nitroprusside, especially in the setting of renal failure. Some report the smell of bitter almonds after a cyanide exposure.

Pathophysiology

Cyanide is rapidly absorbed and distributed after exposure. Cyanide binds to oxidized or ferric iron (Fe^{3+}) and inhibits oxidative phosphorylation by inhibiting the electron transport chain. This inhibition impairs adenosine triphosphate (ATP) production, which causes the body to resort to anaerobic metabolism. Despite the availability of oxygen, these effects lead to severe tissue hypoxia and a gap metabolic acidosis. Several antioxidants are also inhibited, leading the accumulation of oxygen free radicals resulting in the stimulation of N-methyl-D-aspartate (NMDA) receptors and the inhibition of the formation of gamma-aminobutyric acid (GABA), leading to neural insult and death. Cyanide may also bind to ferrous iron (Fe^{2+}), which is important for oxygen transport and may worsen cellular hypoxia.

Medical Screening

A. *Chief complaint:* Unresponsive; inhalation injury
B. Signs and symptoms
1. Headache
2. Confusion
3. Seizures
4. Dysrhythmias
5. Tachycardia and hypertension (HTN), then bradycardia and hypotension later
6. Tachypnea initially, then bradypnea
7. Gastrointestinal (GI) distress
8. Skin irritation

C. Focused assessment
1. Airway, breathing, circulation (ABC)
2. Mental status
3. Cardiovascular and respiratory exam
4. Neurologic exam

Medical Decision-Making/Differential Diagnoses

A. Always consider other exposures.
B. Monitor mental status.
C. Venous blood may resemble arterial blood on blood gas analysis.
D. Carbon monoxide poisoning
E. Cardiotoxins
F. Sepsis

Diagnostic Testing

A. Comprehensive metabolic panel (CMP)—calculate anion gap.
B. Arterial blood gas (ABG)
C. Lactate
D. Cyanide level
E. EKG
F. Pregnancy test, if indicated

Management

A. Procedures
1. Use complete personnel protective equipment (PPE), if concern for dermal exposure.
2. Decontaminate the patient's skin with water, remove all clothing, if concern for dermal exposure
3. Manage airway and ventilation, intubation is often indicated
4. Evaluate with CO-oximeter, if available

B. Pharmacologic therapies
1. Administer high-flow oxygen, even if not hypoxic.
2. Support perfusion with crystalloids, then vasopressors, if needed.
3. Administer activated charcoal if oral ingestion.
4. Administer hydroxocobalamin (Cyanokit) 70 mg/kg, up to 5 g, as soon as possible, may repeat once if needed.
a. Converts cyanide to cyanocobalamin (vitamin B12)
b. May cause transient hypertension and red flushing of the skin, and discoloration of the urine
c. May interfere with CO-oximeter readings
5. If hydroxocobalamin is not available, the cyanide kit is an option, though it is no longer manufactured.
a. Converts cyanide to methemoglobin
b. Amyl nitrite
c. Sodium nitrite
d. Sodium thiosulfate

C. Consultation and collaboration
1. Consult poison control or toxicology.

Patient Disposition

A. Transition of care information
  1. Admit or transfer for inpatient intensive care.
  2. Monitor mental status and vital signs.

Age and Developmental Considerations

A. Prevention and education
  1. Stress the importance of protective equipment when working with cyanide.
  2. Importance of smoke detectors in structures

Hallucinogens

Hallucinations are defined as perceptions or experiences that do not have a physical stimulus or source. Hallucinogens stimulate serotonergic and dopaminergic receptors and antagonize glutamate receptors causing distortions in sensory input, mood, and emotions. Common hallucinogens, or psychedelics, include phencyclidine (PCP), tryptamines, psilocybin, mescaline, lysergic acid diethylamide (LSD) or acid, salvia, and kratom. These may be in a natural form or synthetic. PCP is similar to ketamine and was initially used as an anesthetic. Due to its unpredictability and side effects, its medical use stopped in the 1960s. When used, it is often smoked or taken orally. Psilocybin is the active compound found in some mushrooms. Mescaline can be found in a few types of cacti and structurally are similar to amphetamines. LSD is often consumed orally. Salvia is a member of the mint family and is sometimes referred to as diviner's sage, magic mint, or sage of seers. Salvia leaves are often chewed or smoked. The leaves of the kratom tree may be chewed, smoked, or made into a tea. Most recently, kratom has been popularized as an option for alleviating symptoms of opioid withdrawals.

Pathophysiology

Mainly due to the serotonergic effects, users of these substances experience changes in thought and mood, which can be euphoric, cause dissociation, or may lead to dysphoria, acute panic attacks, and even delirium. Users may have some sympathetic stimulation due to the inhibition of the reuptake of norepinephrine and dopamine. This inhibition may lead to tachycardia, mydriasis, elevated blood pressure, and hyperactivity. All these effects are dose-dependent; the more consumed, the greater the effect. PCP also blocks N-methyl-D-aspartate (NMDA) receptors, which increases its effectiveness. Salvia, unlike other agents in this category, has no effect on serotonin receptors; it achieves its main effect by activating kappa opioid receptors. Kratom contains several chemicals, mostly alkaloids, and has agonist properties to mu and delta opioid receptors. In addition to its psychedelic effects, kratom may cause euphoria, has analgesic properties, and has similar side effects as true opioids.

Usually, the effects of these chemicals are short-lived, except for kratom; these substances are not considered to be addictive. However, some patients may experience flashbacks months or years later after using certain hallucinogens. It is common for patients to have other effects because of other substances or chemicals mixed with the hallucinogen.

Medical Screening

A. *Chief complaint:* Altered mental status (AMS); hallucinations; feelings of dissociation or euphoria

B. Signs and symptoms (depend on time elapsed since ingestion/exposure)
  1. Euphoria
  2. Hallucinations
  3. Agitation
  4. Tachycardia
  5. Hypertension
  6. Hyperthermia
  7. Mydriasis

C. Focused assessment
  1. Airway, breathing, circulation (ABC)
  2. Mental status
  3. Cardiovascular and respiratory exam
  4. Psychiatric exam

Medical Decision-Making/Differential Diagnoses

A. Always consider other ingestants.
B. Monitor mental status.
C. Anticholinergic exposure
D. Sympathomimetic exposure

Diagnostic Testing

A. Basic metabolic panel (BMP)
B. Creatine phosphokinase (CK), if hyperthermic
C. Urine drug screen—utility varies
D. Ethanol level
E. EKG
F. Pregnancy test, if indicated

Management

A. Procedures
  1. Maintain safety.

B. Pharmacologic therapies
  1. Use benzodiazepines (e.g., midazolam) to control agitation, if needed.
  2. Consider the use of an antipsychotic, if benzodiazepines are ineffective.
  3. Ketamine may be an option if benzodiazepines are ineffective.

C. Consultation and collaboration
  1. Consult poison control or toxicology.

Patient Disposition

A. Transition of care information
  1. Admit or transfer for inpatient care for those with acute delirium.
  2. Others may be safe to discharge home with a responsible adult, once back to baseline.
  3. Monitor mental status and vital signs.

Age and Developmental Considerations

A. Prevention and education
  1. Keep all medications and supplements secure, out of reach of children.
  2. Read contents of all medications, including over-the-counter (OTC) product.
  3. Consult clinician or pharmacists with questions about medications and supplements.

Heavy Metals

The term "heavy metal" is used to describe elements that have a high density and are toxic at low concentrations. Sometimes referred to as toxic metals, in addition to iron, this group includes lead, mercury, and arsenic. Of this group, lead is one of the most common metals encountered. With the removal of lead from gasoline, paint, plastics, and other products, the risk of toxicity in the United States is low. Lead is still found in older buildings and water pipes, and in products made in other countries. Most toxic exposures occur over time due to repeated exposures. Children and pregnant women are at higher risk for lead toxicity.

Historically, arsenic has been known as a common agent used during intentional poisoning. Nowadays, most arsenic exposures are environmental or occupational. Arsenic is found in coal and is used in the production of glass, paint, rodenticides, and insecticides. Mercury has a long history of medicinal uses, most recently as a preservative in some immunizations. Mercury is used in the manufacturing of some paints, plastics, and fluorescent lights. Unfortunately, mercury is a common environmental pollutant in some areas leading to restrictions in the consumption of certain fish due to high mercury levels.

Pathophysiology

When exposed to lead, it is absorbed easily and binds to red blood cells, and is easily distributed throughout the body. Structurally, lead is very similar to calcium and interferes with many calcium-dependent cellular activities. The neurologic and hematopoietic systems are the most effected, but renal, cardiovascular, and gastrointestinal (GI) insult may occur. Anemias, developmental delays, and eventually encephalopathy and death may result. Arsenic binds to red blood cells and transport proteins and interferes with energy production, leads to free radical production, which can cause oxidative lung injury, and eventually cellular death. Capillary permeability increases and this can lead to GI and cerebral edema. Mercury has no physiologic function and interrupts many cellular functions including various enzymes and proteins. The cardiovascular and renal systems are impacted by mercury exposure the most.

Medical Screening

A. *Chief complaint:* Developmental delay, altered mental status (AMS), seizures; GI distress
B. Signs and symptoms
   1. AMS
   2. Ataxia
   3. Seizures
   4. Neuropathies
   5. Anemias
   6. Nausea/vomiting/diarrhea (N/V/D)
      a. "Rice water–like" diarrhea—classic for arsenic poisoning
   7. Abdominal pain
   8. Respiratory distress
   9. Tachycardia and/or arrhythmias
C. Focused assessment
   1. Airway, breathing, circulation (ABC)
   2. Mental status
   3. Cardiovascular and respiratory examination
   4. Abdominal examination
   5. Psychiatric examination

Medical Decision-Making/Differential Diagnoses

A. Always consider other ingestants.
B. Monitor mental status, airway, and perfusion.
C. Meningitis/Encephalitis
D. Guillain-Barré syndrome
E. Attention deficit hyperactivity disorder (ADHD)
F. Gastroenteritis

Diagnostic Testing

A. Complete blood count (CBC)
B. Comprehensive metabolic panel (CMP)
C. Urinalysis (UA)
D. Lead, arsenic, and/or mercury levels
   1. Arsenic and mercury require a 24-hour urine collection.
E. 12 lead EKG
F. CT head, if AMS
G. Pregnancy test, if indicated
H. Long bone x-rays may reveal "lead lines" in chronic lead exposures

Management

A. Procedures
   1. GI decontamination—consult with a toxicologist first.
B. Pharmacologic therapies
   1. Administer benzodiazepines, for example, midazolam, to manage hyperactivity and seizures.
   2. Support perfusion and urine output with crystalloids, if needed.
   3. Arrhythmias should be treated using advanced cardiac life support (ACLS) guidelines.
C. Consultation and collaboration
   1. Consult poison control or toxicology.

Patient Disposition

A. Transition of care information
   1. Admit or transfer for inpatient intensive care and consideration of chelation therapy.
   2. Monitor mental status, airway, vital signs.

Age and Developmental Considerations

A. Prevention and education
   1. Keep all chemicals and substances secure, out of reach of children.
   2. Use protective equipment when handling or cleaning up chemicals.
   3. If home exposure, patient should not return until the home is decontaminated.

Organophosphates

Pesticides and nerve agents (e.g., sarin, soman, VX) are organophosphates, which may be encountered in emergency care settings. In most scenarios, the exposure is accidental due to occupational exposure in agricultural

TABLE 43.1 CHOLINERGIC CRISIS MNEMONICS

Sludge:		Dumbels:	
	Salivation		**D**iarrhea/Diaphoresis
	Lacrimation		**U**rination
	Urinary incontinence		**M**iosis
	Diarrhea		**B**radycardia/ Bronchorrhea/ Bronchospasms
	GI distress		**E**mesis
	Emesis/ Expectoration		**L**acrimation
			Salivation

GI, gastrointestinal.

settings, but it can be purposeful, or the result of an act of terrorism. These substances are easily absorbed through the skin, gastrointestinal tract, and respiratory tree. This increases their effectiveness as pesticides; with human exposure, they can also be fatal.

Pathophysiology

Organophosphates inhibit cholinesterases, which allows acetylcholine to accumulate and leads to overstimulation of nicotinic and muscarinic receptors throughout the peripheral and central nervous systems, causing a cholinergic crisis. Nicotinic stimulation leads to cardiovascular stimulation, muscle fasciculations, and potential paralysis. The muscarinic effects cause loss of bodily fluids, bronchospasms, and bradycardia. These effects are summarized by the mnemonics of SLUDGE and DUMBELS (Table 43.1). Death often results from loss of airway control from the bronchorrhea and respiratory arrest from diaphragmatic paralysis. Some agents undergo a process referred to as aging, which is the irreversible binding of the chemical to the cholinesterase; this leads to prolonged stimulation of the receptors.

Medical Screening

A. *Chief complaint:* Vomiting; diarrhea; increased urination; diaphoresis

B. Signs and symptoms
- **1.** Increased secretions
- **2.** Respiratory distress
- **3.** Tremors

C. Focused assessment
- **1.** Airway, breathing, circulation (ABC)
- **2.** Mental status
- **3.** Cardiovascular and respiratory examination
- **4.** Abdominal examination
- **5.** Psychiatric examination

Medical Decision-Making/Differential Diagnoses

A. Always consider other ingestants.

B. Monitor mental status, airway, and perfusion.

Diagnostic Testing

A. Basic metabolic panel (BMP)

B. Venous blood gas (VBG)

C. Lactate

D. Urinalysis (UA)

E. Plasma cholinesterase levels—do not wait on results to treat

F. Pregnancy test, if indicated

Management

A. Procedures
- **1.** Use complete personal protective equipment (PPE).
- **2.** Decontaminate the patient's skin with water, remove all clothing.
- **3.** Elevate the head of the bed.
- **4.** Manage airway and ventilation, as needed.
  - **a.** Suction airway as needed.
  - **b.** If rapid sequence intubation is needed, consider an alternative neuromuscular blocking agent to succinylcholine, as it may have a prolonged effect.

B. Pharmacologic therapies
- **1.** Administer atropine as needed to control secretions (no max dose)
  - **a.** Titrate dose up as needed.
  - **b.** *Pediatrics:* Alter dosage based on current guidelines
  - **c.** An infusion may be required.
  - **d.** Goal is to dry up secretions and resolve respiratory distress.
- **2.** Administer benzodiazepines to manage hyperactivity and seizures.
- **3.** Administer pralidoxime (2-PAM) to bind to the chemical complex and allow normal function to return.
  - **a.** *Pediatrics:* Alter dosage based on current guidelines
  - **b.** May redose hourly and may require an infusion
- **4.** Support perfusion and urine output with crystalloids, if needed.

C. Consultation and collaboration
- **1.** Consult poison control or toxicology.

Patient Disposition

A. Transition of care information
- **1.** Admit or transfer for inpatient intensive care.
- **2.** Monitor mental status, airway, vital signs.

Age and Developmental Considerations

A. Prevention and education
- **1.** Keep all chemicals and substances secure, out of reach of children.
- **2.** Use protective equipment when handling chemicals.

Additional Reading

Additional Reading for this chapter are online only and can be found at https://connect.springerpub.com/content/reference-book/978-0-8261-6091-5/part/part05/toc-part/ch43.

44. Substance Use Disorder

RENEÉ SEMONIN HOLLERAN

Learning Objectives

- Define substance use disorder (SUD).
- Identify patients at risks for developing SUD.
- Discuss the interventions available for SUD for patients seen in the ED.

Substance use disorder (SUD) occurs when the use of substances, such as alcohol, or drugs, such as opioids, cause clinically significant health problems, disabilities, or inability to meet responsibilities such as working, going school, or caring for one's home duties (www.samhsa.gov/find-help/disorders). Drug classes that are involved in SUD include alcohol, cannabis, hallucinogens such as phencyclidine, inhalants, opioids, sedatives, hypnotics, anxiolytics, stimulants, and other unknown substances. In 2019, the National Survey on Drug Use and Health reported that 20.4 million Americans over the age of 12 suffered from a SUD (www.samhsa.gov/data/sites/default/files/reports/rpt29393/2019NSDUHFFRPDFWHTML/2019NSDUHFFR1PDFW090120.pdf). Opioid use disorder (OUD) was found in 1.6 million people including those with a prescription for pain medication.

EDs are a commonplace for patients with a SUD to present.[1] Patients may present going through withdrawal requiring immediate treatment to prevent possible life-threatening consequences or suffering from the consequences of a drug overdose.[2] There is always the potential for violence and aggression related to the care of these patients.

The management of the patient with SUD can be challenging. It requires assessment of the source of SUD, the types of medication that may be used for SUD management in the ED, and identification and referral to community resources as indicated.

Assessment for Substance Use Disorder[3–7]

Screening Tools

A. *SBRIT Assessment Screening:* Screening, Brief Intervention, Referral, and Treatment

B. *CAGE:*

1. Have you felt you needed to **C**ut down on your drinking?
2. Have people **A**nnoyed you by criticizing your drinking?
3. Have you ever felt **G**uilty about drinking?
4. Have you ever felt you needed a drink first thing in the morning (**E**ye-opener) to steady your nerves or to get rid of a hangover?

C. *National Institute on Drug Abuse (NIDA) Drug Screening Tool (NIDA-Modified ASSIST (NMASSIST):* This tool evaluates the use of the following substances a scale that asks how often in the past year a person has used a substance (never; once or twice; monthly, weekly, daily, or almost daily, www.drugabuse.gov/nmassist/step/0).

1. Alcohol
2. Tobacco products
3. Prescription drugs for nonmedical use
4. Illegal drugs

D. Review the state Prescription Drug Monitoring Program Data Red Flags

1. Multiple prescribers
2. Multiple pharmacies
3. Morphine Milligram Equivalents (MME) greater than 100 mg/d (this may vary from state to state)

E. Other risk behaviors

1. Diversion
2. Overlapping prescriptions
3. Hoarding
4. Provider and/or ED "shopping"

F. Opioid Risk Tool (core-rems.org/wp-content/uploads/2019/05/ORT-OUD-tool.pdf) (Answer Yes or No) (Low risk 0–3; moderate risk 4–7; high risk 8 and greater).

1. Family history of substance abuse
   a. Alcohol
   b. Illegal drugs
   c. Prescription drugs
2. Personal history of substance abuse
   a. Alcohol
   b. Illegal drugs
   c. Prescription drugs
3. Personal history of sexual abuse
4. Personal history of psychological diseases
   a. Attention-deficit hyperactivity disorder (ADHD), obsessive-compulsive disorder (OCD), bipolar, schizophrenia
   b. Depression

Physical Examination

A. *Vital signs*

B. *Level of consciousness*

C. Ears, nose, and throat; cardiovascular; respiratory; gastrointestinal; neurologic; and integumentary.

D. *Symptoms of specific substances*
 1. Alcohol
  a. Cardiomyopathy
  b. Hypertension
  c. Arrhythmia
  d. Gastrointestinal bleeding
  e. Hepatitis/cirrhosis
  f. Thrombocytopenia
 2. Opioids
  a. Respiratory depression
  b. Constipation
  c. Injection site infections
 3. Cannabis
  a. Tachycardia
  b. Hyperemesis

E. *Symptoms of drug withdrawal* (*Note:* Always consider the potential for life-threatening symptoms and the risk of suicidal ideation.)
 1. Irritability
 2. Anxiety
 3. Delirium
 4. Insomnia
 5. Seizures

Interventions for Substance Use Disorder in the Emergency Department[5–7]

A. Patient and staff safety is first priority.
 1. Place patient in a safe environment for both the patient and the staff.
 2. Rule out intoxication.
 3. Rule out drug withdrawal.
 4. Evaluation of patient's current psychological status

B. Management of overdose

C. Assess and stabilize airway, breathing, and circulation; this is the first step in overdose management related to SUD.

D. Administer appropriate medication to manage overdose. Apart from a few drugs, there are limited reversal agents for overdoses related to SUD.

E. Opioid overdose
 1. *Naloxone:* Can be administered intravenous, intramuscular, subcutaneous, through an endotracheal tube or nasal spray; amount of medication will be dependent on the amount of opioid used and the patient response to the medication

F. Benzodiazepines overdose
 1. Flumazenil, though controversial, given by IV. Doses determined by what type of benzodiazepine was taken

G. Medications for opioid withdrawal (www.uspharmacist.com/article/managing-opioid-overdose-in-the-hospital-setting)
 1. Clonidine for tachycardia, hypertension, piloerection
 2. Diazepam, lorazepam, hydrazine for agitation/anxiety
 3. Loperamide for diarrhea
 4. Dicyclomine for abdominal cramps
 5. Ondansetron, prochlorperazine for nausea and vomiting (N/V)
 6. Trazodone or temazepam for insomnia

H. Buprenorphine use for opioid withdrawal in the ED[3,8]
 1. *Buprenorphine:* Partial agonist with high affinity and low intrinsic activity for the mu-opioid receptor
 2. Reduces opioid cravings, however, it is a potent medication 25 to 100 times more potent than morphine. It can cause sedation, miosis, and mild respiratory depression. It is an effective analgesic for moderate to severe pain.
 3. Sublingual administration is recommended.

I. Methadone is a full mu-opioid receptor, for treatment of addiction or opioid abuse; requires inpatient or licensed approved program to initiate.
 1. Used as a first-line medication for heroin detoxification.
 2. Detoxification with methadone can cause fewer withdrawal symptoms, reduced use of heroin, and improved treatment retention for SUD and OUD.
 3. Patient needs to be cautioned about respiratory depression.

J. Medication-assisted treatment (MAT) must also include assisting therapies such as mental health referral, attend mutual support groups (Narcotics Anonymous, Alcoholics Anonymous); patient needs to be seen within 48 to 72 hours for reassessment to assure that the patient is taking the appropriate dose of medication.

Characteristics of Substance Use Disorder

A. Frequent visits to EDs for medication refills
B. Treatment for overdose
C. Treatment for alcohol or drug withdrawal
D. Requesting specific medications including route and dosage
E. Not interested in alternative methods for SUD
F. Rehearsal of "textbook" presentation

Risk Factors for the Development of Substance Use Disorder

A. Chronic pain
B. Physical disability
C. Chronic illnesses
D. Polypharmacy
E. Mental illnesses such as depression and anxiety
F. Social isolation
G. Family history or current active use
H. Witnessing family members, friends, or peers using substances
I. Serious and unexpected life changes
J. *Genetics:* The National Center on Addiction and Substance Abuse estimates that 50% to 75% risk for developing a SUD is related to genetics.
K. Physical or sexual abuse
L. Use of substances such as alcohol early in life

Substances of Abuse[1,2,9]

A. *Alcohol:* One of the most common substances used and abused in the world.

B. *Cannabis:* Can be complicated by the legality of the substance in the state in which the emergency nurse practitioner (ENP) practices.
C. *Opioids:* This includes both prescribed and illicit opioid substances such as heroin.
D. Psychostimulants, such as methamphetamines.
E. *Nicotine:* Including cigarettes, e-cigarettes, and other tobacco products

References

References for this chapter are online only and can be found at https://connect.springerpub.com/content/reference-book/978-0-8261-6091-5/part/part05/toc-part/ch44.

VI. Emergency Medical Services, Patient Transport, and Disaster Preparedness

45. Emergency Medical Services

RONALD D. MEADOR

Learning Objectives

- Explain emergency medical services (EMS) systems and components.
- Describe the levels of EMS personnel education, training, and skills as it pertains to patient care and transport.
- Contrast the different levels and modalities of EMS patient transport.
- Apply the EMS Scope of Practice and Care Delivery Model.
- Demonstrate the role of the emergency nurse practitioner (ENP) in relation to EMS systems.

Emergency medical services (EMS) is an integrated system of resources that provides out-of-hospital medical care and transport. Prior to 1960, EMS in the United States consisted of a patchwork of systems provided by hospitals, fire departments, volunteer groups, or undertakers. They were sometimes staffed by physicians or minimally trained or untrained personnel and were born from lessons learned during the Civil War.[1] President Lyndon B. Johnson's Commission on Highway Safety published a report in 1965, which identified the great public health burden of motor vehicle crashes and stated that a coordinated national highway safety program should be a major priority.[2] Subsequently, in 1966, the National Academy of Sciences–National Research Council published a report titled "Accidental Death and Disability: The Neglected Disease of Modern Society." This landmark report documented the absence of quality emergency care which included: (1) no treatment protocols; (2) few trained medical personnel; (3) inefficient transportation; (4) lack of modern communications and equipment; (5) the abdication of responsibility by political authorities; and (6) the lack of research evaluating prehospital care.[3] The recommendations of both reports were incorporated into the Highway Safety Act of 1966, which mandated emergency medical care and transportation of the injured and the inception of EMS systems. Congress enacted the EMS Systems Act of 1973, which created a grant program to further the development of regional EMS systems. This act designated the Department of Health, Education, and Welfare as the lead EMS agency within the federal government. It authorized grants to develop a comprehensive EMS system throughout the country for feasibility studies and planning, the establishment and initial operation of EMS systems, and the expansion and improvement of current systems.[4] This act became a decisive factor in the nationwide development of regional EMS systems and was a pivotal component in the development of the modern emergency medical care system in the United States. This chapter will discuss the structure and function of the EMS systems in the United States and its interaction with the emergency nurse practitioner (ENP) optimizing the continuum of emergency patient care.

Emergency Medical Systems[5–17]

A. *Definition:* A consolidated system of components designed to provide a coordinated, timely, and effective response to a medical emergency.

B. Structure of EMS systems (Figure 45.1)
  1. Public and private agencies and organizations
  2. Communications and transportation networks
  3. Human resources and training
  4. Trauma systems, hospitals, trauma centers, and specialty care centers
  5. Rehabilitation facilities
  6. Public information and education
  7. Trained professionals
     a. Volunteer and career prehospital personnel
     b. Physicians, advanced practice providers, nurses, and therapists)
     c. Administrators and government officials

C. EMS agency geographical settings
  1. *Urban/suburban:* Systems that serve communities with moderate to high population densities, confined geographical borders, and have receiving EDs and specialty emergency care resources (e.g., cardiac catheterization, stroke, and trauma centers).
  2. *Rural:* Systems that serve communities with lower population densities often spread over large geographic areas with limited emergency care resources.

D. EMS provider definitions and scope of practice
  1. *Emergency medical first responder (EMFR):* The initial level of EMS certification. Personnel have a limited scope of practice and have the least amount of comprehensive education, clinical experience, or clinical skills of EMS providers.
     a. Basic Life Support (BLS) including
        i. Patient assessment
        ii. Bag-valve-mask (BVM) ventilation
        iii. Cardiopulmonary resuscitation (CPR)
        iv. Automatic external defibrillator (AED)
        v. Oxygen therapy by nonrebreather mask

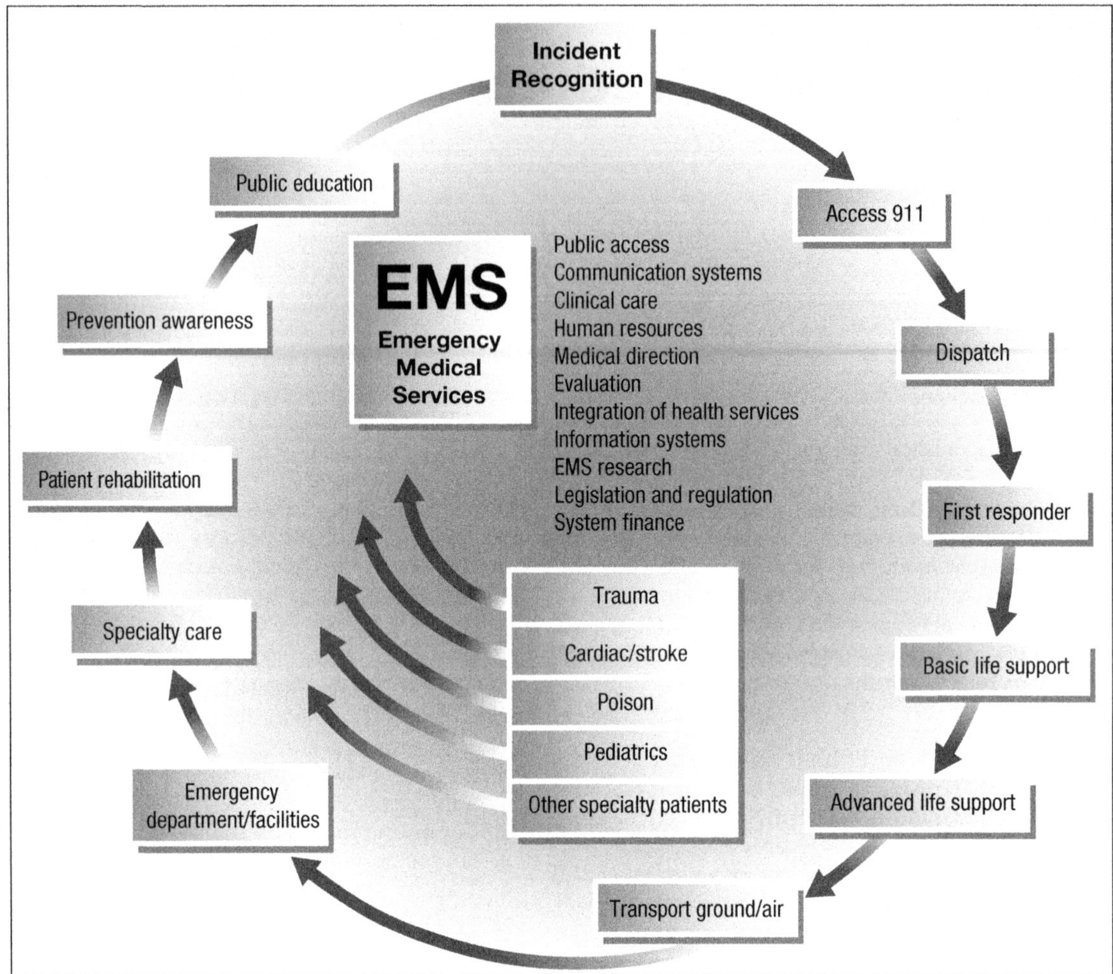

FIGURE 45.1 Elements of comprehensive Emergency Medical Services (EMS) system.
Source: Reprinted from National Highway Traffic Safety Administration. *Guide for Interfacility Patient Transfer* (Report no. DOT HS 810 599). U.S. Department of Transportation; 2006: 5. Copyright 2006 by the U.S. Department of Transportation.[17]

vi. Treatment of external hemorrhaging
vii. Manual cervical spinal restriction
viii. Vital sign (VS) assessment including blood pressure
ix. Initiate immediate on-scene lifesaving care

b. Await additional EMS response and assist higher-level personnel at the scene and during transport

c. EMFRs include, but are not limited to, firefighters, police, life guards, ski patrol, park rangers, event staff, disaster relief, security guards, athletic trainers, Community Emergency Response Teams, emergency management personnel, flight attendants, and so on.

2. *Emergency medical technician (EMT):* Second level of EMS certification and personnel have a limited scope of practice and more comprehensive education, clinical experience, and clinical skills than emergency first responders.

a. BLS skills include those of the EMR in addition to:

i. *Airway adjuncts:* Oral and nasal airways
ii. Long bone immobilization
iii. Joint immobilization
iv. Assistance with self-administration of epinephrine auto-injectors and oral glucose

b. Provide care and transportation

c. Perform interventions with basic equipment typically found on an ambulance under medical direction, which may be provided by the ENP

d. Link from scene to the emergency healthcare system

3. *Advanced emergency medical technician (AEMT):* Third level of EMS certification and personnel have a more advanced scope of practice and have more comprehensive education, clinical experience, and clinical skills than emergency medical technicians.

a. BLS including skills of EMR and EMT in addition to:

i. Supraglottic airway device
ii. Intravenous therapy
iii. Intraosseous therapy

iv. Suctioning of intubated patient
v. Use of continuous positive airway pressure (CPAP)
vi. Medication administration
(1) Intravenous fluid bolus
(2) Sublingual nitroglycerin
(3) Fifty percent dextrose and glucagon for hypoglycemia
(4) Naloxone for opioid overdose
(5) Nitrous oxide for analgesia
(6) Inhaled beta-agonists for respiratory emergencies

b. Provide care and transportation under medical direction

c. Perform interventions with basic and advanced equipment typically found on an ambulance

d. Link from scene to emergency health care system

4. *Paramedic:* Fourth and highest level of EMS certification and personnel have the broadest scope of practice, most education, clinical experience, and clinical skills than all previous levels.

a. BLS skills of previous levels plus Advanced Life Support (ALS) including
i. Advanced cardiac life support including defibrillation, cardioversion, transcutaneous pacing, and cardiac medication
ii. EKG acquisition and interpretation
iii. Manual removal of foreign bodies by direct laryngoscopy
iv. Endotracheal intubation
v. Surgical/needle cricothyrotomy
vi. Emergency childbirth
vii. Needle chest decompression
viii. Gastric decompression
ix. Capnography
x. Emergency medication administration

b. Allied health professional whose primary focus is to provide advanced emergency care and transport under medical direction

c. Possesses complex knowledge and skills to perform interventions with basic and advanced equipment found on an ambulance

d. Link from scene to the emergency health care system

5. *Critical care transport paramedic*: This level of training is not recognized by the National EMS Scope of Practice Model and requirements and privileges vary by agency and state.

E. EMS staffing types

1. Volunteer-based EMS systems utilize noncompensated personnel who freely offers to take part in the delivery of EMS services.

2. Career-based EMS systems utilize compensated personnel in the delivery of EMS services.

3. Combination-based EMS systems utilize both volunteer and career personnel in the delivery of EMS services.

F. EMS response types

1. *Uniformed response:* ALS unit is always dispatched.

a. *Advantage:* ALS responders are always present.

b. *Disadvantage:* Dilution of resources by allocating ALS resources to non-ALS calls

2. *Tiered response:* First responders, BLS units, and/or ALS units are dispatched depending on how the caller answers a series of questions asked by the emergency medical dispatcher.

a. *Advantage:* No dilution of resources as ALS resources are only dispatched when necessary and available for other calls that require ALS resources

b. *Disadvantage:* Requires multiple resources levels

G. EMS agency design types

1. *Multiple-Role EMS Agency:* An agency that cross-trains its personnel to provide various services such as fire-based EMS agency or a public safety agency where personnel provide law enforcement, fire, and EMS services.

2. *Single-Role EMS Agency:* Only provides EMS services and can be municipal or privately operated.

3. *Hospital-Based EMS Agency:* An agency associated with a public or private, for-profit, or not-for-profit hospital system that provides oversight and operational responsibility.

4. *Private EMS Agency:* Individually or corporately owned, provide emergent and nonemergent ambulance services, and may be for-profit or not-for-profit.

5. *Third-Service EMS Agency:* Provides ambulance services in a manner separate, but alongside, fire and law enforcement services where oversight and operational responsibilities are associated with a municipality.

6. *Public Utility EMS Agency:* Provides ambulance services by a contractual agreement between a governmental body and a private agency to provide some component of the system. For example, the governmental agency may own the equipment, apparatus, supplies, and perform billing and a private EMS service will provide the EMS personnel.

H. EMS service levels and transport modalities

1. Ground ambulance transports include patient transport on land and water.

a. BLS includes
i. The provision of medically necessary supplies and services
ii. BLS transportation as defined by the state where the transport occurs

b. ALS, Level 1 (ALS1) includes
i. The provision of medically necessary supplies and services
ii. The provision of an ALS assessment or at least one ALS intervention
iii. An ALS assessment must be performed by an advanced EMT or a paramedic in accordance with state and local laws.

c. ALS, Level 2 (ALS2) includes
i. The provision of medically necessary supplies and services
ii. At least one or more medications by intravenous push/bolus or by continuous infusion excluding crystalloid fluids, or
iii. At least one of these ALS2 procedures
(1) Defibrillation/cardioversion

(2) Endotracheal intubation
(3) Central venous line
(4) Cardiac pacing
(5) Chest decompression needle
(6) Intraosseous line
(7) Surgical airway

d. Specialty care transport (SCT) includes
i. The provision of medically necessary supplies and services at a level of services beyond the scope of and EMT-P and
ii. Provided by one or more professionals in an appropriate specialty (emergency or critical care nursing, emergency medicine, respiratory or cardiovascular care, or a paramedic with specialized training)

e. Paramedic intercept (PI) occurs when the transporting ambulance service only provides BLS and ALS services are required.

2. Air medical transport includes patient transport by fixed-wing (airplane) or rotary-wing (helicopter) aircraft and utilizes the same levels of care as ground ambulances defined above.

I. EMS resource deployment models
1. *Static:* All resources are deployed from a fixed location.
2. *Dynamic:* Resources are deployed from changing locations based on retrospective call volume analysis to statistically predict where the next request for service may occur. This also known as systems status management (SSM).
3. *Hybrid:* Uses a combination fixed and dynamic locations and resources may be rotated as call volume dictates to minimize response times.

J. Emergency medical dispatch (EMD)
1. 911 communications centers are referred to as public safety answering points (PSAPs) and are commonly operated by fire or law enforcement.
2. Incoming transport requests are routed to the appropriate dispatcher who deploys the appropriate resources based on caller questioning and provides appropriate prearrival instructions.
3. EMD programs use finite chief complaints lists that have predetermined questions that dictate resource deployment, the level of deployment (emergency or nonemergent), and appropriate prearrival instructions for the specific chief complaint.

K. Types of EMS services
1. Prevention/public education focuses on prevention of problems that could result in EMS utilization, such as preventable injuries, heart attacks, and strokes. Public education includes first aid classes, AED, and instruction on when to request EMS assistance.
2. Triage of EMS requests needs thorough determination of nature, severity, and resources required from a 911 caller.
3. Ambulance response and transport
4. Prearrival instructions from emergency medical dispatchers (EMD) to guide callers on how to begin treatment and assist responding ambulances in locating the scene.
5. Assessment and treatment
6. Event coverage to provide medical support for public and private events (e.g., sporting events, festivals, concerts).
7. Disaster services for manmade and natural events through threat assessment, planning, activation, and delivery of medical resources and services.
8. Interfacility transport of emergent and nonemergent patients
9. Air medical transport
10. Hazardous materials response medical support
11. Tactical medical response support of law enforcement
12. Community paramedicine to provide services such as monitoring and support of home health services

L. EMS accreditation
1. Center for Public Safety Excellence (CPSE)
2. Commission on Accreditation of Medical Transport Systems (CAAMTS)
3. Non-emergency Medical Transport Accreditation Commission (NEMTAC)
4. National Accreditation Alliance for Medical Transportation Applications (NAAMTA)

EMS Care Delivery[6,11,18–20]

A. Definitions
1. *Scope of practice:* Parameters of various duties or services that may be provided by an individual with specific credentials. Whether regulated by rule, statute, or court decision, it represents the limits of services an individual may legally perform.
2. *Education:* All cognitive, psychomotor, and affective learning that individuals have undergone.
3. *Certification:* External verification of competencies that an individual has achieved typically via examination
4. *Licensure:* Permission granted to an individual by the state to perform certain restricted activities
5. *Credentialing:* Local process by which an individual is permitted by a medical director to practice in a specific setting
6. *Standard of care:* A diagnostic and treatment process followed for a certain medical, traumatic, or psychological process that a clinician should utilize based on the best scientific evidence available

B. National EMS Scope of Practice Model establishes a framework that determines the range of skills and roles that an individual possessing a state EMS license is authorized to perform. Components include education, certification, licensure, and credentialing.

C. Under the Scope of Practice Model an individual may perform a skill or function in a role in which that person is:
1. Trained to perform a skill or role (educated), and
2. Demonstrated competence in that skill or role (certified), and
3. Legally authorized by the state to perform the skill or role (licensed), and
4. Authorized by the medical director to perform the skill or role (credentialed)

D. State government role

1. Authority and responsibility to regulate EMS within its borders and determine the scope of practice of state-licensed EMS personnel.
2. National EMS Scope of Practice Model is a guideline to improve consistency but has no regulatory influence unless adopted by the individual state.

E. Scope of practice versus standard of care
1. Scope of practice does not define the standard of care and is not a practice guideline or protocol.
2. Scope of practice defines what can be legally done and not what should be done.
3. Standard of care is the treatment of a specific condition based on best scientific evidence and defines what should be done.

F. Provision of care
1. Protocols
a. Written physician authorized-treatment guidelines for management of a specific medical condition
b. Define the scope of prehospital care.
c. May be developed and/or mandated by state or regional oversight committees
d. EMS providers must adhere to system protocols unless otherwise advised by online medical direction
2. Standing orders
a. Specific medical orders contained within protocols such as
i. Defibrillation
ii. Advanced airway placement
iii. Medication administration
iv. Certain surgical procedures
3. Online medical direction
a. Patient management through direct contact with a physician by radio, phone, or other communication devices
b. Direct consultation on specific or unusual patient care situations
c. Does not have to be the organization's medical director but must be a physician at a predesignated medical facility.
4. Offline medical direction
a. Development, dissemination, and enforcement of written protocols
b. Protocols and standing orders are examples of offline medical directions
c. EMS provider acts as agent of medical director
d. Accomplished through two methods:
i. Prospective methods such as training, testing, certification, protocol development, operational policies and procedures, and legislative activities
ii. Retrospective methods such as medical audits, review of care, process improvement, the direction of remedial education, and limitation of patient care functions.

G. EMS performance improvement[6,18,21,22–25]
1. *Quality improvement (QI):* Systematic and continuous actions that lead to measurable improvement in healthcare
a. *Prospective:* Front-end training and education
b. *Concurrent:* Direct observation during care delivery
c. *Retrospective:* Chart audits, case reviews, outcomes reviews
2. *Six sigma*: Provides a framework (DMAIC) for managing an organization's overall process for improvement projects
a. Define
b. Measure
c. Analyze
d. Improve
e. Control
3. *Performance measures:* Evidence-based performance assessments for sentinel patient conditions that are time sensitive, treatment sensitive, or both
a. Out-of-hospital cardiac arrest (OHCA)
b. ST-segment elevation acute myocardial infarction (STEMI)
c. Acute stroke
d. Severe trauma
4. *Benchmarking:* Process of seeking out and implementing best practices at best costs
5. *Evidence-based practice:* Development and implementation of structures and processes to access, appraise, and integrate research evidence into practice.

EMS Education[1,4,6,7,10,11,18,19,26]

A. National EMS Education Standards define competencies, clinical behaviors, and judgments that must be met by entry-level EMS personnel to meet practice guidelines defined in the National EMS Scope of Practice Model.

B. National EMS Education Standards consist of four components:
1. *Competency:* Minimum competency for entry-level personnel at each level and applies to patients of all ages, unless a specific age group is specified.
2. *Knowledge required to achieve competency:* Elaboration of the knowledge within each competency that entry-level personnel needs to master to achieve competency.
3. *Clinical behaviors/judgments:* Clinical behaviors and judgments essential for entry-level personnel at each level.
4. *Educational infrastructure:* Support standards necessary for conducting EMS training programs at each level.

C. Assumptions of National EMS Education Standards (https://www.ems.gov/projects/ems-education-standards.html)
1. *Progression:* Personnel at each level is responsible for the knowledge, judgments, and behaviors at their level and at the preceding levels.
2. *Depth of knowledge:* Amount of detail a student needs to know about a particular topic within their level.

3. *Breadth of knowledge:* Number of topics or issues a student needs to learn in a particular competency at their level.

D. EMS Education Program Accreditation

1. Commission on Accreditation of Allied Health Education Programs (CAAHEP)

Legal Aspects of Emergency Medical Systems[11,17,18,20,26]

A. *Negligence:* Act or omission by a medical professional that results in patient injury

1. Duty to act
2. Breach of duty
3. Breach of duty was cause of patient injury
4. Damages occurred from patient injury

B. *Liability:* Legal responsibility for one's actions or omissions.

1. *Direct:* Liability imposed directly on an individual due to their negligence, default, or legal undertaking.
2. *Indirect:* Liability that arises from a legal obligation owed to an injured party for damages that occurred from another's failure to perform or a negligent act.

Role of the ENP[27,28]

A. There is currently no consensus statement from neither the American Academy of Nurse practitioners (AANP) nor the American Nurse Credentialing Center (ANCC) regarding nurse practitioners in the patient transport setting.

B. The Consensus Model for APRN Regulation: Licensure, Accreditation, Certification Education does not limit the scope of practice of APRNs to a specific setting, rather it is based on the needs of the patient (https://ncsbn.org/aprn-consensus.htm).

C. The ENP may receive patients from EMS systems in the ED setting.

D. The ENPs may utilize the EMS system for the transfer and transport of ED patients to other facilities.

E. The ENP may be called upon to participate in the transport of an emergency patient within the EMS system.

References

References for this chapter are online only and can be found at https://connect.springerpub.com/content/reference-book/978-0-8261-6091-5/part/part06/toc-part/ch45.

46. Patient Transfer and Transport

RONALD D. MEADOR

Learning Objectives

- Contrast the fundamental concepts of patient transfer versus patient transport.
- Discuss the elements of interfacility patient transfer and the steps necessary to maximize patient outcomes during transport.
- Describe the components of the Emergency Medical Treatment and Labor Act (EMTALA) as it relates to interfacility transfer of unstable patients.
- Describe the necessity of addressing all key components fully for all interfacility patient transfer documentation.
- Discuss the role of the emergency nurse practitioner (ENP) in the transfer and transport of patients who require transport from one facility to another.

Interfacility patient transfer (IPT) is a pivotal aspect of patient care frequently utilized to improve patient management and outcomes. More than 500,000 IPTs occur each year in the United States. IPTs are highly complex operations involving a multitude of interdependent processes and critical steps, which present varying degrees of unpredictability. The complexity of this operation creates the potential for critical errors that could result in adverse patient outcomes from a cascade of patient handoff situations. A detailed knowledge of the numerous factors involved in patient transfer is required to optimize patient outcomes and mitigate legal liability. The decision to transfer a patient is based on its potential benefits weighed against its potential risks. Emergency care providers frequently engage in IPTs and should be well versed in all complex processes and critical steps involved in successfully transferring a patient.[1–3]

Communication

A. Pretransport
  1. Transferring provider to receiving provider
  2. Primary transferring nurse to charge or receiving nurse
  3. Transferring facility administrator to receiving facility administrator as indicated
  4. Transferring and/or receiving provider to transport personnel
    a. Treatment orders
    b. Transfer orders

B. Intratransport
  1. Contact with transferring and receiving facility as indicated
  2. Online medical direction of transport service
  3. Standing or offline medical direction

C. Posttransport
  1. Report to receiving personnel
  2. Follow-up to referring personnel
  3. Medical audits
  4. Ongoing monitoring to evaluate system effectiveness

Definitions[1–6]

A. *Facility:* Licensed healthcare entity

B. *Integration:* Consolidation and coordination of distinct entities into a unified, harmonious process

C. *Emergency medical condition:* Medical condition of sufficient severity that lack of immediate medical attention could result in:
  1. Placing the health of an individual—or in the case of a pregnant woman, an unborn child—in serious jeopardy
  2. Serious impairment of bodily functions
  3. Serious dysfunction of any bodily organ or part

D. *Stabilization:* Provide medical treatment of a condition as necessary to reasonably assure that no material deterioration of the condition is likely to result from or occur during transfer.

E. *Transfer:* Comprehensive, multistep process involving the movement of a patient from one location to another
  1. *Intrafacility:* Patient movement within a facility
  2. *Interfacility:* Patient movement between facilities

F. *Transport:* Physical process of moving a patient from one location to another
  1. *Air medical transport:* Any rotor-wing (helicopter) or fixed-wing (airplane) transport vehicle
  2. *Surface medical transport:* Any transport vehicle other than that included in air transport

Documentation[1,4,6–12]

A. Complete, accurate, and legible patient care reports

B. Transfer form elements
  1. Patient condition
    a. Risks of transfer outweighed by benefits of transfer

b. Vital signs at time of departure to receiving facility

2. Reason for transfer
   a. A medical necessity exists because the needs of the patient exceeds the capacities of the sending facility.
   b. Patient request
3. Receiving facility acceptance
   a. Name of receiving facility
   b. Name of individual at receiving facility authorized to accept transfers
   c. Name of accepting provider
4. Transfer risks
5. Transfer benefits
6. Transport mode
7. Patient consent

C. Transfer checklist elements
1. Completed certification of transfer form
2. Correct patient identification
3. Prehospital record if appropriate
4. Sending facility records
5. Radiologic studies
6. Patient valuables
7. Transfer records
   a. Patient demographics including next of kin
   b. Patient condition on admission to sending facility
   c. History of present illness or mechanism of injury as applicable
   d. Diagnosis
   e. Diagnostic study results
   f. Treatments and patient response to treatments
   g. Medications administered and patient response including adverse reactions
   h. Patient status at time of transfer
   i. Order to transfer
   j. Name and contact number of transferring clinician
   k. Receiving provider and facility
8. Transport records
   a. Service completing transfer
      i. National Emergency Medical Service Information System
      ii. National Highway Traffic Safety Administration
   b. Facility documentation
      i. Patient demographics
      ii. Vital signs
      iii. Care provided
      iv. Name and signature of transporting personnel
      v. Patient status at time of departure from sending facility
      vi. Patient status at time of arrival at receiving facility

Elements of Patient Transfer[1–10,13–16]

A. Legal considerations
1. Emergency Medical Treatment and Labor Act EMTALA
   a. Designed to prevent hospitals from refusing to treat or transferring patients based on ability to pay
   b. Only applies to hospitals that accept Medicare reimbursement
   c. Facility requirements under EMTALA
      i. Medical screening exam (MSE) to determine whether an emergency medical condition exists without regard to ability to pay
      ii. If an emergency medical condition exists, provision of treatment within the scope of practice of the emergency nurse practitioner (ENP) and other medical personnel until the patient is stabilized or transferred if the facility does not have the capability to treat the emergency medical condition.
      iii. Facilities with specialized capabilities are obligated to accept transfers if they possess the capabilities to treat without regard to ability to pay.
   d. EMTALA does not govern the transfer of stable patients if the attending provider determines that no material deterioration will occur during the transfer between facilities.
   e. Conditions for transfer of unstable patients
      i. Patient or patient advocate provides written request for transfer despite facility EMTALA obligation to provide stabilization.
      ii. Clinician certifies that medical benefits of transfer outweigh patient risk.
   f. Transferring clinician/facility is responsible for patient care until arrival at receiving facility.
   g. Requirement for transfer
      i. Transferring facility must provide all medical treatments within its capacity and scope of practice of the providers at the referring facility.
      ii. Receiving facility must accept transfer and have adequate space and qualified personnel.
      iii. Transferring facility must provide copies of all medical records.
      iv. Qualified personnel with the most appropriate equipment available must accompany the patient during transfer.
2. Certification of medical necessity (CMN)
   a. Requirement of the Centers for Medicare & Medicaid Services (CMS) payment for ambulance transport
   b. Medical necessity is established when the patient's condition contraindicates the transport other than by ambulance because it would endanger the patient's health.
3. Health Insurance Portability and Accountability Act (HIPAA)
   a. Sets standards for use, disclosure, transmission, and storage of protected health information (PHI)
   b. Affects services transporting and facilities transferring medical information from one facility to another
4. Federal, state, and interstate regulations

a. Federal Aviation Administration (FAA) regulations
i. 14 CFR Part 91—General operating flight rules
ii. 14 CFR Part 135—Commuter and on-demand operations
5. State regulation (varies from state to state)
a. Emergency medical service (EMS) scope of practice
b. Protocols
c. Communications
d. Medical oversight
e. Roles and responsibilities regarding interfacility transfers
6. Interstate regulations
a. Remote areas that do not have access to comprehensive or specialty care within their own state create referral patterns that cross state lines
b. Certain metropolitan areas serve more than one state.
c. May require official agreements between states as regulations vary by state as discussed above

B. Clinician considerations
1. Identification of transfer-eligible patients
a. Inadequate resources to provide adequate patient care and expertise
b. Need for medical subspecialties
c. Lack of adequate nursing services (e.g., intensive care services, dialysis)
d. Lack of diagnostic or interventional equipment
2. Pretransfer stabilization and preparation
a. Adequate resuscitation and stabilization to maximum resources and skilled providers available
i. Airway
(1) Positioning
(2) Artificial airways
(a) Oropharyngeal
(b) Nasopharyngeal
(c) Supraglottic
(d) Endotracheal
(3) Suctioning
(4) Gastric decompression
ii. Breathing
(1) Positioning
(2) Supplemental oxygen
(3) Assisted ventilation with bag-valve mask
(4) Mechanical ventilation
(5) Chest decompression
(a) Needle thoracostomy
(b) Chest tube thoracostomy
iii. Circulation
(1) Management of external hemorrhaging
(2) Intravenous access
(3) Crystalloid fluid replacement
(4) Colloid fluid replacement
(5) Cardiac rhythm monitoring
(6) Bladder decompression for monitoring
iv. Spinal motion restriction
(1) Cervical collar
(2) Cervical traction
(3) Appropriate use of a backboard
v. Fracture care
(1) Flexible, vacuum, board splint, SAM splint
(2) Nonflexible, plaster, fiberglass
(a) Plaster should be bivalved before fixed-wing transport.
(3) Air splints, caution in air transport
(4) Traction
(5) Ensure access to distal pulses
vi. Wound care
(1) Control of external hemorrhaging
(2) Do not delay transport for wound closure.
(3) Dressings as indicated
(4) Tetanus and antibiotics as indicated
(5) Burn care to current recommendations
vii. Psychosocial support
viii. Diagnostic studies
(1) Serologic
(2) Urine
(3) Imaging
3. Identification of risk versus benefit stratification; match potential patient needs with appropriate transferring providers.
a. Stable with no risk of deterioration
i. Require oxygen
ii. Vital sign monitoring
iii. Maintenance of saline lock
iv. Basic emergency medical care
b. Stable with low risk for deterioration
i. Intravenous fluids infusion
ii. Limited IV medications, such as analgesics
iii. Pulse oximetry
iv. Advanced emergency care
c. Stable with moderation risk for deterioration
i. Three-lead EKG monitoring
ii. Basic cardiac medications, such as nitroglycerin or heparin
iii. More advanced emergency care
d. Stable with high risk for deterioration
i. Advanced airway management
ii. Ventilator management
iii. Vasoactive medications
iv. Required initial stabilization
v. Critical care
e. Unstable with clinical deterioration
i. Unable to stabilize at sending facility
ii. Currently deteriorating or likely to deteriorate
iii. Invasive monitoring
iv. Balloon pumps
v. Postresuscitation
4. Identification of legal considerations
a. Facility guidelines
i. Transfer guidelines within a specific facility
ii. Facility policies and procedures and staff bylaws that designate who is responsible for

accepting and transferring patients on behalf of the facility
iii. Identification of who is responsible for performing facility MSE
iv. Auto accept policies for specific patient populations

b. Regional guidelines
i. Guidelines for interfacility transfer of patients within specific geographical areas within a state
ii. Designated facilities for higher level of care of specific patient populations, that is, trauma, psychiatry, invasive cardiology
iii. Often established by regional advisories committees or by agreements between facilities within a given geographical area

c. State guidelines
i. Guidelines for interfacility transfer of patients within a state or between states
ii. Often established by state departments of health or state legislatures in administrative codes

d. National guidelines
i. EMTALA

5. Identification of appropriate destination facility
a. Has appropriate resources that the sending facility lacks
b. Has adequate bed availability

6. Negotiation of transfer
a. Acceptance by appropriate provider at receiving facility
i. Auto accept facilities
ii. Nonauto accept facilities
b. Appropriate administrative approval
c. Appropriate order for patient transfer meeting all legal requirements
d. Informed consent of patient or legal representative, where applicable)

7. Identification of appropriate mode of transfer
a. Ground
b. Air

8. Identification of appropriate level of care/equipment needed
a. Basic life support (BLS)
b. Advanced life support (ALS)
c. Critical care transport (CCT)
d. Specialty care transport (SCT)
e. Identification of appropriate personnel
i. Emergency medical technician
ii. Paramedic
iii. Nurse
iv. Respiratory therapist
v. Perfusionist
vi. Advanced practice provider
vii. Physician
f. Identification of risk categories
i. *Medical:* Patient decompensation
ii. *Technical:* Equipment failure
iii. *Human:* Medication, procedural, cognitive errors
g. Consideration of physiologic alterations during transport
i. Noise
(1) Wind
(2) Rotor-blade or propeller
(3) Engine
(4) Monitoring equipment
ii. Vibration
(1) Uneven roads
(2) Vehicle suspension
(3) Rotor-blade or propeller
(4) Engine
(5) Air turbulence
iii. Acceleration, deceleration, and gravitational forces
(1) Radial acceleration/deceleration
(2) Linear acceleration/deceleration
iv. Temperature and humidity
(1) Cold and heat extremes
(2) Humidity change with altitude
v. Altitude
(1) Types of hypoxia
(a) *Hypoxic hypoxia:* As altitude increases, the partial pressure of oxygen decreases and alveolar gas exchange is impaired.
(b) *Hypemic hypoxia:* Impaired oxygen-carrying capacity due to factors such as anemia, hemorrhage, hemoglobin abnormalities, sulfa drugs, nitrites, and carbon monoxide
(c) *Stagnant hypoxia:* Decreased blood flow from heart failure, arterial constriction, and forms of distributive shock
(d) *Histotoxic hypoxia:* Cells are unable to utilize oxygen from substances such as alcohol, opiates, and cyanide.
(2) Gas laws and pressure changes
(a) *Boyle's Law*
- At constant temperature, pressure is inversely proportional to volume.
- As altitude increases, pressure decreases and volume within body cavities or closed containers increases.
(b) *Charles' Law*
- At constant pressure, volume is directly proportional to absolute temperature for a fixed mass of gas.
- Inspired tidal volume increases as temperature increases.
- Volume of oxygen in a cylinder decreases as the temperature decreases and therefore, as altitude increases, temperature decreases and volume of oxygen in a cylinder decreases.

(c) *Ideal Gas Law*
- Combination of Boyle and Charles' Laws
- Used in calculating the volume of oxygen in a cylinder to determine if enough oxygen is available for a given patient transport

(d) *Dalton's Law*
- Sum of partial pressures of a mixture of gases is equal to the total pressure exerted by the mixture.
- As altitude increases and pressure decreases, the delivered concentration of anesthetic gases increases.

(e) *Henry's Law*
- At constant temperature, the amount of dissolved gas in a liquid is directly proportional to the partial pressures of that gas.
- As altitude increases and pressure decreases, the delivered concentration of anesthetic gases increases.

(3) Third space loss
(4) Motion sickness

C. Administrative considerations
1. CMN for ambulance transfer as applicable
2. Interfacility transfer agreements
3. Interfacility transfer guidelines
a. Medical and administrative authority regarding transfers
b. Guideline to determine transfer
i. Patients that require transfer
ii. Most appropriate facility to transfer to
iii. Mode of transport
iv. Minimum equipment and personnel
c. Protocols or standing orders for transport personnel
d. System to arrange transfer and transport
e. Transfer forms
f. Policy regarding special circumstances that occur during transport
4. Compliance with local, state, and federal guidelines
5. Personnel training and education regarding applicable laws

D. Financial considerations
1. EMTALA transfer violations
a. Termination of the hospital or provider's Medicare provider agreement
b. $25,000 per violation for facilities with less than 100 beds
c. $50,000 per violation for facilities with greater than 100 beds
d. $50,000 per violation for providers
2. Facility may be liable for personal injury damages in civil court.
3. Receiving facility may bring suit against the sending facility for financial loss.

Role of the Emergency Nurse Practitioner[1,4,7,8,11,12]

A. The principal goal of the ENP is ensuring the health and well-being of the ED patient who requires transfer to another facility.
B. Follow all applicable laws regarding patient transfer
C. Be responsible for informing the patient or responsible party of the risks and benefit of transfer and ensure adequate documentation of discussion.
D. Use best judgment in compliance with medical staff bylaws regarding patient condition, timing of transfer, mode of transport, level of care needed during transport, and the appropriate destination facility.
E. Accurately complete all pertinent patient care records prior to patient transfer to ensure optimal continuity of care and reducing the potential for handoff errors.

References

References for this chapter are online only and can be found at https://connect.springerpub.com/content/reference-book/978-0-8261-6091-5/part/part06/toc-part/ch46.

47. Crisis and Disaster Management

ERIC ROBERTS | ANDREW ROTJAN

Learning Objectives

- Explain the goals of crisis and disaster management.
- Identify components of an effective emergency operations plan (EOP).
- Define Incident Command System terminology.
- Distinguish between the responsibilities of each position within the Incident Command System.
- Create a strategy for personal readiness during a disaster through an understanding of individual healthcare clinician responsibilities.
- Explain the effects of disasters on the mental health of individuals and families.
- Recognize the unique effects of disasters on the mental health of healthcare workers.
- Employ mental health triage to appropriately connect those in need with available resources.
- Define and apply psychologic first aid.
- Implement self-care strategies to facilitate wellness in disaster response.
- Explain the impact of crisis standards of care on mental health during disasters.
- Recognize how disasters have an impact on the bereavement of individuals that experience loss.

Crises and disasters pose a challenge to healthcare systems. They present with conditions that may overwhelm standard operations and therefore require unique preparation and response. They produce situations that demand a coordinated and deliberate response. The goal of crisis and disaster management is to recognize these challenges and respond in ways to maximize resource utilization for the benefit of minimizing loss of life and property. Outcomes are best achieved when facilities work with community partners to anticipate risks, vulnerabilities, and demands that may be made on resources. In doing this, effective emergency operation plans may be developed. Crisis and disaster response requires an approach that considers prevention, protection, mitigation, response, and recovery to maximize outcomes during events that require integrated tactics. The roles of the individual, facility, and community must be considered from the perspective of moving beyond standard operations to address unique variables that place a strain on the healthcare system.

Organizational preparation is essential. This preparation is best accomplished through the development and execution of a strategic emergency operations plan (EOP). The EOP is individualized to the unique threats and needs of an institution. This plan designates the roles and responsibilities of individuals within the organization. To minimize chaos and maximize effectiveness during a crisis or disaster, these roles are well established within a structured Incident Command System. While the broad-scale organizational structure is addressed, it is essential that individuals understand their personal duties to the organization, community, and self. Individuals have unique roles in all phases before, during, and after a crisis or disaster response. Ensuring individual and organizational readiness will ultimately determine the effectiveness of crisis and disaster response.

Disaster Mental Health Considerations

Disasters place individuals, families, and responders at risk for compromised mental health. The exceptional physical, emotional, and financial stress of a disaster often leaves those involved with unique needs that must be understood and managed. The personal effect of a disaster is unique to the individual and varies. For this reason, it is important to understand risk factors for impaired emotional response. As the impact is unique so also is the required response.

Effect of Disasters on the Mental Health of Individuals

A. There is already a strain on mental health services in the United States.[1]

1. Disasters may add additional strain to access of services causing extended delay in care.

2. Employ mental health triage to appropriately connect those in need with available resources.

a. PsySTART[1,2]

i. Evidence-based rapid mental health triage and incident management system

ii. Rapid individual and population-level triage

iii. Matches appropriate levels of care

iv. Does not require mental health professional to complete

v. Measures impact of extreme stressors and what happened to the person based on extreme exposure, traumatic loss, secondary impacts, injury/illness, panic

vi. Stratified assessment results

(1) *Low risk:* Do not currently present with risk factors; provide psychologic first aid
(2) *Moderate risk:* Presumptive risk factors; require crisis intervention, secondary screening
(3) *High risk:* One or more risk factors; require emergency care, immediate crisis intervention
(4) Danger to self and/or others; are evaluated for danger

B. Recognize high-risk populations[3]
  1. Children
  2. Older adults
  3. Those with preexisting mental health disorders
  4. Rescue personnel
  5. Emergency medicine clinicians

C. Mental health reactions may differ by type of disaster. Common psychologic reaction to bioterrorism includes the following[3]:
  1. Horror, anger, panic
  2. Magical thinking about microbes and viruses
  3. Fear of invisible agents
  4. Arousal symptoms to infection
  5. Anger at terrorists or the government
  6. Scapegoating
  7. Paranoia, social isolation, demoralization

D. Implementation strategies
  1. Mental health operations should be integrated into the Incident Command System (ICS).[1]
  2. Preincident stress inoculation
    a. *Resilience planning:* Develop a mechanism for adapting well in face of adversity, trauma, tragedy, threats of stress; ensure family stability; develop social support, and develop capacity to tolerate stress and uncertainty[1]
    b. Self-triage
    c. Internet-based interventions, including cognitive behavioral therapy, stress, and coping strategies, mindfulness exercise, and problem-solving strategies[4]
  3. Develop mental health training for:
    a. Spiritual care staff
    b. Healthcare clinicians
    c. The public
  4. Disaster mental health response principles[5]
    a. Interventions must be taken *to* survivors as most will not seek help.
    b. Survivors and bereaved are particularly susceptible to efforts that appear voyeuristic.
    c. Never separate children from families.
    d. Limit exposure to death and mutilated.
    e. Give accurate, truthful information.
    f. Protect victim privacy and limit exposure to the media.
    g. Use naturally occurring support systems.
    h. Avoid medicalizing reactions.
    i. Minimize retraumatization.
    j. Mandatory psychologic debriefing is clinically indicated.
  5. Psychologic first aid[5]
    a. Addresses five essential elements
      i. Safety
      ii. Calming
      iii. Connectedness
      iv. Self-efficacy
      v. Hope
    b. Core actions
      i. Contact and engage.
      ii. Provide safety and comfort.
      iii. Stabilize if needed.
      iv. Assess current needs and concerns.
      v. Provide practical assistance.
      vi. Connect with social supports.
      vii. Provide information on coping.
      viii. Link with collaborative services.
  6. Develop behavioral coping component of risk communication.
  7. Anticipate and deploy mental health resources in the most efficient manner.
  8. Planning
    a. Types of disasters most likely in a community
    b. Awareness of county and state mental health disaster plan
    c. Anticipate the type of expertise needed in response.
    d. Preidentify qualified mental health professionals.

Effect of Disasters on the Mental Health of Families and Populations

A. Unique attributes of disasters[3]
  1. Individuals may have to make decisions that involve life and death consequences for family members.
  2. Consequences of decisions may be realized rapidly at the bedside.
  3. Some disasters require social distancing as an implication of healthcare response (e.g., infectious disease), resulting in feelings of isolation.
  4. When crisis standards of care (CSC) are implemented on a large scale, perception of inequality may prevail
  5. Mass panic may be felt if:[1]
    a. There is a belief that there is little chance of escape from the effects of a disaster.
    b. The risk is perceived as having a significant impact.
    c. There are limited resources available.
    d. There is a perception that the response is ineffective.
    e. The authorities are perceived as lacking credibility.

B. *Traumatic grief/traumatic bereavement:* Results when the death of a loved one occurs in traumatic context
  1. CSC may precipitate widespread traumatic grief.
  2. May affect bereaved relatives who did not experience the disaster more significantly than those who survived the event but were not left bereaved

C. Risk factors
  1. Experiencing traumatic loss
  2. Seeing many dead or injured
  3. Hearing cries of pain

4. Being trapped or unable to evacuate
5. Experiencing persistent stressors
6. Home loss
7. Disaster induced relocation

D. Potential reactions and implications
1. Marital discord
2. Parent–child problems
3. Separation anxiety
4. Posttraumatic stress disorder (PTSD)
5. Engagement in high-risk behaviors
6. Severe depression
7. Suicidality

E. Implementation strategies
1. Rapid triage (PsySTART)
2. Allocate limited resources to those at highest risk.

Unique Effects of Disasters on the Mental Health of Healthcare Workers

A. Healthcare workers are responsible for the success of disaster response while being vulnerable themselves.

B. On the front lines, healthcare workers face exceptional stress.
1. Witnessing trauma from the disaster
2. Addressing ethical principles of CSC
3. Confronting the impact of the disaster on themselves and their families

C. Important to understand the risk and approach to maintaining the mental health of healthcare workers.[1]

D. Unique risks in disasters[1]
1. CSC provides stress relative to quantity and quality of patient loss.
2. CSC shifts focus on needs of individual patient to those of the greatest good for the most people.
3. Disasters may result in mass causalities.
   a. May threaten the mental health of workers
   b. May present direct healthcare risk to the worker themselves, increasing mental health stress
4. High mortality rates
5. Death of pediatric patients

E. Mental health response to CSC
1. The concept of mental health operations should be integrated into the Incident Command System and other response plans. Development of a mental health plan should include:
   a. Triggers for mental health resources
   b. How to address the full continuum of those affected
      i. Those with preexisting mental illness
      ii. Those directly affected by CSC
      iii. Affected healthcare workers
      iv. The general public
2. Comprehensive programs should be developed for healthcare workers that integrate personal coping and agency preparedness. These should include:
   a. Preincident stress inoculation
   b. Development of personal resilience plans
   c. Psychologic first aid
   d. Self-triage
   e. Internet-based interventions for those who desire further support

F. Recognition of common stress reactions by disaster workers[3]
1. Psychologic reactions
   a. Denial
   b. Anxiety and fear
   c. Worry about the safety of self or others
   d. Anger
   e. Irritability
   f. Restlessness
   g. Sadness, grief, depression, or moodiness
   h. Distressing dream
   i. Guilt
   j. Hopelessness
   k. Feeling isolated
   l. Apathy
2. Behavioral reactions
   a. Change in activity
   b. Decreased efficiency and effectiveness
   c. Difficulty communicating
   d. Outbursts of anger
   e. Inability to rest
   f. Change in eating habits
   g. Change in sleeping patterns
   h. Change in patterns of intimacy
   i. Change in job performance
   j. Periods of crying
   k. Increased use of alcohol, tobacco, and drugs
   l. Social withdrawal
   m. Vigilance about safety
   n. Avoidance of activities
   o. Proneness to accidents
3. Cognitive reactions
   a. Memory problems
   b. Disorientation
   c. Confusion
   d. Slowness of thinking and comprehension
   e. Difficulty calculating, prioritizing, making decisions
   f. Poor concentration
   g. Limited attention span
   h. Loss of objectivity
   i. Unable to stop thinking about disaster
   j. Blaming
4. Physical reactions
   a. Increased heart, respiratory rate, blood pressure
   b. Nausea and diarrhea
   c. Change in appetite, weight loss, or gain
   d. Sweating
   e. Tremor
   f. Tunnel vision
   g. Headaches
   h. Soreness in muscles
   i. Low back pain
   j. Exaggerated startle reaction
   k. Fatigue
   l. Menstrual cycle change
   m. Change in sexual desire
   n. Decreased resistance to infection
   o. Flair of allergies
   p. Hair loss
5. Risk factors for PTSD in disaster workers

a. Younger age of worker
b. Single marital status
c. Prior psychiatric impairment
d. History of childhood sexual abuse
e. Injury during a disaster event
f. Lack of perceived safety during the event
g. Lesser social support
h. Low self-worth

G. Implementation strategies
1. *Self-care:* Before disaster response
a. *Self-awareness:* Relief workers dealing with excessive stress before disaster response are more susceptible to stress during the response.
b. *Resilience may be impacted by preparation:* Understand unique challenges such as nature of the disaster, cultural issues, disaster history of the area
c. Help disaster responder's family prepare for worker's absence.
i. Financial planning
ii. Childcare
2. *Self-care:* During disaster response
a. Workers clearly benefit from praise and recognition for their good work.
b. Encourage to work with their limits
c. Recognize their own vulnerability
d. Recognize signs of distress
i. Compassion fatigue
ii. Disturbance in sleep
iii. Body aches
iv. Changes in appetite
v. Gastrointestinal (GI) distress
vi. Clock-watching
vii. Depersonalization
viii. Irritability
ix. Pessimism
x. Cynicism
e. Get sufficient sleep.
f. Eat nutritiously and consistently.
g. Exercise.
h. Build sense of community with fellow disaster workers.
i. Mindfulness and relaxation techniques
3. *Self-care:* After disaster response
a. Give sufficient time to recover.
b. Avoid discussing gruesome, highly distressing experiences.
c. Focus on positive results of disaster work.
4. Crisis intervention when appropriate
a. Active listening
i. Allow silence.
ii. Attend nonverbally.
iii. Paraphrase.
iv. Reflect feelings.
v. Allow expression of emotions.
b. Problem-solve
i. Identify and define the problem.
ii. Assess the survivor's function and coping.
iii. Evaluate available resources.
iv. Develop and implement a plan.

Emergency Operations Plan

An EOP is a detailed proposal that outlines a strategic response to emergencies that may occur within the organization or community. These emergencies may affect the demands of the organization, or its ability to provide services. Disasters and crises are generally abrupt events that require prompt action for which preplanning is essential. The EOP is developed in anticipation of how an agency may be vulnerable during a disaster, how operations may be affected, and how resources may be deployed to affect the greatest outcomes. An effective plan addresses five phases of emergency management: prevention, protection, mitigation, response, and recovery.[6]

A. *Comprehensive Emergency Management:* The scope of the EOP should include an all-hazards approach, addressing capacity and capabilities across a full spectrum of emergencies with a focus on these critical elements[7]:
1. Communications
2. Resources and assets
3. Safety and security
4. Staff responsibilities
5. Utilities
6. Clinical support activities

B. *Prevention and Protection:* A component of the plan should include measures that a hospital, healthcare system, or public health agency should take to build capacity, create plans, and identify resources that may be used in the event of an emergency.[6]
1. Core capabilities essential for execution[6]
a. *Intelligence and information sharing:* A mechanism should be in place for sharing with partner organizations when a physical or virtual threat exists.
b. *Interdiction and disruption:* Contemplate ways to intercept, divert, or delay a potential threat.
c. *Screening, search, and detection:* Active and passive surveillance should be used to monitor for threats and hazards.
d. Access control and identification verification should be used to control entry to critical locations and systems.
e. Cybersecurity should be employed to protect electronic communication and information systems.
f. Physical protective measures ensure restricted access to key operational activities and infrastructure.
g. Risk management for protection programs and actives helps identify and prioritize risks and ensure operational readiness.
h. Supply chain integrity and security should be maintained to ensure transportation of requisite materials.
2. Implementation strategies
a. Train, qualify, and certify personnel to ensure that they have the knowledge, expertise, and capability to perform the duties of their assigned role.

b. *Develop simulation exercises:* These enable personnel to understand their capabilities and limitations before an incident.[8]

c. Employee education

d. Public education

e. Develop policies

f. *Create inventories, stockpile supplies, and equipment:* Acquiring, storing, and inventorying

g. Resource management, identify:

h. The capability and category of essential resources

i. How the resource may be widely used, shared, and deployed

ii. Establish mutual aid agreements with community agencies that delineate a legal basis for shared resources.

iii. Determine how and when to reassign existing resources from nonessential tasks.

iv. Develop contracts to acquire resources from vendors in a rapid fashion when needed.

C. *Mitigation:* Consists of measures that a hospital, healthcare system, or public agency may take in advance to lessen the severity and impact of a potential emergency or critical incident.[6,9] The intention is to prevent illness, injury, death, and limit the loss of property.

1. Core capabilities, essential for execution

a. *Community resilience:* Empower others to take necessary actions to adapt, withstand, and recover from crises or disasters.

b. *Long-term vulnerability reduction:* Build systems and infrastructure to reduce vulnerability to threats.

c. *Risk and disaster resilience assessment:* Complete a risk assessment that will inform the organization on how and where to take action.

d. Threats and hazards should be identified for their frequency and significance.

2. Essential concepts

a. *Disaster risk reduction*: Aims to reduce the damage caused by natural hazards like earthquakes, floods, droughts, and hurricanes through implementation of preventative measures.[9]

b. *Disaster risk management*: Seeks to correct or reduce disaster risks that are already present[9]

c. *Structural considerations*: Requires qualified and experienced structural engineers.[9] Plan should include:

i. Contract with engineers for planning and response

ii. Inventory and classification of buildings

iii. Vulnerability assessment

iv. Compliance with building codes

v. Determination of public safety risks

vi. Prioritization of structural reinforcement needs

vii. List of vulnerable structures

d. *Nonstructural considerations:* Help ensure that the operation of the facility is not compromised because of the impact of a disaster on the following:[9]

i. Fuel tanks

ii. Compressed gas

iii. Generators

iv. Equipment and supplies

v. Electrical lines

vi. Information technology

vii. Hazardous materials

3. Implementation strategies

a. Give consideration to how structural and nonstructural components may affect continuity of patient care.

b. Develop and implementing strategies to address potential threats.

D. *Hazard vulnerability analysis (HVA):* An HVA is a written document that allows an organization to recognize internal and external threats to the facility and well as to operations. It provides an opportunity to prioritize planning.[1,10]

1. An HVA will help a healthcare facility plan for specific events by allowing management to screen for risk and plan for strategic response.

2. A hazard may be any threat that could cause injury, fatality, property, infrastructure, or environmental damage or impair operations.

3. It may include an assessment of vulnerabilities to

a. Natural events (e.g., earthquake, flood, hurricane, tornado)

b. Technology events (e.g., electrical/power shortage, loss of backup generators, fire, heating/ventilation/air conditioning [HVAC] failure, structural failure)

c. Human events (e.g., mass causality events, infectious disease, bomb threat, infant abduction)

4. It should be developed by an intradisciplinary team.

5. An identified hazard should be considered for risk to humans, property, and business operations.

6. The HVA should be prioritized and reviewed annually and any time a new threat is realized.

E. *Response:* Includes activities a hospital, healthcare system, or public health agency takes immediately before, during, and after a disaster or emergency occurs.[6] The emphasis should be on saving and sustaining lives, stabilizing the incident, meeting basic human needs, restoring basic services, restoring functionality, establishing a safe environment, and supporting transition to recovery. Disaster response plans should be developed with the premise that the organization may have to operate autonomously for the first 96 hours of a crisis or disaster.

1. Core capabilities, essential for execution:

a. Critical transportation should focus on evacuation of people and animals from impacted areas as well as delivery of vital response personnel and equipment into affected sites.

b. Environmental response, health, and safety. Measures should be taken to ensure the health and safety of the public and workers.

c. Fatality management services should include recovery and victim identification.

d. Consideration should be given to access for fire management and suppression.
e. Logistics and supply chain management will allow for the delivery of essential provisions and equipment necessary to save lives, meet basic human needs, stabilize the incident, as well as for meeting the needs of survivors.
f. Mass care services will focus on providing life-sustaining services to the affected population. This includes feeding, sheltering, temporary housing, and distribution of emergency supplies.
g. Mass search and rescue operations may be necessary to locate and rescue any affected people.
h. On-scene security, protection, and law enforcement are necessary to ensure a safe environment in the affected area.
i. Operational communications should focus on the ability to connect the emergency responders and the affected population as well as reestablishing information sharing networks.
j. Public health, healthcare, and EMS should be protected from additional disease and injury as they complete triage and stabilization of victims and begin definitive care.
k. Situational awareness. Information should be made available and frequently updated to inform decision-making. This includes the nature and extent of the hazard, developing effects, as well as the status of the response.

2. Implementation strategies:
   a. Alert
   b. Assess, size up
   c. Mobilize
   d. Develop implementation plan
   e. Activate systems (Incident Command System [ICS], emergency operations center)
   f. Refine assessment
   g. Set priorities
   h. In disasters, care and resources must be rationed including access to inpatient beds and diagnostic studies.[11]
   i. Communication
3. Triage area
   a. Should include patient identification and establish mechanism for tracking
   b. May incorporate registration
4. Patient flow
   a. Should take into consideration the potential need for decontamination or isolation
   b. Should be moved to designated zoned treatment areas in focused areas of the department after triage. These areas should be organized into small healthcare teams[11]
5. Treatment areas[11]
   a. Should allow treatment teams to focus on a limited number of patients
   b. Minimizes chaos
   c. Performance can be enhanced and clinician time optimized.
6. *Command postactivation:* Should be triggered by leadership involved in the initial response when it is recognized that an event will overwhelm existing resources.[1,8] This allows for a proactive, coordinated management response to meet the needs of the event. Triggers that may become overwhelmed include:
   a. Space
   b. Staff
   c. Supplies
7. Resource allocation concepts:
   a. *Surge capacity*: The ability to evaluate and care for a significantly increased volume of patients.[1] This will challenge or exceeds normal operating capacity.
   b. *Surge capability*: The ability to manage patients requiring unusual or highly specialized medical evaluation and care that are not normally available at the location where they are needed (pediatric care at nonpediatric facility or burn care at a nonburn center).[1]
   c. *Conventional capacity*: The space, staff, and supplies used are consistent with daily practices of the institution.[1]
   d. *Contingency capacity*: The space, staff, and supplies used are not consistent with daily practices, but are functionally equivalent.[1]
   e. *Crisis capacity*: The space, staff, and supplies not routinely engaged during standard care are adapted to meet the needs of the crisis or disaster to provide sufficient care.[1]
8. Implementation of surge response[1]
   a. Develop situational awareness after an incident occurs.
   b. Assess the situation relative to the available resources.
   c. Incident command should advise on development of response strategies, anticipating any resource deficits.
   d. If a resource is scarce, implement adaptive strategies.
   e. Allocation and reallocation of resources may be necessary.
   f. Response strategies should be analyzed at regular intervals and each of these elements repeated until incident concludes.

F. *Recovery:* Activities undertaken after an emergency or disaster to restore minimum services and move toward long-term restoration.[6] These should be focused on clinical, financial, and information systems operations. It should begin with an accurate assessment of populations and operations affected.

1. Core capabilities, essential for execution:
   a. *Economic recovery:* This may include the development of new business or employment opportunities.
   b. *Health and social services:* This includes behavioral health.
   c. Infrastructure
   d. *Natural and cultural resources:* Historic properties should be preserved.
2. Implementation strategies
   1. Return operations to normal.
   2. Detail damage assessment.

3. Ensure care and shelter continues.
4. Identify funding assistance.
5. Remove debris.

Incident Command System[12]

The Incident Command System (ICS) is a management tool that can be implemented to respond during a crisis and disaster for the purpose of minimizing chaos, facilitating communication, and maximizing resource allocation. The goal of ICS is to get the right resources to the right place at the right time. This is accomplished by providing accurate information, requiring strict accountability, and planning to optimize control of the incident. It is scalable, allowing for small-scale or complex events. Conceptual underpinnings of ICS include the following:

A. *Common terminology:* Plain language should be used to identify functions, resource descriptions, and position titles to minimize miscommunication when working incidents that involve multiple agencies.[8,12] This should be applied to organizational functions, resource descriptions, and incident facilities.

B. *Modular organization:* The ICS structure should be staffed based on the size, complexity, and hazard environment.[8,12] Only activate agencies, positions, and resources that are needed for the specific incident.

C. *Unified command:* When multiple agencies are involved in the same response, they should work together, sharing resources.[8,12] Each participating partner maintains authority, responsibility, and accountability for its personnel and resources while jointly managing incident activities.

D. *Management by objectives:* The command staff establishes objectives that drive the incident.[8,12] These should include the following:

1. Specific, measurable objectives for an incident
2. Strategies, tactics, tasks, and activities to achieve the objectives
3. Assignments, plans, procedures, and protocols to accomplish tasks
4. Documenting of results for each objective and facilitate corrective actions

E. *Chain of command:* Defines orderly line of authority that may be needed to perform incident objectives.[8,12] This clarifies reporting relationships for management of personnel to minimize confusion as well as conflicting directives.

F. *Incident action plan:* Concise means of communicating incident objectives, tactics, and assignments for operational and support activities.[8,12]

1. May be formal or informal
2. Are required for all incidents but may not all be written plans
3. Are important to unify response and provide for effective, efficient, and safe operations.

G. *Manageable span of control:* Controls the number of individuals under a single supervisor.[8,12] The recommended range is three to seven, with five being optimal.

1. Enables leadership to effectively manage subordinates under their control.
2. Influenced by type of incident, hazards, experience of supervisor and subordinates.

H. *Predestinated incident facilities:* May facilitate response and management of recourses by controlling environment.[8] This may include the following:

1. *Incident Command Post (ICP):* houses command staff
2. *Staging areas:* Location in which personnel, supplies, and equipment await assignment
3. Mass casualty triage areas
4. Points of distribution
5. Emergency shelters

Incident Command System Positions

A. Incident Commander[8,12]
   1. Responsible for overall direction and guidance of staff
   2. Evaluates the overall requirements of the incident
   3. Determines the overall direction for the team
   4. Establishes priorities
   5. Ensures security
   6. Approves action plans
   7. Coordinates with key stakeholders
   8. Authorizes release of information
   9. Captures lessons learned and best practices
   10. May delegate authority

B. Public Information Officer[8,12]
   1. Responsible for developing and releasing information to the media, incident personnel, and appropriate agencies
   2. Monitors media and sources of public information to collect relevant information
   3. Transmits relevant information to appropriate personnel
   4. Ensures that all messaging is consistent

C. Safety Officer[8,12]
   1. Monitors incident operations and advises the incident commander
   2. Assesses, communicates, and mitigates hazardous environments
   3. Develops incident safety plan making recommendations for actions necessary to ensure personnel safety
   4. Has the authority to suspend, alter, delay, or terminate operations

D. Liaison Officer[8,12]
   1. Serves as the point of contact to and from other agencies
   2. Provides input on policies, resource availability, and incident-related matters
   3. May have assistants

E. Operations section[8,12]
   1. Have primary responsibility to manage the tactical operations
      a. Focuses on
         i. Saving lives
         ii. Reducing immediate hazards
         iii. Protecting property
         iv. Establishing situational control
         v. Restoring normal operations
      b. Develops objectives that are operationalized through planning and coordination with other functions of ICS

F. Planning section[8,12]
1. Responsible for overall accountability of the incident
2. Collect and document information about the response
3. Resource management
a. Identify requirements to meet incident objectives
b. Develop strategy
c. Determine tactics for use
d. Facilitates incident planning meetings
e. Keeps incident commander informed
f. Disseminates incident status information and analyzes the situation as it changes
g. Safeguards all incident documents

G. Logistics section[8,12]
1. Supports the incident by managing facilities, services, and materials
2. Resource management
a. Order and acquire
b. Mobilize
c. Track and report
i. Helps staff prepare to receive and use resource
ii. Facilitates safety and security
iii. Monitors location
iv. Enables coordination and movement
v. *Demobilize:* Orderly, safe, and efficient return of a resource to original location and status
(1) Coordinate with the planning section to determine whether resource should be reassigned rather than demobilized.
vi. Reimburse and restock
d. Coordinates with community resources
e. Oversees technology support, food, and medical care for responders

H. Finance section[8,12]
1. Manages the overall financial aspect of the incident including all procurement, compensation claims, and resource costs.
a. *Reimbursement:* Rectifying expenses incurred by resource clinicians; may be paid or unpaid (providing reciprocal services)
b. Important for establishing and maintaining resource readiness
2. Records personnel time
3. Negotiate leases and maintenance of vendor contracts
4. Determine mechanism for:
a. Collecting bills
b. Validating costs
c. Replacing or repairing damaged equipment
d. Accessing reimbursement programs

Individual Clinician Responsibilities[1]

Emergency medicine clinicians are exceptionally positioned for a role in crisis and disaster response. Given their background in emergency evaluation and treatment, these clinicians are typically frontline responders. They have a unique relationship with the emergency medical service agencies, hospital leadership, and other medical specialties, positioning them to play a key role in communications during a disaster and in the delivery of initial care.[11] Therefore, it is important for clinicians to understand and prepare for these responsibilities. It is imperative that they:

A. Take an active interest in disaster preparedness and response plan.
B. Maintain training on the National Incident Management System (NIMS) including specific training to individual roles within the ICS.
C. Be familiar with crisis standards of care indicators, triggers, and implementation protocols.
D. Understand how crisis and disaster notification will occur, individual responsibilities, and identified areas for reporting or responding. This includes awareness of mechanisms for communicating within the ICS.
1. *Check-in:* Understand where to report to receive assignment.
2. *Recordkeeping:* Follow incident procedures for documenting activities.
3. *Communication:* Observe radio and telephone procedures; use plain language.
4. Check-out:
a. Follow procedures before leaving the incident area.
b. Complete all work in progress unless otherwise directed.
c. Ensure records are up to date; return equipment.
d. Brief incoming personnel
E. Understand personal role in triage and expansion of surge capacity[11]
1. Emergency clinicians are expected to play a role in providing triage, emergency stabilization, and disposition of disaster victims.
2. An immediate role in surge capacity may be that of working to free up space within the ED for disaster victims. This includes helping to relocate patients that are awaiting admission.
3. They may be called upon to establish decontamination areas may need to be established.
4. They may be asked to provide medical treatment in established surge areas outside the ED.
F. Monitor personal stress during and after an incident.
G. Understand when and how to access mental health services for themselves and others.

Mass Casualty Situations and Triage

During times of healthcare crisis and disaster, it is imperative that resources are mobilized and utilized in a manner that will provide the best outcome to the greatest number of people in need. This can only be accomplished by anticipating the needs of the population, as well as actively employing strategies during the crisis that put the right people in the right place to receive care. This requires an understanding of how unique attributes of disasters may lend themselves to unique needs in response. Clinicians must also be competent in disaster-specific triage. While triage occurs daily in times of standard care, disaster triage employs strategies for rapidly sorting large numbers of people, populations that must get expedited access to often limited resources.

Medical Care in Mass Casualty Situations

A. Continuum of medical care
  1. *Conventional care:* Business as usual for all patients[13]
  2. *Contingency care:* Functionally equivalent care[13]
    a. Usual care may be adapted.
      i. For example, triage may occur outside of the ED.
      ii. Critical care may be delivered in a postanesthesia unit.
      iii. Inpatient care may be shifted to hallways.
  3. Crisis care[13]
    a. Usual care cannot be delivered due to lack of resources.
    b. Care should be delivered to best obtainable outcome, depending on the resource limitation.
    c. Associated with increased risk in morbidity and mortality
      i. Risk may be reduced with preplanned strategies for resource allocation and use.
  4. Goals should be to deliver conventional and contingency care.
    a. If delivering crisis care, return to delivering contingency and conventional as soon as possible

B. *Disaster planning:* A systems approach to disaster planning and response is required to integrate all of the values and response capabilities necessary to achieve the best outcomes for the community as a whole.[13]
  1. *Clinical Care Committee:* Hospitals should establish disaster care committees. These should be interdisciplinary to include representatives from administrative leadership, facilities, nursing, pharmacy, respiratory therapy, infection prevention, critical care, emergency medicine, emergency medical services (EMS), ethics liaison, specialty clinicians. This team should participate in strategic response planning and influence preparation, mitigation, and response strategies.
  2. All-hazards planning approach is an integrated approach to emergency preparedness that focuses on capacities and capabilities that are critical to preparedness for a full spectrum of emergencies or disasters.[1] Planning should consider all hazards and threats and address common operational functions in a basic, overarching plan. For example, general tasks of evacuation and shelter in place operations and apply to a broad spectrum of threats. This approach allows planners to identify common tasks and those responsible for the tasks.[14]
  3. Types of disasters
    a. Chemical or hazardous material
    b. Biological
    c. Radiological
    d. Nuclear
    e. Explosive or incendiary
    f. Infectious disease
      i. Influenza
      ii. Ebola
      iii. COVID
    g. Mass shootings
    h. Hurricane
    i. Earthquake
    j. Power outage
    k. Flood or tsunami
    l. Tornado
    m. Fire
    n. Technological
    o. Transportation
      i. Aviation
      ii. Motor vehicle
      iii. Aquatic
      iv. Rail
  4. *Disaster training:* Most ethical and legal conflicts can be avoided with disaster training and familiarity with disaster plans and therefore should be mandatory for all practicing clinicians.[15] The following are established training courses to facilitate disaster training:
    a. National Disaster Life Support Consortium
      i. Basic Disaster Life Support
      ii. Advanced Disaster Life Support
      iii. Core Disaster Life Support
    b. Advanced Trauma Life Support
    c. Federal Emergency Management Agency (FEMA) courses available
  5. *Education, training, and drills:* Disaster plans must be disseminated so that stakeholders and responders can develop the knowledge, skills, and abilities needed to perform the tasks identified in the plan.[14] It is essential for personnel to become familiar with priorities, goals, objectives, and course of actions of disaster plans. The effectiveness of the plan can be evaluated by implementing exercises and drills.[14]
    a. Who
      i. Individual
      ii. Departmental
      iii. Institutional planning
      iv. Local and community planning
      v. State planning
    b. Types
      i. Tabletop
      ii. Computer simulation
      iii. In-situ simulation
        (1) Gather real-time data
    c. When
      i. Recommendation is for at least two times a year.
    d. How
      i. Drill a disaster plan.
    e. Afterward
      i. After-action reports
      ii. Debriefs
      iii. Lessons learned
      iv. Modify plan
  6. Barriers to preparedness
    a. Cost
    b. Time
    c. Staff buy-in
    d. Denial
    e. Exposes institutional risks and flaws
    f. Concern for impact on real-time patient care

C. Resource allocation considerations[13]
 1. Space
  a. Clinicians should be familiar with their hospital's surge plan that may consider:
   i. Rapid discharge protocols
   ii. Rapid transition of admitted patients to inpatient units
   iii. Cancelation of elective surgical procedures
   iv. Preidentified alternate care locations
   v. Outdoor field triage and treatment locations with tents
 2. Personnel and staff
  a. Sufficient available staff
  b. Trained appropriate in disaster plans
  c. Ability to call in clinicians, including subspecialty clinicians
   i. Text message
    (1) Most reliable
   ii. Phone chain
    (1) Relies on:
     (a) Cell towers
     (b) Available bandwidth
   iii. Pager
    (1) Semireliable
    (2) Check system for simultaneous page versus sequential paging.
    (3) Numeric versus alphanumeric paging
   iv. Email
    (1) May require power
    (2) May rely on cell towers
    (3) Local internet provider services to be intact
  d. Ability for responding clinicians to get to the ED
   i. Personal injury
   ii. Concern for the family may inhibit their response.
    (1) Some hospitals create family care centers to employees can focus on patients
   iii. Destruction of personal vehicles or collapse of public transit system related to traffic, mass gatherings, and so on
    (1) Personnel should consider multiple routes and alternate transportation based on various disaster types.
    (2) Hospital may be able to communicate best route.
  e. Use of inpatient teams in the ED
  f. Flexibility of staff to perform alternate tasks and extend capacity (e.g., scribing notes, order entry, runner)
 3. Supplies
  a. Dependent on size of facility and preplanning
  b. Variable based on role within the community
  c. Access to stockpiles
 4. Special populations and events
  a. Isolation rooms and personal protective equipment (PPE)
  b. Decontamination rooms
  c. Burn care
  d. Pediatric services
  e. Ability to transfer to alternate sites

Triage Considerations

Triage is often initially considered by making resource allocation decisions on an individual basis. Clinicians should gain experience in deciding when usual models of care should be abandoned in favor of more limited interventions. Proactive triage should consider resources in relation to the overall event.[13]

A. *Primary triage:* Performed at the first assessment and prior to any interventions.[13]
 1. For example, in the prehospital setting, ambulance bay, waiting room, and so on
 2. Clinicians should have proper training in triage methodology.
 3. Need to be able to assess life threats such as airway compromise, hemodynamic instability, subtle penetrating wounds to the trunk
 4. Clinicians should recognize that not every patient may be cared for, and some will need palliative care for comfort and not resuscitative care for survival.

B. *Secondary triage:* Performed after the initial assessments and initial interventions.[7]
 1. Usually performed by emergency and surgical clinicians to prioritize diagnostic studies and treatment

C. *Tertiary triage:* Performed after or during the provision of definitive diagnosis and medical care.[13]
 1. Unlikely to be performed in the ED
 2. Assesses need for resource allocation to patient to support care
 3. Attempts to be proactive to reallocate resources when needed
  a. For example:
   i. Decision regarding use of ventilatory support in a previously more stable patient
   ii. Decision to continue with surgical evaluation after initial laparotomy

Ethical Decision-Making in Resource Allocation[15]

A. Emergency clinicians have an obligation to plan and practice triage prior to an event to include the following principles:
 1. Fairness
  a. Process treats all patients with similar needs equally.
 2. Duty to care
  a. Clinicians have a duty to provide care to all patients to the best of their ability when accounting for available resources.
 3. Duty to steward resources
  a. Clinicians should aim to have the best outcomes for the greatest number of patients with the available resources.
 4. Transparency
  a. Process and criteria should be transparent.
  b. This can be extremely difficult to communicate with patients and/or the public.
 5. Consistency
  a. The same triage process should be applied to all patients in the same manner, by all triaging clinicians.
 6. Proportionality

a. Resources should be restricted in proportion to demand of the resource as well as the duration of need of the resource.

7. Accountability

a. Emergency clinicians need to be able to support triage decisions.

Triage Methods

A. Sort-Assess-Lifesaving Interventions-Treatment and/or Transport (SALT)[16]

1. Sort

a. Ask those who can walk to relocate to a designated area.

i. Assess third.

b. Ask those remaining to follow a command (e.g., wave).

i. Assess second.

c. Patients who remain still or have an obvious life threat

i. Assess first.

2. Assess

a. Initial assessment should be restricted to lifesaving interventions.

i. Hemorrhage control

ii. Direct pressure

iii. Tourniquets

iv. Other devices

b. Basic airway management

i. Airway repositioning

ii. Head-tilt, chin lift

c. Lifesaving interventions

i. Nasopharyngeal airways

ii. Oropharyngeal airways

iii. Consider two rescue breaths in pediatric patients.

iv. Chest decompression for suspected tension pneumothorax

(1) Large-bore catheter placed midclavicular line of the affected side in the second intercostal space, above the third rib)

v. Autoinjector antidotes

(1) Organophosphate toxicity

(2) Mark I kits (2-PAM chloride/atropine)

vi. Anaphylaxis

(1) Epinephrine

3. Continued assessment

a. Assess the following:

i. Obeys commands or makes purposeful movements

ii. Has a peripheral pulse

iii. Not in respiratory distress

iv. Major hemorrhage controlled

(1) If ALL (a,b,c,d) are yes AND the patient has minor injuries, the patient can be triaged as MINIMAL.

(2) Patient should be triaged as DELAYED if more significant injuries exist.

(3) If ANY (a,b,c,d) are answered NO and they are likely to survive with available resources, then patient is triaged as IMMEDIATE.

v. If unlikely to survive with available resources, the patient should be triaged as EXPECTANT.

B. Simple Triage and Rapid Transport (START; modified START/JUMP START)[17]

1. Assessment

a. Can patient walk?

i. Yes

(1) Triage GREEN

ii. NO

(1) Assess breathing without any airway maneuvers (e.g., head-tilt/chin lift, jaw thrust): *Is the patient breathing?*

(2) NO

(a) Open airway: *Is the patient breathing?*

(b) If NO, patient is tagged BLACK.

(c) If YES, patient is tagged RED.

(3) YES

b. Assess respiratory rate: *Is the respiratory rate >30 breaths per minute?*

i. If YES, patient is tagged RED.

ii. If NO, assess RADIAL pulse.

c. Assess radial pulse: *Is the pulse present?*

i. If NO, patient is tagged RED.

ii. If YES, assess the patient's level of consciousness.

d. Assess level of consciousness: *Is the patient responsive?*

i. If NO, patient is tagged RED.

ii. If YES, patient is tagged YELLOW.

C. Simple Triage Scoring System (STSS)[18]

1. Designed for ED use to triage patients with suspected infection

a. Useful for pandemic influenza

2. Evaluate the following objective data to risk-stratify patients:

a. Respiratory rate (RR) >30 breaths per minute

b. Shock index >1 (heart rate [HR] > blood pressure [BP])

c. Low oxygen saturation

d. Altered mental status (AMS)

e. Age ≥65

3. Each category is assigned one point; the more points a patient has, the more care and resources the patient will need, and therefore is tagged as IMMEDIATE.

D. Fast Triage in Burns (FTB)[19]

1. Assess extent of deep burns.

2. If >50% body surface area (BSA): >95% risk of death; symptomatic treatment only

a. These patients are tagged BLACK.

3. If between 5% and 50%, assess SYSTOLIC blood pressure (SBP)

a. If SBP <60 mmHg (and no pulse present on the radial, femoral, or carotid arteries), there is a >95% risk of death; symptomatic treatment only.

i. These patients are tagged BLACK.

b. If SBP >60 mmHg (pulse is present in at least one carotid artery), then assess TOTAL BSA Burned

i. If >50% BSA burned, there is a 50% to 95% risk of death and urgent intervention and priority evacuation is required.

(a) These patients are tagged RED.

ii. If <50% BSA burned, there is a 5% to 50% risk of mortality and medical intervention and secondary priority evacuation is required.

(a) These patients are tagged YELLOW.

(b) If these patients have evidence of Inhalation injury (charring of naso/oral cavities, angioedema, hoarseness, respiratory failure, or burns sustained in closed spaces), they are tagged RED.

4. If <5%, there is a <5% mortality risk and the patient can wait.

a. These patients are tagged GREEN.

E. CareFlight Triage[20]

1. Assess: *Can patient walk?*

a. YES, then triage as DELAYED.

b. No, then assess: *Does patient obey commands?*

i. YES, then assess: *is the radial pulse palpable?*

(a) YES, patient is triaged as URGENT.

(b) NO, patient is triaged as IMMEDIATE.

ii. NO, then assess: *Does patient breathe with an open airway?*

(a) YES, patient is triaged as IMMEDIATE.

(b) NO, patient is triaged as unsalvageable.

F. Move, Assess, Sort, Send (MASS Triage)[20]

1. Adapted from the military

2. Supported by the National Disaster Life Support (NDLS) program

G. Comparing triage methods[20]

1. CareFlight Triage and START Triage

a. CareFlight assesses ability to obey commands first and does not assess RR.

b. CareFlight appears to have greater specificity.

2. SALT and START Triage

a. SALT is less likely to overtriage.

b. Both SALT and START frequently undertriage.

c. Both have high specificity for predicting death.

d. Neither has good sensitivity to determine patient's level of triage.

Overview of Treatment Considerations[13]

A. Focus on most benefit with the least use of resources.

B. Anticipated resource shortages

1. Oxygen

2. Medications

3. Hemodynamic support

a. Blood products

b. IV fluids

4. Life support technology

a. Ventilators

b. Extracorporeal membrane oxygenation circuits (ECMO)

c. Dialysis circuits

C. General principles

1. Less time dedicated to intensive interventions should be performed as number of patients increase.

2. Rapid treatment interventions should be employed that provide large benefit.

a. Hemorrhage control

b. Basic airway adjunct placement

c. Needle decompression

3. Triage should be adapted to incident.

a. Smaller incidents allow clinicians to focus resources on more critically injured.

b. Larger incidents shift focus to care for the moderately injured, and interventions should be brief and targeted.

4. Diagnostic testing should be reduced and utilized for lifesaving procedures.

a. Blood gas evaluation

b. Hemoglobin evaluation

c. Electrolyte evaluation

i. Important in burn and crush injury patients

ii. Consideration for critical hyperkalemia

d. Point-of-care ultrasound (POCUS)

i. Quickly identify life-threats and need for intervention

ii. May be used for operative triage

e. Chest/abdominal to locate foreign bodies

Legal Considerations[13,15,21]

A. Prior to implementation of crisis standards of care (CSC):

1. States, institutions, personnel should understand what protections may be available to them.

a. May be role and/or location-dependent

2. Reimbursement and financing during disaster response should also be evaluated and understood prior to an event.

B. Professionals need to act as professionals.

1. No protections for poor or careless decision-making or misconduct

C. Institutions and facilities have a "Duty to Plan" for disasters

D. Need to be self-sufficient for 96 hours

Special Considerations

A. Patient identification and tracking, electronic medical record (EMR), and documentation

1. Patient identification and tracking

a. Electronic registration

i. Predetermined disaster nomenclature

(1) Use of state names

(a) e.g., Disaster, Alabama; Disaster, Alaska

(2) Use of colors

(a) e.g., Disaster, Ruby; Disaster, Teal

ii. Test in EMR to ensure visibility of tracking board and computer screen.

iii. Discuss with IT for downstream impacts on medical record

b. Updating tracking board to reflect patient location

i. May require additional personnel

(1) Do not need to be medically trained

ii. Determine whether disaster treatment beds or alternate care locations are preloaded into EMR

iii. Radio-frequency identification (RFID) tagging may play a role in locating patients in the future.

(a) Costly
(b) Potentially could run out of tags
(c) System failures

c. Whiteboard or chalkboard
i. Requires dedicated personnel to maintain and track patients

2. Documentation
a. Preplan disaster documentation (paper versus electronic)
i. *If electronic:* predetermined disaster note fields
ii. Plan for equipment failure.
b. Consider keeping paper documentation attached to patient.
c. Documentation follows patient.

3. Order entry
a. Radiology usually necessary to complete test
b. Laboratory usually does not need electronic order.
i. Consider paper order versus verbal.
c. Medications usually do not require electronic order entry.
i. Consider paper versus verbal.

B. Communicating diagnostic results
1. Laboratory results
a. EMR
b. Paper printouts
c. Phone call or radio
d. Runner
e. Identify clinician caring for patient (may be different than ordering clinician).
2. Radiology results
a. Wet reads versus preliminary results versus final results
b. EMR
c. Paper
d. Phone call or radio
e. Runner
f. Identify clinician caring for patient (may be different than ordering clinician).

C. Telemedicine
1. Subspecialty access to smaller hospitals or field hospitals

D. *Caring for specialty populations:* Special populations are those who may be at increased risk for morbidity and mortality outside a fully functional healthcare environment.[21] It is also important to recognize that these populations may be resource-intensive, presenting challenges that must be recognized in planning.
1. Chronic illness
2. Chronic care facility residents
3. Technology-dependent patients
4. Geriatric population
5. Patients with end-stage renal disease on dialysis

References and Additional Reading

References and Additional Reading for this chapter are online only and can be found at https://connect.springerpub.com/content/reference-book/978-0-8261-6091-5/part/part06/toc-part/ch47.

48. Chemical and Biological Weapons

MELANIE GIBBONS HALLMAN

Learning Objectives

- Describe the basic physiologic effects and mechanisms of action for chemical and biological agents potentially used in acts of terrorism or resulting from manmade and natural disasters.
- Compare and contrast common signs and symptoms of exposure to chemical and biological agents.
- Demonstrate evaluation and medical management of patients exposed to specific chemical and biological agents.
- Develop admission and discharge plans for patients sustaining exposure to specific chemical and biological agents.
- Identify key personnel and authorities requiring a report of patient(s) with known or potential exposure to specific chemical and biological agents.

Introduction to Chemical Agents

Chemical agents exist in solid, liquid, or gaseous forms and are classified by their effects (nerve agents, choking agents, blister agents, and blood agents). Chemical substances are used in terrorism because they impose injury and incapacitation and may be lethal. They act rapidly and leave characteristic signs aiding in their identification. Chemical agents may enter a host by inhalation, ingestion, absorption, or injection. Their acquisition and production are simple, and they are easily distributed by wind, explosives, contaminated water and food, and spraying mechanisms. A chemical attack should be suspected when large numbers of animals, fish, or birds die, or patterns of illness or casualties are reported. Changes in plants and unusual odors in the area where the patient was located prior to treatment are also reasons for suspicion of chemical exposure.

APPROACH TO CHEMICAL AGENTS

Blister Agents

Blister agents (e.g., sulfur mustard, phosgene oxime, Lewisite) or vesicants result in burns and blisters on contact and may damage multiple organs including the eyes and respiratory system.

Introduction

A. *Dissemination:* Liquid, vapor (form varies by ambient temperature)

B. *Routes of entry:* Inhalation, ingestion, and/or absorption (rapid onset)

C. Personal protective equipment (PPE)

1. Head and face covered
2. National Institute for Occupational Safety and Health (NIOSH)–approved powered air-purifying respirator (PAPR) mask; or combination of 99.97% high-efficiency particulate air/organic vapor/acid gas respirator cartridges
3. Chemical-resistant suit, double-layer protective gloves, boots

D. Decontamination

1. Sulfur mustard decontamination should be limited to thorough, gentle washing of exposed skin with large amounts of soap and water.
2. Do not scrub vigorously, avoid 0.5% sodium hypochlorite solution.
3. Flush eyes for at least 15 minutes with water.

E. Pathophysiology

1. Sulfur mustard and Lewisite are cytotoxic alkylating agents.
2. Sulfur mustard reacts with DNA, RNA, and proteins resulting in interruption of cell function.
3. Mustard also causes mild cholinergic activity.
4. Skin contact usually causes the development of bullae but does not contain the chemical agent.

Medical Screening

A. *Chief complaints:* Varies by agent: anxious, distressed patient; eye irritation, sometimes eye pain and swelling; hoarseness; skin sloughing and significant pain in Phosgene and Lewisite exposures.

B. Signs and symptoms—vary by specific chemical:

1. *Mustard agents:* Erythema, blistering, eye irritation and swelling, respiratory failure, lethargy (symptoms may take up to 48 hours to develop if organ damage has occurred; death may result within hours). Mustard agents do not cause immediate pain.
2. *Phosgene oxime:* Significantly corrosive, causes severe pain and deep skin lesions.
3. *Lewisite:* Eye and skin pain, vision loss, erythema of the skin, pain, irritation of mucous membranes, dysphonia, airway sloughing (immediate onset of symptoms, may worsen over several hours)

C. *Past medical history:* Respiratory comorbidities significant

Physical Examination

A. *General:* Anxious patient with eye complaints, pain may vary from none to severe depending on exposure to specific agents; hoarse voice.
B. *Skin:* Burning, irritation, erythema, wheals, vesicles, bullae, tissue necrosis
   1. *Sulfur mustard:* Vesicles may have a string-of-pearls appearance
   2. *Lewisite:* Single vesicle with erythematous base
   3. *Phosgene oxime:* Dermal blanching followed by wheal development, but no vesicle develops
C. *Eyes:* Ocular pain, injection, tearing, photophobia, blepharospasm, conjunctivitis, iritis, eyelid edema, corneal clouding, vision changes
D. *Ears, nose, and throat (ENT):* Nasal irritation, rhinorrhea, sinus irritation, epistaxis, sore throat, hoarseness
E. *Cardiac:* Lewisite increases vascular permeability, may result in third-spacing leading to hypotension.
F. *Pulmonary:* Cough (may be barking), dyspnea, airway necrosis and sloughing, pulmonary edema, acute respiratory distress syndrome (ARDS), respiratory failure, chemical pneumonitis
G. *Neurological:* Mental status change, seizures
H. *Gastrointestinal:* Nausea, vomiting, diarrhea, constipation
I. *Musculoskeletal:* Bone marrow suppression

Differential Diagnoses

A. Contact dermatitis
B. Radiation exposure

Diagnostic Testing

A. Complete blood count (CBC) (leukocytosis; in bone marrow suppression—anemia, leukopenia, thrombocytopenia)
B. Glucose
C. Electrolytes (to monitor GI effects)
D. Renal function studies (blood urea nitrogen [BUN], creatinine)
E. Chest x-ray (CXR; focal or diffuse pneumonitis, pulmonary edema)
F. Pulse oximetry
G. Arterial blood gases (ABG)
H. Gram stain and culture (if secondary bacterial infection suspected)
I. Urinalysis (to assess for thiodiglycol from mustard gas exposure)

Management

A. Treat as thermal burn.
B. *Procedures:* Anticipate intubation and ventilator support with positive end-expiratory pressure (PEEP).
C. Pharmacologic therapies
   1. Consider topical antibiotic ointment (double antibiotic ointment, silver sulfadiazine cream) for treatment of blisters. Leave small blisters intact, unroof large lesions).
   2. Systemic antibiotics may be necessary for greater degrees of skin irritation.
   3. Ocular antibiotics for eye involvement
   4. Bronchospasms may be treated with systemic steroids and inhaled bronchodilator.
   5. Antitussives for cough
   6. Pulmonary antibiotics may be needed for more significant respiratory involvement.
   7. Ciliary spasms may be treated with topical anticholinergics.
   8. GI antispasmodics for GI spasms
   9. Pain management medications
D. Nonpharmacologic therapies
   1. Sterile dressings for burns
   2. Eye and skin exposure to Lewisite can be treated with British anti-Lewisite (BAL) solution in ocular and topical forms (may no longer exist); dimercaprol 2 to 3 mg/kg intramuscularly (IM) every 4 hours for Lewisite exposure
   3. Intubation may be necessary for airway burns. Supportive therapy including airway management, hemodynamic support may be required.
   4. *Consultation and collaboration:* Notify the Centers for Disease Control and Prevention (CDC) immediately.

Patient Disposition

A. *Transition of care information:* Admit to critical care for burns >20% total body surface area (TBSA).

Blood Agents

Blood agents (e.g., hydrogen, cyanide, cyanogen chloride) enter via the respiratory system and prevent oxygenation to organs and tissues. Sometimes detectable by smell, patients may describe the smell of bitter almonds when exposed to hydrogen cyanide. Death may occur in minutes if exposed to a large dose or if untreated. Other causes of cyanide poisoning include domestic fires, industrial exposure, medical treatment for cancer and administration of sodium nitroprusside, and ingestion of foods containing cyanogens (e.g., pits and seeds of peaches, pears, apples, plums, apricots, bitter almonds).

Introduction

A. *Dissemination:* Liquid, aerosol, or gas
B. *Routes of entry:* Inhalation, ingestion, or absorption
C. Personal protective equipment (PPE)
   1. Head and face covered
   2. National Institute for Occupational Safety and Health (NIOSH)–approved powered air-purifying respirator (PAPR); or combination 99.97% high-efficiency particulate air/organic vapor/acid gas respirator cartridges
   3. Chemical-resistant suit, double-layer protective gloves, boots
D. Decontamination:
   1. Remove from source.
   2. Limit to thorough, gentle washing of exposed skin and wounds with large amounts of soap and water
   3. Do not scrub vigorously, avoid 0.5% sodium hypochlorite solution.
   4. Flush eyes minimum of 15 minutes with water. In cases of ingestion of cyanide within 60 minutes of presentation for treatment, a single dose of activated charcoal may be administered orally.

5. If the patient has diminished mental status, intubation should be achieved before administering activated charcoal.
6. Adult dosing is 50 g; for children, the dose is 1 g/kg up to 50 mg maximum
7. Encourage self-decontamination for both adults and children when feasible.
8. Encourage parents or family members to assist in the decontamination process for infants and younger children.

E. Pathophysiology
1. Cyanide inhibits mitochondrial cytochrome oxidase blocking cellular respiration, resulting in anaerobic metabolism and lactic acidosis, hypoxia, syncope, seizures, dysrhythmias, respiratory failure, and death.

Medical Screening

A. *Common chief complaint:* Anxious patient complaining of headache, dizziness, confusion, and shortness of breath. 60% report scent of bitter almonds, metallic taste.
B. Signs and symptoms (similar to nerve agents)
1. Inhalation results in rapid onset of air hunger, vomiting, frothy sputum, upper airway irritation, nausea, vomiting, confusion, seizures, dizziness, lightheadedness, headaches, syncope, respiratory arrest leading to cardiac arrest, death.
2. Ingestion results in slower onset of symptoms.
C. *Medication history:* Not specifically contributory
D. *Past medical history:* Gather occupational history if the exposure occurred at work

Physical Examination

A. *General:* Likely significant distress or unconscious; may present in cardiopulmonary arrest
B. *Skin:* Flushing "cherry red appearance" (early), cyanosis (late, and less likely in hydrogen cyanide), diaphoresis, vesicles, itching, and swelling may be present
C. *Eyes:* Eye irritation (cyanogen chloride)
D. *ENT:* Mucus membrane irritation (cyanogen chloride)
E. *Neck:* No specific changes
F. *Cardiac:* Tachycardia, hypertension (early), bradycardia, hypotension (late), atrioventricular block, ventricular dysrhythmias
G. *Pulmonary:* Gasping respirations, dyspnea, tachypnea (early), bradypnea (late), pulmonary edema, watery productive cough (cyanogen chloride)
H. *Neurological:* Anxiety, may be unresponsive, seizures, coma
I. *GI:* Abdominal pain, vomiting (ingestion of cyanide salts)

Differential Diagnoses

A. Cyanide poisoning
B. Carbon monoxide poisoning
C. Tricyclic antidepressant overdose
D. Salicylate poisoning
E. Organophosphate poisoning
F. Methemoglobinemia
G. Strychnine poisoning
H. Hydrogen sulfide gas poisoning
I. Phosphine poisoning
J. Arsine poisoning
K. Chlorine exposure

Diagnostic Testing

A. Test for elevated blood cyanide concentration.
B. Serum lactate (lactic acidosis)
C. Arterial blood gases (ABG; metabolic acidosis)
D. Venous blood gases (elevated venous oxygen levels)
E. Carboxyhemoglobin
F. Methemoglobin
G. Complete blood count (CBC)
H. Fingerstick blood glucose (to rule out hypoglycemia as cause of confusion)
I. Serum electrolytes
J. Blood urea nitrogen (BUN)
K. Creatinine
L. Calcium
M. Urinalysis (UA; hemoglobinuria/rhabdomyolysis)
N. Acetaminophen and salicylate levels
O. EKG (assess for prolonged QT and QRS intervals)
P. Pregnancy test for females of childbearing age
Q. Chest x-ray (CXR; pulmonary edema)

Management

A. Procedures
1. Maintain respiratory and circulatory support awaiting antidote administration.
2. Anticipate intubation and ventilator support.

B. Pharmacologic therapies—two options to be given immediately barring contraindications:
1. *First choice:* Sodium thiosulfate + hydroxocobalamin
2. *Second choice:* Cyanide antidote kit given in following order:
a. Amyl nitrite + sodium nitrite
b. *CAUTION:* Amyl nitrite or sodium nitrite contraindicated in cases of concurrent carbon monoxide poisoning.
3. If facility does not have hydroxocobalamin or a cyanide antidote kit, or dicobalt edetate may be administered if the patient has no contraindications for either drug.

C. Treat bronchospasms with bronchodilators. Lactic acidosis may be treated with sodium bicarbonate. If hemolysis develops, add 50 to 100 mEq of sodium bicarbonate to one liter of D51/4 normal saline and infuse to maintain urine output at 2 to 3 mL/kg/hour, maintain urine pH >7.5 until no hemoglobin remains in urine. Treat anemia with blood transfusions. Treat seizures with benzodiazepines. Consider hyperbaric oxygen therapy.

D. Nonpharmacologic therapies
1. 100% oxygen, airway support
2. Irrigate eyes and skin exposures with lukewarm water.
3. Consider hemodialysis for treatment of renal failure.

E. Consultation and collaboration
1. Medical toxicologist, poison control center

Patient Disposition

A. *Transition of care information:* Admit to ICU.
B. Prevention and education

1. Patient and public education about sources of cyanide could assist to decrease accidental toxicity.

C. Patient and family education and counseling
1. If patient survives, long-term effects may include neurologic sequelae.
2. Patients receiving hydroxocobalamin should be advised to avoid sunlight until erythema has resolved.
3. They may also develop red urine that should dissipate over time.

D. Pediatric considerations
1. Treat stridor with racemic epinephrine solution in 2.5 mL water nebulizer.
2. Pathophysiology and manifestations of cyanide poisoning are similar for children and adults.
3. Dosing for sodium nitrite should be managed according to the patient's hemoglobin.
4. Consult poison control for dosing assistance.
5. Allow pediatric patients to remain with an adult family member during decontamination and care when possible.

Nerve Agents

Nerve agents (e.g., tabun, sarin, soman, VX) are markedly toxic, hazardous, and unpredictable in liquid and vapor states. Effects are dependent on chemical concentration, and the length and route of exposure. Small exposures may not be noticed for up to 18 hours postexposure. Sarin and VX are odorless. Soman may smell like camphor, and Tabun may smell like rotting fruit.

Introduction

A. *Dissemination*: Gas or liquid; often aerosolized as a vapor

B. *Routes of entry:* inhalation, absorption

C. Personal protective equipment (PPE)
1. Level C, head and face covered (Table 48.1)
2. National Institute for Occupational Safety and Health (NIOSH)–approved powered air-purifying respirator (PAPR) or combination 99.97% high-efficiency particulate air/organic vapor/acid gas respirator cartridges
3. Chemical-resistant suit, double-layer protective gloves, boots

D. Decontamination
1. Prehospital or a location bordering the hospital
2. Remove all clothing, jewelry, and any devices or bandages applied in the field.
3. Gently wash with generous amounts of soap and water to avoid breaking skin thus further absorption of the chemical.
4. Carefully bag contaminated materials for strategic disposal.

E. Pathophysiology
1. Interferes with the central nervous system (CNS)
2. Classified as organophosphates, these chemicals bind and inhibit acetylcholinesterase, an enzyme that normally breaks down the neurotransmitter acetylcholine, resulting in accumulation of acetylcholine at all cholinergic receptors.
3. Increased levels of acetylcholine causes hyperstimulation of central and peripheral muscarinic receptors and nicotinic receptors.

Medical Screening

A. *Common chief complaints:* Difficulty breathing often accompanied by wheezing; chest pain, increased salivation, urination, and runny nose; nausea, vomiting, diarrhea; blurred vision; muscle twitching and weakness evolving to paralysis

B. *Signs and symptoms:* Pinpoint pupils, rhinorrhea, respiratory arrest, diaphoresis, weakness, confusion, slurred speech, abdominal pain, nausea, vomiting, and diarrhea; headache, drooling, trembling, twitching, paralysis, abdominal pain, depression, visual complaints, and seizures

C. SLUDGEM acronym to recall signs and symptoms of nerve agents
1. **S**: salivation
2. **L**: lacrimation
3. **U**: urination
4. **D**: defecation
5. **G**: gastric distress
6. **E**: emesis
7. **M:** miosis

D. *Past medical history:* Respiratory comorbidities significant

E. *Focused assessment:* Degree of symptoms dependent on chemical concentration; length and amount of exposure
1. *General:* Agitation, muscle fasciculations, facial twitching, "wet" sweating patient with copious secretions from eyes, nose, mouth, and urinary tract
2. *Skin:* Copious sweating
3. *Eyes:* Pinpoint pupils
4. *Ears, nose, throat (ENT):* Excessive tearing, runny nose, salivation

TABLE 48.1 PERSONAL PROTECTIVE EQUIPMENT CLASSIFICATION

LEVEL	DESCRIPTION
Level A	Totally encapsulating chemical suit with self-containing breathing apparatus. Highest level of protection from gases, vapors, aerosols, liquids, and solids.
Level B	Independent breathing apparatus with chemical-resistant outer clothing. Offers protection from vapors, aerosols, liquids, and solids.
Level C	Chemical-resistant clothing with air purifiers (minimum standard when providing care in ED to a contaminated patient). Offers protection from vapors, aerosols, liquids, and solids.
Level D	Standard work uniform designed to protect from nuisance exposures, gown, gloves, eye and face shield. Offers minimal protection against solids.

5. *Cardiac:* Bradycardia
6. *Pulmonary:* Dyspnea, possible wheezing, periods of apnea, copious upper and lower mucoid respiratory secretions, severe tightness in chest
7. *Neurological:* Muscle twitching, trembling, evolving flaccid paralysis, seizures, extreme headache, unresponsiveness, coma
8. *Genitourinary:* Increased urination
9. *GI:* Nausea, vomiting, diarrhea
10. *Musculoskeletal:* Chest tightness, muscle fasciculation, weakness

Differential Diagnoses

A. Cholinergic toxicity
B. Organophosphate
C. Biologic weapon
D. Neurotoxin
E. Pesticide

Diagnostic Testing

A. Complete blood count (CBC), serum cholinesterase
   1. Decreased activity of erythrocyte cholinesterase or plasma cholinesterase may indicate nerve agent exposure.
B. Comprehensive metabolic panel (CMP) to monitor for dehydration and electrolyte imbalance

Management

A. *Do not approach/contact patient unless wearing proper personal protective equipment (PPE).*
B. Procedures
   1. Anticipate early intubation.
   2. Consider urinary catheterization to monitor intake and output.
C. Pharmacologic therapies
   1. Administer atropine for bradycardia.
   2. If symptoms are severe, use Nerve Agent Antidote Kits.
   3. Seizure prophylaxis medications may be necessary.
   4. Oximes to free bound acetylcholinesterase and to facilitate paralysis reversal
   5. Anticholinergics as antagonists to antagonize muscarinic effects
   6. *Specific antidotes:* Atropine (may require significant quantities) once symptoms stabilized, pralidoxime (2-PAM, Protopam) to regenerate enzyme activity at affected sites, reverse paralysis
   7. Benzodiazepines to treat seizures
D. Nonpharmacologic therapies
   1. Support airway and anticipated assisted ventilation.
   2. Decontaminate skin with soap and water.
   3. Flush eyes with normal saline or eyewash for 15 minutes.
   4. Do not induce vomiting in cases of ingestion.
   5. In cases of respiratory failure, intubate early and administer positive pressure ventilation.
   6. Frequent suctioning may be needed to manage copious secretions.
E. Consultation and collaboration
   1. Notify the Centers for Disease Control and Prevention (CDC) immediately.
   2. If law enforcement and Emergency Medical Services (EMS) are unaware, inform immediately.

Patient Disposition

A. Transition of care information
   1. Admit to ICU.

Age and Developmental Considerations

A. Prevention and education
   1. Counseling and psychologic support may be necessary for patient and family support system for an extended time after exposure.
B. Patient and family education and counseling
   1. Recovery may take several months, and paralysis may be permanent.
   2. Neuropsychiatric changes may linger for several months or more, polyneuropathy and cognitive changes may persist.
   3. Prolonged seizures possible
C. Pediatric considerations
   1. When children and their adult caregivers require decontamination, attempt to keep them together for the process to decrease psychologic trauma.
   2. Offer continuous reassurance.
   3. Reunite children with parents if separated in process.
   4. Keep older children informed of process.
   5. Use warm water for decontamination to avoid hypothermia in children and infants.

Pulmonary and Choking Agents

Phosgene and chlorine are common industrial chemicals used in chemical warfare. These chemicals are choking agents and predominantly affect the respiratory system causing cellular damage of pulmonary capillaries and alveoli leading to pulmonary edema. They evaporate quickly, often within hours. Most pulmonary and choking agents are found in industry and many found in homes. Some agents may be identified by odor or appearance. Phosgene may smell like freshly cut hay.

Introduction

A. *Dissemination:* Liquid, gas
B. *Routes of entry:* Inhalation
C. Personal protective equipment (PPE)
   1. Head and face covered
   2. National Institute for Occupational Safety and Health (NIOSH)–approved powered air-purifying respirator (PAPR); or combination 99.97% high-efficiency particulate air/organic vapor/acid gas respirator cartridges
   3. Chemical-resistant suit, double-layer protective gloves, boots
D. Decontamination
   1. Remove from hazardous gas.
   2. No decontamination required

E. Pathophysiology
  1. Local irritation or swelling of mucous membranes and respiratory tract
  2. Deposits in peripheral airways, damages alveolar-capillary membrane leading to pulmonary edema and impaired oxygenation

Medical Screening

A. *Common chief complaints:* Eye pain and injection, watery eyes, sore throat, cough, and headache
B. *Signs and symptoms:* Chest tightness, coughing (bronchial irritation), hemoptysis, choking, hypoxia, hypotension, irritation of eyes, nose (rhinorrhea), mouth (increased oral secretions), and of the entire respiratory system. Pulmonary edema may be a delayed effect. Laryngeal spasms may result and be lethal. A postexposure latent period of up to 24 hours may occur. The higher the dose of exposure, the earlier and more severe the symptoms.
C. *Past medical history:* Pre-existing respiratory comorbidities are significant to the outcome.
D. Focused assessment
  1. *General:* Anxious, severe distress, eyes watering and reddened, coughing, chest tightness, dyspnea
  2. *Skin:* Patient may complain of burning sensation on exposed skin
  3. *Eyes:* Painful, injected, watery eyes
  4. *ENT:* Rhinitis, laryngospasms, drooling
  5. *Cardiac:* Tachycardia, hypotension (late)
  6. *Pulmonary:* Cough, pulmonary edema (delayed), tachypnea, crackles
  7. *Neurological:* Headache
  8. *Genitourinary:* Nonspecific exam though nausea and vomiting may present in some patients
  9. *GI:* None specific, nausea/vomiting may present in some individuals

Differential Diagnoses

A. Riot control agents (e.g., pepper spray)
B. Nerve agents
C. Vesicant agents

Diagnostic Testing

A. No specific clinical testing exists.
B. Chest x-ray (CXR)
C. Arterial blood gases (ABG)
D. Complete blood count (CBC) to monitor pulmonary edema

Management

A. *Procedures:* Anticipate intubation.
B. Pharmacologic therapies
  1. No antidote exists.
  2. Antibiotics to treat secondary bacterial infections
  3. IV steroids, nebulized bronchodilators for bronchospasms, supplemental oxygen
C. Nonpharmacologic therapies
  1. High-flow oxygen, frequent suctioning, good pulmonary toilet, bed rest to decrease burden of activity on pulmonary function. If intubation necessary, add positive end-expiratory pressure (PEEP).
  2. If secondary hypotension develops, vasopressors to treat
  3. Avoid high volumes of IV crystalloid or colloid solutions as they may worsen pulmonary edema.
D. *Consultation and collaboration:* Notify Centers for Disease Control and Prevention (CDC), consult pulmonary service.

Patient Disposition

A. Transition of care information
  1. Admit to ICU for severe symptoms.
  2. Admit to observation for monitoring development of latent symptoms, particularly pulmonary edema.

TABLE 48.2 CATEGORIES OF BIOLOGICAL AGENTS

CATEGORY	DESCRIPTION	EASE OF SPREAD	EXAMPLES
A	Highest priority, includes toxins that pose highest threat, requires stockpiling of medication, may require extensive public health efforts, has potential for mass casualties.	Easily spread person-to-person	Anthrax, plague, smallpox
B	Biologic agents with some potential for dissemination and agents of concern for food and water supply. Lower public awareness, require less public health support. Moderate morbidity and low mortality rates.	Moderately easy to spread	*Salmonella*, *Escherichia coli*, *Shigella*
C	Biologic agents that may pose future threat. Readily available agents, easily produced and disseminated, potential for high morbidity and mortality rates; agents could have a major health impact.		Emerging infectious diseases, Nipah virus, Hanta virus

B. Prevention and education
  1. Use of activated charcoal in chemical protective mask may absorb chemical, thus preventing exposure.

INTRODUCTION TO BIOLOGICAL AGENTS

Biological agents are viruses, bacteria, *Rickettsia*, and other toxins that occur naturally but may be altered to accelerate spread of disease and resistance to medications. Because they occur naturally, it may be difficult to determine whether they are associated with a terrorist attack. Symptoms of exposure are the same whether naturally occurring or delayed. Awareness of an attack may be attributed to the time necessary for disease symptoms to develop after exposure to the biological agent. Many of these agents are contagious and result in epidemics. Clinicians are often the first to recognize the possibility of a biological attack. The Centers for Disease Control and Prevention (CDC) maintains a Strategic National Stockpile of pharmaceuticals and healthcare supplies to activate when local supplies run out during an act of terrorism (Strategic National Stockpile).

Three categories have been designated for the biological agents to assist public health authorities in preparing for biological terrorism (Table 48.2). Categorization is based on ease of spread of agents and severity of illness resulting; and may change based on emerging threats (CDC, Bioterrorism Agents/Diseases).

APPROACH TO BACTERIAL AGENTS

Anthrax (*Bacillus anthracis*)—Category A

Introduction

A. *Etiology:* Found in soil, can create spores, typically a disease of animals, spores can remain active in water up to 2 years
B. *Dissemination:* Aerosolized spores; not transmitted human-to-human
C. Routes of entry
  1. *Inhalation (most deadly route):* Breathing spores from infected animals
  2. Ingestion (of contaminated meat)
  3. Absorption
  4. Injection
  5. Direct contact (cutaneous)
D. Personal protective equipment (PPE)
  1. At hospital, universal precautions (hand hygiene, gown, gloves, mask, face shield)
  2. If risk for aerosolized powder contamination, N95 mask or equivalent, or powered air-purifying respirator (PAPR)
  3. Contact isolation if inhalational or cutaneous anthrax.
E. *Decontamination:* If suspicious substance noted on patient's clothing or skin, this is achieved by removal of contaminated clothing, jewelry, and copious irrigation with water
F. Pathophysiology
  1. *Bacillus anthracis* is aerobic, gram-positive, spore-forming bacterium
  2. Spores phagocytosed in host lungs, transported by macrophages to lymphoid tissue
  3. Spores incubate for 1 to 6 days, germinate and multiply causing bacteremia.
G. *Prevalence:* Found on almost all continents and in nearly every country

Medical Screening

A. *Common chief complaint:* Nonproductive cough, chest pain, fever
B. Signs and symptoms:
  1. *Cutaneous:* Fever, malaise, headache, blisters, black lesions
  2. *Inhalation:* Flu-like symptoms, lymphadenopathy, fever, chills, nausea; may progress to respiratory distress, shock, or death
  3. *Gastrointestinal:* Significant abdominal pain, dehydration, fever, vomiting, hematochezia
C. *Past medical history:* Potential for worsened impact of symptoms in patients with preexisting pulmonary, GI diseases, and immunosuppressed states

Physical Examination

A. *General:* Symptoms of anxiety, confusion, or decreased level of consciousness; temperature may be elevated; may complain of pain
B. *Skin:* Cutaneous anthrax—ulcer with black eschar, significant local edema with associated lymphadenopathy.
C. *Ears, nose, and throat (ENT):* Oral ulceration may present with ingestion of the bacteria.
D. *Cardiac:* Tachycardia often present
E. *Pulmonary:* Inhalation anthrax—chest x-ray (CXR) may reveal widened mediastinum, pleural effusions; breath sounds may be normal or decreased depending on the amount of exposure and time elapsed since exposure
F. *Neurological:* Inhalational anthrax—meningeal signs, hemorrhagic meningitis
G. *Gastrointestinal:* GI anthrax—bloody diarrhea, acute (tender) abdomen possibly with associated ascites; bowel sounds may be hyperactive if diarrhea present, or hypoactive

Differential Diagnoses

A. Cutaneous anthrax
  1. Tularemia
  2. Plague
  3. Cellulitis
  4. Spider bite
B. Inhalation anthrax
  1. Community-acquired pneumonia (CAP)
  2. Mycoplasma pneumonia
  3. Influenza
  4. Legionnaire's disease
  5. Q fever
  6. Viral pneumonia
  7. Histoplasmosis
  8. Coccidioidomycosis

C. *CT scan:* Peribronchial thickening, mediastinal, and hilar region lymphadenopathy, pleural effusion seen in inhalation anthrax

D. *Labs:* Blood cultures will be positive for anthrax; white blood cell (WBC) elevated on complete blood count (CBC); later in infection hypocalcemia, hyperkalemia, and hyperglycemia may develop

Diagnostic Testing

A. Lab specimens
   1. Isolation of *B. anthracis* from blood culture, affected tissue, ulcer fluid, or site
   2. Serum chemistries, CBC with differential
   3. Diagnostic imaging—CT scan of chest/thorax

Management

A. *Procedures:* Provide supplemental oxygen, anticipate intubation in patient's exhibiting respiratory compromise

B. Pharmacologic therapies
   1. IV hydration as tolerated (especially helpful in patients with significant GI effects)
   2. Antibiotics including 60 days of ciprofloxacin, tetracyclines, doxycycline, penicillin

C. *Nonpharmacologic therapies:* Pleural fluid drainage

D. Consultation and collaboration
   1. Case of inhalation anthrax considered bioterrorism until ruled out
   2. Mandatory immediate local and state health department notification; report to the Centers for Disease Control and Prevention (CDC), hospital infection control officer.

Patient Disposition

A. *Transition of care information:* Patient will be admitted; patient may require transfer to higher level of care

B. Prevention and education
   1. Antibiotic therapy may be prescribed for 60 days or longer and should not be discontinued unless advised by the treating clinician.
   2. Pain treatment including short-term narcotics may be necessary in some cases.
   3. Anthrax vaccine for prevention

C. *Pediatric considerations:* Amoxicillin alternative for children and pregnant/lactating women

Botulism (*Clostridium botulinum* Toxin)—Category A

Introduction

A. Etiology
   1. Naturally occurring potent neurotoxin that can be used as weapon
   2. Usually found in undercooked or improperly canned food
   3. Highly toxic and if untreated may lead to death
   4. A neuroparalytic illness, descending flaccid paralysis (motor/autonomic) always beginning with cranial nerves; absence of sensory nerve dysfunction

B. *Dissemination:* Liquid or aerosol

C. *Routes of entry:* Ingestion, inhalation, and injection (less commonly may enter via wounds)

D. Personal protective equipment (PPE)
   1. At hospital universal precautions (hand hygiene, gown, gloves, mask, and face shield)
   2. If risk for aerosolized powder contamination, N95 mask or equivalent, or powered air-purifying respirator (PAPR)

E. *Decontamination:* If wound botulism, may require wound debridement to remove bacteria

F. Pathophysiology
   1. Botulism toxin heavy chains permanently bind acetylcholine containing neurons.
   2. Light chains interfere with acetylcholine exocytosis
   3. Toxin then binds to presynaptic nerve terminal
   4. Receptor binding irreversible
   5. Affects neuromuscular junction only
   6. Not spread person-to-person

G. *Prevalence:* Rare, potentially fatal

Medical Screening

A. *Common chief complaint:* Malaise, weakness (descending from head/face to feet), abdominal cramping, nausea, vomiting, diarrhea; anxiety

B. Signs and symptoms
   1. Adult
      a. Onset 4 to 36 hours. Varies by dose and exposure route.
      b. Lethargy, weakness, dizziness, double vision, blurred vision, ptosis, dry mouth, dysphagia, difficulty speaking
      c. More significant symptoms include difficulty breathing, muscle weakness (descending flaccid paralysis, cranial nerves first), distended abdomen, abdominal pain, nausea, vomiting, constipation
   2. Infant
      a. Neck and peripheral weakness, weakened sucking and crying abilities, poor feeding, respiratory failure, constipation
      b. Descending paralysis may develop.

Physical Examination

A. *General:* Distress, uncomfortable; tachypnea in later stages

B. *Eyes:* Vision complaints, pupil dilation (late)

C. *ENT (ear, nose, and throat):* Dysphagia

D. *Neck:* Weakness especially in infants

E. *Cardiac:* Tachycardia may be present.

F. *Pulmonary:* Increased work of breathing may be present in more advanced stages of exposure.

G. *Neurological:* Cranial nerve palsies; eyelid drooping, decreased gag reflex, complete loss (late); speech interference; decreased deep tendon reflexes; worsening descending flaccid paralysis

H. *Genitourinary:* Bladder distention, urinary retention

I. *Gastrointestinal:* Abdominal pain, nausea, vomiting, constipation

J. *Musculoskeletal:* Skeletal muscle weakness

Differential Diagnoses

A. Guillain-Barré syndrome

B. Miller-Fisher syndrome

C. Myasthenia gravis

Diagnostic Testing

A. Diagnosis confirmed by culture of stool, wound, or food (days to complete—don't wait to begin treatment if suspect botulism)
B. Complete blood count (CBC)
C. Electrolytes
D. Liver function tests (LFTs)
E. Urinalysis (UA, no characteristic abnormalities)
F. Cerebrospinal fluid (CSF) studies (typically normal, borderline elevation of protein may be present)
G. Tensilon test (to rule out myasthenia gravis)
H. Mouse bioassay is gold standard.
I. CT or MRI to rule out cerebrovascular accident
J. Abdominal radiographs (constipation may be present)

Management

A. Procedures
  1. Lumbar puncture
  2. Anticipate early intubation and ventilator support (may require for weeks to months).
  3. If wound botulism, may require wound debridement and antibiotic therapy
B. Pharmacologic therapies
  1. Botulinal antitoxin (available from Centers for Disease Control and Prevention [CDC]) will not reverse paralysis, may halt progression; early supportive care
  2. Early antitoxin therapy is crucial; can prevent progression and shorten duration of illness.
  3. Begin antitoxin administration as soon as available.
  4. Do not wait for laboratory confirmation of botulism to begin the antitoxin (CDC, Botulism, Information for Health Professionals)
  5. Pain management medications
C. *Nonpharmacologic therapies:* Supplemental oxygen, IV hydration with crystalloid fluids
D. Consultation and collaboration
  1. If botulism suspected, immediately call the state public health department to report. If no answer, contact the CDC at (770) 488-7100; available 24/7.

Patient Disposition

A. Transition of care information
  1. Admit to ICU for definitive care.
  2. Consult internal medicine, neurology, and infectious disease services.
  3. If wound botulism, consult wound care services.
  4. Isolation is not necessary.
B. Prevention and education: Proper home canning procedures
C. Patient and family education and counseling
  1. Death may occur from respiratory failure or symptoms related to prolonged paralysis.
  2. Expect prolonged recovery period after regeneration of new neuromuscular connections.
  3. If patient survives, potential for persistent fatigue and dyspnea.
  4. Refer to family counseling services.
D. *Pediatric considerations:* Avoid honey in infants <1 year of age.

Brucellosis (*Brucella* Species)—Category B

Introduction

A. Etiology
  1. Infectious bacterial disease of sheep, cattle, goats, pigs, dogs
  2. Humans may contract the disease when in contact with infected animals.
B. *Dissemination:* Aerosol or liquid
C. *Routes of entry:* Inhalation, broken skin, ingestion
D. Personal protective equipment
  1. At hospital universal precautions (hand hygiene, gown, gloves, mask, face shield)
  2. If risk for aerosolized powder contamination, N95 mask or equivalent, or powered air-purifying respirator (PAPR)
E. *Decontamination:* Gentle washing with soap and water
F. Pathophysiology
  1. Parasite commonly from cows, pigs, goats, dogs; releases endotoxin when it dies
  2. Incubation period 1 to 4 weeks
  3. Fatal in <5% if treated
G. *Prevalence:* <100 cases in the United States each year

Medical Screening

A. *Common chief complaint:* Abrupt or insidious development of fever and multiple nonspecific complaints over days to weeks without other objective findings and known to animal tissues and body fluids
B. *Signs and symptoms:* Fever, night sweats, malaise, anorexia, arthralgia, fatigue, depression, dyspepsia, cough, headache, dizziness

Physical Examination

A. *General:* Ill-appearing, febrile
B. *Skin:* A macular/maculopapular or scarlatiniform rash; ulcerations, petechiae, purpura, abscesses possible
C. *Eyes:* Symptoms of uveitis, corneal ulcers, papilledema, optic neuritis
D. *Cardiac:* Findings consistent with endocarditis
E. *Pulmonary:* Cough, pulmonary congestion; findings consistent with lobar pneumonia, pleural effusion, pneumonitis
F. *Neurological:* Meningeal signs in approximately 7% of cases
G. *Genitourinary:* Symptoms of orchitis, epididymitis
H. *Gastrointestinal:* Tenderness over spleen, pancreas, liver, peritonitis
I. *Musculoskeletal:* Tenderness of sacroiliac joints and large joints of extremities

Medical Decision-Making and Differential Diagnoses

A. Lab abnormalities may include anemia, leukopenia, thrombocytopenia, disseminated intravascular coagulation (DIC)
B. Differential diagnosis includes
  1. Tuberculosis (TB)
  2. Malaria
  3. Typhoid

4. Septic arthritis
5. Rheumatoid arthritis
6. HIV

Diagnostic Testing

A. Complete blood count (CBC)
B. Serum comprehensive metabolic
C. Serum coagulation studies
D. Blood cultures
E. Cultures of organ tissues, bone marrow
F. Serum agglutination (SAT): Rose Bengal SAT is rapid screening test
G. Chest x-ray (CXR), abdominal film (hepatic calcification in persistent infection)
H. MRI if spinal cord involvement suspected, bone scan, CT scan

Management

A. Pharmacologic therapies
   1. *In uncomplicated cases (adults):* Doxycycline
   2. *Pregnant women:* Rifampin plus trimethoprim-sulfamethoxazole (TMP-SMX); avoid TMP-SMX 1 week prior to delivery
   3. *Children <8 years:* Oral TMP-SMX plus rifampin
   4. *Children >8 years:* Doxycycline plus rifampin

B. *Nonpharmacologic therapies:* Symptoms support
C. *Consultation and collaboration:* CDC notification, infectious disease specialist

Patient Disposition

A. Transition of care information
   1. Admission to infectious disease service with consults to specialists for organ systems affected
   2. Not easy to determine acute versus persistent disease by serology
   3. Posthospitalization follow-up with infectious disease clinician, health department

B. Prevention and education
   1. Regular vaccination of livestock and slaughter of infected animals are successful prevention techniques
   2. Pasteurization of milk

C. Patient and family education and counseling
   1. Brucellosis infection in pregnancy associated with risk of spontaneous abortion, early delivery, and intrauterine infection

D. Pediatric considerations
   1. Complications of the disease are more prevalent in adults, infection generally more benign in children than adults.

Epsilon Toxin (*Clostridium perfringens*)—Category B

Introduction

A. Etiology
   1. Commonly found in environment and intestines of humans and animals (raw meat, poultry, dried or precooked foods)
   2. Prefers low-oxygen environments, can survive in high temperatures, multiplies rapidly
   3. Eating contaminated food produces a toxin in the intestine resulting in illness

B. *Dissemination:* High numbers of spores in food
C. *Routes of entry:* Ingestion
D. *Personal protective equipment (PPE):* Standard precautions; gloves, gown, mask, eye shield
E. *Decontamination:* No specific decontamination required
F. Pathophysiology
   1. Infection of tissue with anaerobic spore-forming bacilli with production of gas in tissues
   2. A normal inhabitant of large intestines of humans and animals, also found in soil

G. Prevalence
   1. A common source of illness from meats and other foods not kept at proper hot or cold temperatures
   2. Most commonly seen in large portions of food prepared for large groups of people

Medical Screening

A. *Chief complaint:* Sudden onset of abdominal cramps, nausea, and watery diarrhea
B. Signs and symptoms (onset within 6–24 hours)
   1. Sudden onset diarrhea, abdominal cramps, lasts <24 hours
   2. Fever and vomiting not commonly associated
   3. Very young and elderly are at the highest risk of infection, experiencing more severe symptoms (complications, e.g., dehydration, hypotension) that last longer (1–2 weeks)

C. *Past medical history:* History of deep contaminated wound, surgery, trauma

Physical Examination

A. *General:* Minimal or no fever, ill-appearing
B. *Skin:* Subcutaneous crepitus, worsening wound with foul drainage may be present; local swelling, ischemic skin changes that may be pale or bluish in color; edema at may be present at wound sites; gas gangrene may develop with copper-color bullae that may be hemorrhagic when opened
C. *Cardiac:* Hypotension, tachycardia
D. *Genitourinary:* Symptoms and labs consistent with renal failure
E. *Gastrointestinal:* Watery, profuse diarrhea; tense abdomen
F. *Musculoskeletal:* Diffuse edema may be present. X-rays of swollen areas may reveal gas in the soft tissues.

Differential Diagnoses

A. Cellulitis
B. Fasciitis
C. Myositis
D. Toxic shock

Diagnostic Testing

A. Fecal testing (to determine type and number of bacteria)

B. X-ray shows air in fascial planes.
C. Wound smear reveals gram-positive encapsulated rods
D. Complete blood count (CBC); leukocytosis

Management

A. *Procedures:* Extensive debridement in operating room for gas gangrene
B. Pharmacologic therapies
  1. Oral or IV rehydration, electrolyte replacement
  2. Penicillin
  3. Alternatives chloramphenicol, cefoxitin, clindamycin, metronidazole
C. *Nonpharmacologic therapies:* Hyperbaric oxygen treatment especially for gas gangrene

Patient Disposition

A. *Transition of care information:* Admission for hemodynamic stabilization and definitive care
B. Prevention and education
  1. Cook and keep food at the correct temperature, serve meats hot and within 2 hours of cooking.
  2. Refrigerate leftovers, reheat properly. Discard food left out too long.
C. *Patient and family education and counseling:* Infection not transferred person-to-person

Plague (*Yersinia pestis*)—Category A

Introduction

A. Two types—bubonic plague (most common form) and pneumonic plague
B. Etiology
  1. Bites from infected rats, fleas, other mammals
  2. Bacteria can remain live for years and are stable in water.
  3. Sunlight exposure for several hours will kill plague
C. *Dissemination:* Aerosol (pneumonic); blood (bubonic)
D. Routes of entry
  1. Inhalation, ingestion, and injection
  2. *Bubonic plague:* bacteria transmitted from rats by fleas who then bite humans
  3. *Pneumonic plague:* aerosol inhaled in the respiratory tract; consumption of contaminated food
E. Personal protective equipment (PPE)
  1. At hospital universal precautions (hand hygiene, gown, gloves, mask, and face shield)
  2. If the risk for aerosolized powder contamination, N95 mask or equivalent, or powered air-purifying respirator (PAPR)
F. *Decontamination:* Respiratory droplet precautions; disposable mask, gown, gloves, eye protection
G. *Pathophysiology:* Gram-negative rod; incubation pneumonic plague 2 to 3 days; bubonic plague 2 to 10 days
H. Prevalence
  1. 80% to 90% of all plague cases are bubonic plague with relatively low mortality rate.
  2. Pneumonic plague is rare, with mortality rate of 50% if treated and 100% if untreated.

Medical Screening

A. *Chief complaint:* Sudden onset fever, chills, weakness, and headache
B. *Signs and symptoms:* Determined by the type of plague
  1. Bubonic plague
    a. Sudden weakness, high fever, lymphadenopathy (may be tender and erythematous)
    b. May evolve to sepsis and lung involvement
  2. Pneumonic plague
    a. Chills, high fever, headache, hemoptysis, hypertension spike, rapid deterioration of breathing, airway obstruction, discoloration of skin (blue tint)
    b. Respiratory failure, circulatory collapse, and hemorrhage lead to death.
    c. Meningitis, pharyngitis, and tonsillitis with corresponding cervical lymphadenitis may present in some patients.
C. *Past medical history:* Symptoms significant in immunocompromised and pediatric, geriatric patients

Physical Examination

A. *General:* Rapid onset fever, chills, malaise, headache; may appear very uncomfortable/anxious; may report flea bites or travel to an area where plague is common; may ooze blood from orifices and skin
B. *Skin:* Temperature may be elevated (especially bubonic); distal necrosis of fingers and toes may be present in advanced cases
C. *Eyes:* Nonspecific but if advanced, may bleed from eyes
D. *ENT (ear, nose, and throat):* Painful, erythematous, warm lymphadenopathy (bubonic), may involve multiple lymph regions/chains
E. *Neck:* Regional lymphadenopathy (bubonic)
F. *Cardiac:* Tachycardia, hypotension
G. *Pulmonary:* Chest pain, dyspnea, cough, hemoptysis (pneumonic); adventitious breath sounds, especially wheezing
H. *Gastrointestinal:* Nausea, vomiting, diarrhea (septicemia)
I. *Musculoskeletal:* Nonspecific

Medical Decision-Making and Differential Diagnoses

A. Question patients who present with fever and painful lymphadenopathy about recent travel to endemic disease.
B. Strict droplet precautions until pneumonia ruled out, negative sputum cultures, and have received 48 hours of antimicrobial therapy.
C. Differential diagnosis includes
  1. Tularemia
  2. Cat-scratch disease
  3. Lymphogranuloma venereum
  4. Chancroid
  5. Tuberculosis (TB)
  6. Streptococcal adenitis
  7. Meningitis
  8. Encephalitis
  9. Sepsis

Diagnostic Testing

A. Radiographs and routine serum testing not helpful for diagnosis

B. Isolation of organism by culture, serologic testing, or rapid testing

1. Complete blood count (CBC) (white blood cells may vary from 3,000 to 100,000. WBC >20,000 and thrombocytopenia present in 50% of cases)

2. Electrolytes

3. Blood urea nitrogen (BUN)

4. Creatinine

5. Chest x-ray (CXR) for pneumonic plague may reveal bronchopneumonia, consolidation, cavities, or pleural effusions

6. Hilar or mediastinal adenopathy raises suspicion for pneumonic plague

7. Sputum may be clear initially and progress to purulent and bloody containing gram-negative rods on Gram staining

8. Cerebrospinal fluid (CSF) may reveal low glucose and increased protein concentrations, and neutrophilic pleocytosis

Management

A. Procedures

1. Lumbar puncture in cases of suspected meningitis

2. Anticipate intubation in advanced cases.

B. Pharmacologic therapies

1. Antibiotics should be started within 18 hours of onset of symptoms and for 7 to 10 days duration.

2. Drug of choice is streptomycin.

3. In cases of mass casualties, doxycycline or ciprofloxacin are the antibiotics of choice.

4. Gentamicin, tetracyclines, and chloramphenicol are effective alternatives.

5. Pain management medications

C. *Nonpharmacologic therapies:* Supplemental oxygen, IV hydration to treat dehydration

D. *Consultation and collaboration:* Infectious disease service

Patient Disposition

A. *Transition of care information:* Patient will be admitted to ICU on isolation.

B. Prevention and education

1. Reduce exposure.

2. Avoid handling sick or dead animals in endemic areas.

3. Rodent control, flea control, insect repellents

4. A killed whole vaccine is available only to military personnel deployed to areas where endemic plague exists

C. Patient and family education and counseling

1. Postexposure prophylaxis with doxycycline 100 mg twice daily for 7 days for individuals having unprotected face-to-face contact before patient received 48 hours of antimicrobial therapy. Levofloxacin 500 mg daily for 10 days for patients unable to take doxycycline

D. Pediatric considerations

1. Postexposure prophylaxis with 4mg/kg trimethoprim twice daily for 7 days (for pregnant women one tablet double-strength trimethoprim-sulfamethoxazole [TMP-SMX] twice daily for 7 days)

E. Required reporting to Centers for Disease Control and Prevention (CDC), World Health Organization (WHO)

Tularemia (*Francisella tularensis*)—Category A

Introduction

A. Etiology

1. An infection of rodents and rabbits

2. This bacterium can live for several weeks in decaying animals, water, soil, and hay.

3. Detection is difficult since symptoms are similar to respiratory illnesses and diseases caused by ticks.

B. *Dissemination:* Solid or aerosol

C. Routes of entry:

1. Inhalation (agricultural dusts)

2. Ingestion (contaminated water)

3. Injection (bites from ticks, deer flies, and insects)

4. Can be transmitted by handling infected animal carcasses

D. Personal protective equipment (PPE)

1. At hospital universal precautions (hand hygiene, gown, gloves, mask, and face shield)

2. If risk for aerosolized powder contamination, N95 mask or equivalent, or powered air-purifying respirator (PAPR)

E. *Decontamination:* Disinfect contaminated clothing and linens per standard hospital procedure.

F. Pathophysiology

1. Gram-negative coccobacillus transmitted by a tick bite in 50% of cases

2. Can also be used as biologic weapon

G. Prevalence

1. Incidence of exposure peaks in summer and fall.

2. Most common in the United States in Arkansas, Missouri, and Oklahoma

Medical Screening

A. *Common chief complaint:* Fever, cough, headache, chest pain, unilateral eye pain

B. *Signs and Symptoms:* Abrupt fever, headache, myalgias, arthralgias, nonproductive cough, evolving weakness, pneumonia (symptom onset 3–14 days postexposure)

C. *Past medical history:* May report recent travel to endemic area

Physical Examination

A. *General:* Elevated body temperature, moderate distress, achiness

B. *Skin:* May have single, painful necrotic lesion, eschar

C. *Eyes:* Purulent discharge may be present, ulcerative conjunctivitis; usually unilateral complaint.

D. *ENT (ear, nose, and throat):* Oropharyngeal exudate

E. *Neck:* Tender lymphadenopathy, may be ulcerated, erythemic (multiple areas of lymph nodes may be involved)

F. *Cardiac:* Tachycardia, hypotension

G. *Pulmonary:* Wheezing, rhonchi, cough (pneumonic)
H. *Musculoskeletal:* Generalized progressive weakness

Differential Diagnoses

A. Staphylococcal or streptococcal infection
B. Anthrax
C. HIV
D. Cytomegalovirus (CMV)
E. Epstein-Barr virus (EBV)
F. Toxoplasmosis
G. Cat-scratch fever
H. Plague
I. Brucellosis
J. Influenza

Diagnostic Testing

A. Notify lab that tularemia is expected (biosafety 2 and 3 conditions).
B. Culture of swabs or scrapings from skin lesions
C. Lymph node biopsies
D. Pharynx, sputum, gastric secretions
E. Blood cultures (often negative)
F. Direct fluorescent antibody testing
G. Immunohistochemical staining
H. Polymerase chain reaction (PCR)
I. Complete blood count (CBC) with differential
J. Serum chemistries
K. Urinalysis (UA), urine myoglobin (survey for rhabdomyolysis)
L. Chest radiograph (patchy infiltrates indicative of pneumonic)

Management

A. Procedures
  1. Lymph node biopsy
  2. Anticipate intubation if significant respiratory decline.
B. Pharmacologic therapies
  1. Early antibiotic therapy is crucial, can prevent progression and shorten duration of illness.
  2. Streptomycin is the drug of choice, alternatives include gentamicin (10-day course), doxycycline (14-day course), ciprofloxacin (not Food and Drug Administration [FDA] approved, but proven efficacy); narcotic pain management may be necessary.
C. *Nonpharmacologic therapies:* IV hydration, supplemental oxygen
D. *Consultation and collaboration:* Centers for Disease Control and Prevention (CDC) notification

Patient Disposition

A. *Transition of care:* Patient will be admitted, isolation not necessary
B. *Prevention and education:* Insect repellent, use of gloves for contact with dead or dying animals, avoid mowing over dead animals
C. *Patient and family education and counseling:* Infection is not transmitted person-to-person, use standard precautions

FOOD SAFETY THREATS (*SALMONELLA, ESCHERICHIA COLI,* AND *SHIGELLA*)—CATEGORY B

Escherichia coli (E. coli)

Introduction

A. *Etiology:* Bacteria found in the environment, foods, and animal and human intestines
B. *Routes of entry:* Ingestion
C. *Personal protective equipment (PPE):* Standard precautions; gloves, gown, mask, eye shield

Medical Screening

A. *Common chief complaint:* Diarrhea (may be bloody), abdominal pain, nausea, vomiting, fever
B. Signs and symptoms:
  1. Individual symptoms may be mild to severe, even deadly
  2. Shiga toxin–producing *E. coli* (STEC) mild to moderate fever <101°F, extreme stomach cramps, vomiting, diarrhea (frequently bloody)
  3. Onset usually 3 to 4 days after ingestion
  4. Symptoms often resolve within 5 to 7 days.
  5. Approximately 10% of patients with STEC infection develop hemolytic uremic syndrome (HUS) about 7 days after initial symptoms begin while diarrhea is decreasing.
  6. Symptoms of HUS include decreased urination, fatigue, pallor.
  7. Lab findings include low platelet count, anemia, renal failure.
  8. HUS requires hospitalization for monitoring of renal function.
  9. Recovery may occur within weeks, however, permanent damage or death may result.

Physical Examination

A. *General: E. coli* infections may result in a myriad of symptoms related to the system that is primarily infected. Headache, vomiting, diarrhea, confusion, lethargy, fever or hypothermia, developing septic shock, meningitis, pneumonia, and urinary tract infections (UTI).
B. *Skin:* Pallor, cyanosis
C. *Eyes:* May be sunken depending on hydration status; in neonates jaundice may present
D. *Cardiac:* Tachycardia, hypotension
E. *Pulmonary:* Increased work of breathing, tachypnea, crackles on auscultation
F. *Neurological:* Confusion, as symptoms advance may develop seizures
G. *Genitourinary:* Uremia
H. *Gastrointestinal:* Vomiting, diarrhea (may be bloody), dehydration

Differential Diagnoses

A. *Enterobacter* infections
B. *Klebsiella* infections
C. *Proteus* infections

D. *Providencia* infections
E. *Pseudomonas aeruginosa* infections
F. *Serratia*
G. Shigellosis
H. Group B *Streptococcus* infections

Diagnostic Testing

A. Stool culture for STEC 0157
B. Complete blood count (CBC) for leukocytosis
C. Blood cultures
D. Sputum Gram stain
E. Comprehensive metabolic panel (CMP) electrolytes
F. Urinalysis and urine culture
G. Chest x-ray (CXR) or chest CT, CT abdomen/pelvis to evaluate kidneys and observe for abscess or obstruction
H. Lumbar puncture if meningitis suspected

Management

A. Based on site(s) of infection and severity
B. Pharmacologic therapies
   1. *E. coli* meningitis—third-generation cephalosporins
   2. *E. coli* pneumonia—third-generation cephalosporins or fluoroquinolones
   3. *E. coli* enteric infections—doxycycline, trimethoprim-sulfamethoxazole (TMP/SMZ, fluoroquinolones, rifaximin and rifamycin
C. *Nonpharmacologic therapies:* Supportive care for dehydration, oxygenation, vital signs; diarrhea management

Patient Disposition

A. Admission versus discharge with follow-up based on the severity of symptoms, age, comorbidities.
B. *Prevention and education:* Abundant supplies of clean, fresh water and effective feces disposal are crucial to avoiding transmission of *E. coli.*
C. *Patient and family education and counseling:* Contact clinician for diarrhea lasting more than 3 days or accompanied by high fever, blood in stools, inability to keep liquids down, extremely decreased urine output.

Glanders (*Burkholderia pseudomallei*)—Category B

Introduction

A. Etiology
   1. A gram-negative bacillus that causes systemic infection resulting in abscesses
   2. Rare in humans, usually occurring in equines and other mammals
   3. Left untreated, glanders septicemia is usually fatal within 10 days
   4. Chronic infections may result from this disease affecting the liver, lungs, spleen, and skin of the extremities
B. *Dissemination:* Aerosolized
C. *Routes of entry:* Inhalation, cut or scratch on skin
D. *Personal protective equipment (PPE):* Standard precautions including gloves, gown, mask, eye shield
E. *Decontamination:* Wash gently with soap and water; mask patient; place in isolation
F. *Pathophysiology:* Gram-negative bacillus; incubation 10 to 14 days

Medical Screening

A. *Common chief complaint:* Fever, chills, diaphoresis, headache
B. Signs and symptoms
   1. Fever, rigors, headache, diaphoresis, myalgia's and muscle spasms, pleuritic chest pain, rhinitis, photophobia, occasionally excessive tearing, diarrhea
   2. Localized skin ulceration and lymphadenopathy; if respiratory manifestation excessive mucus production in the eyes, nose, and respiratory tract may develop

Physical Examination

A. *General:* Ill, uncomfortable appearance; possibly malodorous
B. *Skin:* Generalized papular or pustular rash
C. *Eyes:* Lacrimation
D. *Ears, nose, and throat (ENT):* Nasal discharge, ulceration
E. *Neck:* Cervical lymphadenopathy
F. *Pulmonary:* Adventitious breath sounds related to pneumonia, bronchopneumonia, lobar pneumonia
G. *Gastrointestinal:* Splenomegaly

Differential Diagnoses

A. Bacterial pneumonia
B. Plague
C. Smallpox
D. Malaria
E. Mycoplasma pneumonia
F. Typhoid fever
G. Viral pneumonia

Diagnostic Testing

A. Culture of blood, sputum, urine, or skin lesions
B. Exudate reveals scan small bacilli using methylene blue stain.
C. Complete blood count (CBC), mild leukocytosis with left shift
D. Chest x-ray (CXR), miliary nodules, small multiple lung abscesses, bronchopneumonia, lobar pneumonia, necrotizing nodular lesions

Management

A. Pharmacologic therapies
   1. Sulfadiazine is effective.
   2. Tetracyclines, ciprofloxacin, streptomycin, novobiocin, gentamicin, imipenem, ceftazidime, and sulfonamides are usually effective
B. *Reportable disease:* Notify local health department immediately.

Patient Disposition

A. Admit for definitive treatment and monitoring.
B. *Prevention and education:* No vaccine, postexposure prophylaxis with Septra, environmental decontamination with 0.5% hypochlorite

Melioidosis (*Burkholderia pseudomallei*)—Category B

Introduction

A. Etiology

1. Distributed widely in contaminated water and soil spread to humans through direct contact with a contaminated source
2. Predominant in tropical climates

B. Dissemination

1. Direct contact with contaminated soil and surface waters by humans and animals
2. Infection categorized as acute or localized infection, pulmonary infection, septicemia, or disseminated infection (abscesses of organs including the liver, lung, spleen, and prostate)
3. Infections of the bones, viscera, lymph nodes, skin and brain may also occur.
4. Person-to-person transmission is rare.

C. Time from exposure to symptoms typically occurs between 2 to 4 weeks but may take years to develop. Localized infection may occur through a break in skin integrity and present as a skin abscess, ulcer, or nodule. Infection may lie latent decades and reactivate, similar to tuberculosis.

D. *Routes of entry:* Inhalation of contaminated dust or water; ingestion of contaminated water, compromised skin in contact with contaminated soil

E. *Personal protective equipment (PPE):* Standard precautions; gloves, gown, mask, eye shield

F. *Decontamination:* Gentle washing with soap and water

G. *Pathophysiology:* Caused by a gram-negative saprophyte

H. *Prevalence:* Rare in the United States, peaks during wet seasons

Medical Screening

A. *Common chief complaint:* Nonhealing skin infection, respiratory infection/pneumonia

B. *Signs and symptoms:* Fever, headache, generalized myalgia, arthralgia, anorexia, weight loss, abdominal pain, respiratory distress, chest pain, confusion, and seizure. Septic shock common in more than half of the cases.

C. *Past medical history:* Can occur in healthy people. Higher risk of clinical disease in individuals with diabetes, alcohol abuse, and chronic renal disease. Risk higher in children with beta thalassemia major.

Physical Examination

A. *General:* Fever, confusion

B. *Skin:* Flushing, jaundice urticaria may present in early stages.

C. *Eyes:* May be jaundiced

D. *Ears, nose, and throat (ENT):* Sore throat

E. *Neck:* Cervical lymphadenopathy may be present.

F. *Cardiac:* Tachycardia related to fever, possibly dehydration

G. *Pulmonary:* Dyspnea

H. *Neurological:* Confusion, agitation

I. *Gastrointestinal:* Diffuse abdominal tenderness

J. *Musculoskeletal:* Rigors, myalgias, muscle tenderness

Diagnostic Testing

A. Isolation of bacteria for culture from blood, urine, sputum, skin lesions, and abscesses

B. Detecting an antibody response to the bacteria

C. Culture is the most accurate method for diagnosis.

D. Sputum and abscess Gram stains may reveal gram-negative bacilli with a "safety pin" appearance

E. Chest x-ray (CXR) in pneumonia may display diffuse, patchy lobar or multilobar consolidation, necrotizing lesions, pleural effusions

F. CT and ultrasound helpful for locating abscesses

G. Serology not helpful for diagnosis

Management

A. Pharmacologic therapies

1. IV ceftazidime or meropenem
2. Oral trimethoprim-sulfamethoxazole (TMP-SMZ) or amoxicillin/clavulanic acid

B. *Reportable disease:* Notify local health department immediately.

Patient Disposition

A. Admit for isolation, definitive treatment, and monitoring.

B. *Prevention and education:* Persons with open skin wounds and impaired immunity should avoid contact with soil and standing water.

Psittacosis (*Chlamydia psittaci*)—Category B

Introduction

A. Etiology

1. A bacteria primarily infecting many types of birds and poultry
2. Sometimes referred to as "parrot fever"
3. Time of exposure to symptoms is 5 to 7 days
4. More common in adults

B. *Dissemination:* Aerosol; direct contact with infected birds who shed bacteria in urine, feces, and respiratory secretions. Rarely, maybe disseminated person-to-person.

C. *Routes of entry:* Inhalation of dust from infected secretions, injection via bird bites, and beak-to-mouth contact.

D. *Personal protective equipment (PPE):* Standard precautions; gloves, gown, mask, eye shield

E. Pathophysiology

1. *C. psittaci* attaches to epithelial cells of the respiratory tract
2. The infection spreads to the blood stream and results in secondary bacteremia within lung tissues

F. *Prevalence:* More common in young and middle-aged adults

Medical Screening

A. *Common chief complaint:* Abrupt onset headache, fever, dry cough

B. Signs and symptoms

1. Symptoms are widely variable, ranging from asymptomatic to systemic illness.
2. Most common presentation is upper respiratory tract infection (URI) often accompanied by abrupt onset of fever and chills, headache, myalgias, and nonproductive cough.
3. CXR may indicate lobar or interstitial pneumonia.
4. Fever without increased heart rate may be present, with rash (infrequently) and splenomegaly on examination.
5. Complications may include respiratory failure, significant pneumonia, endocarditis, myocarditis, hepatitis, arthritis, encephalitis, and sepsis.
6. Less common symptoms include pharyngitis, diarrhea, and altered mental status (AMS).

Physical Examination

A. *Skin:* Horder spots on face, macular rash
B. *Eyes:* Photophobia
C. *Cardiac:* Bradycardia
D. *Pulmonary:* Rales, pleural rub
E. *Neurological:* Headache
F. *Genitourinary (GU):* Acute glomerulonephritis possible
G. *Gastrointestinal:* Occasional splenomegaly, hepatomegaly
H. *Musculoskeletal:* Occasionally rhabdomyolysis may develop

Differential Diagnoses

A. Psittacosis
B. Atypical pneumonia (chlamydia, mycoplasma, legionella)
C. Influenza
D. Endocarditis
E. Septicemia
F. *Coxiella burnetii* infection
G. Leptospirosis
H. Brucellosis

Diagnostic Testing

A. Serum testing for antibodies to the bacteria
   1. Microimmunofluorescent (MIF) antibody test, the most sensitive and specific, only available in specialized labs
B. Cultures discouraged
   1. Highly infectious when cultured
C. Complete blood count (CBC)
   1. Usually no elevation of white blood cells (WBC), but differential "left shift"
   2. Significant leukocytosis
   3. Elevated C-reactive protein (CRP) and erythrocyte sedimentation rates
D. Liver function tests (LFTs)
   1. Aspartate aminotransferase (AST) mildly elevated, low serum albumin
E. Electrolytes
   1. Hyponatremia, mild elevation of serum creatinine, and blood urea nitrogen (BUN) common
F. Occasional elevated creatinine kinase (CK) levels
G. CXR—normal or lower lobe changes, rarely pleural effusions
H. Pulmonary CT

Management

A. Pharmacologic therapies
   1. Doxycycline drug of choice
   2. Alternatives include Macrolides (e.g., erythromycin, azithromycin).
B. Report infection to health department.

Patient Disposition

A. Admit to ICU if symptoms are severe or in acute respiratory failure.
B. Standard infection control for droplet transmission
C. Consult infectious disease service.
D. Patients with minimal symptoms may be discharged but should follow-up with a healthcare clinician within 48 hours
E. Prevention and education
   1. No vaccine available
   2. Not necessary to destroy pet birds (can be isolated and treated with antibiotics)
   3. Contact and respiratory PPE for employees of poultry processing plants

Q Fever (*Coxiella burnetii*)—Category B

Introduction

A. Etiology
   1. "Q" Query fever is a natural bacterial disease of sheep, cattle, and goats.
   2. An incapacitating agent; simple production and storage
   3. The bacteria is resistant to heat, drying, and many disinfectants and can survive for long periods in the environment.
   4. High risk for women who are pregnant even if asymptomatic
   5. A post-Q fever syndrome may develop in $<20\%$ of patients characterized by fatigue, significant headaches, photophobia, myalgia, arthralgia, night sweats, and sleep disturbance.
   6. A chronic form of the infection may develop after infection with Q fever within weeks following recovery from initial infection.
   7. Manifestations include endocarditis, aneurysms, and infections of the bone, liver, and reproductive organs.
B. Dissemination
   1. Aerosol, vector, food supply
   2. Excreted in milk, urine and feces, placenta, and amniotic fluids of infected animals
   3. Tick bites, eating or drinking unpasteurized dairy products, and person-to-person transmission are rare
C. *Routes of entry*: Inhalation, ingestion, direct contact with nonintact skin
D. *Personal protective equipment (PPE):* Standard precautions; gloves, gown, mask, eye shield

E. Pathophysiology
  1. Attaches to host macrophages, enters the cell and fuses with lysosomes
  2. The organism multiplies and ruptures the host cell.
  3. Infected macrophages are transported systemically.

Medical Screening

A. Important to include in history if the patient has an occupation that would expose them to infected livestock
B. Signs and symptoms
  1. Combinations of extremely high fever, prolonged fever, chills, nonproductive cough, chest pain, significant headache, malaise, myalgia, nausea, vomiting, diarrhea (incubation 10–20 days; lasts 2 days to 2 weeks).
  2. Complications may include significant pneumonia, granulomatous hepatitis, myocarditis, or central nervous system sequelae.

Physical Examination

A. *General:* Ill-appearing, high fever, pleuritic chest pain
B. *Skin:* Occasional maculopapular rash on the trunk
C. *Eyes:* Occasional jaundice
D. *Cardiac:* Occasional pericardial rub, heart failure, tachycardia
E. *Pulmonary:* Nonspecific adventitious breath sounds, dyspnea, tachypnea, occasionally pleural effusion
F. *Neurological:* Occasionally meningeal signs, nuchal rigidity
G. *Gastrointestinal:* Hepatomegaly, rare jaundice

Differential Diagnoses

A. Tickborne illness
B. Acute interstitial pneumonitis
C. Arbovirus encephalitis
D. Bacterial endocarditis
E. Brucellosis

Diagnostic Testing

A. Rapid confirmation by (polymerase chain reaction [PCR]) with serum antibody titers
B. Serologic testing of whole blood, serum, and/or tissue biopsies from site of active infection within the first 2 weeks of illness.
C. Patients who are immunosuppressed and those who were pregnant when infected should have routine serology to monitor for development of chronic Q fever for approximately 2 years following initial infection.
D. Complete blood count (CBC) (low platelet count, normal leukocytes count)
E. Chemistry panel (elevated liver enzymes)
F. Not all patients will exhibit abnormal serology.
G. CT scan of the brain indicated if neurologic symptoms present
H. Chest x-ray (CXR) may reveal atypical pneumonia.

Management

A. Do not withhold treatment awaiting definitive test results. Treat if clinical suspicion for Q fever exists since test results may be negative for 2 weeks following initial infection.
B. Pharmacologic therapies
  1. Doxycycline
  2. Alternatives include ciprofloxacin, tetracycline, moxifloxacin, clarithromycin, and rifampin
  3. For symptomatic pregnant women: trimethoprim/sulfamethoxazole up to 32 weeks' gestation.
C. Collaboration and consultation: infectious disease service

Patient Disposition

A. Admission versus outpatient management determined by the seriousness of symptoms
B. Discharge instructions
  1. Repeat serologic testing at 3 months and 6 months to monitor for persistent infection
  2. Retinal examinations every 6 months if patient treated with hydroxychloroquine
  3. Photosensitivity associated with doxycycline
C. *Prevention and education:* Consume only pasteurized milk and milk products
D. Patient and family education and counseling
  1. 20% of patients diagnosed with Q fever develop post-Q fever fatigue syndrome after acute illness passes
  2. Similar to symptoms of chronic fatigue syndrome
E. Pediatric considerations
  1. Treat with doxycycline for children 8 years of age or older.
  2. *Less than 8 years old:* Treat with trimethoprim-sulfamethoxazole (TMP/SMZ).

Salmonella

Introduction

A. Etiology
  1. Majority of infections result from food sources
  2. More common in summer
  3. Breastfed infants less likely to contract *Salmonella* infection
  4. Use of gastric acid reduction medications increases risk of Salmonella infection.
B. *Dissemination:* Direct contact with feces of animals or humans, by eating contaminated foods (meat, eggs, and vegetables).
C. *Routes of entry:* Ingestion
D. *Personal protective equipment (PPE):* Standard precautions; gloves, gown, mask, eye shield
E. *Pathophysiology:* Gram-negative facultative intracellular anaerobes that affect the intestinal tract

Medical Screening

A. *Chief complaint:* Fever, chills, headache, abdominal pain, nausea, vomiting, diarrhea for 6 to 12 hours
B. Signs and symptoms
  1. Most patients develop fever, diarrhea (may be bloody), abdominal cramps within 12 to 72 hours of infection
  2. Fewer patients experience nausea, vomiting, headache
  3. Illness lasts 4 to 7 days

4. Most patients do not require treatment beyond oral rehydration with gastrointestinal (GI) symptoms resolving in 5 to 7 days
5. Dehydration may develop and require hospitalization.
6. Risk of bacteremia (requiring antibiotics), meningitis, osteomyelitis, and even death
7. Infants, elderly, immunocompromised at highest risk for serious illness
8. For severe infections, use of fluoroquinolones, third-generation cephalosporin, or ampicillin. Resistance to antimicrobial drugs is not uncommon.

Physical Examination

A. *General:* Ill-appearing, symptoms of malaise
B. *Skin:* May be tenting, dry due to dehydration
C. *Eyes:* May be dull, sunken
D. *Ears, nose, and throat (ENT):* Dry mucosa, hoarse voice
E. *Cardiac:* Tachycardia related to dehydration status
F. *Pulmonary:* Tachypnea related to dehydration and fever
G. *Neurological:* May complain of headache
H. *Genitourinary:* Decreased urine output
I. *Gastrointestinal:* Abdominal cramping, bloating

Differential Diagnoses

A. *Campylobacter* infections
B. *Cyclospora* infection
C. *E. coli* infections
D. *Listeria monocytogenes* infection
E. Shigellosis
F. *Vibrio* infections
G. *Yersinia enterocolitica*

Diagnostic Testing

A. Culture of stool or blood

Management

A. *Pharmacologic therapies:* Antibiotics recommended in presence of sepsis, severe diarrhea, excessive fever, infants, elderly, and if immunocompromised

Patient Disposition

A. Admission for rehydration and correction of electrolyte imbalances
B. Prevention and education
1. Patients with severe illness may require several months for bowel activity to return to normal.
2. Other long-term effects may include reactive arthritis, eye irritation, and dysuria.

Shigella—A Highly Contagious Infection

Introduction

A. *Etiology:* Common in developing countries where sanitation is poor. From human feces often transmitted by flies.
B. *Dissemination:* Food, drinking and recreational water, surfaces contaminated with *Shigella*
C. *Routes of entry:* Ingestion
D. *Personal protective equipment (PPE):* Standard precautions; gloves, gown, mask, eye shield
E. *Decontamination:* No formal decontamination
F. Pathophysiology
1. Gram-negative, nonmotile, facultatively anaerobic, non-spore-forming rods
2. Causes bacterial invasion of the colonic epithelium and inflammatory colitis
3. Local release of cytokines and inflammatory elements
4. Colitis in the rectosigmoid mucosa results in loose watery blood-tinged mucoid stools.

Medical Screening

A. *Common chief complaint:* Watery diarrhea, nausea, fever, chills, abdominal cramping, mild to moderate dehydration
B. Signs and symptoms:
1. Diarrhea (often bloody mucoid), fever, crampy abdominal pain, dehydration, and frequent urge to defecate
2. Symptoms typically begin 24 to 48 hours after exposure and usually up to 7 days but sometimes longer for bowel function to return to normal.
3. Rarely, a form of postinfectious arthritis may develop.

Physical Examination

A. *General:* Febrile, toxic, or ill-appearing, restless or uncomfortable behavior
B. *Skin:* May be tented or dry if dehydrated
C. *Eyes:* If dehydrated, sunken appearance may be present especially in children
D. *ENT (ear, nose, and throat):* Oral mucosa may be tacky or dry if dehydrated
E. *Cardiac:* Tachycardia may be present if dehydrated, hypotension
F. *Pulmonary:* Tachypnea possible
G. *Neurological:* Confusion or lethargy may be present if electrolyte imbalance or dehydration are significant
H. *Gastrointestinal:* Tenderness in lower abdomen and distention may present, normal or hyperactive bowel sounds

Differential Diagnoses

A. *Escherichia coli*
B. *Salmonella enteritidis*
C. *Yersinia enterocolitica*
D. *Campylobacter* species
E. *Entamoeba histolytica*

Diagnostic Testing

A. Stool specimen for culture
B. Comprehensive metabolic panel (CMP)
C. Complete blood count (CBC)

Management

A. Pharmacologic therapies
1. Do not prescribe antidiarrheal agents for patients with shigellosis.
2. *Antibiotics:* Ampicillin, amoxicillin, third-generation cephalosporins, ciprofloxacin, azithromycin

B. *Nonpharmacologic therapies:* Oral rehydration solution, Pedialyte for children

Patient Disposition

A. Discharge instructions

1. Strict handwashing; do not touch your mouth without thoroughly washing hands first.

2. Wrap soiled diapers and dispose in the trash.

3. Avoid sex with a person who recently had diarrhea.

4. Educate about dehydration and reinforce with written instructions for rehydration and reasons to return to the ED.

5. Do not take drugs that slow down the GI tract like loperamide (Imodium).

6. This can make your diarrhea worse. Shigella is resistant to some antibiotics.

7. Patient should return to the ED if symptoms worsen or are not significantly improved in 5 days.

B. *Transition of care information:* If dehydration is significant or electrolyte imbalance present, hospitalize for IV rehydration and electrolyte replacement.

C. Prevention and education

1. Strict handwashing, keep hands away from mouth, don't have sex until you have been diarrhea and feverfree for at least 1 week, do not take anti-diarrheal medications for this infection.

2. Do not return to school or work until diarrhea has resolved.

D. *Pediatric considerations:* Children <4 years of age at risk for convulsions in setting of high fever and family history of seizures.

Staphylococcal Enterotoxin B—Category B

Introduction

A. Etiology

1. Staph enterotoxin B is a toxin produced by *Staphylococcus aureus* that causes gastrointestinal illness.

2. *Staphylococcus* bacteria is easily destroyed during cooking, but the toxins produced by the bacteria are heat-resistant and not easily eliminated during cooking.

B. *Dissemination:* Not transferred person-to-person

C. *Routes of entry:* Ingestion of contaminated food or water, or inhalation of fine mist

D. *Personal protective equipment (PPE):* Standard precautions; gloves, gown, mask, eye shield

E. Pathophysiology

1. Mediated stimulation of T lymphocytes within the host's immune system results in massive amounts of cytokines

2. The host's inflammatory response mediates many toxic effects of the infection.

Medical Screening

A. Signs and symptoms

1. Rapid onset between 30 minutes to 6 hours and lasting up to 24 hours

2. Gastrointestinal distress symptoms including nausea, vomiting, abdominal cramping, and diarrhea.

3. Not typically tested unless an outbreak occurs.

4. Even low doses inhaled may cause fever, cough, difficulty breathing, headache, nausea, and vomiting.

Physical Examination

A. *General:* Ill-appearing, acute, crampy abdominal pain, myalgias

B. *Cardiac:* Hypotension, tachycardia, may complain of substernal chest pain

C. *Pulmonary:* Dyspnea, occasional pulmonary edema

D. *Gastrointestinal:* Hyperperistalsis, watery diarrhea, diffuse, abdominal pain

Differential Diagnoses

A. Acute pericarditis

B. Adult respiratory distress syndrome

C. Cyanide poisoning

D. Nerve agent exposure

E. Acute pancreatitis

F. Acute gastroenteritis

G. Small bowel obstruction

Diagnostic Testing

A. Stool or emesis cultures for Staph toxins or cultured from contaminated food

B. Antibody titers rise dramatically at 10 to 20 days postexposure.

Management

A. Pharmacologic therapies

1. Treated with oral or IV fluid rehydration

2. Antibiotics are not useful for this infection.

3. Antiemetics may be helpful.

Patient Disposition

A. Admission if dehydration, hypoxia, or respiratory distress are present

B. Notify health department if multiple patients present with similar symptoms.

C. Notify local Federal Bureau of Investigation (FBI) branch if terrorist attack suspected.

D. Prevention and education

1. Safe handling of food, thorough hand hygiene before and after preparing food

2. Covering any open wounds on hands and wrists, maintaining a consistently clean environment in food serving areas

3. Do not keep food out more than two hours and 40 degrees or cooler if cold food, 140 degrees or warmer if hot food.

Typhus Fever (*Rickettsia prowazekii*)—Category B

Introduction

A. Etiology

1. Spread by human head and body lice

2. Symptoms typically begin 7 to 14 days post-exposure.

3. *Note:* There is also a similar fleaborne typhus (murine typhus caused by *Rickettsia typhi*) but not discussed in this chapter

B. *Dissemination:* Lice can spread human-to-human by close contact, sharing clothes, sleeping in bed of infected person

C. *Routes of entry:* Excoriated skin

D. *Personal protective equipment (PPE):* Gown, gloves

E. *Decontamination:* With pesticides

F. Pathophysiology
   1. Louse deposits *R. prowazekii* infection into human during a blood meal.
   2. Infection spreads through blood steam and/or lymphatic system.

G. *Prevalence:* More common in cold weather, humidity, poor hygiene; rare worldwide

Medical Screening

A. *Common chief complaint:* Abrupt onset fever, headache

B. *Signs and symptoms:* Fever, headache, tachypnea, chills, muscle tenderness, late rash begins on trunk spreads to extremities, abdominal tenderness, joint pain, nonproductive cough, nausea

Physical Examination

A. *Skin:* Rash on trunk and extremities, may become petechial in severe illness; eschar may be present in more advanced cases

B. *Cardiac:* Relative bradycardia

C. *Respiratory:* Tachypnea, cough

D. *Neurological:* Confusion, drowsiness, coma, seizures, focal neurologic signs

E. *Gastrointestinal:* Occasional mild splenomegaly and mild hepatomegaly

F. *Lymphatics:* Generalized tender lymphadenopathy

Differential Diagnoses

A. Anthrax

B. Brucellosis

C. Dengue

D. Epstein-Barr virus

E. Kawasaki disease

Diagnostic Testing

A. Complete blood count (CBC), leukopenia, mildly elevated white blood cells (WBC), thrombocytopenia

B. Comprehensive metabolic panel (CMP), hyponatremia, mildly elevated transaminase, low albumin

C. Urinalysis (UA)

D. Chest x-ray (CXR) may reveal subtle abnormalities.

E. *Serum:* Indirect immunofluorescent antibody test is definitive.

Management

A. Pharmacologic therapies
   1. Doxycycline drug of choice
   2. Chloramphenicol also effective
   3. Infected individuals and those in close contact with them should be treated with long-acting insecticides.

Patient Disposition

A. Admission for patients unable to maintain oral hydration or unable to take oral antibiotics. Outpatient care for uncomplicated cases.

B. Prevention and education
   1. Delousing with long-acting pesticides when exposed to lice (may require two separate applications/treatments)
   2. Precautions to avoid flying squirrels and their nests

C. *Patient and family education and counseling*: Response to antibiotics usually rapid, within 48 hours of the start time.

VIRAL AGENTS

Smallpox (*Variola major*)—Category A

Introduction

A. A highly infective viral infection that is easily transmitted as an aerosol. More common during cool, dry winter months. Host is infectious upon development of rash until all eschar is gone.

B. *Dissemination:* Spreads easily, aerosol, contact with infected humans or contaminated objects

C. *Routes of entry*: Inhalation, absorption

D. *Personal protective equipment (PPE):* Standard, contact, and airborne precautions including National Institute for Occupational Safety and Health (NIOSH)–approved N95 particulate respirator.

E. Pathophysiology
   1. Virus replicates within cell cytoplasm without need of a nucleus.
   2. Initially replicates within respiratory tract epithelial cells

F. *Prevalence:* Highly unusual worldwide since early 1970s

Medical Screening

A. *Common chief complaint:* Initially lesions in the mouth that spread to face then to extremities, fever, chills, malaise, nausea, vomiting, and headache.

B. Signs and symptoms
   1. Initially high fever (as high as 104°F)
   2. Significant lethargy, severe headache, backache, and abdominal pain
   3. Vomiting
   4. Rash on tongue and mouth that evolves to open sores
   5. Full body rash begins as red bumps then evolves to itchy blisters.
   6. The blister opens, and scabs develop. Scabs fall off after 1 to 2 weeks.

Physical Examination

A. *General:* Patient may be alert or present with decreased level of consciousness, fever >101°F, uncomfortable, moderate to severe distress

B. *Skin:* Popular/vesicular lesions in mouth, throat, face, extremities
C. *Pulmonary:* Wheezing, rhonchi if pneumonia has developed

Differential Diagnoses
A. Acute leukemia
B. Allergic dermatitis
C. Chickenpox
D. Drug reactions
E. Erythema multiforme

Diagnostic Testing
A. Specimen collection from vesicle (personal protective equipment [PPE] and collector who has been previously immunized)
B. Chest radiograph (assess for pneumonia)
C. Direct fluorescent antibody test, polymerase chain reaction (PCR) test, or electron microscopy to test for varicella-zoster (VZV)
D. Lumbar puncture to exclude meningococcemia
E. Viral swab of the pharynx

Management
A. Immediate contact/droplet isolation
B. Isolate anyone who came in contact with the patient within 17 days prior to illness.
C. Mandatory notification of local and state health department; considered a major health threat.
D. Mandatory immediate notification of Centers for Disease Control and Prevention (CDC) and for specimen management.
E. *Procedures:* Respiratory and contact isolation precautions
F. Pharmacologic therapies
  1. Prevention via smallpox vaccine
  2. Supportive therapy and antibiotics for secondary bacterial infections
  3. Pain management medications as indicated

G. *Nonpharmacologic therapies*: IV hydration, supplemental oxygen as needed
H. Consult infectious disease service.

Patient Disposition
A. Admit to strict contact/droplet isolation.
B. *Prevention and education:* Place all exposed persons in quarantine immediately.

Viral Hemorrhagic Fevers—Filoviruses and Arenaviruses

Introduction
A. Filoviruses include Ebola and Marburg—Category A
B. Arenaviruses include Lassa and Machupo—Category A
C. Etiology
  1. Associated with fever and bleeding
  2. Transmission varies by individual virus; transmitted by human contact or mosquito bites
  3. Incubation 2 to 21 days

D. *Dissemination:* Solid, liquid, aerosol
E. *Routes of entry:* Inhalation, ingestion, injection (insect bites), absorption (via nonintact skin)
F. Personal protective equipment (PPE)
  1. Standard, contact, and airborne precautions to include NIOSH-approved N95 particulate respirator
  2. Goggles or face shield
  3. An impermeable gown
  4. Double gloves
  5. Shoe and leg covers
  6. Single-use head covers
  7. Lassa, Ebola, Marburg, and Congo-Crimean hemorrhagic fever viruses may be particularly prone to aerosol nosocomial spread

G. *Pathophysiology:* Hemorrhagic fever viruses are extremely viremic and result in increased vascular permeability.

Medical Screening
A. Common chief complaint
  1. Flu-like symptoms, bruising, may bleed from orifices
  2. Moderate to severe discomfort
  3. May report recent travel to an endemic region

B. Signs and symptoms
  1. Significant fever
  2. Fatigue, dizziness, myalgias, weakness, malaise
  3. Serious illness may result in bleeding beneath skin, in organs, or from mouth, eyes, ears
  4. Bloody diarrhea may be present.
  5. Signs of shock, nervous system malfunction, coma, confusion, seizures
  6. Renal failure may occur.
  7. May experience significant complications from VHF infections (retinitis, orchitis, hepatitis, transverse myelitis, uveitis, deafness, spontaneous abortion, renal insufficiency)

Physical Examination
A. *General:* May be lethargic or comatose
B. *Skin:* Bruising, oozing blood; petechial rash
C. *Eyes:* May bleed from orifices
D. *Cardiac:* Tachycardia, hypotension

Differential Diagnoses
A. Typhoid fever
B. Meningococcemia
C. Rickettsial infections
D. Acute leukemia
E. Idiopathic thrombocytopenic purpura

Diagnostic Testing
A. Complete blood count (CBC) may reveal leukopenia and thrombocytopenia.
B. Comprehensive metabolic panel (CMP) potential for hypokalemia, hypocalcemia, hyponatremia, elevated creatinine, elevated anion gap acidosis, and elevated hepatic transaminases
C. Prothrombin time/partial thromboplastin time (PT/PTT) prolonged clotting times
D. Disseminated intravascular coagulation (DIC) profile
E. Reverse transcription-polymerase chain reaction (RT-PCR) is the most common method to detect Ebola in serum.

Management

A. *Procedures:* Anticipate intubation for respiratory compromise

B. Pharmacologic therapies

1. Supportive care including hydration and blood pressure maintenance
2. Ribavirin may be helpful.

C. *Nonpharmacologic therapies:* Warmed large-bore IVs for hydration and blood products as indicated, supplemental oxygen

D. *Collaboration and consultation:* Immediate notification of local and state health departments and mandatory notification of CDC

E. Consult facility infectious disease specialist.

Patient Disposition

A. Patient must be admitted or transferred to CDC-approved facility by CDC-directed transfer mechanism and entity.

B. *Prevention and education:* Isolate patient contacts immediately.

BIOLOGIC TOXINS

Ricin Toxin from *Ricinus communis* (Castor Beans)—Category B

Introduction

A. Etiology

1. Toxins evolve from plants (castor beans = Ricin, fungi), animals, bacteria.
2. Significantly lethal, noncontagious, rapid-acting
3. Very stable when released into environment
4. Patients typically exhibit symptoms at scene of toxin release.
5. Symptoms may progress over 1 to 12 hours.
6. Similar actions as chemical agents, but usually more potent
7. Death may occur in 3 to 6 days.

B. *Dissemination:* Solid, liquid, aerosol

C. *Routes of entry:* Inhalation, ingestion, injection

D. *Personal protective equipment (PPE):* Standard precautions; gloves, gown, mask, eye shield

E. Decontamination

1. Remove clothing, gently irrigate exposed skin with copious water and mild soap, do not scrub the skin.
2. Do not induce vomiting, keep patient NPO.

F. Pathophysiology

1. Ricin is composed of two hemagglutinins and two toxins.
2. The B-chain toxin binds to host cell surfaces and affects cell entry while the A-chain toxin inhibits cell protein synthesis and leads to cell death.

Medical Screening

A. *Common chief complaint:* Fever, cough, nausea, chest tightness, diaphoresis (inhalation route); diarrhea (may be bloody), nausea, vomiting (ingestion route)

B. Signs and symptoms

1. Fever, generalized weakness, myalgias, arthralgias, dizziness, mouth and throat dryness, blurred vision, respiratory failure, hypotension
2. Inhalation symptoms include dyspnea, chest tightness, fluid in the lungs.
3. Ingestion symptoms include abdominal pain, vomiting, diarrhea, dehydration.

Physical Examination

A. *General:* May be lethargic to comatose; moderate to severe distress

B. *Skin:* Developing cyanosis, urticarial

C. *Ears, nose, and throat (ENT):* Oral or upper airway edema; tongue swelling possible

D. *Cardiac:* Tachycardia, hypotension; symptoms of developing shock

E. *Pulmonary:* Potential for developing hypoxia, dyspnea, tachypnea

F. *Gastrointestinal:* Vomiting, diarrhea, dehydration; in severe exposure hematemesis, bloody diarrhea, or melena

Differential Diagnoses

A. Staphylococcal enterotoxin B

B. Q fever

C. Tularemia

D. Pneumonic plague

E. Cholera

F. Necrotizing fasciitis

G. Acute arsenic toxicity

Diagnostic Testing

A. Urinalysis for ricin (must be processed at a Centers for Disease Control and Prevention [CDC]-approved facility)

B. Complete blood count (CBC), electrolytes, blood type and screen, blood urea nitrogen (BUN) and creatinine

C. Amylase, lipase, liver function tests (LFTs), lactic acid

D. Cultures of blood, urine, and sputum

E. Coagulation studies if hemorrhagic

F. Arterial blood gases (ABG)

G. Chest x-ray (CXR) or chest CT to evaluate respiratory distress

Management

A. *Pharmacologic therapies:* There is no antidote

B. Nonpharmacologic therapies

1. IV hydration with warmed normal saline and blood products
2. Supplemental oxygen
3. Anticipate intubation

C. *Consultation and collaboration:* Notify CDC immediately.

Patient Disposition

A. Admission to ICU

Water Safety Threats (*Vibrio cholerae*, *Cryptosporidium parvum*)—Category B

Introduction

A. Etiology

1. Sporadic, often water-related outbreaks resulting in self-limited diarrhea

2. Can cause serious, life-threatening illness in immunocompromised patients
3. Children suffering malnutrition and diarrhea in developing countries
4. More frequently seen in children
5. Incubation period typically 7 to 10 days
6. Typically resolves without treatment in 10 to 14 days

B. *Dissemination:* Spread by an infected human or animal via food or contaminated drinking or swimming water source
C. *Routes of entry:* Fecal to oral route
D. Personal protective equipment Standard and contact isolation
E. Pathophysiology
1. *Vibrio* species produce extracellular cytotoxins and enzymes that can cause extensive tissue damage and resulting sepsis.
2. Parasitic infection thought to interfere with architecture of villi causing inflammatory changes resulting in intestinal malabsorption
3. As parasites increase, small intestine dysfunction occurs.
4. Migration to the biliary system may result in strictures and cholangitis
5. Infected persons may be asymptomatic.
6. Pulmonary infestation possible

F. Prevalence
1. 30% of childhood infections are asymptomatic, but more commonly seen in children than adults
2. Immunocompromised patients at higher risk for developing disease
3. May prove fatal in elderly who become dehydrated
4. More common in countries with poor sanitation

Medical Screening

A. *Common chief complaint:* Diarrhea, abdominal cramping, and fatigue
B. Signs and symptoms
1. Ranges from asymptomatic to severe
2. Malaise, watery diarrhea, nausea, anorexia, abdominal cramping, low-grade fever
3. Profound weight loss possible with persistent severe diarrhea

C. *Medication history:* Diuretic use may predispose to dehydration
D. *Past medical history:* More severe in immunocompromised patients

Physical Examination

A. *General:* Ill-appearing, severe dehydration, malaise; fever in pediatric patients
B. *Skin:* Longitudinal tenting
C. *Eyes:* Sunken appearance; sunken fontanelles in neonates
D. *Ears, nose, and throat (ENT):* Dry mucosa
E. *Cardiac:* Tachycardia, thread pulses, hypotension
F. *Pulmonary:* Tachypnea, hypercapnia
G. *Neurological:* In pediatric patient drowsiness and even coma
H. *Gastrointestinal:* Vomiting, watery diarrhea; abdominal distention may be present in severe cases.
I. *Musculoskeletal:* Muscle spasms may present with severe electrolyte imbalances.

Differential Diagnoses

A. *E. coli* infection
B. Pediatric gastroenteritis
C. Rotavirus

Diagnostic Testing

A. Comprehensive metabolic panel (CMP) (hyponatremia, hypoglycemia, hypokalemia, acidosis; calcium and magnesium levels may be high due to hemoconcentration)
B. Complete blood count (CBC)
C. Liver function test (LFT)
D. Serum alkaline phosphatase (elevated with biliary involvement)
E. Ultrasound/CT (may reveal gallbladder enlargement and wall thickening with dilated intra- and extrahepatic biliary ducts)
F. Stool specimen (ova and parasites not helpful for definitive diagnosis), duodenal aspirates, respiratory secretions, or GI biopsy for definitive diagnosis
G. Modified acid-fast stains usually necessary
H. Polymerase chain reaction (PCR) is the method of choice.

Management

A. Hydration and electrolyte balance
B. Pharmacologic therapies
1. Antibiotic therapy postrehydration and cease of vomiting
2. Single-dose IV tetracycline, doxycycline, furazolidone, or ciprofloxacin are often effective.

C. Nonpharmacologic therapies
1. Careful measures and maintenance of intake and output including replacing volume lost in diarrhea is especially important.
2. Correction of electrolyte imbalances

Patient Disposition

A. Admission for IV rehydration, IV antibiotics, and correction of electrolyte imbalances

Additional Resources

Strategic National Stockpile: http://www.bt.cdc.gov/stockpile/
World Health Organization: http://www.who.com
Additional Resource Information to Collect for Your Area of Practice: FEMA.
To report an incident: CDC (770)488-7100; available 24/7.
Phone numbers for Local, Regional, and State Department of Public Health.

Additional Reading

Additional Reading for this chapter are online only and can be found at https://connect.springerpub.com/content/reference-book/978-0-8261-6091-5/part/part06/toc-part/ch48.

VII. Special Patient Populations

49. The Pregnant Patient

TRACY BROWN

Learning Objectives

- Evaluate and treat pregnancy complications seen in pregnant patients under 20 weeks' gestation.
- Evaluate and treat pregnancy complications seen in pregnant patients over 20 weeks' gestation.
- Care for a pregnant patient experiencing delivery and the complications associated with the event.
- Tailor treatment of nonobstetric abdominal pain in a pregnant patient for best mother and fetus outcomes.
- Tailor care of a pregnant patient experiencing emergent conditions such as traumatic injury, burns, poisonings, and resuscitative care, for best mother and fetus outcomes.
- Account for pregnancy or breastfeeding in a patient when initiating pharmacologic management of a condition.

Both traditional and pregnancy-related emergencies are seen in women of reproductive age. Caring for women during pregnancy and into the postpartum breastfeeding state, has to encompass traditional problems both medical and traumatic that are seen in the nonpregnant population. Treatment for traditional emergencies that occur while a woman is pregnant or breastfeeding sometimes requires alternative interventions or alternative drug therapy. Pregnancy itself comes with a unique set of problems that require clinician care in handling. While obstetrics is a specialty unto itself, knowledge in the obstetric realm by all clinicians is crucial to the successful care of both a mother and her unborn child or breastfeeding newborn. In the United States, obstetric care is not found at every institution, putting emergency nurse practitioners (ENPs) in such settings on the front line of care, without direct assistance. As emergency medicine clinicians, ENPs often care for many diverse populations in sometimes very remote locations. This chapter covers obstetric-related emergency care, common emergency complaints with pregnancy considerations, as well as a multitude of less frequent emergent complaints that require nontraditional treatment for successful outcomes for both mother and fetus. Some treatments covered are not seen on ENP credentialing list. Legal implications in providing and performing the treatments need to be considered. The knowledge to provide key emergent lifesaving interventions has been provided in this chapter. ENP readers will need to make ethical decisions related to the use of this knowledge should they find themselves in one of these emergent situations without backup.

APPROACH TO THE PREGNANT PATIENT

Abdominal Pain in Pregnancy <20 Weeks' Gestation

Medical Screening

A. Chief complaint: A bdominal pain[1,2]

B. Signs and symptoms

1. Pain in any region
2. Referred pain to shoulder or back
3. Development of contractions
4. Fever, case specific
5. Hypotension, case specific
6. Tachycardia, case specific
7. Nausea and/or vomiting
8. Dysuria, frequency, hematuria

C. Focused assessment

1. Location of pain
2. Quality and pattern of pain
3. Pregnancy history (e.g., gravida [G], para [P], estimated date of confinement [EDC]); fundal height examination
4. Contraction pattern, quality if pertinent

Diagnostic Testing

A. *Laboratory studies (order as indicated):* Complete blood count (CBC), metabolic panel (MP), liver functions, urine analysis (UA), MP, qualitative beta human chorionic gonadotropin (b-HCG), wet prep, pH and ferning test, drug screen

B. *Imaging:* Ultrasound (US), transvaginal or transdermal pending suspected diagnosis. CT, risk versus benefit must be considered before using.

C. Monitoring of uterine activity for any contraction pattern

Medical Decision-Making, Differential Diagnoses, and Treatment

A. Ectopic pregnancy [2]

1. Stabilization needs addressed, including hemodynamic resuscitation
2. Consultation and transfer of care to obstetric specialist necessary for implementation of pharmacologic or surgical management

B. Nonobstetric diagnosis (Table 49.1)

TABLE 49.1 NONOBSTETRIC CAUSES OF ABDOMINAL PAIN IN PREGNANCY[1]

	PRESENTATION	CONSIDERATIONS
Appendicitis	Most common s/s remain RLQ pain at or near McBurney's point. N/V follows onset of pain and is associated with it.	Increased morbidity and mortality to fetus due to peritonitis, abscess formation, and perforation. Delay in dx due to pregnancy. Increase in rupture rates in pregnancy. More prominent in second trimester.[3,4]
Cholelithiasis/ Cholecystitis	RUQ pain with or without radiation to other location, may include back or shoulder.	Changes in hormone levels during pregnancy will increase possible stone development. Second trimester best time for removal since uterus has not yet obstructed to gallbladder. Decreased risk of preterm labor and need for tocolytic therapy in these patients.
Urinary Tract Infection	Either asymptomatic or including lower abdominal pain, dysuria, urinary frequency, and/or urgency.	Asymptomatic bacteremia must be treated with antibiotic therapy specific to cultures and pregnancy-safe antibiotics. Options include nitrofurantoin or fosfomycin. Many cases of ESBL have been found susceptible to these antibiotics. Adverse outcomes include low birth weight and preterm delivery.
Pyelonephritis	Lower abdominal pain, lower back pain, dysuria, urinary frequency and/or urgency, fever, chills, costovertebral angle tenderness, nausea, and vomiting.	While nonpregnant women may be treated outpatient, inpatient therapy is recommended in pregnancy with IV antibiotics. Transition to oral therapy can take place after patient has been afebrile for 24–48 hours with symptom improvement.[5] Algorithms on treatment for inpatient care are found in the literature.[6] Complications include bacteremia, septic shock, renal insufficiency or failure, anemia, and ARDS. Adverse outcomes include preterm delivery. Tocolysis and steroid therapy may be required.[6]
Nephrolithiasis	Severe flank/low back pain, abdominal pain. Fever (rare).	Renal ultrasound used for identification of stone. Normal ureteral dilation in pregnancy allows for easy passage of most stones. Pain management must be determined based on risk versus benefit and stage of pregnancy.[7] Tamsulosin is a pregnancy category B medication that may be beneficial in pregnancy.[8]
Ovarian Torsion	Lower abdominal pain in one of the lower quadrants. Cramp-type pain.	More common in pregnant patients. Ovarian cysts over 5 cm must be removed to prevent torsion. Progesterone usage required until 10 weeks' gestation if corpus luteal cyst removed.[9]

ARDS, acute respiratory distress syndrome; dx, diagnosis; ESBL, extended spectrum beta-lactamase; N/V, nausea and vomiting; RLQ, right lower quadrant; RUQ, right upper quadrant; s/s, signs and symptoms.

Abdominal Pain in Pregnancy >20 Weeks' Gestation

Medical Screening

A. Chief complaint: Abdominal pain[1]
- **1.** Signs and symptoms
  - **a.** Pain in any region
  - **b.** Referred pain to shoulder or back
  - **c.** Development of contractions
  - **d.** Fever, case specific
  - **e.** Hypotension, case specific
  - **f.** Tachycardia, case specific
  - **g.** Nausea and/or vomiting
  - **h.** Dysuria, frequency, hematuria
  - **i.** Vaginal complaints
- **2.** Focused assessment
  - **a.** Location of pain
  - **b.** Quality and pattern of pain
  - **c.** Pregnancy history (e.g., G, P, EDC). Fundal height examination
  - **d.** Contraction pattern and quality if pertinent

B. Diagnostic testing
- **1.** Laboratory studies:
  - **a.** CBC
  - **b.** MP
  - **c.** Liver function studies
  - **d.** Urinalysis (UA)
  - **e.** Wet prep
  - **f.** pH and ferning test
  - **g.** Drug screen
- **2.** Imaging:
  - **a.** US transdermal abdominal
  - **b.** CT, risk versus benefit must be considered before using.
  - **c.** MRI is now identified in the literature as alternative to radiation exposure (not noted to be mainstream approach).

d. External fetal monitoring for uterine activity and fetal heart rate patterns

Medical Decision-Making, Differential Diagnoses, and Treatment

A. Preterm labor[10]

1. Stabilization needs addressed

2. Identify and treat cause associated with preterm labor.

3. IV hydration, 5% dextrose in normal saline (D5NS) or dextrose in lactated Ringer's (D5LR)

4. Tocolytic drugs

a. Terbutaline sulfate, SC every 20 minutes to maximum of three doses[11]

b. Indomethacin, loading dose then dose every 4, 6, or 8 hours for 24 to 48 hours pending dosages used. Must not be used over 48 hours, can result in the ductus arteriosus closing prematurely.[11]

c. Magnesium sulfate, recommended loading dose over 30 minutes then recommended dose in a continuous infusion. Therapeutic levels should remain between 4 and 7 mEq/L.[11] Pharmacologic therapies should be based on evidenced-based recommendations from recognized sources, for example, the CDC, or guidelines specific to the environment where the clinician practices.

5. When membranes are ruptured, use sterile speculum for exam and do not perform bimanual examination.

6. Consultation and transfer of care to obstetric specialist for ongoing management

7. Pharmaceutical fetal maturity intervention

a. Betamethasone intramuscularly (IM), drug of choice (DOC)[12]

b. Dexamethasone IM q12h x 4 doses[12]

B. Nonobstetric diagnosis (see Table 49.1)

C. Precipitous delivery (Table 49.2)

D. Intra-amniotic infection

1. Consider problem when pyelonephritis is initially suspected.

2. Presentation may also include premature rupture of membranes, foul odor to fluid, uterine tenderness, no bacteria on UA.

3. OB consultation and hospital admission required

Nonobstetric Abdominal Pain

A. *Chief complaint:* Nonobstetric abdominal pain complaint

B. Summary of nonobstetric causes of abdominal pain in pregnancy can be found in Table 49.1[1]

C. Management of a pregnant patient with any nonobstetric cause of abdominal pain should be handled the same as a non-pregnant patient.

1. Patient stabilization is top priority in the ED.

2. Consultation with surgery, gastroenterology, urology, or nephrology should be included along with the obstetric specialist and an intensivist if needed.

TABLE 49.2 SPECIFIC DELIVERY CONSIDERATIONS[13,14]

SITUATION	CONSIDERATIONS
Normal delivery	Equipment includes towels, bulb syringe, and cord clamps. Support perineum and slide over the head. Use counter pressure on the exposed occiput to prevent explosive delivery resulting in periurethral tears. Dry infant aggressively on the back for 3 minutes. Cord clamping is no longer indicated immediately unless fetal resuscitation is required.[15–17] When clamping the cord, use 2 cord clamps 4–5 cm from the abdominal wall of the baby. Cut the cord between the 2 clamps.
Placental delivery	Signs of placental separation (about 5 minutes following delivery of baby) Sudden increase in blood from vault Uterus becomes elevated in the abdomen Presenting cord lengthens Utilize gentle traction and fundal message to facilitate delivery. Complications of forcing delivery include the cord breaking resulting in severe hemorrhage and even uterine inversion. Assess for three vessel cord and intact placenta
Nuchal Cord	Options for resolving a cord around the neck Reduce cord over the top of the head. Deliver the baby through the cord. Clamp the cord in place and cut cord before delivery.
Meconium stained fluid	Suctioning of infant prior to delivery of the chest helps to minimize the contaminants inhaled into the lungs. Wipe nose and mouth quickly, the bulb suctioning (nares and mouth).
Shoulder dystocia (*traditional delivery Lithotomy position in a delivery bed*)	Utilization of McRobert's maneuver and supra pubic pressure. Hyperflexion of the legs to rotate pelvis Apply pressure just above the pubic bone to push shoulder out from behind the symphysis pubis.
Shoulder dystocia (*result of delivery location*)	Turn patient on their side. Support superior leg. Deliver via R-S method: Guide head toward Rectum to deliver superior shoulder and then toward the suprapubic bone to deliver the inferior shoulder

3. Pregnancy considerations involve
   a. Antibiotic selection
   b. Imaging choices—ultrasound (US) being preferred over CT
   c. Surgical versus nonsurgical interventions
4. Plan of care will depend on the trimester of the pregnancy.

D. Normal abdominal changes in pregnancy result in a dulling effect of pain.
1. Occurs as a result of stretching and moving of the anterior abdominal wall resulting in potential decreased irritation of the peritoneum that would otherwise cause pain.
2. Typical guarding and rebound examination findings may be absent as a result.
3. As progression of the pregnancy develops, examination becomes difficult. Placing the patient on her side to displace the uterus may be found helpful during examination. There is a historic theory that during the course of pregnancy the location of the organs (appendix specifically) migrates upward. This has been proven false.
4. Associated symptoms such as nausea and vomiting may be a result of normal pregnancy.
5. Leukocytosis is commonly seen with pregnancy and thus is not always associated with infection.
6. Elevated alkaline phosphate is seen as a normal variant in pregnancy, thus elevation may not be reliable as a diagnostic tool in cholelithiasis and cholecystitis.

Vaginal Bleeding <20 Weeks' Gestation

Medical Screening

A. *Chief complaint:* Vaginal bleeding <20 weeks' gestation[2,12,18]

B. Signs and symptoms
1. Bleeding history including quality and quantity
2. Any pain or lack of pain in the abdomen associated with onset of bleeding
3. Weakness and fatigue
4. Hypotension
5. Tachycardia

C. Focused assessment
1. Appearance, quality, and quantity of bleeding on examination (history best obtained by identifying the number of pads used)
2. Hemodynamic stability
3. History surrounding onset
4. Speculum examination

Diagnostic Testing

A. Laboratory studies (ordered as indicated)
1. CBC
2. MP
3. Beta human chorionic gonadotropin (b-HCG)
4. Type and cross
5. Coagulation panel
6. Kleihauer–Betke test
7. Fibrinogen
8. Fibrinogen degradation products
9. Gestational trophoblast disease pathology testing on products of conception
10. *US:* Transvaginal or transdermal pending suspected diagnosis

Medical Decision-Making, Differential Diagnoses, and Treatment

A. Abortion[18]
1. *Threatened:* Identified intrauterine pregnancy with closed cervix
   a. Traditional recommendations include decreased activity and pelvic rest.
   b. Rh immunoglobulin as indicated
2. *Missed:* Identified nonviable intrauterine pregnancy with a closed cervix. Fetal demise is identified or no fetal development (blighted ovum, now termed embryonic gestation).
   a. There are three options of care:
      i. Natural course without medical intervention; can have more pain and bleeding
      ii. Pharmaceutic intervention with misoprostol. Current dosing options include 600 to 800 mcg intravaginal, repeat in 24 hours as needed. The medication may be given in a 600-mcg dose sublingual and then repeated q3h x 2.[19]
      iii. Dilation and suction curettage, requires OB consultation
   b. Rh immunoglobulin as indicated
3. *Inevitable:* Cervical dilatation and in some cases the presence of conception products at cervical os.
   a. The same three options apply regarding care.
   b. Curettage may be performed in the operating room (OR) by consultant. The literature does discuss the procedure being done in the ED with IV sedation and/or the use of a paracervical block. Note privileging from credentialing committee is required to perform this procedure.[12]
   c. If products are visible at cervical os, usage of ring forceps to gently guide the products of conception out can complete the process.
   d. Rh immunoglobulin as indicated
4. *Incomplete:* Passage of part of the products of conception. Ultrasound will identify evidence of remaining products.
   a. The use of misoprostol as a one-time dose of 600 micrograms has been found effective to complete the process.[20]
   b. Most common practice is curettage as noted above.
   c. Rh immunoglobulin as indicated
5. *Complete:* All tissue has passed (6 weeks' gestation or less). Ultrasound will confirm diagnosis.
   a. Patient is usually able to identify significant decrease in severity of symptoms.
   b. Rh immunoglobulin as indicated
6. *Septic:* Another type of abortion with a pelvic infection. The infection is usually from retained products of conception.
   a. Fever and vaginal discharge can be seen with the other symptoms.

b. Fluid resuscitation may be indicated if sepsis is identified.

c. Antibiotic therapy is indicated to treat both normal vaginal flora and bacteria associated with sexually transmitted diseases. Options include the following:

i. Ampicillin/sulbactam IV or clindamycin IV[2]

ii. And gentamycin IV[2]

d. OB consultation for product extraction is indicated.

e. Rh immunoglobulin as indicated

i. *Rh immunoglobulin usage:* The American College of Obstetricians and Gynecologists (ACOG) have published no formal recommendations in the first trimester for at-risk cases. Traditionally, a 50 mcgRh immunoglobulin dose has been used in pregnancies under 12 weeks' gestation, if used at all. Fetal–maternal hemorrhage has been documented as early as 7 weeks' gestation. With this finding, some clinicians will use a full 300 mcg dose. Over 12 weeks' gestation the full 300 mcg dose is indicated.

f. *Ongoing care:* Patient education should be provided on identifying signs and symptoms concerning possible infection and bleeding. Pelvic rest is recommended. Repeat b-hCG testing is done in some cases to identify an ongoing pregnancy or the completion of the abortion process. OB follow-up in clinic is necessary in all cases. A 2-week follow-up is the standard time frame after a completed abortion.

B. Gestational trophoblast disease, hydatidiform mole (molar pregnancy)[2]

1. Two types of moles

a. *Complete moles.* No actual fetus present (most common type).

b. *Partial moles:* A nonviable fetus—deformed—is present.

2. The trophoblasts will produce b-hCG, thus patients will have positive pregnancy tests. This may contribute to the hyperemesis seen with the diagnosis.

3. Vaginal bleeding seen in up to 95% of the cases

4. Moles can continue into the second trimester.

5. Patients who develop pregnancy-induced hypertension/preeclampsia before 24 weeks will need evaluation for the diagnosis.

6. Incidence in the diagnosis is increased in the Asian population and those having previously been diagnosed with a molar pregnancy.

7. Any tissue expelled prior to OB intervention should be sent to pathology.

8. If ultrasound findings, high b-hCG levels, or large uterine size suggests the diagnosis, OB consultation is required.

C. *Implantation bleeding:* Usually spotting in nature but can mimic menstrual bleeding. Noted around 5 to 6 weeks after last menses. Emergent diagnosis needs to be ruled out first. Accurate history is important.

D. Vaginal infections, see Vulvovaginitis section.

E. Cervical lesions

1. These will be visualized on speculum examination. Lesions, ulcerations, and polyps may be seen. Cultures may be required for identification. OB consultation or outpatient follow-up is indicated.

2. Friable cervix

a. Common in pregnancy. As a result, spotting is frequently seen after intercourse or sex toy usage. History-taking is important in these cases.

Vaginal Bleeding >20 Weeks' Gestation

Medical Screening

A. *Chief complaint:* Vaginal bleeding >20 weeks' gestation[12,13]

B. Signs and symptoms

1. Bleeding history to include quality and quantity
2. Any pain or lack of pain in the abdomen associated with the onset of bleeding
3. Weakness and fatigue
4. Hypotension
5. Tachycardia
6. Visible signs of abdominal trauma (as indicated)

C. Focused assessment

1. Appearance and quality of bleeding, usually identified with the number of pads used
2. Hemodynamic stability
3. *Uterus examination:* Boundaries, firmness, tenderness, and height as it relates to gestational age (12 weeks: just above symphysis pubis; 20 weeks: umbilicus; 36 weeks: just below the xiphoid process)
4. Fetal positioning
5. Speculum examination
6. History surrounding onset

Diagnostic Testing

A. Laboratory studies (ordered as indicated):

1. CBC
2. MP
3. Qualitative beta human chorionic gonadotropin (b-hCG)
4. Blood type and cross match (two units available immediately)
5. Coagulation panel
6. Kleihauer–Betke
7. Fibrinogen
8. Fibrinogen degradation products
9. Lamellar body count, or institutional equivalent (for fetal lung maturity)

a. Lamellar body count is the only commercial laboratory study available test left on the market. Some institutions may still have other testing methods they are using, for example, phosphatidylglycerol (PG), optical density at 650 nm, foam stability index (FSI), surfactant/albumin ratio, or lecithin/sphingomyelin ratio.[21]

10. *US:* Transvaginal versus transdermal pending suspected diagnosis

Medical Decision-Making, Differential Diagnoses, and Treatment

A. Placenta previa

1. Traditional ED thought is to avoid speculum and bimanual examination and consult OB. Ultrasound can now identify placental location to make diagnosis if it has not been identified during routine prenatal care. The type of previa is referred to as either a complete previa (placenta is seen covering the cervical os) or an incomplete previa (placenta seen within 2 cm of the cervical os), based on ultrasound findings.[12]
2. Speculum examination with or without an extremely gentle digital examination notes a complete previa as one that completely covers the cervical os. A marginal previa is when the placenta is at the edge of the os. And a low-lying placenta is diagnosed by the ability to feel the edge of the placenta on digital examination.
3. Digital examination was traditionally only done in the operating room (OR) in case of complications so emergent cesarean section could be performed.
4. ED care will focus on hemodynamic stability and OB consultation. If patient is having contractions, tocolytic therapy and steroids for fetal lung development as indicated.

B. Abruptio placenta

1. There are three grades of abruption:
   a. *Grade 1:* Minimal or no vaginal bleeding with minimal pain and no compromise to the fetus
   b. *Grade 2:* Bleeding is mild to moderate with the presence of contractions and some fetal distress.
   c. *Grade 3:* Bleeding is severe or concealed bleeding with severe contractions and fetal distress or demise.
2. US will only identify severe placental abruption.
3. Fetal monitoring is utilized for evaluation and ongoing monitoring.
4. Uterine boundary marking on initial presentation is helpful when multiple team members will be involved in ongoing examination.
5. Risk factors for spontaneous abruption include hypertension, cocaine use, and smoking.
6. The diagnoses may not present for up to 5 days in trauma patients.[22-24]

C. Uterine rupture

1. Emergent cesarean section and uterine repair is the definitive treatment. In some cases, immediate hysterectomy is required.
2. Rapid intervention for hypovolemic shock and preparation for operative management is required in the ED.
3. Abdominal examination will identify a boggy uterus and, in some cases, palpable fetal parts.
4. When obvious findings on examination are not seen, ultrasound can be used. Sensitivity is only 25% for the diagnosis but with a 98% specificity.[25]
5. When no definite diagnosis can be identified either by physical or diagnostic evaluation, early fetal monitoring is recommended. Uterine irritability and fetal distress are indicators of the diagnosis with fetal monitoring.

Vulvovaginal Pain, Irritation, and Vaginal Discharge

Medical Screening

A. *Chief complaint:* Vulvovaginal pain, irritation, vaginal discharge[26,27,28]

B. Signs and symptoms

1. Vaginal pain
2. Skin irritation with or without urination
3. Lesions or wounds
4. Rash
5. Vaginal discharge
6. Foul odor
7. Fever and/or chills

C. Focused assessment

1. Visual perineal findings
2. Speculum examination

Diagnostic Testing

A. Laboratory studies:

1. UA
2. Vaginal cultures
3. Wet prep

Medical Decision-Making, Differential Diagnoses, and Treatment

A. Gonorrhea

1. *Antibiotic treatment for nonpregnant patients:* Ceftriaxone given intramuscularly with azithromycin (current recommendations based potential resistance issues associated with doxycycline)[29]
2. *Pregnancy considerations:* Traditional therapy should be used. Doxycycline should *not* be used. Retesting is recommended within 3 months of treatment and again during the last trimester if the patient is at high risk.[30]
3. *Lactation considerations:* No formal considerations in the literature. Ceftriaxone and azithromycin have low levels in breast milk. Dosing either doesn't affect the infant or is lower than standard infant dosing.[31]

B. Chlamydia

1. Antibiotic treatment for nonpregnant patients: azithromycin single dose OR doxycycline[32]
2. Pregnancy considerations: azithromycin treatment regimen only. Doxycycline should *not* be used. If unable to use azithromycin, amoxicillin or erythromycin regimens are an alternative. Retesting required within 3 weeks of completing treatment. Ocular infection in infants can result if infection is present.[30]
3. Lactation considerations: azithromycin and amoxicillin regimens are recommended. Other medications are contraindicated in lactation.

C. Bacterial vaginosis (BV)

1. *Antibiotic treatment for nonpregnant patients:* Metronidazole or metronidazole in one dose. Tinidazole is an alternative but more expensive.[33]
2. *Pregnancy considerations:* Statistically significant risk in premature births have been identified, and thus treatment of infection is recommended.[34] Metronidazole PO days, metronidazole, or clindamycin.[33] Teratogenic

effects are noted per the manufacturer of the drug; however, the Centers for Disease Control (CDC) no longer follows the practice of not using medication in first trimester of pregnancy.[27]

3. *Lactation considerations:* Vaginal dosing recommended since oral dosing can cause gastrointestinal (GI) issues in infants. Oral clindamycin will affect GI flora in infants resulting in candidiasis infections and antibiotic-associated colitis.[28] The use of other azole medications requires pumping and discarding of breast milk during administration and for 3 days after.[35]

D. *Trichomonas vaginalis*

1. *Antibiotic treatment for nonpregnant patient:* Metronidazole OR metronidazole 1 x dose. Tinidazole is an alternative but more expensive.[33]

2. *Pregnancy dosing and considerations:* Metronidazole 1 dose or BID dosing for 5 to 7 days frequency used because of the drugs' nausea and vomiting side effects. Do not use tinidazole in pregnancy as data on drug usage in pregnancy not available to safely use drug. PO treatment required since vaginal creams do not always kill off bacteria. *Trichomonas* infections carry over 40% increased risk of premature delivery and premature rupture of membranes.[36] Metronidazole does have placenta permeability.[37]

3. *Lactation considerations:* Metronidazole dosing is decreased since the drug crosses over to breast milk. This keeps drug levels at acceptable limits.[38]

E. Candidiasis

1. *Pharmacologic treatment for nonpregnant patient:* antifungal treatment, fluconazole tab. Uncomplicated infections do not require a repeat dose. Complicated and recurrent infections may require 2 to 3 doses, each dose being 72 hours apart.[39] Fluconazole has been found to remain at effective levels in vaginal secretions for up to 72 hours. Topical treatment is also an option but tends to be less utilized because of the mess. Cure rates of the two approaches are very similar. Sexual partner treatment is not necessary.

2. *Pregnancy considerations:* Azole drug class is avoided in first trimester because of lack of data. Vaginal treatment is preferred with the use of topical clotrimazole or miconazole.[39]

3. *Lactation considerations:* Oral and vaginal therapy is acceptable with fluconazole. Fluconazole is found in breast milk, but no adverse effects have been seen and the drug is used in infants. Nystatin is not found in breast milk and therefore may be used.[40]

F. Pelvic inflammatory disease (PID)

1. This is a rare diagnosis in pregnancy given the uterus becomes sealed off from bacterial entry with the development of the mucous plug. The diagnosis can be seen in the first 12 weeks.[41]

2. Antibiotic treatment in nonpregnant patient may be found in Chapter 18, Table 18.1.

3. *Pregnancy considerations:* Hospitalization is required. First-line therapy is cefoxitin 2 G IV q6h or cefotetan 2 G IV q12h AND azithromycin 1 gm PO (instead of doxycycline).

4. *Lactation considerations:* Antibiotic choice will first need to be based on inpatient versus outpatient treatment. There are several combinations of therapies noted in the table previously mentioned. A published case study notes the use of daptomycin for a multi-drug-resistant methicillin-resistant *Staphylococcus aureus* (MRSA) pelvic infection in a breastfeeding patient. The daily dose of daptomycin was as recommended based on evidence-based recommendations. Breast milk drug levels were tested and found to be extremely low. The molecule has a large molecular weight and a high affinity for binding with protein may account for the low levels seen in the breast milk. The use of the drug may want to be considered in other MRSA-based infections.[42]

LABOR AND DELIVERY COMPLICATIONS

Breech Delivery[13,14]

A. Signs and symptoms
   1. History of rupture of membranes
   2. History of contractions

B. Focused assessment
   1. Digital examination to evaluate for presenting part
   2. Leopold's maneuver to determine fetal position

C. Diagnostic testing
   1. *Laboratory studies:* Labs obtained for emergent delivery at the individual institution
   2. *Imaging:* Ultrasound for purpose of identifying the position of the legs
   3. Doppler for fetal heart rate evaluation

D. Medical Decision-Making, Differential Diagnosis, and Treatment
   1. Treatment involves emergent OB consultation for delivery. Emergent cesarean delivery has been the typical practice for many years.
      a. Emergent patient positioning to maintain fetal heart rate
      b. Emergent IV establishment and additional OR preparation
      c. Transport to the OR
   2. Plan B for those practicing at a facility that does not provide obstetric services and the patient presents ready to deliver and the fetus is in the breech position.
      a. Determine lower extremity positioning. Easiest position for delivery is having lower extremities straight with feet next to the head (frank breech position).
      b. Allow delivery of buttock until the back of the knees can be reached.
      c. Gentle pressure to the back of each knee will cause a flexion response by the fetus to bend the extremity allowing for the delivery of the leg.
      d. Each upper extremity can be guided out one at a time.

e. The head will want to stay trapped with the occiput behind the symphysis pubis. Flexion of the head will be needed for delivery. Lowering the fetus downward will assist with the process. Putting a finger in the mouth to guide the chin down will aid in flexion. Suprapubic pressure will guide the occiput around the symphysis pubis.

Compound Presentation[13,14]

Signs and Symptoms

A. History of rupture of membranes
B. Complaint of something in vaginal vault
C. Protrusion of an extremity
D. Abdominal pain depending on the presence of contractions

Focused Assessment

A. Digital examination to evaluate for presenting part and presence of umbilical cord
B. Pulsation of umbilical cord
C. Leopold's maneuver to determine fetal position

Diagnostic Testing

A. *Laboratory studies:* Labs obtained for emergent delivery at the individual institution
B. *Imaging:* Ultrasound for purpose of identifying fetal heart activity and fetal positioning
C. Doppler for fetal heart rate evaluation

Medical Decision-Making, Differential Diagnoses, and Treatment

A. Emergent cesarean section for fetus with heart activity
   1. Emergent patient positioning, IV establishment and additional operating room (OR) preparation, transport to the OR
   2. Patient should be placed in knee chest position to aid in decompressing the cord at impingement site from fetus.
   3. Clinician should perform digital vaginal exam to aid in holding presenting part off cord to stop compression.
B. Preparation for delivery of fetal demise (see Fetal Demise)

Fetal Demise[43]

Signs and Symptoms

A. Absence of fetal movement at home
B. Absence of heart tones on arrival to the hospital
C. Trauma to mother as to make diagnosis obvious on visual inspection of the mother

Focused Assessment

A. Examination centered on definitive confirmation of fetal demise
B. Asses for any maternal emergent diagnosis that may or may not have played a role in the demise of the fetus.

Diagnostic Testing

A. Laboratory studies (as indicated)
   1. CBC
   2. MP
   3. Coagulation panel
   4. Liver functions studies
   5. UA
   6. Pathology testing as indicated based on delivery findings, trauma-associated studies, etc.
B. *Imaging:* US for purpose of identifying fetal heart activity
C. Doppler for fetal heart rate evaluation

Medical Decision-Making, Differential Diagnoses, and Treatment

A. Evaluate and anticipate severity of the grief response.
B. Disposition of patient needs to include both medical follow-up and emotional support. Include information on fetal loss support groups in the region.

Hyperemesis Gravidarum[2]

Diagnosis: Intractable Vomiting Resulting in Dehydration, Weight Loss, and Electrolyte Disturbances

A. Signs and symptoms
   1. Nausea and vomiting
   2. Hypotension
   3. Tachycardia
   4. Dry skin and mucosa
   5. Weakness and/or fatigue
   6. Absence of abdominal pain
   7. Symptoms consistent with hypokalemia
B. Focused assessment
   1. Evaluation of electrolyte disturbances
   2. Additional findings on physical examination not seen with diagnosis, to include abdominal pain, workup needs to focus on another diagnosis

Diagnostic Testing

A. Laboratory studies (as indicated):
   1. CBC
   2. MP (including blood urea nitrogen [BUN]/ creatinine)
   3. UA
B. Any studies needed to evaluate and/or rule out another diagnosis

Medical Decision-Making, Differential Diagnoses, and Treatment

A. Treat dehydration to resolve ketonuria (seen early in starvation). IV 5% dextrose in normal saline (D5NS) or 5% dextrose in lactated Ringer's (D5LR) is given till ketonuria has resolved.
B. NPO until nausea and vomiting are resolved
C. Antiemetics for symptoms. Typically, ondansetron or promethazine are used, both are equally effective.[44]
D. Patient is safe for discharge home when tolerating oral intake. Prescription needed for an antiemetic that the patient can tolerate at home.

Postpartum Hemorrhage[45]

Signs and Symptoms

A. Ongoing vaginal bleeding or recurrence of vaginal bleeding
B. Hypotension
C. Tachycardia
D. Uterine atony
E. Incomplete placenta on delivery
F. Physical injuries associated with delivery
  1. Focused assessment
G. *Causes of the following:* Uterine atony, vaginal lacerations, perineal lacerations, retained placenta, placental fragments not delivered

Diagnostic Testing

A. Laboratory studies (as indicated):
  1. CBC
  2. MP
  3. Coagulation panel
  4. Blood type and cross matching
B. Imaging: ultrasound to identify any retained placental fragments

Medical Decision-Making, Differential Diagnoses, and Treatment

A. Uterine message to stimulate contraction of the uterus
B. Oxytocin, 10 to 40 to 1,000 mL bag of lactated Ringer's solution (LR) and run at 150 mL/hour, no IV access, may be IM given[13]
C. Methylergonovine, IM (do not give IV)[13]
D. Emergent hysterectomy
E. Administer 1g of TXA IV

Preeclampsia and Eclampsia[46,47]

A. Diagnosis made by having systolic blood pressure (SBP) ≥140 and diastolic blood pressure (DBP) ≥90 with proteinuria or without proteinuria but with at least one sign or symptom of significant end-organ dysfunction.[48]

Signs and Symptoms

A. Headache
B. Vision changes: spots (scotamata), flashing lights (photopsia), blurred vision
C. Lower extremity edema
D. Hand and face swelling
E. Hyperreflexia
F. Seizure activity
G. Shortness of breath
H. Decreased urinary output
I. Proteinuria
J. Hypertension (HTN), anything above 140/90[44]

Focused Assessment

A. Central nervous system (CNS) hyperactivity to include reflexes
B. Fetal lung development in preparation for early delivery
C. Leopold's maneuver for fetal positioning

Diagnostic Testing

A. Laboratory studies (standard)
  1. CBC
  2. MP
  3. Magnesium level
  4. UA
  5. Liver function studies
  6. Fetal lung development testing (see vaginal bleeding >20 weeks)
B. *Laboratory studies (to consider):* Based on patient's complications
C. *Imaging:* US if fetal position identification is needed

Medical Decision-Making, Differential Diagnoses, and Treatment

A. Definitive treatment is delivery.
  1. Steroid therapy for fetal maturity (see preterm labor)
  2. Treatment of hypertension
  3. *Hydralazine:* Initial dosing IV, repeat dosing IV every 20 minutes until DBP to 90 or total of recommended medication. Drug may also be titrated in an infusion format.[48]
  4. *Labetalol:* May also be given in infusion format (not for use in asthmatic patients)[48]
B. CNS depressant for decreasing seizure threshold and hypertension
  1. *Magnesium sulfate:* In recommended loading dose over 30 minutes then continuous infusion. Therapeutic levels should be monitored and based upon evidence-based recommendations.[48]
C. *Postpartum presentation of preeclampsia/eclampsia:* The critical time period for presentation of symptoms is 5 days to 1 week postpartum.[49,50] Admission and treatment with magnesium sulfate for patients with severe hypertension or if the hypertension is new but mild with any headache or visual changes.[51]

Preeclampsia With Severe Features[47]

A. Diagnosis is made by having SBP ≥160 and DBP ≥110 with proteinuria or SBP ≥140 and DBP ≥90 with at least one sign or symptom of significant end-organ dysfunction.[52]

Signs and Symptoms

A. Those included in traditional preeclampsia/eclampsia
B. Altered mental status (AMS)
C. Chest pain
D. Renal insufficiency with serum creatinine >1.1
E. Pulmonary edema
F. Platelets <100,000/microliter
G. Severe right upper quadrant (RUQ) pain not responding to medication and not associated with another diagnosis and/or serum transaminase levels 2x the high end of normal limits
H. Focused assessment (see above)

Diagnostic Testing

A. *Laboratory studies (standard):* See above.
B. Laboratory studies (to consider)

1. *Coagulation panel:* Patients with complications
2. *Troponin:* It has been found in several clinical studies that troponin will elevate in preeclampsia. Only initial studies have been performed and ongoing investigation is needed.[53]

C. *Imaging:* See above.

Medical Decision-Making, Differential Diagnoses, and Treatment

A. See above.
B. Additional treatment based on patient's complications

Prolapsed Cord[13,14]

Signs and Symptoms

A. History of rupture of membranes
B. Complaint of something in vaginal vault
C. Protrusion of the cord from the vaginal vault
D. Abdominal pain depending on the presence of contractions

Focused Assessment

A. Digital exam to evaluate for cord in vault if not visible
B. Pulsation of umbilical cord
C. Leopold's maneuver to determine fetal position

Diagnostic Testing

A. *Laboratory studies:* Labs obtained for emergent delivery at the individual institution
B. *Imaging:* Ultrasound for purpose of identifying fetal heart activity
C. Doppler for fetal heart rate evaluation

Medical Decision-Making, Differential Diagnoses, and Treatment

A. Emergent cesarean section for fetus with heart activity
   1. Emergent patient positioning, IV establishment and additional operating room (OR) preparation, transport to the OR
   2. Patient should be placed in knee chest position to aid in decompressing the cord at impingement site from fetus.
   3. Clinician should perform digital vaginal exam to aid in holding presenting part off cord to stop compression.

B. Preparation for delivery of fetal demise (see Fetal Demise)

RASH DEVELOPMENT OR EXPOSURE IN PREGNANCY

Herpes Simplex Virus[23,54]

Diagnosis Information and Exposure Concerns

A. The genital rash seen in herpes simplex virus (HSV) involves 2 mm ulcers that are pruritic and can be extremely painful. Patients may also have fever, dysuria, and lymphadenopathy in the inguinal region.

B. There are three types of the disease
   1. *Primary:* No antibodies found in the serum, first outbreak of the genital rash
   2. *Nonprimary:* Positive antibodies found in the serum, first genital outbreak
   3. *Recurrent:* Positive antibodies, prior genital rash outbreaks

C. While diagnosis is easily made with history and examination, confirmation needs to occur with laboratory testing. In pregnancy, the testing will be based on the presentation and the history of the disease. Specific testing varies with the institution to confirm the diagnosis within each type.

D. All pregnant patients with no prior history of the diagnosis need to have a vesicle serologically tested (polymerase chain reaction [PCR] or culture) to make definitive diagnosis.

E. Fetal transmission often occurs during delivery and is referred to as vertical transmission. The fetus gets exposed to sloughing viral cells in the birth canal. Highest transmission rates are with a primary genital herpes infection.[55]

Management

A. Acyclovir × 7 to 10 days. Treatment may be extended if the lesions are still present.[55]

B. *Delivery options:* Patients with a history of genital herpes who have active lesions or prodromal symptoms should be offered cesarean section per the Centers for Disease Control and Prevention (CDC) and American College of Obstetricians and Gynecologists (ACOG) recommendations, once in labor, or if they have had rupture of membranes.[30,56]

Pruritic Urticarial Papules and Plaques of Pregnancy

Diagnosis Information and Signs and Symptoms

A. *Rash location:* Trunk, breasts, and thighs along striae
B. Itching is involved.
C. Typically seen in late in the last trimester. Usually more prominent in first pregnancies
D. One theory for the development of the problem is related to the maternal immune system response to fetal antigens in the bloodstream.[57]
E. Another theory to the problem is associated with triggering inflammatory changes from dermal antigens. Previous thought on the problem centered around hormone changes in pregnancy, but that has not been proven.[57]

Management

A. Topical use of high-dose corticosteroid topical preparations
B. Oral steroids in short treatment course are an option for severe problems.[57]

Syphilis[26,58]

Diagnosis Information and Exposure Concerns

A. Two stages of the disease process are identified with the presence of a rash.

1. Primary syphilis stage includes a papule painless-type rash that the ulcerates, converting to the classic chancre.
2. Secondary syphilis stage includes a maculopapular-type rash that is classically seen on the mucous membranes, palms of hands, and soles of feet.

Management

A. Only penicillin will eradicate the infection. Usually, treatment is provided on an outpatient basis. Some clinicians will administer the initial dose of penicillin in labor and delivery department to permit fetal monitoring for 24 hours.[58] A reaction to penicillin called Jarisch–Herxheimer can result in preterm labor. See chapter 22.

B. Penicillin G benzathine 2.4 million units given IM (intramuscularly) × 1 dose is the normal practice of treatment for primary, secondary, or early latent disease. Pharmacokinetic studies of pregnant women and penicillin levels have questioned the eradication of the disease and thus a second dose 1 week later is seen in some practices.[58]

C. No other antibiotic will kill syphilis, as a result, those patients with penicillin allergies undergo desensitization in order to receive the medication.[58]

Varicella Zoster, Chickenpox, and Shingles

Diagnosis Information and Exposure Concerns

A. Incidence of varicella (chickenpox) disease is unchanged by pregnancy; however, severity of disease seems to be greater.

B. Standard incubation period is 10 to 21 days after exposure for pregnant patients as well.

C. The concerning complication with exposure to varicella zoster in pregnancy has to do with development of herpes zoster in infancy, neonatal varicella, and the fetal development of congenital varicella syndrome, which results in neurologic, limb, and ocular abnormalities among other problems.[59]

D. Exposure

1. Person-to-person transmission of varicella (chickenpox) is up to 90% in unvaccinated people who are exposed in close contact situations.[59]
2. Acquiring of varicella (chickenpox) from zoster (shingles) exposure is possible but in susceptible people and the transmission rate is low. Direct, close exposure to the lesion fluid is required.[59]

E. Fetal transfer of infection

1. *Varicella (chickenpox):* Perinatal infection of the fetus is from transplacental exposure. Immediate postnatal infection can be from traditional droplet exposure or direct contact with active disease.
2. *Zoster (shingles):* Rare transmission to the fetus. This may be a result of two factors, the first being the serum viral load being much lower with zoster versus varicella. The second factor is the presence of maternal antibodies to varicella as a result of previous vaccination or disease.[60]
3. If maternal development of varicella (chickenpox) is near the time of delivery or immediately after, can result in neonatal varicella.

F. Secondary transmission is a very rare development of infection from exposure to someone who recently received the varicella vaccine within the last 10 to 21 days. The vaccinated person may also have developed the disease from the vaccine.[59]

Management

A. *Treatment of varicella (chickenpox):* Acyclovir PO 5x a day for 7 days

1. Secondary transmission treatment is the same.
2. Treatment needs to start within 24 hours for best effectiveness.[59]

B. *Treatment of zoster (shingles):* Acyclovir PO 5x a day for 7 days

1. When to treat varies in the literature. One school of thought is to start treatment at the first onset of lesions. The other treatment idea is to only treat if the patient has developed over 50 lesions and/or has in the presence of acute neuritis.[54,59]

C. Acyclovir is transmitted through breast milk and thus maternal benefits versus risk to the newborn should be evaluated before treatment.[61]

SPECIAL SITUATIONS AND CONSIDERATIONS

Burns

A. The Parkland Formula is readily used around the world for fluid replacement: %TBSA (total body surface area) burn × weight in kilograms (kg) in the first 24 hours, half in the first 8 hours, and the second half in the last 16 hours.[62] The formula is not as effective with pediatric patients and pregnant patients because of the increased body surface area (BSA). Pregnant patients also have an increase in circulating blood volume 50% more than nonpregnant patients. These factors need to be considered in the fluid resuscitation of the pregnant patient. There is no direct formula cited in the literature specific to pregnant patients.[63] A case study review by LD Pacheco involving a 34-week pregnant patient, identified IV fluid (IVF) resuscitation volumes being double what the Parkland Burn Formula recommended to treat the patient's hypovolemic state during the first 24 hours.[64]

B. A mortality rate of 100% has previously been identified once burns reach 40% with the pregnant population.[65] A recent study, out of India, noted 100% mortality rate is now seen with 70% BSA burn or greater.[66] BSA burn of 50% to 70% has an 83% mortality, and BSA burn of 30% to 40% is down to 44% mortality.

C. There may be an upside to being pregnant at the time of a significant burn injury. A team out of Morocco has used amniochorionic membrane to cover burned areas. Multiple types of growth factors and cytokines are found in human amniochorionic membranes, aiding in the healing process and reducing the bacterial count. Reduced scarring and inflammation has also been noted.[67]

Clotting Emergencies[68-70]

A. The risk of clotting emergencies is five times higher in pregnancy.[71] The most important risk of thrombosis is from stasis of blood, the triad of the problem noted below. Proteins that inhibit coagulation during the clotting cascade are decreased in numbers during pregnancy. The inability to inhibit clotting with the proteins is known as thrombophilias. There are many proteins involved, but for ED purposes we will not go into detail. About 30% to 60% of pregnant women with deep vein thrombosis (DVT) have a silent pulmonary embolism (PE); 70% of those with a PE also have a DVT.

B. Pulmonary Emboli Rule-out Criteria (PERC) and Well's Criteria in pregnancy: These latest evaluation tools are not accurate because of normal physiologic changes in pregnancy. The Wells Criteria has not been validated in the pregnant population, which was excluded in the initial validation study and in subsequent studies to date.[72] There has been discussion in the past of PERC modification to account for a pregnant patient's physiologic changes. As yet, no research has been seen on validation of such a tool.

C. *D-dimer usage in pregnancy:* The d-dimer test is found to not be accurate due to known elevation in the result from emergent pregnant conditions along with progressive elevation with pregnancy length and the number of babies being carried.[73,74]

D. *Virchow Triad:* Changes in pregnancy, increasing risk of blood stasis in the lower extremities

1. Compression of iliac veins by the uterus
2. Vein dilation from hormone changes
3. Immobilization

E. Risk factors seen in an ED presentation

1. Over 35 years old
2. Dehydration
3. Immobilization for extended periods of time with travel
4. Obesity
5. Sickle cell disease
6. Smoking
7. Prior history of thromboembolic
8. Infection or inflammation
9. Thrombophilia, accounting for 50% of all events in pregnancy[75]

F. Detailed signs and symptoms of DVT and PE are noted in Chapter 17.

G. DVT evaluation is performed by lower extremity venous US. If negative but evaluation suspicious for diagnosis, repeat of study should take place in 3 to 5 days. Running a d-dimer level can be done with reassurance that if it is not elevated, the patient does not have a DVT. If elevated, a repeat US is once again recommended.

H. *PE evaluation:* There are several different thoughts on the type of imaging to evaluate for PE. Radiation exposure is at the forefront of the argument. CT imaging remains a risk versus benefit decision. Ventilation–perfusion (VQ) scan risk centers around the ionized contrast dose. It has been determined that there are no reports of thyroid dysfunction in the fetus with a single-dose exposure.[76] Below is an easy method of evaluating while keeping radiation exposure in mind. If a patient has symptoms suspicious for a PE diagnosis, evaluate as follows:

1. *Laboratory studies:* CBC, chem, coagulation studies, fibrinogen, and fibrinogen split products may also be considered.
2. Lower extremity venous Doppler, given that this is most often the cause of the PE. If positive, patient can be treated for the problem, avoiding radiation exposure during imaging.
3. If ultrasound is negative, proceed to chest x-ray (CXR) baseline imaging. If the imaging is abnormal, CT angiogram (CTA) scan should be used as the diagnostic imaging of choice to distinguish differential diagnosis from PE. If the CXR is negative, a VQ scan be done for minimal radiation exposure.
4. If there is a high degree of concern for PE and the CTA results are negative, it is recommended to proceed to VQ scan. Recent studies have called into question the accuracy of CTA in diagnosing PE in pregnant patients. Because of normal physiologic changes in pregnancy, poor timing of the injection of contrast is responsible for up to 35% of nondiagnostic CTAs. Dilutional effects, increased vena cava pressure, and chest cavity negative pressure elevation are also cited for poor imaging and artifact.[77,78]

I. Treatment: Pharmacologic therapies should be based on evidenced-based recommendations from recognized sources, for example, the CDC (Centers for Disease Control and Prevention), or guidelines specific to the environment where the clinician practices.

1. *Low molecular weight heparin (LMWH):* Dosing of enoxaparin is 1 mg/kg subq q12h. This is the DOC in pregnant patients.
2. *Unfractionated heparin (UFH):* The dosing is 10,000 units or greater subq q12h, with dosing being titrated to a PTT (partial thromboplastin time) therapeutic range of 1.5 to 2.5 drawn 6 hours after dose administration.
3. *Tissue plasma activator (T-PA):* Used for massive pulmonary emboli. The drug does not cross the placental barrier and is thus safe in pregnancy.[79,80] The agent should be used when risk of mortality is high. Postpartum hemorrhage and abruptio placenta are of concern when T-PA is used close to delivery.
4. Filter placement and clot retrieval should be left up to the specialist. Maternal risk for clot retrieval is minimal. Stillbirths range from 20% to 40%.[80]

Drug Therapy in Pregnant and Lactating Patients[81]

Table 49.3 summarizes common drug therapies in pregnant and lactating patients according to the established Food and Drug Administration (FDA) pregnancy and lactation classification categories:

A. *Category A:* Adequate and well-controlled studies have failed to demonstrate a risk to the fetus in the first trimester of pregnancy (and there is no evidence of risk in later trimesters).

B. *Category B:* Animal reproduction studies have failed to demonstrate risk to the fetus, and there are no adequate and well-controlled studies in pregnant women.

C. *Category C:* Animal reproduction studies have shown an adverse effect on the fetus and there are no adequate and well-controlled studies in humans, but potential benefits may warrant use of the drug in pregnant women despite potential risks.

D. *Category D:* There is positive evidence of human fetal risk based on adverse reaction data from investigational or marketing experience or studies in humans, but potential benefits may warrant use of the drug in pregnant women despite potential risks.

E. *Category X:* Studies in animals or humans have demonstrated fetal abnormalities and/or there is positive evidence of human fetal risk based on adverse reaction data from investigational or marketing experience, and the risk involves in the use of the drug in pregnant women clearly outweigh potential benefits.

2015 Revision to Food and Drug Administration Drug Categorizations

A new categorization system was adopted by the FDA in 2015. The new system encompasses a large amount of data surrounding the medication and its effects, requiring significant reading and interpretation of the information. Since it remains not widely used at this time, the previous classification system has been used for clinician familiarity in Table 49.3. A recent research study, however, has identified the new system as a possible detriment to the use of drugs within certain former drug classes, when using the new system.[82] The complexity of the new system is believed by some to possibly lead to varying interpretations as to when to use a medication. The lettering system, however, was believed by some to be overly simplistic.[83] New sections included in the revised drug categorization include:

A. Pregnancy
  1. Pregnancy exposure registry
    a. If the drug has registry information, it must be listed on the product.
  2. Risk summary
    a. Risk statement based on human data
      i. Include clinical trials, exposure registry data, large epidemiologic studies
      ii. Include incidence, effect of dose, effect of exposure duration, effects of gestational timing exposure
    b. Risk statement based on animal data
      i. Include species effects (number and type)
      ii. Timing of exposure

TABLE 49.3 DRUG THERAPY IN PREGNANCY AND LACTATION

DRUG/DRUG CLASS (NAME BRAND/EXAMPLE)	PREGNANCY AND LACTATION CLASSIFICATION	BARRIER CROSSING	CONSIDERATIONS/EXCLUSIONS TO USE
Allergic Reaction			
Diphenhydramine/Benadryl	B/X	PP BMS	Avoid near delivery. Do not use in lactation r/t infant antihistamine EXPOSURE (PG 435). DOC in pregnancy if mother needs antihistamine treatment
Methylprednisolone, e.g., Solumedrol	C/X	PP BMS	First trimester: cleft palate. Lactation: suppress growth
Dexamethasone/Decadron	2cd, 3rd tri / L	PP BMS	First trimester: cleft palate, and other osteogenesis problems. Lactation: suppress growth.
Analgesics			
Acetaminophen/Tylenol	B/L	PP BM	No identifiable complications. Breast milk levels are very small, noted to be less than infant doing. Toxic levels in overdosing will affect fetus.
Aspirin	D/L*	PP BMS	Low dose ASA for use with preeclampsia has shown no increased risk to the fetus.[95]* High-dose ASA in lactation for risk of rash, platelet abnormalities, and bleeding. Risk of Reye's syndrome in breastfeeding infants is unknown.

(continued)

TABLE 49.3 DRUG THERAPY IN PREGNANCY AND LACTATION (*CONTINUED*)

DRUG/DRUG CLASS (NAME BRAND/EXAMPLE)	PREGNANCY AND LACTATION CLASSIFICATION	BARRIER CROSSING	CONSIDERATIONS/EXCLUSIONS TO USE
NSAIDs/Ibuprofen, Advil, Aleve	C*/L*/P*	PP BMS	Aleve is not rated. P* = Do not use any in third trimester. First-trimester use increases malformation risk and miscarriage. L* = low levels of meds found in breast milk are lower than dosing used for infant care.
Fentanyl	C/D/L*	PP BMS	L* = congenital issues, respiratory depression and withdrawals. Transient neonatal muscular rigidity when used in labor. Small amounts found in breast milk. Abstain from breastfeeding for 24–72 hours after dose pending route of administration.
Morphine	C/L*	PP BMS	Respiratory depression and withdrawals postdelivery. No increased risk of major or minor defects have yet to be seen. L* = levels in infant remain detectable 4+ days after last maternal dose when maternal levels are not detected.
Hydromorphone/Dilaudid	C/L*	PP BMS	Respiratory depression and withdrawals postdelivery. No increased risk of major or minor defects have yet to be seen. L8 = risk of apneic spells that resolve with narcan.
Hydrocodone	C/L*	PP BMS	Respiratory depression and withdrawals postdelivery. No increased risk of major or minor defects have yet to be seen. L* = hypersomnolence.
Codeine	C/L*	PP BMS	Respiratory depression and withdrawals post -delivery. No increased risk of major or minor defects have yet to be seen. L* = concern for apneic episodes
Antibiotics			
Antimicrobials (e.g., nitrofurantoin, macrodantin)	B/L	Unknown BM	No known placenta permeability, or if so not effected. Breast milk levels extremely low.
Aminoglycosides (e.g., tobramycin, streptomycin, neomycin)	D/L	PP BM	Nephrotoxicity, ototoxicity. Breast milk levels extremely low.
Cephalosporins (e.g., cefazolin, cefdinir, cefepime, ceftriaxone, cephalexin)	B/L	PP BM	Lower blood level concentrations in fetus. Breast milk levels too low to result in side effects.
Fluoroquinolones (e.g., ciprofloxacin, moxifloxacin, levofloxacin)	C/L	PP BM	Potential carcinogenic effects. Low levels of drug in breast milk.
Glycopeptides (e.g., vancomycin)	B-C/Unknown	PP BM	Listed B in oral form. Ototoxicity and nephrotoxicity possible, thus monitoring is recommended. Conflicting data in the literature, infant affects unknown.
Lincosamides (e.g., clindamycin)	B/L*	PP BM	Avoid vaginal forms in pregnancy given high absorption rate. L* = lactation for gastrointestinal flora affects in neonates. Unlikely vaginal cream form will result in same outcomes.
Macrolides (e.g., erythromycin, azithromycin, clarithromycin)	B-B-C/L	PP BM	Clarithromycin is class C. Animal studies have identified cardiovascular changes, spontaneous abortions, cleft palate, and delayed growth of fetus. Breast milk levels very small, questionable gastrointestinal flora changes
Nitroimidazoles (e.g., metronidazole)	B*/L/P*	PP BM	P* = Contraindicated in the first trimester. Questionable increase in preterm births. Potential dose to neonates is lower than receiving independent treatment.

(*continued*)

TABLE 49.3 DRUG THERAPY IN PREGNANCY AND LACTATION (*CONTINUED*)

DRUG/DRUG CLASS (NAME BRAND/EXAMPLE)	PREGNANCY AND LACTATION CLASSIFICATION	BARRIER CROSSING	CONSIDERATIONS/EXCLUSIONS TO USE
Penicillins (e.g., penicillin VK, penicillin G, amoxicillin, ampicillin, dicloxicillin, imipenem)*	B-C*/L	PP BM	P* = Imipenem is class C. Animal studies noted increased abortion of pregnancy. Breast milk levels are in small amounts. Questionable gut flora effects not fully evaluated.
Penicillin combinations (e.g., pcn/clavubinate [Augmentin])	B/L	PP BM	While there are no teterogenic effects in animal studies, there is a questionable increased risk in neonates of necrotizing enterocolitis if used if premature rupture of membranes occurs.
Sulfonamides (e.g., TMP/SMX [Bactrim])	C/L*	PP BM	While TMP is a class B drug it is not used in isolated form, SMX portion of combination is sulfa based and is class C. L* = If the infant is premature, bilirubin levels can be affected.
Tetracyclines (e.g., doxycycline, minocycline)	D/X	PP BM	Dental discoloration, there have been some studies suggesting no significant dental discoloration with the use of doxycycline. Drug is still listed as class D; dental discoloration remains a concern in breastfeeding as well.
Antivirals			
Acyclovir	B	PP BM	Suppressive therapy results in decreased C-section deliveries. No adverse reactions seen with breastfeeding.
Valtrex	B	PP BM	No good controlled studies in humans. No adverse reactions seen with breastfeeding.
Antifungals			
Nystatin	A/C /L	PP -	Most formulations of nystatin are classified as category C. Nystatin vaginal inserts are classified as category A. May be used on the breast during breastfeeding (allow 10 minutes after application)
Fluconazole/Diflucan	C/D/L	PP BM	Low dose (150 mg) for vaginal candidiasis is still class C. High doses have now been listed as class D; rare congenital defects have now been associated with use. Used in infants as well.
Anticoagulants			
Warfarin/Coumadin	X/not classified	PP BM	Spontaneous abortion, stillbirth, hemorrhage.[89] Research suggests minimal risk to breast-fed infants.
Heparin	C/Unknown	PP ?	DOC in pregnancy but extended use may lead to osteopenia in the mother. Has not been studied in lactation.
Low molecular weight heparin/Lovenox	B/Unknown	PP ?	Enoxaprin has been linked to death and valvular clotting with mechanical heart valve patients. Excretion in breast milk unknown/believed to be low if any. Does not cross the placental barrier. Not linked to teterogenic effects in fetus.
TPA	C/not discussed	No PP ?	Despite no placenta permeability, drug listed as C because of increasing bleeding in other pregnancy complications. Nonstatistical increase in cranial bleeding (symptomatic) with pregnant and immediate postpartum patients.[17,85]
Plavix	Not rated/?	PP BM	Animal studies have not shown any harm. Stop usage 5–7 days prior to delivery. Infant effects in lactation are unknown.
Antiemetics[84]			
Chlorpromazine/Thorazine	C/L*	PP BM	Routes: po, iv, pr. Very low breast milk levels; L* = Monitor for drowsiness.

(*continued*)

TABLE 49.3 DRUG THERAPY IN PREGNANCY AND LACTATION (*CONTINUED*)

DRUG/DRUG CLASS (NAME BRAND/EXAMPLE)	PREGNANCY AND LACTATION CLASSIFICATION	BARRIER CROSSING	CONSIDERATIONS/EXCLUSIONS TO USE
Hydroxyzine/Atarax	C/L*	PP BM	Routes: po. Animal studies have shown cleft palate risk. Decreased milk supply potential. Prolonged use may affect infant.
Meclizine	B/L*	Unknown SBM	Large doses can affect milk supply and may affect infant.
Metoclopramide/Reglan	B/L*	PP BM	Routes: po, iv. Side effects include fatigue, irritability, and depression. Has been used to increase breast milk production.
Ondansetron/Zofran	B/L*	Unknown BM	Routes: po, iv. Does enter breast milk but effects on infant is unknown.
Promethazine/Phenergan	C/L*	PP BM	Routes: po, iv, pr. Possible increased risk of miscarriage in first trimester. Prolonged use monitor infant for drowsiness.
Prochlorperazine/Compazine	Not assigned/X	Unknown SBM	Routes: po, iv, pr. Animal studies identified sperm aberrations. Withdrawal symptoms in neonates. No clear recommendation for use in lactation.
Trimethobenzamide/Tigan	C/no data	SPP SBM	Increased stillbirths in animals. No human trials. Molecular size suggests ability to cross placenta and be excreted in breast milk.
Antihypertensives			
ACE Inhibitor (e.g., Lisinopril)	D/Unknown	PP ?	Renal damage in fetus. Pulmonary hypoplasia in fetus, skull anomalies, growth retardation in second and third trimester. No breastfeeding data.
Angiotensin II Receptor Blockers (ARB) (e.g., valsartan, losartan)	D/Unknown	PP ?	Spontaneous abortion, newborn renal dysfunction. No breastfeeding data
Beta Blockers (e.g., Metoprolol, Labetalol, Propranolol)	C/L	SPP BM	Some questions concerning placenta perfusion, but no definitive data in the US. Breast mild levels vary between drugs. Propranolol is the DOC for breastfeeding, lowest level of drug in breast milk.
Ca Channel Blocker (e.g., Nifedipine, Nitroprusside, Verapamil)	B-C*/L	PP BM	P* = Nitroprusside converts to cyanide in the human body and should not be used in pregnancy/lactation. Teratogenic effects in animals. Rest of drug class is commonly used during pregnancy and lactation to treat hypertension, arrhythmia, and preeclampsia. Excreted in breast milk in low levels/minimal risk identified.
Diabetes			
Glucophage/Metformin	B/L	PP* BM	Placental perfusion is by active transport. New research shows drug may be used after the first trimester with insulin. Very low breast mild transmission. Now used for Type 2 diabetes mellitus control in breastfeeding mothers[96,97]
Insulin—short acting (e.g., regular, aspart, lispro)	B/L	PP BM	Breast-fed infants may have decreased risk in development of Type 1 diabetes mellitus.[98]
Insulin—long-acting (e.g., NPH, detemir, glargine)	C (NPH no class listing) /L	PP BM	NPH - DOC. NPH has no class listing. Detemir and glargine are used for better postprandial control.
Gastroesophageal Reflux			
Calcium Carbonate (e.g., Tums)	C*/Unknown	PP	P* = Animal study complications. Regarded safe in humans.
Aluminum and Magnesium Hydroxide (e.g., MAALOX)	B/L	PP BM	Because of the known tocolytic action these are avoided by some clinicians. Low breast milk levels.
Simethicone (e.g., Mylanta)	C/Unknown	Not PP	Complications in animals. Does not cross placenta thus safe in humans.

(*continued*)

TABLE 49.3 DRUG THERAPY IN PREGNANCY AND LACTATION (*CONTINUED*)

DRUG/DRUG CLASS (NAME BRAND/EXAMPLE)	PREGNANCY AND LACTATION CLASSIFICATION	BARRIER CROSSING	CONSIDERATIONS/EXCLUSIONS TO USE
H2 Blockers (e.g., Tagamet, Zantac)	B-C	PP	Insufficient data on the first trimester usage. Avoid nizatidine (Axid) due to spontaneous abortion risk and increased risk of fetal deaths found in animals.
Proton Pump Inhibitors (e.g., protonix, prevacid, Prilosec)	B-C*/L	PP BM	Prilosec is class C due to fetal reabsorption in animals. Small levels in breast milk, in high doses gynecomastia may be seen.
Pulmonary Disease			
Albuterol	C/?	PP ?	Effects in animal studies isolated to mice. Risk versus benefit decision and avoidance of excessive use should be considered. No isolated data but other similar medications have low levels in breast milk. There is low bioavailability in serum levels with inhaled bronchodilators.
Ipratropium bromide (Atrovent)	B/?	SPP No info	Animal studies for both inhaled and oral show no identifiable fetal defects. Low maternal blood levels in inhaled form, so presumed breast milk levels to be low.
Levalbuterol (Xopenex)	C/no data	PP No data	Teratogenic effects to include cleft palate in some animal studies.
Magnesium	D/L	PPBM	Positive fetal risk in humans.
Terbutaline	B-C/L	PP BM	Some data says to avoid in first trimester. Drug used as tocolytic. Very little excretion into breast milk.
Resuscitation Medications			
Adenosine	C/not discussed	PP ?	Half life of medication prevents medication from accumulating
Amiodarone	D/not discussed	PP ?	Possible congenital hypothyroidism in newborn. Transient bradycardia and prolonged QT in newborn
Atropine	C/not discussed	PP ?	No fetal abnormalities. Possible fetal tachycardia.
Dobutamine	C/not discussed	PP ?	No fetal effects in animal trials. No human studies.
Dopamine	C/not discussed	PP ?	No embryotoxic or teratogenic effects in animals. Few studies in humans.
Epinephrine	C/not discussed	PP ?	No definitive human teratogenic effects. May decrease uterine blood flow.
Lidocaine	B/not discussed	PP ?	No risk to fetus has been identified.
Norepinephrine	C/not discussed	PP	No studies available.
Sodium Bicarbonate	C/not discussed	PP ?	No studies available.
Contrast Agents			
Iodine or Gadolinium agents	B/X	PP BM	Very small amount will cross placenta. Lactation: small amount secreted. Dumping breast milk for 24 hours after contrasted studies is recommended.[99]

A, FDA Pregnancy Category A; ASA, drug caution code; B, FDA Pregnancy Category B; BM, breast milk transfer; C, FDA Pregnancy Category C; D, FDA Pregnancy Category D; DOC, drug of choice; iv, intravenously; L, Lactation safe; P, pregnancy; PP, placenta permeability; po, orally; pr, rectally; SBM, suspected breast milk transfer; SPP, suspected placenta permeability; X, not lactation safe.

Permeability and transfer capability can be suspected due to many factors including molecular weight of the drug.

iii. Doses in terms of human equivalents
iv. Outcomes of pregnant animals and offspring
c. Risk statement based on pharmacology
3. Clinical considerations
a. Disease-associated material and/or embryo/fetal risk
b. Dose adjustments during pregnancy and the postpartum period
c. Material adverse reactions
d. Fetal/neonatal adverse reactions
e. Labor or delivery

B. Lactation considerations
C. Female and male reproduction potentials

Use of Drug Databases for Drug Selection in Pregnant Patients

Databases with or without smartphone applications are helpful in the selection of an appropriate drug in these special populations. LactMed, a database of medication effects in lactation, for example, can now be found throughout the literature cited as a reference. LactMed, specifically, was developed by the National Institutes of Health (NIH).

Poisonings[100]

A. Specialist consultation should always be included when poisoning is involved. The Poison Control Center has one number nationwide: 1-800-222-1222. Your phone call goes to the nearest call center associated with your area code and can be routed to the center nearest you as needed. The implementation of care and specialty considerations with pregnant patients can be guided by the group of specialists in the field of toxicology. Consultation with OB is needed as well. If your institution does not provide obstetric capability, make sure to follow toxicology guidelines, which may include transferring to a facility with obstetric care.

B. *Acetaminophen:* Crosses the placental barrier, which in toxic doses can also cause liver damage to the fetus. N-acetylcysteine (NAC) is used in the overdose of acetaminophen. The chemical has been deemed safe in pregnancy and also found to cross the placental barrier and may affect toxic metabolite levels in the fetus. The IV formulation is preferred over oral, therapeutic levels are noted to be 10 to 100 times greater.[101] The drug is most successful when begun within 16 hours of toxic ingestion.[102] There has been discussion that cesarean section delivery of near-term or term fetus for direct administration of NAC to the neonate may be more successful.[100]

C. *Salicylates:* Toxic levels in adults of 90 mg/dL or 60 mg/dL (chronic overdoses) are standard levels to warrant hemodialysis for treatment, with or without symptoms associated with toxic levels. It has been identified, however, that levels noted on the fetal side are much higher due to protein binding differences. As a result, a much lower maternal level of around 40 mg/dl should be considered for hemodialysis to preserve the fetus. Possible cesarean section may be considered for direct treatment of the fetus.[80]

D. *Iron:* There are no specific changes to treatment of iron overdose cases. Iron does not cross the placental barrier. See Chapter 47 for additional information.

E. *Snakebites (rattlesnake, copperheads, and cottonmouths):*[100] The adverse effects of using antivenom during pregnancy are unknown. Administration decisions involve a risk versus benefit decision. Snake venom results in bleeding problems in the victim. Pregnant patients will need to be monitored for additional sources of bleeding, including vaginal bleeding that may result in miscarriage. Fetal monitoring is recommended to evaluate for fetal bradycardia and uterine contractions that may develop as a result of bleeding.

F. Spider envenomation

1. Black widow spider envenomation signs and symptoms can be consistent with those of preeclampsia or an emergent abdominal problem. Good history-taking is essential to treat emergency appropriately. Symptom relief is the usual recommendation. Patient will need tetanus immunization updated, which is safe in pregnancy.
2. Brown recluse spider envenomation treatment involves symptomatic care of the local reaction. There is no change with the pregnant patient.
3. The neurotoxins of each spider are similar, and area treated with the same antivenom. There is disagreement throughout the literature, however, on the use of antivenom in the pregnant patient. Alpha-latrotoxin is not believed to cross the placental barrier given the size of the molecule.[103]

G. Scorpion envenomation

1. Only 30 of the 1,500 species of scorpions are considered dangerous to humans.[104] *Centruroides sculpturatus* is the only one of the 30 found in the Unites States. There is an antivenom for this species of scorpion.[105]
2. Knowledge about the treatment of pregnant patients with antivenom derives from studies on animal subjects.[102–106] Some antivenoms for scorpions, in other areas of the world can trigger abortions because of 5-hydroxytryptamine found in the formulas.[106] Anascorp, used in the United States, does not contain this compound. The Anascorp package insert lists it as pregnancy class C.[107] It is unknown if the antitoxin is found in breast milk.
3. Specific care in the United States is centered around symptomatic treatment of the adrenergic crises that develops. Care specific to pregnant patients involves choosing medications to combat the adrenergic changes. Because blood volumes in pregnant patient increase dramatically, choose medications that are easy to control so as to prevent hypotensive events.

Resuscitation[108–110]

A. Physiologic changes to consider

1. Respiratory system and oxygenation
2. Upper airway edema creates a Mallampait 4 intubation

a. Displacement of the abdominal contents from the gravid uterus results in a decrease in vital capacity and physiologic oxygen reserves.

b. Rapid onset of hypoxia related to above factors

c. There is a 20% increase in oxygenation consumption at term.

d. The fetus has a greater oxygenation saturation affinity that the mother at any partial pressure.

3. Circulatory changes

a. Gravid uterus will compress the vena cava, decreasing venous return.

b. Infradiaphramatic vessels also have a decrease in return, making IV sites in the femoral areas and lower extremities poor choices for medication administration.

c. Fetal circulation typically houses 25% of the circulating volume from the extensive vasculature.

d. Physiologic anemia

B. Aids for success

1. Best chance for fetal survival is maternal survival.

2. Respiratory system and oxygenation

a. Be prepared for backup plan when attempting endotracheal intubation. Have additional equipment ready, including alternative airway, bougie, and even surgical airway kit.

b. Place mother in sniffing position as seen with neonates using a towel under the shoulders to aid in proper positioning for best chance for intubation success.

c. Keep mother on a nasal cannula at 15 L throughout intubation process to aid in preventing hypoxia.

d. Initial vent settings are the same as a nonpregnant patient. Adjust based on blood gas results to avoid alkalosis, which can decrease uterine blood flow.

e. Normal $PaCO_2$ for a nonpregnant patient is 40 mmHg, which seen in a pregnant patient is suggestive of respiratory acidosis from inadequate ventilation. In pregnancy, the normal $PaCO_2$ is down around 30 mmHg.

3. Circulatory success

a. Keep patient rolled to the left side at the pelvis and lower lumbar area to displace the gravid uterus, entire back board tilted when spinal trauma may be involved.

b. Use upper extremities or central line sites above the heart for medication administration to ensure better circulation of the medication during resuscitation process.

c. Standard resuscitation dosages are used in pregnancy, there is no evidence to support changing the dose relative to the increase in blood volume.[110]

C. Perimortem cesarean section

1. This procedure is now referred to as a resuscitation hysterotomy, which shows the highest promise for success if begun by the fourth minute following maternal arrest. The goal is to have the fetus delivered by the fifth minute. Accordingly, this becomes an ER procedure, and in some countries an in-the-field procedure.[108,111] Some successful case studies have shown the procedure to improve chances of resuscitation of the mother.[112–114]

2. Ideal situation is to have the most experienced OB physician do the procedure. The experience of the current generation is in the horizontal approach, previous generations, the classic vertical as well. The type of approach used should be what the OB is most comfortable doing.[115]

3. Equipment[116,117]

a. *Minimal:* Scalpel, scissors, and gloves

b. *Optimal:* C-section or abdominal ex-lap kit, emergency thoracotomy kit can also be used. If no kit available scalpel, large scissors, hemostats, sterile gauze, suction, betadine, sterile attire.

4. Steps in a cesarean section below have been taken from references on how to perform the procedure from all over the world. The steps are simplified under the assumption that the clinician is not an OB surgeon and has never seen the procedure.[109,116–118]

a. *Onset of arrest:* Let team know the plan for fetal delivery and the start timer at 4 minutes. If Foley placement is possible, do it at this time to have the bladder decompressed. Prep abdomen—not an absolute—utilize betadine or chlorhexidine before the 4-minute mark.

b. Other team member will take over CPR and basic advanced cardiovascular life support (ACLS) protocol

c. Midline vertical incision from just below the xiphoid to the symphysis pubis using a scalpel down to the peritoneal through all the subcutaneous tissue; #10 blade is easiest

d. Punch hole with fingers through the peritoneal wall just below the umbilicus. Extend the opening either by pulling apart the tissue with hands or use scissors to cut it open along the midline.

e. Lift uterus out of the cavity for easy visualization—not absolutely necessary—assure bladder is pulled out of the way if not decompressed with a Foley.

f. Small vertical incision along uterine wall. Use fingers to hold up uterine wall and then use scissors to extend the incision without cutting fetus. Stop cutting before shiny tissue (hyper-translucent) near the base of the uterus is reached. If the placenta is in the way, cut through it.

g. Delivery of fetus: expect resuscitative efforts. Suction nose prior to mouth. Clamp cord in two places and cut cord between the two clamps.

h. *Delivery of placenta:* Do not pull cord too hard. Pack uterus and abdominal cavity.

i. Continue resuscitation of the mother.

j. If resuscitation is successful, it is best if an OB physician closes the uterus.

5. *Critical point:* Do not wait. Begin immediately thinking of the resuscitative hysterotomy at the onset of the code of the mother.

6. *Legal:* If the mother dies, perimortem cesarean section can be interpreted as a wrongful dissection (mutilation of a corpse). If the mother lives, it can be considered battery. The argument has always been

that the procedure is done to save a life.[115] There are now laws in many states protecting the performing physician from prosecution under the Good Samaritan Law. No physician in the United States has ever been prosecuted for performing the procedure. The emergent exception rule applies to operating without consent.[119] The legal issue for nurse practitioners is practicing outside your scope of practice. With the change in thought and renaming of the procedure to resuscitative hysterotomy, it may one day be considered to be part of the scope of ACLS.

D. Complications of resuscitation

1. Maternal

a. Increased problems associated with rib fractures because of location of organs and uterus late in pregnancy

b. Fetus

i. Central nervous system (CNS) toxicity from medications

ii. Hypoxia and acidemia from decreased placental perfusion

iii. Electrical shock can result in transient dysrhythmias.

E. Latest advances

1. Therapeutic hypothermia postresuscitation is found to be successful in maternal arrest as well.[120]

2. Fibrolytic therapy for pulmonary emboli in cardiac arrest can be used. Emergent cesarean section complications are possible.

Trauma[19,22]

A. Laboratory studies

1. CBC with differential

2. Blood type and cross match for a minimum of two units with Rh identification

3. Complete MP

4. Coagulation panel

5. Liver function studies

6. Fibrinogen and fibrinogen degradation products

7. Kleihauer–Betke

B. Imaging considerations

1. Ultrasound FAST scan (focused assessment for sonography in trauma) provides sensitivity and specificity to identify intraperitoneal fluid is similar for both pregnant and nonpregnant patients.[19,121]

2. Evaluation of the fetus is also done with this diagnostic tool.

3. CT imaging usage with trauma in pregnancy requires risk versus benefit analysis in decision-making. As expected, radiation exposure to the fetus is significantly increased with abdomen and abdominal/pelvis imaging because of direct exposure to the fetus. Use of CT imaging for evaluation of other portions of the anatomy exposes the fetus to significantly less radiation with use of shielding of the abdomen. The latest research on CT imaging with regard to head CT usage for identifying intracranial hemorrhage suggests that the dosing to the fetus is minimal given the distance away from the fetus.[122]

4. *Radiographic imaging:* Far less radiation exposure for the fetus. When not imaging pelvis or lumbar regions, screening of the fetus can be done to significantly affect the quantity of exposure.[123]

C. Alternative diagnostic studies

1. Open diagnostic peritoneal lavage is safe in pregnancy. Consider when ultrasound has not revealed injury and patient remains unstable.[19,124–126] This study will need to be performed by credentialed clinicians.

2. Retroperitoneal and uterine injury identification are the limitations to the study.

D. Packaging and transport[11]

1. *Early intubation:* See resuscitation section regarding changes.

2. *Aggressive fluid resuscitation:* See resuscitation section regarding changes.

3. *Backboard tilting:* See resuscitation section regarding changes.

E. Evaluation and treatment considerations related to normal pregnancy changes

1. The symphysis pubis becomes widened around the seventh month 4 to 8 mm beyond normal. The sacroiliac joint space is also affected.[19] These changes must be kept in mind when evaluating pelvic radiographs.

2. Ureteral compression from gravid uterus can result in the appearance of hydronephrosis on radiographic imaging.[127]

a. Additional information in resuscitation section

F. Safety considerations

1. *Seat belts:* Education in placement of waist strap below gravid abdomen across thighs and shoulder strap above gravid uterus

2. Do not advise patients to turn off airbag systems.

3. *Domestic violence:* Increased incidence in pregnancy. Early identification for patient safety (see Chapter 58).

G. *Radiation exposure in pregnancy:* The individual modalities are discussed as they pertain to the emergency being discussed for ease of use of text. It is important to note that the increased risk of severe mental retardation as a result of radiation exposure in a fetus is between 8 and 15 weeks' gestation.[128]

References

References for this chapter are online only and can be found at https://connect.springerpub.com/content/reference-book/978-0-8261-6091-5/part/part07/toc-part/ch49.

50. The Pediatric Patient

LAURA L. KUENSTING

Learning Objectives

- Identify genetic, anatomic, and physiologic differences in infants and children.
- Use growth and developmental achievements to guide interventions for infants and children.
- Differentiate the pathophysiology of various systems between infants, children, and adults.
- Select recommended interventions and treatments for medical conditions in infants and children.
- Formulate differential diagnoses for common pediatric medical conditions.

Care of the Child in the ED

The care provided to children in the ED should include the caregiver and family. Separating children from their caregiver or family may cause additional psychological and physiological stress in the stressful environment of the ED.

A fundamental understanding of growth and developmental stages is needed when caring for children in the ED. Communicating with them based on understanding cognitive and emotional development may enhance their cooperation (Table 50.1). Chronological age may

TABLE 50.1 COGNITIVE, EMOTIONAL, AND COMMUNICATION CONSIDERATIONS

AGE	STAGE	KEY COGNITIVE/EMOTIONAL CONSIDERATIONS	KEY COMMUNICATION CONSIDERATIONS
0–11 months	Infant	Crying is a response to stress Caregiver presence Encourage touching, holding Soothing techniques (e.g., pacifiers, swaddling)	Face-to-face interaction Soft speech, talking, singing Give caregiver a "job" Least invasive to most invasive in approach
1–3 years	Toddler	Crying is a response to stress Caregiver presence Use of play Maintain routine Syllogistic reasoning (i.e., based on previous experiences)	Avoid words with more than one meaning Use concrete words (explain in terms the child may already be familiar with, e.g., "makes a loud noise like a vacuum cleaner") Give caregiver a "job" Least invasive to most invasive in approach
4–5 years	Preschooler	Caregiver presence Provide choices Syllogistic reasoning Fantasy thinker (cannot distinguish between reality and fantasy)	Words taken literally Avoid unfamiliar words (e.g., "stitches," say instead "magic string") Use concrete words Describe in familiar terms (i.e., based on experiences they may have already had) Least invasive to most invasive in approach
6–11 years	School-aged	Caregiver presence Provide choices Probability reasoning (e.g., if A=B and B=C, then A=C)	Age-appropriate explanations Allow participation in care Head-to-toe approach
12–13 years	Preadolescent	Optional caregiver presence Include in decision-making Probability reasoning	Honest explanations/answers to questions Allow participation in care Head-to-toe approach
14–17 years	Adolescent	Optional caregiver or friend presence Privacy is important. Include in decision-making Probability reasoning or abstract thinking	Honest explanations/answers to questions Set limits (boundaries) Allow participation in care Use of electronic technologies Head-to-toe approach

not be a primary indicator of developmental level; therefore, knowledge of general cognitive and developmental stages is imperative. Children are not educated about procedures that are common in the ED; however, cooperation can be enhanced when a clinician understands how to communication with them.

General Approach to the Pediatric Patient Presenting to the ED for Care

Children With Genetic Alterations

A. Currently, over 23,000 genetic traits have been identified in humans; about one-third of hospitalized children have a genetic disease.[1]

B. Genetic testing is commonly used to determine pharmacologic therapies and genetic therapy (a direct alteration of genes) and is becoming increasingly effective for some diseases.[1]

C. Chromosomal alterations, congenital malformations, and genomic imprinting are the primary result of genetic alterations in children

D. Common chromosomal alterations

1. Down syndrome
   - **a.** The most common autosomal aneuploidy (body does not contain 23 pairs of chromosomes)
   - **b.** The aneuploid cell contains three copies of one chromosome (trisomy) on the 21st chromosome.[1]
   - **c.** A mosaic may occur when the trisomic cells are attenuated, resulting in less severe symptoms.
   - **d.** Prevalence, characteristics, and risk factors are outlined in Table 50.2.
2. Sex chromosome conditions
   - **a.** Trisomy X, Turner syndrome, and Klinefelter syndrome are sex chromosome aneuploidies and are generally less severe than autosomal aneuploidies.
     - **i.** In trisomy X, instead of two X chromosomes, these females have three or more X chromosomes.
     - **ii.** In Turner syndrome, there is one X chromosome not paired with another X or Y chromosome. These females have 45 chromosomes instead of 46 (also known as 45, X).
     - **iii.** In Klinefelter syndrome, individuals have two X chromosomes and one Y chromosome (47, XXY).
   - **b.** Characteristics and considerations for each sex chromosome condition are listed in Table 50.3.
3. Congenital malformations
   - **a.** About 2% of newborns will have a congenital malformation present at birth.[1] These congenital

TABLE 50.2 KEY DOWN SYNDROME INFORMATION

Prevalence	One in 800 live births 1%–3% are mosaics
Characteristics	IQ between 25 and 70 Facial alterations: low nasal bridge, epicanthal folds, protruding tongue, flat and low-set ears Hypotonia Short stature Congenital heart defect common in one-third to one-half of children with trisomy 21 Average life expectancy is about 60 years
Risk factors	Increased risk for trisomy 21 with maternal age (>35 years) Increased risk for respiratory infections Increased risk for leukemia Increased risk for Alzheimer's disease by age 40

TABLE 50.3 SEX CHROMOSOME CHARACTERISTICS AND CONSIDERATIONS

CONDITION	PREVALENCE	CHARACTERISTICS	RISK FACTORS
Trisomy X (XXX)	One in 1,000 female newborns	Female No overt physical characteristics Possible sterility Menstrual irregularities	Increased cognitive deficits with each additional X chromosome
Turner syndrome (45, X)	One in 2,500 female newborns	Female Sterile Physical alterations: Short stature, about 50% have neck webbing, widely spaced nipples, 15%–20% have coarctation of the aorta, foot edema (in newborns), sparse body hair Cognitive alterations: Normal IQ, but spatial and math reasoning may be compromised	Adolescent will require estrogen to develop secondary sex characteristics, and possibly growth hormone to increase stature
Klinefelter syndrome (47, XXY)	One in 1,000 male newborns	Male appearance Sterile Physical alterations: 50% will develop gynecomastia, small testes, sparse body hair, high-pitched voice, elevated stature Cognitive alterations: Moderate cognitive impairment	Degree of physical and mental alterations increases with each additional X chromosome

diseases may include cleft lip/palate, clubfoot, heart defect, hydrocephaly, neural tube defect, and gastrointestinal (GI) defect (e.g., pyloric stenosis).

b. Some are surgically repaired without further comorbidities, while others may be associated with other disorders such as trisomy 13, trisomy 18, or trisomy 21.[1]

c. Environmental exposures may also contribute to congenital malformations (e.g., maternal rubella infection may cause a congenital heart defect).

4. Genomic imprinting

a. Genetic material is inherited from two copies of each autosomal gene (one from mother and one from father). Some autosomes may contain an inactivated copy from the mother or the father; this condition is called imprinting.[2] While not well understood, the resulting phenotype is a chromosome deletion.

b. The common conditions resulting from imprinting are Prader–Willi and Angelman syndromes, Beckwith–Wiedemann syndrome, and Russell–Silver syndrome. Characteristics and conditions from imprinting are given in Table 50.4.

Children With Immune Emergencies

A. The innate immune function in neonates is initially depressed since the neonate was contained in a sterile environment until birth.[3] Those who were preterm with respiratory distress syndrome are usually deficient in at least one type of collectin (surfactant), which compromises innate immunity against respiratory tract infection. In general, chemotaxis from the neutrophils and monocytes may not be efficient; therefore, neonates are susceptible to cutaneous abscess and candidiasis.[3] Neonates are also deficient in complement and tend to develop severe, overwhelming sepsis or meningitis when there are no maternal antibodies available in the presence of some bacteria.[3]

B. The young infant immune system undergoes rapid development within the first 3 months of life; however, until some adaptive immunity is acquired, the infant is susceptible to serious bacterial infection (SBI). An infant fever is defined as ≥38°C (100.4°F) and is the early systemic response caused by the release of endogenous pyrogens (fever-causing cytokines) acting on the hypothalamus.[3]

1. A normal hypothalamus has internal mechanisms to control the height of the fever from reaching brain-damaging heights of 41.6°C (107°F) or higher. A fever may provide beneficial effects, such as nonspecific immunity, and may provide an environment of elevated body temperature that is incompatible with some microorganisms (e.g., syphilis, gonorrhea); nonetheless, a fever may also provide some harmful effects by enhancing the person's susceptibility to the effects of Gram-negative endotoxins.[3]

2. A true fever may cause discomfort, and treatment with antipyretics may be indicated.

a. Treatments such as sponge bathing, tepid baths, and other exogenous sources of reducing body temperature have not been demonstrated to be effective in reducing an endogenous (true) fever or discomfort.

C. While the most common SBIs in the young infant are urinary tract infection (UTI) and occult bacteremia, viral infections are the most common cause of fever (Ishimine, cited in[4]).

1. An SBI in the young infant may also cause meningitis and pneumonia. The most common viral and bacterial pathogens for young infant fever are listed in Table 50.5. Viral infections often provide opportunity for bacteria proliferation in a young infant's immature immune system and may preclude an SBI.

D. The febrile young infant (<3 months of age)

1. Evaluation must include a history of symptom development and prenatal history, especially maternal infections requiring antibiotic treatment. The birth history, including complications, and postnatal care is also necessary.[4]

TABLE 50.4 GENETIC IMPRINTING CHARACTERISTICS AND CONSIDERATIONS

CONDITION	PREVALENCE	CHARACTERISTICS	RISK FACTORS
Prader–Willi syndrome (chromosome 15 deletion from father)	One in 15,000 births	Physical alterations: Short stature, hypotonia, small hands/feet, obesity, hypogonadism Cognitive alterations: Mild to moderate intellectual disability	Morbid obesity
Angelman syndrome (chromosome 15 deletion from mother)	One in 15,000 births	Severe intellectual disability Excessive happiness (laughter) Ataxic gait	Seizures
Beckwith–Wiedemann syndrome (chromosome 11 overexpression from father or mother)	One in 10–15,000 births	LGA Neonatal hypoglycemia Physical alterations: Large tongue, earlobe creases, omphalocele (at birth), asymmetrical overgrowth of a limb or one side of the face/trunk	Elevated risk for cancer, especially Wilm's tumor or hepatoblastoma
Russell–Silver syndrome (chromosome 11 downregulation from father or mother)	One in 30–100,000 births	Physical alterations: Growth retardation, short stature, leg length discrepancy, small, triangular face	Delayed development Hypogonadism function Testicular cancer Uterine or vaginal dysgenesis Metabolic syndrome

LGA, large for gestational age.

TABLE 50.5 SERIOUS BACTERIAL INFECTIONS (SBIs) CONDITIONS AND COMMON PATHOGENS

SBI CONDITION	COMMON PATHOGENS
Bacteremia	Group B *Streptococcus*
Meningitis	*Escherichia coli*
UTI	*Listeria monocytogenes*
Pneumonia	*Staphylococcus aureus*
	Enterococcus species
	HSV
	CMV
	Varicella-zoster virus
	RSV
	Candida species

CMV, cytomegalovirus; HSV, herpes simplex virus; RSV, respiratory syncytial virus; UTI, urinary tract infection.

2. Physical exam will be limited since young infants may or may not appear toxic and there are no specific or localizing symptoms.[4] Because of this, a "septic workup" is recommended to include:
   a. Blood culture
   b. Complete blood count (CBC) with manual differential
   c. Urine culture (suprapubic or urinary catheter)
   d. Urinalysis (UA)
   e. Lumbar puncture (LP) may be considered if infant is <60 days and considered low risk. Cerebrospinal fluid (CSF); if CSF pleocytosis, then also an HSV (herpes simplex virus) polymerase chain reaction (PCR)
   f. Chest x-ray (CXR, if respiratory symptoms)
   g. Stool culture (if diarrhea)
3. Hospitalization for at least 48 to 72 hours is often recommended in the young infant.
   a. Empiric, parenteral antibiotics initiated: Ampicillin and gentamycin OR ampicillin and cefotaxime (ceftriaxone is not recommended in infants <30 days of age)
   b. If there is CSF pleocytosis, prolonged rupture of membranes, maternal HSV infection, fetal scalp electrode use, mucocutaneous lesion, or seizure activity, then acyclovir is a recommended addition.[4]

E. The febrile older infant and toddler (>4 months of age)
1. The older infant or toddler is still at risk for SBI, and an infection may present as a fever without a source (FWS).
2. While fever may be of viral etiology, there are three SBIs causing fever without other clinical symptoms: bacteremia, UTI, and pneumonia.[4]
3. When an older infant or toddler presents with FWS, a key indicator in an otherwise healthy child is their toxic or nontoxic appearance.
   a. *Toxic appearance:* Hospitalization, septic workup, and empiric antibiotics are recommended.[4]
      i. Antibiotic selection should include broad-spectrum drugs with CSF-penetrating properties (e.g., ceftriaxone or cefotaxime AND vancomycin) until culture susceptibilities are available.
   b. *Well-appearing:* One of three management strategies are recommended (Table 50.6).
      i. If empiric antibiotic therapy is initiated, consider broad-spectrum with CSF-penetrating properties (e.g., parenteral ampicillin, ceftriaxone or cefotaxime, AND vancomycin[4]).

TABLE 50.6 MANAGEMENT OF FEVER WITHOUT A SOURCE (FWS) IN THE OLDER INFANT AND TODDLER

ROCHESTER CRITERIA		
PHYSICAL EXAM	**DIAGNOSTIC PARAMETERS**	**PLAN**
Low risk: Well-appearing Term infant No prior antibiotics (including perinatal) No hospitalization No underlying disease High risk: Ill-appearing Well-appearing but does not meet diagnostic parameters	Low risk: WBC: 5,000–15,000/μL Bands: <1,500/μL UA: <10 WBCs/hpf Stool: <5 WBCs/hpf High risk: Does not meet low-risk criteria	Low risk: Discharge to home with follow-up in 24 hours High risk: Hospitalize Begin empiric, parenteral antibiotics
BOSTON CRITERIA		
PHYSICAL EXAM	**DIAGNOSTIC PARAMETERS**	**PLAN**
Low risk: Well-appearing No antibiotics or immunizations in prior 48 hours No dehydration No ear, soft tissue, or bone infections High risk: Ill-appearing Well-appearing but does not meet diagnostic parameters	Low risk: WBC: <20,000/μL CSF: WBC < 10/μL UA: <10 WBCs/hpf CXR: No infiltrate High risk: Does not meet low-risk criteria	Low risk: Discharge home after ceftriaxone (50 mg/kg) IM Follow-up in 24 hours High risk: Hospitalize Begin empiric, parenteral antibiotics

(continued)

TABLE 50.6 MANAGEMENT OF FEVER WITHOUT A SOURCE (FWS) IN THE OLDER INFANT AND TODDLER (CONTINUED)

PHILADELPHIA CRITERIA		
PHYSICAL EXAM	**DIAGNOSTIC PARAMETERS**	**PLAN**
Low risk: Well-appearing Unremarkable physical exam High risk: Ill-appearing Well-appearing but does not meet diagnostic parameters	Low risk: WBC: <15,000/µL Band/neutrophil ratio: <0.2 UA: <10 WBCs/hpf and gram-negative stain CSF: WBC < 8/µL and gram-negative Stool: No blood and few or no WBCs on smear CXR: No infiltrate Highrisk: Does not meet low-risk criteria	Low risk: Discharge to home with follow-up in 24 hours No antibiotics High risk: Hospitalize Begin empiric, parenteral antibiotics

CSF, cerebrospinal fluid; CXR, chest x-ray; IM, intramuscularly; UA, urinalysis; WBC, white blood count.

F. The febrile neutropenic child
  1. Neutropenia is defined as an absolute neutrophil count (ANC) of <500 neutrophils/mm^3, or <1,000 neutrophils/mm^3 with further decline anticipated.[4]
  2. In children, cancer and its therapies are the primary cause of neutropenia.
  3. Fever in neutropenic children may be due to infectious, allergic, and hypersensitivity reactions to medications, blood transfusions, graft-versus-host disease, thrombosis, and paraneoplastic etiologies.[4]
  4. Diagnostic studies are imperative and include two blood culture specimens (from peripheral and central venous catheter [CVC] sites if there is a CVC site).
    a. Empiric parenteral antibiotic therapy should begin immediately and be bactericidal, have few side effects, limit the potential for resistant organisms, and based on the institution's most encountered pathogens and rates of antibiotic resistance.[4]

Children With Neurologic Emergencies

A. Neurologic conditions in children evolve any time before birth and through adolescence.

B. Pediatric neurologic conditions that require emergent neurology consultation include[5]:
  1. High suspicion of stroke
  2. Autoimmune encephalitis
  3. Acute demyelinating encephalomyelitis
  4. Acute peripheral neurologic deficit, including acute flaccid myelitis, Guillain-Barré syndrome, and acute brachial neuritis
  5. Transverse myelitis
  6. Any suspected seizures in a child <1 year
  7. Reported or witnessed seizure activity with loss of normal mental or physical functions or other systemic functions
  8. Newly documented neurologic deficits/symptoms or a first-time seizure that cannot be followed up in a timely manner
  9. Refractory status epilepticus, convulsive or nonconvulsive

C. Structural malformations may include neural tube defects such as anencephaly, encephalocele, meningocele, and myelomeningocele.
  1. Hydrocephalus and Arnold-Chiari malformations are generally associated with myelomeningocele.
  2. Craniosynostosis is malformation of the skull, while microcephaly, cortical dysplasia, and congenital hydrocephalus are malformation of brain development.

D. The function of the brain may be affected by static encephalopathies (e.g., cerebral palsy [CP], inborn errors of metabolism [IEM]), acute encephalopathies (e.g., drug-induced or infectious), cerebrovascular disease (e.g., stroke), or seizure disorder (e.g., epilepsy[6]).

E. CP
  1. A static encephalopathy affecting brain function, CP is a disorder of movement, muscle tone, or posture caused by an injury or abnormal development in the brain before, during, and up to 1 year after birth.[6]
  2. Diagnosis occurs by 3 years of age but usually between 12 and 18 months of age and is a clinical diagnosis based on motor development.
  3. Severity depends on the (gestational) age at the time of injury, type, and severity of the injury resulting in spasticity, dystonia, ataxia, or a combination of these.[6] There may or may not be cognitive delay.

F. IEM
  1. Another IEM is an inherited metabolic disorder affecting amino acid, lipid, and carbohydrate metabolism leading to diffuse brain dysfunction.[6]
  2. May not be apparent until childhood or adulthood; newborn and infant identification is important to prevent brain injury.
  3. Newborns are screened for approximately 35 genetic and metabolic conditions, but these are state-dependent and are not a comprehensive screening for all disorders. There are three groups of IEM.
    a. Group 1 results in the accumulation of toxic compounds.
    b. Group 2 includes disorders in energy metabolism.

c. Group 3 includes alterations in the synthesis or catabolism of complex molecules.[7]

4. An IEM should be considered when a previously healthy newborn becomes acutely ill, presenting with a feeding intolerance, history of vomiting, altered mental status, failure to thrive (FTT), or neurologic deterioration. Neurologic symptoms such as ataxia, lethargy, seizures, encephalopathy, or neurologic delays may be suggestive of an IEM.

5. Diagnostic studies

a. Complete blood count (CBC), electrolytes, glucose, ammonia blood gas, uric acid, lactate, acyl carnitine profile, plasma, and urine amino acids and urine organic acids[8]

6. Consultation with and referral to a genetic or metabolic specialist is essential when IEM is suspected or confirmed.

G. Stroke

1. Perinatal stroke may be ischemic or hemorrhagic and can occur between 20 weeks' gestation and up to 28 days after birth.[6]

2. Intraventricular hemorrhage (IVH) is a complication of prematurity with up to 75% of affected infants developing hydrocephalus, CP, and/or cognitive disability.

3. Diagnosis may not occur until later infancy or early childhood and is confirmed with neuroimaging.[6]

4. Ischemic stroke in children is rare but may result from embolism, arteriopathy, or sinovenous thrombosis; however, children do not have the typical adult risk factors for stroke (e.g., atherosclerosis or hypertension).[9]

5. Hemorrhagic stroke in children usually results from arteriovenous malformations or aneurysm, and is rare.

H. Seizures

1. Abnormal discharge of electrical activity in the brain and epilepsy is the occurrence of at least two unprovoked seizures more than 24 hours apart.[6]

2. Generalized seizures involve both hemispheres of the brain and may include a loss of consciousness, tonic-clonic, tonic, clonic, myoclonic, myoclonic-atonic, or epileptic spasm activities. Generalized seizures are likely to have a genetic component.[6]

3. Childhood absence epilepsy (formerly petit mal seizures) is a type of generalized epilepsy occurring between 4 and 10 years of age and includes a sudden onset and termination of an impairment of consciousness for about 10 seconds. Seizures may occur hundreds of times per day.[6]

4. Other epilepsy syndromes include neonatal seizures (rhythmic eye movements, chewing, and swimming movements), febrile seizures (associated with fever and are benign), complex febrile seizures (lasting longer than 15 minutes and have focal characteristics), and infantile spasms (sudden flexion or extension of the neck, trunk, and extremities occurring in clusters) occurring at 4 to 8 months of age.

5. Treatment

a. Lorazepam is considered first-line therapy for pediatric seizure (outside of the neonatal period) actively occurring in the ED.

b. If seizure activity persists, additional antiepileptic medications such as phenobarbital or fosphenytoin are recommended. For seizures refractory to standard management, a drug-induced coma by a continuous infusion of barbiturates (i.e., pentobarbital, thiopental, benzodiazepine, or anesthetic agents) may be necessary.[5,10]

c. The underlying cause of the seizure must be identified, and if this is a first-time seizure, the child will require history and physical exam, laboratory, and imaging such as a CT scan when indicated.

d. Seizures may require prompt diagnostic evaluation and a therapeutic plan in consultation with a neurologist.

I. General senses

1. Alterations in sensory functions involve the general and special senses.[11]

2. Dysfunction in the general senses includes pain, abnormal temperature regulation, and sleep disturbances, while the special senses include tactile, proprioceptive, and vestibular dysfunctions originating from the senses of vision, hearing, touch, smell, and taste.[11]

J. Pain considerations

1. Infants and children have the neurobiologic, anatomic, and functional ability to feel pain.[11] In fact, a fetus's nociceptor function is established at 15 to 20 weeks' gestation, requiring analgesia for painful fetal procedures.

TABLE 50.7 COMMON PEDIATRIC PAIN SCALES

SCALE	TYPE	RECOMMENDED AGE	SCORE	CONSIDERATIONS
FLACC	Observational	2 months through 7 years	0–10	Recently validated up to 16 years; may be useful in the cognitively impaired child
FACES	Self-report	3 years and older	0–5 or 0–10	May not reflect the appropriate face for the child to identify with; does not consider different ethnic backgrounds and associated faces for pain; numeric score does not correspond to numeric rating scale
NRS	Self-report	8 years and older	0–10	Dependent on the child's understanding of numeracy

FLACC, faces, legs, activity, cry, and consolability; FACES, Wong-Baker FACES Pain Rating Scale; NRS, numeric rating scale.

2. In the preterm infant, repeated painful procedures or prolonged exposure to analgesics may permanently alter developing synaptic and neuronal pain pathways, causing irreversible hypersensitivity to pain, delayed postnatal growth, and poor early neurodevelopment in cognitive and motor functions.[11]
3. Infant and pediatric pain can be assessed with a variety of validated pain assessment tools; however, self-report tools have been demonstrated as reliable, but are dependent on family and ethnic cultures, prior pain experiences, and societal norms (Table 50.7).
4. All children should have their pain assessed and treated using recommended pediatric dosing and appropriate monitoring. The child's age and previous experiences related to pain need to be considered. Older children (aged 5–18 years) tend to have a lower pain threshold than adults.[11] Again, it is important, just as with the adult patient with pain in the ED, that each child receives individual attention related to the assessment and treatment of their pain.
5. Other methods to help children manage pain include comfort positioning, distraction techniques, guided imagery, music, use of sucrose in infants, application of topical anesthetics such as EMLA, and other marketed devices specific for the pediatric population.

K. Thermoregulation considerations
1. Young, term infants produce body heat through brown adipose tissue (BAT) metabolism and cannot shiver or sweat due to a nonshivering thermogenesis.
2. Increased glucose and free fatty acid oxidation occurs at a rate 50 times greater than that in white adipose tissue (WAT), protecting against obesity and metabolic syndrome.[12] Infants do not conserve or expel heat well due to their greater body surface area to body weight ratio and little subcutaneous fat (for insulation).
3. Older infants and children also have a greater body surface area to weight ratio, fewer sweat glands and lower sweating rate, higher peripheral blood flow when heated, and greater vasoconstriction in a cold environment or vasodilation in a warm environment when compared to an adult.[11]
4. Heat loss occurs through conduction and convection, requiring hats, clothing, and blankets to assist with thermoregulation. Heat expulsion can be assisted with bathing to facilitate cooling from evaporation on skin.
5. Hyperthermia
a. Occurs when normal thermoregulatory mechanisms (i.e., sweating) have been exceeded or impeded in the presence of an external heat source.
b. Heat cramps, heat exhaustion, heat stroke, malignant hyperthermia, drug-induced hyperthermia, neuroleptic malignant syndrome, and possibly sudden infant death syndrome (SIDS) can occur.
c. In the case of SIDS, evidence is evolving to suggest heat stress decreases minute ventilation and may be a contributing factor.[13] Regardless, a medical emergency occurs when the body temperature rises without an endogenous source or control from the hypothalamus. External and rapid cooling measures, such as ice to the groin and axilla, cool parenteral fluids, and cooling blankets, must be provided to reduce the body temperature since antipyretics are not helpful in this situation.

L. Sleep considerations
1. Pediatric sleep patterns change with age. Newborns sleep 16 to 18 hours per day, with total sleep time decreasing slightly from birth to 1 year. Within the age range of 3 to 5, the child sleeps 8 to 10 hours at night.
2. Sleep disorders can occur and include causes such as obstructive sleep apnea syndrome (OSAS). Adolescent sleep deprivation is associated with obesity, depression, anxiety disorders, poor academic performance, and safety issues.[11]

M. Special senses
1. The somatosensory system includes peripheral receptors and the central nervous system pathways receiving information from the special senses of sight, hearing, smell, and taste.[11]
2. Conditions altering these senses in children generally include those causing alterations in adults. Untreated conditions in children can permanently alter the developing senses.

Children With Psychiatric Emergencies

A. Every mental disorder has a range of symptoms that vary in intensity depending on the brain structures and function.[14] When managing these children in the ED, the emergency nurse practitioner (ENP) should be familiar with updated *Diagnostic and Statistical Manual of Mental Disorders*, Fifth Edition *(DSM-5)*. Just as adult patients, children can suffer from mental disorders and will be brought to the ED by families or others for evaluation and treatment.

B. Bipolar II and attention deficit hyperactivity disorder (ADHD)
1. In children, bipolar II and ADHD include symptoms of increased behavioral activity, excessive talking, restlessness, and distractibility.
a. Misdiagnosing bipolar II as ADHD with a prescribed treatment of a stimulant drug may exacerbate the child's bipolar II symptoms.
b. When ADHD is misdiagnosed as bipolar II, treatment is ineffective.[14]
c. The *DSM-5* now includes a category called "disruptive mood dysregulation disorder" (DMDD) to reduce the misdiagnosis of children for bipolar disorder, ADHD, conduct disorder (CD), and oppositional defiant disorder (ODD). The use of DMDD as a diagnosis for children aged 6 to 10 years who display only some of the symptoms of bipolar II, such as frequent temper outbursts, irritability, and bad moods, is recommended.[14]

C. Suicidal ideation assessment
1. Past history of suicidal ideation
2. Changes in behavior, withdrawal from family and friends, personality changes
3. Concerns expressed about the child by a friend. Not uncommon for the child to disclose a suicidal plan to a friend

4. Stressors such as a relationship breakup, change in a family, bullying, generation of personality changes, or recognition of gender changes

5. Referral to a mental health specialist for adequate assessment and accurate diagnosis of the child's condition is encouraged.

Children With Endocrine Emergencies

A. Alterations in hormonal function are caused by hyper- or hyposecretion of various hormones.

B. *Hypothalamic–pituitary system:* Disease in the posterior pituitary causes abnormal secretion of antidiuretic hormone (ADH), with an excess resulting in water retention and a hypo-osmolar state (e.g., syndrome of inappropriate antidiuretic hormone [SIADH]) or a deficiency resulting in water loss and hyperosmolarity (e.g., diabetes insipidus [DI]).[15]

C. *Anterior pituitary:* Conditions such as hypopituitarism where low levels of growth hormone or insulin-like growth factor (IGF-1) affect the growth of children; hyperpituitarism from a primary adenoma; hypersecretion of growth hormone (e.g., acromegaly); and hypersecretion of prolactin (e.g., amenorrhea, galactorrhea, and infertility in females)

D. Alterations in thyroid function result from its primary dysfunction or from a secondary cause such as pituitary or hypothalamic dysfunction. Hyperthyroidism (e.g., Grave's disease) and hypothyroidism (e.g., Hashimoto disease, congenital hypothyroidism, and thyroid carcinoma) are considered a primary cause for dysfunction. The parathyroid may also have hyper- and hypoparathyroidism causes for dysfunction. [15]

E. Diabetes mellitus (DM)

1. Group of metabolic diseases characterized by hyperglycemia resulting from a defect in insulin secretion, insulin resistance, or both[15]

2. DM type 1 involves beta-cell destruction leading to absolute insulin failure and is one of the most common childhood diseases. The peak onset is 11 to 13 years of age and in those who are generally of normal or underweight. The cause is theorized to occur as an autoimmune response targeting the beta cells in the islets of Langerhans (usually to a recent viral infection or environmental trigger) in genetically susceptible individuals.[15]

3. History and physical exam usually reveals nausea and vomiting, polyuria, polydipsia, polyphagia, and weight loss.

4. Diagnostic evaluation should include a complete blood count (CBC), electrolytes, blood urea nitrogen (BUN), creatinine, calcium, magnesium, phosphate, pH (arterial or venous blood gas), serum ketones, urinalysis, osmolality, and hemoglobin A1c (HbA1c).

5. In diabetic ketoacidosis (DKA), a blood glucose >200 mg/dL with ketoacidosis (ketonemia and ketonuria) is present. Leukocytosis is not a reliable indicator of infection in children with DM type 1 since stress hormones (epinephrine and cortisol) may mimic infection. Antibiotics are only indicated if fever is present and cultures are obtained. If respiratory symptoms are present, a chest x-ray (CXR) is indicated; a baseline EKG may detect any electrophysiologic changes occurring.[16]

a. If DKA is present, fluid and electrolyte replacement is a priority. Assessing for the anion gap helps to quantify the unmeasured ketones and lactate, calculated as:

i. Anion gap = $[Na^+ + K^+] - [Cl^- + HCO_3]$ or $[Na^+] - [Cl^- + HCO_3^-]$[16]

6. A bolus of insulin is not recommended (the goal is to gradually replace); therefore, insulin is initiated 1 to 2 hours after initial fluid replacement at a rate of 0.1 unit/kg/hour.[16]

7. Glucose supplementation prevents hypoglycemia as it provides a substrate for the insulin to bind to as normal glucose metabolism is restored.

8. Glucose (5% dextrose) should be added to fluids when the serum glucose drops below 250 mg/dL to maintain the serum glucose between 200 to 250 mg/dL; 10% dextrose should be initiated if the serum glucose is <200 mg/dL.[16] Glucose can be removed when the child is ready to eat, and the insulin is stopped.

9. Electrolyte replacement is also an important part of correcting the effects of DKA since hyperglycemia suppresses serum sodium (Na) due to the movement of water into the extracellular spaces causing a dilutional hyponatremia.[16] Generally, normal saline (0.9%) or Ringer's lactate is used for the first 4 to 6 hours, followed by 0.45% normal saline with additional electrolytes. Calculation for correcting Na concentration is:

a. Corrected $Na^+ = [Na^+] + [1.6 \times (\text{plasma glucose mg/dL} - 100)] / 100$[16]

b. Failure of the Na level to rise is a worrisome sign and is associated with cerebral edema, the most common cause of death in pediatric DKA (Wolfsdorf, cited in Briars, 2015).[16]

10. Additional electrolytes, such as potassium (K^+), phosphorous, calcium (Ca^+), and bicarbonate must also be considered. Insulin administration should not begin until severe hypokalemia is corrected because an intracellular shift of K+ back into cells will occur with the correction of acidosis and supplementation of insulin. Continuous EKG monitoring is necessary to detect changes in T waves, widening QT intervals, or the presence of U waves (with hypokalemia). Replacing phosphate with 20 mEq/L of K^+ phosphate plus 20 mEq/L of K^+ chloride decreases the amount of chloride given, resulting in a hyperchloremic metabolic acidosis to reduce the complication of tetany.[16] Monitoring Ca^+ and phosphorous levels at least every 12 hours is recommended.[16] Bicarbonate is only needed in severe cases of DKA, as most cases will reverse the acidosis with fluid replacement and insulin administration. Consultation with an endocrinologist or intensivist is necessary if considering the administration of bicarbonate.

11. DM type 2 (insulin resistance) is becoming increasingly prevalent in obese children because of genetic and environmental influences.[15] Obesity is one of the most important contributors to insulin resistance; however, a family history of DM type 2 is almost always present in at least one parent or first-degree relative.[16] Children will present with hyperglycemia and glycosuria without ketonuria. Children with DM type 2 have no evidence of autoimmunity, but will have normal to elevated fasting insulin and C-peptide levels.[16] Polycystic ovarian syndrome (PCOS), lipid disorders, and hypertension may occur in children with DM type 2.[16] Treatment is generally aimed at weight reduction, lipid management, and occasionally medication management.

12. Hypoglycemia may occur from exogenous (medications, alcohol, or exercise), endogenous (pancreatic tumor or inherited disorder), or functional (liver disease) causes.[15] Those with DM type 2 are at less risk for hypoglycemia because they have some intact glucose counter-regulatory mechanisms (e.g., catecholamines, cortisol, glucagon, and growth hormone). Treatment for hypoglycemia is immediate replacement of glucose. Hyperglycemia may result in DKA, as previously discussed, and is a serious complication from insulin deficiency and an increase in insulin counter-regulatory mechanisms. In children, DKA occurs in approximately 30% of those with DM type 1 and in about 5% of those with DM type 2, known as ketosis-prone type 2 diabetes (KPD).[15]

F. Congenital adrenal hyperplasia (CAH)

1. CAH is part of the newborn screening; symptoms become apparent within the first few weeks of life.

2. About 95% of all cases are from 21-hydroxylase deficiency (21-HD), with males presenting in a salt-wasting crisis or a shock state at 1 to 2 weeks of age, before newborn screening results are available. The 21-HD missing enzyme decreases cortisol and aldosterone production by the adrenal glands and results in an adrenal insufficiency (AI) state.

a. As the pituitary does not receive enough cortisol, more cholesterol is delivered, with the extra cholesterol being converted to androgen. More androgens create ambiguous genitalia; therefore, CAH is more easily recognized in females.

b. In aldosterone deficiency, electrolyte deficiencies such as hyponatremia, hyperkalemia, hypocalcemia, and/or hypercalcemia may be present. In cortisol deficiency, anemia, acidosis, lymphocytosis, and/or eosinophilia may be present.

3. Immediate treatment for AI includes glucocorticoid replacement (usually a hydrocortisone 1–2 mg/kg IV bolus, then 25–50 mg/kg divided every 6–8 hours), correction of electrolyte or metabolic abnormalities, volume replacement, and correction of any precipitating events.

4. Diagnostic studies include initial cortisol levels, neuroimaging to evaluate for pituitary hemorrhage or tumor, and ACTH stimulation testing (administration of ACTH followed by cortisol levels at specific time intervals). Only if the cortisol response to the ACTH stimulation test is <9 mcg/dL, are glucocorticoids administered. Continuous cardiorespiratory monitoring, admission to a pediatric ICU (PICU), and consultation with an endocrinologist are indicated in a child with AI.

Children With Nutritional Emergencies

The hypothalamus regulates body temperature, food intake, and energy metabolism. The hypothalamus also assists in the regulation of reward, pleasure, memory, and addictive behavior.[12] Higher brain centers can override hypothalamic control of food intake and satiety, resulting in increased and decreased consumption of food and increased or decreased fat stores.

A. Malnutrition

1. A lack of nourishment due to decreased calories, protein, vitamins, or minerals from an inadequate diet, alterations in digestion, chronic disease, or a combination of these defines malnutrition.[12]

2. Starvation is a reduction in energy intake leading to weight loss.[12]

a. A ketotic state will occur until adipose tissue has been used for energy.

b. Treatment for malnutrition and starvation occurs with enteral or parenteral nutrition.

B. Eating disorders

1. Anorexia nervosa, bulimia nervosa, and binge eating disorders are related to a distorted body image with a desire for thinness and fear of fatness.[12]

a. These disorders are considered psychiatric disorders and are included in the *Diagnostic and Statistical Manual of Mental Disorders*, Fifth Edition (*DSM-5*). They usually occur in adolescent females but can occur in males. Table 50.8 includes complications related to malnutrition and weight changes involving all organ systems, which may be life-threatening.[12]

C. Failure to thrive is described in children whose current weight or weight gain is less than that of a child with similar age and gender.

1. Causes of failure to thrive may result from a medical problem.

2. May also be caused by neglect and abuse

3. Signs and symptoms

a. Growth that has stopped or slowed

b. Weight loss

c. Delayed social skills

d. Delayed physical skills; for example, an infant who should be able to roll over and cannot

e. Assessment

f. Denver Developmental Screening Test

g. Evaluation of social environment

4. Management

a. Blood and urine tests to rule out a medical problem

b. X-rays to determine growth issues

c. Nutritional education and counseling

d. Notification of appropriate agencies

Children With Reproductive Emergencies

A. Puberty is the sexual maturation of an individual during adolescence.

1. Girls' puberty occurs between 8 and 12 years of age with breast development (thelarche); obesity may induce earlier puberty.

TABLE 50.8 EATING DISORDERS AND COMPLICATIONS

EATING DISORDER	CRITERIA	COMPLICATIONS
Anorexia nervosa	■ Persistent restriction of energy intake resulting in low body weight ■ Intense fear of gaining weight or persistent behavior interfering with weight gain ■ Disturbance in the way one's body weight or shape is experienced ■ Subtypes: Restricting or binge-eating/purging	Gastrointestinal ■ Dysphagia, slowed gastric emptying, early satiety, nausea and bloating, constipation, elevated transaminases Cardiac ■ Dysrhythmias, left ventricular hypertrophy, mitral valve prolapse, sudden cardiac death Pulmonary ■ Aspiration pneumonia Hematologic ■ Anemia, leukopenia, thrombocytopenia Musculoskeletal ■ Osteoporosis, increased risk for stress fractures Endocrine ■ Hypogonadal; females with low estrogen and loss of menses; males with low testosterone, low libido, loss of muscle strength; hypothyroidism, hypercortisolism, hypoglycemia, impaired temperature regulation Neurologic ■ Brain atrophy, cognitive impairment Dermatologic ■ Xerosis, hair thinning, acrocyanosis
Bulimia nervosa	■ Recurrent episodes of binge eating at least once per week for 3 months ■ Recurrent, inappropriate compensatory behavior to prevent weight gain at least once per week for 3 months (e.g., self-induced vomiting, misuse of laxatives or diuretics; fasting, excessive exercise) ■ Self-evaluation is unduly influenced by body shape and weight ■ Disturbance does not occur exclusively during episodes of anorexia nervosa	Self-induced vomiting ■ Persistent gastric acid reflux, dysphagia, dyspepsia, and chronic induced vomiting ■ Electrolyte and acid–base disorders, metabolic alkalosis, hypokalemia ■ Tooth erosion ■ Vocal cord inflammation and hoarse voice ■ Parotid gland enlargement Laxative abuse ■ Hypokalemic metabolic alkalosis ■ Diarrhea, hemorrhoids, rectal prolapse ■ Hyperphosphatemia
Binge eating disorder	Recurrent episodes of binge eating ■ Eating, in a discrete period, an amount of food larger than most people would be able to eat ■ Lack of control of overeating during the episode Binge eating episodes are associated with three or more ■ Eating more rapidly than normal ■ Eating until uncomfortably full ■ Eating large amounts even though not hungry ■ Eating alone due to embarrassment of how much eaten ■ Feeling disgusted with oneself, depressed, or guilty afterward ■ Marked distress during binge eating ■ Binge eating occurs at least once per week for 3 months. ■ Binge eating is not associated with recurrent use of inappropriate compensatory behaviors.	

2. Boys' puberty begins about 11 years of age; can occur earlier with increased weight and body mass index.[11]

a. First sign of puberty is enlargement of the testes and thinning of the scrotal skin.[17]

3. Dependent upon estrogen, puberty is a time of rapid skeletal growth, with most of the bone development and mineralization occurring during adolescence. Inadequate estrogen circulation may predispose a child to inadequate bone density (osteoporosis) into their adulthood.

B. Delayed puberty

1. *Girls:* Delayed puberty is diagnosed when thelarche does not occur until 13 years of age or later, but the clinical diagnosis can be made if menarche is absent by age 15 or 16 years.[18]

a. If a female has not had routine genital assessment during well-child exams, hymenal imperfections, specifically an imperforate hymen, may prevent signs of menarche. Hence, a visual examination of the female genitalia (anatomy) is important.

2. *Boys:* Puberty is delayed if there are no clinical signs of puberty by age 14 years.[17] While physiologic delay (familial delay) is common, there are times when hormonal therapy in small doses may be needed. In addition, further testing may be indicated for genetic disorders not detected earlier in life. If delayed puberty is suspected, consultation with an endocrinologist is warranted.

C. Precocious puberty

1. Precocious puberty is defined as the onset of clinical signs of puberty (breast or pubic hair development) before the age of 8 years in girls and 9 years in boys.[17,18]

2. Precocity causes premature closure of the epiphysis of long bones resulting in short stature.

3. All cases of precocious puberty require a thorough evaluation by an endocrinologist.

4. Treatment for all forms of precocious puberty includes removing the underlying cause or administering the appropriate hormones.[11]

D. Dysmenorrhea and amenorrhea

1. *Dysmenorrhea:* Pelvic pain associated with the onset of menses.

a. A primary dysmenorrhea involves painful menstruation without evidence of pelvic disease and secondary dysmenorrhea is related to a pathologic pelvic disorder such as ovarian cysts, adenomyosis, or endometriosis.[11]

b. The administration of NSAIDs is the treatment of choice due to the COX enzyme activity and subsequent prostaglandin production.[11] For those not responding to NSAIDs, hormonal contraception is indicated.

2. *Amenorrhea.* Lack of menstruation caused by chromosomal abnormalities, hypothalamic dysfunction, polycystic ovarian syndrome, prolactinemia, hypothyroidism, malnutrition, and ovarian failure[11]

a. Primary amenorrhea is the failure of menarche by age 13 years without the development of secondary sex characteristics, or by age 15 years regardless of secondary sex characteristic development.

b. Secondary amenorrhea is the absence of regular menses for 3 months, or irregular menses for 6 months, in women who have previously menstruated.[11]

c. Treatment includes the correction of underlying disorders and possibly phimosis and paraphimosis.

3. Disorders of the foreskin include foreskin tightness affecting its ability to move over the glans penis.

4. *Phimosis:* Condition in which the foreskin cannot be easily retracted over the glans and is commonly caused by poor hygiene or chronic infection; whereas, paraphimosis is the opposite, when the foreskin is retracted and cannot be moved over the glans (Rodway & McCance, 2019).

5. *Paraphimosis:* Foreskin is retracted and cannot be moved over the glans.[17] Paraphimosis can constrict the penis, causing edema of the glans.

6. Both conditions can become a surgical emergency if phimosis creates urinary obstruction or paraphimosis causes necrosis of the glans.17

E. Testicular torsion

1. Rotation of the testes, twisting blood vessels in the spermatic cord; primarily occurs in adolescent males[17]

2. Physical examination reveals scrotal swelling, diffuse tenderness, and an absent cremasteric reflex on the side of the torsed testes.

3. Diagnostic testing includes a UA and color Doppler ultrasonography.

4. Testicular torsion is a surgical emergency, with the best outcomes when surgery is performed within 6 hours of the onset of symptoms.[17]

F. Gynecomastia

1. The incidence of gynecomastia is greatest in adolescent males and usually affects the left breast. [17]

2. Gynecomastia results from idiopathic or systemic hormonal alterations, usually involving an imbalance between estrogen and testosterone.

3. Physical exam reveals breast enlargement that is firm, palpable, and at least two centimeters in diameter beneath the areola.

4. Diagnostics may include fine needle aspiration, cytology, mammography, ultrasound, or biopsy as all unilateral breast enlargement in males warrants an evaluation for malignancy.[17]

5. Treatment is dependent upon the cause.

Children With Hematologic Emergencies

A. The primary function of red blood cells (RBC) is to deliver oxygen, electrolytes, and nutrients, while removing waste products in tissues under aerobic conditions.[19] Plasma constitutes a major portion of the blood, with approximately 90% of plasma is water, 8% is solutes such as albumin, 1% electrolytes, and the remaining 1% being other components such as hormones.[19,20] In addition, blood is identified by groups A, B, AB, and O, and Rh types: positive or negative. In neonates and young infants, all antibodies originate from the mother and is why group O negative blood is used for transfusion of packed red blood cells (PRBC) when needed.[19] In older infants and children, transfusion with group- and type-specific PRBCs is preferred. Hematopoiesis occurs in the liver and spleen of a fetus, but only in the bone marrow after birth.[20]

B. Anemia

1. *Aplastic anemia:* A rare but life-threatening disease of bone marrow failure, occurring as either congenital (20%) or acquired (80%), caused by idiopathic, constitutional, or iatrogenic factors.[19]

2. *Pancytopenia:* May be caused by aplastic anemia, viral infection, drug exposure, toxic exposure, myelodysplastic syndrome, or a congenital abnormality and should be included in a list of differential diagnoses when a neonate, infant, or young child presents with anemia.[19]

a. A transfusion of 10 to 20 mL per kg body weight of PRBCs is warranted with a hemoglobin value <7 gm/dL in a neonate, <10 gm/dL in infants and children with an oxygen requirement, or <12 gm/dL in infants and children on ventilatory support.[19] Otherwise, other treatments for anemia are based on its etiology (i.e., beta thalassemia, iron deficiency, sickle cell, and anemia of chronic disease).

C. Glucose-6-phosphate dehydrogenase (G6PD) deficiency

1. Classified as a hemolytic anemia, G6PD-deficient RBCs are at risk for hemolysis.

2. The G6PD is an enzyme important in maintaining the integrity of the RBC wall.

a. With G6PD deficiency, reactive oxygen radicals damage the RBC membrane resulting in hemolysis, which is not detected as an anemia unless an exogenous challenge (e.g., infection) is presented.[19]

b. Neonatal jaundice may be a manifestation of G6PD deficiency, but most children will be asymptomatic until illness, ingestion of fava beans, antimalarial or sulfa-containing medications, aspirin, quinolones, and other antimicrobials are introduced.[19]

3. Treatment is targeted at correcting the anemia and removal of the exogenous cause.

D. Sickle cell disease

1. A hereditary hemoglobinopathy, hemoglobin S (HbS) occurs because of a genetic mutation in ß-globin.[21] When deoxygenation occurs, the HbS molecule will structurally deform into a concave shape while becoming more adhesive to the endothelium of blood vessels (i.e., sickled cells). Occlusion of blood flow occurs as the HbS accumulates, particularly in the microvasculature, thus causing further deoxygenation of the blood as circulation becomes compromised.

2. Clinical manifestations are variable.

a. Vaso-occlusive (pain) crisis (i.e., swelling of hands and feet in younger children; or a deep, throbbing pain in the lower back, shoulders, elbows, femur, and knees in older children)

b. Acute chest syndrome (i.e., chest pain, fever, and respiratory symptoms with a pulmonary infiltrate evident on chest x-ray [CXR])

c. Acute abdominal pain (resulting from mesenteric vessel sickling or vertebral disease with nerve root compression)

d. Stroke (i.e., brain infarction, a leading complication)

e. Priapism

f. Splenic sequestration (a leading cause of death)

g. Infection (the most common cause of death due to functional asplenia)

3. Treatment for sickle cell anemia is related to hemolysis.

a. Severe pain crises should be aggressively treated with hydration (e.g., parenteral, isotonic fluids) to increase vascular space for blood flow and with analgesias (e.g., NSAIDs and morphine), since pain increases oxygen demand; however, care is needed to avoid fluid overload and cardiac failure.

b. Unless hypoxic, supplemental oxygen is of little value and can suppress erythropoiesis and reticulocyte formation.[22]

c. In stroke or recurrent acute chest syndrome, a transfusion of PRBCs may be indicated. Episodic transfusion may be helpful in the treatment of priapism not responding to other medical therapies.[22]

E. Hemolytic uremic syndrome (HUS)

1. The type of vasculitis characterized by hemolytic anemia, thrombocytopenia, and acute kidney failure is known as HUS.

2. Occurs when bacterial verotoxins (e.g., *Escherichia coli* 0157:H7 or *Shigella dysenteriae*) are absorbed into the intestines, causing extensive damage to erythrocytes and endothelial cells.[23] The endothelial cells in the glomerular arterioles of the kidneys are particularly susceptible to edema, causing the release of clotting factors, which in turn causes fibrinolysis and a resulting decrease in platelets and thrombocytopenia.[23]

a. Decreased glomerular filtration, hematuria, proteinuria, and oliguria may result.

3. Incubation period is 3 to 5 days, and a child may initially present with fever, watery diarrhea, and abdominal pain, but a hemorrhagic colitis can occur 5 to 7 days after diarrhea begins.[23]

4. Diagnostic findings reveal elevated blood urea nitrogen (BUN), creatinine, bilirubin, and potassium levels, but decreased hemoglobin, hematocrit, and platelet counts.

5. Treatment is supportive; serum samples for enzyme-linked immunosorbent assay (ELISA) testing for antibodies to *E. coli* and Shiga toxin should be obtained at diagnosis and 2 weeks later.[23]

F. Henoch-Schoenlein purpura (HSP)

1. Vasculitis resulting from the immune response to a viral infection, environmental trigger, or medication and is the most common vasculitis in children.[23]

2. History of a recent upper respiratory infection, some fever and fatigue, followed by nonblanching, nonpruritic, palpable, purpuric lesions in an otherwise well-appearing child. Transient arthritis and intermittent abdominal pain may occur; hematuria, proteinuria, and hypertension may represent nephrotic syndrome, a feared complication from HSP.[23]

3. Treatment is supportive with acetaminophen, but in cases of severe abdominal or arthritic pain, oral corticosteroids of 1 to 2 mg/kg/d for 2 weeks are recommended.[23] Close follow-up is needed, and hospitalization is recommended for those children with signs of renal impairment.[23]

G. Immune thrombocytopenic purpura (ITP)

1. Acquired, viral-mediated autoimmune disorder; ITP accelerates platelet destruction by coating circulating platelets with IgG, IgA, or IgM autoantibodies, which are removed from the circulation system by the spleen.

2. Antibodies affect platelet development in the bone marrow, resulting in decreased platelet production.[23]

3. Common in children between 2 and 6 years of age with a history of a recent viral illness. These children are well-appearing, with a sudden onset of petechiae, purpura, or spontaneous bleeding from mucus membranes.

4. Diagnostic evaluation usually reveals a normal CBC, with a platelet count <100,000 mm^3.[23]

5. Most cases of ITP will resolve spontaneously and without treatment, but treatment is based on whether it is acute or chronic.
   a. Follow evidence-based guidelines when prescribing.
   b. For acute ITP, oral corticosteroids, tapering dose based on platelet counts.
   c. For severe thrombocytopenia, IV immunoglobulin (IVIG) is recommended.[23]
   d. For chronic ITP, regular administration of IVIG, WinRho-D, or a splenectomy may be indicated.[23]
   e. Medications enhancing bleeding (e.g., NSAIDs) or injectable medications should be avoided while the child has ITP, and the child should avoid contact sports or similar activities which may provoke bleeding.

H. Hemophilia

1. A bleeding disorder and inherited X-linked recessive condition resulting in a secondary hemostasis where fibrin clot formation is unstable and bleeding becomes difficult to control. Intrinsic and extrinsic pathways of a clotting cascade are activated to secure a platelet plug for containing the bleed, but children with hemophilia are deficient in one of the factors necessary for hemostasis.[24] Factor VIII (hemophilia A) or IX (hemophilia B) deficiency are most common and often diagnosed at birth from a family history of the disease, intracranial hemorrhage or cephalohematoma, excessive bleeding from puncture sites or the umbilicus, or unusual bleeding from circumcision.

2. Diagnostic studies should include a CBC, blood smear, prothrombin time (PT), international normalized ratio (INR), partial thromboplastin time (PTT), fibrinogen, and bleeding time.[24] Hemophilia is likely when a normal PT, platelet count, fibrinogen, and bleeding time are accompanied by a prolonged PTT.

3. Treatment is coagulation factor replacement, including 100% replacement of Factor VIII IV for major bleeding (100 units/kg); 50% to 60% replacement for joint or muscle bleeding (50–75 units/kg); and 30% to 50% replacement for mucocutaneous bleeding (25–50 units/kg); whereas Factor IX replacement is 100% (100 units/kg) for major bleeding; 50% to 80% (40–80 units/kg) for hemarthrosis; and 30% to 50% (25–50 units/kg) for mucocutaneous bleeding.[24] Intracranial, tracheal, and peritoneal bleeding can be life-threatening and requires daily factor replacement for a minimum of 14 days. Those with mild to moderate hemophilia A may be treated with desmopressin acetate (DDAVP®) parenterally (0.3 mcg/kg for 3 doses) or intranasally (150 mcg for children <50kg; or 300 mcg for children >50 kg).

4. To prevent unexpected bleeding, parents of children with hemophilia should be taught to avoid medications inhibiting platelet or coagulation factors, avoid contact sports, and vaccinate their child for Hepatitis A and B.[24]

Children With Cardiovascular and Lymphatic Emergencies

A. Growth and developmental changes affect a child's cardiovascular function into adulthood. The number and size of myocardial cells and collagen change from stiff (type I) to compliant (type II) in the first several years of life.[25] In neonates, excitation–contraction coupling occurs primarily from extracellular calcium (unlike adults who utilize intracellular calcium). The number and size of myocytes, collagen changes, and calcium utilization contribute to pediatric cardiac muscle stiffness; consequently, heart rate rather than stroke volume is responsible for cardiac output in infants and young children.

B. Hydrostatic and oncotic pressures affect blood flow throughout the cardiovascular system. Hydrostatic forces push fluid out while oncotic pressures pull fluid in, resulting in a steady lymphatic flow. Edema occurs when total lymphatic flow exceeds the capability of the lymphatic forces, obstructions are present, or central venous pressures are elevated.[25]

C. Neural control of pressures, flow, and vascular amenability by central nervous system (CNS)-mediated reflexes are affected by development, disease, and trauma.[25]

D. Congenital heart disease (CHD) begins in utero and results in a shunt lesion, left-side obstruction, right-side obstruction, or conotruncal lesion (Table 50.9).

TABLE 50.9 CONGENITAL HEART DISEASE

TYPE OF LESION	NAME OF LESION	PATHOPHYSIOLOGY	PRESENTATION
Shunt lesion	PDA	Small vessel connecting left main pulmonary artery to the descending aorta to allow for fetal circulation. After birth, if patent, left-to-right shunting increases pulmonary blood flow, left atrial dilation, and left ventricular overload. Typically closes during 2–14 days of age	Machinery-type murmur, if large, symptoms of congestive heart failure (CHF), pulmonary hypertension, wide pulse pressure, bounding peripheral pulses
	ASD	An opening in the atrial septum. Left-to-right shunting between atria can result in right atrial dilation, right ventricular overload, and increased pulmonary flow	Possibly a soft, systolic ejection murmur; otherwise, asymptomatic. Slender body. CHF may occur in ages 20 through 30 years

(continued)

TABLE 50.9 CONGENITAL HEART DISEASE (*CONTINUED*)

TYPE OF LESION	NAME OF LESION	PATHOPHYSIOLOGY	PRESENTATION
Shunt lesion (cont.)	VSD	Left-to-right shunting across an opening in the ventricular septum resulting in left atrial dilation, left ventricular overload, and increased pulmonary blood flow	Size-dependent, but often failure-to-thrive, frequent respiratory infections, and CHF symptoms
	AVC	Left-to-right shunting from three components: ASD, VSD, and abnormal formation of the AV valves	Depends on type of AVC. A small or partial AVC may be relatively asymptomatic. A large VSD will likely have CHF symptoms. Holistic murmur, tachypnea, and poor weight gain are likely with moderate to severe mitral valve regurgitation
	TA	Arterial trunk failed to separate and divide into an aorta and pulmonary artery. A single atrial vessel originates, overrides the ventricular septum, supplies the coronary and pulmonary arteries, and systemic circulations. A VSD is always present, and the truncal valve is abnormal (i.e., two to six leaflets). May be associated with DiGeorge syndrome	If undetected in utero, the infant presents in a cardiogenic shock state due to low cardiac output. Often CHF symptoms occur, bounding peripheral pulses, and cyanosis (if pulmonary stenosis is present)
	TAPVR	Drainage of the pulmonary veins into a systemic venous structure or right atrium instead of the left atrium. Can be partial or complete. Unobstructed TAPVR has left-to-right shunting with increased pulmonary flow and right AV dilation. Obstructed TAPVR creates pulmonary hypertension and pulmonary edema, including CHF	Unobstructed TAPVR may present with CHF symptoms, mild cyanosis, inadequate growth, and frequent pulmonary infections. Positive snowman's sign on chest x-ray by 4 months of age. Obstructed TAPVR may have marked cyanosis and respiratory distress during the neonatal period. Chest x-ray has normal size, but there is evidence of pulmonary edema
Left-side obstruction	COA	A narrowing of the aorta, usually near the ductus arteriosus, which can be associated with bicuspid aortic valve, VSD, or mitral stenosis. May be associated with Turner's syndrome	Neonatal presentation results from acute onset obstruction once the ductus arteriosus closes, resulting in CHF and shock. Infant or childhood presentation results from chronic LV pressure and includes hypertension and thoracic aortic collateral development. Hallmark findings are significant differences between systolic and diastolic pressures (15 mmHg or more) between upper and lower extremities, and differences in the quality of pulses (i.e., weaker in the lower extremities)
	IAA	Lack of continuity between the ascending and descending aorta. Three types: A, interruption is distal to the left subclavian artery; B (most common), interruption is between the carotid and subclavian arteries; and C, interruption is between carotid arteries	Cardiovascular collapse occurs upon closure of the ductus arteriosus in the immediate neonatal period. LV failure with pulmonary edema can result from chronically obstructed blood flow until surgically corrected
	AS	Thickened tissue occurring above, below, or at the level of the aortic valve	In utero, mild symptoms may be LVH. After birth, moderate LVH, normal LV size, but asymptomatic. Severe AS will present with a neonate in CHF; cardiac output is significantly compromised without a patent ductus arteriosus
Right-side obstruction	PS	Thickened tissue occurring above, below, or at the level of the pulmonic valve, causing a rise in RV pressure. Right-to-left shunting occurs	Neonates with severe PS will be cyanotic and critically ill. Children with mild to moderate PS are usually asymptomatic. Exercise intolerance and fatigue may be initial symptoms

(*continued*)

TABLE 50.9 CONGENITAL HEART DISEASE (*CONTINUED*)

TYPE OF LESION	NAME OF LESION	PATHOPHYSIOLOGY	PRESENTATION
Right-side obstruction (cont.)	TOF	Four characteristics: VSD, PS (RV outflow obstruction), overriding aorta, and RVH. Associated intracardiac defects can include ASD and defects in the left superior vena cava	Most common cyanotic CHD and is dependent on the degree of pulmonary obstruction. Characteristic murmur is harsh at the left sternal border. A boot-shaped heart on chest x-ray. Most children are asymptomatic until surgical repair (about 6 months of age)
	Absent pulmonary valve	A variant form of TOF. Usually accompanied by a VSD, pulmonary outflow obstruction, and dilated pulmonary arteries. The RV is markedly hypertrophied and pulmonary arteries are markedly dilated	Infants present with extreme respiratory distress, cyanosis, wheezing, and tachypnea. One-third of infants will die
	SV	One or two ventricles. In two ventricles, one ventricle is dominant due to hypoplasia of the other, or the AV valve does not allow for partitioning of the two ventricles. Also, often atresia of the AV or semilunar valves occurs. Complete mixing of venous returns occurs. Congenital defects include tricuspid atresia, pulmonary atresia with intact ventricular septum and hypoplastic RV, double-inlet LV, and hypoplastic left heart syndrome	Dependent on pulmonary blood flow. Severe cases present with CHF and hypoxemia, usually without poor blood pressure or metabolic acidosis. Excessive pulmonary flow occurs with less systemic circulation resulting in shock and death
	Pulmonary atresia (with intact ventricular septum)	The pulmonic valve is imperforate, and pulmonary blood flow is ductal-dependent. Considered a variant of SV pathology. An enlarged RV is present, and an ASD is essential for survival because of right-to-left shunting. Coronary artery anatomical changes are common	Usual presentation at the time of ductus arteriosus closure with significant metabolic acidosis and decreased cardiac output. A soft, pansystolic murmur heard at the left lower sternal border
Conotruncal lesion	TGV	The aorta originates from the RV and the pulmonary artery originates from the LV. Often associated with VSD, but less often with coarctation or obstruction to LV flow outflow. Anomalies of the coronary arteries is possible	Severe hypoxia and cyanosis until surgical correction is completed. A lethal defect if not corrected in the first few days to week of life

AS, aortic stenosis; ASD, atrial septal defect; AVC, atrioventricular canal; CHF, congestive heart failure; COA, coarctation of the aorta; IAA, interrupted aortic arch; LV, left ventricular; LVH, left ventricular hypertrophy; PDA, patent ductus arteriosus; PS, pulmonary stenosis; RV, right ventricular; RVH, right ventricular hypertrophy; SV, single ventricle; TA, truncus arteriosus; TAPVR, total anomalous pulmonary venous return; TGV, transposition of the great vessels; TOF, tetrology of Fallot; VSD, ventricular septal defect.

Children With Pulmonary Emergencies

A. Upper and lower airway differences exist between children and adults until approximately 8 years of age. Upper airway differences include the head, which is larger in proportion to the body and increases airway obstruction when the child is in supine position and without support under the shoulders. Small nasal airways increase resistance to air flow and are exponentially affected by increased secretions, edema, or blood. While the ethmoid and maxillary sinuses are present at birth, the frontal sinuses are not developed until 5 to 7 years of age. Increased secretions from the sinuses may cause upper airway difficulty and present a risk for aspiration into lower airways in the younger child. The nasopharynx consists of the Eustachian tubes, adenoids, and tonsils, which are subject to obstructive nasal breathing and complications from repeated infections. The oropharynx contains the soft palate extending to the tip of the epiglottis and includes the tongue, which can cause obstruction in the relaxed, supine-lying infant or child. The larynx, including the vocal cords, is located between the pharynx and the trachea, with its narrowest point at the cricoid cartilage (the only complete cartilaginous ring). Uncuffed endotracheal tubes have long been recommended to decrease the risk of acquired subglottic stenosis with prolonged or repeated intubations.

B. Cricoid cartilage in a newborn is located near the C4 area, in a school-aged child around C5, and by adulthood around the C6 area. This variation affects the angle at which visualization of the vocal cords for intubation may occur.

C. The epiglottis is relatively round and floppy in children, whereas in adults a firm, leaf-shaped structure is present. For this reason, a straight Miller laryngoscope blade is more likely to lift the epiglottis.[26]

D. The chest wall is less ossified in infants, and the ribs are positioned in a more horizontal plane than an adult whose ribs are fully ossified and are positioned in more downward plane.

E. Cartilaginous ribs and less muscle mass attribute to increased chest wall compliance, making retractions much more notable in children. Lower airway differences include the trachea, which bifurcates into the right and left mainstem bronchi. When compared to the left, the right mainstem bronchus is larger with less of an angle at the bifurcation, thereby contributing to easier aspiration of material. Also, the trachea is of smaller diameter, with weaker cartilage, in infants and young children, resulting in an increased resistance to flow and potential collapse of the airways (atelectasis) during expiration. Edema and secretions increase the already high resistance to flow by a power of four in children when compared to the same amount of edema or secretions in the adult. In the lungs, segmental bronchi create branches in each lung lobe. In infancy, a lung has nearly 20 segmental bronchi, with approximately 50 million alveoli for gas exchange to occur. By adulthood, there are about 25 segmental bronchi and 500 million alveoli.[26]

F. Apparent life-threatening event

1. An apparent life-threatening event (ALTE) is alarming to the observer. The National Institutes of Health (NIH) characterize the condition as a combination of apnea spell(s), color change, change in muscle tone, choking, or gagging.[26]

2. This condition was previously known as "near-miss sudden infant death syndrome." Etiology varies, and in most cases is unknown despite diagnostic testing. The average age of occurrence is about 10 weeks, and usually the infant has a "normal" appearance upon arrival in the ED.

G. Asthma

1. An airway obstruction resulting from inflamed airways becoming hyperresponsive (broncho constricted) and edematous (swollen). Current evidence-based recommendations by the National Heart, Lung, and Blood Institute (NHLBI)[27] include a short-acting $beta_2$ agonist (SABA) and oral (or IV) corticosteroids (1-2 mg/kg/24 hours) within the first hour of an acute exacerbation.

2. A mild exacerbation may result in discharge after 60 minutes of observation following the last SABA with the child remaining symptom-free, maintaining oxygen saturations on room air, able to eat or drink without difficulty, and forced expiratory volume in one second (FEV_1) is 70% or more of predicted value.

3. Inpatient admission is warranted if symptoms continue, there is an oxygen requirement, SABA is required more than every 2 hours, or there is a history of a pediatric ICU admission for asthma.[26]

H. Bronchiolitis

1. Bronchiolitis is a common viral respiratory infection in infants and young children characterized by edema, secretions, and bronchiolar epithelium changes.

2. The infection begins in the upper airways (i.e., rhinorrhea, congestion, and low-grade fever), but travels to the lower airways within 2 to 5 days.

3. Cough and wheezing begin, but air trapping and hyperinflation may occur from bronchiolar changes, and the mismatch of pulmonary ventilation and perfusion can result in hypoxemia.

4. Atelectasis occurs when the bronchioles become completely obstructed and trapped air becomes absorbed. Edema, secretions, and atelectasis contribute to increased resistance to flow and place the infant or child at risk for respiratory distress and failure.

5. Currently, evidence-based practice guidelines recommend diagnosis based on history; there is limited evidence to support the use of diagnostics.[28]

6. Supportive therapy is recommended.

I. Pneumonia

1. Pneumonia is an infection and inflammation of the lower airways and a major cause of morbidity and mortality in infants and children.

2. Common etiologies are viruses, then bacteria and atypical microorganisms.

3. Children generally present with fever and respiratory symptoms; however, bacterial pneumonia should be suspected in children <2 years of age with tachypnea and a fever >38°C (100.4°F).

TABLE 50.10 ANTIMICROBIAL THERAPY FOR PEDIATRIC PNEUMONIA

AGE	RECOMMENDED ANTIMICROBIAL	ALTERNATIVES
Birth to 1 month	Ampicillin and gentamicin (IV)	Cefotaxime may be considered.
1 month to 3 months (well-appearing)	High-dose amoxicillin (PO)	Sulfamethoxazole-trimethoprim, amoxicillin-clavulanic acid, or macrolide. Parenteral ceftriaxone for the first dose, then amoxicillin
1 month to 3 months (ill-appearing)	Cefotaxime or cefuroxime (IV)	Add macrolide if pertussis or chlamydia suspected
4 months to 5 years	High-dose amoxicillin (PO)	Sulfamethoxazole-trimethoprim, amoxicillin-clavulanic acid, or macrolide
6 years to adolescence	Macrolide (PO)	Amoxicillin-clavulanic acid or cephalosporin if *S. pneumoniae* suspected

4. Diagnosis of pneumonia is made clinically, but even a negative CXR does not rule out the diagnosis of pneumonia. While viral etiologies do not require antibiotics, bacterial and atypical microorganisms do (Table 50.10).

Children With Renal and Urologic Emergencies

A. At birth, all nephrons of the kidney are present. The kidney reaches an adult size by adolescence. Small amounts of urine are in the bladder at birth, yet the neonate may not void for 12 to 24 hours. Renal blood flow increases at birth, but shorter loops result in more dilute urine up to 6 months of age. While the immature kidney is less responsive to antidiuretic hormone, the glomerular filtration rate (GFR) is at adult levels by 2-years of age.[29] Consequently, infants and young children are at an increased risk for fluid imbalance and acidosis. An infant's daily exchange of 600 to 700 mL is nearly 50% of extracellular volume, making control of fluid balance a challenge.

B. Acute poststreptococcal glomerulonephritis

1. Acute poststreptococcal glomerulonephritis (PSGN) is relatively common in children 5 to 15 years of age. The condition occurs 1 to 2 weeks after pharyngitis or up to 6 weeks after an impetigo infection with strains of group A beta-hemolytic streptococci (or possibly *Staphylococcus*). Often, the antigen or antigen–antibody complexes become trapped within the glomerulus. The glomerulus becomes thickened, and the GFR decreases. Membrane permeability is altered, causing hematuria and proteinuria to occur along with mild hypertension because of fluid retention.[29]

2. Acute treatment is directed by the severity of the illness. Focus to prevent hypertension and edema. Restriction of salt and water can help prevent these conditions. Loop diuretics also help to manage hypertension and edema. In the acute phase, admission is advised to manage these potential complications.

3. A renal biopsy may be needed, depending on the severity of the disease. Indications for renal dialysis include hyperkalemia and uremia.

4. Physical activity should be restricted until the child is feeling better.

C. Nephroblastoma (Wilms tumor)

1. Wilms tumor is an embryonal tumor of the kidney resulting from an abnormal proliferation of renal stem cells. Most children with the tumor are between 1 and 5 years of age, female, and Black rather than White. Most Wilms tumors present as an enlarging, asymptomatic upper abdominal mass in an otherwise healthy child.[29] Most tumors are discovered by the parent when dressing or bathing the child.

2. *Physical exam:* A firm, nontender mass is palpated on one (or both) side(s) of the abdomen. Surgical intervention is needed for staging and subsequent treatment, but survival is 85% to 90% 4 years post tumor.

D. Urinary tract infection (UTI)

1. UTI occurs anywhere along the urinary tract (urethra, bladder, ureter, and kidney). During the neonatal period, uncircumcised males and infants with congenital renal abnormalities are at increased risk.[29] Females are more likely to acquire a UTI after 1 year of age and have an increased risk during adolescence. The pathophysiology in children is like that of adults; however, symptoms are nonspecific.

2. Risk factors for pediatric UTIs include younger age, female sex, uncircumcised boys, and non-Black race. Consider a possible UTI with a medical history of premature birth, sexually active, genitourinary abnormalities, chronic constipation, and immunocompromised.

3. Clinical evaluation will be determined by the child's age. It is noted that neonatal patients should have sterile urine obtained through catheterization or suprapubic aspiration. In infants and children, a catheter urine culture should be obtained. In school-aged children and adolescents, a catheter collected urine is better, but clean catch urine samples may be obtained.

4. Possible urosepsis should always be considered. Infants and children with a febrile UTI may have an indication for hospital admission. These indications include age younger than 2 months, unstable vital signs, immunocompromised, ill-appearing or lethargic, unable to tolerate oral medications, known genitourinary abnormality, failure of outpatient treatment, and family or caregiver who cannot provide the care for the ill child.

5. In children 2 to 24 months of age, antimicrobial treatment can be oral over the course of 2 to 4 days for uncomplicated UTI, but parenteral antibiotics until clinically improved is recommended for more complicated cases.[30] Antibiotics should be used as indicated, without putting the child at risk of developing antibiotic resistance. The emergency nurse practitioner (ENP) needs to be aware of current guidelines.

Children With Gastrointestinal Emergencies

A. The gastrointestinal tract originates at the mouth and ends at the anus. Disorders of the GI tract in children include congenital anomalies with structural and functional alterations, enzyme deficiencies, and infection, all of which can affect motility, digestion, nutrition, growth, and development.

B. Esophageal atresia/tracheoesophageal fistula

1. Esophageal atresia (EA) is the term used when the esophagus ends as a pouch. Usually, EA has a fistula between the esophagus and the trachea (tracheoesophageal fistula [TEF]); however, either defect can occur alone. EA is suspected at birth when the neonate has drooling, cannot swallow secretions, or has choking with feeding, respiratory distress, and an inability to pass an orogastric tube.

2. Radiographic evaluation confirms the diagnosis. Pulmonary complications can occur from aspiration and chemical irritation.

3. Following diagnosis, a tube with continuous suction should be placed into the pouch, the head of the bed elevated, and the neonate should not be fed until surgical repair is completed.[31]

C. Pyloric stenosis

1. The most common cause of intestinal obstruction in infancy is a narrowing of the pylorus due to thickening, causing obstruction resulting in vomiting. This condition occurs in the first few weeks of life, is twice as likely in males than females, Whites more often than Blacks, and full-term more often than premature infants. The usual presentation is a well-appearing, weight-gaining neonate with a sudden onset of projectile vomiting within 20 minutes of feeding. Hunger after the vomiting is another sign. Constipation occurs due to little food being digested. The neonate is difficult to console because of hunger and the discomfort of vomiting and esophagitis. Sometimes, a small palpable, olive-sized mass is in the right upper quadrant (RUQ).

2. Ultrasound is the diagnostic of choice for definitive diagnosis.

3. Surgical repair is the definitive treatment.

D. Malrotation

1. Most common congenital anomaly of the small intestine.[31] The small intestine is not posteriorly fixated as it should be and is only fixated at the origin of the superior mesenteric artery. If rotation does not occur, the colon remains in the RUQ where a membrane (or band) called a periduodenal band may press on and obstruct the duodenum.[31] The nonfixated loops of the intestine can then twist upon themselves (volvulus). This twisting can partially or completely occlude the superior mesenteric artery, causing necrosis of the midgut. Most cases of malrotation (volvulus) develop in the neonatal period, but some develop during childhood or adulthood.

2. Symptoms include bilious vomiting after feeding and gastric distention after feeding. Dehydration and electrolyte imbalance occur due to vomiting. Fever can occur. Diarrhea and bloody stools are congruent with progressive volvulus and necrosis.[31]

3. Diagnosis is based on clinical history and presentation, radiographic diagnostics, and exploratory surgery with correction of the defect(s).

E. Gastroesophageal reflux disease (GERD)

1. GERD is the passage of gastric contents into the esophagus independent of swallowing, irritating the esophagus, and if untreated, can cause injury to the esophagus.[31]

2. Clinical presentations include excessive vomiting, anorexia, inconsolable crying, choking/gagging, insomnia, dysphagia, and/or abdominal pain. Extraesophageal symptoms include cough and wheezing, laryngitis, pharyngitis, dental issues, sinusitis, and recurrent otitis media.[31] Mild GERD in infancy is resolved by nonpharmacologic treatment: small frequent feedings, frequent burping, position changes, and thickened feedings. For children and adolescents, weight loss, smoking cessation, sleeping position changes, and avoidance of caffeine, chocolate, alcohol, and spicy foods may be encouraged.[31]

3. Medications are prescribed to treat esophagitis, including proton pump inhibitors and prokinetic agents.

4. Definitive treatment is a fundoplication surgical procedure.

F. Intussusception

1. Intussusception is the invagination of intestine into itself, causing a temporary obstruction. This condition is the most common cause of small bowel obstruction in children, with most cases occurring under the age of 5 years and more often in males than females.[31]

2. Children present with abdominal pain causing the knees to be drawn up to the chest at intervals in an otherwise asymptomatic, healthy child. Lethargy can be a significant symptom. Other symptoms may include an abdominal mass (sausage-shaped and palpable), vomiting, and bloody (currant-jelly) stoolst. Diagnosis is based on clinical history and findings.

3. Abdominal radiographs, CT, point of care ultrasound (PoCUS) of the abdomen can assist in the diagnosis.

4. Air-contrast or gastrogaffin enema can be effective in reducing the obstruction; surgical reduction may be required for treatment.

5. Because of the possibility of reoccurrence, admitting for observation should be considered.

G. Gastroenteritis (GE) and dehydration

1. *In infants, water accounts for about 70% of their lean body mass (LBM):* Intracellular fluid (45%), extracellular fluid (25%), interstitial fluid (19%), and plasma (6%).[32]

2. In children under 5, LBM is approximately 60% water, but by 5 years of age, the LBM is essentially that of an adult, with extracellular fluid consisting of 20% water and 50% within the intracellular compartments.

3. Because of the higher water/LBM ratios in infants and children and greater excretion of fluids per day, the risk of dehydration is increased when compared to adults.[32]

4. GE

a. *Isonatremic dehydration (Na: 130–150 mEq/L):* Water and salt concentrations are usually balanced in stool; however, vomiting decreases oral intake, resulting in additional water loss and contributes to a more hypernatremic dehydration (Na: >150 mEq/L).

b. GE may evolve into a hypernatremic dehydration. It may also result from excessive sweating, certain medications, significant thermal injury, or renal disease.

c. Hyponatremic dehydration (Na: <130 mEq/L) can result from loss of fluid and salt in stool or sweat.

5. Diagnostic testing

a. For mild to moderate dehydration due to GE, serum diagnostics are not recommended.[32]

b. A clinical dehydration score may be used to determine the severity of dehydration.[33] The use of the mnemonic "GETT" may be useful in remembering the significant clinical findings for scoring.

6. Treatment

a. Fluid and electrolyte replacement

b. In mild to moderate dehydration, oral rehydration therapy with an oral rehydrating solution

(ORS) is the preferred method for replacement, with 50 to 100 mL/kg ORS over 2 to 4 hours. In addition, for children:

i. *10 kg:* Add 60 to 120 mL ORS for each episode of vomiting or diarrhea occurring during the replacement phase.

ii. *≥10 kg:* Add 120 to 240 mL ORS for each episode of vomiting or diarrhea occurring during the replacement phase.

iii. Beverages such as Gatorade are insufficient for GE as this formulation is specific for the prevention of dehydration from sweating.

iv. Fluids such as soda, apple juice, or chicken broth contain high amounts of carbohydrates, sodium, and have high osmolarities, thus worsening dehydration and the electrolyte imbalance. An oral antiemetic may be considered in the case of repeated vomiting, but antidiarrheal medications are not recommended.[32]

c. In more moderate to severe dehydration, parenteral fluid administration is necessary.

i. For isonatremic and hyponatremic dehydration states, fluid replacement with normal saline is preferred, but Ringer's lactate may be more beneficial in hypernatremic (or hyperchloremic) dehydration and in the case of dehydration caused by thermal injury.

ii. A 20 mL/kg fluid bolus repeated as needed is given for the initial replacement therapy. Glucose is avoided in the initial replacement phase unless there is a documented hypoglycemia, but 5% glucose is added for ongoing maintenance.

iii. Potassium may be added (20 mEq/L) once adequate renal function is established.

iv. The Holliday and Segar Maintenance Fluid Calculation (cited in[37]) determines the volume of fluid required for maintenance therapy based on the average kilocalories used per day

(1) *3 to 10 kg:* 100 mL/kg/day at a rate of 4 mL/kg/hour

(2) *10 to 20 kg:* 1,000 mL + 50 mL for each kg over 10 at a rate of 40 mL/hour + 2 mL/hour for each kg over 10

(3) *20 to 70 kg:* 1,500 mL + 20 mL for each kg over 20 at a rate of 60 mL/hour + 1 mL/hour for each kg over 20

d. Return of a child's normal diet should occur as soon as possible. Assuring follow-up care with a medical clinician the next day is important to evaluate if rehydration has been successful.

Children With Musculoskeletal Emergencies

A. In children, musculoskeletal disorders can be congenital, hereditary, or acquired and can be acute or chronic. Bone growth in children begins in utero and continues until adult stature is reached at the end of puberty. Primary ossification begins in the diaphysis where bone develops and at the secondary ossification centers located in the epiphysis.[34] The physes, located on each epiphyseal plate of the bones, are the center for constant endochondral ossification and determine the growth and sensitivity to injury during childhood. Growth hormone must be constantly secreted by the pituitary gland to stimulate growth at the physes.[35] The apophyses are secondary growth plates located in areas where the muscle–tendon elements attach to bones. While the apophyses do not enhance growth of the long bones, the apophyses and physes are made of similar growth cartilage.[34]

B. Once skeletal maturity occurs, bone cells continue to be destroyed and restored. In children, this process is rapidly occurring, which allows for bone healing to be achieved more quickly in the case of injury; however, there is evidence demonstrating the importance of vitamin D and its role in bone healing for children and adults.[35]

C. Skeletal development begins with the axial skeleton. A newborn has a kyphosed spine, and lordosis (curvature) of the spine occurs with developmental milestones, such as head control (cervical spine) and sitting (lumbar spine) during infancy. Likewise, the extremities grow during childhood but are dependent on spinal growth which also has a role in preventing premature fusion of the physes. Rotation and alignment of the long bones occur between 8 and 12 years of age. Furthermore, growth of muscle occurs in concert with growth of the skeleton. The facial and respiratory muscle groups are well developed at birth, but muscle groups such as the pelvic muscles take several years to develop.[35]

D. Osteogenesis imperfecta (OI)

1. Also known as brittle bone disease, OI is a collagen-related dysplasia. An error in the synthesis of collagen occurs as a result of a genetic alteration in the triple helix (matching two alpha chains and one beta chain).

2. The severity of OI is dependent upon the severity of the genetic anomaly and metabolic abnormalities, such as thyroxine levels.

3. A child with OI presents with osteoporosis, fractures, triangular facies, poor dentition and possible bony deformations, vascular weakness (aneurysms), and blue sclerae.[35] Serum alkaline phosphatase levels are elevated in all forms of OI.

4. Careful positioning and handling during infancy can help prevent fractures. Prompt splinting of fractures and correction of deformities assist in minimizing the disabilities incurred from OI.

E. Osteomyelitis

1. Infection in the bone when bacteria enter the bone through the bloodstream and lodges in the medullary cavity at the end of the venous loops beneath the epiphyseal plate

2. Infection develops because there are no phagocytic cells present to remove bacteria.[35]

3. Neonates and infants are commonly infected by *Staphylococcus aureus*; however, Group B *Streptococcus* and *Escherichia coli* can occur. In older children, *S. aureus* and methicillin-resistant *S. aureus* (MRSA) are the most common organisms for infection.[35]

4. Infants

a. Illness is characterized by fever and failure to move the extremity. In children aged 1 year to puberty, fever, and systemic signs of toxicity can occur.

b. Often, the child experiences an abrupt onset of swelling, fever, tenderness, and a decreased ability to move or bear weight on the extremity.

c. An elevated white blood cell (WBC) count, erythrocyte sedimentation rate, and C-reactive protein are indicators for osteomyelitis when accompanied by these symptoms.

d. A bone scan can be positive for osteomyelitis within 48 hours of symptom onset.

5. Adolescents

a. The vertebrae may be involved with back pain as the only symptom. Parenteral antibiotics should be administered after culture and sensitivity studies are performed; however, a combination of oral and parenteral antibiotics over 6 weeks may be used in reliable patients and families. A tuberculin skin test is recommended because *Mycobacterium tuberculosis* is sometimes the causative organism.[35]

b. Immobilization may assist in pain control.

F. Legg-Calvé-Perthes disease

1. Legg-Calvé-Perthes disease (LCPD), also known as Perthes disease, generally occurs between 3 and 10 years of age and is more common in boys. The natural course of Perthes disease is 2 to 5 years.

a. In the first stage, the soft tissue of the hip is swollen, edematous, hyperemic, and there is fluid in the joint. As the joint space widens, the joint capsule enlarges.

b. After several weeks, fragmentation occurs (the second stage) where the epiphysis of the femoral head loses blood supply resulting in the metaphyseal bone on the femoral neck and epiphyseal plate to soften from decalcification.

c. The third stage (healing) can last 2 to 3 years as the dead femoral head is replaced by callus, eventually becoming flattened, with the femoral neck becoming short and wide.

d. In the last stage (healed), remodeling occurs and spongy bone becomes evident.[35]

2. The onset of symptoms is insidious; referred knee pain may result in a misdiagnosis. The inner thigh and groin can be painful with motion. A typical finding includes spasm on inward rotation of the hip with a limited internal rotation, flexion, and abduction.[35] An abnormal gait is evident, with the trunk bent toward the affected side. If muscle atrophy occurs (such as in the case of prolonged symptoms), a limb length discrepancy can occur.

3. Diagnosis is confirmed with a plain film.

4. Treatment involves keeping the femoral head in the socket and some motion to maintain the articular cartilage. Anti-inflammatory medications and crutches may be helpful during the active phase of the disease. Orthopedic follow-up is recommended.

G. Osgood-Schlatter disease

1. Osgood-Schlatter disease (OSD) is a tendonitis of the anterior patellar tendon (with the patella imbedded in the tendon). This condition occurs more often in boys, and in athletic preadolescent or adolescent individuals. Avascular necrosis of the tibial tubercle causes a hypertrophic cartilage formation during repair.[35] The hypertrophied cartilage causes a pronounced and tender area near or at the tibial tubercle, especially after physical activity.

2. Diagnosis is made on plain film evaluation.

3. Treatment is aimed at reducing stress and inflammation at the tubercle with 4 to 8 weeks of rest and anti-inflammatory medications. If pain is not relieved after a rest period and anti-inflammatory treatment, then casting or bracing may need to be considered.[35]

H. Slipped capital femoral epiphysis

1. A slipped capital femoral epiphysis (SCFE) is a separation of the physis on the proximal femoral head. The epiphysis begins to slip posteriorly, and avascular necrosis of the femoral head begins to occur. This condition typically occurs between 12 and 15 years of age in African American or Hispanic males, and in those who are obese.[36]

2. Symptoms include complaints of acute or chronic hip, thigh, or knee pain and limited internal rotation. The child has an observed external rotation of the hip. As the condition progresses, a limb length discrepancy occurs. If the condition is acute, severe pain and a dramatic change in gait occurs .[36]

3. To establish a diagnosis of SCFE, plain films of the pelvis and a "frog-leg" view are recommended, which demonstrate the appearance of an "ice cream slipping off a cone." Compare to the contralateral side.[36]

4. Once diagnosed, strict non-weight-bearing orders are recommended until surgical correction can be done.

I. Toxic synovitis

1. Toxic (transient) synovitis (TS) is an inflammatory condition affecting large joint spaces, especially the hip (but can be the knee). This condition usually occurs between 3 and 8 years of age and lasts a few days to weeks. While the etiology is unknown, it is suspected to result from a previous viral infection, trauma, or allergic reaction.

2. Children present typically present with mild fever, acute joint pain, limping (antalgic) gait, and refusal to bear weight. On physical examination, there is mild limitation on abduction and internal rotation of the femoral head.

3. Differential diagnoses include septic arthritis (SA), osteomyelitis, trauma, or neoplasm. Children with osteomyelitis or SA are much more toxic-appearing.

4. Common serum diagnostic findings include a complete blood count (WBCs may be elevated), C-reactive protein (mildly elevated), and erythrocyte sedimentation rate (more than 40 mm/hour).[36]

5. Plain films evaluate for trauma or bony abnormality but are not definitive for TS. Ultrasound assists in the evaluation for excessive joint fluid, and if found, can be aspirated by an interventional radiologist for analysis to rule out SA. In TS, joint fluid analysis is unremarkable. An MRI or bone scan can evaluate for osteomyelitis or neoplasm.[36]

6. Treatment for TS is regular dosing of oral anti-inflammatory medication for a week, and symptomatic care such as ice and elevation of the affected extremity.

J. SA

1. SA is a bacterial infection in the synovial fluid of a joint. Rapid destruction of articular cartilage (within 6 hours) can occur.[37] The joints most affected are the hip, knee, elbow, and ankle. Osteomyelitis is often a precursor to SA due to the intraarticular location of metaphyseal bone.[37] Peak incidence is in children 3 years or younger, and males are affected twice as often as females.[37] In neonates, group B ß-hemolytic *Streptococcus* is common, *Kingella kingae* is frequent in children under 4 years of age with a history of an upper respiratory infection, but *S. aureus* is the most common organism for almost all children.[37]

2. In SA, neonates may have an inconsolable cry or be difficult to arouse, have decreased oral feeding, and fail to spontaneously move a limb. Children with SA complain of acute joint pain and refuse or have difficulty using the extremity. Generally, a history of upper respiratory infection or soft-tissue infection is present.

3. The infected joint is painful, erythematous, warm, and swollen.[37] Joint range of motion is painful and limited. If the hip is affected, the child will lay with the hip in external rotation, adduction, and mild flexion.[37] A fever >38°C (100°F) and ill appearance may be present.

4. A complete blood count may be normal, but the C-reactive protein and erythrocyte sedimentation rates will be elevated. Ultrasound is the most useful radiographic evaluation for joint effusion, and culture from aspirated joint fluid will likely identify a pathogen.[37]

5. Parenteral antibiotics are initiated as soon as cultures are obtained. Immediate orthopedic consultation is recommended for surgical irrigation and drainage.

Children With Dermatologic Emergencies

A. Dermatologic pathologies in children have some similarities to adults; however, there may be different etiologies and patterns of distribution. With all skin pathologies, a history, appearance, and pattern of distribution are important factors when formulating a diagnosis.

B. Atopic dermatitis

1. Atopic dermatitis (AD), also known as eczema, has a prevalence of 25% in children when compared to 2% to 3% in the adult population.[38] The onset of AD occurs as early as 2 months of age, with most cases occurring in the first 5 years of life. The exact cause is unknown, but is suspected to be a combination of genetic predisposition and an altered skin barrier function. AD has a variety of clinical features, including frequent exacerbations, severe pruritis, and a characteristic appearance of redness, mild swelling, and severe pruritis.[38] As barrier function becomes increasingly impaired, skin becomes more dry, sensitive, pruritic, and inflamed. Of these, pruritis is the hallmark sign of AD.

2. *Infants and young children:* AD rash appears on the face, scalp, trunk, and extensor surfaces.

3. *Older children and adults:* Rash is more commonly found on the neck, antecubital and popliteal fossa, hands, and feet. Lichenification is more common in adolescents and adults due to scarring from chronic scratching.

4. There are no specific laboratory diagnostics to assist in diagnosis and treatment for AD, as this is a clinical diagnosis.

5. Acute treatment recommendations include topical and/or oral anti-inflammatory agents, such as topical corticosteroids, calcineurin inhibitors, and diphenhydramine.

6. Maintenance of the condition involves the avoidance of triggers and the enhancement of skin hydration to include emollients. For those children developing skin infections from scratching, bleach baths are recommended.[38]

C. Impetigo contagiosum

1. Impetigo is a common skin infection usually caused by *S. aureus* and less commonly by *Streptococcus pyogenes*, or both. Impetigo is more common in summer, with hot, humid conditions, and an increase in skin-to-skin human contacts. Exfoliative toxins from the bacteria cause a blister formation and may result in a nonbullous or bullous type of the infection. As vesicular lesions form and rupture, a honey-colored crust appears. Often lesions are located on the face around the mouth and nose, but hands and other exposed skin may be involved.[38]

2. Topical mupirocin and fusidic acid are recommended for uncomplicated lesions, but systemic antibiotics may need to be added for complicated cases. If methicillin-resistant *S. aureus* is suspected, ß lactam antibiotics should be avoided.[38]

3. Complications from untreated impetigo include glomerulonephritis, necrotizing fasciitis, and septic shock.

4. Prevention education should include good handwashing and isolating the child's washcloth and towels, drinking, and eating utensils.

D. Staphylococcal scalded skin syndrome

1. Staphylococcal scalded-skin syndrome (SSSS) is the most serious skin infection affecting infants and children under 5 years of age. The condition is caused by virulent group II *Staphylococci* producing an exfoliative toxin. The toxin affects the adhesion matrix just below the granular layer of the epidermis, causing a separation of the skin.[38] Interestingly, *Staphylococci* are not found in the skin lesions themselves, but toxin is delivered to the skin from other sites via blood circulation. Adults have circulating anti-staphylococcal antibodies, which allows them to metabolize and excrete the toxin.

2. Diagnostics include culture and histologic or exfoliative cytology to be done to differentiate SSSS from Stevens–Johnson syndrome and toxic epidermal necrolysis associated with drug reactions.[38]

3. Neonates are at highest risk due to their immature immune systems and lack of immunity.

4. Symptoms include an acute onset of fever, malaise, rhinorrhea, difficult consolability, generalized erythema, and exquisite tenderness of the skin. Erythema begins on the face, travels to the trunk, then out to the extremities except for the palms, soles, and mucus membranes.[38] Within 24 to 48 hours, blisters and bullae develop, giving the child a "scalded" appearance. Severe pain requires analgesics; fluid loss from ruptured lesions and water evaporation warrant fluid replacement; and oral or parenteral antibiotics are needed.

5. In severe cases, the skin of the entire body may slough; therefore, treatment of children with SSSS by a burn team may mitigate exposure to secondary infection and enhance healing without scarring, especially to eyes and lips.

References and Additional Reading

References and Additional Reading for this chapter are online only and can be found at https://connect.springerpub.com/content/reference-book/978-0-8261-6091-5/part/part07/toc-part/ch50.

51. The Geriatric Patient

RENEÉ SEMONIN HOLLERAN

Learning Objectives

- Identify common age-related physiologic and cognitive changes in the geriatric patient.
- Use evidence-based guidelines to provide a comprehensive evaluation of the geriatric patient's physical function, cognitive function, and psychological and social situation.
- Identify common medical and traumatic geriatric emergencies.
- Provide pain management in the geriatric patient.
- Utilize the Beers Criteria for medication recommendations when prescribing for the geriatric patient
- Formulate a transition of care for the geriatric patient including a summary of the visit, notification of the patient's caregiver, or place of residence such as a skilled care facility, and written instructions.
- Identify community resources to provide care for the geriatric patient and family.
- Assure a safe environment for the geriatric patient within the ED.
- Initiate palliative or end-of-life (EOL) care when indicated based on the patient's Advance Directives or Physician's Orders for Life Sustaining Treatment (POLST) forms.

It is estimated that patients over the age of 65 years represent 15% of the population in the United States. This percentage is predicted to increase to 20% in 2030 and to double by 2050.[1,2] Visits to the EDs by geriatric patients increased by 24.5% between 2001 and 2009.[2]

Geriatric patients use the ED for many of the same reasons that other age groups do. However, they tend to use the ED at a higher rate, remain longer in the ED, and require more medical interventions and nursing care. Because the majority of older patients have more than one medical problem, take multiple medications, and suffer from diseases commonly associated with aging, it is more challenging to provide safe and competent care—especially in the ED environment—to this patient population.[3,4]

Important concepts related to the care of the geriatric patient in the ED include the following[5–7]:

- Geriatric patients who present to the ED generally have complex complaints.
- The disease process is not always clear as in other age groups. Common indicators of critical illnesses and injuries, including changes in vital signs, physical examination signs, and changes in laboratory findings, as well as imaging, are not always present in the geriatric patient.[7]
- The comorbid factors of aging must always be considered when evaluating the geriatric patient.
- Polypharmacy is common in geriatric patients. Medications [including over-the-counter (OTC), herbs, or other remedies] may be the source of some problems.
- Recognition of age-related changes such as cognitive impairment and frailty is important.
- Baseline assessment of functional status is important to know when evaluating a new problem.
- Geriatric patients experience decreased physiologic reserve, which places them at greater risk of morbidity and/or mortality from infections, and common pain complaints such as chest and abdominal pain.
- Diagnostic tests may have different values in the geriatric patient or be "normal" for that particular patient.
- The geriatric patient may have limited social support or access to needed resources which can affect their physical and mental care.
- It has been estimated that 23% of geriatric patients are undertriaged related to illness and injury when presenting to the ED.[7]
- An ED visit can be an opportunity to assess and intervene in a geriatric patient and their families' lives.

In 2010, Geriatric Competencies for Emergency Residents (EM) was published and was based on an expert consensus process.[8] This document addresses eight domains and 26 competencies specific to the management of the geriatric patients in the ED. Table 51.1 contains the EM resident's domains and competencies. These competencies provide a helpful foundation for the assessment and management of the geriatric patient in the ED.

General Approach to the Geriatric Patient

Physiological and Cognitive Changes in the Geriatric Patient[1,3,6,8,9–13]

A. Airway
  1. Tooth decay and loose teeth, increased risk of obstruction
  2. Presence of dentures or other oral appliances
  3. Oropharyngeal tumors
  4. Decreased gag reflex, increased risk of aspiration
  5. Limited cervical range of motion due to disease processes such as osteoarthritis, ankylosing spondylosis; rigidity from neuromuscular disease such as

TABLE 51.1 GERIATRIC COMPETENCIES FOR EMERGENCY RESIDENTS (EM): DOMAINS AND COMPETENCIES

DOMAIN	COMPETENCIES
I. Atypical presentation of diseases	**1.** Generate an age-specific differential diagnosis for elder patients presenting to the ED with general weakness, dizziness, falls, or altered mental status. **2.** Generate a differential diagnosis recognizing that signs and symptoms such as pain and fever may be absent or less prominent in elders with acute coronary syndromes, acute abdomens, or infectious processes. **3.** Document consideration of adverse reactions to medications, including drug–drug and drug–disease interactions, as part of the initial differential diagnosis.
II. Trauma including falls	**4.** In patients who have fallen, evaluate for precipitating causes of falls such as medications, alcohol use/abuse, gait or balance instability, medical illness, and/or deterioration of medical condition. **5.** Assess for gait instability in all ambulatory fallers; if present, ensure appropriate disposition and follow-up including attempt to reach primary care provider. **6.** Demonstrate ability to recognize patterns of trauma (physical/sexual, psychological, neglect/abandonment) that are consistent with elder abuse. Manage the abused patient in accordance with the rules of the state and institution. **7.** Institute appropriate early monitoring and testing with the understanding that elders may present with muted signs and symptoms (e.g., absent pain and neurologic changes) and are at risk for occult shock.
III. Cognitive and behavioral disorders	**8.** Assess whether an elder is able to give an accurate history, participate in determining the plan of care, and understand discharge instructions. **9.** Assess and document current mental status and any change from baseline in every elder, with special attention to determining if delirium exists or has been superimposed on dementia. **10.** Emergently evaluate and formulate an age-specific differential diagnosis for elders with new cognitive or behavioral impairment, including self-neglect; initiate a diagnostic workup to determine the etiology; and initiate treatment. **11.** Assess and correct (if appropriate) causative factors in agitated elders such as untreated pain, hypoxia, hypoglycemia, use of irritating tethers (defined as monitor leads, blood pressure cuff, pulse oximetry, intravenous access, and Foley catheter), environmental factors (light, temperature), and disorientation.
IV. Emergency intervention modifications	**12.** Recommend therapy based on the actual benefit to risk ratio, including but not limited to acute myocardial infarction, stroke, and sepsis, so that age alone does not exclude elders from any therapy. **13.** Identify and implement measures that protect elders from developing iatrogenic complications common to the ED including invasive bladder catheterization, spinal immobilization, and central line placement.
V. Medication management	**14.** Prescribe appropriate drugs and dosages considering the current medication, acute and chronic diagnoses, functional status, and knowledge of age-related physiologic changes (renal function, central nervous system sensitivity). **15.** Search for interactions and document reasons for use when prescribing drugs that present high risk either alone or in drug–drug or drug–disease interactions (e.g., benzodiazepines, digoxin, insulin, NSAIDs, opioids, and warfarin). **16.** Explain all newly prescribed drugs to elders and caregivers at discharge, assuring that they understand how and why the drug should be taken, the possible side effects, and how and when the drug should be stopped.
VI. Transitions of care	**17.** Document history obtained from skilled nursing or extended care facilities of the acute events necessitating ED transfer including goals of visit, medical history, medications, allergies, cognitive and functional status, advance care plan, and responsible PCP. **18.** Provide skilled nursing or extended care facilities and/or PCP with ED visit summary and plan of care, including follow-up when appropriate. **19.** With recognition of unique vulnerabilities in elders, assess and document suitability for discharge considering the ED diagnosis, including cognitive function, the ability in ambulatory patients to ambulate safely, availability of appropriate nutrition / social support, and the availability of access to appropriate follow-up therapies. **20.** Select and document the rationale for the most appropriate available disposition (home, extended care facility, hospital) with the least risk of the many complications commonly occurring in elders during inpatient hospitalizations. **21.** Rapidly establish and document an elder's goals of care for those with a serious or life-threatening condition and manage accordingly. **22.** Assess and provide ED management for pain and key nonpain symptoms based on the patient's goals of care. **23.** Know how to access hospice care and how to manage elders in hospice care while in the ED.
VIII. Effect of comorbid conditions	**24.** Assess and document the presence of comorbid conditions (e.g., pressure ulcers, cognitive status, falls in the past year, ability to walk and transfer, renal function, and social support) and include them in your medical decision-making and plan of care. **25.** Develop plans of care that anticipate and monitor for predictable complications in the patient's condition (e.g., gastrointestinal bleed causing ischemia). **26.** Communicate with patients with hearing/sight impairments, speech difficulties, aphasia, and cognitive disorders (e.g., using family / friend, writing).

EM, emergency medicine; NSAIDs, nonsteroidal anti-inflammatory drugs; PCP, primary care physician.

Source: With permission from Hogan TM, Losman ED, et al. Development of geriatric competencies for emergency medicine residents using an expert consensus process. *Acad Emerg Med.* 2010 Mar;17(3):316–24. doi: 10.1111/j.1553–2712.2010.00684.x., Table 3.[8]

Parkinson's disease; multiple cervical surgeries with fusion, and hardware placement
6. Increased airway resistance

B. Respiratory
1. Decreased respiratory muscle strength
2. Decreased elasticity of lung tissue, which contributes to decreased vital capacity
3. Diminished cough reflex
4. Increased anterior/posterior diameter; chest deformities, kyphosis
5. Underlying pulmonary diseases such as chronic obstructive pulmonary disease (COPD), lung scarring, and fibrosis
6. Inability to tolerate a supine position

C. Cardiovascular
1. Stiffening of the arterial vascular and myocardium, which can lead to higher baseline blood pressure.
2. A stressor such as an infection or inappropriate medication dose can cause a precipitous drop in blood pressure.
3. Decreased peripheral blood flow
4. Reduction in total body water can cause dehydration.
5. Diastolic function is prolonged.
6. Systolic murmurs are more common with aging.

D. Renal
1. Decrease in creatinine clearance occurs with age
2. Decrease in creatinine clearance affects the kidneys' ability to clear medications
3. Serum creatinine should not be used to estimate renal function. It is recommended that glomerular filtration rate (GFR) should be calculated for a more accurate GFR. Crockroft-Gault equation should be used, especially when prescribing medication (www.kidney.org/professionals/KDOQI/gfr_calculatorCoc).
4. Decrease in ability to retain sodium and water will place the patient at risk for dehydration.
5. Impaired thirst response and poor oral intake can put patients at risk of reduction in total body water resulting in physical, motor, and cognitive impairments.

E. Neurologic
1. Cognitive changes should not be attributed to age alone.
2. Delirium is a sign of acute illness in the elderly.
3. Medications, alcohol, and other illicit drugs can cause confusion and delirium.
4. Dementia may be missed in an ED depending on the reason for the patient's visit.
5. ED should have tools to identify and manage dementia. Seven A's of dementia:
   a. *Anosognosia:* Loss of awareness of the disease
   b. *Agnosia:* Loss of recognition through senses
   c. *Aphasia:* Loss of language
   d. *Apraxia:* Loss of purposeful action
   e. Altered perception
   f. *Amnesia:* Loss of memory
   g. *Apathy:* Loss of initiative

F. Eyes, hearing, taste
1. Visual changes such as the development of cataracts place patients at risk of falling.
2. Arcus senilis is a common variation in older patients' eyes, which is a benign peripheral ring of opacification that does not interfere with vision.
3. Patient may have cataracts, glaucoma, or macular degeneration, which can place the patient at risk of falling or increase inability to read and take medications correctly.
4. High-frequency sounds become harder to hear (presbycusis). Sensorineural hearing loss can occur from trauma, medications, or other chronic medical problems.
5. Taste begins to change after the age of 50. Decrease in saliva production leads to dry mouth. Atrophic changes in the mouth place patients at risk of pain and development of ulcers. All can interfere with the patient's ability to eat and overall nutrition.

G. Musculoskeletal/frailty/impaired mobility
1. Bone density declines with age as well as loss of height.
2. Joint changes include narrowing of the joint space and inflammation.
3. Frailty is described as a decline in physiologic reserves and a resistance to stressors. It can be evaluated by grip strength, walking speed, and weight loss; this loss can contribute to impaired mobility and poor outcomes to disease processes.

H. Skin
1. The skin becomes thinner and loses its elasticity.
2. Skin becomes drier, and itching is a frequent complaint and can lead patients to an increased risk of infections.
3. The thinner skin due to loss and loosening of subcutaneous fat places patients at risk for skin breakdown, tearing, and pressure sores, especially with immobility.
4. Decrease in blood supply to the skin
5. Decreased ability to sweat
6. Obesity

I. Gastrointestinal
1. Esophageal emptying time is increased.
2. Dysphagia
3. Decrease in liver size
4. Constipation is a common problem and may become an unhealthy focus.
5. Increased risk for stool impactions

J. Immunosenescence
1. Aging causes a decrease in both humoral and cellular immunity.
2. Physical barriers to infection become impaired, skin fragility, mobility of respiratory cilia, poor nutrition, and decreased mobility place the patient at risk of infection. Presence of indwelling catheters or other medical devices increases the risk of infection.
3. Older patients generally will have atypical presentations of infection (i.e., afebrile, white blood cell count may be inaccurate marker of infection, leukocyturia, and bacteria may be normal findings).

K. Pharmacokinetics and pharmacodynamics
1. Responses to medications change with aging.
2. Decrease in total body water and circulating plasma proteins and an increase in total body fat

concentrations will impact how the drug is absorbed and metabolized.

3. Renal function is affected by age and acute illness-related medications use.

Assessing the Geriatric Patient in the ED

A. *Focused history:* History of the present illness/chief complaint: CLIENT OUTCOMES and SAMPLE mnemonics[11]:

1. *C:* Character of the symptoms related to the chief complaint
2. *L:* Location of the problem including radiation if indicated
3. *I:* Impact of the systems on the patient's ability to function, activities of daily life and on the patient's quality of life
4. *E:* Expectations of care in the ED
5. *N:* Neglect or abuse that includes signs of physical abuse or neglect, emotional abuse, signs of anxiety or fear related to caregiver, illness or injury matches the chief complaint
6. *T:* Timing, which includes onset, duration, frequency of symptoms. Are symptoms related to a longstanding illness (i.e., heart failure)?
7. *O:* Other symptoms or problems that may be occurring
8. *U:* Understanding of what is happening by the patient, family, caregivers
9. *T:* Treatment, current medications, interventions (i.e., left ventricular assist device [LVAD], pacemakers, implantable cardioverter defibrillator [ICD], feeding tubes, catheters)
10. *C:* Complementary alternative medicine and interventions (i.e., aromatherapy, acupuncture, herbal medications)
11. *O:* Options for care that may influence the patient's care (i.e., Advanced Directives, POLST [Physician's Orders for Life Sustaining Treatment] form)
12. *M:* Modulating factors that precipitate, aggravate, or alleviate symptoms
13. *E:* Exposure to infectious agents, toxic material, possible ingestion. Does the patient live in a community setting with others and may have been exposed to an illness?
14. *S:* Spirituality, including patient's religious beliefs or beliefs related to patient's current state of health
15. *S:* Symptoms associated with the illness or injury
16. *A:* Allergies and vaccination status (i.e., pneumococcal, shingles)
17. *M:* Medication prescribed or OTC
18. *P:* Past medical history including hospitalizations—especially the most recent—and surgeries.
19. *L:* Last oral intake
20. *E:* Events related to the illness or injury

B. Primary assessment (refer to Physiological and Cognitive Changes in the Geriatric Patient)[11–13]

1. Airway
2. Breathing
3. Circulation
4. Disability
5. Exposure

C. Secondary assessment (refer to Physiological and Cognitive Changes in the Geriatric Patient)[11–13]

1. Medical History
2. Comorbidities
3. Medications
4. Head-to-toe assessment
5. Presence of catheters, feeding tubes, LVAD, ICD, pacemaker, and so on.
6. Inspect posterior surfaces.

D. *Cognitive assessment:* Multiple assessments available. The environment where the clinician is employed needs to select the most appropriate for that department. Below are three of the most recognized tools.[14]

1. Mini-Mental State Examination (MMSE) www.heartinstitutehd.com/Misc/Forms/MMSE.1276128605.pdf
2. Mini-Cog mini-cog.com/wp-content/uploads/2018/03/Standardized-English-Mini-Cog-1-19-16-EN_v1-low-1.pdf
3. MOCA (Montreal Cognitive Assessment) www.parkinsons.va.gov/resources/MOCA-Test-English.pdf

E. *Delirium assessment*[5,15,16]: An acute altered mental status generally caused by reversible conditions. It is important to quickly identify the acuity of the condition and intervene as needed.

1. *Causes:* Medications, over the counter and prescribed; metabolic such as hyponatremia, thyroid dysfunction; cerebral injury, cerebrovascular accident (CVA), hemorrhage; pain; urinary retention; constipation; dehydration; ED environment; and a combination of many things
2. *Interventions:* Avoid physical and pharmacological restraints; provide comfort measures such as food, drink, warmth; assure safe mobility; manage toileting; provide frequent orientation; make sure patient has sensory glasses, hearing aids to correct sensory impairments; and provide an environment that allows for limited noise and family presence.
3. Use a simple assessment test such as what is the day of the week; what is the date; spell WORLD backward; what is the year.
4. Transition to care is imperative when delirium is identified (see Transition of Care).

F. *Functional assessment:* Made up of multiple components. The focus of functional assessment is to identify the patient's baseline function because it will have an impact on the care the patient receives in the ED and after admission or discharge. There are several tools that can be initiated in the triage area.[15]

1. Location of where the patient lives: Home, assisted living, skilled care facility
2. Environmental obstacles
3. Gait, balance, mobility
4. *Mobility aids:* Canes, wheelchair, motorized chairs
5. History of falls:
   a. Presents to the ED with the complaint of an acute fall
   b. Two or more falls in the last 12 months
   c. *Cause of falls:* Environment, medications, medical problems
6. Muscle strength

7. Feet and footwear
8. "Timed Up and Go" test www.cdc.gov/steadi/pdf/TUG_Test-print.pdf
9. "Chair test" www.cdc.gov/steadi/pdf/STEADI-Assessment-30Sec-508.pdf

Geriatric Medical and Trauma Emergencies[3,15–19]

A. *Atypical presentations:* Geriatric patients' complaints may be nonspecific. Signs and symptoms of acute illness and injury are not always clear and do not proceed as in other age groups due to physiological changes and other problems related to age as well as polypharmacy and cognitive changes such as dementia and delirium. The presence of other illnesses such as COPD, congestive heart failure, and diabetes can complicate disease presentations. Many geriatric patients cannot mount a febrile response to infections, so when an increased temperature would be expected in an ill person, it may not be present. Symptoms that may be observed include delirium, frequent falls, incontinence, lack of appetite, and failure to thrive. Patients with pre-existing dementia may be at greater risk of complications from infection. When treating geriatric patients with infectious diseases, it is important to keep in mind that repetitive exposure to antimicrobials can place the patient at risk to *Clostridium difficile* and the development of multidrug-resistant microbes.

B. *Pneumonia*[17–19]

1. Community-acquired pneumonia (CAP) is an acute infection of the lower respiratory tract. Symptoms such as cough, shortness of breath (SOB), pleuritic chest pain, and fever may not be seen in the older patient. Instead, they present with delirium and tachypnea. Microorganisms that cause pneumonia in the United States include *Streptococcus pneumoniae* (accounts for almost 50%), *Haemophilus influenzae, Legionella pneumophila, Staphylococcus aureus, Chlamydia pneumoniae,* and gram-negative bacilli such as *Klebsiella pneumoniae* and *Escherichia coli.* Where the patient resides needs to be included in considering the cause of the pneumonia.
2. *Assessment*[19] *history:* Age of the patient, place of residence, coexisting illnesses (e.g., active malignancy, liver disease, congestive heart failure (CHF), cerebrovascular disease, chronic kidney disease).
   a. *Physical exam:* Mental status, respiratory rate, systolic blood pressure, pulse rate, and temperature
   b. *Laboratory:* Arterial pH <7.35, blood urea nitrogen (BUN) > 11 mmol/L or 30 mg/dL, Na <130 mmol/L, glucose >14 mmol/L or 250 mg/dL, hematocrit <30%; PaO_2 <60 mmHg, pleural effusion on chest radiograph.
3. *Treatment:* See Thoracic Emergencies including management using IDSA (Infectious Disease Society of America www.idsociety.org/practiceguidelines#/date_na_dt/DESC/0/+/).

C. *Urinary tract infections (UTIs)*[17,19]

1. Common reason why elderly patients are seen in the ED. Risk factors related to age include diseases such as Parkinson's disease, which can cause a neurogenic bladder; in women, postmenopausal changes in the vagina and the use of diapers or other methods to manage incontinence.
2. *Assessment:* The classic is an altered mental status (AMS). Acute dysuria may be present and is more specific to an acute UTI. Other symptoms may include urinary incontinence, diarrhea, loss of appetite, nausea, and vomiting. *E. coli* (most common), *Enterococcus, Proteus mirabilis,* and *K. pneumoniae* are responsible for infections.
3. *Treatment:* Obtain clean catch urine with culture. Treatment with antimicrobials in the elderly in the outpatient setting can be considered when two of the following are present: fever greater than 38°C; acute dysuria, frequency, suprapubic pain, CVA tenderness; pyuria; or a positive urinary culture. New treatment guidelines were published by the American Urological Association (www.auanet.org/guidelines/recurrent-uti">https://www.auanet.org/guidelines/recurrent-uti). See Chapter 18: Renal, Genitourinary, and Reproductive Conditions.

D. *Sepsis*[18,19]: Defined as life-threatening organ dysfunction caused by the elderly patient's response to infection. There is a spectrum of disease severity from bacteremia to septic shock. The older patient is at greater risk than other age groups to suffer from sepsis and septic shock. More than half of the patients diagnosed with sepsis are over the age of 65. The most common causes of sepsis in the elderly patient include urinary tract, respiratory, and bloodstream infections. Increasing age, chronic illnesses, and nursing home residences are additional factors that have been found to increase the risk of sepsis. See Chapter 22: Infectious Diseases.

1. *Assessment:* Atypical presentations of infections can make it challenging to identify sepsis in the geriatric patient. Older adults may not be febrile; atypical symptoms such as confusion may be indicative of pneumonia. Patients with dementia may not be able to express their discomfort. It is important to listen to caregivers about the changes that have been noted in the patient. Other risk factors to consider include the presence of urinary catheters, feeding tubes, comorbid conditions such as COPD and diabetes, recent hospitalizations, recent exposure to antibiotics, and a history of multiple drug-resistant organisms.
2. *Treatment:* Use of the Surviving Sepsis Guidelines www.survivingsepsis.org/GUIDELINES/Pages/default.aspx. Important to consider the physiological changes related to aging, particularly the impact of pharmacokinetics and pharmacodynamics of the medications selected to treat the infection. Drug absorption and renal function are affected by age. Patients with sepsis may present with delirium and pain related to the disease process. Nonpharmacologic management may be a safer alternative to medications, especially the use of benzodiazepines.

E. *Abdominal pain*[16,20]: Common causes of abdominal pain in the geriatric patient include constipation, bowel obstruction, biliary disease, diverticulitis, and gastritis. Potentially life-threatening causes include gastrointestinal bleeding, aortic dissection, mesenteric ischemic, volvulus, and aneurysmal rupture. See Chapter 16: Vascular Emergencies (AAA) and Chapter 17: Medical Emergencies of the Stomach, Esophagus, and Duodenum.

1. *Assessment:* Important to rule out extraabdominal causes, including myocardial infarction, heart failure, pericarditis, lower lobe pneumonia, pulmonary embolus, pneumothorax, diabetic ketoacidosis, cellulitis, prostatitis, uterine prolapse, acute leukemia, and drug withdrawal. Differences to consider in the geriatric patient include atypical presentation such as a lack of fever or atypical pain pattern. Always review the patient's medication list. Polypharmacy can be a cause of abdominal pain.
2. *Treatment:* Laboratory tests complete blood count (CBC), serum chemistries, lipase, amylase, and a urinalysis. Additional tests may be indicated based on the patient's chief complaint and could include serum lactate, blood cultures, arterial blood gases (ABG), and type and crossmatch.
3. *Imaging:* Abdominal radiograph, chest radiograph, CT scan, ultrasound, MRI, and angiography.
4. See Chapter 6. Analgesia is an important component in the management of abdominal pain, and many times this is not appropriately managed in the geriatric patient.[20] An early consultation with surgery when indicated—especially with high-risk patients—for example, when a ruptured aortic aneurysm is suspected.

F. *Chest pain*[21–23]: Age increases the mortality and morbidity in the geriatric population. Life-threatening causes of chest pain in the elderly include acute coronary syndrome (ACS), aortic dissection, pulmonary embolus, pneumothorax, and esophageal rupture.

1. *Assessment:* Chest pain in the elderly often presents with other complaints including SOB, diaphoresis, nausea and vomiting, and syncope. SOB assessment should include asking about lifetime exposure to environmental or chemical toxins; worsening symptoms related to exercise or overall daily function; orthopnea; smoking history; and recent hospitalization or a procedure. Assess for S_3, use of abdominal muscle during breathing, peripheral edema, or presence of rashes wounds or scars. Diagnosis of an aortic dissection in the elderly should include a high index of suspicion. The risk of a pulmonary embolism increases over the age of 70. Geriatric patients are at significant risk of developing cardiac arrhythmia, especially atrial fibrillation.
2. *Treatment:* The management of these emergencies is similar to younger patients with the need for an immediate EKG, chest radiograph, CT pulmonary angiogram (CTPA), and labs as indicated. The need to consider the physiological changes related to age and the comorbidities will help in the management of the geriatric patient with chest pain. Management of atrial fibrillation will involve rate control and oral anticoagulation. Considerations for the initiation of oral anticoagulation in the elderly include age of the patient-older age patients are at a higher risk of bleeding/frailty; renal function; risk of an ischemic stroke; and ethnicity (Asian patients have increased risk of intracranial hemorrhage, major bleed). In addition, Advanced Directives may need to be considered depending on the potential outcome related to the cause of the chest pain. See Chapter 14: Cardiovascular Emergencies and Chapter 15: Thoracic Respiratory Emergencies.

G. *Neurological emergencies*[24–28]: The neurological changes related to aging—as well as common comorbidities such as hypertension and cardiovascular disease—can cause increased mortality and morbidity related to neurological emergencies in the geriatric patient. Acute ischemic stroke, transient ischemic attack (TIA), intracerebral hemorrhage, chronic subdural hematoma, traumatic brain injuries (TBIs), seizures, and central nervous system infections are some of the neurological emergencies that may present in the geriatric patient. Geriatric patients have a high incidence of new-onset seizures and central nervous infections. These may be missed due to attribution of symptoms—such as altered mental status, muscular weakness, changes in speech, as well as lack of fever—to other causes.[27]

1. *Assessment:* Risk factors include hypertension (HTN), smoking, diabetes hyperlipidemia, atrial fibrillation, and previous stroke or other neurological diseases, use of anticoagulation medications, recent head injury, or history of neurological disease such as seizures. Presenting symptoms may include altered mental status, motor weakness, sensory loss, aphasia, dysarthria, neglect, dizziness, vertigo, visual fields deficits, lack of balance, falls, neck stiffness, severe headache, neck stiffness, or nausea and vomiting. For the patient with suspected acute stroke or TIA, a National Institutes of Health (NIH) Stroke Scale should be included in the initial assessment. Etiologies for elderly patients with seizures may include a stroke, intracranial hemorrhage (ICH), infection, TBI, metabolic problems such as hyponatremia, cerebral anoxia, and medication withdrawal.
2. *Treatment:* Check for hypoxia and hypoglycemia; EKG to determine the risk of arrhythmias; brain imaging; vascular imaging; therapeutic interventions for stenosis. Management will be based upon diagnosis including medications such as rt-PA; reversal of anticoagulants when indicated; and intracranial decompression. For the treatment of seizures in the elderly, lower doses of medication may be more appropriate due to physiological and pharmacodynamic changes in the elderly (see Chapter 26).

H. *Behavioral emergencies*[26–29]: Behavioral emergencies that may present in the geriatric patient include agitation, anxiety/panic, delirium, dementia, depression, and psychosis. Geriatric patients have been found to be in one of the highest risk groups for suicide. They are also at risk of completing a suicide attempt. Suicide in the elderly patient generally can occur without warning, and the attempts are more lethal in character.

1. *Assessment:* In the geriatric patient, it is important to take an accurate history as well as perform a comprehensive physical exam in order to rule out illnesses or injuries as to the cause of their behaviors. Hypoglycemia, hyponatremia, thyrotoxicosis, anemia, hypoxia from lung diseases, and UTIs are only a limited number of illnesses that can mimic a behavioral emergency. Pain, alcohol or drug use, or withdrawal are other examples. Polypharmacy continues

to be a serious source of possible physical and psychological behavioral changes. Finally, trauma should always be considered. For example, a TBI postfall. Laboratory and imaging should be focused on excluding illness or injury. If drug or alcohol intoxication is suspected, urine and serum drug screening should be included in laboratory tests. Other screening tools that should be considered based on the patient's chief complaint include the CAGE Questionnaire Adapted to Include Drugs (CAGE-AID) screening tool for alcohol and substance abuse disorders, Geriatric Depression Scale, and Geriatric Anxiety Inventory-Short Form. Assess for patients at risk of suicide and access to a method, family history of suicide, physical illness, chronic pain, previous attempts, male gender, white race, and a stressful life event.

2. *Treatment:* Depending on the particular behavioral emergency, patient safety is of primary importance. Medications and interventions are determined by the particular behavioral emergency. The American Psychiatric Association published guidelines for the treatment of psychosis and agitation for patients with dementia (psychiatryonline.org/guidelines). Behavioral emergencies in the elderly require a team approach. EDs need to have a plan of care that includes mental health resources. An appropriate plan of care involving the patient, family, or place of residence needs to be developed and communicated. At times, a geriatric patient may need to be admitted and the legal status of the need for admission must be considered. Is the admission voluntary or involuntary? Follow-up care needs to be identified and appropriate resources such as social workers, psychologists, and psychiatrists notified as soon as possible (see Chapter 23).

I. *Geriatric trauma*[30–35]: Age influences the outcome of the injured patient. Frailty can lead to decreased reserve and resistance to stressors to all physiological systems. Patients may also suffer from multiple comorbidities such as cardiovascular and pulmonary diseases. There is not one specific "cutoff" for age that describes a geriatric patient. Age range can be from 45 to 80 years. All do agree that age contributes to increased mortality and morbidity related to trauma. The frailty of the injured patient needs to be assessed and considered when managing the injured geriatric patient. Falls are the most common cause of injury in the elderly. Motor vehicle crashes and pedestrians' injuries are other sources of trauma. Ground-level falls can easily precipitate a functional decline if short-term adverse outcomes are not identified and mitigated. Adverse events postfall may include another fall, an ED revisit, or death within a year after the initial event.

1. *Assessment*[13,30–35]: Primary and secondary survey with focus on the physiological changes related to age. Identify comorbidities that may interfere with the initial resuscitation and long-term care. Loss of physiologic reserve related to age can increase overall complications, decreased functionality and independence, and increased morbidity and mortality. The Ohio geriatric triage criteria are used for patients over the age of 70 to identify the need for care in a trauma center. The criteria include[30] Glasgow Coma Scale (GCS) <14 in the presence of a TBI; systolic blood pressure (BP), 100 mmHg; fall from any height with evidence of a TBI; multiple system injuries; struck by a moving vehicle; and presence of any long bone fracture after motor vehicle trauma. Groin pain can be a significant indication of a hip fracture. Obtain current medication list so that appropriate medications are included as needed (see Chapters 24 and 25).

2. *Treatment:* Resuscitation based on the age of the patient and the physiological changes related to age; early recognition for the need to transfer the patient to a trauma center, especially one that specifically manages geriatric trauma; imaging based on mechanism of injury with a low threshold of suspicion for finding injuries; hip fractures can have serious effects on function and quality of life and there is a high risk of death within 1 year of the injury; female patients are at greater risk of hip fractures and the average age is 80; pain management in the elderly may be underassessed and undermanaged, which can lead to additional stress. Prevention strategies should be initiated for patients who are not admitted from the ED. Fall risk assessment has been recommended before discharge along with a referral for an evaluation where the patient lives. Suggested interventions for patients at risk include minimize medications, provide individual exercise programs, identify and treat vision problems, manage postural hypotension, manage heart arrhythmia and heart rate, supplement vitamin D, recommend appropriate footwear, modify home environment (e.g., grab bars), and provide patient and caregivers education and information.[32]

J. *Elder abuse*[35]: It is estimated that one in 10 people over the age of 60 suffer some sort of elderly abuse (www.ncoa.org/public-policy-action/elder-justice/elder-abuse-facts/#intraPageNav1). Elder abuse can include physical, sexual, and psychological abuse, neglect, and financial exploitation. The ED can play an important role in the identification and notification of appropriate authorities to help assure the safety of a geriatric patient at risk.

1. *Assessment:* Risk factors for elder abuse may include functional dependence or disability, poor mental or physical health, low socioeconomic status, history of family violence, substance abuse, caregiver stress, and family or friend dependence on an elderly adult. Important to observe and note the interactions of the patient and his or her caregivers. For example, is the elderly patient fearful or hostile toward the caregiver? Does the caregiver seem not to know about the patient's current medical problems? Is the risk that both the patient and the caregiver are participating in substance abuse (drugs or alcohol)? History of unexplained injuries to the ED and delay from the time of an injury or illness until treatment in the ED are other possible signs of elder abuse or neglect. Physical signs of abuse or neglect may include bruising in atypical patterns, scars on extremities suggestive of restraints, traumatic alopecia, genital or rectal trauma, evidence of a sexually transmitted disease, malnutrition, dehydration, dirty clothing, and poor hygiene. Emergency medical service (EMS) providers can be important sources of information related to the conditions in which the elderly patient lives and if the illness or injury matches the history.

2. *Treatment:* Labs and imaging based on suspicion of repeated injury or lack of adequate nutrition resulting in dehydration and anemia. Documentation of the history and physical assessment is an important part of identifying elder abuse and neglect. The chart may be a part of the investigation and assist in the identification of elder abuse or neglect. The ED clinician needs to treat any acute injuries or illnesses, assure that the patient is safe, which may involve arranging for admission of the patient, and notify the appropriate authorities. Adult Protective Services (APS) is generally where this is reported. In some states, reporting elder abuse and neglect is mandatory. It is important to have a team approach to this issue, just as is done with suspected pediatric abuse and neglect.

Pain Management in the Geriatric Patient[36–39]

A. *Presentation:* Pain management is challenging in the geriatric patient in the ED. Many geriatric patients' pain is not well assessed or treated even though pain remains one of the primary complaints that causes the older patient to come to the ED in the first place. Patients who are cognitively impaired such as those with severe dementia make it difficult to adequately assess and identify the source of his or her pain. Pain contributes to problems with sleep and interferes with appetite and overall function. It can lead to social isolation. Unresolved pain can contribute to decreased functioning, cause depression, and contribute to an untimely death. Chronic pain can lead to frequent visits to the ED. Geriatric patients can suffer from nociceptive pain related to an acute injury or illness. Many have neuropathic pain related to chronic illnesses such as diabetes. It is always important to evaluate the adverse effects of polypharmacy on the management of pain. Disease comorbidities such a renal and liver impairments can decrease the capability of using medications such as acetaminophen or NSAIDs for pain management. There continue to be uneducated prejudices related to the use of opioids in the elderly. Unfortunately, many alternative methods to manage pain such as thermotherapy, distraction, acupuncture, and massage are not even considered.

B. *Assessment:* Pain assessment in the geriatric patient can be challenging because of the atypical presentation of illnesses and injuries. Cognitive impairment may interfere with the patient's ability to use pain scores. Many older patients are stoic about pain as a part of aging. The Verbal Descriptor Scale (pallipedia.org/verbal-descriptor-scale/) and the Numeric Rating Scales (www.physio-pedia.com/Numeric_Pain_Rating_Scale) are two of the most common pain assessment scales used in the ED. Pain assessment in patients with cognitive impairment can be assessed using facial expressions (grimacing), verbal expressions (moaning), aggressive or combative behaviors, body movements (refusal to move a painful area), refusing food, and changes in mental status (crying, irritability, confusion).[36] Once the medication has been administered, pain levels should always be reassessed. Substance abuse disorder always needs to be considered when assessing pain, especially when one is not familiar with the patient or with patients who frequently visit the ED.[39] Substance abuse may include both alcohol and medications. Symptoms of substance abuse in older patients may include cognitive changes (confusion, drowsiness, daytime drowsiness); social and behavioral changes (withdrawal from usual social activities and family discord); physical symptoms (unexplained injuries, unexplained bruises, malnutrition); physical symptoms (nausea and vomiting, tremors); and psychiatric symptoms (sleep disturbances, irritability, and anxiety).[39]

C. *Treatment:* Pain management should be based on protocols taking into consideration the effects of specific medications on the geriatric patient. Alternative methods should be incorporated as often as possible. Battlefield acupuncture is a method that can be easily learned and used for acute pain and has been found to be of use for some patients in the ED.[40] Geriatric patients experiencing severe pain at the end of life can present to the ED for care. It would be helpful to be familiar with medications, dosing, and methods of administration for these patients (see the section Palliative and End of Life Care in the ED).

Medication Prescribing for the Geriatric Patient[40–43]

A. *Presentation:* Adverse drug reactions (ADRs) are a cause of geriatric patients seeking care in the ED. Many older patients are on multiple medications known as polypharmacy. The definition of polypharmacy is the use of multiple medications. The cutoff can range from 5 to 20 medications. In addition to prescribed medications, many patients take OTC medications including dietary supplements.[40] It has been estimated that many elderly patients are also taking medications—whether prescribed or OTC—that are not appropriate for their age group and place them at risk of an ADR, which could lead to a visit to the ED. This can also occur with prescriptions or medication recommendations from the ED as well.

B. *Assessment:* The physiological and pharmacodynamic impacts of aging need to be considered when prescribing medications in the ED. When prescribing medications, the prescriber needs to consider the geriatric patient's lean body mass, renal dysfunction, liver dysfunction and protein binding, effect on the central nervous system, nutrition status and diet, living conditions, social support, and most important of all, the ability to understand why and how to take the prescribed medication from the ED.

C. *Treatment:* The Beers Criteria has been published by the American Geriatric Society (AGS) since 2011. The AGS produces updates on a 3-year cycle. Its focus is to provide a comprehensive, systematic review and grading of the evidence on drug-related problems and adverse events in older adults related to the use of appropriate medications for adults 65 years and older in all ambulatory, acute, and institutionalized settings of care, except for the palliative care and hospice settings. The prescriber should consult the most recent Beers Criteria for potentially inappropriate medications for the geriatric patient (www.nwrcwa.org/files/2019/04/

Potentially-Inappropriate-Medications-for-Seniors.pdf).[43] Drugs that have been recommended to be used with caution are listed in Table 4 in the document. Trimethoprim-sulfamethoxazole is an important one to note since many older patients present to the ED with symptoms of UTI.[43]

1. Calculate the geriatric patients' Cockcroft-Gault formula for creatinine clearance for medications eliminated through the kidneys.
2. Protocols should be in place for prescribing for the geriatric patient.
3. Consult a pharmacist for guidance when prescribing for the geriatric patient in the ED.

Geriatric ED and Transition of Care[4,44–47]

A. Risk factors for increased risk of death or readmission to the ICU shortly after discharge from the ED include[47] cognitive impairment and systolic blood pressure >120 mmHg and pulse rate <90 beats per minute. Quality indicators to be evaluated for the care of the geriatric patient in the ED should include readmission of patients >65 years of age, geriatric transfers from long-term care facilities, admission upgrade with 24 hours of being seen in the ED, geriatric abuse and neglect, cardiopulmonary arrest, deaths, falls, use of urinary catheters, medication management problems, delirium and restraint use, and transition of care.

B. *Geriatric ED*[46]: Focused on the care of the geriatric patient. Provision of a safe and comfortable environment including exam chairs that can recline, arm rests that support the patient to safely get up, extra-thick mattresses, moisture-proof upholstery, nonslip fall mats, assist devices to get in and out of beds, close appropriately equipped bathroom, soft colors, adequate lighting, and space for families.

C. *Available resources*[4,46]

1. Practice Management/Geriatric-Videos: American Geriatrics Society Clinical Practice Guideline for Postoperative Delirium in Older Adults (geriatrics careonline.org/ProductAbstract/ american-geriatrics-society-clinical-practice-guideline-for-postoperative-deliriumin-older-adults/CL018)
2. The Geriatrics for Specialty Residents Toolkit: Emergency Medicine (geriatricscareonline.org/toc/the-geriatrics-for-specialty-residents-toolkit-emergency-medicine/TK008)
3. ENA comprehensive geriatric online course consisting of 17 modules (www.ena.org/education/education/GENE/Documents/Modules.pdf)
4. Geriatric education for emergency medical services (geriatricscareonline.org/ ProductAbstract/geriatric_education_for_emergency_medical_services/B017)

D. *Transition of care*[4,44,45]: Involves verifying that the patient has a primary care physician or medical home, involving the patient's support system in the plan of care by providing education and management of the patient's illness or injury, completing medication reconciliation, especially if medications are going to be changed or added to, accessing accurate information that is needed to address the reason why the patient presented to the ED, and addressing palliative care needs as indicated. It is important that the ED involves the relevant agencies concerned with the care of geriatric patients within their communities, including the Area of Agency on Aging, senior centers, churches, and the local AARP. When possible, a care transition model should be in place that may be composed of nurses, social workers, pharmacists, and other members as needed. This will help assist in the best care for the patient and the most appropriate use of ED resources.

1. Protocols should be in place for the transition of care from the ED. The following components should be included[4]: complaint related to the ED visit, test results and interpretation of the results, what therapy was provided in the ED and the patient's response, consultation notes if one was performed, working discharge diagnosis, copy of ED clinician's notes any changes in current medications, new prescriptions based on the presenting chief complaints (should include an explanation of the changes), and follow-up plan of care.
2. All documents need to be Health Insurance Portability and Accountability Act (HIPAA) compliant; copied discharge instructions should be provided to family and care providers.
3. If the patient is provided with discharge documents, information should be in a font that is readable.
4. A follow-up call to the patient, care provider, or place of residence within 24 hours of discharge for continuity of care (see Patient Disposition)

Palliative and End of Life Care in the ED[4,48,49]

A. *Presentation:* The ED continues to be a place where patients and families turn to for end-of-life care. Patients may also present with an illness or injury that requires a palliative care consult. Some of these presentations include a massive stroke, cardiac arrest, or surgical emergency such as a ruptured aneurysm. Patients may also be brought to the ED by a family that cannot manage the progressive symptoms of dementia. Challenges to end of life and palliative care in the ED include lack of access to a palliative care team, incomplete medical records related to the patient's illness or injury, absence of the presence of Advanced Directives or Physician Orders for Life Sustaining Orders (POLST), and the ED environment, which is primarily focused on saving lives.

B. *Screening:* A screening tool that has two questions has been found to be of use in the ED[48]:

1. Does the patient have a life-limiting illness or injury? For example, end-stage renal disease, end-stage cancer, septic shock.
2. Does the patient have two or more unmet palliative care needs? For example, frequent ED visits, uncontrolled symptoms, uncertainty about goals of care.
3. Protocols should be developed or available for providing end-of-life and palliative care in the ED and include pain management, non-pain management, comfort care, coordination with an in-house palliative care team, local hospice agency, and support staff for the family.

References

References for this chapter are online only and can be found at https://connect.springerpub.com/content/reference-book/978-0-8261-6091-5/part/part07/toc-part/ch51.

52. Rural/Austere Patient Population

JOHN F. L. JAMISON

Learning Objectives

- Define what constitutes a rural or austere emergency care environment.
- Identify and discuss important geographical and environmental factors.
- Discuss unique population, injury, and illness patterns typically seen in rural environments.
- Demonstrate resource and priority management for patient care.
- Explain training and educational needs for continued competency.
- Demonstrate utilization of local and regional resources.
- Interpret management of interfacility transfers and admissions.

Rural and Austere Emergency Care

Rural and austere emergency care provides a unique, challenging, and rewarding care setting for the emergency nurse practitioner (ENP). Rural healthcare settings vary widely, from small remote critical access facilities to larger but geographically isolated regional hospitals. Austere healthcare environments exist in any situation where healthcare needs outstrip available resources. Austere care conditions are typically experienced during remote medical operations, mass casualty events, and natural disasters. To be successful, ENPs working in rural and austere environments must be confident and adaptable to provide competent and autonomous care with limited resources and support. ENPs working in rural and austere environments may also, at times, be the highest level of care and need to have excellent assessment skills, strong knowledge of emergency conditions, and a high level of comfort with procedures to manage cases until additional resources are available.

The core principle of rural and austere emergency medical care is resource management. The ENP should be familiar with their own in-house resources and capabilities as well as resources and services offered at other community, regional, and tertiary care centers. The ENP must know how to access and ensure resources and procedures are in place for specialty consults and transfer of patients to higher-level care as indicated. Finally, the ENP has to be familiar with interfacility transport options and how weather, geography, and the patient's status can impact the mode of transport and the ability to safely transfer the patient. As the healthcare team leader in the rural and austere environment, the ability of the ENP to effectively orchestrate all these variables will have a significant impact on patient outcomes.

Definitions

Rural or austere emergency care applies to any situation or location with limited resources and/or access to definitive care.

A. Location

1. Disaster response zones
   a. Natural disasters
      i. Hurricanes, tornados, flooding, earthquakes, blizzards
         (1) Usually disrupts or damages infrastructure, communications, and access to public services such as water, gas, and electricity. Can cause significant health and safety risks due to environmental contaminations or toxic chemical releases. Often overwhelms local resources.
   b. Manmade disasters
      i. Building collapses, mining and construction accidents, mass shootings, industrial or manufacturing complex fires or explosions
         (1) Usually very localized events with little impact beyond the immediate area. Often have specialized hazards requiring specialized response teams. The situations are often dynamic, fast-moving, and can be chaotic. Prolonged rescue and extraction may require on-site relocation of clinicians to the scene. Family, friends, and bystanders can become additional psychologic victims.
2. Locations geographically isolated by terrain or distance
   a. These areas have unique problems related to accessing care and arranging transfers. The ENP often needs to make early and aggressive decisions about transferring acutely ill patients and must understand the availability and limitations of transport options. The ENP needs to be able to anticipatorily judge the risks and benefits of transfer. The ENP must also be prepared to possibly stabilize, manage, and care for these patients for an extended amount of time before the transfer can be accomplished.

i. *Terrain:* Areas isolated by terrain are usually in mountainous regions but can also include areas surrounded by large bodies of water or other natural barriers. These areas typically have limited and often difficult access by road and are often adversely affected by severe weather. Many of these areas also experience seasonal influx for recreational or tourist activities.

(1) *Examples:* Aspen, Colorado; Jackson Hole, Wyoming (Yellowstone Park); Key West, Florida, and the Florida Keys.

ii. *Distance:* Geographic isolation due to distance comes in several forms. The areas are isolated from regional and tertiary resources by pure distance and/or lack of direct travel access and roads.

(1) *Example:* A prime example of isolation are the rural Indian Health Service (IHS) facilities in the southwest United States. In addition to having terrain-related geographic issues, they also have distance issues both in their pure distance from resources and their lack of direct road access. For the most remote facilities, it can be as much as 10 hours by ground transport to higher-level care and 3 hours for aeromedical resources to respond to and reach the facility.

3. Urban and semiurban areas with severe economic depression and disparity

a. Areas do not always have to be geographically isolated to be considered rural or austere environments. Facilities (even in large urban locations) that are located in areas of severe socioeconomic depression or disparity can experience the same problems with access to care and resources that more traditional rural and austere locations face. The populations in these areas tend to be uninsured or underinsured and have significantly greater healthcare issues and comorbidities than the average population. The populations in these areas often have health disparities that are exacerbated by physically demanding jobs, lack of quality healthy food choices, and lack of routine preventative healthcare.

i. *Examples:* The nontypical rural and austere areas include the large farming communities of the western United States, depressed industrial cities and towns of the Northeast, and mining towns in the southeast.

4. Resource availability

a. Lack of infrastructure

i. In rural and austere areas, the ENP may encounter a lack of infrastructure that they normally take for granted. Examples include limited and sometimes impossible road access, underdeveloped electrical or plumbing services that may be prone to failure, and possible lack of or limited internet service that many people and clinicians rely on for access to medical resources.

b. Lack of clinicians and general healthcare services

i. Healthcare clinicians and specialty services tend to be geographically clustered in regional and metropolitan population areas. The ENP working in a critical access facility that provides safety net services may find primary care and diagnostic services lacking and specialty services of every kind nonexistent. One of the primary recruitment tools for these locations is federal student loan repayment to clinicians for primary care services. As an expert generalist, the ENP may be one of the most qualified clinicians for hundreds of miles.

ii. Access to obstetrics, pediatrics, surgery, cardiology, neurology, ICUs, and other definitive care services

iii. Facilities in rural and austere areas lack the overall economic support base to support most specialty services. It is also not feasible or practical to transfer every acutely ill patient to a tertiary care facility. The ENP needs to be knowledgeable of local capabilities and referral resources and have the confidence to make appropriate decisions between transfer and observation of patients. The ENP also needs to have the capability to advocate for appropriate patient transfers that the receiving facility may be reluctant to accept. This reluctance may be due to a lack of understanding about the limited capabilities of the rural or austere facility; therefore, the ENP must have a clear understanding of why the patient requires a higher level of care and be able to clearly articulate this to the referral facility.

Scope of Care

A. Scope of care for ENPs is unique and complicated by many factors.

1. The ENP needs to be an expert generalist.

a. Most medical specialists are knowledgeable within their field of expertise but can find it difficult to manage unrelated medical issues due to a highly specialized skill set at the expense of a strong generalized medical skill set. Emergency medicine is a unique specialty where clinicians are required to have both a strong specialized and generalized skill set to manage any patient complaint or situation that might present. This skill range is especially true for rural and austere clinicians where back-up resources may be limited or unavailable. The ENP should take pride in this unique specialization as an expert generalist and strive to improve their knowledge and skills in all areas.

2. The ENP may be the only clinician available and requested to provide primary, emergency, and inpatient care services.

a. In smaller or more remote facilities, the ENP may be required to rotate through or concurrently provide coverage for admitted/observation patients and primary care clinics, in addition to covering emergency care. The well-prepared ENP should have the necessary knowledge to function in these areas. However, each area will have unique processes and management considerations the clinician will need to become familiar with. Scope of practice issues will need to be considered, and the ENP who wants to work in a rural or austere location may need additional training or specialty certification to increase their scope of practice.

3. Exposure to low-volume, high-risk situations and procedures requires frequent training and education to maintain skills and knowledge.

a. The ED is an inherently unpredictable and chaotic environment. The ENP must be prepared to handle patient resuscitation and procedures under less than ideal conditions. Situations often involve critical and high-risk activities that the ENP, especially in the rural setting, may rarely perform. The ENP needs to actively pursue opportunities to refresh and maintain their knowledge and skills.

b. Examples of high-risk, low-volume lifesaving interventions the ENP may be expected to perform include:

i. Rapid sequence induction (RSI) and endotracheal intubation
ii. Central line placement
iii. Needle decompression or tube thoracotomy (chest tube placement)
iv. Surgical cricothyroidotomy
v. Paracentesis or pericardiocentesis
vi. Emergency childbirth and neonatal resuscitation
vii. Anesthesia and procedural sedation

4. Limited availability and training of medical support staff

a. Another limited resource in rural and austere areas is support personnel. Ancillary staff typically come from the limited local population, where training and education opportunities may have been limited. Staff may work in multiple clinical roles and have limited experience beyond the facility. Travel and locum personnel brought in to supplement local staffing may have difficulty adapting to the limited resources available and be unfamiliar with facility capabilities and indications for transfer. The ENP needs to function as a leader to provide guidance and support.

B. *Diagnostic and treatment capability*

1. Available lab tests and turnaround time

a. Most facilities have at least basic in-house laboratory testing, but may lack the ability to directly process common but less critical lab work, thereby requiring it to be sent outside of the facility for processing. Austere environments are even more limited, but with the availability of portable handheld equipment, critical lab results can be obtained if carefully planned for. Timely access to results can also be problematic. Older in-house equipment may not process specimens as fast as the ENP is accustomed to, and laboratory studies that are sent out can take hours to days to get results.

2. Imagining services and technicians

a. The ability to obtain x-ray images has become ubiquitous and available in most environments. Bedside ultrasound is also becoming increasingly common. However, in rural and austere environments, advanced imaging such as CT, MRI, and technical ultrasound services may be limited or unavailable, requiring patient transfer. Even when the services are available, there may be delays related to needing to call in staff from home during nonpeak hours. The ENP with additional training in diagnostic capabilities, such as ultrasound, can improve the rapid identification of serious pathology, allowing the patient to obtain more timely definitive care.

3. Availability of ancillary services such as respiratory therapists, pharmacists, and laboratory staff

a. Specialized staffing and services that are taken for granted in the urban setting are usually limited in the rural and austere setting. The ENP must anticipate and know how to work around these barriers. Examples include:

i. Staff callouts resulting in low or unavailable staffing for nurses, radiology, laboratory, respiratory therapy, and so on necessitates a back-up plan. The ENP will need to assess whether the patient can be safely evaluated and treated without these services, followed up as needed on an outpatient basis, or transferred for additional evaluation.

ii. After-hours pharmacy services

(1) Consider whether the patient can wait until the next day for needed medications.

(2) Consider whether the facility can dispense full prescriptions or temporary "go packs" of medications for patients; what medications are available for dispensing.

(3) Consider whether the facility is at greater risk for medication errors with low-volume, high-risk medications due to reduced pharmacist involvement in order placement.

4. Quantity and quality of monitoring and diagnostic equipment

a. It is not unusual for rural and austere environments to have limited availability of diagnostic and monitoring equipment, which can often be one or more generations older than the current equipment in use in urbanized areas. This equipment is quite functional, but may require the ENP to have a better understanding of diagnostic interpretation and equipment limitations. Newer generations of equipment may have much-improved sensitivity, specificity, accuracy, and automation that clinicians in more urban areas have come to expect. The ENP may have to interpret lower quality or resolution radiology images or hard-copy films without the benefit of digital enhancement. EKG machines may provide no or unreliable interpretation assistance due to lack of older diagnostic algorithms. The ENP may also have to prioritize which patients receive monitoring and diagnostic testing to provide the best outcome for all patients.

5. Limited supplies and medication choices

   a. In major metropolitan and urban facilities, there may be a seemingly endless supply of disposable items and equipment and access to just about any needed medication. In rural and austere facilities or environments, the ENP must be aware of medication availability and potential need for resource management. Excessive use or waste of even ubiquitous items, such as gauze and syringes, can quickly deplete available stock, especially during a high-volume event. This is an even greater issue with more limited types of supplies such as chest-tube trays. Basic medications usually have good availability, but some medication quantities, varieties, and alternatives may be limited, requiring the ENP to adapt to what is available rather than relying on their usual preference.

C. *Locality considerations:* In addition to generally being remote, rural and austere environments can have one or more of the following considerations related to their locality.

1. Geography and accessibility

   a. Rough and impassible terrain with limited roads may inhibit access and availability of assistance.

   b. Limited access roads and geographic hazards can potentially isolate the facility from ground and aeromedical access.

   c. *Examples:* The Florida Keys, the Rocky Mountains and other mountainous areas, the north versus south rims of the Grand Canyon

2. Extremes of weather

   a. Any location can experience extremes of weather, including hurricanes, tornadoes, tropical storms, extreme heat, blizzards, or sustained snowstorms.

   b. In addition to being prepared to manage patients for extended periods without assistance, the ENP must also be prepared to accurately assess and manage various weather-related medical problems and injuries that may be common or specific to their location.

3. Demographics of local population

   a. Demographics of the local population has a large impact on the types of cases seen and the typical care needed.

   b. People in rural and austere areas are often low-income, have multiple risk factors for disease, and suffer from a higher than average degree of chronic comorbid health conditions. Smoking, drug use, alcohol abuse, and a lack of regular primary care also tend to be present at a higher rate as compared to more urban areas.

   c. The employment opportunities available in rural and austere areas are primarily industrial or agricultural, where patients may be routinely exposed to hazardous chemicals and pesticides.

4. Seasonal and special event visitors

   a. Many rural areas are popular for outdoor recreation or experience seasonally related or special event influxes of visitors.

   b. Depending on the nature of the event or activity, the influx of visitors has the potential to overwhelm local resources.

   c. Activities and events can vary in size and nature. These can range from small influxes for seasonal sports and recreation or organizational gatherings to large music, film, and art festivals or annual national rallies.

5. Access to and distance from regional or tertiary and definitive care services

   a. Availability and accessibility to higher-level and specialty care services can vary from a short drive to a major metropolitan area with extensive services to multihour drives to the closest regional medical facility with limited services.

   b. It is important to be familiar with local resources and which alternatives are available should the closest or preferred facility not be available or accessible.

   c. These factors have a major impact on transfer decisions when considering patient stability and mode of transport.

Access to Definitive Care and Specialty Services

A. Knowing what your local, regional, tertiary, and definitive care services are

1. Location and availability

   a. Consider whether the closest facility is the most appropriate.

   b. Consider whether your facility has transfer agreements with a partner facility or if the patient or patient's insurance have a preferred destination.

   c. Consider whether the patient is already under a specialist care for their condition and where that specialist has admitting privileges.

2. Referral and transfer procedures

   a. Determine if transfers handled via a transfer center or directly with the receiving facility, clinician, or specialty service.

   b. Confirm availability of a bed and accepting clinician at the receiving facility.

   c. Get patient consent and complete the Emergency Medical Treatment and Active Labor Act (EMTALA) transfer certification form.

   d. Complete the medical record and transfer packet.

3. *Specialty populations:* Obstetrics, neonatal, pediatrics, psychiatric

   a. Services for specialty populations are not as readily available as other services and may have capacity issues affecting the ability to transfer the patient.

b. Specialty populations may require specialty transport services, increasing the complexity of transfer.

4. *Specialty diagnostics and assessment:* CT, MRI, trauma, cath lab, neurosurgery

a. Patient condition, prognosis, and urgency can impact transfer and disposition considerations for patients requiring urgent or emergent diagnostic services unavailable at the rural or austere facility.

b. Disposition options can include

i. Transfer for diagnostic procedure and return to the rural facility for disposition.

ii. Transfer to receiving ED for additional evaluation and disposition.

iii. Transfer and admit for definitive care and treatment.

B. *Transfer and referral considerations*

1. Make the decision to transfer early and get the process started.

a. In addition to transport time, arranging for a receiving facility and transport services can potentially add hours to the diagnostic and treatment process. The sooner that a patient is identified as needing admission or transfer, the sooner the process can be initiated and the more effectively the patient's transfer and care can be managed.

2. EMTALA

a. The federal EMTALA regulation has specific requirements for transferring patients that can result in large fines for the clinician and the sending facility if regulations are not followed.

3. Gain patient acceptance at regional tertiary care facilities for transfers.

a. After determining that a patient needs to be transferred, the next most important step is getting the patient accepted by a clinician at a receiving facility.

b. It can occasionally be difficult to locate an available facility and a clinician willing to accept the patient. Having patient information well organized and being able to state the patient's case and reason for transfer clearly and succinctly will facilitate transfer acceptance.

4. Ambulance diversion to available higher-level care

a. Determine if protocols are in place if the rural facility is on diversion to incoming ambulance traffic.

b. Determine if protocols are in place to allow for an ambulance patient to be safely diverted to another facility to avoid the need for a transfer (e.g., a stable open fracture requiring surgery).

c. Ambulance diversions can be an EMTALA violation if the patient cannot be safely transported to a more distant facility.

5. Treat and refer to outpatient follow-up versus transfer and admit to inpatient status

a. Consider whether a patient can be safely discharged for follow-up diagnostics and specialty evaluation the next day.

b. Consider whether ill but noncritical patients can be safely discharged to return if their symptoms worsen.

6. Local management via observation admission versus discharge and serial follow-up evaluation

a. Determine if the patient can be held and treated in the ED for a short period of time until they can be safely discharged.

b. Determine if the patient's treatment can be safely managed with discharge and return visits for serial evaluation and treatment (e.g., wound checks, repeat IV or intramuscular [IM] antibiotic).

C. *Management of available resources is a critical concept.*

1. Relatively minor events can quickly overwhelm resources and become a mass causality event. As an example, something as simple as a motor vehicle crash with 2 or 3 serious injuries can potentially overwhelm resources in a rural or austere facility.

2. Triage needs to be performed with management of supply utilization and transfer prioritization.

a. The ENP needs to be aware of resource limitations, such as staff, blood products, and infrequently used interventional supplies that may be used up by acute needs. The ENP may also need to prioritize which patients need to be transferred first based on acuity or who will reap the most benefit if enough transfer resources are not immediately available.

3. Maintain an organized overview of the operational flow.

a. As a nurse, the ENP is used to providing direct care, but as one of the senior medical personnel, the ENP needs to be able to step back to organize and direct the care of the patient.

b. The most important thing is to not lose sight of the big picture by focusing on a single issue or event. For example:

i. Being overly focused on a dramatic extremity injury and missing the subtle but more life-threatening chest injury

ii. Getting overwhelmed by many minor patients from an accident and failing to evaluate and intervene in a timely manner for the walk-in patient having a heart attack

D. *Transport and transfer considerations*

1. EMTALA

a. Requires EDs to provide a medical screening exam and stabilization of emergency medical conditions for all patients who present for care.

b. Requires patients to be seen and evaluated by an on-call specialist if available.

c. Requires certification by clinician that the benefits of transfer outweigh the risk.

d. Each violation can result in a $50,000 fine for both the clinician and the facility.

2. Stable versus unstable versus decompensating

a. Patient stability affects the decision to transfer and the mode of transport to use. Stable patients can typically be transferred with monitoring and basic care. Unstable patients need to have the risk of further decompensation weighed against the benefit of transfer considered and will need a higher level of medical transport service. Patients that are decompensating should not be transferred until they can be stabilized to the point at which they have the greatest chance of surviving transfer.

3. Risks and benefits of transfer and transport
   a. The main benefits of transfer are access to higher levels specialized care to reduce morbidity and mortality.
   b. Transfers are inherently risky in many ways. The primary risks are the patient decompensation or additional accident or injury during the transport.
   c. *Timing of transfers and transport:* Transfers should generally be expedited to improve patient outcomes, but in some cases delaying transfer can benefit the patient. Examples include:
      i. *Pregnancy and labor:* Decision of transport versus wait and deliver. If a patient cannot safely make it to the receiving facility without delivering, it is better to prepare for delivery and call for specialty transport to transfer the mother and infant after delivery.
      ii. *Unstable patients with labile vital signs:* Patients that are likely to acutely decompensate during transport put both the patient and transportation crew at risk. Every effort needs to be made to maximize patient stability prior to transport.
      iii. *Respiratory distress without definitive airway:* Patients with severe respiratory distress or potential airway compromise and risk for respiratory arrest need to have a definitive airway prior to transfer.
4. Deciding on mode of transport
   a. Consider type of care and management the patient requires en route.
   b. Air versus ground transport
      i. Ground transport is more readily available, safer, more cost-effective, and less affected by weather than aeromedical transport.
      ii. Aeromedical transport units have expanded training and scope of care and often have additional medications and blood products. Aeromedical transport is significantly faster at transport distances over 150 miles.
   c. Mode of transport
      i. *Private vehicle:* Should be used rarely and with caution, but can be appropriate for a small group of patients that are stable and do not require active medical management enroute
      ii. *Basic life support (BLS) ambulance:* Staffed with emergency medical technicians (EMTs) who can provide oxygen and basic vital sign monitoring, but no advanced skills, monitoring, or interventions
      iii. *Advanced life support (ALS) ambulance:* Staffed by paramedics who can provide BLS services as well as cardiac monitoring, airway management, limited medication monitoring and administration, and some advanced skills such as basic ventilator monitoring
      iv. *Critical care transport (ground/air):* Staffed by highly trained medical transport crews, typically a nurse and a paramedic, but can include an advanced practice clinician, physician, respiratory therapist, or other specially trained clinicians. These are highly skilled medical transport crews with additional specialty training. These crews can typically manage all types of patients and provide advanced interventions and monitoring, ventilator management, specialty medication management, and blood product administration.
      v. *Specialty teams (OB/pediatric/neonatal):* Highly specialized critical care transport crews with extensive training in managing certain high-risk patients that require special knowledge and experience

E. *Special situations*

1. Emergency medical services online medical control
   a. *Role and responsibility:* Emergency medical service (EMS) operations and crews are regulated by their state health department much the way nurses are regulated by the state board of nursing. Oversite is provided by a medical director who determines training priorities, does chart reviews, and establishes written protocols and the relationship with a base hospital for patient care consultation. Within state regulations and their scope of practice certification level, EMS crews provide care and treatment via offline (written protocol) and online (base hospital) medical direction. Medical crews can request online medical direction from either their assigned base hospital or the receiving facility. The ENP becomes involved when the EMS crew calls for medical direction orders or consult and the ENP is the most qualified clinician available. The situation is comparable to that of the ENP consulting an attending physician. Coordinating patient care and medical orders with EMS crews is within the scope of practice of an RN, but some states also require additional training and certification for nurses to interact with EMS crews via online medical direction.
   b. *Familiarity with protocols:* EMS crews receive the same basic training and education; however, their scope of practice can vary greatly from state to state, within regions, and even between EMS services within the same geographic location. The EMS crew's scope of practice is delineated by their protocols, and they may have limited ability to deviate from these protocols. Some crews may also operate under guidelines instead of protocols, which usually give them more latitude in their patient care management. EDs should maintain copies of protocols for EMS crews they provide medical control for and other EMS services that regularly interact with their facility. Regulations and protocols spell out which medications crews can carry and use, as well as treatment expectations for different

patients and situations. Being familiar with the protocols will help the ENP better interact with the EMS crews to provide better patient care.

c. *Familiarity with crews and capabilities:* As with any healthcare clinician, different EMS crews and services have varying levels or training, experience, and skills. Getting familiar with the crews that regularly come to your facility can identify those that may need a bit more oversight, as well as guide recommendations for additional training and continuing medical education.

d. *Paid versus volunteer versus private services:* EMS crews work for one of three types of service. Each service has its own set of characteristics and purpose.

i. *Paid:* Paid services are typically municipally supported organizations that provide 24-hour EMS coverage for their communities. They are often fire service based, but can also be dedicated third service units that provide EMS only. These crews are typically high volume and receive a high degree of continuing training/education as well as medical director oversite. They are also typically the best-equipped crews. This setup is what most people imagine when they think about EMS.

ii. *Volunteer:* Volunteer crews are citizens with regular jobs who dedicate some of their time to serving their community. Some can get municipal support, but most rely on community support through fundraising. Some agencies can be mixed services, with a small full-time paid cadre supplemented by volunteers. Volunteer agencies typically operate in larger rural areas and some suburbs; they are also more common in the eastern United States. Due to typically lower volumes and part-time volunteer status, some crews may have rather limited experience despite many years of service.

iii. *Private:* Private EMS for-profit agencies work on a contract basis. Some work as dedicated EMS or as transport clinicians for fire services. They are often composed of local or regional "mom and pop" operations, but as with healthcare consolidation in general, many have been acquired by large ambulance service corporations such as American Medical Response or Rural-Metro. There are also several larger private EMS agencies that contract and function like a regional third service EMS operation. Examples of these services include Acadian Ambulance Service, REMSA (Regional Emergency Medical Services Authority), and Sunstar EMS. In addition, private EMS services provide the primary interfacility transport service in most locations, although in some locations, the community EMS organization also provides transfer services.

(1) *Certification level:* EMS crews are certified at one of four levels that define their scope of practice within their protocols. Designations can vary by state. The descriptions and designations are based on the National Highway Traffic Safety Administration (NHTSA) Office of EMS Scope of Practice and National Registry of Emergency Medical Technicians (NREMT) certification levels.

(i) *Emergency medical responder (EMR):* First responders have the lowest level of training. They are trained in CPR, hemorrhage control, simple splinting, simple airway assistance. Clinicians with this certification level are typically found on non-EMS volunteer fire units and in-house industrial emergency response teams.

(ii) *EMT:* EMTs are the core basic level EMS clinician. In addition to the EMR training and skills, EMTs also have training in additional basic airway management, immobilization, and other patient treatments.

(iii) *Advanced EMT (AEMT):* AEMTs can start IVs and have additional limited medication and advanced airway management training. AEMTs are typically encountered in rural areas with limited paramedic service or as paramedic students gaining additional experience while completing their paramedic program.

(iv) *Nationally registered paramedic (NRP):* Paramedic is the highest level of EMS licensure. Paramedics have training in advanced cardiac life support (ACLS), 12-lead EKGs, advanced airway management, and other skills. They also carry a limited medication supply for use in treating and stabling patients during the transport to the ED. Some paramedics may also have additional training certification in RSI, chest tube and central line placement, management of additional drugs for transport, and other advanced skills.

2. *Local hazards:* Every location has its own unique hazards and ED visit patterns. Learning and preparing for these hazards will increase the ENP's effectiveness in providing care.

a. *Farm equipment and injuries:* Farming and agriculture operations involve several types of hazardous equipment and chemicals and large animals that can cause unique trauma injuries requiring adaptation to normal treatment interventions. Patients may have an extended period from injury to definitive care management.

b. *Wilderness emergencies and injuries:* Most wilderness emergencies and injuries are routine but complicated by difficulty accessing the patient. They can also be complicated by prolonged extrication times or environmental factors leading to dehydration, hypothermia, heatstroke, or metabolic derangements.

c. *Hazmat and industrial hazards:* Industrial and chemical manufacturing located in rural areas are usually geographically isolated because of their dangerous nature; mining can also be a hazardous local industry. The ENP should be familiar with the potential local hazards and special treatment requirements that may be required.

d. *Seasonal tourist/weather/special events:* Being aware of seasonal influxes, pending extreme weather, and special events will help the ENP prepare for the increased demand and manage treatment capabilities at the facility.

3. *Special resources, training, and support:* There are many resources, training, and support services that can assist the ENP in providing quality care.

a. *Specialty consults and definitive care resources:* The ENP should have an on-site or on-call emergency physician available for consultation. Additionally, there should be an agreement in place with a tertiary facility to provide consultation services if there are no on-call specialists available.

b. *Poison control center:* The National Poison Control number (1-800-222-1222) is an excellent toxicology resource.

c. *Telemedicine and e-ICU resources:* Modern telemedicine and e-ICU resources when available can provide expedited patient assessment and consultation for psychiatry, neurology, cardiology, and other types of patients requiring additional services.

d. *Hazmat and fire service:* Fire department training includes training on managing hazardous materials situations and special training on potential local hazardous material situations.

e. *CME and electronic resources:* The proliferation of the internet has allowed for rapid dissemination of the most up-to-date medical information. There are many high-quality free sites for retrieving information and education. In addition to conferences, continuing medical education is also readily available in various digital formats.

f. *EMS and critical care transport crews:* Having a mutual relationship with the local EMS and critical transport crews can benefit both patients and clinicians. Combined training can maximize resources and enhance teamwork in mutual assistance situations.

Additional Reading

Additional Reading for this chapter are online only and can be found at https://connect.springerpub.com/content/reference-book/978-0-8261-6091-5/part/part07/toc-part/ch52.

53. Sexual and Gender Minority Patients in the Emergency Department

RICK RAMIREZ

Author's Note: For the purpose of this chapter, LGBTQIA patients are identified as Sexual and Gender Minorities (SGM).

Learning Objectives

- Identify key definitions and healthcare points related to SGM patients.
- Identify methods of "inclusive safe-space" promotion in the ED setting for the SGM population.
- Recognize bias, stigma, and fear of clinician-related gaps in knowledge and understanding related to the SGM population.
- Define key history taking and assessment techniques for patient comfort and safety.
- Recognize specific healthcare disparities related to the SGM population.
- Evaluate how gender-affirming therapies and lifestyle choices can affect and skew patient assessment and diagnostic test interpretation within the ED setting.
- Provide sound explanation into healthcare aspects, support, and follow-up during the ED visit.
- Demonstrate the role of the emergency nurse practitioner (ENP) as an advocate for the SGM population.

This chapter covers a wide array of topics related to the care of the SGM population but is not an exhaustive examination of the extreme specifics related to the breadth of SGM healthcare, nor does it substitute for interpersonal cultural-care training of this very unique population.

A. The ED is a fast-paced, intense, oftentimes protocol-driven, and overcrowded unit. The emergency nurse practitioner (ENP) is often found in a variety of roles, from triage, to direct patient care, to ensuring appropriate follow-up for patients evaluated.

B. In this fast-paced environment, patient sexual and gender identity recognition often goes unnoticed, leaving the SGM patient feeling untrusting and uncared for by their clinician.

1. Approximately 4.5% of Americans identify as LGBT.[1]

2. More than 1 million persons who identify as LGBT are U.S. military veterans.[2] Of those, approximately 150,000 active and veteran military identify as transgender.[3]

3. SGM populations are at risk for poorer health outcomes and decreased access to care related to health insurance needs and services, compared to their heterosexual counterparts.[4] There is also a paucity of healthcare-related research specific to this population, creating healthcare challenges and competent medical care for the SGM community.[5]

4. ED clinicians do not ask SGM-related questions due to perceived lack of medical relevance to care. In contrast, ED patients note that SGM-related questions are appropriate in all circumstances to provide care in a holistic manner.[6] It is important for the ENP to initiate a consistent interview process for all patients. That includes incorporation of questions pertaining to gender identity and pronouns to help establish patient trust.[7]

C. Members of the SGM population often do not seek out care because of fear of being outed, bias, stigma, and prior delays or denial of care they, or their friends, have experienced.[8]

1. Nearly 33% of transgender patients admit to a delay in seeking out healthcare because of negative past experience, and one-fifth of transgender patients admit to being refused healthcare altogether related to their identity.[8]

2. In a 2011 study published by the *Journal of the American Medical Association*, medical schools spent a median of 5 hours of instruction on SGM health,[9] whereas schools of nursing often fail to place SGM content in their advanced practice curriculum, leaving the nurse practitioner (NP) with a paucity of, or no source of information into the care of this population.[10]

a. 91% of NPs do not receive SGM-specific content or courses in their educational programs. If the ENP does receive content, it is limited to a few hours.[11]

3. Health-related disparities based on sexual orientation and gender identity are rooted in, and reflect, historical stigma of the SGM population.

a. Most patients in this population experience gaps in clinician knowledge and bias from an early age, which shapes how they perceive and interact with the healthcare system for the rest of their lives.
b. Despite Freud believing in 1935 that homosexuality should not be classified as a mental illness, American psychoanalysis broke with Freud and in 1952 listed homosexuality as a "sociopathic personality disorder" in the newly created *Diagnostics and Statistical Manual of Mental Disorders* (*DSM*) in 1952.[12,13]
c. Research concluded that homosexuality was not associated with psychopathology,[14] which in turn caused a cascade of research into the arena, eventually becoming the mainstream view of mental health professionals in the United States. Yet, SGM patients continue to experience hardships related to their healthcare, such as lack of appropriate healthcare access, lack of knowledgable clinicians, and lack of feeling safe with their clinicians, often causing SGM persons to seek care in the ED.[13]
d. Transgender persons may or may not undergo gender-affirming hormone therapies. These include the use of prescription or nonprescription hormone replacement (e.g., estrogen, spironolactone, testosterone, leuprolide, anabolic steroids).[15]
e. Transgender persons may or may not undergo partial or complete gender-affirming surgical procedures. These are termed "Top Surgery" (i.e., the removal or addition of breast tissue) or genitourinary reconstruction or "Bottom Surgery" (i.e., vaginoplasty, phalloplasty, scrotoplasty, metaoidioplasty, hysterectomy, oophorectomy, salpingo-oophorectomy, orchiectomy, vaginectomy, penile prosthesis, testicular prosthesis, urethroplasty, vulvoplasty).[15–19]

Definitions

According to the Healthcare Equality Index, SGM patients are at increased risk for substandard, intensive, or even abusive care related to stigmatization.[20] It is well known that the SGM population is more likely to delay seeking care, be more likely to be dependent on social and illicit substances, is at increased risk of intimate partner violence (IPV), and has a higher risk of depression and suicidal ideations.[5] One of the first steps to bridging this gap is to be knowledgeable about SGM identity terminology and the meaning of being LGBTQQIAAP (Table 53.1).

TABLE 53.1 LGBTQQIAAP TERMINOLOGY

LETTER	TERM	DEFINITION
L	Lesbian	A person who identifies as a female who is sexually or emotionally attracted to other persons who identify as female **1.** Cisgender female: A person who was assigned female at birth and who currently identifies as female
G	Gay	A person who identifies as a male who is sexually or emotionally attracted to other persons who identify as male **1.** Cisgender male: A person who was assigned male at birth and currently identifies as male
B	Bisexual	A person who identifies as either male or female who is sexually or attracted to both male and female identities
T	Transgender	A person whose gender identity does not align with the gender they were assigned at birth **1.** Transman (transmale, FTM): A person who was assigned female at birth but currently identifies their gender as male **2.** Transwoman (transfemale, MTF): A person who was assigned male at birth but currently identifies their gender as female **3.** Genderqueer: A person whose gender identity falls outside of the traditional binary (male/female) construct **4.** Genderfluid: A person who can simultaneously identify as male or female and flow between the two definitions **5.** Nonbinary: A person whose gender does not conform to the idea that there are two genders or that a person must fit into a category **6.** Transgender people may be attracted to women (gynephilic), attracted to men (androphilic), or identify as heterosexual, gay, lesbian, bisexual, asexual, pansexual, or queer
Q2	Queer Questioning	Queer is considered by many in the SGM community to be derogatory, however, many still refer to themselves as Queer, which is an umbrella term encompassing most of the SGM types **1.** Drag Queen: A person who was born and appears male who impersonates women as a means of gender expressions or entertainment **2.** Drag King: A person who was born and appears female who impersonates men as a means of gender expression or entertainment **3.** Transvestite (Tranny): Former term (and now derogatory) to identify persons who identified as a male who dressed in clothing designed for females as a form of expression Questioning: Simply means that the person does not know what gender identity they are or what gender they are attracted to
I	Intersex	The term used for a variety of conditions in which a person is born with reproductive or sexual anatomy that does not fit the typical definitions of male or female
A2	Asexual Ally	A person who lacks sexual attraction or desire for other people. An Ally is typically a heterosexual person who supports and advocates for the SGM community
P	Pansexual	A person who self-identifies as a specific gender who is sexually and/or emotionally attracted to others regardless of their sexual orientation, genders, or expression

Note: FTM, female to male; MTF, male to female.

TABLE 53.2 BASIC GENDER IDENTITY AND PRONOUN USE

GENDER IDENTITY	PRONOUN IDENTITY	PRONOUNS
Cisgender male	Masculine pronouns	He/him/his/himself
Cisgender female	Feminine pronouns	She/her/hers/herself
Transgender and nonbinary	Inclusive or gender-neutral pronouns	They/them/theirs/themselves/ze/hir/hirs/hirself

After confirming legal names of patients, a model the ENP can adapt and utilize to discern this is to ask, "What name would you like to be addressed as?" or "What name can I use in your care today?" and "What do you consider your sexual orientation to be?" or "Who are you attracted to?" or "Describe your sexual identify."[7,15] The ENP should be aware that data concerning one's sexuality may change over time.

Once sexual orientation and/or gender identity is confirmed, the next step to affirming confidence and care is to ask the patient, "What pronouns do you use?" Pronoun use is, at times, very tricky as the patient may mix or match pronoun use to how they identify. However, a basic understanding is summarized in Table 53.2.

Finally, asking the question about sexual partners is crucial, especially in the setting of IPV, sexually transmitted infections (STIs), or who their partner is. Initial questions to ask are, "Have you had intimate contact with anyone in the past year," "What gender(s) do you have sexual contact with," "How many partners have you had in the past year," "How many new partners have you had in the past year," "Do you feel safe in your environment/home?" Asking these questions without identifying gender or orientation allows the patient to feel more open and accepted in the presence of the ENP.

General Approach to the Sexual and Gender Minority Patient in the Emergency Department

Authors Note: The below statements are general in nature and may be adapted for SGM patients of any age group across the life span.

Introduction

A. Legal name
B. Preferred name
C. Gender identity
 1. Cisgender male/female
 2. Transgender male/female
 3. Nonbinary/genderfluid/intersex
D. Pronouns
 1. He/him/his, she/her/hers, they/them/theirs, and so on
E. Sexual orientation/identification
 1. L, G, B, T, Q, I, A, P, and so on
F. Chief complaint
G. Medical history, medications, surgical history
 1. Transgender gender-affirming therapies
  a. Feminizing hormones (e.g., estradiol-oral/transdermal/parenteral, spironolactone, progestins, and leuprolide in the suppression of endogenous hormones during puberty).[21]
  b. Masculinizing hormones (e.g., testosterone, 5-alpha reductase inhibitors, aromatase inhibitors, methylprogesterone, other anabolic steroids, and perhaps intrauterine device placement).[21,22]
  c. Top surgery (e.g., mastectomy [bilateral] or breast augmentation)
  d. Bottom surgery (e.g., sexual organ [anatomic] inventory, hysterectomy, phalloplasty, oophorectomy, salpingo-oophorectomy, orchiectomy, vaginectomy).[16,17,19]
 2. Complete sexual history and screening for IPV, sex trafficking, STIs, and nonaccidental trauma.
 3. Home/environment safety
 4. Family/partner safety
 5. Forced actions
 6. Danger Assessment Tool for Domestic Abuse[23]

General Medical and Trauma-Related Chief Complaints

A. Assessed and cared for using evidence-based practice guidelines
B. *Example:* Chest pain (CP)
 1. EKG, laboratory studies (order as indicated): complete blood count (CBC), metabolic panel (MP), liver functions, troponin (Trop I), urinalysis (UA), qualitative beta-human chorionic gonadotropin (b-HCG) if potential or indicated, urine drug screen if potential or indicated. Chest x-ray (CXR), chest CT scan if potential or indicated, and so on.
C. *Example:* Motor vehicle crash (MVC)
 1. Designate trauma level based on prehospital or patient report. Assume trauma protocols. Laboratory studies (order as indicated): CBC, MP, liver functions, UA, b-HCG if potential or indicated, urine drug screen if potential or indicated. CXR, pelvic radiograph (pelvic x-ray), chest CT scan if potential or indicated, and so on.
D. Assess use of gender-affirming medical therapies.
 1. Estrogen
  a. Ethinyl estradiol is no longer used because of its side-effect profile.[21]
  b. May increase risk for venous thromboembolism (VTE), hypertension (HTN), cancer, diabetes, fluid retention, impaired conversion of T4 to T3, pulmonary embolism (PE), myocardial infarction (MI), cerebrovascular accident (CVA), irregular bleeding, weight gain, headache, depression, skin rash. hypocalcemia, hypertriglyceridemia, pancreatitis, gastroenteritis, liver dysfunction, mastalgia, diabetes mellitus exacerbation[15,24,25]

c. Oral, transdermal estradiol, and parenteral estradiol valerate are preferred agents.[21]

2. Spironolactone (used for antiandrogen effects)
   a. Increases risk of electrolyte imbalances, hyperkalemia, rash, Stevens–Johnson syndrome, amenorrhea, decreased libido, gout, hyperglycemia, hypocalcemia, hypomagnesemia, hyponatremia, hepatotoxicity, renal insufficiency and failure, volume depletion[15,26]
3. Testosterone
   a. May be given intramuscularly, topically, or implanted pellets subcutaneously
   b. May cause polycythemia, liver dysfunction, hormonal induced acne/cystic acne, cardiovascular issues, prostrate growth, mood swings, HTN, skin blisters, benign prostatic hypertrophy, edema, peripheral vascular disease, headache, vertigo, acne, hypokalemia, hypertriglyceridemia, elevated thyroid-stimulating hormone levels, gynecomastia, hepatic dysfunction, increase in serum prolactin, obstructive sleep apnea exacerbation, endometrial and vaginal atrophy, renal dysfunction[15,21,24]
4. 5-alpha reductase inhibitors
   a. May cause orthostatic hypotension, peripheral edema, decreased libido, gynecomastia, breast tenderness, anorgasmia, aspermia, depressions, suicidal ideation[27]

Sexually Transmitted Infections

A. The Centers for Disease Control and Prevention (CDC) notes approximately 20 million new STIs per year, with SGM patients disproportionately affected.[24]

B. Medical screening
1. Sexual health screening in the SGM population
   a. Who do you have intercourse with?
   b. What gender(s) do you have intercourse with (e.g., male, female, transmale, transfemale, intersex, nonbinary)?
   c. What type of intercourse do you participate in (e.g., oral, vaginal, anal, other)?
   d. How many sexual partners have you had in the past 12 months?
   e. Are you or your partner(s) trying to become pregnant?
   f. Do you use intercourse barriers or contraceptive medications/devices (always/sometimes/never, with all/some/no partners, medications/methods)?
   g. What do you do use for STI/HIV protection (e.g., condoms, pre-exposure prophylaxis [PrEP], others)?
   h. Last time tested for STIs/HIV?
   i. Pain with intercourse?
   j. Do you use any type of intercourse-enhancing devices, toys, substances (illicit or prescription)?
   k. Have you or your partner(s) ever had or been treated for an STI?
   l. Home, environment, context safety questions
   m. Inquiry into current prescription and over-the-counter medications and herbs. Inquiry into gender-affirming medication treatments.
      i. Studies have shown that antiretroviral therapy medications (i.e., protease inhibitors [PIs], non-nucleoside reverse transcriptase inhibitors [NNRTIs]), specifically Efavirenz, negatively affect estradiol and medroxyprogesterone metabolism.[28,29]
2. Nonaccidental trauma and human trafficking screenings
   a. Do you exchange money or substances for intercourse?[15,24]
3. Physical assessment
   a. Discuss the need to perform physical assessment.
   b. Take into consideration the patient's sexual/gender identity.
   c. Take an anatomic inventory.
   d. Patients may not identify with the sexual organs they have. Take this into consideration and discuss with the patient using cultural competence methods of communication prior to the examination. Use the patient's preferred adjective descriptions of organs when discussing the examination if possible.

Physical Trauma

A. SGM patients are at increased risk (18%) of physical, intimate partner, and sexual violence as compared to their heterosexual counterparts, with prevalence significantly higher in bisexual and gay men.[24,30]

B. Over 11% of SGM screened positive for IPV, physical, or sexual violence based on orientation or gender identification alone[30]; 47% of transgender people are assaulted and 50% of all SGM populations who have died from physical, intimate partner, or sexual violence were transfemale[30,31]; 20% of SGM youth have had forceful sexual encounters with 11% of those attacks based solely on status as SGM.[32]

C. Medical screening
1. Primary and secondary trauma surveys
   a. Airway
      i. Airway assessment with cervical spine precautions
      ii. Address airway concerns/compromise.
      iii. Assess for bruising/missing teeth, and so on.
      iv. Breathing
      v. Inspection/palpation/auscultation
      vi. Address breathing compromise or abnormal findings.
   b. Circulation
      i. Inspect pulse and quality. Assess for signs of nonaccidental trauma/bleeding.
      ii. Address hemorrhage.
         (1) Hemorrhage may occur in relation to gender-related violence. Violence can occur in many forms, including penetration, sharp force, and blunt trauma. These types of trauma can occur at any point on the body.

2. Disability
   a. Assess the neurological status.
3. Exposure
   a. Completely expose the patient to evaluate for injuries.
   b. Acknowledge gender identity and take anatomic inventory.
   c. Transmales may have uterine or vaginal trauma/bleeding. Transfemales may demonstrate blood at the penile meatus or have a floating prostate on digital rectal examination.[30]
   d. Use appropriate screening tools to identify human trafficking victims.[32]

Sexual and Gender Minority Mental Health Emergencies

A. SGMs are marginalized and at increased risk of discrimination, psychological abuse, stigmatization, and paucity of acceptance within peers, family, and self.[30]
B. SGM youth have significantly increased rates of suicidal ideas, suicidal actions, illicit substance abuse, smoking, alcohol use, and decrease access to social support and services[30,32]; 40% of undomiciled youth identify as SGM, which has either been forced or voluntary based on social constructs within the family.[32]
C. SGM of advanced age are increasingly marginalized, contributing to isolation, abuse, depressions, neglect, and suicidal actions.[33]
D. Medical screening
E. Psychiatric screening
   1. Identify homicidal/suicidal ideas and/or evidence of hallucinations.
   2. Identify previous homicidal/suicidal thoughts/actions.
      a. Active and veteran members of the military have increased rates of psychiatric processes including posttraumatic stress disorder, anxiety, depressions, suicidal ideation, and military sexual trauma.[2]
   3. Rule out organic causes.
      a. CBC, MP, urinalysis (UA), urine drug screen, urine hCG (if indicated)
      b. Salicylate, acetaminophen, ethanol serum levels (if indicated)
      c. *Neuroimaging:* CT, magnetic resonance imaging (if indicated)
      d. EKG/echocardiogram (if indicated)
      e. Lumbar puncture (if indicated)
   4. Assess for withdrawal symptoms.
   5. Assess for psychosis.
   6. Altered mental status (AMS) or personality
      a. Disorientation/confusion/paranoia
      b. Hallucinations
   7. Abnormal vital signs/focal neurological signs
      a. Use "SAD PERSONS" score to correlate for hospitalization.
   8. Identify risk factors and access to firearms.
   9. Identify safety within the home/friendships/relationships.
   10. Identify symptoms of anhedonia, depression, hopelessness.
   11. Identify social support variances.
      a. Family structure and safety
      b. Signs of bullying, neglect, nonaccidental trauma, discrimination
      c. Undomiciled status
      d. Economic hardship
      e. Forced sexual acts
      f. Family/friends use of illicit substances
F. Consult psychiatric services for assessment and intervention.[30,32–34]

Toxicology

A. SGM populations have documented increased rates of smoking, alcohol, and illicit substance use as compared to their heterosexual counterparts. Illicit substances can include (but are not limited to) cocaine, 3,4-methylenedioxymethamphetamine (MDMA, Ecstasy, Molly, "rolling"), marijuana, lysergic acid diethylamide (LSD), heroin, amyl nitrates ("poppers"), methamphetamine, sedatives, hallucinogens, analgesics, and so on.[30]
B. Medical screening
   1. Assess airway and control if necessary.
   2. Assess breathing and intervene as necessary.
   3. Assess circulation.
      a. Vital signs may be elevated related to the type of substance used.
   4. Identify at-risk behaviors.
   5. Identify timing of ingestion.
   6. Identify coingestions.
   7. Screen for suicidal/homicidal ideations.
   8. Screen for hallucinations.
   9. Identify the length of symptoms.
C. Diagnostic labs
   1. CBC, MP, salicylate/acetaminophen/ethanol levels, urine drug screen (will not produce results of all illicit substances)
D. Utilize Screening, Brief Intervention, and Referral to Treatment (SBIRT) to identify, evaluate, intervene, and decrease substance use.
   1. Reinforces healthy actions/behaviors
E. Identify physically or mentally unstable patients and admit per hospital protocols as needed.

References

References for this chapter are online only and can be found at https://connect.springerpub.com/content/reference-book/978-0-8261-6091-5/part/part07/toc-part/ch53.

54. Vulnerable Populations in the Emergency Setting

MELANIE GIBBONS HALLMAN | LEIGH HART | PATRICIA M. SPECK

Learning Objectives

- Define vulnerable populations with sensitivity to trauma as a universal experience.
- Describe the impact of lived experience on health outcomes for vulnerable populations.
- Identify principles of trauma-informed care for micro-, mezzo-, and macrosystems in emergency care provision that contribute to safe environments that are transparent and patient centered.

General Approach to Vulnerable Populations in the ED

A. The ED is a primary source of healthcare for many culturally diverse and vulnerable populations.

B. The social determinants of health (Figure 54.1) influence longevity and are the conditions in which people live, work, and age.

1. The determinants include economic stability, neighborhood and physical environment, education, food, community and social context, and healthcare system.

C. The increased understanding of the relationship between stress and lifelong impact on health provides insight into the possibility of significant trauma in the lived experience of every patient. Rhetorically, how does a lively, happy baby become homeless, uninsured, disabled or an un/documented e/immigrant? The emerging evidence points to stress from unstable families, communities under stress, and systems that deny liberty to the vulnerable.

Overview of Vulnerable Populations

A. Vulnerable populations are persons experiencing poor health without resources in the micro-, mezzo-, and macrosystems to address their personal needs.

1. Microlevel resources refer to those of the individual or the individual's family.
2. Mezzolevel resources refer to local institutions and community resources and equity in access.
3. Macrolevel resources are the government systems' resources, where structural gaps may prevent access and equity in morbidity and mortality, akin to the social determinants of health discussed later.

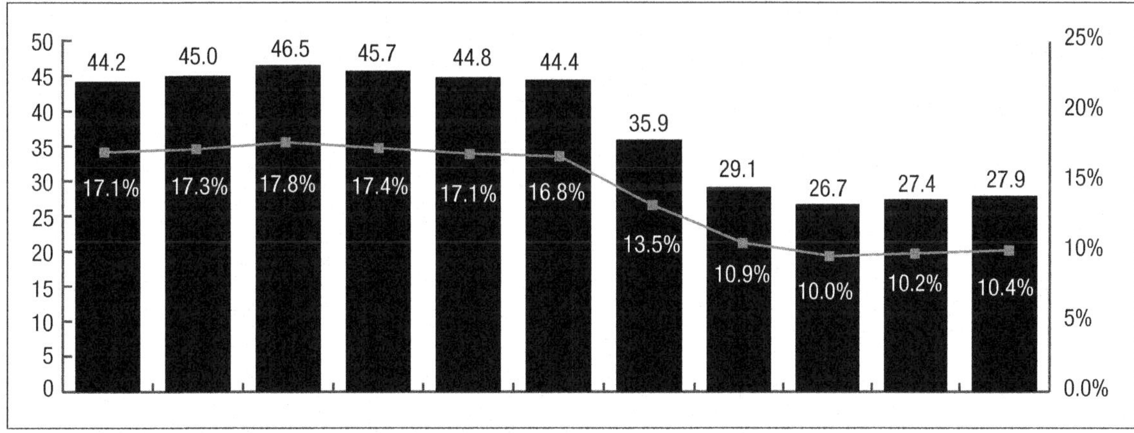

FIGURE 54.1 Kaiser Foundation social determinants of health.
Source: Reproduced with permission from the Kaiser Family Foundation. https://www.kff.org/disparities-policy/issue-brief/beyond-health-care-the-role-of-social-determinants-in-promoting-health-and-health-equity/[1]

B. Lack of resources is influenced by socioeconomic status, age, gender, race and ethnicity, English language proficiency, and medical issues and disabilities.

1. Their vulnerabilities place persons at risk for the big five illnesses of cardiac disease, diabetes, stroke, chronic obstructive pulmonary disease (COPD), and hypertension (HTN).
2. The vulnerable populations remain at risk for acute and chronic illnesses, exposure to environmental disasters, and unable to protect themselves in a public health emergency that exposes vulnerability at micro-, mezzo-, and macrosystems.

C. EDs provide a safety net for healthcare of vulnerable populations. In the 1990s, the Substance Abuse and Mental Health Services Administration (SAMHSA) prepared a consensus document related to guidance for a trauma-informed approach by healthcare institutions. Since then the growing awareness of trauma as a universal experience has resulted in principles of trauma-informed care.

D. Key assumptions include "three Es"—the event, the experience of the event, and the effect.

1. Event includes "an actual or extreme threat of physical or psychological harm."
2. The experience "helps to determine whether it is a traumatic event."
3. Adverse effects may be immediate or delayed or a combination of both. The individual may not recognize the connection. The impact is the individual is unable to cope with daily challenges of living, resulting in an inability "to trust and benefit from relationships; to manage cognitive processes . . . ; or to control the expression of emotions."

E. "A program, organization, or system that is trauma-informed realizes the widespread impact of trauma and understands potential paths for recovery; recognizes the signs and symptoms of trauma in clients, families, staff, and others involved with the system; and responds by fully integrating knowledge about trauma into policies, procedures, and practices, and seeks to actively resist re-traumatization" (SAMHSA, p. 8).

F. There are six key principles of a trauma-informed approach:

1. Safety
2. Trustworthiness and transparency
3. Peer support
4. Collaboration and mutuality
5. Empowerment, voice, and choice
6. Cultural, historical, and gender-based issues

G. These key principles are designed to resist traumatization in patients as well as clinicians and staff. In a trauma-informed approach to patient-centered care, the assessment strategy is modified to enhance inclusion of social determinants of health (Table 54.1). In a coordinated community response, clinicians and institutions collaborate with community resources in a shared decision-making between patient and clinician. The micro-, mezzo-, and macroapproaches to all patients improve safety and create an actionable trauma-informed approach to vulnerable populations.

H. Many times, vulnerable populations experience addictions and seek care in the ED. Often their health is not routinely addressed in primary care. The reasons for this vary, but they may be homeless, uninsured, immigrant, or disabled. Hence, the patient may be in crisis. The cause may be unknown to the ED clinician initially without a drug screen, and the presentation of the patient may be complicated because of addictions, self-medication, or recreational drug use. The healthcare clinician must remain aware of possible drug interactions as they proceed with emergent treatment. Table 54.2 provides potential drug interactions in the ED setting.

TABLE 54.1 EXAMPLES OF VULNERABILITIES CATEGORIZED USING SOCIAL DETERMINANTS OF HEALTH [a]

ACUTE AND CHRONIC ILLNESSES MEDICAL HISTORY (MICRO)	ENVIRONMENTAL RISKS (MEZZO)	PUBLIC HEALTH AND EMERGENCIES (MACRO)
Cancer diagnoses	Water	Access to healthcare
Liver disease	Food insecurity	Equity in healthcare
Cardiac disease	Housing insecurity	Social support
Pulmonary disease	Employment insecurity	Weather-related events
Metabolic disease	Financial resources	Personal disasters
End-stage disease	Transportation	
Addictions[b]	Community strife	
	Education	

[a]This table lists challenges to vulnerable populations but is not comprehensive.

[b]Considerations with drug interactions are expanded in Table 54.2.

TABLE 54.2 MEDICATION CONSIDERATIONS FOR SPECIAL POPULATIONS EXPERIENCING ADDICTIONS

MEDICATION	SPECIAL CONSIDERATION(S)
Albuterol	May be used to enhance crack cocaine effects
Anticholinergics	May cause serious hyperpyrexia, especially if used in warm climates with diuretics
Beta-blockers	Caution in cocaine toxicity, may exacerbate coronary spasm. If used, it is recommended to use a beta-blocker with alpha- and beta-blocking activity and to add a vasodilator such as NTG or a calcium channel blocker Abrupt discontinuation can result in rebound hypertension
Bupropion (Wellbutrin)	Can be made into a powder used to get high
Clonidine	May prolong the effects of heroin and opioids
Diuretics	May exacerbate dehydration and electrolyte imbalances
NSAID	May exacerbate heart failure related to fluid retention
Promethazine	May be used in methadone maintenance patients to potentiate a "high" feeling
Pseudoephedrine	Used in the creation of methamphetamine
Quetiapine (Seroquel)	Used to enhance the effects of heroine

NTG, nitroglycerine.

VULNERABLE POPULATIONS COMMONLY CARED FOR IN THE ED

E/Immigrants and Undocumented Individuals

Definition

A. Persons leave their homes for a variety of reasons. Safety and opportunity drive populations of people to new lives. However, the reasons provided are as varied as the persons leaving their home. Though often confused, there are distinctions between emigration, immigration, and migration. The definitions for the three types of migration follow:

1. *Emigrate*: To leave one's country or region to settle in another
   a. Each year many people emigrate from Europe.
2. *Immigrate*: To enter and settle in a country of which one is not a native, usually for permanent residence
   a. There are many reasons to immigrate to the United States.
3. *Migrate*: To go from one country, region, or place to another, especially periodically
   a. Rural populations have migrated to urban areas.

B. Aliens are persons used for work who are not citizens of the country in which they reside.

C. Population movements are cataloged in a variety of ways by governments, depending on the nature of human movement. These terms are predicated on reasons for leaving one's home country as well as the work while in the foreign land. Documentation of movement between borders of persons is unique to the country and may include quarantine. At this time, no country allows persons to arrive without documentation and assessment for disease transmission; however, persons arrive without documentation, and recently there has been an uptick in sexually transmitted and communicable diseases credited to undocumented emigration.

1. *Asylum*: Under U.S. law, a status that may be granted to an alien physically present in the United States, whom has been determined, among other requirements, to satisfy the U.S. statutory definition of a refugee. After a continuous year in asylum status, an alien may petition for adjustment to permanent resident status. Only 10,000 such requests may be approved in any fiscal year.
2. *Displaced*: An individual who has been forced or obliged to flee or leave their home temporarlly and who expects to return eventually.
   a. Internally displaced persons (IDPs) have relocated within their country, while externally displaced persons have crossed an international border. Depending upon their ability to return, and whether they are subject to persecution in their home country, externally displaced persons may be entitled to recognition as refugees under the United National High Commissioner on Refugees's (UNHCR) mandate.
3. *Refugee*: Under the Immigration and Nationality Act, any person who is outside any country of such person's nationality or, in the case of a person having no nationality, is outside any country in which such person last habitually resided, and who is unable or unwilling to return to, and is unable or unwilling to avail themself of the protection of that country because of persecution or a well-founded fear of persecution on account of race, religion, nationality, membership in a particular social group, or political opinion.

Epidemiology of E/Immigrants and Undocumented Individuals

A. In 2019, an estimated 11 million non-English-speaking impoverished, uninsured, and undocumented e/immigrants resided in the United States.
B. Undocumented e/immigrants account for approximately 25% of the uninsured population.
C. Many undocumented e/immigrants have experienced excessive violence, political and criminal torment, and sought refuge when entering the United States without seeking legal asylum.
D. Undocumented e/immigrants are subject to violence and repeat injury and often avoid reporting crimes to authorities for fear of retaliation or exposure of their undocumented status.
E. Undocumented e/immigrants are often victims of domestic violence, human trafficking, and exposure to dangerous and illegal work environments.

Special Considerations

A. Social determinants of health (macro)
- **1.** Undocumented e/immigrants are ineligible for most federal, state, and local health benefits, leaving them heavily dependent to seek healthcare in EDs.
- **2.** These individuals are only partially assisted by the Affordable Care Act of 2010, even when "lawfully present."
- **3.** The federal government failed to establish laws related to e/immigration. However, the U-Visa is part of the Victims of Trafficking and Violence Protection Act of 2000 and offers a structured mechanism to attain legal residency when a victim of crime is willing to partner with legal authorities to prosecute criminal cases where a patient's citizenship status impedes communication and care.

B. Trauma-informed care considerations (mezzo and micro)
- **1.** In a transparent relationship, the emergency clinician should carefully explain the confidentiality of the patient–clinician relationship and provide details about the U-Visa, offering referral to social work or local legal aid agencies for access to psychosocial support and asylum programs.
- **2.** Past events in an e/immigrant's life experience often results in depression, anxiety, and posttraumatic disorders, long-term pain complaints, and overall reduced physical function. Creating a safe environment in the institution will diminish resistance to care for the patient and their family.
- **3.** Many fear prosecution related to e/immigration, which causes them to avoid enrolling themselves or their children in available health support options.
- **4.** Straightforward, clear communication between undocumented patients and emergency nurse practitioners (ENPs) is crucial to building trust, conveying compassion, and assuring fair treatment for vulnerable populations to improve the quality, safety, and satisfaction of patient care.
- **5.** To create a sense of safety, both clinical and social aspects of care must be considered when evaluating and planning discharge care for e/immigrants.

C. Medical (micro)
- **1.** Clinicians must assure that equitable high-quality ED care, clear communication, safety assessment, strategic discharge education, and timely referral to community and federal resources are implemented.
- **2.** Non-English-proficient patients are more likely to repeat ED visits within 72 hours of discharge. This likelihood raises concern for the quality of ED care provided and discharge education provided.
- **3.** Schulson et al.[2] found that low-English proficient patients treated in EDs were more likely to have a higher rate of testing and hospital admissions.
- **4.** Victims of human trafficking are often difficult to identify due to distrust of legal authorities, and fear of retaliation and potential deportation. Clinicians should attempt to assess patients without visitors present, attempt to form a relationship of trust, and offer resource options for use when the victim chooses to seek assistance. ENPs should inform likely victims of trafficking of the T-Visa program, which offers temporary visas to victims of trafficking who agree to assist legal authorities in prosecution of traffickers. T-Visas have potential to become permanent visas in many cases.
- **5.** Early identification of language barriers is of utmost importance to assure safety, quality, and patient satisfaction. Professional interpreters should be consulted early in the patient care encounter. Title VI of the 1964 Civil Rights Act of the Department of Health and Human Services mandates that low-English-speaking patients should be referred knowledgeable legal advocates to avoid misinterpretation of information provided by the healthcare team.

Persons Experiencing Homelessness

A. The U.S. Department of Housing and Urban Development's (HUD, 2020) current definition of homelessness:
- **1.** An individual who lacks a fixed, regular, and adequate nighttime residence; as well an individual who has a primary nighttime residence that is a supervised publicly or privately operated shelter designed to provide temporary living accommodations, an institution that provides a temporary residence for individuals intended to be institutionalized; or a public or private place not designed for, or ordinarily used as, a regular sleeping accommodation for human beings.
- **2.** To further explain, individuals who lack resources and support networks to obtain permanent housing meet HUD's definition of homeless.

B. Categories of homeless include experiences of those who:
- **1.** Are trading sex for housing
- **2.** Are staying with friends, but cannot stay there for >14 days
- **3.** Are being trafficked
- **4.** Left home because of physical, emotional, or financial abuse or threats of abuse and have no safe, alternative housing

C. Epidemiology of homelessness

1. Majority male
2. Female homeless patients are ususally caring for children.
3. Numbers may be underreported and not include the housing of insecure individuals.
4. Homeless population cycles from ED to hospital admission. The lack of community health resources facilitates this cycle and results in a continual deterioration of health status.
5. Experience higher rates of 30-day ED and/or hospital readmission
6. Suffer higher mortality rates, higher rates of chronic illness, higher rates of infection, substance abuse, and mental illness
7. At higher risk for assaults and violence
8. Though shelters provide resources and respite, they may place homeless at increased risk for mental health issues, access to illicit substances, and sexually transmitted diseases.
9. Lesbian, gay, and transgender individuals experience worse health outcomes than their heterosexual counterparts living in a homeless environment.
10. May be difficult to identify while receiving care in the ED.
11. Homelessness may befall a person at any point during a lifetime.
12. Evidence of changing demographics
    a. Increase of average age of homeless from 37 to 50 years.
    b. Due to the prevalence of chronic and acute illness, 50 years of age is considered elderly in a homeless person.
13. Deficiency in amount of research focused on homeless pediatric and adolescent populations

Special Considerations

A. The following are some examples of special considerations for vulnerable populations:
1. Social determinants of health (macro- and mezzosystems)
2. *Transportation:* May come in by ambulance following incidents in public or lack of transportation
3. Trust/safety deficits
4. Difficulty managing wounds and chronic illnesses such as diabetes, asthma, and chronic obstructive pulmonary disease (COPD) due to lack of resources, including balanced nutrition
5. Face barriers to care, including difficult choices between available resources, food and shelter, and their medical needs
6. Concerns for safety, hunger, and lack of shelter may be precipitating factors for ED visits, relying on the ED to meet these needs in times of resource depletion.
7. Consider significant lack of resources for follow-up care when developing discharge plans.

B. Trauma-informed care considerations (mezzo and micro)
1. Must gain patient's trust early in interaction
2. Higher rates of
    a. Schizophrenia
    b. Depression
    c. Substance abuse
    d. Burn injuries
    e. Pediatric immunization delay
3. Medical (micro)
    a. Experience higher rates of
        i. Cardiovascular disease
        ii. Hypertension (HTN)
        iii. Mental health issues
        iv. Tuberculosis (TB)
        v. Violent injuries
    b. Need a trust/safety pact agreed upon by patient and clinician; if not agreed upon, have an assistant present during the physical examination.
    c. Often have difficulty obtaining and storing medication
    d. May share medications with other people due to sporadic access to healthcare and funding.
    e. At risk for medication interactions and misuse of common medications
4. ENPs should maintain an updated list of community resources for food, shelter, medication support, and primary medical care available to support a variety of vulnerable and homeless patients. Secure housing decreases ED visits and improves health outcomes.

Resources

A. There is significant need for specialized education for emergency clinicians focused on providing care to the homeless population, including accessing community resources. This education is notably absent in most emergency-specific curricula.

B. Recommended that healthcare personnel compile and maintain a current list of reduced fee healthcare resources available for the community in which they work.

C. A series of guidelines for the care of common medical conditions in the homeless population can be found at the National Council for Caring for the Homeless website.
1. *Adapting your practice:* Treatments and recommendations for caring for the homeless (www.nhchc.org/resources/clinical/adapted-clinical-guidelines/)
2. Also includes resources for caring for specific diseases in the homeless population

Persons Who Are Uninsured

Definition

A. The uninsured are persons who lack health insurance (Centers for Disease Control and Prevention [CDC], U.S. Census).

Epidemiology of the Uninsured

A. The number of ED visits by uninsured persons remained consistent from 2006 to 2013. By 2018, the number of ED visits increased by 25.6 million visits per year in spite of a 91.5% insured population.
1. Nearly three-quarters of uninsured populations had at least one full-time worker.

2. 83% had full- or part-time workers in the family.
3. 80% of the uninsured experienced incomes 400% below poverty levels.
4. The preponderance of persons identified to be uninsured are nonelderly adult males working frequently uninsured for long periods of time. Despite speculation, the number of patients and their reasons for presenting to EDs for care are very similar between adults who are insured and those who are uninsured.
a. Figure 54.2 represents a longitudinal view of uninsured populations.

Special Considerations

A. The following are some examples of special considerations for vulnerable populations.
B. Social determinants of health (macro)
1. The Emergency Medical Treatment and Labor Act (EMTALA) is a macroapproach to ensure equity and access to care by ensuring all individuals the right to receive emergency care regardless of their ability to pay, but does not provide protection from financial responsibility for care rendered. The stigma of being uninsured may pose barriers to emergency care for vulnerable populations.
C. Trauma-informed care considerations (primarily mezzo and micro)
1. Uninsured persons fear financial burden and will delay care. The medical system's trauma-informed approach would provide financial advice and consider financial limitations of the patient. Medical systems can assist the patient in creating financial stability by including a question about the patient's need for financial help with appropriate referral to community organizations.
2. In trauma-informed care, the mezzoapproach is to create systems to support the patient who is uninsured.
3. The micro approach to trauma-informed care related to safety and transparency ensures that patients have the choice and the voice in the acceptance of their individual planned treatments and approaches.
D. Medical (micro)
1. ENPs should be cognizant of the expense incurred for all diagnostic tests that they order, especially for those patients who will be paying the cost of the visit and diagnostics themselves. In trauma-informed care, full transparency for financial burden is necessary for patients to accept or decline a clinician's recommendations. For example, sutures that dissolve and Steri-Strips are an option for lacerations, making a return visit unnecessary unless a worsening condition develops.
2. ENPs should be aware of options for medications offered by local pharmacies and community support options at no cost or reduced cost for patients. Generic drugs should be prescribed when feasible to increase affordability and to increase success of adherence with discharge plans.

Persons With Disabilities

Definition of Disability

A. A disability is a physical or mental condition that limits a person's movements, senses, or activities.
B. The following are types of disabilities explained in this chapter:
1. Visual impairment
2. Hearing impairment

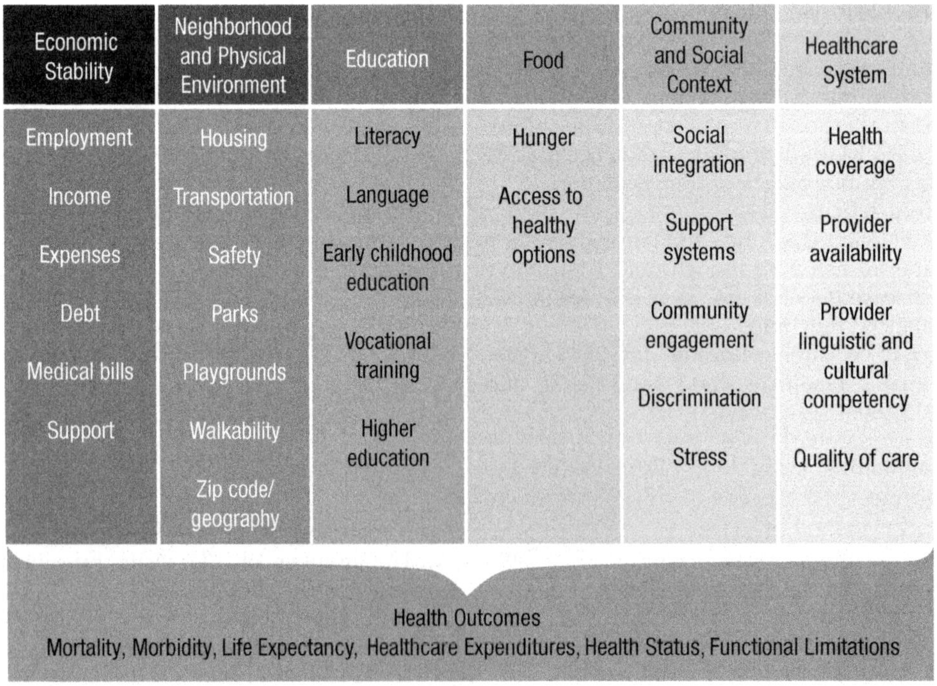

Economic Stability	Neighborhood and Physical Environment	Education	Food	Community and Social Context	Healthcare System
Employment Income Expenses Debt Medical bills Support	Housing Transportation Safety Parks Playgrounds Walkability Zip code/ geography	Literacy Language Early childhood education Vocational training Higher education	Hunger Access to healthy options	Social integration Support systems Community engagement Discrimination Stress	Health coverage Provider availability Provider linguistic and cultural competency Quality of care

Health Outcomes
Mortality, Morbidity, Life Expectancy, Healthcare Expenditures, Health Status, Functional Limitations

FIGURE 54.2 Kaiser Foundation uninsured population 2008 to 2018.
Source: Reproduced with permission from the Kaiser Family Foundation. https://www.kff.org/uninsured/issue-brief/key-facts-about-the-uninsured-population/[3]

3. Motor disabilities
4. Mental and intellectual disabilities

C. The variety and combinations of disabilities reported by ED patients are numerous and include both physical and behavioral diagnoses.

Epidemiology of Disability

A. Data from the Medical Expenditure Panel Survey (MEPS) revealed that adults with disabilities account for 17% of the adult population but reflect 40% of ED visits. The Centers for Disease Control and Prevention (CDC) reports[4]:

B. One in five adults or >53 million people in the United States have a disability of one form or another, with state-level estimates ranging from 1 in 6 (16.4%; Minnesota) to nearly 1 in 3 (31.5%; Alabama).

C. The most common functional disability type was mobility disability, reported by about one in eight adults.

D. Over a third of adults ≥65 years of age reported any disability.

E. Adults 45 to 64 years of age were more likely than other age groups of adults to report a cognitive disability.

F. Individuals reporting a higher household income or education level were less likely to report having a disability, compared to individuals in lower income or education levels.

G. Women were more likely to report any disability when compared with men (24.4% versus 19.8%). This likelihood was also seen for most of the disability types.

H. Disability was more frequently reported by non-Hispanic black (29.0%) and Hispanic (25.9%) adults than by white non-Hispanic (20.6%) adults.

Special Considerations

A. Social determinants of health (macro)

1. Hospitals and institutions serving persons affected by social determinants of health and with disabilities design facilities that accommodate and are compliant with the Americans with Disabilities Act (ADA).
2. Growing awareness about the connection between social determinants of health and disease in organizations provides opportunities for community stakeholders to participate in organizational improvements.

B. Trauma-informed care considerations (mezzo and micro)

1. Policies and procedures developed with community stakeholders promise to improve safety through transparent processes and provide opportunity for voice and choice.
2. Community participation in healthcare organization change, with the goal of reaching a trauma-informed approach to care, has the potential to heal communities experiencing social determinants of health.
3. Supporting employees and staff as they embrace trauma-informed care principles

C. Medical (micro)

1. Care of patients with disabilities often requires additional time and the ENP should take this into consideration when establishing patient load in the ED.
2. Frequent supervision of these patients is necessary.
3. ENPs should introduce themselves to the patient to assess abilities and limitations, including the ability to communicate and follow commands.
4. Caregivers often automatically assume communication for a patient with disabilities despite the patient being able to communicate and function with some independence.
5. Caregivers should be incorporated into the communicative patient's care with permission of the patient to uphold confidentiality requirements when possible.
6. Clear, detailed communication and patient permission, when possible, are essential to good patient/clinician and caregiver relationships.

Visually Impaired

A. Clearly speak your name and role in their care.

B. Always speak to the patient and advise them of what you are doing before you touch them, especially during the physical examination.

C. Provide clear, detailed instructions regarding normal and abnormal diagnostic and physical findings, medications, and discharge instructions.

Hearing Impaired

A. Establish if the patient reads lips, has a hearing aid, uses other methods of communication, or exclusively uses sign language.

B. If sign language is the patient's primary means of communication, access an interpreter for the patient if they do not have a significant other with them to interpret or if they prefer an interpreter instead of their significant other.

C. Elicit feedback from the patient to make certain that your communication has been clearly received and understood.

D. Use clearly written instructions as an additional mode of communication, especially in discussing findings from diagnostics, pertinent physical examination findings, and discharge instructions.

Motor Disabilities

A. Remove any physical barriers that may interfere with their care (e.g., cane, wheelchair).

B. Assure that the patient has a means to request assistance for moving about to avoid unnecessary falls.

Mental and Intellectual Disabilities

A. Tailor communication to best meet the patient's ability and comfort for communication. Allow the patient to manage as much communication as possible.

B. Include the patient's legal guardian in communications, especially for those who need an intermediary to assist or provide their care. Be certain that the intermediary clearly understands all details of the plan of care and discharge medications and instructions and can restate the information to you. Provide all information in writing to bolster understanding. Caregivers and intermediaries must be aware of any conditions to anticipate and monitor for, and what expected responses are from medications and therapies prescribed.

C. The more profound the disability, the greater instruction caregivers will need.

D. Anxiety and behavior fluctuations are common in patients with mental and intellectual disabilities. Show compassion and allow the patient to express themself in a safe manner.
E. Respectfully communicate to the patient when you are going to touch them, especially while performing the physical exam.
F. Potential risks for patients with disabilities are plentiful and diverse and must be considered and discussed with all parties essential to the patient's care to best protect the patient and ensure quality care.
G. Consideration should be given to the patient's physical and/or mental disability when ordering diagnostic tests. Patient mobility, medical and emotional stability, and staff availability should be considered when selecting diagnostic orders.
H. EDs provide care for individuals with mental health diagnoses. ENPs should assess for contextual factors possibly exacerbating existing mental health diagnoses and be aware that these are sometimes treated by self-medication with recreational drugs and substances.
I. Individuals with autism spectrum disorder (ASD) may require assistance from the ED when caregivers are unable to manage their needs. Many ASD patients suffer from anxiety and depression as well as other mental health diagnoses.
J. There are no medication treatments for ASD. Cognitive interventions should be attempted prior to or concurrently with medications when possible.
K. It is ethically and medically essential that prior to administration of medications commonly prescribed in the ED for mental health crises that benefits, risks, and potential extrapyramidal side effects, including initiation or worsening of akathisia, be discussed with the patient and/or significant others and caregivers. Prescribing the lowest effective dose and assessing response is key to least side effects and best outcomes.
L. Early referral for follow-up by a mental health specialist is best, but can be challenging to arrange if the patient is not already associated.

References

References for this chapter are online only and can be found at https://connect.springerpub.com/content/reference-book/978-0-8261-6091-5/part/part07/toc-part/ch54

55. Victims of Violence: Interpersonal Violence, Intimate Partner Violence, and Sexual Assault

KATHLEEN S. JORDAN

Learning Objectives

Interpersonal Violence: Abuse and Neglect

- Describe child and elder abuse as a public health problem in the United States in terms of incidence, prevalence, and the effect on individuals, families, and society at large.
- Identify risk factors for the recognition and reporting of child and elder abuse in the ED.
- Based on current evidence, describe essential clinical data the advanced practice clinician should obtain that may indicate child or elder abuse.
- Discuss evidence-based treatment for specific injuries associated with child and elder abuse.
- Describe essential documentation elements of child and elder abuse for medicolegal purposes.

Intimate Partner Violence

- Discuss the incidence and prevalence of intimate partner violence as a major public health problem in the United States.
- Define the mechanisms of injury that are classified as intimate partner violence.
- Identify appropriate screening questions to be used to identify patients who are potential survivors of intimate partner violence.
- Identify special populations who are at risk of intimate partner violence.
- Discuss the identification and management of patients who have sustained nonfatal strangulation in an intimate partner relationship.

Sexual Assault

- Describe sexual violence as a major public health problem in the United States in terms of incidence, prevalence, and the effect on individuals, families, and society at large.
- Define the acts that constitute sexual violence.
- Discuss factors that may increase an individual's vulnerability and risk of sexual violence.
- Based on current evidence, describe essential clinical data the advanced practice clinician should obtain from a survivor of a sexual assault.
- Discuss evidence-based treatment for a survivor of sexual assault in the ED.
- Discuss the ED diagnosis and treatment of pediatric sexual assault.
- Describe the ED management of an individual who is suspected/confirmed to be a victim of human trafficking.

Interpersonal Violence: Abuse and Neglect

Interpersonal violence is a significant public health problem affecting people at all ages and stages of life. Violence against another person regardless of their age or stage of life has substantial impact on individuals, their families, and society at large. Each year, millions of people experience the physical, mental, and economic consequences of violence in the United States. Violence-related injuries adversely affect the health and welfare of all people through premature death, disability, medical costs, and lost productivity. This section includes an overview of the different forms of interpersonal violence that involve children and elders. Emphasis is on the critical role that the advanced practice clinician in emergency care plays in prevention, identification of those individuals at risk, medical decision-making/differential diagnoses, and evidence-based interventions.

Advanced Practice Clinicians as Mandatory Reporters

Advanced practice clinicians in all 50 states, the District of Columbia, and the U.S. territories are required to report suspected abuse and neglect of children, elders, and other vulnerable populations to an appropriate agency, such as protective services or a law enforcement agency.[5] Most U.S. states have also enacted mandatory reporting laws related to intimate partner violence. As mandatory reporters, ED advanced practice clinicians must make a report under all circumstances when they have a reasonable suspicion that a child, elder, or vulnerable person has been abused or neglected. In the situation that the abused person is transferred to another

ED for a higher level of care, the clinician who initially examines the individual is still responsible to make a report.

Mandatory reporters are required to report the facts and circumstances that led them to suspect the abuse or neglect. This report and disclosure of patient information does not constitute any violation or conflict between privacy laws. The mandated reporter does not have to provide the burden of proof that abuse or neglect has occurred; their only requirement is that there is a reasonable suspicion of abuse and/or neglect. As a mandated reporter, immunity from civil, criminal, and professional litigation and licensure actions is granted. If a mandatory reporter willfully fails to make a report of interpersonal violence when legally required to do so, professional or legal disciplinary action may result.

Child Abuse and Neglect

Crimes against children, including child abuse and neglect, are described as one of the greatest threats facing the health, welfare, and social well-being of children in the United States. The 2020 published statistics by the U.S. Department of Health and Human Services (HHS) describe approximately four million reports of alleged child abuse and neglect involving 7.2 million children made in a 1-year period. Approximately 2.2 million of these alleged child maltreatment cases were investigated and 25% were substantiated and received postresponse services.[6] These figures account for 550,000 defenseless and powerless children who lack the ability for self-protection. During this one-year period, there were 1,580 pediatric fatalities included in this population.[6]

Despite mandatory reporting laws, child maltreatment is greatly underrecognized and underreported by healthcare clinicians. ED use for pediatric health care is escalating. It is estimated that 22% of all patients evaluated in EDs in the United States are under the age of 18 years old. Between the years 2001 and 2010, there was a 14.4% increase in ED visits by pediatric patients in the United States. These statistics mandate the need for all ED clinicians to have the knowledge and skill set to maintain quality and safety for optimal pediatric patient outcomes.

As the entryway into the healthcare system, many pediatric patients evaluated in the ED have experienced some form of child maltreatment. In the majority of cases, these children come to the ED without a declaration of maltreatment and the signs and symptoms are of a subtle nature. Emergency healthcare clinicians must develop an expert knowledge base and skill set to identify children who are at risk of maltreatment so that interventions to ensure their safety and protection can be implemented.

Definition of Child Abuse and Neglect

The Centers for Disease Control and Prevention (CDC) broadly defines child maltreatment as words or overt actions of commission or omission by a parent or other caregiver (e.g., clergy, coach, teacher) that cause harm, potential harm, or threat of harm to a child.[7,8]

A. *Acts of commission:* Deliberate and intentional, although the actual harm/injury to a child might not be the intended consequence. Intention only applies to caregiver acts—not the consequences of those acts. The following types of abuse involve acts of commission:

1. *Physical abuse:* Defined as any nonaccidental physical injury inflicted upon a child by a person responsible for the care of that child. Physical abuse includes actions such as striking, kicking, shaking, burning, or biting the child, or any other action that results in a physical injury to the child. This abuse also includes injuries resulting from harsh discipline through corporal punishment.

2. *Sexual abuse:* Defined as the involvement of a child in sexual activity that he or she does not fully comprehend, is unable to give informed consent to, is developmentally unprepared for, or violates the laws or social taboos of society. The age of consent varies among jurisdictions and ranges between 16 and 18 years. The most common age among all jurisdictions is 16. The term sexual exploitation is used when a child is allowed to engage in prostitution or in the production of child pornography. In most states, the definition of sexual abuse includes human trafficking, including sex trafficking or trafficking of children for sexual purposes.

3. *Emotional abuse:* Defined as injury to the psychological capacity or emotional stability of a child. Manifestations in the child may include changes in behavior, emotional response, or cognition, anxiety, depression, withdrawal, or aggressive behavior.

4. *Caregiver-fabricated illness:* Defined as a form of child maltreatment caused by a caregiver who falsifies and/or induces a child's illness, leading to unnecessary and potentially harmful medical investigations and/or treatment. This condition can result in significant morbidity and mortality. Historically, this condition has been labeled as Munchausen syndrome by proxy, pediatric condition falsification, factitious disorder (illness) by proxy, child abuse in the medical setting, and medical child abuse.

B. Acts of omission

1. *Neglect:* Defined as the failure of the parent or other caregiver to provide needed food, clothing, shelter, medical care, or supervision to the degree that the child's health, safety, and well-being are threatened with harm. Accounts for 75% of all reports of child maltreatment. Specific types of neglect include the following:

a. *Physical neglect:* Abandoning the child or refusing to accept custody, failure to provide for basic needs including nutrition, hygiene, or appropriate clothing

b. *Medical neglect:* Delaying or denying recommended healthcare for the child

c. *Emotional neglect:* Isolating the child, not providing affection or emotional support, or exposing the child to domestic violence or substance abuse

d. *Inadequate supervision:* Leaving the child unsupervised, not protecting the child from safety hazards, not providing adequate caregivers, or engaging in harmful behaviors

e. *Educational neglect:* Failing to enroll the child in school or homeschool, ignoring special needs, or permitting chronic absenteeism from school

Risk Factors for Child Maltreatment

It is estimated that only one-third of all children who experience maltreatment are ever identified and reported to child protective agencies. In the majority of cases, these children come to the ED without a declaration of maltreatment and the signs and symptoms are of a subtle nature. It is recommended by specialty organizations involved with the care of children that clinicians possess a strong knowledge base and screen children for maltreatment as an integral part of their clinical decision-making/differential diagnoses. ED clinicians must maintain a high index of suspicion for child maltreatment in order to have the knowledge and skill set to recognize children in a high-risk situation. Box 55.1 outlines factors that place children in this high-risk situation.[9]

History and Physical Examination

A. *Chief complaint:* Variable, ranging from subtle and non-acute to life-threatening. There may or may not be a disclosure of abuse. Red flags in the history that should raise the index of suspicion for abuse include the following:

1. Lack of an explanation or a vague explanation of the injury
2. Denial of trauma in a child with an obvious injury
3. Inconsistency in the history provided to explain the injury
4. Pattern, age, or severity of the injury is inconsistent with the child's physical or developmental level
5. Unexplained or unexpected delay in seeking medical care[11]

B. *Physical examination:* An immediate evaluation must be conducted to determine the presence of acute life-threatening trauma and the need for intervention. All children evaluated for abuse must be completely undressed and in a hospital gown. A complete head-to-toe exam must be performed so that any potential abusive injuries or signs of neglect are not missed.

1. *General appearance:* Dress, cleanliness, behavior, emotional state, and affect
2. Head, eyes, ears, and mouth
   - **a.** *Head:* Inspection and palpation of the scalp for traumatic wounds or patches of alopecia, fullness or sunken anterior fontanelle in infants
   - **b.** *Eyes:* Inspection and palpation of the eyes for orbital and periorbital trauma. Dilation for fundoscopic examination for retinal hemorrhage
   - **c.** *Ears:* Inspection of the ears for trauma to the pinna, the back of the ear, the hairline behind the ears, hemotympanum, cerebral spinal fluid otorrhea
   - **d.** *Mouth:* Inspection of the mouth for trauma to the lips, buccal mucosa, gums, palate, teeth, or frenulum
   - **e.** *Neck:* Inspect for ligature marks or other evidence of choking
   - **f.** *Chest:* Inspection for symmetry and signs of external trauma. Palpate for costochondral tenderness or chest deformity
   - **g.** *Abdomen:* Inspect for signs of external trauma, distention. Auscultate for bowel sounds. Palpate for tenderness or masses
   - **h.** *Back:* Inspect for signs of external trauma. Palpate for costovertebral (CVA), paraspinal, or spinal tenderness
   - **i.** *Extremities:* Inspect for external trauma. Palpate for deformities, tenderness, or crepitus
   - **j.** *Neurologic:* Evaluate mental status, behavior, level of consciousness, developmental abilities and developmental stage

BOX 55.1 CHILD MALTREATMENT SCREENING: RISK FACTORS

CHILD RISK FACTORS

Premature birth
Congenital birth anomalies
Low birth weight
Physical/cognitive/emotional disability
Chronic or serious childhood illness or trauma
Aggression or behavioral problems

PARENTAL/FAMILY RISK FACTORS

Personality Factors
- External locus of control
- Poor impulse control
- Depression/anxiety
- Low tolerance for frustration
- Feelings of insecurity
- Lack of trust
- Insecure attachment with own parents
- Childhood history of abuse
- High parental conflict, domestic violence

Family Structure
- Single parent with lack of support
- High number of children in household
- Social isolation
- Parental psychopathology
- Substance abuse
- Separation/divorce, especially high-conflict divorce
- Poor parent–child interaction
- Negative attitudes and attributions about child's behavior
- Inaccurate knowledge and expectations about child development and behavior

SOCIAL/ENVIRONMENTAL RISK FACTORS

Low socioeconomic status
Stressful life events
Lack of access to medical care, health insurance, adequate child care, and social services
Parental unemployment
Exposure to racism/discrimination
Poor schools
Exposure to environmental toxins
Dangerous/violent neighborhood
Community violence

Source: U.S. Department of Health and Human Services. Retrieved from https://www.cdc.gov/violenceprevention/childabuseandneglect/riskprotectivefactors.html)[10]

Differential Diagnoses

There are few single injuries that are specifically pathognomonic for abuse. There are four general questions that must be considered when evaluating a child for potential abuse:

A. Is the history consistent with the mechanism of injury?
B. Is the injury consistent with the developmental level of the child?
C. Is there any other medical explanation for this injury or finding (e.g., illness or genetic condition)?
D. Is there corroborative information that supports concern for maltreatment?
E. Physical examination findings that suggest abuse [9,11,12]
  1. Any injury in a preambulatory infant
  2. Injuries to multiple organ systems
  3. Injuries in various stages of healing
  4. Patterned injuries
  5. Injuries to nonbony or other atypical locations
  6. Significant injuries that are unexplained
  7. Evidence of child neglect
F. Physical findings that may be confused with abuse
  1. Hematologic disorders
    a. Hemophilia
    b. Idiopathic thrombocytopenic purpura
    c. Von Willebrand disease
    d. Henoch–Schonlein purpura (HSP)
    e. Other coagulopathies
  2. Dermatologic
    a. Mongolian spots
    b. Impetigo
    c. Staph scalded skin syndrome
  3. Metabolic conditions
    a. Osteogenesis imperfecta
    b. Rickets
    c. Ehlers–Danlos syndrome
  4. Cultural practices
    a. Cultural practices that cause physical or psychological injury must be reported as a mandated.
    b. Ecchymosis secondary to cupping or coining
    c. Use of folk remedies
  5. Newborn period
    a. Retinal hemorrhages up to 6 weeks after birth
    b. Petechiae and bruising up to 1 week after birth
    c. Clavicle fractures
    d. Vaginal discharge
    e. Mongolian spots
  6. Straddle injuries
  7. Genital complaints (e.g., vaginal discharge, pinworms, Group A strep, lichen sclerosis)
    a. Urethral prolapse

Specific Injuries

A. Bruises
  1. Most common and readily visible but may be missed as a sentinel injury; may be the only external indicator of a more serious underlying injury.
  2. Pattern in abused children differs from those in nonabused children; the head and face are the most common sites of bruising in abused children. Abused children frequently have more bruises and may also have defensive bruises. May represent an object pattern (e.g., hand, fist, belt, looped cord).
  3. There is a strong correlation between bruising and mobility in infants and toddlers; bruises are rare in preambulatory children. Any body part is vulnerable to bruising by abuse. The mnemonic "TEN 4" identifies bruises that are of concern for abuse (Table 55.1).

TABLE 55.1 TEN 4 MNEMONIC FOR BRUISES OF CONCERN

T	Torso
E	Ear
N	Neck
4	Any bruise in an infant under 4 months or age or any bruise in the above areas in a child under the age of 4 years

  4. The age of a bruise cannot be accurately determined, but bruises show a predictive pattern as they heal, ranging from red-purple for a fresh bruise to yellow-brown as they heal. Accurate documentation of bruises in the medical record should include the color, shape, size, and measurements. Photo documentation and diagrams add valuable data.

B. Bites
  1. May be inflicted by an adult, another child, an animal, or the patient.
  2. Evaluation of the bite mark should include the size, dentition characteristics within the wound, location, presence of puncture marks, arch form, and intercanine distance. If the distance between the maxillary canine teeth exceeds 3 cm, it is indicative that the bite was inflicted by an adult.

C. Burns
  1. Inflicted burns are typically more severe than accidental burns and commonly associated with a delay in seeking care.
  2. Inflicted immersion burns typically have sharp lines of demarcation and often involve the genitals and lower extremities.
  3. Contact burns are inflicted with hot solids, including curling irons, radiators, stoves, cigarettes, or irons.

D. Skeletal injuries
  1. Second most common injury caused by abuse; any bone can be fractured as a result of physical abuse. Some fracture types are highly suggestive of abuse (Table 55.2).
  2. Rib fractures in children less than 3 years of age are strongly associated with physical abuse. Most commonly due to compressive forces, these fractures are often multiple, can be unilateral or bilateral, and can occur anywhere along the rib cage, although are most frequently located posteriorly.
  3. Red flags for abusive fractures include the following:
    a. Fractures in nonambulatory infants and children
    b. Children with multiple fractures
    c. Infants and children with rib fractures
    d. Infants and toddlers with midshaft humerus or femur fractures
    e. Fracture inconsistent with the history

E. Thoracoabdominal injuries
  1. Abdominal trauma is the second most common cause of mortality due to abuse.

TABLE 55.2 SPECIFICITY OF ABUSIVE FRACTURES

HIGHLY SPECIFIC	MODERATELY SPECIFIC	COMMON, LOW SPECIFICITY
Classic metaphyseal fractures	Multiple fractures	Clavicle fractures
Rib fractures (especially posteromedial)	Fractures of different ages	Long bone shaft fractures
Scapular fractures	Epiphyseal separations	Linear skull fractures
Sternal fractures	Vertebral body fractures	
Spinous process fractures	Digital fractures	
	Complex skull fractures	

2. Most thoracoabdominal injuries are due to inflicted blows or crush injury. Both solid and hollow organs are at risk for injury.
3. There may be no external signs of abdominal trauma, despite severe internal organ injury. Initial manifestations may be nonspecific and include abdominal pain and distention, nausea, vomiting, and fever.
4. Pulmonary injuries include contusions, lacerations resulting in pneumothorax, hemorrhagic effusions or pneumomediastinum, and pulmonary edema associated with suffocation or head trauma.

F. Head injuries
1. Abusive head trauma (AHT) is the leading cause of child abuse fatality. Defined as an injury to the skull or intracranial contents of an infant or young child (<5 years of age) due to inflicted blunt trauma or violent shaking. Crying in a young infant is the most commonly cited precipitating factor.
2. Presenting symptoms are variable and may lead to misdiagnosis; these include vomiting, poor feeding, fussiness/irritability, lethargy, seizures, apnea, cardiac arrest.
3. AHT is associated with subdural hemorrhage, retinal hemorrhage, hypoxic ischemic encephalopathy, and cutaneous, skeletal, and visceral injuries.

G. Caregiver-fabricated illness
1. Ninety-eight percent of perpetrators are biologic mother; mortality is up to 9%.
2. Examples include lying about symptoms such as persistent vomiting; giving poisons, ipecac, salts, or insulin to induce apnea, seizures, emesis, or diarrhea; inducing skin rashes or lesions. May be history of unusual death in a sibling (Box 55.2).

BOX 55.2 RISK FACTORS FOR CAREGIVER-FABRICATED ILLNESS

- Experienced physicians caring for the child are perplexed by the case.
- Child has received care at multiple different sites.
- Child's symptoms are persistent, recurrent, and do not respond to therapy.
- Child's symptoms never occur when witnesses are present.
- Symptoms resolve in a monitored environment.
- Mother is overly attentive and enthusiastic about additional tests.
- Mother has a medical or para-medical background.
- Laboratory results do not correlate with the case.

Diagnostic Testing

The selection and extent of diagnostic testing is based on variables including the type and severity of the injury, age of the child, developmental level of the child, and physical examination findings. Recommended guidelines for diagnostic tests for children under the age of 2 years of age with suspected AHT and their siblings are listed in Table 55.3.[12,13]

A. Labs
1. *Bleeding evaluation:* Complete blood count (CBC), with differential, platelet count, international normalized ratio (INR), prothrombin time (PT), partial thromboplastin time (aPTT)
2. *Chemistry:* Serum electrolytes, including calcium, phosphate and alkaline phosphatase, liver enzymes, pancreatic enzymes, urinalysis
3. *Toxicology:* Urine and /or serum panels for drugs, alcohol, or other toxic substances

B. Diagnostic imaging
1. *Plain film x-rays:* The skeletal survey is considered the best method for detecting acute and old fractures in children who have been abused. This technique requires 21 views. In children over the age of 2 years, specific x-ray selection is based on clinical findings.
2. *CT:* Head CT is indicated in all children with suspected acute brain injury and bony injury to the skull or face. Chest and/or abdominal CT is indicated to determine the presence of fluid/blood and the extent of lung injury.
3. *MRI:* Brain MRI offers the most complete soft tissue image of the brain, best for evaluation of subacute or chronic injury.
4. *Ultrasound:* Focused assessment with sonography for trauma (FAST) to determine the presence of intraabdominal fluid/blood in an unstable patient

Documentation

A. Accurate and detailed documentation should include the following:
1. Presenting chief complaint, verbatim using quotations
2. Medical and social history
3. Physical examination findings (include diagrams and/or photo documentation)

TABLE 55.3 CLINICAL GUIDELINES FOR SUSPECTED ABUSIVE HEAD TRAUMA 0–2 YEARS OF AGE

Imaging	Head CT and skeletal series Abdominal CT—signs of intraabdominal trauma or elevated LFTs
Labs	CBC, PT/PTT, INR, CMP, amylase, lipase UA: urine toxicology screen Isolate bruises: CBC, PT/PTT, INR
Sibling evaluation	Skeletal survey and fundoscopic exam in twin or sibling under 2 years of age

CBC, complete blood count; CMP, comprehensive metabolic panel; INR, international normalized ratio; LFT, liver function test; PT, prothrombin time; PTT, partial thromboplastin time; UA, urinalysis.

4. Diagnostic impressions
5. Details of patient management

Treatment and Disposition

A. Ensure the safety and protection of the child if patient is discharged
B. Initiate interprofessional consultations
C. Neurology/neurosurgery/orthopedics/trauma as indicated
D. Social work
E. Law enforcement
F. Child protective services

Elder Abuse

Elder abuse, neglect, and financial exploitation are common societal problems of increasing incidence and prevalence partly due to aging demographics. An elder adult is defined as someone aged 60 or 65 years or older (varies with jurisdiction).[1] In the United States, it is estimated that 500,000 to 1 million elder adults are abused, neglected, or exploited annually. These statistics are likely an underestimation of the true significance of this problem. Many elder adults are reluctant to tell police, family, or friends about their situation due to fear, shame, or their physical and/or psychological inability to disclose. In addition, many others who are aware of the abuse or neglect of the older person fail to report. Therefore, elder abuse remains unrecognized and underreported. All healthcare clinicians are mandatory reporters of elder abuse and neglect. Community-dwelling elders are protected in all states by state adult protective services. Elders who reside in institutional settings are protected by state long-term care ombudsman programs. Both of these agencies serve to provide support and advocacy for the aging population.

Definition of Elder Abuse

Elder abuse is broadly defined as an act of commission or omission resulting in harm or the potential for harm of an older adult by someone in a relationship of responsibility toward that person.[2] By definition, perpetrators of elder abuse only include those individuals who are expected to be responsible for that person, such as caretakers. Elder abuse is further classified as follows:

A. *Physical abuse:* Willful infliction of pain or injury or the improper use of physical or chemical restraints
B. *Sexual abuse:* Willful nonconsensual sexual contact of any kind
C. *Emotional or psychological abuse:* Willful infliction of anguish, emotional pain, or distress
D. *Caregiver neglect:* Deprivation of food, clothing, hygiene, medical care, shelter, or supervision
E. *Self-neglect:* Failure or unwillingness of a vulnerable elder adult with diminished capacity to perform essential self-care care tasks and/or self-protection
F. *Abandonment:* Desertion of an elder adult by a caregiver or caretaker
G. *Financial exploitation:* Nonconsensual appropriation of an elder adult's resources, property, and/or assets for the benefit of another by someone with responsibility and duty towards that person

Risk Factors for Elder Abuse

Elder abuse often goes undisclosed and therefore is underreported. In 1992, the American Medical Association proposed that clinicians in all practice settings screen individuals aged 65 years and older for abuse. Several risk factors and warning signs have been identified as red flags for elder abuse (Box 55.3).[2]

Physical Examination

A. *Chief complaint:* If the patient is cognitively able, it is best to interview the patient in private. Be astute to behavioral signs and symptoms suggestive of abuse or neglect including depression, fear, withdrawal, confusion, anxiety, and low self-esteem.
B. *Examination:* Findings vary from subtle and nondiagnostic to highly suspicious. The patient must be

BOX 55.3 RISK FACTORS ASSOCIATED WITH ELDER ABUSE

Elder Risk Factors

- Advanced age
- Female gender
- Disability in self-care
- Cognitive impairment
- Physical dependency
- Lack of social support
- Substance abuse
- Psychiatric disorders
- Social isolation
- Low education and income levels
- Family stress
- Family stress
- Unfavorable caregiver characteristics (e.g., mental illness, substance abuse, financial dependency, violent tendencies)

undressed, and a complete physical examination must be performed so as to not miss any suspicious injuries. Red flags for abusive injuries include the following:

1. *General appearance:* Poor personal hygiene, inappropriate or soiled clothing, dehydration, malnutrition
2. *Skin findings:* Skin tears, abrasions, lacerations, bruising, or burns that are not correlated with mechanism of injury or in unusual locations (e.g., inner arms or inner thighs, mastoid area, palms, soles, and buttocks)
   a. Multiple injuries in various stages of healing
   b. Signs indicative of inappropriate restraints (e.g., rope burns on wrists and ankles)
3. *Fractures:* Spiral fractures of long bones, defensive fractures, fractures of the wrists, hip, or vertebrae
4. *Pressure ulcers*
5. *Indicators of sexual abuse*
   a. Pain, soreness, or itching in the anogenital area
   b. Vaginal or rectal bleeding
   c. Bruises or lacerations on the vulva, abdomen, or breasts
   d. Sexually transmitted infections (STIs)

Differential Diagnoses

A. Geriatric patients have many underlying medical conditions that may be suspicious for abuse and astute screening in the ED is critical to differentiate these causes. Physical examination findings may not be specific or pathognomonic for elder abuse.

B. Laboratory/diagnostic imaging

1. The selection and extent of diagnostic testing is based on correlation of the screening history and physical examination findings.
2. Common laboratory abnormalities in an abused elder include the following:
   a. Hypernatremia (Na >45 mmol/L)
   b. Elevated blood urea nitrogen (BUN)/creatinine ratios >20
   c. Elevated uric acid
   d. Elevated hemoglobin
   e. Low serum albumin <3.5 g/dL
   f. Elevated creatine kinase (CK)
   g. Urine myoglobin

Documentation

A. Accurate and detailed documentation should include the following:

1. Presenting chief complaint, verbatim using quotations
2. Medical and social history
3. Physical examination findings (include diagrams and/or photo documentation)
4. Diagnostic impressions
5. Details of patient management

Treatment and Disposition

A. Medical problems and injuries must be stabilized and treated with possible in-patient admission.

B. Ensure the safety and protection of the patient if patient is discharged.

C. Initiate interprofessional consultations.

1. Neurology/neurosurgery/orthopedics/trauma as indicated
2. Social work
3. Law enforcement
4. Adult protective services

Intimate Partner Violence

Intimate partner violence (IPV) is a significant public health problem that affects over 32 million individuals in the United States.[1] IPV is associated with high morbidity and mortality rates, including life-threatening injuries and death, as well as other physical and mental health problems of both an immediate and long-term nature. Violence in an intimate relationship occurs in every racial, socioeconomic, ethnic, cultural, geographic, religious, and educational group. The majority of IVP survivors are women, but men are also affected. Statistically, it is estimated that more than one in three women and one in four men experience IPV during their lifetime.[1] Approximately 50% of female homicide victims are killed by a current or former male intimate partner.[2]

Intimate Partner Violence Defined

By definition, IPV refers to physical and/or sexual violence, psychological aggression (including coercion), or stalking by a current or former intimate partner. The term intimate partner is used to describe an individual who is, was, or wishes to be in a close or dating relationship with an adult or adolescent of the same or opposite sex. There are four main classifications of IPV[14,15]:

A. *Physical violence:* The intentional use of physical force with the potential for causing death, disability, injury, or harm. This classification also includes coercing other people to commit physical acts of violence on a targeted individual or group.

B. *Sexual violence:* This claissification includes any unwanted sexual contact or sexual experience, attempted or completed rape, or penetration of the individual and includes the use of drugs and/or alcohol to facilitate this violence. Sexual violence also includes sexual experiences that are not of a physical nature (e.g., exposure to pornography, sexual harassment).

C. *Stalking and cyberstalking:* Refers to a pattern of repeated, unwanted attention or contact that causes fear or concern for one's own safety or the safety of someone else (e.g., family member or friend).

D. *Psychological aggression:* The use of verbal or nonverbal communication with the intent to harm another person psychologically (emotionally or mentally) and/or to exert control over another person.

Risk Factors for Intimate Partner Violence

There are certain risk factors that have been identified as high risk for IPV (Table 55.4).[1,2,15] The ED clinician must remain astute to the possibility of IPV as many patients attempt to withhold information and conceal that they are in an abusive relationship. Reasons for this lack of disclosure include fear, shame, embarrassment, finances, or

TABLE 55.4 RISK FACTORS ASSOCIATED WITH INTIMATE PARTNER VIOLENCE

INDIVIDUAL	RELATIONSHIP	COMMUNITY/SOCIETAL
Low self-esteem	Dominance and control of relationship by a male	Poverty
Female	Couples with income, education, or job status disparities	Overcrowding
Substance abuse	Excessive jealousy or possessive behavior	Lack of community resources
Young age		Weak community sanctions against intimate partner violence
Depression/mental health disorders		
Anger/hostility		
Social isolation		
Unemployment		
Emotional dependence and insecurity		
History of abuse		

faith. Red flags that should raise the index of suspicion for IPV include the following:

A. Inconsistent history/explanation of mechanism of injury, particularly involving the head, neck, teeth, or genital area
B. Delay in seeking treatment
C. Frequent ED visits
D. Late initiation of prenatal care
E. Medication nonadherence
F. Overly attentive or verbally abusive partner

Medical Screening

Major medical organizations, including the Joint Commission, the American College of Emergency Physicians (ACEP), U.S. Preventative Services Task Force (USPSTF), and the National Academy of Medicine, advocate screening all women of childbearing age for IPV.[16,17] There are several validated short screening tools appropriate for use in the ED. There is no gold standard for a screening tool that is 100% sensitive or specific. Regardless of the tool selected, screening for IPV should be completed on all adolescent and adult women. Examples of screening questions are listed in Box 55.4.

Chief Complaint

A. Often is vague and nonspecific (e.g., headaches, back pain, excessive fatigue, dizziness, memory loss)
B. *Gynecologic complaints:* Chronic pelvic pain, sexually transmitted infection (STI), unwanted or unplanned pregnancy

BOX 55.4 SCREENING QUESITONS FOR INTIMATE PARTNER VIOLENCE

Are you ever afraid of your partner?
In the last year has your partner hit, punched, kicked, or otherwise hurt you?
In the last year has your partner humiliated you, put you down, or tried to control what you can do?
In the last year has your partner threatened to hurt you?

C. *Psychologic complaints:* Depression, suicidality, anxiety/panic disorders, eating disorders, substance abuse, PTSD
D. *Specific injuries:* Any injury without a valid explanation should raise suspicion.

Physical Examination

An immediate evaluation must be conducted to determine the presence of acute life-threatening trauma and the need for intervention. Various patterns and severity of injuries may be the result of IPV. There are no typical injuries common to all survivors of IPV. Many physical examination findings are of low acuity and include scratches, abrasions, minor bruises, and so on.

All patients evaluated for IPV should be completely undressed and in a hospital gown. A complete head-to-toe exam must be performed so that any potential abusive injuries are not missed. Physical signs of IPV may include:

A. *Injuries indicative of violence:* Bite marks, scratches, broken fingernails, dental injuries, burns, abrasions, bruises, ligature marks, facial/conjunctival petechiae, hoarseness or voice changes
B. *Central pattern of injuries:* Injuries to the head, face, thorax, breasts, and abdomen
C. *Genital injuries:* Bleeding, ecchymosis, abrasions, and lacerations
D. *Defensive injuries:* Forearm bruises or fractures
E. *Multiple injuries:* In various stages of healing

Medical Decision-Making/Differential Diagnoses

Special Populations

A. Pregnancy[18]
  1. IPV during pregnancy has a prevalence of 6% to 22%.
  2. Risk factors include young maternal age/adolescence, unintended pregnancy, delayed/lack of prenatal care, lack of social support.
  3. Effect on the mother and fetus may be life-threatening, and complications include the following:
    a. Gestational hypertension
    b. Vaginal bleeding

c. Urinary tract infections
d. Spontaneous abortion
e. Preterm labor
f. Low birth weight
g. Substance abuse
h. Postpartum depression
i. PTSD

B. Adolescence/teen dating violence[19]
1. Widespread with serious long- and short-term consequences; approximately 20% of females and 14% of males experience some form of IPV before the age of 18.
2. Risk factors include the following:
a. Belief that dating violence is acceptable
b. History of depression, anxiety, or symptoms of trauma
c. Aggressive behavior towards others
d. Substance abuse
e. Early sexual activity or multiple partners
f. Interpersonal conflicts
g. Witness or experience violence in their home

Specific Injuries

A. Strangulation
1. Strong predictor of homicide
2. Terminology
a. *Strangulation:* External pressure applied to the neck compromising blood flow and air movement
b. *Suffocation:* Obstruction of the airway at the nose or mouth, accidentally or intentionally (e.g., sitting on one's chest)
c. *Choking:* Obstruction of the airway with food or an object
3. Estimated that 11 pounds of pressure applied to both carotid arteries for 10 seconds leads to unconsciousness; brain death can result if sustained for 4 to 5 minutes. It is estimated that 33 pounds of pressure is required to close the trachea.[20]
4. There may be a lack of visible injury; however, delayed signs and symptoms may develop.[21]
5. Physical examination[20,21]
a. Loss of consciousness (anoxic brain injury)
b. Visual changes
c. Facial, intraoral, or conjunctival petechiae
d. Ligature marks or neck contusions
e. Soft-tissue swelling and tenderness of the neck
f. Neurologic signs (seizures, mental status changes, amnesia, stroke-like symptoms)
g. Dysphonia/aphonia
h. Dyspnea
i. Subcutaneous emphysema (tracheal/laryngeal rupture)
j. Incontinence
6. Delayed complications[22]
a. May develop over several hours or days
i. Carotid dissection or cerebral infarct
ii. Pneumonia or aspiration pneumonitis
iii. Edematous internal tissue of the airway
iv. Progressive irreversible encephalopathy
v. Neurologic disorders
vi. Spontaneous abortion

Laboratory and Diagnostic Imaging

A. Based on specific injury pattern
B. Strangulation
1. CT angiogram (CTA) of carotid/vertebral arteries is gold standard for evaluation of vessels and bony/cartilaginous structures; less sensitive for soft tissues.[22]
2. CT neck with contrast or MRI of neck is best for soft tissue trauma.
3. MRI/magnetic resonance angiography (MRA) of the brain is most sensitive for anoxic brain injury, stroke symptoms, or intracerebral petechial hemorrhage.

Documentation

A. Accurate and detailed documentation should include the following:
1. Presenting chief complaint, verbatim using quotations
2. Medical and social history
3. Physical examination findings (include diagrams and/or photo documentation)
4. Diagnostic impressions
5. Details of patient management

Treatment and Disposition

A. Based on individual needs of the survivor. Treat physical injuries and provide necessary intervention.
B. Ensure a safety plan if patient is discharged.
C. All patients with a history of nonlethal strangulation should be admitted for observation for delayed manifestations.
D. Initiate interprofessional consultations.
1. Neurology/neurosurgery/orthopedics/trauma
2. Social work
3. Law enforcement
4. Community resources (e.g., domestic violence hotline, shelters)

Sexual Assault

Sexual assault is a major public health problem, with an estimated one in three women and nearly one in six men in the United States having experienced some form of sexual violence during their lifetime. It is estimated that one in five women have experienced completed or attempted rape at some point in their life.[23] Sexual assault can result in both acute and chronic physical and psychological effects for the survivors, including the following:

A. Pregnancy
B. Chronic health problems (e.g., chronic pain, gastrointestinal (GI) disorders, GYN complications)
C. Depression, anxiety, post-traumatic stress disorder (PTSD), suicidality
D. Strained social relationships, isolation

Sexual Assault Defined

Sexual assault is defined as any sexual act committed against someone without that person's freely given consent.[23] It may result from the use of force, the threat of force, or from the survivor's inability or refusal to give consent. The term sexual assault encompasses four acts.

A. *Rape:* Any completed or attempted nonconsensual penetration of the vagina, mouth, or anus through the use of physical force or threats to physically harm another person. This term includes circumstances when the individual is under the influence of alcohol or drugs, or in an altered level of consciousness, that renders them unable to consent.

B. *Forced penetration:* Refers to circumstances in which an individual is physically forced to sexually penetrate or attempt to penetrate another person without that person's consent.

C. *Sexual coercion:* Unwanted sexual penetration that occurs after a person is pressured in a nonphysical way, such as false promises, being lied to, use of influence, or authority

D. *Unwanted sexual contact:* Unwanted sexual touching without penetration, such as fondling or groping

Risk Factors for Sexual Assault

No individual is responsible for being sexually assaulted, however, there are certain high-risk characteristics that increase the likelihood that an individual may be the target of sexual violence. Examples of these risk factors include the following[24]:

A. Adolescents and young adults ages 16 to 24 years
B. Previous history of sexual and/or physical assault
C. Substance use and abuse
D. Multiple sexual partners
E. Delinquency
F. Preference for impersonal sex and sexual risk-taking
G. Childhood history of physical, sexual, or emotional abuse
H. Societal norms that support sexual violence and male or female inferiority

History and Physical Examination

Many sexual assault survivors do not report the assault to law enforcement or seek medical care. All sexual assault patients should be triaged as a high priority. Most authorities agree that an evidentiary examination should not be performed if the sexual assault occurred greater than 72 prior to the exam. This is state specific as some states have expanded this time period to 96 hours post-assault for an evidentiary examination.

A. History
  1. Pain and/or injuries sustained, presence of bleeding, loss of consciousness or memory loss, recent alcohol or drug use
  2. Detailed circumstances surrounding the assault, including date, time, location, use of weapons, force, restraints, or threats
    a. The assailant's description and identifying information
    b. Specifics regarding sexual acts, including actual or attempted penetration of the mouth, vagina, and anus/rectum; condom use, ejaculation
    c. Recent bath/shower, enema, use of toothpaste/mouthwash, removal of tampon or barrier contraceptive device, clothing change
    d. Recent consensual sexual activity before or after the assault, including penetration and condom use
    e. Last menstrual period
    f. Past medical history

Physical Examination

An immediate evaluation must be conducted to determine the presence of acute life-threatening trauma and the need for intervention. All patients should be completely undressed and in a hospital gown. A complete head-to-toe exam must be performed so that any potential abusive injuries are not missed.

A. Emotional state/mental status

B. *Injuries indicative of violence:* Bite marks, scratches, broken fingernails, dental injuries, burns, abrasions, bruises, ligature marks, facial/conjunctival petechiae, hoarseness or voice changes

C. *Central pattern of injuries:* Injuries to the head, face, thorax, breasts, and abdomen

D. *Genital injuries:* Suggested terminology includes the TEARS categorization: tears (any break in the skin), ecchymosis, abrasions, redness, and swelling
  1. In males, be particularly aware of injuries to the penis and scrotum, evaluating for erythema, ecchymosis, excoriation, lacerations, or suction petechiae.
  2. Retained foreign body

E. *Defensive injuries:* Forearm bruises or fractures

Medical Decision-Making/Differential Diagnoses

Diagnostic Testing

A. Labs
  1. *Urine pregnancy test:* Before giving emergency contraception
  2. *Complete blood count (CBC), serum chemistry, liver function studies:* For patients who will receive HIV prophylaxis.
  3. Serum alcohol level and urine toxicology screen if indicated
  4. Urine toxicology for drug-facilitated assault (i.e., "date rape drugs" include ketamine, Rohypnol, and gamma-hydroxybutyric acid [GHB]).
    a. Rohypnol can be detected in the urine for up to 72 hours.
    b. GHB can be detected in the urine for up to 12 hours.
  5. Ensure follow-up or obtain serum specimens for HIV, rapid plasma reagin (RPR), and Hepatitis B.
  6. Testing for sexually transmitted infections (STIs) is elective as guidelines suggest empiric treatment, and testing does not provide definitive evidence that infection was acquired at the time of the assault.

Treatment and Disposition

A. Based on individual needs of the survivor. Treat physical injuries and provide necessary intervention.

B. STI prophylaxis; empiric treatment as recommended by the Centers for Disease Control and Prevention (CDC[25]; Table 55.5)

C. *Emergency contraception:* May be offered once it is ruled out through laboratory testing that the patient is not pregnant or in patients who have had a hysterectomy.

TABLE 55.5 CDC RECOMMENDED REGIMENS FOR SEXUALLY TRANSMITTED INFECTIONS PROPHYLAXIS

Ceftriaxone 500 mg IM (>150 kg 1000 mg IM) single dose
Plus
Metronidazole 2 g PO in a single dose
Plus
Or
Doxycycline 100 mg PO twice daily for 7 days

Source: Centers for Disease Control and Prevention. Sexually transmitted disease: treatment guidelines https://www.cdc.gov/std/treatment/default.htm.[25]

The copper intrauterine device inserted within 5 days of unprotected intercourse (UPI) is the most effective method, with first cycle pregnancy rates of 0.1%.[26]

D. Medications may also be used as listed below.[26] It is recommended that an antiemetic is also prescribed for the patient if emergency contraception is used. There are three common emergency contraceptive regimens available.

1. *Ulipristal:* 30 mg orally in a single dose; preferred treatment over 72 hours, effective up to 120 hours after intercourse and in overweight or obese women
2. *Levonorgestrel (Plan B):* 1.5 mg orally once or 0.75 mg at 1 and 12 hours; available over the counter in the United States, well tolerated but less effective over time and ineffective in women who are overweight
3. *Combined estrogen-progestin:* Less effective, with a high incidence of nausea and vomiting

E. *Hepatitis B vaccine:* Recommended by the CDC post-exposure without hepatitis B immune globulin (HBIG) exposure known. If the assailant is known to be hepatitis B infected, HBIG is recommended. Vaccine is not necessary if the patient has had previous hepatitis B vaccine and documented immunity. If immunity is not known, the CDC recommends a single hepatitis B booster vaccination.[23]

F. *HIV infection:* Postexposure prophylaxis (PEP) with antiviral drugs should be addressed with every patient postsexual assault. Despite the presumed low risk of transmission, it is recommended that consultation with a specialist familiar with PEP regimens be done. Antiviral drugs are most efficacious when started within 4 hours of the assault and should not be prescribed if more than 72 hours have elapsed. The CDC recommends that the patient be given an initial prescription for PEP for 3 to 7 days, with follow-up for further counseling and extension of treatment for 28 days.[23] Patients at higher risk of contracting HIV through a sexual assault include the following:

1. Male on male rape
2. Sexual assaults in a region with a high prevalence of HIV
3. Multiple assailants
4. Anal sexual assault
5. Sexual assault where the survivor has trauma, bleeding, or genital lesions

G. *HPV infection:* Vaccine recommended at the time of initial evaluation after sexual assault in females aged 9 to 26 and males aged 9 to 21 if not previously vaccinated

H. *Psychosocial concerns:* Sexual assault survivors require extensive psychosocial support. Acute crisis counseling should be offered in addition to referrals for outpatient counseling.

Special Populations

Pediatric Sexual Assault

A. *Definition:* The involvement of a child in sexual activity that he or she does not fully comprehend and is unable to give informed consent or that violates the laws or social taboos of society. In the United States, approximately 26% of females and 5% of males have experienced some type of sexual abuse by the time they reach age 17. Sexual abuse accounts for 10% of all cases of child maltreatment in the United States.[27]

B. Sexual abuse offenses include the following:

1. *Touching:* Fondling, forcing a child to touch an adult's sexual organs, an adult touching a child's sexual organs or digital or object penetration of the anus or vagina that does not have a medical purpose
2. *Nontouching:* Indecent exposure, exposing children to pornographic material, deliberately exposing a child to the act of sexual intercourse, or masturbating in front of a child
3. *Sexual exploitation:* Engaging a child for the purposes of prostitution, human trafficking, or using a child to film, photograph, or model pornography

Differential Diagnoses

A. *Triage categorization:* Determine the goals of treatment in the emergency care setting; once a medical screening exam is performed, it may be in the best interest of the child to have their complete medical and forensic evaluation performed at a child advocacy center.[28] All children who are triaged as emergent should be managed in the ED care setting to address their acute needs.

1. Emergent
   - a. Acute medical concerns (e.g., bleeding, pain)
   - b. Need for evidentiary exam (within 72 hours of the last event)
   - c. Need for emergency contraception
   - d. Need for PEP for STIs including HIV
   - e. Human trafficking
2. Urgent
   - a. Reported sexual abuse within the previous 2 weeks without emergent needs
3. Nonurgent
   - a. Disclosure of abuse by child, sexualized behaviors, family concern but contact occurred more than 2 weeks ago and without emergent needs

B. History/chief complaint

1. The diagnosis of sexual abuse relies heavily on the history provided, specifically the disclosure made by the child.

2. Obtain as much detail as possible from the personnel accompanying the child without the child present.
3. Interview the child separately to obtain the information necessary to make the determination as to whether an acute medical emergency exists that needs to be addressed. Reserve the detailed disclosure to a specially trained forensic interviewer.
   a. Consider age and developmental level.
   b. Use direct quotes, medical hearsay permissible

C. Physical examination—anogenital
1. The absence of physical findings does not eliminate sexual abuse—95% of physical examinations do not have any physical evidence of abuse.[28]
2. Perform a complete physical examination with the child in a hospital gown, so no injury is overlooked. Sexually abused children have already experienced the abuse of authority and control and should be allowed to have a supportive, nonoffending caregiver or another supportive adult present.
3. In general, the anogenital exam is limited to inspection of external areas.
4. Never force any part of the exam.
5. Supine frog-leg position to allow for visualization of the labia, ease of labial separation, and traction techniques; confirm abnormalities in the prone-knee chest position.
6. Speculum only in prepubescent girls with concerns for bleeding, mass or foreign body, or sexually active postpubescent girls
7. Sedation only with concerns for significant anogenital bleeding or injury, or foreign body
8. Abnormal findings
   a. Discharge or lesions
   b. Lacerations, abrasions, or bleeding
   c. Ecchymosis
   d. Posterior (inferior) hymenal ring abnormalities
   e. External anal exam abnormalities

D. Documentation
1. Mental/emotional status of child
2. Describe relevant anogenital physical findings using a clock-face orientation.

E. Treatment
1. STIs
   a. Prevalence is low in prepubertal children (<5%).
   b. STIs in children strongly suggest sexual abuse.
      i. Consider perinatal transmission.
   c. Empiric prophylaxis is not recommended in prepubescent children, defer STI treatment until after initial tests are conducted and any positive results are confirmed with follow-up tests.
   d. Consider the need for testing on a case-by-case basis. Those at high risk include
      i. Penetration
      ii. Abused by a stranger
      iii. Abused by someone at high risk/known for STI
      iv. Person in the household with an STI
      v. High rate of STIs in community
      vi. Signs or symptoms of STI
      vii. Prior STI
      viii. Caregiver request for testing
   e. Testing for STIs[27]
      i. Gonorrhea and chlamydia
         (1) *Prepubescent females:* Urine nucleic acid amplification tests (NAAT), follow up positives with a culture **NO DNA Gen probe.
         (2) *Males:* Culture
         (3) *Oropharyngeal and anal:* Culture (do not test for oropharyngeal *Chlamydia*)
      ii. *Trichomonas vaginalis*
         (1) Wet mount
      iii. Herpes simplex virus (HSV)
         (1) Culture or polymerase chain reaction (PCR)
         (2) Type-specific serology
      iv. Syphilis
         (1) Serology
      v. HIV
         (1) Serology

Documentation

A. Accurate and detailed documentation should include
   1. Mental/emotional state of child
B. Presenting chief complaint, verbatim using quotations
C. Medical and social history
D. Physical examination findings (include diagrams and/or photo documentation)
E. Diagnostic impressions
F. Details of patient management

Disposition

A. Ensure the safety and protection of the child if patient is discharged.
B. Initiate interprofessional consultations.
   1. Social work
   2. Law enforcement
   3. Child protective services
   4. *Child advocacy center:* Where the child and nonoffending family members receive support, crisis intervention, and referrals for mental health and medical treatment.

Human Trafficking

Human Trafficking Defined

Also referred to as "modern slavery," defined as "the act of harboring, recruiting, transporting, providing or obtaining a person for completed labor or commercial sex acts through the use of force, fraud or coercion" (U.S. Department of State, 2013). It is difficult to determine the exact incidence and prevalence of human trafficking because of the illegal and concealed nature of this problem but is considered the fastest growing criminal enterprise in the world. Sex trafficking includes individuals of all ages and both sexes.[3,4]

Risk Factors for Human Trafficking

Women and children are the most vulnerable to being trafficked, although men are also at risk. Females 12 to

16 years of age are at the highest risk, particularly those in the foster care system. Other factors that place an individual at risk are listed in Box 55.5.[4]

Medical Screening

Individuals that are trafficked rarely identify themselves due to a variety of reasons, including fear, embarrassment, distrust, feelings of hopelessness, and threats. As such many patients are not identified as victims of trafficking while in the ED. Human trafficking victims may present to the ED with vague physical symptoms, including headache, fatigue, back pain, or dizziness. Medical care may be delayed (e.g., pregnancy), and the patients may present with severe injuries or advanced illness. A high index of suspicion must be maintained. Use of screening questions (Box 55.6) is recommended.

A. *History/chief complaint:* See Box 55.3 for examples of screening questions.[3,4]

1. Potential clinical indicators of human trafficking include the following:

a. Shares a scripted or inconsistent history

b. Stated age is older than visual appearance

c. Is unwilling or hesitant to answer questions; vague responses, appears fearful

i. History of frequent sexually transmitted infections (STIs), pregnancies

d. Accompanied by an overbearing individual who does not permit the patient to answer questions, refuses to give the patient privacy

e. Patient displays excessive concern or fear of displeasing a caregiver or employer.

f. Unwilling to provide demographics; no identification documents

2. *Physical examination:* All patients should be undressed and in a hospital gown so as not to miss any injuries or markings

a. General appearance

i. Appears anxious, fearful, distrustful

ii. Dressed inappropriately for visit or environmental conditions

iii. Appears underweight/malnourished, unkept, poor dental hygiene

iv. Signs of physical abuse or unexplained injuries

v. Appears under the influence of substances

b. Skin

i. Evidence of trauma (e.g., burns, bruises, scarring)

ii. Tattoos or branding, including barcodes, symbols, numbers that indicate what trafficker the patient "belongs to"

c. Head, ears, eyes, nose, throat (HEENT)

i. Traumatic head injuries

ii. Dental/oral injuries

d. Neck

i. Strangulation injuries

e. Genital

i. Traumatic injuries

ii. Evidence of STIs

iii. Retained foreign body

BOX 55.5 RISK FACTORS FOR HUMAN TRAFFICKING

Risk Factors

- Involvement with child welfare or foster care system
- Poverty
- Poor social support
- Female gender
- Low education
- Low self-esteem
- Childhood sexual abuse/trauma
- Substance abuse
- Intimate partner violence
- Homelessness
- Runaway youth
- LGBTQ+

BOX 55.6 SCREENING QUESTIONS FOR HUMAN TRAFFICKING

- Can you leave your job or situation if you want to?
- Can you come and go as you please?
- Have you been physically harmed in any way?
- Have you been forced to have sex or perform sex acts that you do not want to?
- Where do you eat and sleep?
- Are there locks on your doors or windows?
- Is anyone forcing you to do anything that you do not want to do?
- Are you required to ask permission to do things that you want to do?

Documentation

A. Accurate and detailed documentation should include the following:

1. Mental/emotional state of patient

2. Presenting chief complaint, verbatim using quotations

3. Medical and social history

4. Physical examination findings (include diagrams and/or photo documentation)

5. Diagnostic impressions

6. Details of patient management

Disposition

A. To report human trafficking (even if just suspected), contact the National Human Trafficking Hotline (NHTH): call 1-888-373-7888; text Help or INFO or BeFree to 233733; or email help@humantraffickinghotline.org

B. Follow mandatory reporting laws for reportable events (e.g., children and disabled persons).

References and Additional Reading

References and Additional Reading for this chapter are online only and can be found at https://connect.springerpub.com/content/reference-book/978-0-8261-6091-5/part/part07/toc-part/ch55.

56. Palliative and End-of-Life Care

GARRETT K. CHAN

Learning Objectives

- Define and describe palliative care in the ED.
- Identify trajectories of advanced illness and approaching death.
- Discuss the skills and methods that may be used by the emergency nurse practitioner (ENP) to deliver bad or serious news.
- Describe pain management related to palliative to end-of-life care.
- Discuss how to calculate equianalgesic equivalents for opioid management.

Calculating Equianalgesic Doses for Pain Management

Pain is one of the most common causes for patients to present to the ED. When thinking about the use of opioids in pain management, clinicians commonly order opioid doses within their comfort level, yet those doses may not achieve good pain relief.[1] Although there is a chapter in this textbook dedicated to pain management (Chapter 7), choosing appropriate and safe doses for breakthrough pain in patients who are chronically on opioids is common in palliative care. Patients who are on around-the-clock opioids for at least 7 days are thought of to be opioid-tolerant as opposed to opioid-naïve, or those who have not taken opioids around the clock for at least 7 days. The calculation of equianalgesic doses is only for patients who are opioid-tolerant and not for opioid-naïve patients.

There are some considerations emergency nurse practitioners (ENPs) need to be aware of before managing any type of pain crisis in opioid-tolerant patients. Factors include, but are not limited to, the duration and dosing of opioids prior to arrival to the ED, past and current medical and psychiatric history, hepatic and renal function, age and weight of the patient, previous substance abuse history, genetics (i.e., fast metabolizers or slow metabolizers of opioids), allergy and opioid tolerance history, side effects experienced with opioids, the patient's functional level in the presence of chronic and acute pain, and the patient's and family's ability to understand and follow instructions. In addition, the ENP should consider the use of nonopioid medications in pain crises or in procedural situations such as ketamine. In and of itself, ketamine does not provide analgesia, per se, but rather is a hypnotic dissociative medication.

In order to correctly and safely dose patients for adequate analgesia, the ENP needs to understand the concept of equianalgesic dosing. The Pain Assessment and Management Initiative Emergency Department (PAMI-ED) is an initiative of the University of Florida College of Medicine in Jacksonville and has excellent resources and a guide on pain management and dosing of medications on their website. The Pain Management & Dosing Guide from PAMI-ED serves as the reference for the equianalgesic dosing chart depicted in Table 56.1.

The fentanyl patch (Duragesic) Food and Drug Administration (FDA) drug insert states that the equianalgesic dose of 25 mcg/hour is equivalent to 60 mg oral morphine in 24 hours or 30 mg oral oxycodone in 24 hours.[3]

Significance and Precautions Related to Pain Management

Understanding the concept of equianalgesic doses is important for a few reasons. First, patients who have chronic cancer-related pain have been reported to have significant poor pain control and may present to the ED in a pain crisis. Sometimes, the patient may be taking a lower potent opioid such as hydrocodone but may need a higher potent opioid for his or her pain crisis such as morphine. The definition of equianalgesic dose is "that dose at which two opioids (at steady-state) provide approximately the same pain relief."[4] The doses are usually standardized to 10 mg of IV morphine; therefore, the term "morphine milligram equivalent (MME)" is also seen in the literature as another term for equianalgesic doses. Equianalgesic charts compare the relative amount of analgesia, or pain relief, of one opioid dose compared to another opioid dose. For example, in Table 56.2, 10 mg of morphine IV has the same equivalent analgesia as 2 mg of hydromorphone IV. Another example is that 2 mg of hydromorphone IV has the same equivalent analgesia as 20 mg of oxycodone PO.

There are some precautions that ENPs need to be aware of when using equianalgesic charts. First, equianalgesic dosing is an inexact science. Each chart is slightly different from the next chart because most studies that are conducted on establishing equianalgesia are single site studies with small sample sizes and usually with the short-acting preparations and not the extended-release preparations.

Second, the concept of cross-tolerance needs to be taken in consideration. In long-term exposure, a patient

TABLE 56.1 SUMMARY OF PALLIATIVE INTERVENTIONS BY PROGNOSIS

PROGNOSIS:	HOURS	DAYS	WEEKS	MONTHS	YEARS
GOALS:	■ Comfort only	■ Comfort only	■ Prioritize quality of life over longevity	■ Try interventions but stop if they are not effective	■ Full efforts to cure
INTERVENTIONS:	■ Symptom control ■ Consider withholding or withdrawing life-sustaining measures ■ Family presence at the bedside ■ Skillful delivery of serious news ■ Psychosocial and spiritual care, as indicated ■ Cultural considerations for postmortem care	■ Symptom control ■ Consider withholding or withdrawing life-sustaining measures ■ Family presence at the bedside ■ Skillful delivery of serious news ■ Psychosocial and spiritual care, as indicated ■ Clarify patient's goals of care and match interventions to those goals ■ Assess for advance directives ■ Determine how decisions are made within the family	■ Symptom control ■ Skillful delivery of serious news ■ Psychosocial and spiritual care, as indicated ■ Clarify patient's goals of care and match interventions to those goals ■ Assess for advance directives ■ Determine how decisions are made within the family	■ Symptom control ■ Attempt resuscitation; stop if signs of instability persist after reasonable efforts ■ Psychosocial and spiritual care for patient and family, as indicated ■ Assess for caregiver burnout ■ Clarify patient's goals of care and match interventions to those goals ■ Assess for advance directives	■ Full resuscitation efforts; maximal efforts to stabilize; admit to the hospital ■ Symptom control ■ Psychosocial and spiritual care for patient and family, as indicated ■ Assess for caregiver burnout

Source: Emanuel LL, Quest T, eds. The Education in Palliative and End-of-life Care for Emergency Medicine (EPEC™-EM) Curriculum. ©The EPEC Project, 2008; Chan GK. Trajectories of approaching death in the emergency department: clinician narratives of patient transitions to the end of life. *J Pain Symptom Manage*. 2011;42(6):864–881. https://doi.org/10.1016/j.jpainsymman.2011.02.023.[2]

may develop physiological tolerance, and therefore less analgesic effect, to one opioid, for example, morphine. Morphine is in the family of opioids called the phenanthrenes. Other opioids in this family are codeine, oxycodone, hydrocodone, and hydromorphone. So, if the patient develops a physiological tolerance to morphine, because the chemical structure of morphine is shared in the phenanthrenes, the patient may also be physiologically tolerant to other medications in the phenanthrenes family, also known as cross-tolerance. If the patient has cross-tolerance to opioids, the ENP will see that the patient will not receive any analgesic effect when given another medication in the same family.

Third, equianalgesic dosing applies only to pain relief. Careful consideration needs to be taken in the presence of comorbidities such as hepatic or renal failure, drug–drug interactions, side effect profiles, gender differences, among other safe medication practice principles.

Lastly, when doing equianalgesic calculations, the focus should not be solely on the computation. The main goal is adequate pain relief. So, while the calculations can help with a safe starting point, the ENP should focus on pain relief as a major outcome.

Calculation of Equianalgesic Medications

There are many online calculators and equianalgesic tables available. Most of them have different equianalgesic doses but follow the same math equations. One calculation approach, among many others, is the Ratio and Proportion Method[5] that can be applied to equianalgesic dosing calculations.

$$\frac{\dfrac{\text{Opioid \#1}}{\text{Equianalgesic}}}{\dfrac{\text{Opioid \#2}}{\text{Equianalgesic}}} = \frac{\text{Patient's 24-hour oral dose of opioid \#1}}{\text{Patient's 24-hour oral dose of opioid \#2}}$$

Example: A patient with a history of colon cancer comes into the ED with severe abdominal pain over the past 12 hours. In addition to doing the workup to determine the underlying etiology of this pain crisis, the ENP wants to give some medication for the breakthrough pain. The patient is taking two tablets of hydrocodone/acetaminophen 7.5 mg/300 mg every 8 hours. The patient has been taking this dose around the clock, every day, for the past 14 days and so is opioid-tolerant. We want to give hydromorphone IV for her breakthrough pain.

- *Step 1:* Calculate the 24-hour total of the medication currently being taken, also known as the total daily dose (TDD). Note: if the patient is taking multiple opioids (e.g., fentanyl patch and oxycodone oral), the TDD should include all opioids in a 24-hour period.[6] Also, the Centers for Disease Control and Prevention (CDC)[6] notes that patients who take 50 MME a day or higher have twice the risk of overdose than patients who take less than 20 MME a day.

$$\text{Hydrocodone 15 mg PO} \times 3 \text{ (every 8 hours)} = \text{45 mg per 24-hour period}$$

- *Step 2:* Calculate the 24-hour equianalgesic dose, in oral equivalents, for the desired medication using the equianalgesic dosing chart above.

$$\frac{\text{Hydrocodone 25 mg PO}}{\text{Hydromorphone 5 mg PO}} \times \frac{\text{Hydrocodone 45 mg PO in 24 hours}}{\text{Hydromorphone } x \text{ mg PO in 24 hours}}$$

Therefore:

$$25x = 5(45)$$
$$25x = 225$$
$$x = \frac{225}{25}$$
$$x = 9 \text{ mg hydromorphone PO in 24 hour}$$

- *Step 3:* A palliative care expert panel recommends reducing the dose 25% to 50% when converting between opioids due to incomplete cross tolerance.[7]

Hydromorphone 9 mg PO in 24 hours × (0.25 or 0.5)
= 2.25 or 4.59 mg − 2.25 or 4.5
= 4.5 to 6.75 mg PO in 24 hours

- *New opioid:* Hydromorphone 4.5 to 6.75 mg PO in 24 hours. This is the hydromorphone PO TDD. This can be divided into three times per day, so 1.88 mg or 2.81 mg PO (can round to 2 mg to 3 mg) every 8 hours.
- *Optional Step 4:* If the ENP wants to use hydromorphone to treat the breakthrough pain, sometimes called a "rescue dose," take 5% to 15% of the hydromorphone TDD (see Step 3 above[7]). An easy and safe number to calculate is 10%.

Hydromorphone PO total daily dose
= 4.5 to 6.75 mg PO

10% of 4.5 mg or 6.75 mg PO is 0.45 or 0.68 mg PO. An easier number to use is 0.5 mg PO.

- **Optional Step 5:** If using the IV preparation is desired, the equianalgesic table can be used to convert the PO dose to an IV dose using the same Ratio and Proportion Method.

$$\frac{\text{Hydromorphone 5 mg PO}}{\text{Hydromorphone 2 mg IV}} \times \frac{\text{Hydromorphone 0.5 mg PO}}{\text{Hydromorphone } x \text{ mg IV}}$$

Therefore,

$$5x = 2(0.5)$$
$$5x = 1$$
$$x = \frac{1}{5}$$

Where x = 0.2 mg hydromorphone IV bolus for break-through pain

Delivering Bad or Serious News

When ENPs evaluate undifferentiated patients, they may find themselves in a situation where the information necessary to convey may adversely or seriously affect the patient's view of his or her future. Bad news is always "in the eye of the beholder," so we may not know what is perceived as being bad news by the patient or family. Examples of bad news may be a diagnosis of cancer when it is unexpected, or the bad news could be that the patient needs to be admitted for a few days yet is the sole caregiver of a beloved pet at home.

Delivering bad or serious news is an important skill to master for a few reasons.[8] First, it is a frequent but stressful task. Second, people want the truth. Third, there are ethical and legal imperatives such as informed consent that need to be considered. Fourth, delivering bad or serious news badly can have a traumatic and lasting effect on the patient or family. Lastly, by having the accurate information, patients and families can make quality of life decisions. However, it is difficult to deliver bad or serious news as it causes clinicians to experience strong emotions such as anxiety and a feeling of burden. Very few clinicians are educated in delivering bad or serious news.

There are many acronyms that can help a clinician remember the important steps to deliver the serious news in a compassionate and supportive way. One method is called SPIKES.[8]

A. SETTING UP the interview and preparation
  1. Confirm the facts of the situation.
  2. Anticipate and prepare answers to likely questions from the patient/family.
  3. Arrange for some privacy; find the right place in the ED to deliver the news.
  4. Involve significant others.
  5. Sit down.
  6. Make connection with the patient and family.
  7. Manage time constraints and interruptions.
  8. Arrange for a translator, if needed.
  9. Prepare a likely plan of action of next steps. The ENP may need to call a consultant to refer the patient for further workup or treatment.
  10. Give a "warning" that there is difficult news to share. One example could be, "I have some serious news I would like to talk about (the "warning" that you have some difficult news). Is there anyone you would like to be with you when we have this conversation?"

B. Assessing the patient's PERCEPTION
  1. Implement the axiom, "before you tell, ask."
  2. Use open-ended questions to understand the patient or family's perception of the situation. What do they know? What do they think is going on? What has been told to them before?
  3. This step will help you understand the patient's and family's perspective and can build upon the previous information given to them or correct any misinformation in a later step in SPIKES.

C. Obtaining the patient's INVITATION
  1. Ask the patient if they want the information or how they want the information. One example could be, "How would you like me to give you the test results? Would you like for me to share this with you or talk with your loved ones or both?"
  2. Most patients want the news, but some do not want to hear serious or bad news.

D. Giving KNOWLEDGE and information to the patient
  1. In this stage, you should give another warning that bad news is coming so that the shock may be

lessened by being prepared. An example could be, "Unfortunately, I have some bad news to tell you."

2. Give the information to the patient at the level of comprehension and vocabulary of the patient.

3. Use nontechnical words.

4. Avoid excessive bluntness such as, "You have a very bad cancer and unless you get treatment right away, you will die."

5. Give information in small doses and check periodically for understanding.

6. Do not use phrases such as "there is nothing more we can do for you." We can always offer something to patients and families such as aggressive symptom management.

E. Addressing the patient's EMOTIONS with empathy and compassion

1. Responding to emotions is one of the most challenging aspects of delivering bad or serious news.

2. Patient or family responses can range from silence to crying, denial, or anger.

3. Responding with empathy using empathic statements and exploring how someone is feeling is important in offering support to patients and families.

4. Pause and let the patient experience their emotions.

5. An empathic response has four steps[9]:

a. Observe for any emotion by the patient and family.

b. Identify the emotion experienced by having them name it using exploratory questions (see F below).

c. Identify the reason for emotion. It usually is connected to the bad news, but you should verify that is the case.

d. After giving the patient some time to express the emotion, make a connecting statement from the information to the empathic statement. An example could be:

i. *ENP:* I'm sorry to say that the CT shows that the tumor is larger now than a month ago and is causing you more pain [*pause*]. It seems to be growing despite the chemotherapy. (Information)

ii. *Patient:* [*cries*]

iii. *ENP:* [*Moves her chair closer to the patient, offers a tissue, and allows time for silence.*] I know this is not what you wanted to hear. I wish the news were better. (Empathic statement)

6. Examples of an empathic statement would be, "I am sorry to have to tell you this," or "I can see how upsetting this is to you."

7. Examples of exploratory questions are, "Tell me more about how you're feeling," or "Can you explain what you mean when you said ____?"

8. Validating responses to expressions of shock, sadness, anger could be, "I can understand how you felt that way," or "some people have had that same reaction."

F. STRATEGY and SUMMARY

1. Patients who have a clear plan for next steps are less likely to feel anxious or uncertain and may feel supported in their journey.

2. Make sure the patient and family are ready to talk about the plan of action or if they need some time to process the news. When the patient and family are ready for the information, be sure to give the information verbally and in writing.

3. Check to make sure they heard the news accurately and correct any misunderstandings.

4. Do not overestimate the success of treatment or promise something that is not realistic. At the same time, reassure the patient and family that the team is there to support them.

Overview

Providing good palliative and end-of-life care is an essential component of ENP practice. Palliative care is defined as "an approach that improves the quality of life of patients and their families facing the problem associated with life-threatening illness, through the prevention and relief of suffering by means of early identification and impeccable assessment and treatment of pain and other problems, physical, psychosocial and spiritual."[10] Palliative care should be given to patients and families from the moment of presentation with an undifferentiated illness or upon diagnosis even when curative interventions are part of the plan of care; the intensity of palliative care increases in advanced illness. When curative therapies are recognized as no longer beneficial, end-of-life care should be provided to patients. Palliative care is comprehensive care that should be given to all from the time of diagnosis to the death of a patient, and then to families who survive the patient in the form of bereavement care. Palliative care includes physical, psychological, emotional, and spiritual dimensions and has been shown to improve quality of life. Most literature regarding palliative and end-of-life care describes strategies for physical and mental health symptom management, communication, ethical issues, cocreating plans of care, and spiritual support; resources for these topics can be found widely in the literature. This chapter focuses on specific palliative and end-of-life topics for the ENP that are not commonly emphasized in other literature.

Trajectories of Advanced Illness and Approaching Death

In order to provide excellent palliative care to patients and families, it is important to understand the natural history of diseases. In the seminal article by Lunney et al.,[11] the authors found four trajectories of dying: sudden death, terminal illness, organ failure, and frailty. Chan[2] further refined these end-of-life trajectories specifically for emergency medicine and nursing: (a) Dead on arrival, (b) prehospital resuscitation with subsequent ED death, (c) prehospital resuscitation with survival to admission, (d) terminally ill and comes to the ED, (e) frail and hovering around death, (f) sudden death in the ED, and (g) potentially avoidable death by omission or commission.[2] These trajectories help clinicians understand the likelihood of how patients approach death, also known as

TABLE 56.2 EQUIANALGESIC DOSING CHART

OPIOID	PARENTERAL (IV/IM/ SUBCUTANEOUS) IN MG	ENTERAL (ORAL) IN MG
Morphine	10	25
Hydromorphone	2	5
Hydrocodone	--	25
Oxycodone	--	20
Fentanyl IV	150 mcg	--

IM, intramuscularly; IV, intravenous.
Source: http://pami.emergency.med.jax.ufl.edu/.

prognostication. Emergency clinicians are often focused on resuscitation and intense investigation of presenting symptoms while we treat and possibly reverse underlying pathology. However, by understanding the prognosis or how advanced the patient's illness is and probability the patient will approach death, we can offer appropriate interventions that are beneficial given the stage of the disease and patient preferences for their plan of care.

Clinicians often think about prognosis as the likelihood of death or survival in a set timeframe such as the patient has a 10% chance of surviving 6 months. The focus on a percentage can cause the clinician to hesitate to give a prognosis since we do not want to be inaccurate. A more helpful and comfortable approach for patients, families, and clinicians is to think of prognosis in another way. A clinician can think of the probability the patient will die in terms of hours, days, weeks, months, or years. The plan of care and interventions for a patient who has hours to live is very different than if the patient has months to live. The intensity and variety of emergency palliative care services can be escalated when there are only hours or days to live.

In the literature, there has been great interest in sensitizing clinicians to offering palliative care or referring to a palliative care specialist. One method is for the clinician to ask themselves, "Would I be surprised if the patient were to die within the next time period (e.g., 2 days, 1 month, 6 months, 1 year)."[12] While this question is not intended to accurately prognosticate death, it is intended to help clinicians recognize that palliative care services may be warranted to support patients and their families during this time of advanced illness or end-of-life. Table 56.2 illustrates some possible interventions given the prognosis of the patient.

The practice and science of calculating equianalgesic dosing can change, so please refer to current recommendations and guidelines for equianalgesic doses and follow the Food and Drug Administration approved indications, contraindications, and dosing for all medications.

References

References for this chapter are online only and can be found at https://connect.springerpub.com/content/reference-book/978-0-8261-6091-5/part/part07/toc-part/ch56.

Index